CLINICAL ANATOMY FOR STUDENTS:
Problem Solving Approach

CLINICAL ANATOMY FOR STUDENTS: *Problem Solving Approach*

Neeta V Kulkarni MD
Head of the Department of Anatomy
Dr SMCSI Medical College
Karakonam, Trivandrum

Formerly
Professor and Head, Department of Anatomy
Government Medical College
Trivandrum

JAYPEE BROTHERS
MEDICAL PUBLISHERS (P) LTD
New Delhi

Published by

Jitendar P Vij
Jaypee Brothers Medical Publishers (P) Ltd
EMCA House, 23/23B Ansari Road, Daryaganj
New Delhi 110 002, India
Phones: +91-11-23272143, +91-11-23272703, +91-11-23282021, +91-11-23245672
Fax: +91-11-23276490, +91-11-23245683
e-mail: jaypee@jaypeebrothers.com
Visit our website: www.jaypeebrothers.com

Branches

- 2/B, Akruti Society, Jodhpur Gam Road Satellite, **Ahmedabad** 38 0015
  Phone: +91-79-30988717, +91-79-26926233 e-mail: jpamdvd@rediffmail.com
- 202 Batavia Chambers, 8 Kumara Krupa Road, Kumara Park East, **Bangalore** 560 001
  Phones: +91-80-22285971, +91-80-22382956, +91-80-30614073
  Tele Fax : +91-80-22281761 e-mail: jaypeemedpubbgl@eth.net
- 282 IIIrd Floor, Khaleel Shirazi Estate, Fountain Plaza, Pantheon Road, **Chennai** 600 008
  Phones: +91-44-28193265, +91-44-28194897 Fax: +91-44-28193231
  e-mail: jpchen@eth.net
- 4-2-1067/1-3, 1st Floor, Balaji Building, Ramkote Cross Road, **Hyderabad** 500 095
  Phones: +91-40-55610020, +91-40-24758498, +91-40-30940929, Fax: +91-40-24758499
  e-mail: jpmedpub@rediffmail.com
- 1A Indian Mirror Street, Wellington Square, **Kolkata** 700 013
  Phones: +91-33-22456075, +91-33-22451926, +91-33-30901929, Fax: +91-33-22456075
  e-mail: jpbcal@cal.vsnl.net.in
- 106 Amit Industrial Estate, 61 Dr SS Rao Road, Near MGM Hospital, Parel, **Mumbai** 400 012
  Phones: +91-22-24124863, +91-22-24104532, +91-22-30926896, Fax: +91-22-24160828
  e-mail: jpmedpub@bom7.vsnl.net.in
- "KAMALPUSHPA" 38, Reshimbag, Opp. Mohota Science College, Umred Road, **Nagpur** 440 009 (MS)
  Phones: +91-712-3945220, +91-712-2704275, Fax: +91-712-2704275
  e-mail: jpmednagpur@rediffmail.com

Clinical Anatomy for Students: Problem Solving Approach

First Edition: **2007**

ISBN 81-8061-734-3

Typeset at JPBMP typesetting unit

Printed at Ajanta Offset & Packagings Ltd., New Delhi

Dedicated to

- *The Divine guidance, which sustained this adventure*
- *My parents and teachers*
- *Students—past, present and future*
- *Professional colleagues—pre-clinical, para-clinical and clinical*

Foreword

I have great pleasure in writing a foreword to Dr Neeta V Kulkarni's new book: *Clinical Anatomy for Students: Problem Solving Approach.* It is a unique blend of gross, developmental, radiological and clinical anatomy. To emphasize the fact that anatomical knowledge goes hand in hand with bedside medicine, she has given solved examples of clinicoanatomical problems. For example, anatomical relations as a basis of symptoms and signs in various body parts—head, neck and brain, thorax, abdomen and pelvis, upper and lower limbs—have been dealt with very well—which makes the book a valuable companion to the clinicians as well as to imaging departments. It gives a crisp and lucid account of correlative neuroanatomy.

Concept of Functional Anatomy

Nuclear Medicine uses radiolabelled tracers to study organ function, hence knowledge of underlying anatomy is important in the interpretation of the images—planar as well as 3 dimensional images provided by SPECT (Single Photon Emission Computed Tomography) or PET (Positron-Emission Tomography). Hepatobiliary scintigraphy, renography, cisternography (CSF imaging), myocardial, pulmonary and cerebral perfusion imaging, bone scan are examples of combining anatomy with physiology, structure with function. Current trend is to fuse images of structure (CT/MRI) with images of function (perfusion, metabolism, receptor activity, etc.). Hybrid machines, which perform CT/PET images together have come into routine use.

Lymph Nodes and Lymphatic Drainage

Anatomic location of lymph nodes and lymphatic drainage in various body regions has been very adequately described in this book. This subject is of great interest to the clinicians specially in the context of infectious and autoimmune diseases (tuberculosis, HIV/AIDS, sarcoidosis) and malignancy (lymphoma—Hodgkins'and non-Hodgkins) and metastasis from various cancers. Detection of the sentinal node has gained importance in the staging of cancers. The newer technology of PET/CT permits detection and precise localization of disease. Cancer cells take up several times more glucose than the surrounding normal cells. Similarly macrophages and lymphocytes take up more glucose. Hence, a radioactive tracer FDG (fluorodeoxyglucose) is taken up avidly by these cells and in a PET (Positron-Emission Tomography) image, the lesion shows up a *hot-spot* even if anatomically the size of the lesion is 2 mm. In the next edition of this book, I would like to see a FDG PET image fused with a CT image showing the involvement of lymph nodes (not accessible to palpation) and the complete disappearance of the affected lymph node lesions following chemotherapy.

Developmental Defects

While interpreting structural or functional images of various organs clinicians come across many developmental and congenital defects (such as lingual thyroid, thyroglossal cyst, agenesis of a lobe, ectopic parathyroid in the mediastinum, ectopic and horseshoe kidneys, intrahepatic gallbladder, Meckels' diverticulum, congenital heart disease, etc.). Hence, the description of developmental defects in this book is of great value to the clinician. This book includes radiological and CT/MRI images in several sections. I suggest the inclusion of ultrasound images especially in the sections of Thorax, Abdomen, Pelvis and Perineum. 2-D echocardiographic images of the heart should be included as an integral component of teaching anatomy of the heart. Hence, pictures such as ultrasound-guided drainage of a pancreatic pseudocyst will enhance the value of the book.

Visible Human Project (VHP)

In my recent book, "Computers in Medicine: Progress in Medical Informatics" (2005: Tata McGraw Hill Publisher) I have described the Visible Human Project; sponsored by NLM-NIH USA, in which a complete, anatomically detailed, three-dimensional representation of the normal human male and female bodies has been acquired from cadavers by transverse CT, MRI and cryosection images. These sections have been taken at intervals of one millimeter in male and 0.3 mm in female providing 1871 and 5189 cross-sections respectively. This data bank serves as a common reference point for the study of the human anatomy available in the public domain. The data sets are already being applied to a wide range of educational, diagnostic, therapy planning, virtual reality, artistic, mathematical and industrial uses. The VHP was to be the cornerstone for future sets of related digital image libraries including libraries of normal structural variations, collections of diseases and abnormal structures, embryology and pediatrics. The atlas website allows the user to interact with the appropriate imagery to demonstrate functionality, for example the function of the muscles that control and move the mandible bone during the chewing reflex. They illustrate neurovascular relationships through the interactive dissection of anatomic structures and fly-through views. The Next Generation Internet (NGI) has led to a new NLM project "The Anatomy Work Bench" and "Surgery Work Bench" for teaching anatomy and surgery using real time Internet. I am sure that these projects of VHP will be greatly beneficial to the Indian anatomists and students.

It is my expectation and hope that forward looking and innovative anatomists like Dr Neeta V Kulkarni will take the initiative in utilizing the available new technology for teaching purpose in all the 180 Medical Colleges in India without further delay.

The recent launch of EduSat, the Indian Space Research Organization's (ISRO) newest satellite exclusively dedicated to education, is a wonderful new opportunity for medical and nursing education in India. The technology is available and affordable. We need the vision and motivation to employ it forthwith. May this new book trigger that new era, by becoming part of the International digital library.

Dr RD Lele
Hon. Chief Physician and Director, Nuclear Medicine Department, Jaslok Hospital and Research Centre, Mumbai
Hon. Director of Nuclear Medicine and RIA Dept., Lilavati Hospital and Research Centre, Mumbai
Emeritus Professor of Medicine (for life) and Ex-Dean, Grant Medical Collage and Sir JJ Hospitals, Mumbai
Emeritus Professor of the National Academy of Medical Sciences (India)

Preface

It is a well-known fact that is documented right from the Greek era that anatomy provides a firm foundation to the edifice of medical education. However, in the new paradigm, the clinical anatomy provides the keystone to this foundation. It must be appreciated that no part of the human body can be learnt in isolation and that relations of the same structure change from region to region. These anatomical relations may be the basis of the symptoms of a particular disease or of the signs of the disease or of a clinical test (used for diagnosis of a disease) or of a surgical procedure (used to diagnose and/or treat the disease). Traditionally, we are conditioned to equate anatomy to the science of muscles and bones, which gives the beginner an incorrect impression about the potential of the subject. The key to successful and enjoyable learning lies in consciously correlating the basic and clinical anatomy (like for example, understanding anatomical basis of, symptoms and signs of diseases, surgical procedures, contraceptive measures, understanding embryological basis of congenital anomalies, identifying normal structures in radiographs and comparing them with changes in the disease state, etc.). Medical Council of India in its stipulations of 1997 has reduced the duration of the first MBBS course and has recommended problem-based learning in preclinical subjects. This situation demands a fresh approach in which the students are trained to solve clinical problems using the anatomical knowledge gained during the first professional course. To choose essentials of anatomy for first MBBS students from a vast body of anatomical facts posed a challenging task. Reading through the paraclinical and clinical texts besides special interactive sessions with clinical teachers gave an insight (to a certain extent) into how much of anatomy learnt at preclinical level is actually applied to gain sound clinical training. Accordingly, in a few instances, clinically oriented concepts or interpretations are mentioned along with the conventional. The clinical testing of skeletal muscles is included to make the learning of muscles more meaningful. Thus, the problem solving approach creates an imprint on the minds of the students that preclinical anatomy is an integral part of bedside medicine. The presentation of the subject matter throughout the text is logical and reader-friendly. Essentials of anatomy covering all regions of the body are encapsulated in a single volume in order to gain a holistic perception of the anatomical structures. The central theme of this text is, developing skills in anatomical thinking for solving clinical problems. It was indeed a Herculean task to give concrete shape to such a complex theme. Let us hope that students will enjoy learning anatomy when they are able to solve clinical problems given at the end of the sections.

Neeta V Kulkarni

Acknowledgements

I do not remember, at what point of time, 'the adventure bug', to write a book of this type, bit me. Nonetheless, the credit for this largely goes to the fellow anatomists and the students and of course to the inner urge to lift this unsung discipline and bring it in the mainstream medicine. Interaction with the clinical teachers provided a basis on which the core theme was developed. In this regard, Dr YM Fazil Maricker (former Professor and Head of Surgery, Medical College, Trivandrum) deserves special thanks. Being a renowned teacher and an author himself, his suggestions on essential anatomy for a student of surgery, were invaluable. He, in fact, went through the manuscript of quite a few chapters. Equal thanks are due to Dr Ramnarayan (former Professor and Head of Cardiothoracic Surgery, Medical College, Trivandrum), who evaluated the Chapters on heart and great blood vessels authentically. In a lighter vein, let me add, these two surgeons turned out to be better qualified for this job, because their better halves happen to be the anatomists. I would like to extend my sincere thanks to all my coworkers in the department of anatomy, Dr SMCSI Medical College, Karakonam, for their constructive criticism, which led to the continuous assessment and reassessment of the manuscript and the figures. I owe a debt of gratitude to Dr N Vijayashankar (formerly Director of Neuroanatomy in Old Westbury, NY, USA and currently my coworker) for lending me the latest reference books on neuroanatomy and for assisting in proofreading.

Words are inadequate to fully express my gratitude to the generosity of the Department of Radiology, CMC Vellore for the high quality images of normal anatomy and altered anatomy in disease states. My thanks also are due to the Department of ENT, Dr SMCSI Medical College, for providing some rare radiographs.

Anatomy book without expressive illustrations is like a human body without life. My artist, Mr Sivaraman (with whom I had association in various Government Medical Colleges in Kerala), was ever ready to draw the sketches repeatedly. I must confess that the most laborious and time consuming part of the book, was preparing reader-friendly and realistic illustrations.

In computer processing of these illustrations, my husband, Dr VP Kulkarni (former Director of Electronics Research and Development Center, of Govt. of India, Trivandrum) played a pivotal role. I would like to stress here that his comments and suggestions regarding the layout and positioning the labels in the figures have enhanced their educative value.

I would like to appreciate the inspirational support given by my son, Dr Utkarsh and my daughter, Dr Vinee throughout this endless marathon.

I consider it an honor to have Dr RD Lele, a renowned physician and the doyen of nuclear medicine in India and above all a visionary medical educationist (he was my Professor of Medicine in Government Medical College, Nagpur, in mid-sixties), to write a foreword for this book.

Finally (although it should be the first and foremost), I am grateful to Shri Jitendar P Vij (CMD) Jaypee Brothers Medical Publishers P. Ltd for publishing this book. I acknowledge most humbly the king size contribution of Mr Tarun Duneja [young and dynamic General Manager (Publishing) of Jaypee Brothers Medical Publishers, New Delhi] and his team. He has truly understood the importance of Clinical Anatomy in modern medical curriculum. Synthesis of science and art seen in this book is the result of the sincere efforts of his team, especially Mr Sukhdev Prasad and Mr Manoj Pahuja.

Contents

SECTION FOUR: ABDOMEN, PELVIS AND PERINEUM

SECTION FIVE: LOWER EXTREMITY

SECTION SIX: OVERVIEW OF OSTEOLOGY

SECTION ONE

Upper Extremity

1 Pectoral Region

The pectoral or the breast region is the name given to the front of the chest or thorax. This region contains the mammary glands, pectoral muscles, fasciae and pectoral nerves.

SURFACE LANDMARKS

a. Some parts of the osteocartilaginous framework of pectoral region (Figs 1.1 and 1.2) are palpable through the skin. The sternum (breastbone) is located in the midline. All the three parts of sternum (manubrium, body and xiphoid process) are palpable. On each side, the manubrium articulates above with the clavicle and below with the first costal cartilage. The second costal cartilage articulates with the sternal angle, which is the junction of manubrium and body of sternum. The sternal angle is a very important landmark for the clinician during examination of chest, as it indicates the position of second rib from which the rest of the ribs can be counted. The body of sternum articulates with costal cartilages of the third to seventh ribs.

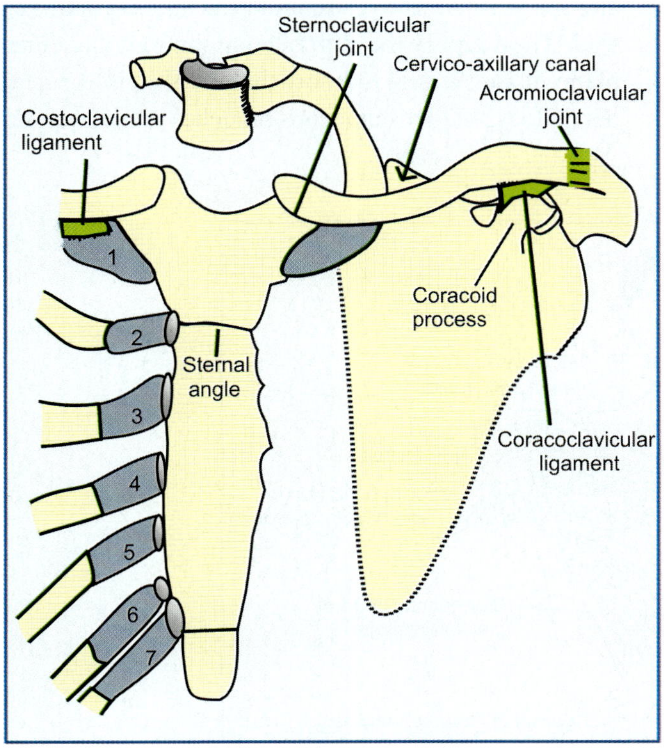

Fig. 1.1: Scheme to depict osteo-cartilaginous framework of pectoral region

b. The clavicle or collarbone is horizontally placed in the upper part of the pectoral region. Being subcutaneous it is palpable in its entire extent. It articulates medially with the manubrium sterni at sternoclavicular joint and laterally with acromion of the scapula at acromioclavicular joint.
c. The coracoid process of scapula projects under the lateral part of the clavicle. It can be felt 2-3 cm below the clavicle on firm pressure of the thumb in the lateral part of infraclavicular fossa or deltopectoral triangle (Fig. 1.2).
d. The anterior axillary fold (produced by pectoralis major muscle) is a visible landmark, as it becomes prominent, when the abducted arm is adducted against resistance.

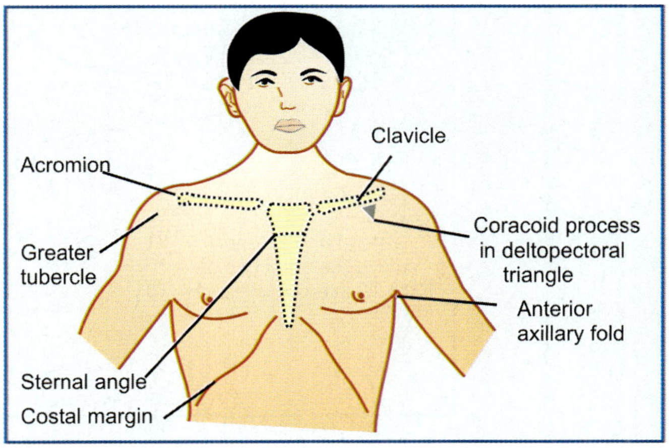

Fig. 1.2: Surface landmarks of pectoral region

SUPERFICIAL FASCIA

a. The main feature of the superficial fascia is the presence of mammary glands.

b. The platysma is seen in the upper part of the pectoral region. This is a thin subcutaneous muscle that takes origin from the deep fascia covering the upper part of pectoralis major and adjacent deltoid muscle. It crosses the clavicle to enter the neck and is inserted in the lower margin of the body of mandible partly and in to the facial muscles around the mouth (Fig. 1.3). In its course through the neck the platysma lies in the superficial fascia overlying the posterior triangle of neck. The facial nerve (seventh cranial nerve) supplies the platysma in the neck.

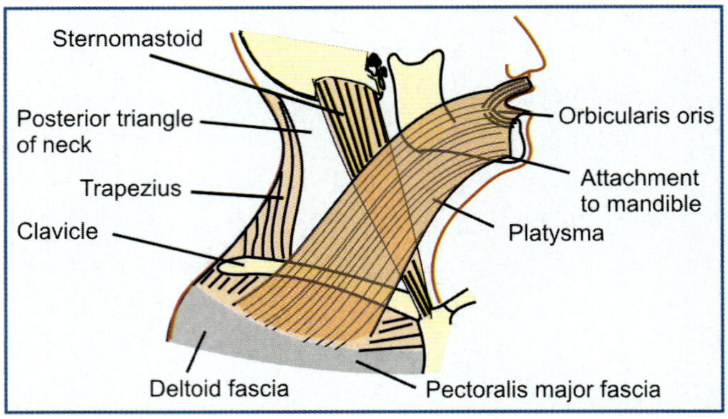

Fig. 1.3: To show origin of platysma from fascia covering pectoralis major and deltoid

CUTANEOUS NERVES (Fig.1.4)

a. The skin above the sternal angle is supplied by the medial, intermediate and lateral supraclavicular nerves (C3, C4), which arise in the neck from the cervical plexus. These nerves descend to the pectoral region by crossing in front of the clavicle or frequently by piercing it. The medial supraclavicular nerve supplies the skin overlying the manubrium. The intermediate nerve supplies the skin over the upper part of pectoralis major muscle and the lateral nerve supplies the skin over the shoulder.

b. The anterior cutaneous branches of the second to the sixth intercostal nerves enter the pectoral region along the lateral margin of sternum after piercing the sternocostal head of pectoralis major muscle and the deep fascia. These branches are accompanied by corresponding arteries, which are the branches of internal thoracic artery. The area of supply of these nerves extends from the anterior median plane to the midclavicular line on each side. The lateral cutaneous nerves are the branches given by the intercostal nerves along a vertical line just behind the anterior axillary fold. They supply the skin beyond the midclavicular plane. It is essential to know that the first intercostal nerve does not give cutaneous branches to the pectoral

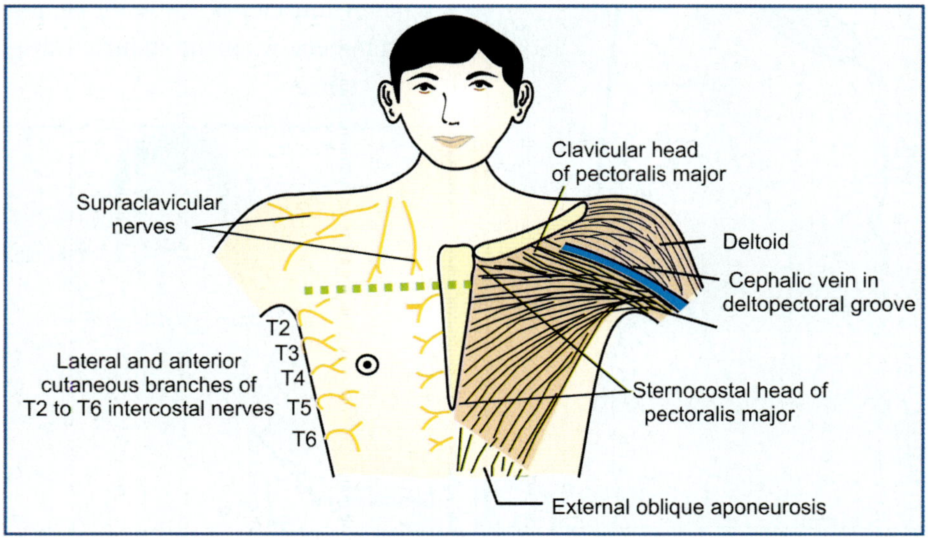

Fig. 1.4: Showing cutaneous nerves of pectoral region on right side and origin of pectoralis major muscle on left side. At the dotted green line discontinuous dermatomes (C4 and T2) meet

region. Thus, from the cutaneous nerve supply we learn that at the level of sternal angle, C4 and T2 dermatomes come close to each other (Fig. 1.5). There is interruption of the sequence of dermatomes at this site because C5 to T1 dermatomes are carried in the upper limb from the trunk during embryonic development.

DEEP FASCIA

The deep fascia of the pectoral region is called pectoral fascia because it covers the pectoralis major muscle. It is continuous with the periosteum of the clavicle and the sternum. It passes over the deltopectoral groove to become continuous with the fascia covering the deltoid. The upper portion of the pectoral fascia gives origin to fibers of platysma (Fig.1.3). At the lower margin of pectoralis major the pectoral fascia and the fascia covering the latissimus dorsi are connected by the axillary fascia, which lies in the floor of the axilla. The suspensory ligament of axilla connects the axillary fascia to the clavipectoral fascia at the lower margin of pectoralis minor.

DELTOPECTORAL TRIANGLE (Fig. 1.4)

The boundaries of this triangle are, the upper margin of pectoralis major medially, anterior margin of deltoid laterally and the clavicle superiorly. The triangle contains the cephalic vein, deltoid branch of thoracoacromial artery and the deltopectoral lymph nodes. In its upper part the coracoid process of scapula is present.

PECTORALIS MAJOR

This is the largest muscle of the pectoral region. It forms the anterior axillary fold.

Origin (Fig. 1.4)

a. Clavicular head takes origin from the anterior surface of the medial half of the clavicle.
b. Sternocostal head arises from the front of the manubrium, body of the sternum and from second to sixth costal cartilages.
c. Aponeurotic fibers arise from the aponeurosis of the external oblique muscle of the anterior abdominal wall.

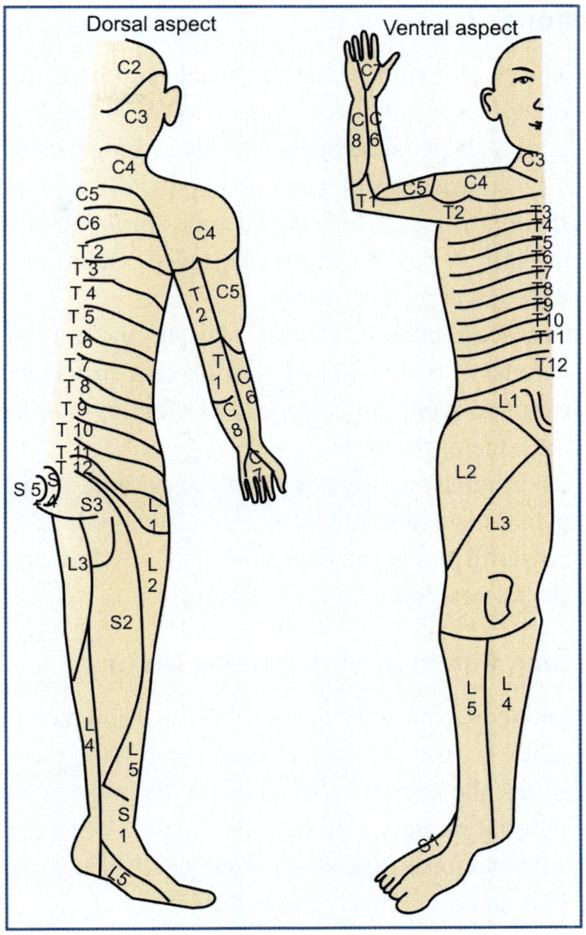

Fig. 1.5: Dermatomes of the ventral and dorsal aspect of the body

Insertion

Pectoralis major is inserted into the lateral lip of the intertubercular sulcus of humerus by a bilaminar U-shaped tendon (the two limbs of the U being called anterior and posterior laminae). The anterior lamina, which is formed by clavicular fibers, is inserted into the lower part of the lateral lip while the posterior lamina formed by aponeurotic fibers is inserted into the upper part of the lateral lip of the intertubercular sulcus. The sternocostal fibers form the base of the U.

Nerve Supply

The medial pectoral (C8, T1) and lateral pectoral (C5, C6, C7) nerves supply the muscle.

Actions

a. The contraction of entire muscle produces medial rotation and adduction, of arm as for example while putting the hand on one's hip and pushing forcibly.
b. The contraction of clavicular part alone produces flexion of arm. This part becomes prominent, when the arm is flexed against resistance, e.g. in pushing the edge of a heavy table.
c. The contraction of sternocostal part alone produces extension of the flexed arm against resistance for example while pulling a heavy table by holding on the edge of the table.
d. In climbing on a rope or a tree, the sternocostal part of pectoralis major and latissimus dorsi produce a very powerful movement of extension the arm from its fully flexed position.

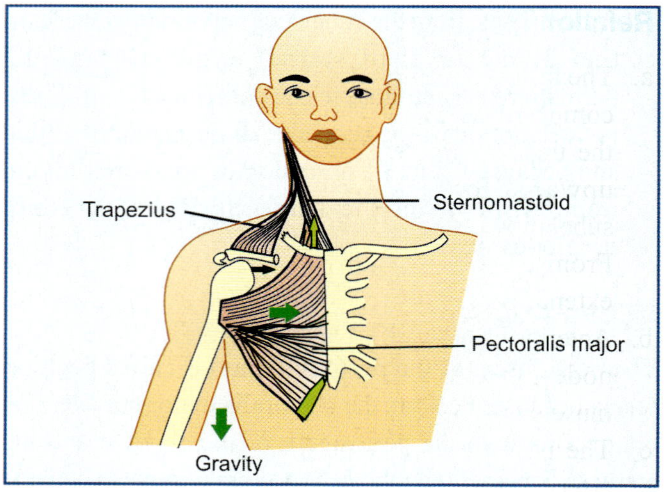

Fig. 1.6: Fracture of right clavicle (Note: The upward displacement of medial fragment and medial displacement of lateral fragment due to muscle pull)

Testing Function of Pectoralis Major

The subject abducts the arm to about 60° and then flexes the elbows. Then the subject attempts to bring the hands together. The examiner watches for the prominence of the anterior axillary fold (another method of testing the muscle function is by asking the subject to place hands on the hips and press firmly inwards).

Clinical Highlights

a. In congenital absence of pectoralis major muscle the anterior axillary fold is absent.
c. In fracture of clavicle (Fig.1.6) the contraction of pectoralis major along with other adductors shifts the lateral fragment of clavicle in medial direction below the medial fragment. The sternomastoid muscle of the neck pulls the medial fragment upward. This results in overriding of the fragments.

PECTORALIS MINOR (Fig.1.7)

This is a triangular muscle in the anterior wall of axilla, placed posterior to the pectoralis major. It has anterior and posterior surfaces and upper or medial and lower or lateral margins.

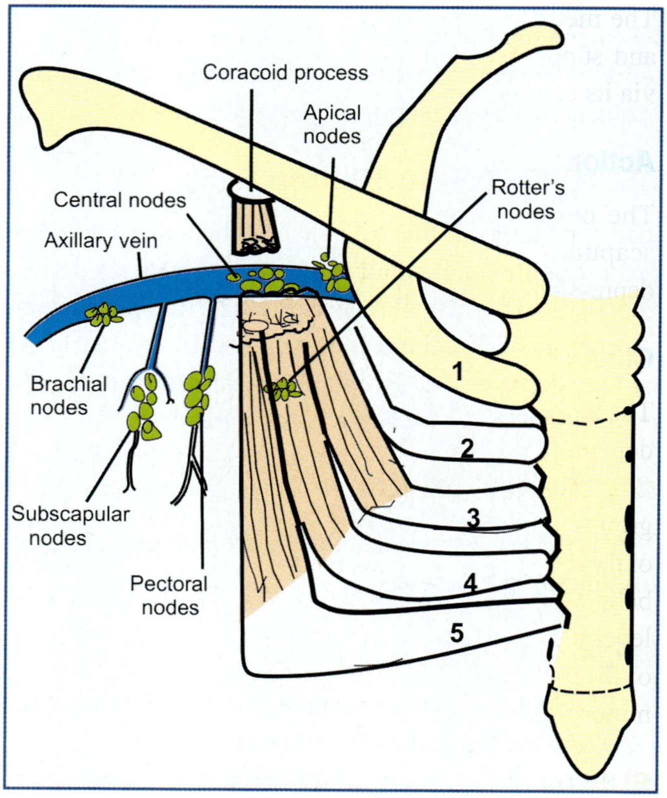

Fig. 1.7: Schematic diagram showing pectoralis minor muscle and axillary lymph nodes

Origin

It takes origin from the outer surfaces of third, fourth and fifth ribs near the costal cartilages.

Insertion

It is inserted into the medial border and upper surface of the coracoid process of scapula.

Relations

a. The fascial relations of the muscle are as follows. It is completely enclosed in the clavipectoral fascia. From the upper margin of the muscle the fascia extends upwards for attachment to the margins of the subclavian groove on the lower surface of clavicle. From the lower margin of the muscle the fascia extends downwards as suspensory ligament of axilla.
b. Anteriorly, muscle is related to the interpectoral lymph nodes (Rotter's nodes) and the pectoralis major muscle.
c. The posterior relations are second part of axillary artery, axillary vein and cords of brachial plexus.
d. Its lower (lateral) margin is related to lateral thoracic vessels and anterior group of axillary lymph nodes.

Nerve Supply

The medial pectoral nerve pierces the pectoralis minor and supplies it. The lateral pectoral nerve sends twigs via its communication with the medial pectoral nerve.

Actions

The pectoralis minor muscle helps in protraction of scapula along with serratus anterior muscle and in depression of scapula along with lower fibers of trapezius.

Clinical Highlights

The axillary lymph nodes are grouped into three levels, depending on their relation to pectoralis minor muscle (Fig. 1.7). Level-I nodes (anterior, posterior and lateral groups) are located below and lateral to the lower margin of the muscle. In level- II nodes the central group is located behind and the interpectoral in front of the muscle. The level -III nodes (apical group) lie above the upper margin of the muscle. In operation of mastectomy the pectoralis minor muscle is an important landmark for the surgeon.

SUBCLAVIUS

This is a small muscle in the uppermost part of the pectoral region. The subclavius takes origin by a narrow tendon from the first costochondral junction and is inserted into the groove on the undersurface of the middle third of clavicle.

Nerve Supply

The muscle receives twigs from the nerve to subclavius, which is a branch of the Erb's point of brachial plexus. This nerve contributes C5 fibers to phrenic nerve through accessory phrenic nerve.

Action

The subclavius steadies the clavicle during movements of the scapula at girdle joints.

CLAVIPECTORAL FASCIA (Fig. 1.8)

This fascia spreads across the gap between the upper margin of pectoralis minor muscle and the clavicle. In this part, it is attached medially to the first rib and laterally to the coracoid process of scapula. Above, it splits to enclose the subclavius muscle and its two layers attach to the lips of subclavian groove on the inferior surface of clavicle. Below it splits to enclose the pectoralis minor, at the lower margin of which the two layers unite to form the suspensory ligament of axilla, which become continuous with the axillary fascia. The four structures that pierce the fascia spanning between the pectoralis

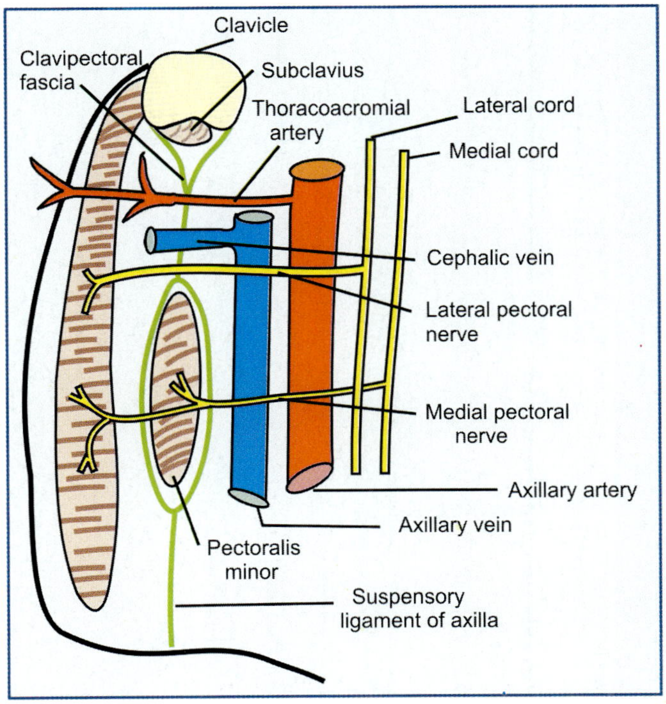

Fig. 1.8: Scheme to depict the disposition of clavipectoral fascia and structures piercing it

minor and the clavicle are, lateral pectoral nerve, thoraco-acromial artery, cephalic vein and lymphatic vessels.

PECTORAL NERVES

There are two pectoral nerves, medial and lateral. The medial pectoral nerve (C8, T1) arises from the medial cord of the brachial plexus. The nerve lies behind the first part of axillary artery initially but it soon curves forwards to receive a communicating ramus from the lateral pectoral nerve in front of the axillary artery. It enters the deep surface of the pectoralis minor muscle, supplies it and enters the substance of the pectoralis major muscle. The lateral pectoral nerve (C5, 6, 7) arises from the lateral cord of the brachial plexus. It travels forwards on the lateral side of axillary artery and pierces the clavipectoral fascia and the clavicular part of pectoralis major, which it supplies.

Breast (Mammary Gland) 2

The breasts or mammary glands are a pair of modified sweat glands, located in the superficial fascia of the pectoral region. Each breast is composed of glandular tissue, which is embedded in fibrofatty stroma and covered with the skin, areola and nipple. The breasts are rudimentary in male. In the female, after the onset of puberty they form secondary sexual character and are the source of nutrition to the newborn.

Development of Breast

In the seven-week embryo, ectodermal milk line appears on the ventral body wall on each side, extending from the limb bud of the upper limb to that of the lower limb. The milk lines in the pectoral region give rise to a pair of glands and the remaining milk lines disintegrate. The female breasts start growing with the onset of puberty.

Congenital Anomalies

a. Accessory nipples (polythelia) may be found anywhere along the milk line that extends from the axilla to the inguinal region (Fig. 2.1).
b. A complete accessory breast (polymastia) may develop along the milk line.
c. Amastia or amazia is bilateral agenesis of breast.
d. Athelia is absence of nipple.
e. In Poland syndrome or anomaly, there is complete or partial absence of glandular tissue with normal nipple, which is usually associated with absence of pectoralis major muscle.

Female Breast

The breast consists of a broad base in contact with chest wall and a pointed apex, which bears the nipple. The base or the deep surface of the breast extends vertically from the level of second to the sixth ribs and in the transverse plane, from the sternal margin to the mid-axillary line. A projection of the glandular tissue from the upper and outer quadrant of the breast, into the axilla, is called axillary tail of Spence (Fig. 2.2), which passes through an opening (foramen of Langer) in the axillary fascia. So, the axillary tail is at a deeper plane compared to the rest of the gland. It is in direct contact with the anterior group of axillary lymph nodes. Due to this proximity, cancer of the axillary

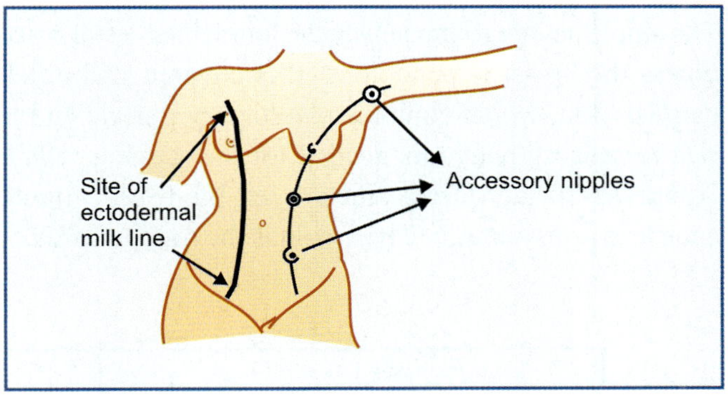

Fig. 2.1: To show developmental source of mammary gland on right side and anomaly of polythelia along milk line on left side

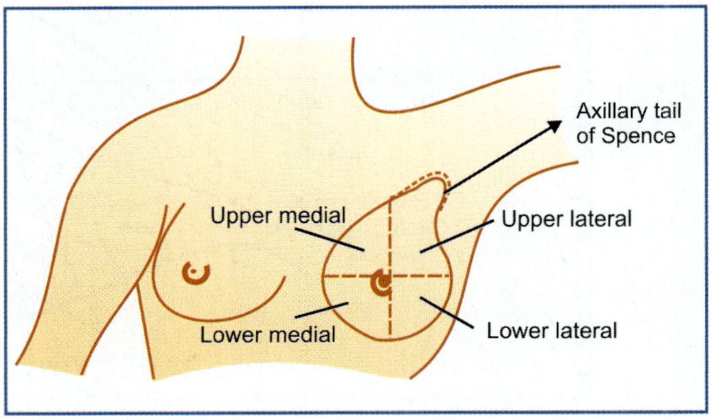

Fig. 2.2: Quadrants of breast (Note that the axillary tail from upper lateral quadrant is deep to deep fascia)

tail may be mistaken for an enlarged anterior lymph node or the nodes may be directly infiltrated from the tail instead of via the lymphatic route.

Base of the Breast (Fig. 2.3)

The base of the breast is in contact with the pectoral fascia, deep to which it rests on three muscles, which form the bed of the mammary gland. The pectoralis major muscle is in contact with the greater part of the base. The serratus anterior is related superolaterally and the aponeurosis of external oblique muscle of the abdomen inferiorly. Between the base and the pectoral fascia, there is a retromammary space filled with loose connective tissue and fat. This space allows some degree of mobility to the breast. When the pus collects in this space it is called retromammary abscess.

Nipple and Areola

The nipple lies approximately in the fourth intercostal space unless the breast is pendulous. It is covered with thick hairless skin, which contains involuntary muscle and is rich in sensory receptors needed for the sucking reflex. About 15-20 lactiferous ducts open by 15-20 minute apertures at its summit. The areola is the rounded area of pigmented skin that encircles the nipple. Permanent darkening of the areola and nipple occurs during first pregnancy. The areola contains involuntary muscles, sebaceous glands and sweat glands. The sebaceous glands enlarge during pregnancy as subcutaneous tubercles (Montgomery tubercles). The oily secretion of these glands is a protective lubricant to nipple during lactation.

Structure (Fig. 2.3)

The breast consists of parenchyma (ducts and secretory acini), connective tissue stroma, adipose tissue, blood vessels and lymphatics. The breast parenchyma is arranged in 15-20 lobes. Each lobe has a main lactiferous duct, which converges towards the nipple. The number of lactiferous ducts is equal to that of the lobes. Each lactiferous duct receives numerous smaller ducts and as it approaches the nipple, it dilates beneath the areola to form the lactiferous sinus, and then narrows again to reach its opening at the summit of the nipple. The lactiferous ducts converge towards the nipple in a radiating manner. Therefore, while draining a breast abscess a radial incision is placed to avoid injury to these ducts. The ligaments of Cooper are the special thickened parts of stromal tissue, which serve to anchor the gland to the overlying skin at certain points. They also connect the base of the gland to

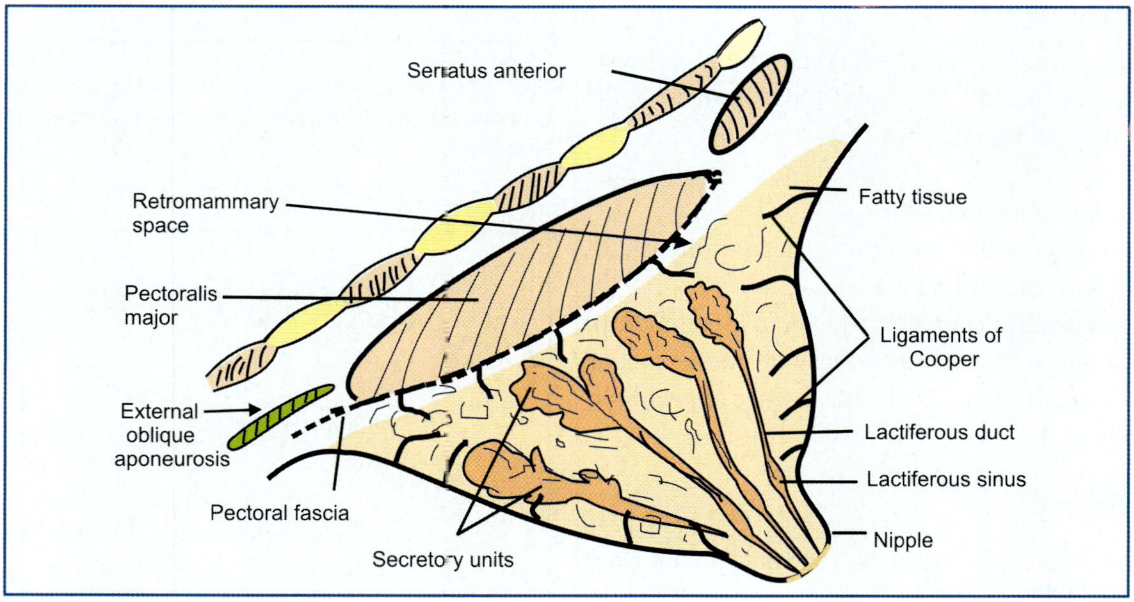

Fig. 2.3: Schematic cross-section depicting structure of the breast and muscles in relation to its base

the pectoral fascia, without hampering the mobility of the normal gland on the contracted pectoralis major muscle (Fig. 2.4).

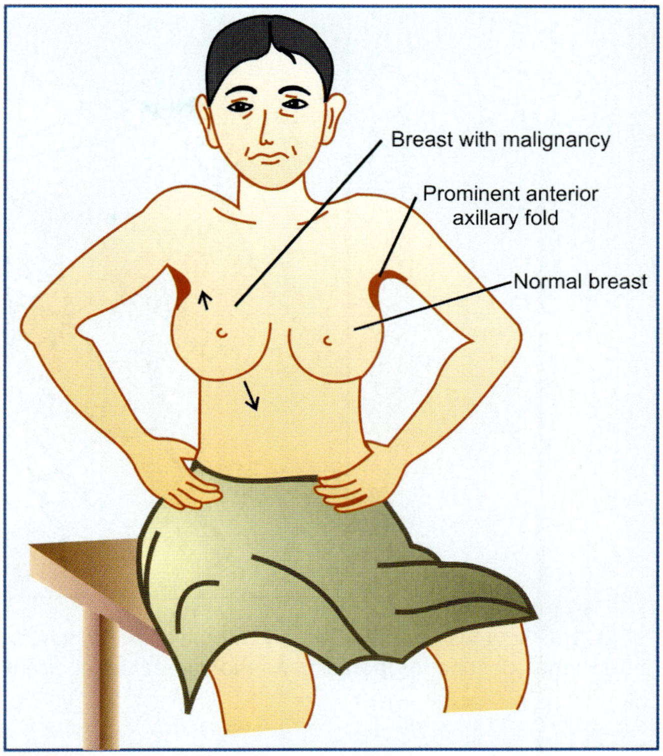

Fig. 2.4: Importance of pectoralis major muscle in clinical examination of breast (The arrows indicate the direction along which the breast is moved on contracted pectoralis major)

Histological Type

Breast is a compound tubuloalveolar gland. According to its modes of secretion, it is classified as both merocrine and apocrine gland. The release of protein molecules without loss of plasma membrane falls under merocrine mode while release of fat globules by loss of apical plasma membrane falls under apocrine mode.

Arterial Supply

The breast receives arteries mainly from four sources (Fig. 2.5).

a. The branches of lateral thoracic artery supply the lateral part of the gland.
b. Twigs from the perforating cutaneous branches of internal mammary artery in the second, third and fourth intercostal spaces supply the medial part of the gland.
c. The pectoral branches of acromiothoracic and superior thoracic artery may provide additional supply the upper part of breast.
d. The posterior intercostal arteries in the second, third and fourth spaces supply the breast from its base.

Venous Drainage

The veins radiate from the circular venous plexus subjacent to the areola. They drain into the surrounding veins namely, axillary, internal thoracic and intercostal veins. The communication of posterior intercostal veins with the internal vertebral venous plexus via intervertebral veins is the basis of spread of cancer to the vertebrae and skull bones (vide infra).

Lymphatic Drainage

The lymph vessels form the major route for the spread of cancer to the adjacent lymph nodes. The lymph vessels are grouped in superficial and deep sets.

a. The superficial lymph vessels (Fig. 2.6) drain the skin overlying the breast except that of nipple and areola. A few lymph vessels from the skin of the upper part of the breast directly reach the supraclavicular nodes by crossing the clavicle while a few terminate in the deltopectoral nodes. The skin of the medial part drains in to the internal mammary (parasternal) nodes of the same side. A few lymphatics crossover to communicate with the lymphatics of the contralateral breast. The skin of the rest of the breast drains into the anterior group of axillary nodes. A few lymphatics from the lower part may communicate with subperitoneal plexuses of abdominal cavity via the rectus sheath.
b. The deep lymph vessels (Fig. 2.7) drain the gland parenchyma and the skin of the nipple and areola. The lymph plexuses in the parenchyma around the lactiferous ducts and in the stroma communicate with the sub-areolar plexus of Sappey. Lymph vessels from the parenchymal plexuses and the subareolar plexus mainly drain into pectotal (anterior) group of axillary nodes. A few drain to the interpectoral or Rotter's nodes and others to the subscapular (posterior) and brachial (lateral) groups of axillary nodes. From here, the lymph passes to the central nodes and finally to the apical nodes. Some vessels from the peripheral

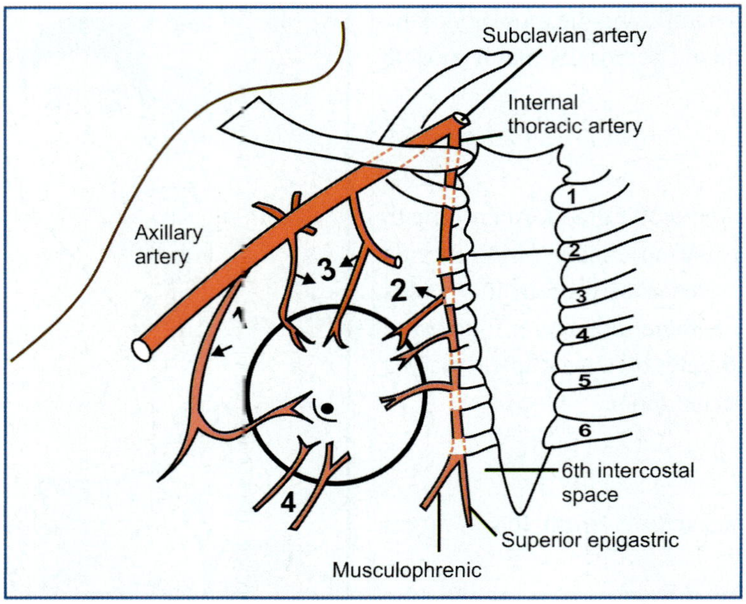

Fig. 2.5: Sources of arterial supply of breast: 1- Branches of lateral thoracic artery. 2- Branches of internal thoracic artery. 3- Branches of superior thoracic and thoraco-acromial arteries. 4 - Branches of 2nd, 3rd and 4th posterior intercostal arteries

part of superior quadrants pass directly into apical group. About 75 percent of lymph from the breast drains in to the axillary nodes. Rest of the parenchyma drains in to the internal mammary (parasternal) nodes. Lymph vessels that leave the deep surface of the breast reach the intercostal nodes located at the posterior ends of the intercostal spaces. A few lymph vessels from the base communicate with those in the rectus sheath and with the subperitoneal lymph plexuses.

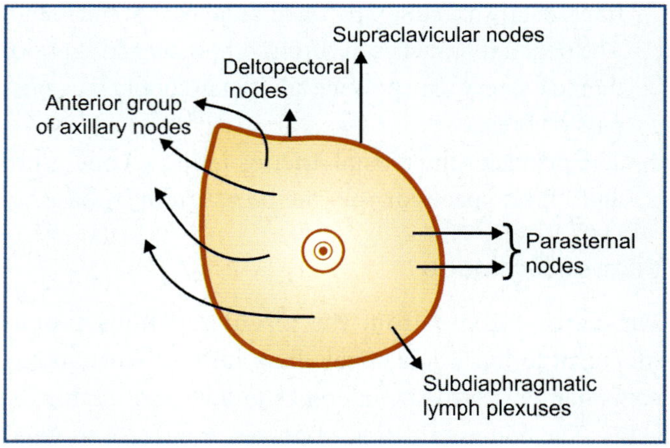

Fig. 2.6: Scheme to depict lymphatic drainage of the skin of breast (excluding areola and nipple)

Clinical Highlights

The breast cancer in women is a global problem. The cancer usually arises from the epithelium of the ducts. The upper outer quadrant of the breast is the most common site. The early symptom of cancer is the presence of a painless hard lump in the breast.

Spread or Metastasis of Breast Cancer

The spread of cancer cells from the lesion in the breast is by three routes, lymphatic, local infiltration and blood borne (all routes have anatomical basis).

a. The lymphatic spread of the cancer to the axillary lymph nodes takes place at a very early stage. Therefore, clinical examination of breast is incomplete without the palpation of axillary lymph nodes. The biopsy of lymph nodes is necessary for confirmation of the diagnosis. For practical purposes the axillary lymph nodes are divided in three levels depending on their relation to the pectoralis minor muscle (Fig. 1.7). Level-I nodes include anterior (pectoral), posterior (subscapular) and lateral (brachial) groups. Level-II nodes include central group and interpectoral or Rotter's nodes. Level-III nodes include apical nodes. The level-I nodes are the first to enlarge in cancer of breast, followed by level-II and Level-III.

b. The local spread produces following effects at three places.
   i. Involvement of the ligaments of Cooper's results in dimpling or puckering of skin. The ligaments of Cooper, at the base of the breast, may be fibrosed, which results in fixation of the breast to the underlying pectoral fascia leading to loss of mobility of the breast. To assess the mobility of the breast the patient is asked to press on the hip as hard as possible (to adduct the arm against resistance), so as to contract the pectoralis major muscle (Fig. 2.4). The breast is then moved in the direction of fibers of the muscle.
   ii. The blockage of cutaneous lymph vessels causes edema of the overlying skin. The points of openings of sweat ducts (sweat pores) do not show edema and hence remain depressed. As a result, the skin over the breast resembles an orange peel (peau d' orange appearance).
   iii. Retraction of the nipple may occur if the cancer cells invade the lactiferous ducts.
c. The cancer cells spread to distant sites as follows.
   i. The cancer cells spread to subdiaphragmatic and hepatic nodes via the subperitoneal lymph plexuses. A few cells may drop in the peritoneal cavity to deposit on any organ usually, the ovary. Secondary deposits through transcoelomic spread, are called Krukenberg's tumors.
   ii. The cancer cells spread to vertebral column, cranial bones, ribs and femur by entering the venous circulation. During rise in intrathoracic pressure (in acts like coughing, straining, etc.) there is reversal of blood flow in the intervertebral veins, which facilitates the spread into the internal vertebral venous plexus and into vertebral bodies (Fig. 2.8) and cranial bones. For this reason radiological examination of the skeleton is mandatory in cases of breast cancer.

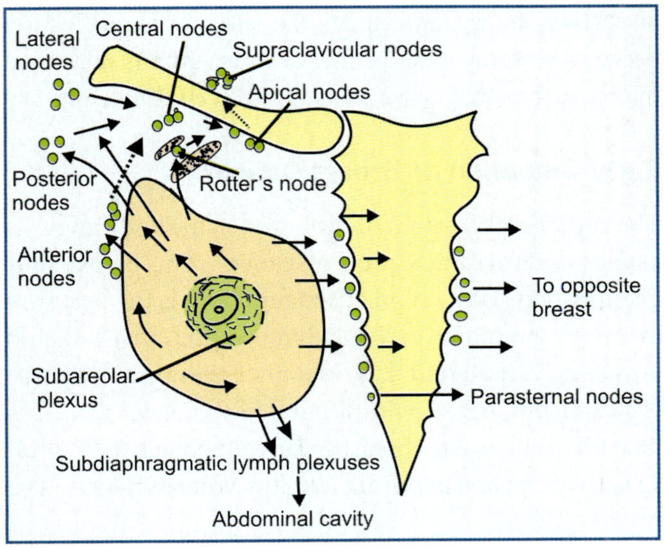

Fig. 2.7: Schematic depiction of lymphatic drainage of breast parenchyma and skin of areola and nipple

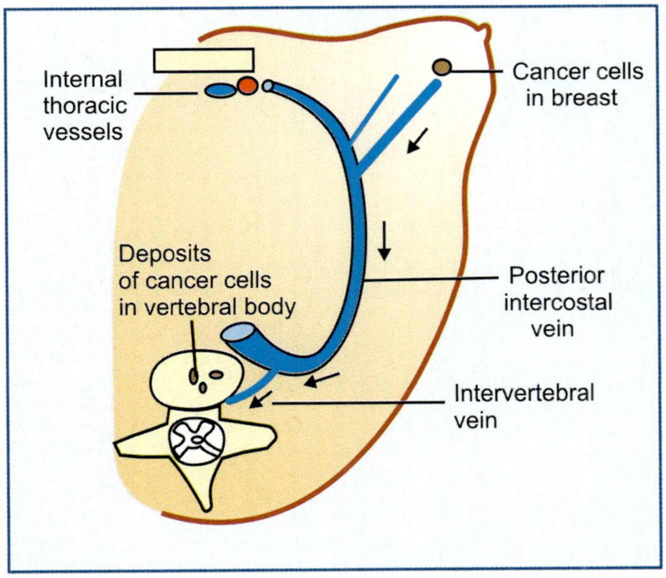

Fig. 2.8: Scheme showing venous route of spread of cancer cells during temporary reversal of blood flow in intervertebral veins

Mastectomy

The surgical removal of breast is known a mastectomy. Treatment of cancer in the majority of cases is by mastectomy, for which knowledge of the anatomy of the breast, pectoral region and axilla is essential. Nowadays radical mastectomy (in which the breast, pectoral muscles, clavipectoral fascia, deltopectoral lymph nodes and axillary fat along with all the axillary lymph nodes are removed) is rarely performed. In its place the standard modified radical mastectomy is preferred. This procedure includes simple mastectomy with removal of axillary lymph nodes (level I and II) and the preservation of pectoral muscles. While dissecting the axillary nodes the surgeon identifies the nerve to serratus anterior, nerve to latissimus dorsi and intercostobrachial nerve so as to avoid cutting them.

Early Detection of Breast Cancer

The superficial position of the breast in the body allows a chance for early detection of cancer. The breast self-examination (BSE) if practised regularly is the best way to detect the tumor early. A lump in the breast should always be viewed seriously. Mammography is a soft tissue X-ray of the breast, with minimum radiation risk. It is taken by placing the breast in direct contact with ultra-sensitive film and exposing it to low voltage X-rays. The presence of macrocalcification is indication of malignancy. This method is useful in locating clinically undetected lesion, especially in patients, who have a family history of breast cancer.

Gynecomastia

Gynecomastia is the abnormal enlargement of male breast. In some individuals it may be idiopathic (without any cause). The pathological causes of gynecomastia are, liver disease, hormone secreting tumors, side effects of drugs and leprosy. Gynecomastia is one of the characteristic features in XXY sex chromosomal anomaly (Klinefelter's syndrome).

3 Axilla

The axilla is a roughly pyramidal space situated between the lateral surface of chest wall and the medial aspect of the upper part of the arm. The anatomy of axilla is important not only because it gives passage to the neurovascular structures of the upper limb but also because it is examined clinically for enlargement of axillary lymph nodes and dissected during surgery for removing lymph nodes in cancer of the breast.

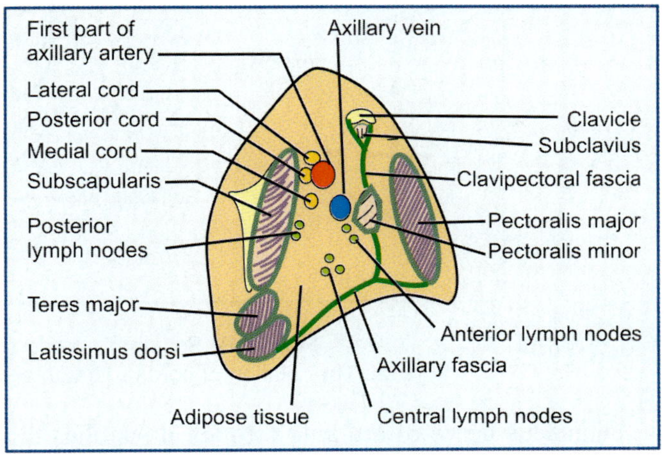

Fig. 3.1A: Parasagittal section of axilla showing its anterior and posterior walls and major contents

CONTENTS OF AXILLA

a. Axillary artery and its six branches
b. Axillary vein and its tributaries
c. Axillary lymph nodes
d. Adipose tissue (axillary pad of fat)
e. Infraclavicular part of brachial plexus (which includes three cords and their thirteen branches), long thoracic nerve and intercostobrachial nerve
f. Axillary tail of Spence.

WALLS OF AXILLA (Figs 3.1A and B)

When the arm is abducted the narrow space of axilla increases in size forming a recognizable armpit bounded by anterior and posterior axillary folds. The axilla has anterior, posterior, medial and lateral walls and a base and an apex.

a. The anterior wall consists of the pectoralis major and deeper to it, pectoralis minor, clavipectoral fascia and subclavius muscle in that order from below upward. The lateral thoracic vessels and anterior or pectoral group of lymph nodes are present inside this wall. The anterior axillary fold formed by lower margin of pectoralis major muscle becomes prominent, when the arm is adducted against resistance.
b. The posterior wall consists of (from above downward) the lateral part of costal surface of scapula covered with subscapularis, teres major and latissimus dorsi muscles. However, as the teres major and latissimus dorsi twist around each other, they come to lie in the same plane. The important relations of the posterior wall are, subscapular vessels, subscapular and thoracodorsal nerves and posterior or subscapular lymph nodes. The posterior axillary fold is formed by the teres major and latissimus dorsi muscles and it becomes prominent, when the arm is adducted against resistance.
c. The medial wall consists of first four ribs with intervening intercostal muscles and the upper four digitations of serratus anterior muscle. This wall is not related to any large vessel. The long thoracic nerve descends on the surface of serratus anterior muscle. The intercostobrachial nerve (lateral cutaneous branch of second intercostal nerve) pierces the serratus anterior to enter the axilla. As it crosses from medial to lateral side of axilla, it passes through the central group of axillary lymph nodes. It joins the medial

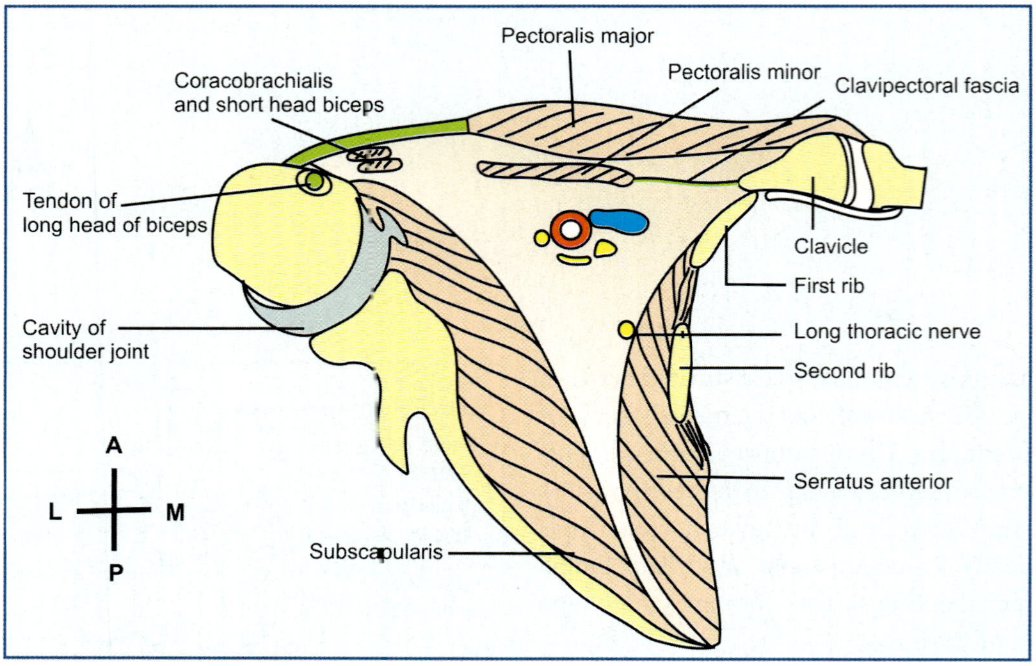

Fig. 3.1B: Schematic cross-section to show the walls of axilla
Note: The relation of cords of brachial plexus to the second part of axillary artery

cutaneous nerve of arm and through it supplies the skin of the axilla and medial aspect of the uppermost part of the arm. Compression of this nerve due to enlarged central lymph nodes, gives rise to pain in its area of supply.

d. The lateral wall is the narrowest and is formed by the bicipital groove of the humerus with tendon long head of biceps brachii. The tendon of coracobrachialis and short head of biceps brachii lie very close to this wall, which is very close to the axillary vessels.
e. The base or the floor is composed of (from below upwards) the skin, superficial fascia and the dome-shaped axillary fascia. The axillary tail of Spence passes through the foramen of Langer in the medial part of axillary fascia to enter into the axilla.
f. The apex or cervicoaxillary canal is the communicating passage between the axilla and the posterior triangle of the neck. The boundaries of the apex are the middle third of clavicle anteriorly, the superior margin of scapula posteriorly and the outer margin of the first rib medially (Fig. 3.2). The structures that pass through the apex are, axillary vessels, cords of brachial plexus, long thoracic nerve and the subclavian lymph trunk.

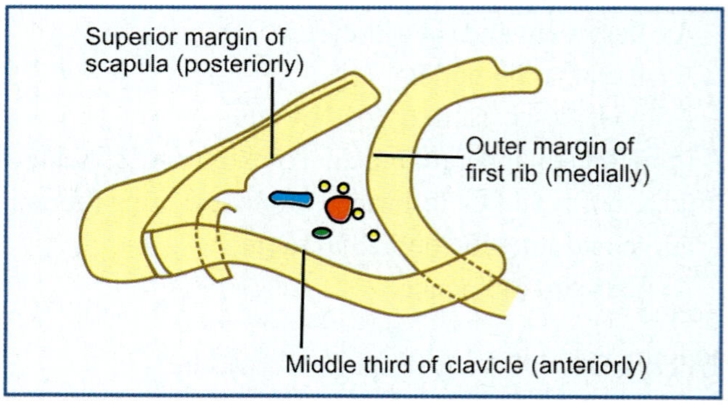

Fig. 3.2: Boundaries of apex of axilla
Contents of the apex—Axillary vessels, cords of brachial plexus, long thoracic nerve and subclavian lymph trunk

Clinical Highlights

The vascular relations of the walls of axilla should be borne in mind while placing an incision on the base of axilla for draining an abscess. The safe site to place the incision is midway between the anterior and posterior margins of the base closer to the medial wall.

Serratus Anterior Muscle

This is a broad and flat muscle of the trunk in the medial wall of the axilla (Fig. 3.3). The serratus anterior arises

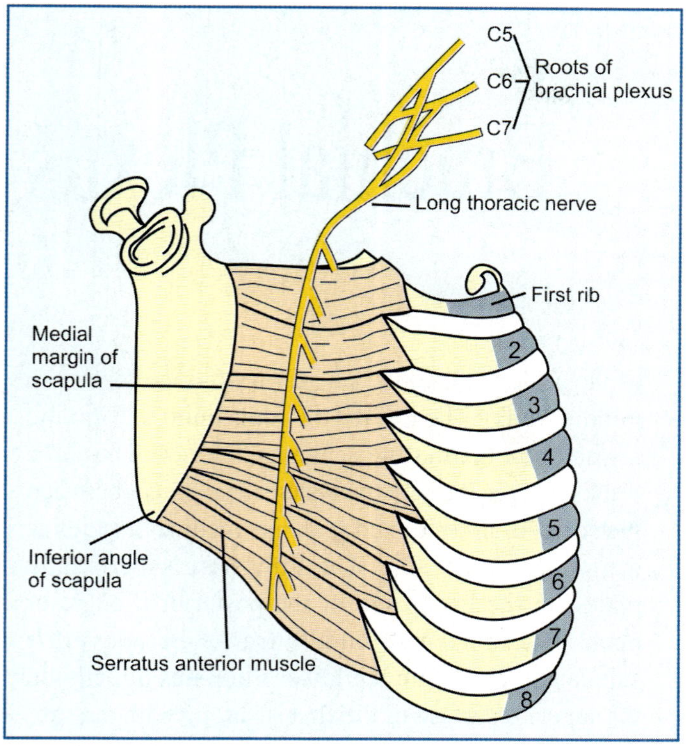

Fig. 3.3: Schematic diagram of serratus anterior muscle and long thoracic nerve in medial wall of axilla

from the anterior aspect of the upper eight ribs by eight fleshy digitations. It passes backwards around the chest wall to be attached to the medial border of the ventral surface of scapula. The first digitation arises from the outer border of the first rib and from the second rib. It is inserted in the superior angle of scapula. The second, third and fourth digitations arise from respective ribs and spread out to be inserted along the entire medial border. The lower four digitations arise from the respective ribs and converge for insertion in the inferior angle of scapula.

Nerve Supply

The long thoracic nerve (nerve of Bell) supplies the serratus anterior muscle. The nerve descends on the superficial surface of the muscle and gives separate twig to each digitation.

Actions

The serratus anterior muscle protracts the scapula with the help of pectoralis minor. Protraction is required during punching and pushing movements hence serratus anterior is called the boxer's muscle. The lateral rotation of scapula is brought about by the lower five digitations with the help of trapezius. It fixes the scapula against the ribs during scapular movements.

Testing Muscle Function

The subject is asked to place the stretched hands on the wall and push forwards (Fig. 3.4). Normally the scapulae will remain fixed to the thoracic cage. If the medial border of scapula is raised during this act it is indicative of weakness or paralysis of serratus anterior.

WINGING OF SCAPULA (Fig.3.4)

If the long thoracic nerve is injured the medial border and inferior angle of scapula are raised from the ribs. This deformity is called winging of scapula (as if the scapula developed a wing). The patient experiences difficulty in abduction of arm above 90°.

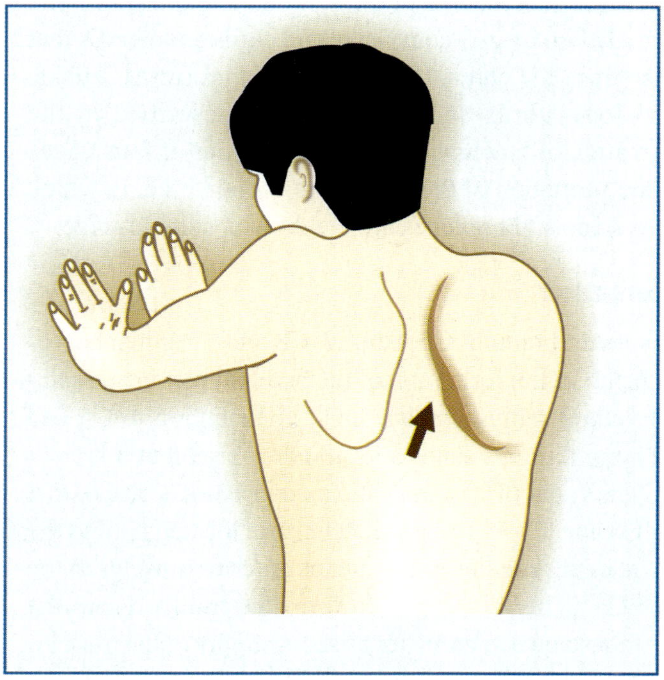

Fig. 3.4: Winging of right scapula on pressing outstretched hands against wall

4 Brachial Plexus

The brachial plexus is a plexus of nerves, which is responsible for the nerve supply of the superior extremity including a few muscles of the trunk. Through connections with the sympathetic ganglia, the branches of the brachial plexus provide pilomotor branches (to arrectores pili of skin), sudomotor branches (to sweat glands) and vasomotor branches (to the smooth muscle of blood vessels) to the skin of the upper limb.

Location and Parts

The brachial plexus lies partly in the posterior triangle of the neck and partly in the axilla. So, it is divisible into the supraclavicular and infraclavicular parts. The supraclavicular part consists of roots, trunks and divisions. The infraclavicular part consists of the cords and nerves that arise from the cords. Usually, five stages (roots, trunks, divisions, cords and branches) are described in the formation of brachial plexus. Descriptions of four stages in the formation of the plexus are encountered, in which cord stage and branches are clubbed in a single stage.

Formation (Fig. 4.1)

The ventral rami of C5, C6, C7, C8 and T1 spinal nerves take part in the formation of the brachial plexus. Usually C4 ventral ramus sends a small contribution to C5 and T2 ventral ramus sends a small contribution to T1.

a. The roots of brachial plexus consist of C5, C6, C7, C8 and T1 ventral rami, which are located behind the scalenus medius and scalenus anterior muscles in the neck. The roots unite to form the trunks. From the root stage two branches arise for supply of the muscles of the upper extremity, namely, dorsal scapular nerve or nerve to rhomboids (C5) and long thoracic nerve or nerve of Bell (C5, C6, C7).
b. There are three trunks. The C5 and C6 roots unite to form the upper trunk (Erb's point) at the lateral margin of the scalenus medius. The C7 root alone forms the middle trunk. The C8 and T1 roots unite to form the lower trunk behind the scalenus anterior. The three trunks emerge through the interscalene space (between the scalenus anterior and scalenus medius muscles as shown in Figure 30.1. The trunks are superficially placed in the lower part of the posterior triangle of neck. The upper and middle trunks lie above the subclavian artery but the lower trunk lies directly on the superior surface of the first rib along with the subclavian artery (Fig. 30.1). The upper trunk gives rise to two branches, namely, suprascapular nerve (C5, C6) and nerve to subclavius. No branches arise form the middle and lower trunks.
c. Each trunk slants obliquely downwards towards the middle third of the clavicle, where it terminates in to anterior and posterior divisions just behind the clavicle.
d. The cords are formed at the cervicoaxillary canal as follows. All the three posterior divisions unite to form the posterior cord. So, the posterior cord should contain fibers of all the roots. But in reality T1 fibers are usually absent, the reason being, the slender posterior division of the lower trunk carries C8 fibers only. The anterior divisions of upper and middle trunks unite to form the lateral cord (C5, C6, and C7). The anterior division of the lower trunk continues as the medial cord (C8, T1). The relations of the cords to the first and second parts of the axillary artery are different. Around the first part, the medial cord is in posterior position while the lateral and posterior cords are in lateral position. However, the cords take up the positions as signified by their names around the second part of the artery.
e. A large number of branches arise from the cords in the axilla.

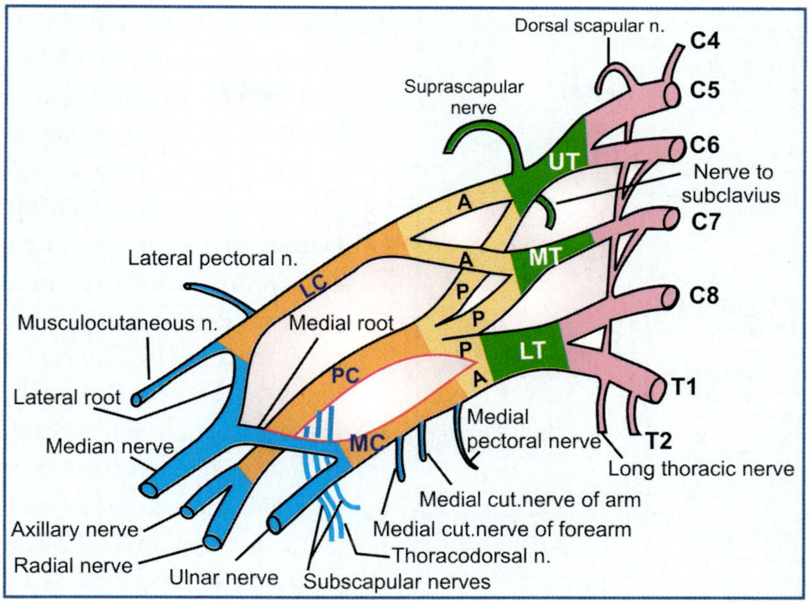

Fig. 4.1: Schematic depiction of stages in the formation of brachial plexus
(UT-Upper trunk, MT-Middle trunk, LT-Lower trunk, LC-Lateral cord, PC-Posterior cord, MC-Medial cord)

Branches of Cords

Cords	*Branches*
Lateral cord (3 branches)	Lateral root of median—C5, C5, C7 Lateral pectoral—C5, C6, C7 Musculocutaneous—C5, C6, C7
Medial cord (5 branches)	Medial root of median—C8, T1 Medial pectoral—C8, T1 Medial cutaneous nerve of arm—C8, T1 Medial cutaneous nerve of forearm—C8, T1 Ulnar nerve—C8, T1
Posterior cord (5 branches)	Upper subscapular—C5, C6 Lower subscapular—C5, C6 Thoracodorsal—C6, C7 or C6, C7, C8 Axillary nerve—C5, C6 Radial nerve—C5, C6, C7, C8, (T1)

Pre-fixation and Post-fixation of Brachial Plexus

Pre-fixed brachial plexus moves one segment higher than usual because the contribution from C4 becomes larger, that from T1 is reduced and that from T2 is absent. Post-fixed brachial plexus moves one segment lower than usual because the contribution from T2 is larger, that from C5 is reduced and that from C4 is absent. Post-fixed brachial plexus will have mechanical disadvantage since the lower trunk has to be more angulated and hence stretched on the upper surface of the first rib. This may give rise to symptoms of compression of the lower trunk.

Connections with Sympathetic Chain (Fig. 4.2)

The ventral rami of the C5 to C8 and T1 spinal nerves receive postganglionic sympathetic fibers from the middle cervical and stellate ganglia of the sympathetic chain via the grey rami communicantes (GRC). In this way the nerves of the plexus carry postganglionic sympathetic fibers to the upper limb. The ventral ramus of T1 presents additional connection to stellate ganglion via the first white ramus communicans (WRC). The preganglionic sympathetic fibers in the first WRC supply the head and face. They synapse in the superior cervical ganglion, from where the postganglionic fibers supply the dilator muscle of the pupil, smooth muscle of the upper eyelid (Müller's muscle) and vasomotor, sudomotor and pilomotor fibers to the skin of the head and face. The WRC of T1 ventral ramus may be avulsed in traumatic injury to the brachial plexus, which may give rise to symptoms associated with loss of sympathetic supply to the face (Horner's syndrome).

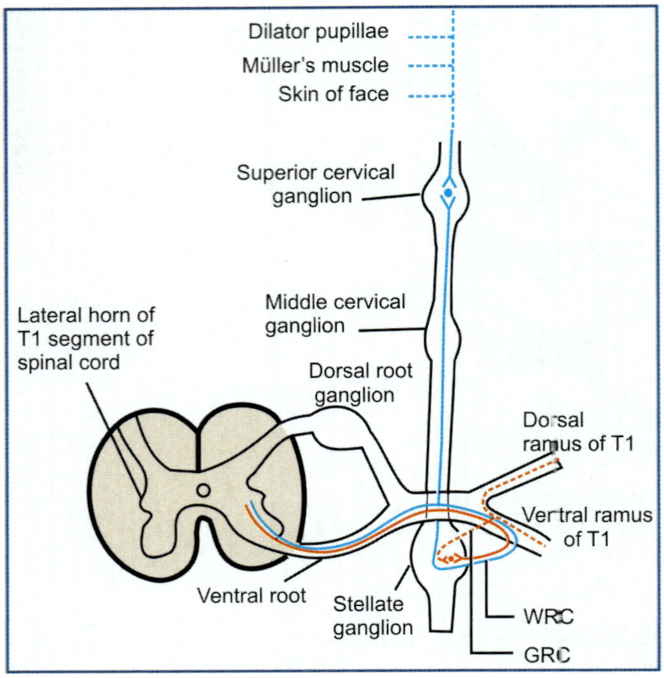

Fig. 4.2: Sympathetic connections of first thoracic spinal nerve. Postganglionic fibers from stellate ganglion supply pilomotor, sudomotor and vasomotor fibers to the skin and those from superior cervical ganglion supply structures in head and neck as shown in figure

Clinical Highlights

The brachial plexus may be damaged due to trauma, compression or malignancy of breast. The traumatic causes of the brachial plexus injury are, forceps delivery, gunshot or stab injuries, fall from a height or automobile accidents. Compression of plexus is usually due to aneurysm (dilatation) of the axillary artery. The plexus may be injured due to radiation of the axilla for breast cancer or by direct infiltration of malignant cells.

a. Total brachial plexus paralysis is a serious injury. The roots of the plexus are avulsed so the upper limb is paralyzed with total loss of sensation. The serratus anterior and rhomboid muscles are also paralyzed. Damage to T1 ventral ramus involving preganglionic sympathetic fibers for head and face (Fig. 4.2) results in Horner's syndrome on the affected side. This syndrome consists of partial ptosis (due to paralysis of Müller's muscle), constriction of pupil (due to paralysis of dilator pupillae), loss of sweating (due to loss of sudomotor supply) and flushing of face (due to loss of vasomotor supply).

b. The upper trunk or Erb's palsy in newborn usually occurs during forceps delivery, during which, there may be forceful separation of neck and shoulder with resultant stretching of the upper trunk (Erb's point). Hence it is also known as obstetrical palsy. It may also happen due to accidental trauma. The Erb's point is described as the meeting point of six nerves (Fig. 4.3), which include ventral rami of C5 and C6, two branches (suprascapular and nerve to subclavius) of upper trunk and two divisions of upper trunk. The upper limb is held in porter's tip or policeman's tip or waiter's tip position, in which the arm is adducted and medially rotated and the forearm is extended and pronated (Fig. 4.3). This happens due to paralysis of following muscles and consequent overaction of antagonist muscles as given in following Table 4.1.

Table 4.1

Position	*Paralysis of*	*Overaction of*
Adduction of arm	Supraspinatus and deltoid	Adductors of shoulder
Medial rotation of arm	Teres minor and infraspinatus	Medial rotators of shoulder
Extension of forearm	Biceps brachii, brachialis and brachioradialis	Extensors of elbow
Pronation of forearm	Biceps brachii and supinator	Pronators of forearm

c. The lesion of lower trunk or Klumpke's paralysis is usually produced by traction on the lower trunk exerted by a cervical rib or forcible hyper-abduction in a fall from a height or malignant infiltration of the lower trunk (as in pancoast tumor of lung or carcinoma breast) or postfixed brachial plexus. This lesion results in complete claw hand (Fig. 4.4), in which there is slow progressive weakness in interossei and lumbricals supplied by C8 and T1 root via branches of ulnar and median nerves. In claw hand the fingers are hyperextended at metacarpophalangeal joints and hyper flexed at interphalangeal joints due to paralysis of interossei and lumbricals. The wrist joint is hyperextended due to paralysis of flexors of wrist and overaction of extensors. There is pain and numbness along the medial side of the arm, forearm and medial one and half fingers. Horner's syndrome may be produced due to injury to the ventral ramus of T1 spinal nerve or first WRC (Fig. 4.2).

d. Injury to posterior cord of brachial plexus results in following functional deficits. The muscles supplied via the branches of posterior cord will be paralyzed.
   i. Loss of extension of shoulder (axillary nerve—posterior fibers of deltoid, subscapular nerve- teres major and thoracodorsal nerve- latissimus dorsi).
   ii. Loss of extension of elbow, wrist and thumb (radial nerve and branches—triceps brachii, extensors of wrist and thumb).
   iii. Loss of shoulder abduction beyond 20° (axillary nerve-deltoid).
   iv. Weakness of supination (deep branch of radial nerve-supinator).
   v. Weakness of medial rotation (subscapular nerve-subscapularis muscle).

Long Thoracic Nerve (Fig. 3.3)

This is also known as the nerve of Bell. It is a branch of the root stage of the brachial plexus. It is a purely motor nerve. The long thoracic nerve begins from C5, C6 and C7 nerve roots in the neck.

Cervical Course

The three roots pass downwards behind the supraclavicular part of the brachial plexus. The C5 and C6 roots separately pierce the scalenus medius muscle and then unite with each other. This common trunk and the C7 root enter the axilla through its apex and unite with each other to form the long thoracic nerve.

Axillary Course

The long thoracic nerve is closely related to the lateral surface of serratus anterior muscle, which forms the medial wall of the axilla. It gives separate twigs to each of the eight digitations of the muscle.

Winging of Scapula or Winged Scapula

The long thoracic nerve may be injured during surgical removal of axillary lymph nodes. This results in paralysis of the serratus anterior muscle leading to a deformity called, winged scapula. In this, the medial border and inferior angle of scapula stand out from the chest wall (Fig. 3.4) and the patient experiences difficulty in abduction of arm above 90°.

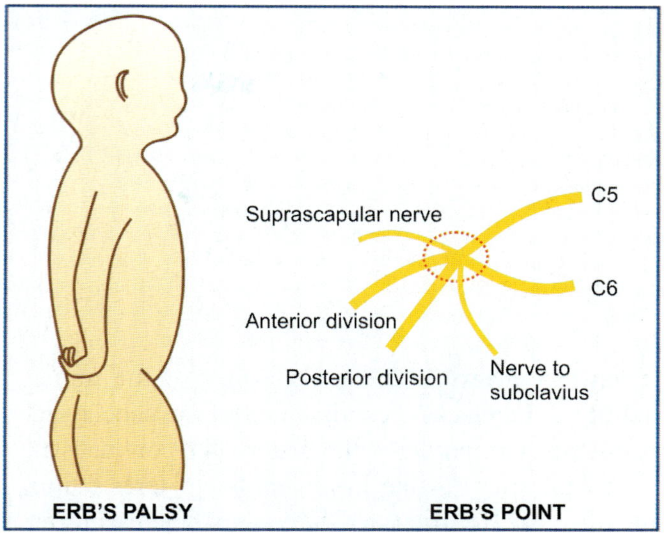

Fig. 4.3: Porter's tip position of right upper limb due to injury to Erb's point

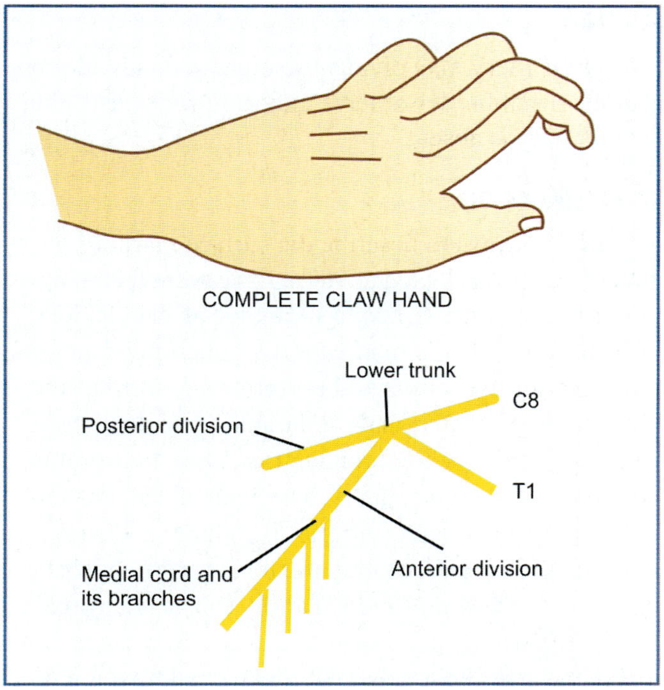

Fig. 4.4: Complete claw hand due to injury to lower trunk of brachial plexus

Axillary Vessels 5

The axillary artery is the main artery of the upper extremity. It begins as a continuation of the subclavian artery at the outer border of the first rib and continues as the brachial artery at the lower border of teres major muscle. The axillary artery and the cords of brachial plexus are wrapped in a fascial sheath derived from the prevertebral fascia of the neck.

Variation

The axillary artery may divide into ulnar and radial arteries at the distal border of teres major. In such cases the brachial artery is absent.

Surface Marking

There are two ways to describe the surface marking.

a. With the arm abducted to 90° and the palm facing up, the first point is marked at midpoint of the clavicle. The second point is marked at the junction of the of the anterior two-thirds and posterior one-third of the line joining the lower ends of the anterior and posterior axillary folds. A line connecting these two points represents the axillary artery. The point of demarcation of axillary and brachial arteries is roughly at the level of the lower end of the posterior axillary fold (Fig. 5.1), where pulsation of artery can be felt against the humerus.
b. With the arm abducted to 90° and the palm facing up the midpoint of clavicle is marked. The second point is marked one cm below the midpoint of the line joining the two epicondyles of humerus (just medial to the tendon of biceps brachii). The upper one-third of the line joining the two points represents the axillary artery and the lower two-thirds the brachial artery.

Course and Subdivisions

As the axillary artery enters the axilla through the apex it is in intimate relation to the medial wall of axilla, which is formed by the first two digitations of serratus anterior. As it courses downwards with a lateral convexity it comes in very intimate relation to the lateral wall of the axilla.

The axillary artery is subdivided into three parts by the pectoralis minor muscle, which crosses it anteriorly (Fig. 5.2). The first part extends from the outer margin of the first rib to the upper margin of pectoralis minor. The second part lies deep or posterior to the pectoralis minor. The third part extends from the lower margin of the pectoralis minor to the lower margin of teres major. The first and second parts of the axillary artery are related to the cords of the brachial plexus and the third part to the branches of the cords.

Relations of First Part (Fig. 5.3)

a. The anterior relations (from superficial to deep) are the skin, superficial fascia and the platysma, the pectoral fascia and the clavicular head of the pectoralis major muscle. Deeper still the clavi-pectoral fascia

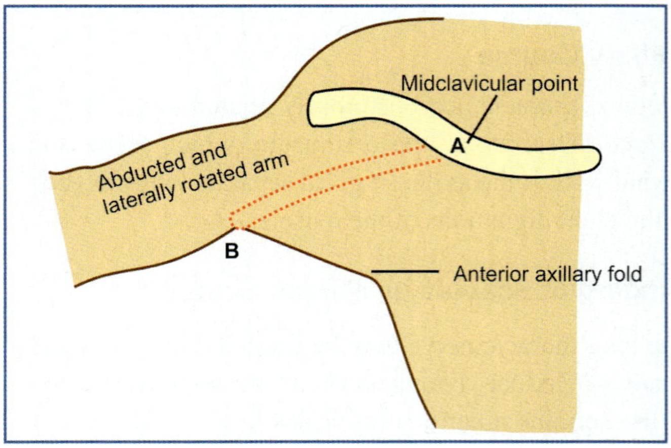

Fig. 5.1: Surface marking of axillary artery (line AB). B- Point at the junction of anterior 2/3rd and posterior 1/3rd of a line joining lower ends of anterior and posterior axillary folds

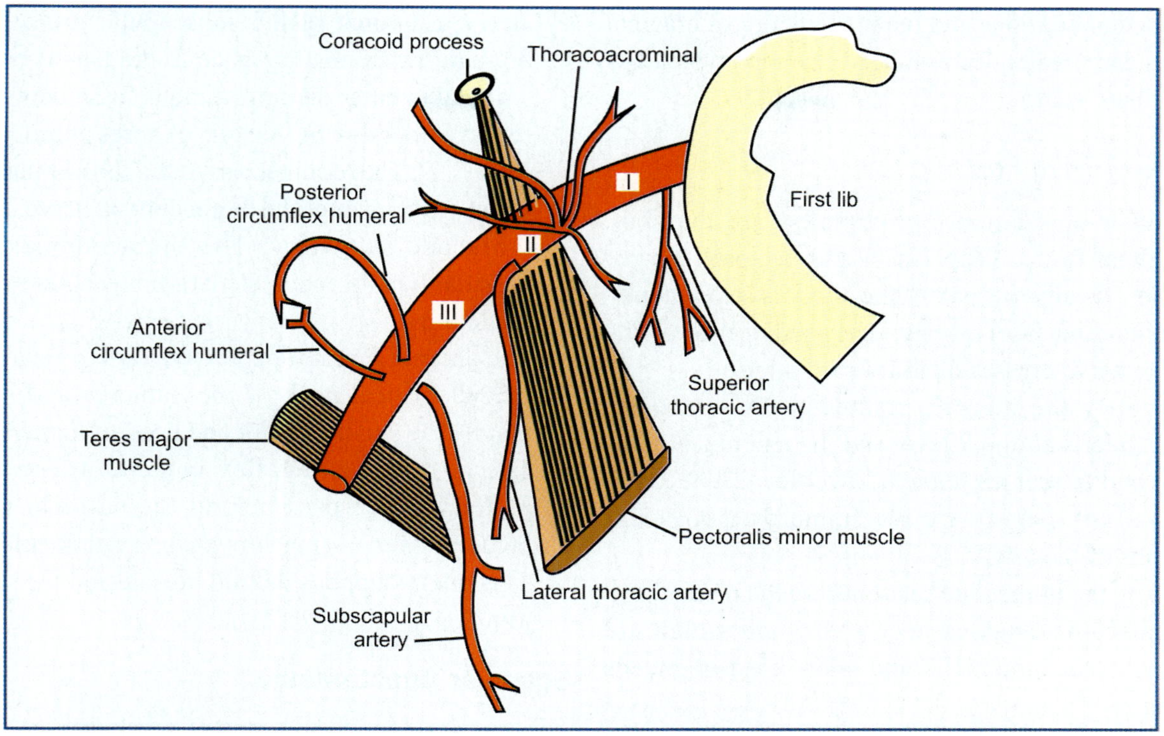

Fig. 5.2: Schematic diagram of extent, parts and branches of axillary artery

and the structures that pierce it lie in front of the artery. The communication between medial and lateral pectoral nerves crosses in front of the first part.

b. The posterior relations are the first two digitations of the serratus anterior muscle, with medial cord of brachial plexus and the long thoracic nerve.
c. The lateral relations are the lateral and posterior cords of brachial plexus and the lateral pectoral nerve.
d. The axillary vein is the medial relation.

Relations of Second Part (Fig. 5.3)

a. The anterior relations (from superficial to deep) are the skin, superficial fascia, the pectoral fascia and the clavicular head of pectoralis major. Deeper to this, the second part is crossed by the pectoralis minor muscle.
b. Posteriorly the artery is related to the subscapularis muscle and the posterior cord of the brachial plexus.
c. Lateral relations are, the coracobrachialis, short head of biceps brachii and the lateral cord of brachial plexus.

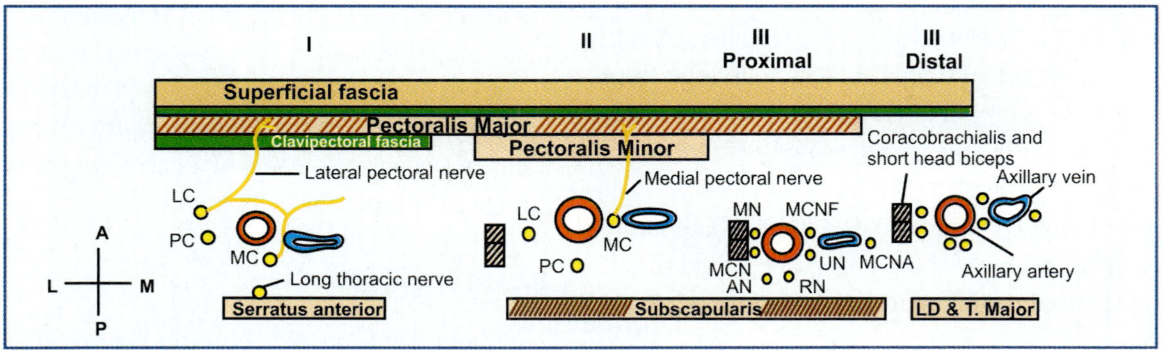

Fig. 5.3: Schematic depiction of relations of various parts of axillary artery. LC-Lateral cord, PC-Posterior cord, MC-Medial cord, MN-Median nerve, MCN-Musculocutaneous nerve, AN-Axillary nerve, RN-Radial nerve, UN-Ulnar nerve, MCNF-Medial cutaneous nerve of forearm, MCNA-Medial cutaneous nerve of arm

d. The medial relations are, the medial cord of brachial plexus and medial pectoral nerve, beyond which lies the axillary vein.

Relations of Third Part (Fig.5.3)

a. The anterior relations, proximally, are the skin, superficial fascia, deep fascia and pectoralis major muscle. Distally this part of the artery is covered only with skin and fasciae only. The medial root of the median nerve crosses the third part anteriorly.
b. Posteriorly the muscles related to this part are, subscapularis at upper level and the tendons of teres major and latissimus dorsi at lower level. The radial and axillary nerves are the immediate posterior relations of the artery.
c. Laterally the immediate relations are the median and the musculocutaneous nerves, beyond which are located coracobrachialis and short head of biceps brachii.
d. Medially, the medial cutaneous nerve of forearm and the ulnar nerve separate the artery and the axillary vein.

Branches (Fig. 5.2)

The first part of the axillary artery gives origin to one branch (superior thoracic), the second part to two branches (thoracoacromial and lateral thoracic) and the third part to three branches (subscapular, anterior and posterior circumflex humeral).

a. The superior thoracic artery supplies the upper two intercostal spaces anteriorly.
b. The thoracoacromial artery pierces the clavipectoral fascia to appear under cover of the clavicular head of pectoralis major. Then it divides into clavicular, deltoid, pectoral and acromial branches, which diverge from each other for supplying the pectoral and shoulder regions. It gives branches to breast and nutrient artery to clavicle.
c. The lateral thoracic artery takes a larger share in the supply of lateral part of the breast and the axilla. It lies along the inferior margin of pectoralis minor muscle.
d. The subscapular artery, the largest branch, courses downwards along the posterior wall of the axilla lying on subscapularis muscle. The circumflex scapular artery, a branch of the subscapular artery, passes through the triangular space at the lateral border of scapula, to enter the infraspinous fossa between two sets of fibers at the origin of teres minor muscle (Fig.11.2). The terminal part of the subscapular artery, which accompanies the thoracodorsal nerve, is called thoracodorsal artery. The thoracodorsal neurovascular bundle enters the latissimus dorsi muscle at the hilum.
e. The anterior circumflex humeral artery runs in front of the surgical neck of the humerus and supplies mainly the shoulder joint and head of humerus.
f. The posterior circumflex humeral artery and the axillary nerve pass behind the surgical neck of humerus after passing through the quadrangular space. This artery supplies deltoid muscle and the shoulder joint.

Scapular Anastomosis (Fig. 5.4)

The branches from the first part of subclavian artery make anastomotic connections with branches of third part of axillary artery around the scapula. Three arteries take part in the anastomosis.

a. The suprascapular artery, a branch of thyrocervical trunk of the first part of the subclavian artery supplies the costal and dorsal surfaces of scapula after it enters the supraspinous fossa by passing over the transverse scapular ligament.
b. Conventionally it is described that the deep transverse cervical artery (a branch of the thyrocervical trunk of the first part of the subclavian artery) takes part in the scapular anastomosis. It is now established that the dorsal scapular artery (a branch of third part of subclavian artery) being more constant than the deep cervical artery, takes part in scapular anastomosis.
c. The circumflex scapular branch of subscapular artery (from the third part of the axillary artery) reaches the dorsal surface of scapula by interrupting the origin of teres minor muscle.

Clinical Highlights

a. The scapular anastomosis brings in to communication the first part of subclavian artery with the third part of axillary artery. Thus, it acts as a collateral channel in case the subclavian or axillary artery is blocked anywhere between the first part of subclavian artery and the third part of the axillary artery, proximal to the origin of its subscapular branch (Fig.5.4). The anastomosis ensures adequate circulation to the upper limb. In such situations the arteries around scapula enlarge to a considerable extent. This may give rise to a clinical sign called 'pulsating scapula'.

b. Aneurysm means localized dilatation of the artery. The axillary aneurysm presents as a soft pulsating mass often palpable through the base of the axilla. Aneurysm may give rise to symptoms and signs due to compression of the nerves of axilla and the axillary vein.

Axillary Vein

According to one description, the union of basilic vein and the venae comitantes accompanying the brachial artery (brachial veins) form the axillary vein at the lower margin of teres major muscle. According to another description, the basilic vein continues as the axillary vein at the same level and the brachial veins open into the axillary vein at the lower margin of the subscapularis. The axillary vein becomes the subclavian vein at the outer border of first rib. It lies medial to the axillary artery throughout its course. The medial cutaneous nerve of the arm is medial to the vein and the medial cutaneous nerve of forearm

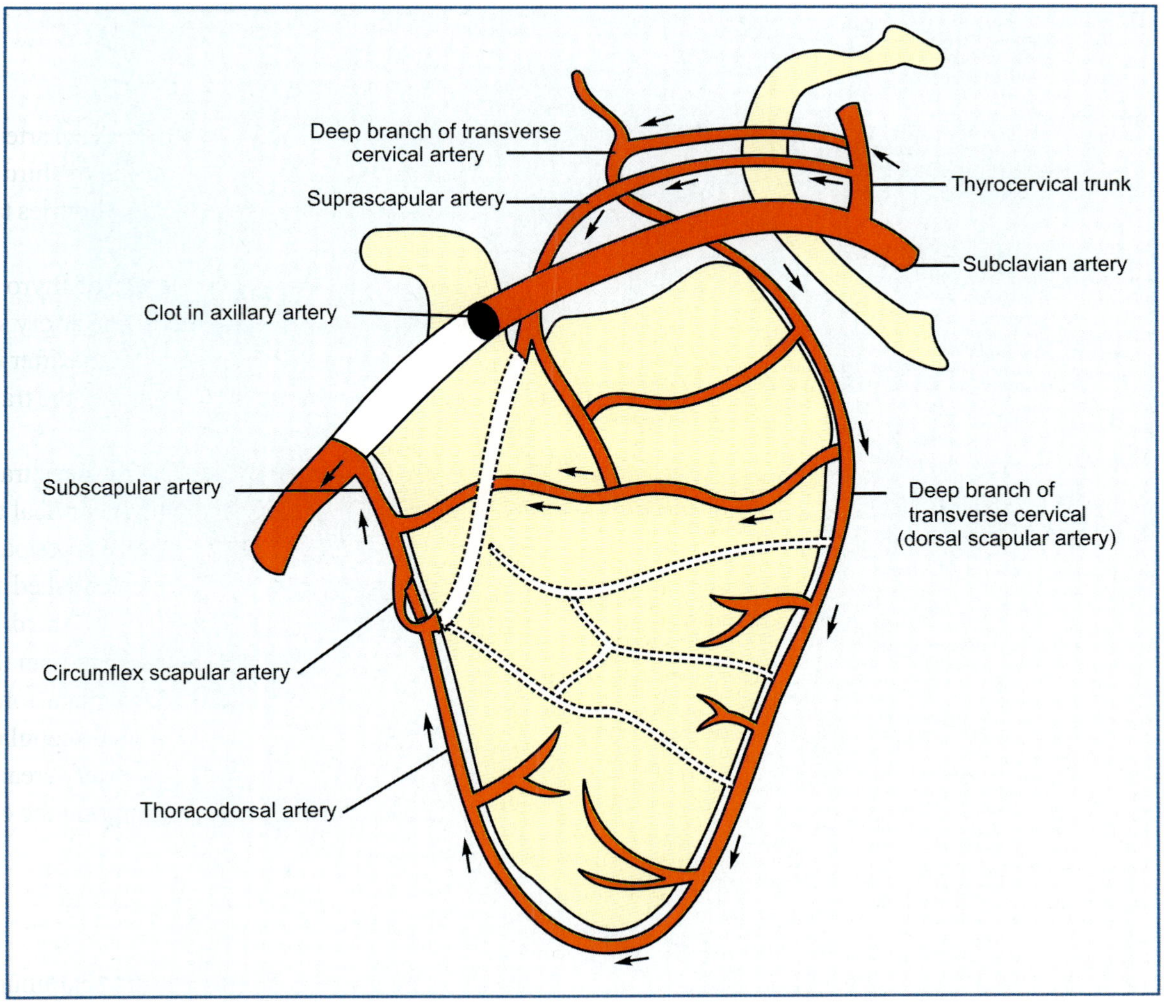

Fig. 5.4: Scapular anastomosis on anterior aspect of right scapula. Arrows indicate direction of blood flow in case of block in third part of axillary artery proximal to origin of its subscapular branch

and the ulnar nerve are lateral to the vein. The veins accompanying the branches of axillary artery are the tributaries of the axillary vein, though the venous pattern may be variable. The cephalic vein from the upper limb is its largest tributary.

Axillary Vein Thrombosis

Thrombosis in the terminal segment of the axillary vein in the apex of axilla may occur due to traction as seen in people, who have to keep the arm hyperabducted for long stretches of time (for example during plastering or painting the ceiling). The apical, central and lateral groups of axillary lymph nodes are very closely related to the axillary vein (Fig. 1.7). These nodes are removed during mastectomy by dissection. If the vein is injured during removal of nodes postoperative thrombosis may occur. This results in venous stasis causing edema of the upper limb and dilatation of superficial veins of the pectoral and shoulder regions.

6 Axillary Lymph Nodes

The axillary lymph nodes (Figs 1.7 and 3.1) are arranged into five principal groups. The area of their drainage includes the entire upper extremity and the thoraco-abdominal walls up to the level of umbilicus on the front and up to the level of iliac crest on the back. The axillary nodes drain nearly 75 percent of the breast tissue.

a. The anterior or pectoral group (Sojius' glands) is located in the anterior wall of the axilla along the course of lateral thoracic vessels. These nodes receive lymph from major portion of breast tissue, anterior chest wall and anterior abdominal wall up to the level of umbilicus. Its efferent vessels mainly go to the central nodes. The part of the mammary gland, which lies deep to the deep fascia (axillary tail of Spence), lies in close contact with these nodes.
b. The posterior or subscapular group is located in the posterior wall of axilla along the subscapular vessels. These nodes receive lymph from the posterior chest wall and posterior abdominal wall up to the level of iliac crest.
c. The lateral or brachial group is located on the lateral wall of axilla along the axillary vein. The lymph nodes of lateral group receive lymph from the entire upper limb. A few vessels accompanying the cephalic vein drain in the deltopectoral nodes and others from lateral aspect of proximal arm terminate directly into the apical nodes. Some lymph vessels accompanying the basilic vein terminate in the epitrochlear (supratrochlear or cubital) nodes, the efferent vessels from which drain in the lateral group. Inflammatory lesion anywhere in the upper limb gives rise to enlarged and painful lateral group of lymph nodes.
d. The central group is composed of three or four large lymph nodes embedded in the fatty tissue along the axillary vein. These nodes receive lymph from anterior, posterior and lateral groups and drain into the apical nodes. The intercostobrachial nerve passes through the central nodes. Therefore, the swollen central nodes may be the cause of pain along the medial side of upper part of arm and the base of axilla.
e. The apical group consists of six to eight lymph nodes lying partly in the apex of the axilla and along the axillary vein in the triangular space between the axillary vein, outer margin of first rib and the upper margin of pectoralis minor muscle. These nodes receive lymph from the central group, deltopectoral or infraclavicular nodes and interpectoral nodes. They receive a few lymphatics directly from the superior peripheral region of the breast and a few from the proximal arm. The apical lymph nodes are the terminal nodes of the upper extremity. Their efferent vessels unite to form the subclavian lymph trunk, which terminates in the jugulovenous junction or the subclavin vein or the jugular lymph trunk or the right lymph trunk on the right side and the thoracic duct on the left side

Special Note

The surgeons include the interpectoral or Rotter's nodes as a sixth group of axillary lymph nodes. The interpectoral nodes are situated between the pectoralis major and minor muscles, closer to the anterior wall of axilla. They receive deep lymphatics from the breast and drain directly in to the apical group or into the central group.

New Classification of Axillary Lymph Nodes

The axillary lymph nodes are divided into three levels depending on their relation to the pectoralis minor muscle (Fig. 1.7). Level-I nodes are below the pectoralis minor muscle and include the lateral, anterior and posterior axillary lymph nodes. Level-II nodes are present either behind or in front of the muscle and include central and

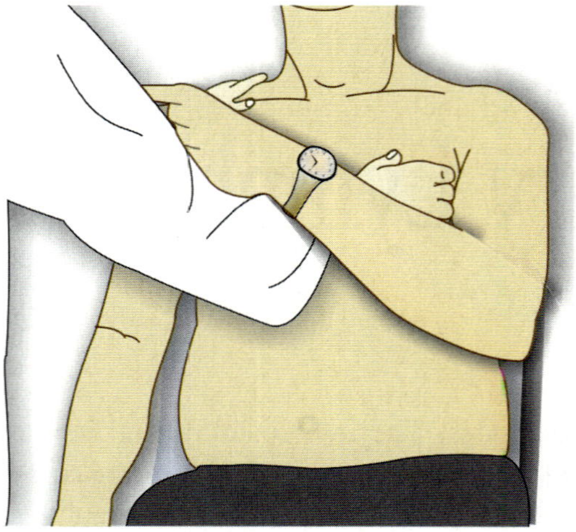

Fig. 6.1: Palpation of pectoral group of axillary lymph nodes

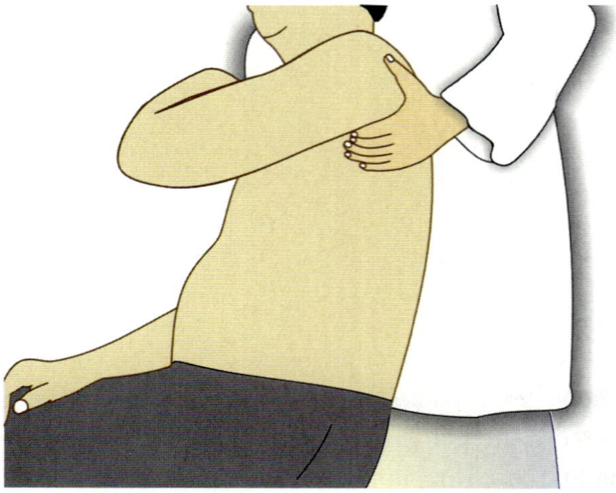

Fig. 6.2: Palpation of subscapular group of axillary lymph nodes

interpectoral nodes of Rotter. Level-III nodes are above the pectoralis minor muscle and include apical group. This leveling of the axillary nodes is very useful during surgery for breast cancer.

Clinical Highlights

a. The enlargement of lymph nodes is called lumphadenopathy. Cancer of the breast causes painless enlargement of the axillary lymph nodes. The painful enlargement is due to any infective focus in the area of drainage of the axillary lymph nodes. The nodes are also enlarged in generalized lymphadenopathy due to other causes like Hodgkin's lymphoma.

b. For palpation of axillary lymph nodes in a patient, the examiner may use his or her right hand for left axilla and left hand for right axilla. The examiner supports the arm of the patient in a slightly abducted position so as to relax the axillary floor and walls. Standing in front of the patient the semiflexed fingers are gently but firmly pushed in the floor of the axilla to palpate the anterior, central, apical and lateral nodes (Fig. 6.1). Standing behind the patient the examiner can feel the posterior nodes (Fig. 6.2).

7 Cutaneous Nerves of Upper Limb

The upper limb is a segmented lever. It consists of upper arm (arm), elbow, forearm, wrist, hand and digits. The upper limb consists of different groups of muscles, nerves and blood vessels enclosed within fascial compartments. The deep fascia and the intermuscular septa help in defining the boundaries of the fascial compartments. The superficial fascia contains the cutaneous nerves and the superficial veins.

Cutaneous Nerves

There are three sources from which cutaneous nerves originate.

a. Supraclavicular nerves (Fig. 1.4) from the cervical plexus.
b. Intercostobrachial nerve (lateral cutaneous branch of the second intercostal nerve).
c. Direct cutaneous nerves from brachial plexus and cutaneous nerves from branches of brachial plexus.

Cutaneous Nerves of Arm

a. Lateral supraclavicular nerve (C3, C4) supplies the area of shoulder overlying the upper part of the deltoid muscle.
b. Intercostobrachial nerve (T2) gives branches to the skin of the floor of axilla and the upper part of the medial side of arm.
c. Upper lateral cutaneous nerve of arm (C5, C6), a branch of axillary nerve, supplies the skin overlying the lower half of deltoid.
d. Lower lateral cutaneous nerve of arm (C5, C6), a branch of radial nerve in spiral groove, supplies the skin on the lateral side of arm below the insertion of deltoid.
e. Posterior cutaneous nerve of arm (C5), branch of radial nerve in the axilla, supplies the skin of the back of arm from the insertion of deltoid to the olecranon.
f. Medial cutaneous nerve of arm (T1) is a branch of medial cord of brachial plexus. It pierces the deep fascia at the middle of the medial side of arm to supply the skin on the lower half of arm.

Cutaneous Nerves of Forearm

a. Posterior cutaneous nerve of forearm (C6, C7, C8), a branch of the radial in the spiral groove, supplies the skin of the lateral side of arm. It travels in the superficial fascia of the middle of the back of the forearm and supplies the skin there.
b. Lateral cutaneous nerve of forearm (C5, C6) is a continuation of musculocutaneous nerve. It supplies the skin covering the anterolateral and posterolateral surfaces of the forearm (extending up to the ball of thumb) and accompanies the cephalic vein (Fig. 8.1).
c. Medial cutaneous nerve of forearm (C8, T1) is a branch of medial cord of brachial plexus. It pierces the deep fascia with the basilic vein (Fig. 8.1) at the level of insertion of coracobrachialis and supplies the skin of the anteromedial and posteromedial surfaces of the forearm.

Cutaneous Nerves of Hand

a. Superficial branch of radial nerve (C6, C7, C8) is one of the terminal branches of radial nerve. It supplies the lateral two-thirds of the dorsum of the hand and dorsal aspects of thumb and lateral 2½ fingers through five dorsal digital nerves (Fig. 23.1). However, there is considerable variation in the area of supply of the radial nerve on the dorsum of hand and digits.
b. Palmar cutaneous and palmar digital branches of median nerve (C6, C7, C8) supply the skin of the palm and the palmar aspect of lateral 3½ fingers including

the skin on the dorsal aspect of the terminal phalanges of the corresponding fingers (Fig. 25.3).

c. Dorsal and palmar cutaneous branches of ulnar nerve (C7, C8, T1) supply the medial side of the hand and the medial 1½ fingers on both aspects (Fig. 25.4).

Comparison of the areas of the cutaneous supply of different nerves reveals that the radial nerve supplies the maximum area. However, it is observed that the areas of sensory loss due to injury to the individual nerve do not coincide with the areas of their cutaneous supply. The reason for this discrepancy is that the cutaneous nerves supplying adjacent areas of skin overlap to a considerable extent. To cite an example, if the radial nerve is injured in the axilla or in the arm the area of sensory loss is invariably confined to a small area on the dorsum of hand between the thumb and index finger. In the case of injury to axillary nerve the sensory loss is found on a small patch of skin on the lower half of deltoid (regimental badge anesthesia) as shown in Figure 12.2.

Dermatomes

A dermatome is an area of skin supplied by a single spinal segment through its dorsal root. In the case of the trunk the dermatomes extend from the posterior to anterior median lines of the trunk. There is a marked overlap in adjacent dermatomes so that injury to a single spinal nerve produces very little sensory loss in the corresponding dermatome. In the case of the upper limb the innervation is through the brachial plexus and not directly from the spinal nerves. So a limb dermatome can be defined as an area of skin supplied by the ventral ramus of a single spinal nerve through the branches of the plexuses. There is marked overlap in the adjacent dermatomes because of the presence of fibers of more than one ventral ramus in different branches of the plexus. Thus, it can be inferred that the area of distribution of any one cutaneous nerve cannot be equated to any one dermatome.

Dermatomes of Upper Limb (Fig. 1.5)

The dermatomes of the upper limb can be understood better if we know the development of the limb. In the embryo the upper limb bud carries within it the ventral rami from C5 to T1 segments of the spinal cord. Each limb bud has ventral and dorsal surfaces and preaxial (cranial) and postaxial (caudal) borders. The upper limb bud undergoes lateral rotation as a result of which the preaxial or cranial border becomes the lateral border and postaxial or caudal border becomes the medial border of the limb. Consequently the thumb becomes the preaxial digit and little finger the postaxial digit. The proximal two dermatomes (C5 and C6) are arranged in numerical sequence along the preaxial border up to the preaxial digit. Similarly distal two dermatomes (C8 and T1) are arranged along the postaxial border from the little finger. The middle dermatome (C7) is present only in the hand and it includes the middle three digits (Fig.1.5). C4 dermatome overlies the shoulder and T2 dermatome covers the base of axilla. Thus the dermatomes are arranged in such a way that the discontinuous dermatomes come to lie side by side on the surfaces of the limbs along the ventral and dorsal axial lines.

Clinical Highlights

Damage to the cutaneous nerves results in anesthesia or sensory loss in the skin (inability to feel the exteroceptive sensations like touch, pain and temperature). A dermatomal sensory loss results if the dorsal roots of a spinal nerve are damaged. So a dermatome does not coincide with the area of supply of any one cutaneous nerve. The neurological examination of the patient with nerve root lesion, for example, compression of C7 root (in acute disc lesion) is incomplete without a thorough examination of dermatomes and areas of cutaneous distribution of upper limb. This is very crucial in differentiating the disease of the nerve root from that of a peripheral nerve. Therefore, a clinician must have a working knowledge of dermatomes of the body. In herpes zoster (shingles), the virus affects the dorsal root ganglion. This typically gives rise to a crop of cutaneous blisters in the dermatome of that particular nerve.

8 Veins of Upper Limb

The upper limb has two sets of veins. The deep veins accompany the arteries as venae comitantes. The superficial veins are located in the superficial fascia and being easily accessible, are often used for drawing blood sample or for giving intravenous injection.

Superficial Veins

The cephalic and basilic veins are the two main superficial or subcutaneous veins in the upper limb. They begin at the dorsal venous network. Other named veins like median cubital vein and the median vein of the forearm are the tributaries of these two main veins.

Dorsal Venous Network (Fig. 8.1B)

The dorsal venous network or arch is located in the superficial fascia on the dorsum of the hand. The dorsal digital veins draining the adjacent sides of the four fingers unite to form three dorsal metacarpal veins, which form a dorsal venous network. The lateral end of this network receives the digital vein from the radial side of index finger and two veins from the two sides of the thumb and this union continues proximally as the cephalic vein. Medially, the dorsal digital vein of the ulnar side of the little finger joins the network and continues as the basilic vein.

Cephalic Vein (Fig. 8.1A)

The cephalic vein begins on the lateral aspect of wrist from the lateral end of the dorsal venous network and terminates in the axillary vein in the axilla. It lies posterior to the styloid process of radius and in the roof of the anatomical snuffbox. It ascends along the posterolateral side of the forearm and turns anteriorly to reach the front of the lateral part of elbow. In this course the cephalic vein is closely related to lateral cutaneous nerve of forearm. In the arm the vein ascends along the lateral side of biceps brachii. At the upper part of the arm (at the level of lower margin of pectoralis major muscle) the cephalic vein pierces the deep fascia and enters the deltopectoral groove, where it is related to the deltoid branch of the thoraco-acromial artery and the deltopectoral lymph nodes. At the infraclavicular fossa (deltopectoral triangle) the vein takes a sharp turn backwards to pierce the clavipectoral fascia and enters the axilla to terminate into the axillary vein.

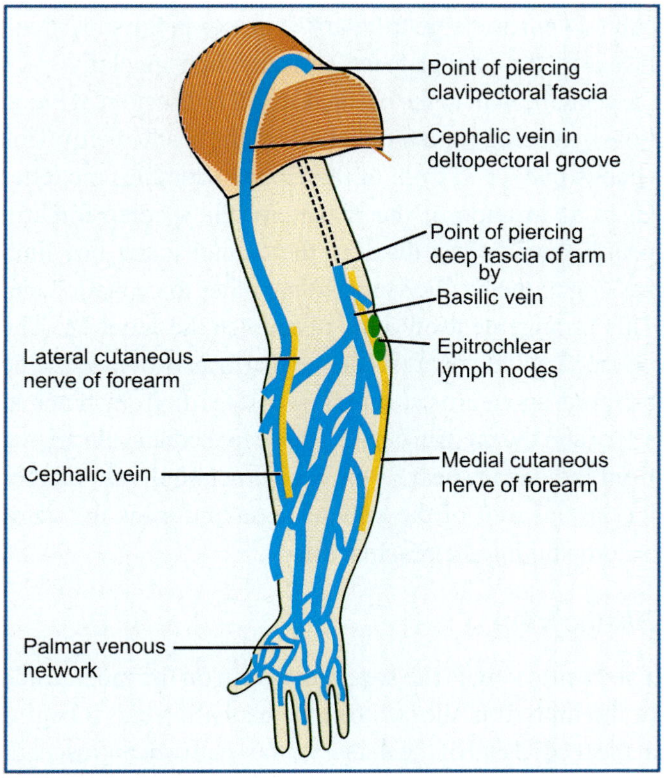

Fig. 8.1A: Superficial veins of upper limb

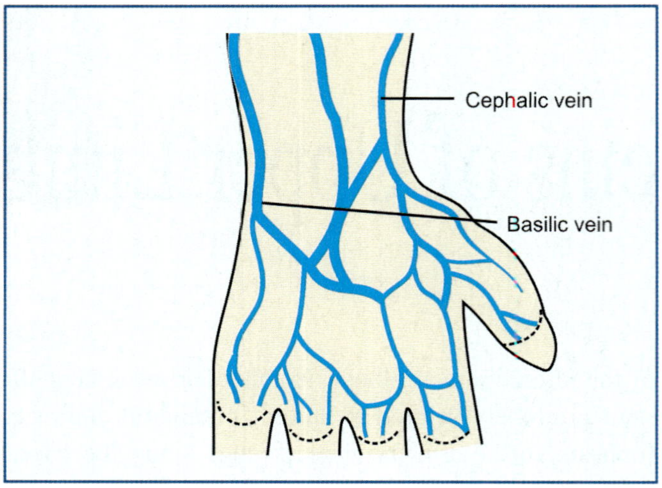

Fig. 8.1B: Origin of superficial veins from dorsal venous network

Tributaries

A large number of tributaries, which collect blood from the hand, forearm and arm open into the cephalic vein. Occasionally, a small communicating vein, which crosses the clavicle superficially, may join the uppermost part of the cephalic vein to the external jugular vein. Median cubital vein is a large tributary. It passes in the superficial fascia of the cubital fossa, upwards and medially from the cephalic vein to the basilic vein (The direction of blood flow in it being from the cephalic to the basilic vein). This venous pattern in front of the elbow resembles the letter H. In a variation of the H pattern, the median forearm vein bifurcates just distal to the cubital fossa, one limb passing to the basilic vein and the other to cephalic vein. This arrangement of veins resembles the letter M. The median cubital vein rests on the platform provided by the bicipital aponeurosis, which separates it from brachial artery and the median nerve. The deep median vein arising from the deep aspect of the median cubital vein pierces the fascial roof of the cubital fossa and joins the veins accompanying the brachial artery.

Basilic Vein

The basilic vein is the superficial vein on the medial side of the limb. It is shorter than the cephalic vein. It begins at the medial end of the dorsal venous network and ascends on the medial side of posterior surface of the forearm. Just below the elbow it moves to the anterior surface of the forearm and crosses the medial part of the front of elbow to enter the arm. The medial cutaneous nerve of the forearm is closely related to it in front of the elbow. The epitrochlear (supratrochlear) or superficial cubital lymph nodes lie by the side of basilic vein just above the elbow. In the arm the basilic vein runs along the medial margin of biceps muscle and at the mid-arm level it pierces the deep fascia of the arm to enter the anterior compartment, where it lies medial to the brachial artery. At the lower border of teres major, the basilic vein unites with the brachial veins (venae comitantes of the brachial artery) to form the axillary vein. However, since the basilic vein is more in line with the axillary vein, some authors describe that basilic vein continues as axillary vein at the lower margin of teres major and that the brachial veins open in the axillary vein.

Tributaries

The basilic vein collects blood from the medial aspect of hand, forearm and arm by numerous tributaries. The median cubital vein is its large tributary. It may also receive median forearm vein from the front of the forearm if it does not join the median cubital vein.

Median Vein of Forearm

This vein on the front of the forearm is also called antebrachial vein. It drains the superficial palmar plexus and travels in the superficial fascia of the front of forearm upward to open into the median cubital vein or the basilic vein.

Clinical Highlights

a. For routine purposes like drawing blood sample for laboratory investigations or for giving intravenous medicines or glucose or for blood transfusion the preferred sites for venipuncture are the median cubital vein (Fig. 16.3) in front of elbow, median vein of forearm and the cephalic vein behind styloid process of radius.
b. The cephalic vein cut-down at deltopectoral groove is preferred, when superior vena caval infusion is necessary.
c. The basilic vein is preferred for inserting a cardiac catheter to reach the right side of the heart. To enter

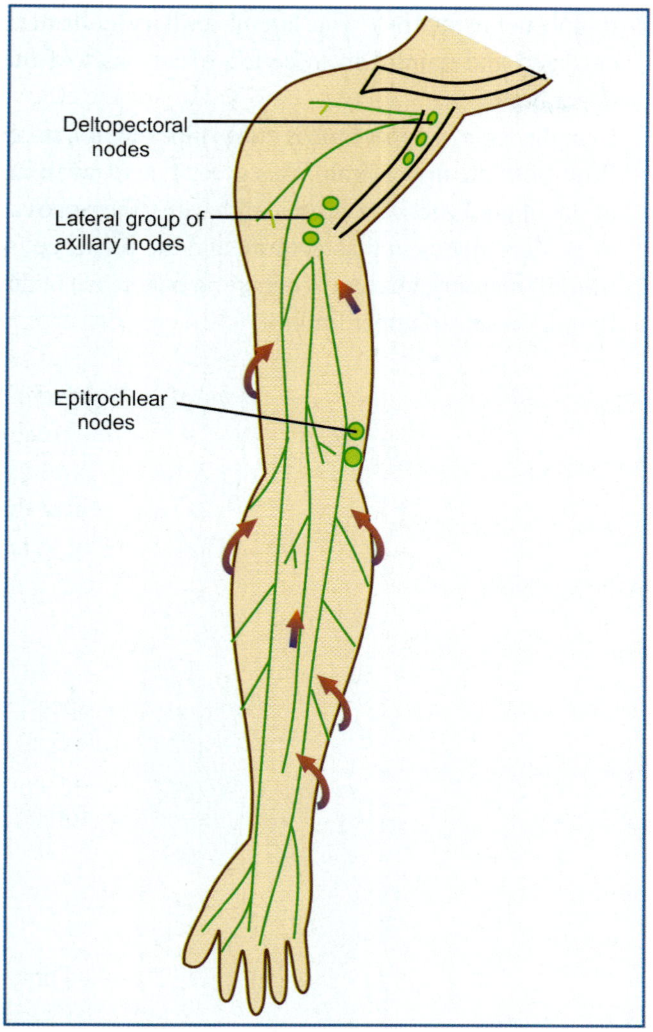

Fig. 8.2: Scheme to depict lymph vessels and nodes of upper limb

the right atrium the catheter passes in succession through the following veins, the basilic, axillary, subclavian, brachiocephalic and finally the superior vena cava. The sharp curve at cephalo-axillary junction and presence of valves at this junction are the two factors because of which cephalic vein is not preferred for this purpose.

d. Patients with chronic renal failure are subjected to hemodialysis at regular intervals to remove accumulated waste products from the blood. For this purpose the cephalic vein is arterialized as follows. A subcutaneous arteriovenous fistula is created at the wrist by anastomosing the cephalic vein to the radial artery. The cephalic vein gradually shows distension and thickening as it is subjected to arterial pressure. This structural change in the cephalic vein is called its arterialization. This enables repeated punctures in it with a wide bored needle. The arterial and venous lines of the cannula are introduced in the cephalic vein, whenever dialysis is necessary. The impure blood is drawn in to the dialysis machine via the venous line and the purified blood is returned to the cephalic vein via the arterial line.

Lymphatic Drainage of Upper Limb

The superficial lymph vessels from the lateral side of the limb and lateral two digits course along the cephalic vein while those from the medial side of the limb and medial three digits follow the basilic vein. Some of the medial vessels terminate in supratrochlear or epitrochlear nodes which are situated just above the medial epicondyle along the basilic vein (Fig. 8.2). When enlarged these nodes can be felt on palpation (Fig. 8.3). Almost all the superficial vessels of the upper limb drain into the lateral group of axillary nodes. A few along the cephalic vein (draining the thumb and lateral side of upper limb), end in the deltopectoral nodes, from where the new lymphatics pierce the clavipectoral fascia to terminate in to the apical group. A few superficial vessels directly pierce the

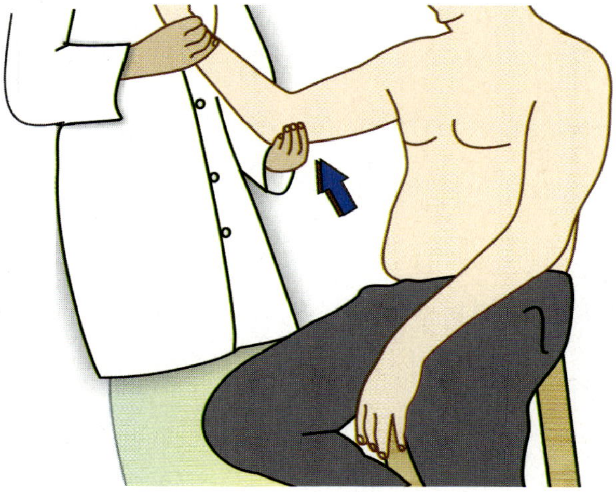

Fig. 8.3: Method of palpation of epitrochlear lymph node

clavipectoral fascia to enter directly in the apical group. The deep lymph vessels of the upper limb, course along the arteries and drain into the lymph nodes of lateral group.

Clinical Highlights

a. Lymphadenopathy is enlargement of lymph nodes. The infections affecting the medial side of hand and forearm may cause painful enlargement of the supratrochlear lymph nodes at first. The lateral axillary nodes are enlarged and painful in infection of any part of the upper limb.
b. Lymphedema of upper limb is due to blockage to lymph flow from the upper limb. This gives rise to swelling of the upper limb. The causes of this are, the removal of axillary nodes in mastectomy and the presence of filarial microorganisms (Wuchereria bancrofti) in the lymph vessels of upper limb.

9 Pectoral Girdle

The pectoral or shoulder girdle consists of two bones, clavicle and scapula. The clavicle articulates with the axial skeleton by the sternoclavicular joint, which is the only link between the upper limb and the trunk. It articulates with the scapula at the acromioclavicular joint. The pectoral girdle is suspended from the cranium and cervical vertebrae by the trapezius muscle.

SPECIAL FEATURE OF PECTORAL GIRDLE

The scapula is a highly mobile bone due to its unique relationship to the posterior thoracic wall. The subscapularis and serratus anterior muscles occupy the interval between the costal surface of scapula and the thoracic wall. There is a loose packing of areolar tissue between serratus anterior and chest wall as well as between the serratus anterior and subscapularis. This unit between the scapula and thoracic wall can be imagined as a scapulothoracic joint. Due to the presence of this pseudojoint the scapula slides over the thoracic wall easily. The scapula is supported by the clavicle and reinforced dynamically by the muscles, which insert into it from the axial skeleton (serratus anterior, trapezius, rhomboideus and levator scapulae). The high mobility of the scapula is responsible for the high mobility of the shoulder joint.

Girdle Joints (Fig. 1.1)

There are two joints in the pectoral girdle, sternoclavicular and acromioclavicular joints, where movements of scapula take place.

Sternoclavicular Joint

This is a saddle type of synovial joint. The articulating ends are the sternal end of the clavicle and the clavicular notch on the manubrium sterni and the first costal cartilage. The anterior and posterior sternoclavicular ligaments reinforce the fibrous capsule. The interclavicular ligament passing through the suprasternal space connects the medial ends of the two clavicles. The articular disk completely divides the joint cavity. The costoclavicular ligament is a powerful ligament that passes from first costochondral junction to the inferior surface of medial end of clavicle. It acts as a fulcrum during the movements of the scapula and prevents dislocation of the joint.

The posterior relations of this joint are important since they are in danger in posterior dislocation of the joint. The brachiocephalic veins and trachea on both sides and the brachiocephalic artery (on the right side) are related posteriorly.

Acromioclavicular Joint

This is a plane synovial joint. The articulating ends are the acromial end of the clavicle and the medial border of the acromion. The joint is divided by incomplete articular disk projecting inside from the upper part of the capsule. The fibrous capsule covers the joint and is strengthened superiorly by the acromioclavicular ligament. The coracoclavicular ligament is the main bond between clavicle and scapula. It is a very powerful ligament as it transmits the weight of the upper limb to the medial two-third of the clavicle. Its two parts are conoid and trapezoid. The conoid part is attached above to conoid tubercle of clavicle and below to the root of coracoid process. The trapezoid part is attached above to the trapezoid line of clavicle and below to the upper surface of coracoid process.

The acromioclavicular joint is prone to dislocation or shoulder separation, in which the fibrous capsule and the coracoclavicular ligament are torn. The scapula falls away from the clavicle and weight transmission to the axial skeleton becomes impossible.

Movements (Fig. 9.1)

The girdle joints allow free sliding of the scapula on the thoracic wall. The elevation and depression of scapula take place around an anteroposterior axis passing through costoclavicular ligament. The protraction and retraction of scapula take place around a vertical axis passing through costoclavicular ligament. Lateral or forward and medial or return rotation of scapula takes place around an axis passing through acromioclavicular joint.

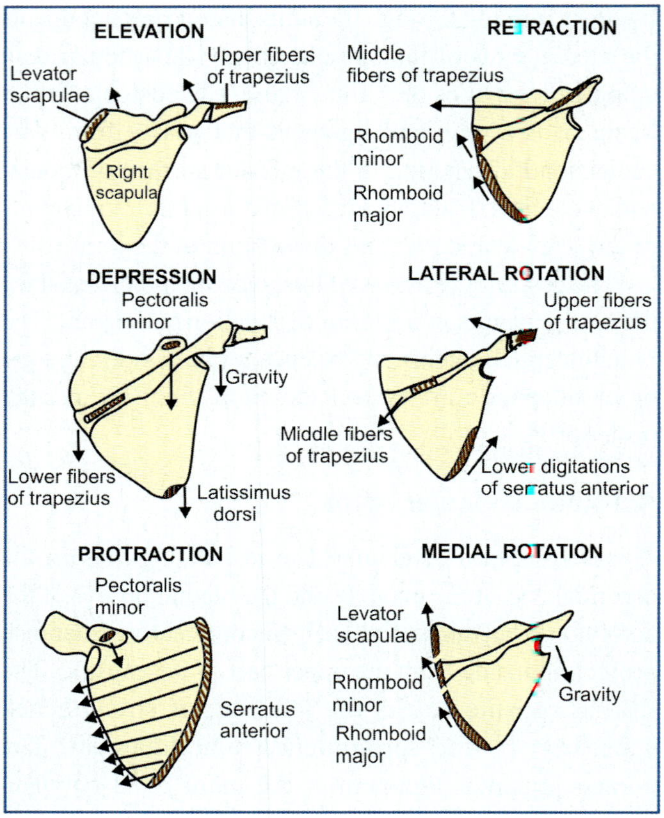

Fig. 9.1: Movements of scapula

Elevation and Depression

When the lateral end of the clavicle is elevated, the scapula is also elevated along with it and the medial end of the clavicle is depressed. When the lateral end of the clavicle is depressed, the scapula is also depressed. The elevation of scapula (shrugging movement) is caused by contraction of the upper fibers of trapezius and the levator scapulae. The depression of the scapula is produced by contraction of pectoralis minor along with lower fibers of trapezius.

Protraction and Retraction

During the protraction and retraction the lateral end of clavicle moves forwards or backwards respectively, along with the scapula. Protraction is the movement used in punching, pushing and reaching forwards. It is produced due to combined action of serratus anterior and pectoralis minor muscles. Retraction is the result of contraction of middle fibers of trapezius and rhomboids.

Rotation

The scapula shows forward or lateral rotation and medial or return rotation. In lateral rotation, as the clavicle rotates upwards along its longitudinal axis, the scapula also rotates so that its acromion is lifted upwards and medially and the inferior angle is turned forwards and laterally. The net effect is on the glenoid cavity, which faces upwards. The forward or lateral rotation of the scapula is an integral part of abduction of shoulder above 90°. This rotation is produced by the lower five digitations of the serratus anterior along with upper and lower fibers of trapezius. Medial or return rotation of scapula is due to the action of the muscles attached to the medial border of scapula assisted by gravity.

10 Muscles of the Back

The superficial muscles on the back of thorax are disposed in two layers. The outer layer is composed of two flat muscles, trapezius and latissimus dorsi. The inner layer consists of muscles attached to the medial border of scapula and the muscles attached to the dorsal surface of scapula.

TRAPEZIUS (Fig. 10.1 Right Side)

Each trapezius muscle is triangular in shape. The muscles of the two sides lie side by side in the midline along their linear attachment to the vertebral column and together form an outline of a diamond or a trapezoid (hence the name trapezius). The trapezius is the only muscle that suspends the pectoral girdle from the cranium.

Origin

The trapezius has a wide origin from the medial third of superior nuchal line, external occipital protuberance, ligamentum nuchae, spine of the seventh cervical vertebra and the supraspinous ligaments and spines of all thoracic vertebrae.

Insertion

a. Upper fibers pass downwards and laterally to insert in the posterior aspect of lateral third of clavicle.
b. Middle fibers pass horizontally to the medial aspect of acromion and crest of the spine of scapula.
c. Lower fibers pass upwards and laterally for attachment to a well-marked deltoid tubercle at the junction of medial and middle thirds of the spine of scapula.

Actions

a. The upper fibers elevate the scapula along with levator scapulae. Its middle fibers cause retraction of scapula along with rhomboids. The upper and lower fibers of trapezius in conjunction with lower five digitations of serratus anterior bring about lateral or forward rotation of scapula.
b. The cervical fibers of trapezius of both sides act together to extend the neck.

Nerve Supply

The spinal part of accessory nerve gives motor supply and the C3 and C4 ventral rami are proprioceptive.

Testing Muscle Function

The subject is asked to raise shoulders towards the ears and simultaneously the examiner depresses the shoulders forcibly. Inability to raise the shoulder is suggestive of the weakness of the muscle.

LATISSIMUS DORSI (Fig. 10.1)

This is a large and flat muscle and is the only muscle that connects the pelvic girdle and the vertebral column to the upper limb. This muscle forms the posterior axillary fold.

Origin

The latissimus dorsi has a wide origin from the lower six thoracic spines and supraspinous ligaments, the spines of lumbar and sacral vertebrae through the posterior lamina of thoracolumbar fascia, outer lip of the posterior part of iliac crest, the lower three or four ribs and by a few slips from the inferior angle of scapula.

Insertion

The muscle converges towards the shoulder region and winds round the teres major muscle in the posterior wall

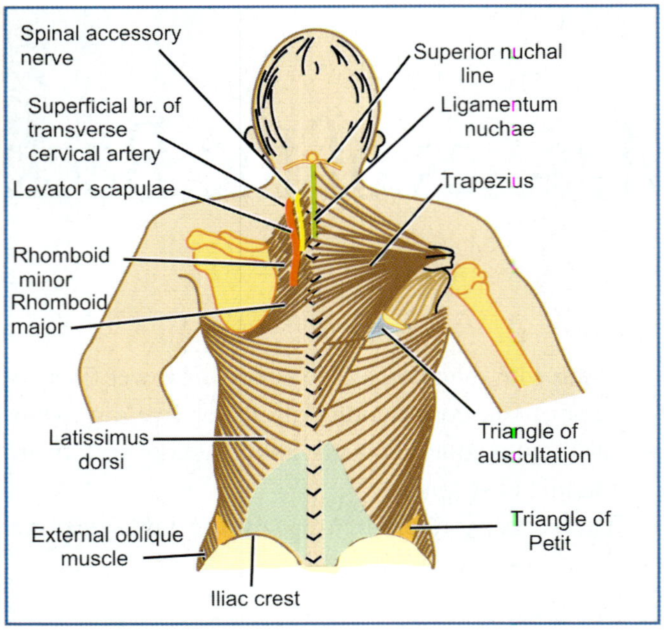

Fig. 10.1: Schematic depiction of superficial muscles of back on right side and some structures deep to thoracic part of trapezius on left side

of axilla, where it gives rise to a narrow flat tendon. The tendon of latissimus dorsi gains insertion in the floor of the intertubercular sulcus of humerus.

Nerve Supply

Thoracodorsal nerve, a branch of posterior cord of brachial plexus, supplies the muscle. The thoracodorsal nerve and thoracodorsal artery (continuation of subscapular artery beyond the origin of circumflex scapular artery) descends in the posterior wall of axilla to enter the latissimus dorsi muscle at a specific point called neurovascular hilum. This is of importance in reconstructive surgery.

Actions

a. The latissimus dorsi brings about adduction and medial rotation of the arm at the shoulder joint.
b. It is responsible for extension of arm at shoulder along with teres major and posterior fibers of deltoid.
c. It elevates the trunk as in climbing (Fig. 10.2) by extending the flexed arms to the side against resistance. This action is in conjunction with pectoralis major muscle.
d. The muscle is active in coughing and sneezing, which are the expiratory processes.

Testing Muscle Function

When the subject is asked to adduct the arm abducted to 90° against resistance the muscle can be felt in the posterior axillary fold. An alternative method is to ask the subject to cough and then feel the contraction of latissimus dorsi.

Triangles Related to Latissimus Dorsi (Fig. 10.1)

a. The triangle of auscultation is located in the back of the thorax. Its boundaries are the upper transverse margin of latissimus dorsi, lateral margin of trapezius and medial margin of scapula. The sixth and seventh ribs and the sixth intercostal space are in the floor of the triangle. The upper part of the lower lobe of the lung lies deep to this triangle on both sides.
b. The triangle of Petit or lumbar triangle is located in the lumbar region. It is bounded by iliac crest, posterior margin of external oblique and anterior margin of

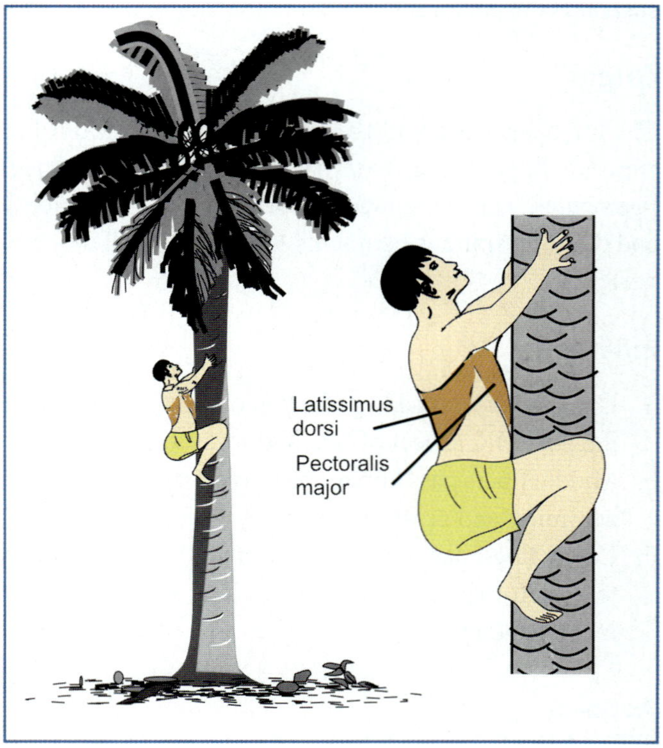

Fig. 10.2: Simultaneous contraction of latissimus dorsi and pectoralis major during climbing on a tree

latissimus dorsi. The internal oblique muscle is in the floor. This triangle is a potential site for herniation of abdominal contents.

Muscles Attached to Medial Border of Scapula (Fig. 10.1)

The levator scapulae and the two rhomboid muscles are attached to the medial or vertebral border of the scapula. Like the trapezius, serratus anterior and pectoralis minor, these muscles attach the scapula to the trunk.

a. The levator scapulae takes origin from the transverse processes of the upper four cervical vertebrae and is inserted into the medial border of scapula opposite the supraspinous fossa. The upper part of this muscle forms part of the floor of the posterior triangle of the neck.
b. The rhomboideus minor takes origin from lower part of ligamentum nuchae and the spines of seventh cervical and the first thoracic vertebrae. It is inserted into the medial border of scapula opposite the root of the spine.
c. The rhomboideus major takes origin from the spines of second to fifth thoracic vertebrae and the intervening supraspinous ligaments. It is inserted into the medial border of the scapula opposite the infraspinous fossa.

Nerve Supply

All the three muscles receive branches from the dorsal scapular nerve (C5). The levator scapulae muscle receives twigs from C3 and C4 ventral rami in the posterior triangle of neck.

Actions

All the three muscles stabilize the scapula during shoulder movements and transmit the body weight to the vertebral column especially during lifting heavy weight. The levator scapulae elevates the scapula along with upper fibers of trapezius. The rhomboid muscles along with middle fibers of trapezius retract the scapula. All the three muscles help in reverse or medial rotation of scapula.

Testing Muscle Function

With hands on the hips the subject tries to force the elbows backwards against resistance.

Dorsal Scapular Nerve (Nerve to Rhomboideus)

This nerve takes origin from the C5 nerve root (first stage of brachial plexus) in the neck. It is a purely motor nerve. Its course can be divided in two parts, cervical (in the posterior triangle of neck) and thoracic (scapular region). The nerve passes through the scalenus medius muscle and comes to lie on the anterior aspect of the levator scapulae muscle in the posterior triangle. Here the deep branch of the transverse cervical artery (or the dorsal scapular artery) joins it. The two descend in the back along the anterior surface of the levator scapulae muscle and the rhomboids, to which it gives motor twigs.

Muscles Attached to Dorsal Surface of Scapula

The supraspinatus and infraspinatus are the two muscles that are attached to the dorsal aspect of scapula (Fig. 15.1).

Attachments

a. The supraspinatus takes origin from the supraspinous fossa of scapula and is inserted in to the upper facet of the greater tubercle of the humerus. It is transversely disposed from origin to insertion.
b. The infraspinatus takes origin from infraspinous fossa of scapula and is inserted in middle facet on the greater tubercle of humerus.

Actions

a. The action of supraspinatus is to initiate the abduction of the shoulder joint.
b. The infraspinatus is the lateral rotator of humerus.

Nerve Supply

Both supraspinatus and infraspinatus receive nerve supply from suprascapular nerve, which begins at Erb's point of brachial plexus.

Testing Muscle Function

a. For supraspinatus the subject is asked to initiate abduction of the arm from the side, against resistance.
b. For infraspinatus the subject keeps the flexed elbow by the side of the trunk. Then the forearm is turned backwards against resistance (this is to test the lateral rotation of arm).

Special Features of Supraspinatus

It is fused with the tendons of infraspinatus, teres minor and subscapularis muscles (SITS muscles) to form rotator cuff around the shoulder joint. The supraspinatus tendon is separated from the coracoacromial arch by the subacromial bursa. At the end of abduction the greater tuberosity of humerus and the attached supraspinatus tendon (along with subacromial bursa) slide under the acromion.

Clinical Highlights

a. The tendon of supraspinatus shows degenerative changes from the age of forty and above. Hence rupture, inflammation and calcium deposits in the tendon are very common. Supraspinatus tendonitis (with or without subacromial bursitis), calcification and rupture are some of the causes of supraspinatus syndrome. This presents with painful arc of abduction, which is characterized by painless abduction upto 60°, painful abduction between 60 to120° and painless beyond this. The mid-abduction pain is due to impingement of inflamed and thickened tendon against the lateral edge of acromion.
b. Patients with ruptured supraspinatus tendon or paralyzed supraspinatus are not able to initiate abduction. But soon the patient learns to overcome this deficiency by tilting the shoulder of affected side away from the body to cover initial abduction after which deltoid takes over.

Suprascapular Nerve

This nerve arises from the upper trunk (Erb's point) of the brachial plexus in the posterior triangle of the neck. Its root value is C5, C6. In its cervical course the nerve descends downwards and laterally along the upper margin of the brachial plexus and then leaves the posterior triangle deep to trapezius. The suprascapular artery, a branch of thyrocervical trunk from the first part of subclavian artery, accompanies the nerve to the scapular region. The suprascapular nerve and vessels reach the superior margin of scapula, where the nerve enters the supraspinous fossa by passing through the foramen formed by the suprascapular notch and the transverse scapular ligament and the artery passes over the ligament to enter the fossa. After supplying the supraspinatus the nerve passes through the spinoglenoid notch to enter the infraspinous fossa, where it supplies the infraspinatus muscle. It also gives articular twigs to the shoulder and the acromioclavicular joints.

Clinical Highlights

In Erb's palsy the suprascapular nerve is injured at its origin. So the muscles supplied by it are paralyzed with resultant loss of initiation of abduction of shoulder joint, weakness of lateral rotation of arm and the weakening of the rotator cuff of the shoulder joint.

11 Deltoid Muscle

The deltoid muscle is triangular in shape. It surrounds the shoulder joint on all sides except inferomedially and is responsible for giving a rounded contour to the shoulder.

Origin (Fig. 11.1)

The origin of deltoid is described as V-shaped (corresponding to the insertion of trapezius). The anterior fibers take origin from the lateral third of the anterior aspect of the clavicle, the middle fibers from the lateral margin of the acromion and posterior fibers from the lower margin of the crest of scapular spine. Only the acromial fibers are multipennate.

Insertion

The insertion of deltoid is in to the V-shaped deltoid tuberosity of the humerus.

Deep Relations

The deltoid muscle covers a large number of structures, which can be grouped as follows:

a. Bony parts include the coracoid process of scapula and the upper end and adjacent part of the shaft of humerus.
b. Joints and ligaments include the shoulder and acromioclavicular joints and the coracoacromial ligament.
c. The subdeltoid and the subacromial bursae.
d. Vessels and nerves are the anterior and posterior circumflex humeral vessels and axillary nerve.
e. The quadrangular and triangular intermuscular spaces
f. The muscles that are attached to coracoid process of scapula, those attached to supraglenoid and infraglenoid tubercles of scapula, those attached to intertubercular sulcus of humerus and those attached to the greater and lesser tubercles of humerus.

Nerve Supply

The axillary nerve supplies the deltoid muscle.

Actions

a. The anterior fibers bring about flexion and medial rotation of arm.
b. The acromial (middle) fibers cause abduction of arm up to 90°.
c. The posterior fibers cause extension and lateral rotation of arm.

Testing Muscle Function

The subject is asked to hold the arm abducted and hold it in abducted position against the resistance. Contracted muscle can be seen and felt.

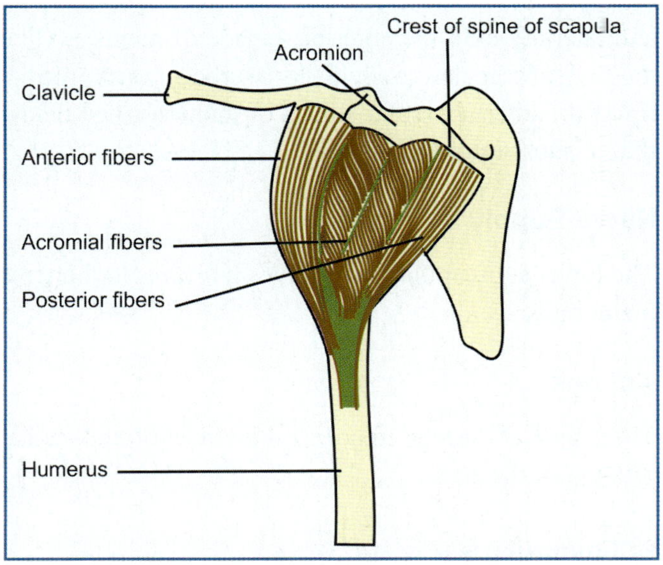

Fig. 11.1: Attachments of deltoid muscle. Note that acromial fibers are multipennate

Effect of Paralysis

There is loss of rounded contour of shoulder due to wasting of deltoid and there is loss of ability to abduct the arm beyond 15-20°.

Teres Minor

This is a narrow muscle that takes origin from the upper two-thirds of the lateral border of the scapula by two sets of fibers. The circumflex scapular artery enters the infraspinous fossa from the upper triangular space between the two sets of fibers (Fig. 11.2). The teres minor is inserted into the lower facet on the greater tubercle of humerus.

Nerve Supply

The axillary nerve supplies the muscle through a branch that has pseudoganglion on it.

Actions

The teres minor is a lateral rotator of arm. Along with infraspinatus and subscapularis it forms a couple, which neutralizes the upward pull of deltoid in initial stages of abduction.

Teres Major (Fig. 11.2)

This muscle arises from the dorsal surface of lateral border of scapula below the teres minor. The fibers pass upwards and laterally onto the anterior surface of humerus (like those of subscapularis muscle). Its insertion is on the medial lip of the intertubercular sulcus of humerus, just below that of subscapularis muscle.

Nerve Supply

The lower subscapular nerve gives branches to the teres major muscle.

Actions

The actions of the teres major are the adduction and medial rotation of the arm.

Subscapularis (Fig. 14.3)

This is a bulky multipennate muscle that fills the subscapular fossa. It takes origin from the medial two-thirds of subscapular fossa (anterior or costal surface of scapula). It is inserted into the lesser tubercle of humerus by a wide tendon that lies immediately anterior to the capsule of shoulder joint. A subscapular bursa is in communication with the cavity of the shoulder joint. Since the muscle is part of the posterior wall of the axilla, its anterior surface is related to the posterior cord of brachial plexus and its branches, second and third parts of the axillary artery and the subscapular artery.

Nerve Supply

The upper and lower subscapular nerves supply the muscle.

Actions

Along with supraspinatus, infraspinatus and teres minor muscles the subscapularis forms the rotator cuff around the shoulder joint to reinforce the capsule. It is a medial rotator of the humerus when the arm is at the side.

Intermuscular Spaces (Fig.11.2)

Three intermuscular spaces are located under cover of the deltoid muscle in the shoulder region. Of these spaces, two are triangular and one is quadrangular.

Quadrangular Space

This space is bounded inferiorly by the teres major muscle and superiorly by subscapularis in front and teres minor behind. The medial aspect of the surgical neck of the humerus is its lateral boundary and the long head of the triceps is its medial boundary.

The space gives passage to the axillary nerve and the posterior circumflex humeral vessels. The sagging part of shoulder joint capsule is seen in the space.

Upper Triangular Space

The apex of the space lies along the lateral margin of the scapula. The teres minor and major form the superior and inferior margins respectively. The long head of the triceps forms the lateral boundary or base. The circumflex scapular artery, a branch of subscapular artery, winds round the lateral margin of scapula (Fig. 11.2) between two sets of fibers of origin of teres minor, to enter the infraspinous fossa.

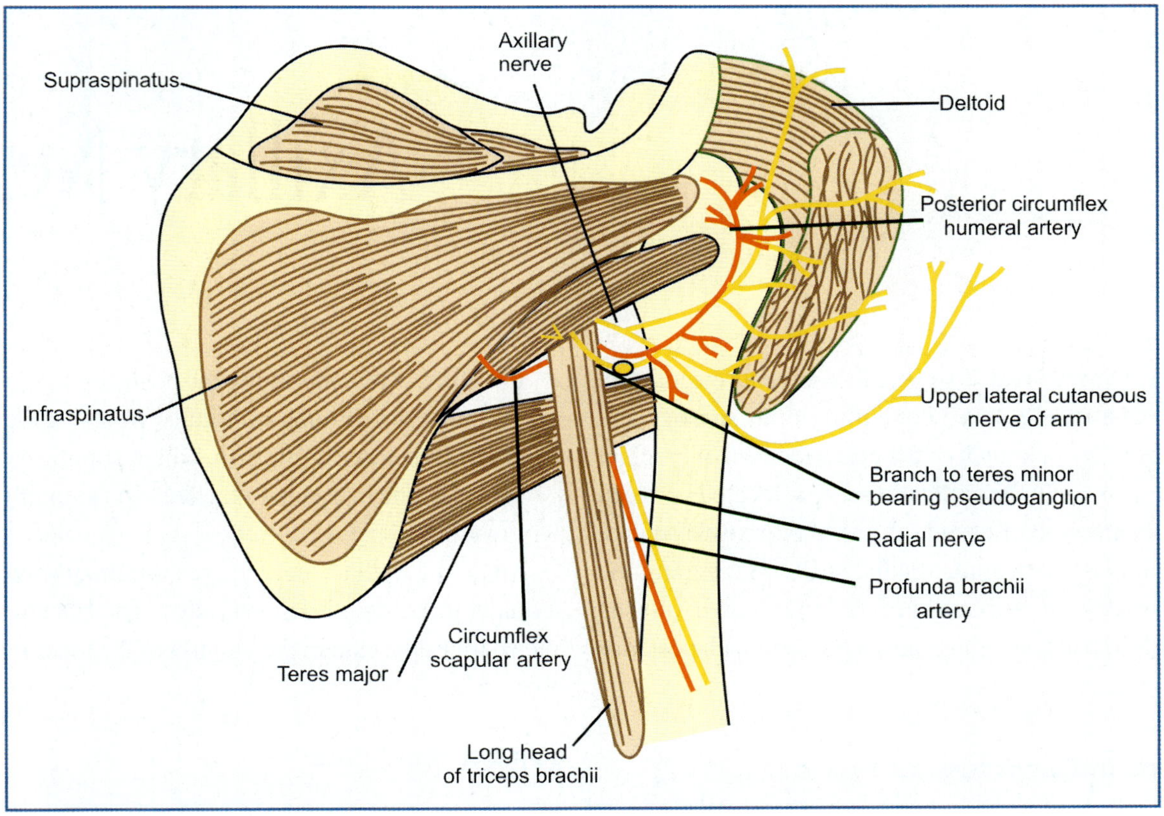

Fig. 11.2: Quadrangular and triangular spaces viewed from posterior aspect. Note: The distribution of axillary nerve

Lower Triangular Space

The superior boundary is the teres major muscle and the medial boundary is the long head of triceps. The shaft of the humerus limits the space laterally. The radial nerve and profunda brachii vessels pass through this space to reach the spiral groove on the back of humerus.

12 Axillary Nerve

The axillary nerve (C5, C6) is also known as circumflex nerve. It is a mixed nerve containing both sensory and motor fibers. It is a branch of the posterior cord of brachial plexus (Fig. 4.1). In the axilla the nerve is located between the axillary artery in front and subscapularis muscle behind. The radial nerve lies on its medial side. On reaching the lower border of subscapularis, the nerve passes backwards into the quadrangular space along with posterior circumflex humeral vessels.

Relations in Quadrangular Space (Fig. 11.2)

The axillary nerve is related to the boundaries of the quadrangular space, teres minor (posteriorly) and subscapularis (anteriorly) above, teres major below, long head of triceps brachii medially and surgical neck of humerus laterally. It is closely related to the infero-medial part of the fibrous capsule of the shoulder joint (Fig. 13.1).

Distribution

a. The trunk of axillary nerve gives off an articular twig to the shoulder joint and divides into anterior and posterior branches.
b. The anterior branch and posterior circumflex humeral vessels wind round the posterior aspect of the surgical neck of the humerus to reach the anterior border of the deltoid muscle. Along its course, the anterior branch gives motor branches to deltoid and a few cutaneous branches through the deltoid to the skin over the lower part of the deltoid.
c. The posterior branch sends a twig to teres minor, which bears a connective tissue swelling called pseudo-ganglion. After supplying the posterior part of deltoid the posterior branch continues as the upper lateral cutaneous nerve of the arm, which supplies a patch of skin over the insertion of the deltoid extending upto its lower half (Fig. 12.1).

Since the axillary nerve gives articular branch to the shoulder joint, supplies the muscles, which act on the joint and supplies the skin in the vicinity of the joint, it is said to obey Hilton's law.

Clinical Highlights

The axillary nerve may be injured in fracture of the surgical neck of humerus or in anterior dislocation of humeral head. This results in following motor and sensory deficiencies:

a. Weakness of deltoid causes inability to abduct the arm
b. Wasting of deltoid causes loss of rounded contour of the shoulder.

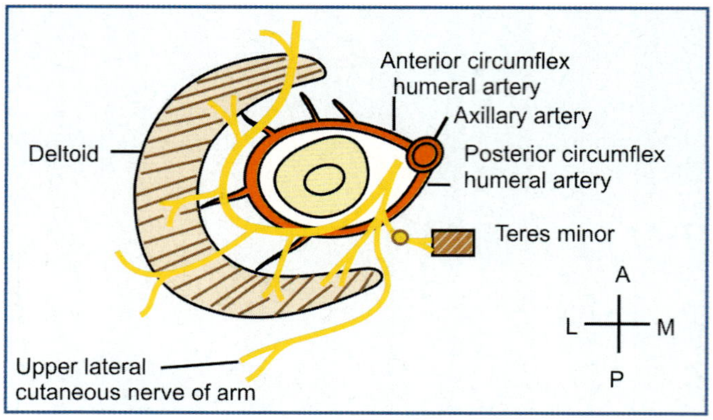

Fig. 12.1: Scheme to show axillary nerve and arterial anastomosis around upper end of humerus

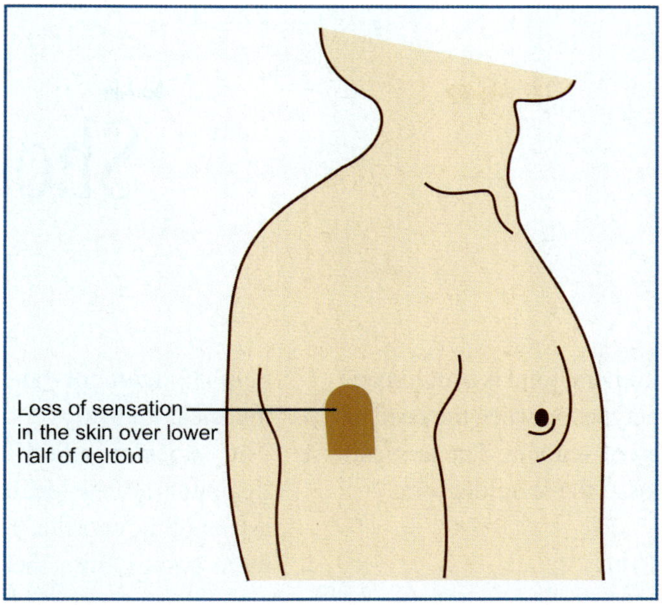

Fig. 12.2: Regimental badge anesthesia in axillary nerve injury

c. Paralysis of teres minor results in weak lateral rotation of arm.
d. Sensory loss on outer aspect of arm over lower half of deltoid, which is known as regimental badge anesthesia (Fig. 12.2).

A patient with dislocation of shoulder joint, experiences pain on movements of the joint. In order to test the integrity of the axillary nerve in such a patient, the abduction cannot be tested. Therefore, sensory loss on the lower half of deltoid is the sign to be looked for.

13 Shoulder Joint

The shoulder joint or the glenohumeral joint is a multiaxial synovial joint of ball and socket type, between the head of humerus and the glenoid cavity of scapula. The arm can be moved freely in all directions at the shoulder joint.

Articular Surfaces (Fig. 13.1)

The large hemispherical head of the humerus articulates with the smaller and shallower glenoid cavity of scapula. Both articulating surfaces are covered with hyaline articular cartilage. The scapular articulating surface is deepened slightly by glenoid labrum, which is a fibrocartilagenous rim attached to the margins of the glenoid cavity. Due to marked disproportion in the sizes of the two articular surfaces only a small part of the head of the humerus comes in contact with the glenoid cavity in any one position of the joint.

Ligaments (Fig. 13.2)

a. The fibrous capsule envelops the joint on all sides. The capsule is very lax. Laterally, it is attached to the anatomical neck of the humerus except inferomedially, where the capsular attachment shifts one cm or more on the humeral shaft. This is the dependent part of the capsule. Medially, the capsule is attached to the margin of glenoid cavity outside the glenoid labrum. Since the capsule is attached to the root of the coracoid process the supraglenoid tubercle of the scapula becomes intracapsular. There are two constant apertures in the fibrous capsule. The aperture for the long head of the biceps branchii is located on the anteroinferior aspect. The aperture of the subscapular bursa is located on the anterior aspect. The incongruity of articulating surfaces and the laxity of the capsule confer great mobility to the joint at the expense of stability. Therefore, the capsule is reinforced with the help of ligaments and tendons of the rotator cuff muscles.
b. The superior, middle and inferior glenohumeral ligaments are the localized thickenings of the anterior aspect of the capsule. The superior glenohumeral ligament passes from the base of the coracoid process and adjacent glenoid labrum to the upper part of the anatomical neck. The middle glenohumeral ligament extends from the anterior margin of the glenoid cavity to the lesser tubercle deep to the insertion of subscapularis. The inferior glenohumeral ligament extends from the anterior and posterior margins of the glenoid cavity to the inferomedial part of the anatomical neck. The part of the capsule, where the superior band of the inferior glenohumeral ligament is attached, is known as axillary pouch. In traumatic anterior dislocation, the inferior glenohumeral ligament is stretched or its attachment to glenoid labrum is torn. This is known as Bankart lesion, which predisposes to recurrent dislocation of the joint.
c. The coracohumeral ligament extends from the base of coracoid process to the upper surface of greater tubercle of humerus. A few tendinous fibers from the insertion of pectoralis minor may become continuous with coracohumeral ligament.
d. The transverse humeral ligament bridges the gap between the greater and lesser tubercles, thus converting the intertubercular sulcus into a canal for the passage of the tendon of long head of the biceps brachii.

Synovial Membrane

The synovial membrane lines the fibrous capsule internally and covers intracapsular part of the anatomical neck of humerus. The intracapsular part of the long tendon of biceps is enveloped in a tubular synovial sheath, which

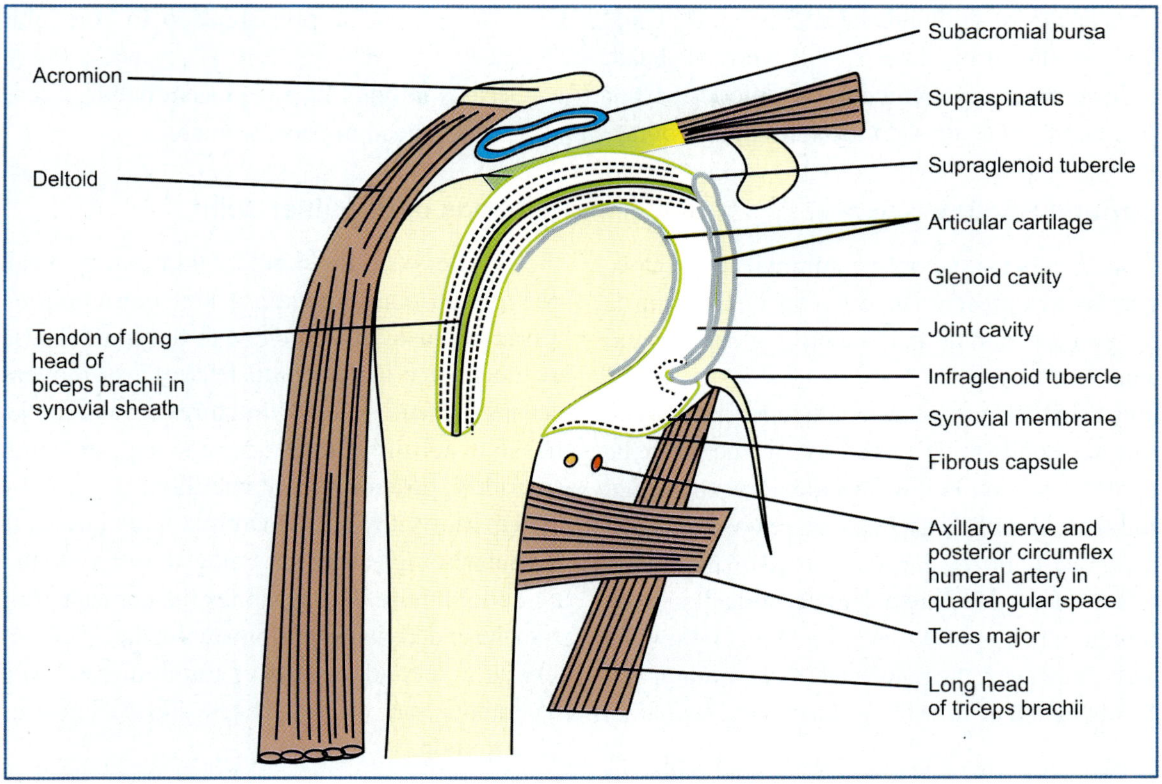

Fig. 13.1: Schematic coronal section through shoulder joint to depict fibrous capsule and synovial membrane

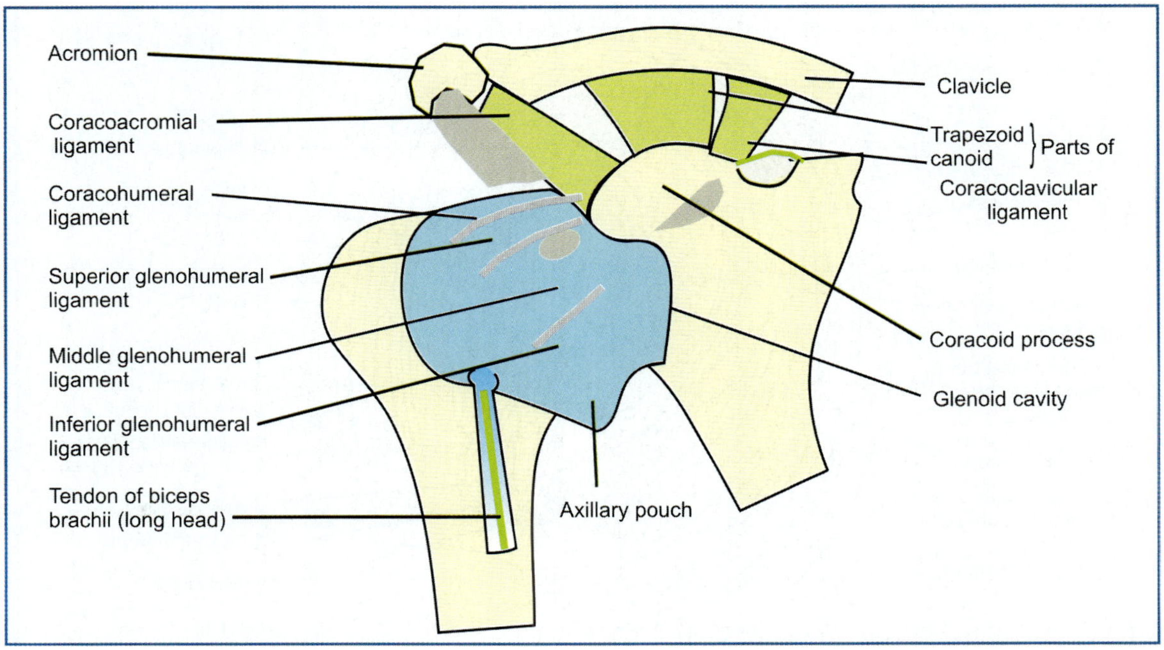

Fig. 13.2: Schematic diagram of anterior aspect of shoulder joint depicting glenohumeral and other ligaments

is carried outside the joint through the intertubercular canal upto the level of the surgical neck. The synovial sheath also protrudes through an opening in the anterior part of the capsule to communicate with the subscapular bursa.

Bursae Around Shoulder Joint (Fig. 13.3)

a. Subscapular bursa is the only communicating bursa, which is always present. Its opening in the joint is located between middle and superior glenohumeral ligaments.
b. Infraspinatus bursa may occasionally open in the joint.
c. Subacromial (subdeltoid) bursa is located between the supraspinatus tendon below and the coracoacromial arch and deltoid muscle above. It is a non-communicating bursa. It is the largest bursa in the body. Inflammation of this bursa (subacromial bursitis) causes pain, when pressure is applied just below the acromion. However, the pain at the same point is not felt after abduction of arm. This is known as Dawbarn's sign.
d. Supra-acromial bursa lies above the acromion.
e. Subcoracoid bursa is below the coracoid process.
f. A bursa may be present deep to coracobrachialis tendon.
g. Occasionally a bursa is present between teres major and long head of triceps brachii.

Relations of Shoulder Joint (Fig. 13.3)

The muscles wrap the shoulder joint snugly on almost all sides. Both communicating and non-communicating bursae are also located close to the joint. These bursae are necessary to facilitate frictionless movements of various musculoskeletal structures around the joint. The massive deltoid muscle covers the joint anteriorly, superiorly, posteriorly and laterally.

Superiorly the coracoacromial arch covers the joint. The subacromial bursa lies below the arch and the adjoining deltoid muscle. It separates the coracoacromial arch from the underlying supraspinatus tendon. This large bursa acts as a secondary socket for humeral head during hyperabduction, when the bursa shifts its position under the acromion.

Posteriorly the joint is related to the infraspinatus and teres minor muscles.

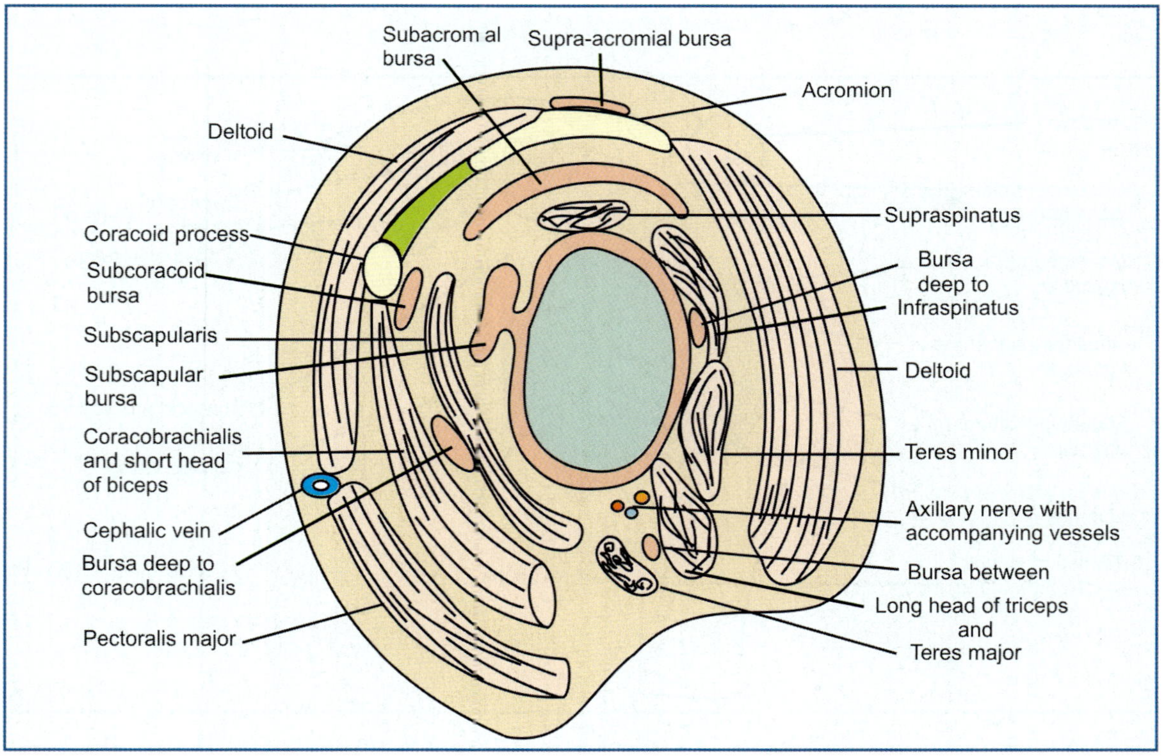

Fig. 13.3: Semidiagrammatic sagittal section through left shoulder joint showing muscles and bursae surrounding it

Immediately anterior to the joint there is the subscapularis tendon. The coracoid process and the origin of conjoint tendon of coracobrachialis and biceps brachii are located in front of the subscapularis.

Inferiorly, the capsule is closely related to the axillary nerve and posterior circumflex humeral vessels in the quadrangular space. The long head of triceps offers the only support for the capsule inferiorly. Hence, the head of humerus is more prone to subglenoid and subcoracoid dislocation. The axillary nerve is in danger of injury.

Stability of Shoulder Joint

a. The musculotendinous rotator cuff provides dynamic stability as its component muscles undergo tonic contractions. The rotator cuff is composed of the tendons of supraspinatus above, infraspinatus and teres minor behind and subscapularis in front. These muscles are known as SITS muscles. The cuff blends with the fibrous capsule. The inferomedial part of the capsule sags down in the quadrangular space, when the arm hangs by the side. This part is the weakest and is maximally stretched during abduction. Rotator cuff syndrome is due to the complete or partial rupture of one or more tendons (usually supraspinatus) of the rotator cuff. The rupture is secondary to prolonged wear and tear.
b. The coracoacromial ligament extends from the tip of the acromion to the lateral surface of coracoid process. These two bony processes and the coracoacromial ligament constitute the coracoacromial arch above the humeral head and provide a secondary socket for the joint. The subacromial bursa intervenes between the arch and the tendon of supraspinatus. The movements of the upper end of humerus in abduction of the arm are smoothened by the presence of the bursa. The coracoacromial arch prevents the upward dislocation of shoulder joint during abduction.

Blood Supply

The articular branches of the anterior and posterior circumflex humeral, suprascapular and the circumflex scapular arteries supply the joint.

Nerve Supply

The articular branches of the suprascapular, axillary and lateral pectoral nerves supply the joint.

Movements

The shoulder joint is multiaxial hence movements take place along three mutually perpendicular mechanical axes.

a. In flexion-extension the axis passes through the center of the humeral head at right angles to the glenoid fossa, but in the plane of the scapula. In flexion the arm crosses the front of the chest. In extension the arm moves backwards and laterally.
b. In adduction-abduction the axis passes through the humeral head and parallel to the glenoid plane but at right angle to the scapular plane. In adduction the arm is by the side of the body while in abduction the arm moves away from the side of the body in lateral and forward direction.
c. Circumduction is a succession of flexion-extension and adduction-abduction in an order.
d. In medial and lateral rotation, the longitudinal axis passes through the humeral head and capitulum. To test the rotation of humerus elbow should be flexed. In medial rotation the hand is carried medially while in lateral rotation the hand is carried laterally.

Analysis of Movement of Abduction (Fig. 13.4)

In abduction movement, the arm is carried away from the trunk laterally till it lies horizontally at right angles to the trunk. The abduction can be further continued to raise the arm to a vertical position above the head so that the arm moves a total of 180°. Abduction takes place in three stages. In the first stage the arm is abducted from neutral position to 15-30° at shoulder joint by contraction of supraspinatus. In the second stage further abduction to 90-120° occurs at the shoulder joint by contraction of acromial fibers of deltoid. The hyperabduction from 90-120 to 180° takes place at the sternoclavicular and acromioclavicular joints by the contraction of trapezius and serratus anterior muscles. The subacromial bursa facilitates abduction above 90°. The greater tuberosity of humerus slips below the bursa deep to the acromion.

Scapulohumeral Rhythm

The fluoroscopic studies of the joint movements have thrown light on newer concept of scapulohumeral rhythm in the analysis of abduction movement. The humerus and scapula move simultaneously in their respective joints during abduction and not successively. For every 15° of

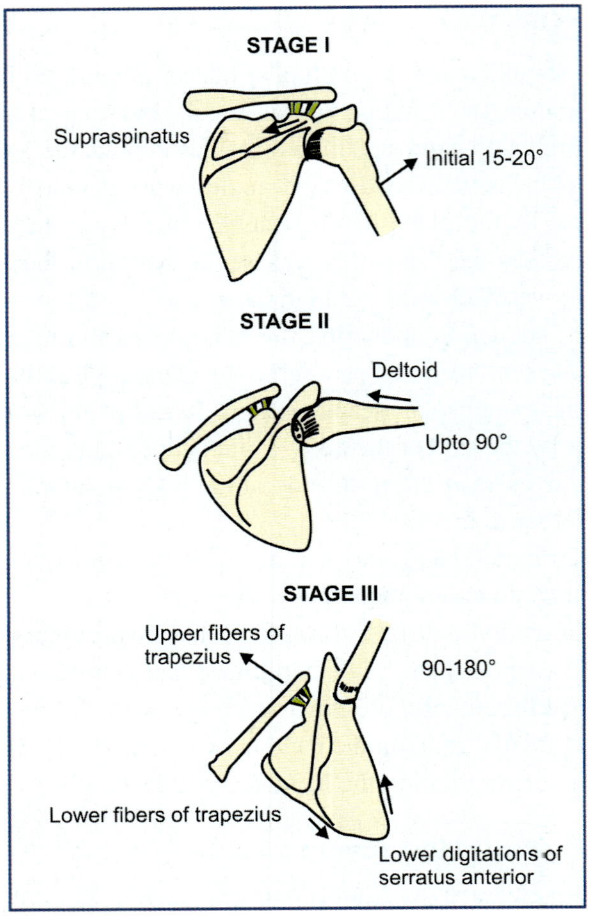

Fig. 13.4: Stages in abduction of shoulder joint

abduction, the shoulder joint contributes 10°, while the girdle joints contribute 5° (in the ratio of 2:1). After 90° of abduction, this ratio is reversed so that in hyperabduction the scapular movements assume greater significance.

Movements of Shoulder Joint

Movement	*Muscles responsible for movement*
1. Flexion	Clavicular head of pectoralis major, anterior fibers of deltoid and coracobrachialis
2. Extension	Posterior fibers of deltoid, teres major and latissimus dorsi
3. Abduction	Supraspinatus and deltoid
4. Adduction	Pectoralis major, latissimus dorsi and teres major
5. Medial rotation	Pectoralis major, teres major, latissimus dorsi, subscapularis
6. Lateral rotation	Infraspinatus, teres minor and posterior fibers of deltoid

Clinical Highlights

a. The painful arc syndrome is also known as impingement syndrome. The condition occurs usually in elderly, who complain of pain in the shoulder (aggravated on attempting certain activities like putting on a jacket). This condition is characterized by mid-abduction pain. The abduction movement up to 60° is painless. Further abduction up to 120° is acutely painful while beyond it is painless. The pain in mid-abduction is due to impingement of the swollen supraspinatus tendon (chronic tendonitis) or of the inflamed subacromial bursa under the coracoacromial arch.

b. Aspiration of fluid from the joint cavity is done by introducing the needle either anteriorly through the deltopectoral groove lateral to the tip of coracoid process or from lateral aspect between the acromion and greater tubercle of humerus.

c. The steps in the anterior or deltopectoral approach to the shoulder joint (Fig. 13.5) are easy to follow with the help of the diagram of the relations of the joint. The skin incision is placed along the anterior margin of the deltoid muscle to expose the deltopectoral groove, in which the cephalic vein is isolated. The pectoralis major and deltoid muscles are retracted from each other to expose the coracoid process and the conjoint tendon (pectoralis minor and short head of biceps brachii) attached to its tip. The conjoint tendon is divided about two cm below the coracoid process to expose the subscapularis tendon, which is cut to reach the capsule of the shoulder joint.

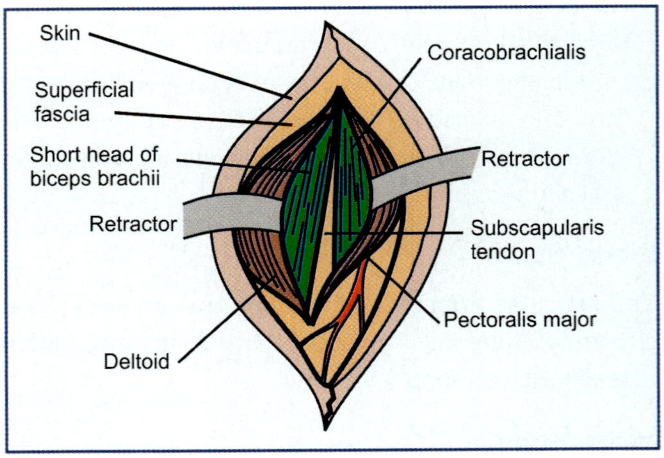

Fig. 13.5: Showing deltopectoral approach to shoulder joint

14 Anterior Compartment of Arm

The arm is the part of the free upper limb, which extends between the shoulder and elbow. It is divisible in anterior and posterior compartments. The deep fascia of the arm surrounds it on all sides like a sleeve. Lateral and medial intermuscular septa extend from the deep fascia to the humerus to divide the arm into anterior and posterior compartments. The septa are attached to the margins of supracondylar ridges of the humerus. Some structures pierce the lateral and medial intermuscular septa to shift from one compartment to the other (Fig. 14.1). The ulnar nerve, ulnar collateral nerve and superior ulnar collateral artery pierce the medial intermuscular septum to enter the posterior compartment. The radial nerve and radial collateral artery pierce the lateral intermuscular septum to enter the anterior compartment.

Contents of Anterior Compartment

a. There are three main muscles, coracobrachialis, biceps brachii and brachialis that belong to the front of the arm (Fig. 14.2). Apart from this, origins of the brachioradialis and extensor carpi radialis longus (ECRL) muscles are located in the lower lateral part of the compartment.

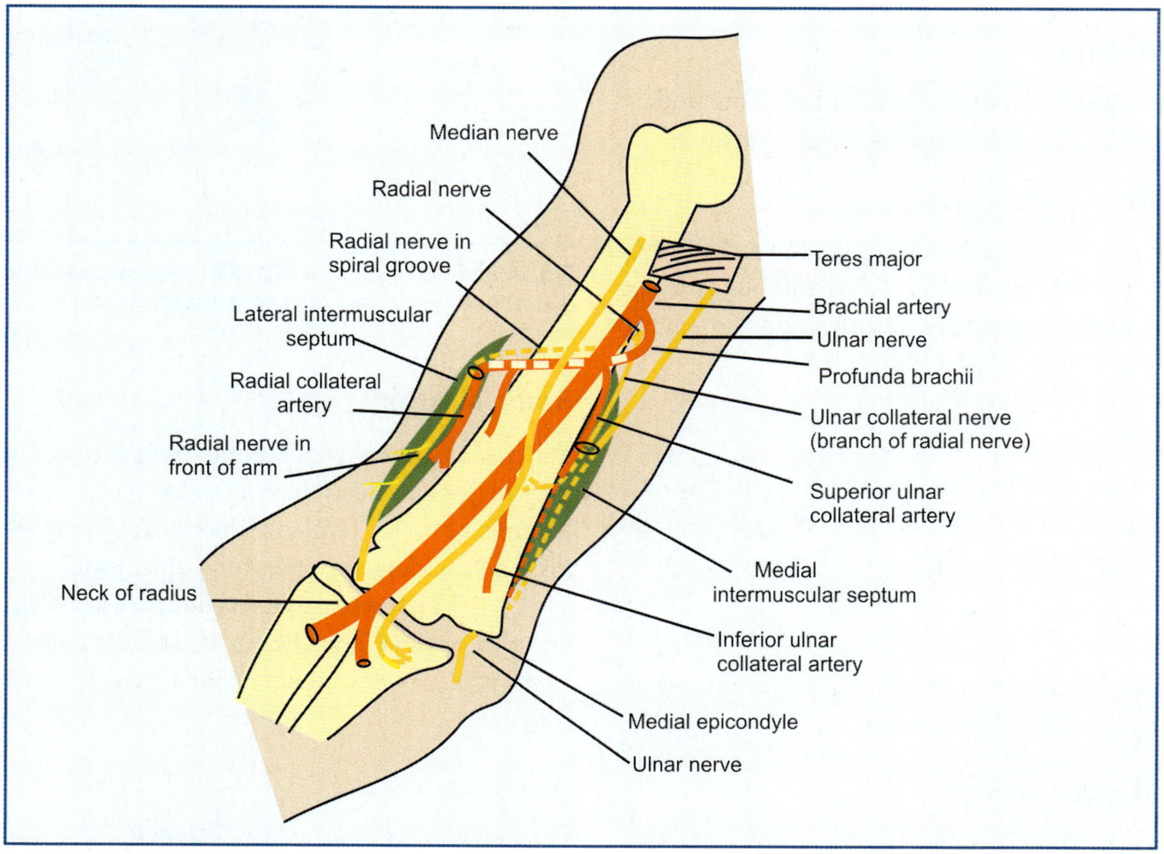

Fig. 14.1: Schematic diagram of major nerves and arteries of anterior compartment of arm

b. The median nerve passes through the entire extent while the ulnar nerve is found in the upper half (medially) and the radial nerve in the lower half (laterally). The musculocutaneous nerve is the nerve of the compartment as it supplies the three main muscles mentioned above. The medial cutaneous nerves of forearm and of arm are present in till they pierce the deep fascia to become superficial.
c. The brachial artery and the venae comitantes are present throughout. The basilic vein enters the compartment by piercing the deep fascia at the level of insertion of coracobrachialis.

Coracobrachialis

The coracobrachialis muscle takes origin from the tip of coracoid process of scapula along with short head of biceps brachii by a conjoint tendon. It is inserted in the middle of medial surface of humerus. It is a short muscle, which is pierced by the musculocutaneous nerve (Fig. 14.2) and also supplied by it.

The coracobrachialis is a weak flexor the arm at shoulder joint.

Biceps Brachii

This muscle being a strong supinator of forearm is described in Chapter 20 along with muscles of supination.

Brachialis

The brachialis muscle arises from the lower half of the anterior surface of the humerus. It passes through the floor of cubital fossa to reach its insertion on the anterior surface of the coronoid process of ulna.

Nerve Supply

The brachialis has dual nerve supply. The musculocutaneous nerve provides motor branches while the radial nerve gives proprioceptive (sensory) fibers.

Action

It is the chief flexor of elbow joint. It flexes the elbow joint in any position of the forearm.

Testing Muscle Function

The subject is asked to flex the elbow against resistance in any position of the forearm.

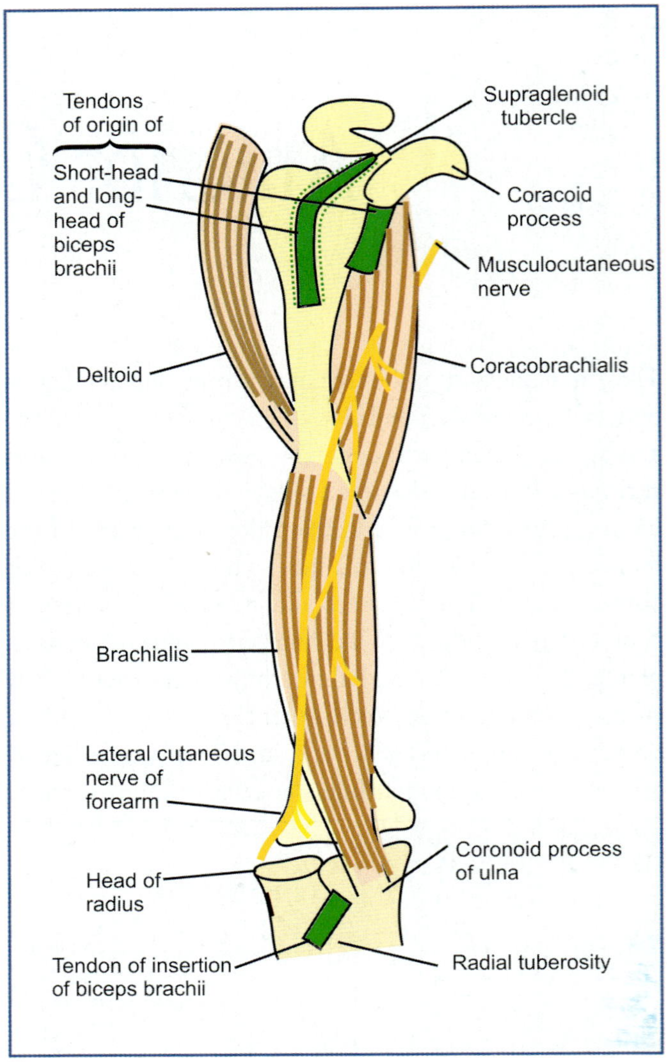

Fig.14.2: Course and branches of musculocutaneous nerve (Note that fleshy part of biceps brachii is not shown in the figure)

Brachial Artery

The brachial artery begins at the level of lower border of teres major muscle as the continuation of axillary artery. It terminates at the level of the neck of radius in the cubital fossa by dividing into radial and ulnar arteries (Figs14.3 and 14.4). Variations in the brachial artery like high division into two or three branches or its absence when axillary artery itself divides in radial and ulnar arteries are fairly common.

Relations in Arm

The brachial artery is accompanied by vena comitantes, which are connected by transverse channels.

a. Anteriorly, the brachial artery is easily accessible because only the skin and fasciae cover it. At the mid-arm level the median nerve crosses anterior to the artery from lateral to medial side.
b. Posteriorly, from above downwards the brachial artery rests on the long head of triceps, medial head of triceps, coracobrachialis and brachialis muscles. The level of insertion of coracobrachialis is the best place to apply pressure by squeezing the artery against the shaft of the humerus (Fig. 14.6). This is necessary if severe hemorrhage takes place from any artery distal to the brachial artery and direct pressure on the bleeding artery fails to stop the hemorrhage (for example in bleeding wounds of the palmar arches).
c. Laterally, the proximal part of the brachial artery is related to the median nerve (before it crosses the artery) and coracobrachialis muscle while its distal part is in relation to biceps brachii muscle.
d. Medially, its proximal part is in relation to the ulnar nerve, medial cutaneous nerve of forearm and the basilic vein while its distal part is related to median nerve.

Relations in Cubital Fossa

The tendon of biceps brachii lies laterally and the brachialis muscle is on the posterior aspect. The median nerve is the medial relation. Anteriorly it is separated from median cubital vein by bicipital aponeurosis.

Brachial Pulse (Fig. 14.5)

It is felt in the cubital fossa medial to the tendon of biceps usually for the purpose of recording blood pressure (Biceps tendon is palpable in flexed position of the elbow).

Branches (Fig.14.3)

a. Profunda brachii is the largest branch. It arises from the posteromedial part of brachial artery just below the lower border of teres major muscle. It immediately leaves along with the radial nerve through the lower

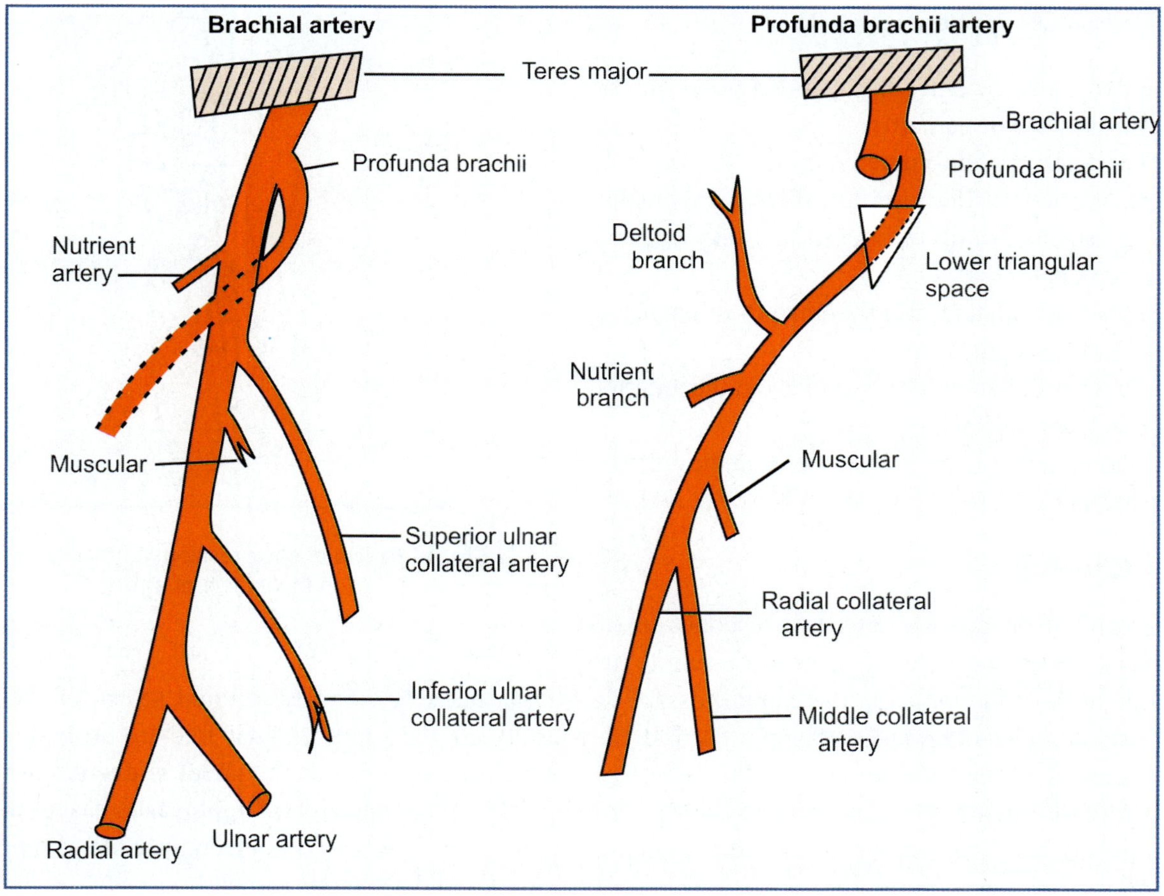

Fig. 14.3: Schematic representation of branches of brachial and profunda brachii arteries

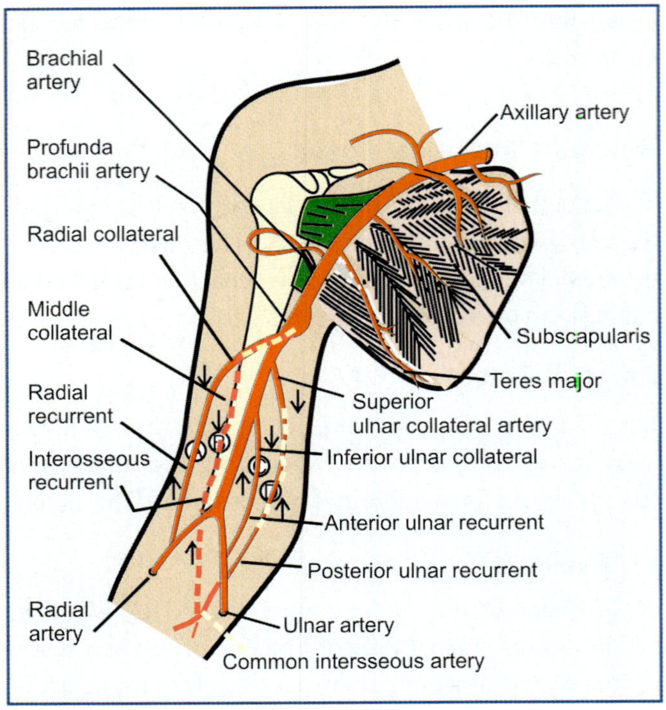

Fig. 14.4: Arterial anastomosis around elbow. Note: The continuity of axillary artery with brachial artery at the lower margin of teres major muscle

triangular space to enter the spiral groove on the posterior surface of humerus.

b. Nutrient artery to the humerus enters the nutrient foramen located near the insertion of coracobrachialis. It is directed downwards towards the non-growing end of the humerus.
c. Superior ulnar collateral artery follows the ulnar nerve to the posterior compartment.
d. Inferior ulnar collateral artery divides in the anterior and posterior branches.
e. Muscular branches supply the muscles in the anterior compartment.

Surface Marking

The upper end of the brachial artery corresponds to the lower end of the axillary artery and its lower end to the level of the neck of the radius in the cubital fossa. The brachial artery corresponds to the lower two-thirds of the line connecting the midclavicular point to the point 1cm below the midpoint of the interepicondylar line of humerus (position of arm similar to surface marking of axillary artery).

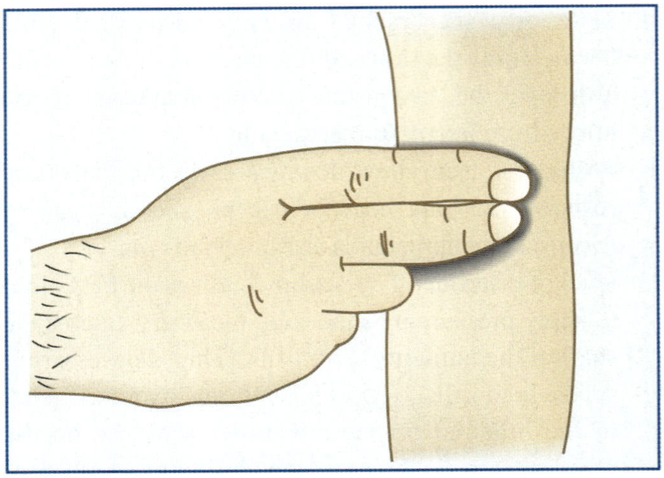

Fig. 14.5: Site of palpation of brachial pulse in cubital fossa

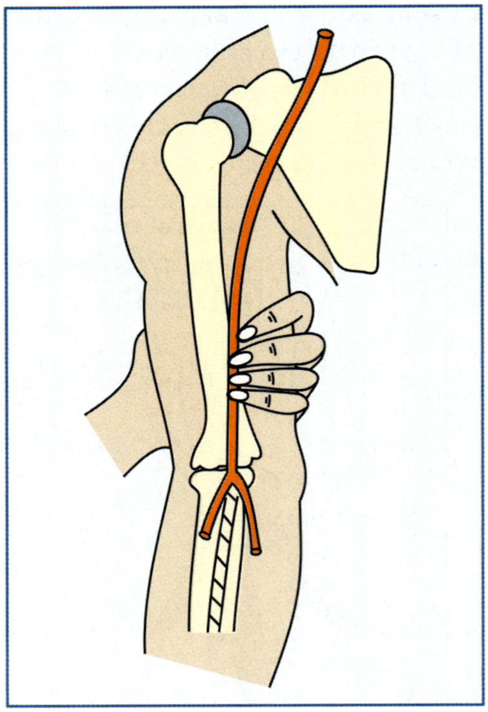

Fig. 14.6: Site of compression of brachial artery in the middle of arm

Clinical Highlights

The causes of compression and spasm of the brachial artery are the supracondylar fracture of the humerus in which the upper bony fragment is displaced anteriorly (Fig. 17.4), application of tight plaster cast or tourniquet to the arm. This results in inadequate blood supply to the muscles in the anterior compartment of forearm. Initially this gives rise to five signs and symptoms **(5 P's)**, **p**allor, **p**ain, **p**uffiness, **p**ulselessness and **p**aralysis. Further reduction in blood supply leads to necrosis and fibrosis of these muscles leading to Volkmann's ischemic contracture, in which there is flexion contracture of the metacarpophalangeal and interphalangeal joints.

Musculocutaneous Nerve (Fig. 14.2)

The musculocutaneous nerve (C5, C6, C7) is the nerve of the anterior compartment of arm. It is a branch of the lateral cord of the brachial plexus in the axilla. It pierces the coracobrachialis muscle on its way to the front of the arm. It courses down lying between the biceps brachii and brachialis muscles and comes out of the intermuscular plane laterally. In the lower part of arm it passes in front of the elbow and pierces the deep fascia to become the lateral cutaneous nerve of forearm a little below the elbow.

Distribution

The musculocutaneous nerve supplies the coracobrachialis, biceps brachii and brachialis muscles. The lateral cutaneous nerve of forearm supplies the skin along the lateral side of the forearm as low down as the ball of the thumb.

Injury to musculocutaneous nerve though rare, produces inability to flex and supinate the forearm strongly. There is loss of biceps tendon reflex and loss of sensation along the lateral aspect of forearm.

Median Nerve (Fig. 14.1)

The median nerve is formed in the axilla by the union of lateral and medial roots from the respective cords of brachial plexus. Initially it is in lateral relation of the brachial artery but it crosses in front of the artery at the level of insertion of coracobrachialis. Below this level it travels downwards to the front of the elbow in medial relation to the artery. The median nerve gives vascular branches to the brachial artery and may supply muscular branch to the pronator teres muscle just above the elbow.

Ulnar Nerve (Fig. 14.1)

The ulnar nerve arises in the axilla from the medial cord of brachial plexus. It is in medial relation to the brachial artery till the midshaft level where it pierces the medial intermuscular septum and leaves the anterior compartment along with superior ulnar collateral branch of brachial artery and the ulnar collateral nerve (branch of radial nerve) to enter the posterior compartment. It passes behind the medial epicondyle to enter the forearm between the two heads of flexor carpi ulnaris. The ulnar nerve does not give any branches in the arm.

15 Posterior Compartment of Arm

The triceps brachii is the only muscle in the posterior compartment. The other contents are, the radial nerve and the profunda brachii artery in the spiral groove and the ulnar nerve in the lower half medially.

Triceps Brachii

The triceps brachii has three heads. The long head takes origin from the extracapsular infraglenoid tubercle of scapula by a tendon. The lateral head arises from a linear oblique ridge on the posterior surface of the shaft of humerus above the level of spiral groove. The medial head has extensive origin from the posterior surface of the shaft of humerus below the level of spiral groove. The nerve to anconeus and middle collateral artery pass downwards in the substance of the medial head. The three heads unite to form a common tendon, which is inserted into the olecranon process of ulna.

The articularis cubiti or subanconeus is a small muscle, which is part of the medial head and is inserted in the fibrous capsule of the elbow joint.

Actions

The triceps brachii is the main extensor of the elbow joint. The long head supports the inferior part of the capsule of the shoulder joint during hyperabduction.

Testing Muscle Function

To test the function of triceps muscle the subject is asked to extend the elbow against resistance.

Nerve Supply

The radial nerve supplies a separate branch to each head of triceps. In the axilla it gives a twig to the long head. Before entening the spiral groove, it gives rise to ulnar collateral nerve that supplies the medial head. The branches for the medial and lateral heads arise in the spiral groove. Thus, the medial head receives two separate branches at two levels.

Spiral or Radial Groove (Fig. 15.1)

The spiral groove is present on the back of the shaft of humerus.

Boundaries

The spiral groove is bounded anteriorly by the middle third of the posterior surface of the shaft of the humerus and posteriorly by the lateral head of triceps. Its upper boundary is the origin of lateral head and its lower boundary is the origin of the medial head of triceps brachii.

Contents

The spiral groove contains the radial nerve and profunda brachii vessels.

Profunda Brachii Artery (Fig. 14.3)

The profunda brachii artery is the first and the large branch of the brachial artery. It arises immediately below the lower border of teres major muscle. It enters the spiral groove through the lower triangular space along with the radial nerve and terminates by dividing in middle collateral and radial collateral arteries at the lower end of the spiral groove.

Branches

a. Muscular branches to triceps brachii muscle.
b. Nutrient branch to the humerus.
c. Deltoid branch ascends to anastomose with a branch of posterior circumflex humeral artery.
d. Middle collateral artery (posterior descending) descends through the substance of medial head of

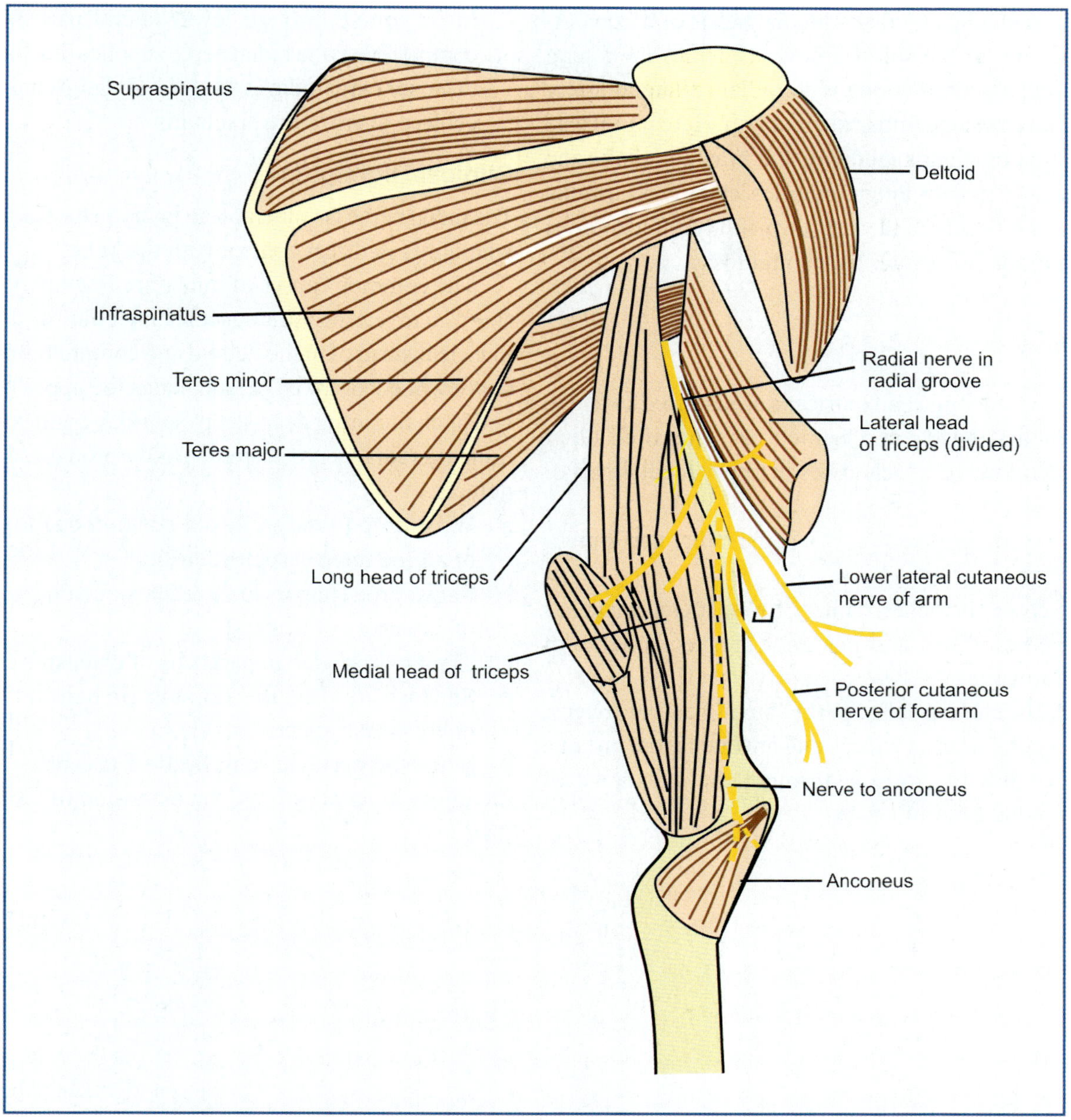

Fig. 15.1: Schematic diagram to show distribution of radial nerve in spiral groove. (Note that lateral head of triceps brachii is divided to expose the radial nerve)

triceps and takes part in elbow anastomosis behind the lateral epicondyle.

e. The radial collateral artery (anterior descending) pierces the lateral intermuscular septum along with radial nerve to enter the anterior compartment, where it travels down to take part in elbow anastomosis in front of the lateral epicondyle.

Radial Nerve

The radial nerve arises in the axilla from the posterior cord of brachial plexus. It is in posterior relation to the initial part of the brachial artery. It soon leaves the medial part of the arm in company with the profunda brachii artery to enter the spiral groove at the back of the humerus. While in the spiral groove in direct contact with the bone, it lies between the lateral and medial heads of triceps. At the lower end of the spiral groove it pierces the lateral intermuscular septum along with radial collateral artery to enter the anterior compartment of arm. Here it is placed between the brachialis medially and brachioradialis and extensor carpi radialis longus muscles laterally. The radial nerve passes in front of the lateral epicondyle under cover of brachioradialis to enter the cubital fossa.

Branches

a. Branches to long head of triceps arises in axilla and to the medial head via a named branch called ulnar collateral nerve which arises in upper medial part of arm.
b. In the spiral groove (Fig. 15.1) the radial nerve gives off:
   i. Sensory branches, namely, lower lateral cutaneous nerve of arm and posterior cutaneous nerve of forearm.
   ii. Muscular branches to the lateral head of triceps, medial head of triceps and anconeus (the last one reaches the muscle through the substance of medial head of triceps).
c. In its course through lower lateral part of anterior compartment, the radial nerve supplies brachioradialis, extensor carpi radialis longus besides giving proprioceptive fibers to the brachialis.

Clinical Highlights

The radial nerve is vulnerable to injury in the spiral groove, where it is in direct contact with the bone.

The common causes of injury are fracture of humeral shaft, inadvertent intramuscular injection in the triceps muscle instead of in the deltoid and compression of radial nerve while a drunken person hangs the upper limb from bed or chair during deep sleep (saturday night palsy). The injury to radial nerve in spiral groove produces following defects:

a. Wrist drop (wrist in flexed position due to paralysis of all the three carpal extensors)
b. Finger drop (fingers in flexed position due to paralysis of extensors of fingers)
c. Thumb drop (due to paralysis of extensors of thumb)
d. Sensory loss on the dorsum of hand at the first interosseous space.

Since the nerve to long head of triceps is spared in the injury at spiral groove the extension of elbow is not lost.

16 Cubital Fossa

The cubital fossa is a triangular intermuscular space seen as a shallow surface depression in front of the elbow.

Boundaries (Fig. 16.1)

a. The base of the cubital fossa is the imaginary line passing through the medial and lateral epicondyles of humerus.
b. The medial margin of the brachioradialis muscle forms its lateral boundary and the lateral margin of pronator teres muscle forms its medial boundary.
c. The apex is the crossing of these two muscles.
d. The floor consists of the brachialis in the upper part and supinator in the lower part.
e. The roof consists of the skin, superficial fascia and the deep fascia strengthened by the bicipital aponeurosis. The latter is crossed superficially by median cubital vein, which is by and large the most favored vein for venipuncture. The bicipital aponeurosis provides a firm platform to steady the vein and also protects the brachial artery and median nerve during venipuncture (Fig. 16.3).

Contents (Fig. 16.2)

The main contents from lateral to medial side, are, the tendon of biceps brachii, brachial artery and median nerve. The radial nerve is present in the superolateral part of the fossa under cover of the brachioradialis.

a. The brachial artery divides into its terminal branches (radial and ulnar) at the level of neck of radius in the cubital fossa.
b. The radial artery, after giving its radial recurrent branch, leaves the cubital fossa through its apex to enter the front of forearm.
c. The ulnar artery gives three named branches, namely, anterior ulnar recurrent, posterior ulnar recurrent and common interosseous. The common interosseous artery divides into anterior and posterior interosseous arteries (the interosseous recurrent is a branch of posterior interosseous artery). The ulnar artery leaves the cubital fossa deep to the deep (ulnar) head of pronator teres.
d. The median nerve gives medially directed muscular branches to pronator teres, flexor carpi radialis, palmaris longus and flexor digitorum superficialis muscles and leaves the fossa between the ulnar (deep) and humeral (superficial) heads of pronator teres (Fig. 16.2).

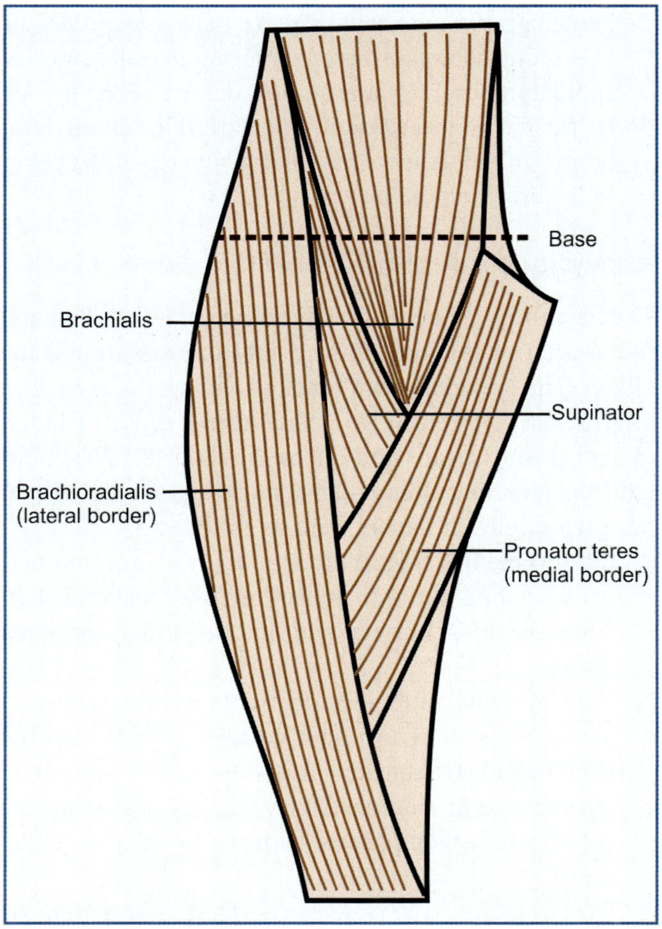

Fig. 16.1: Boundaries and floor of cubital fossa

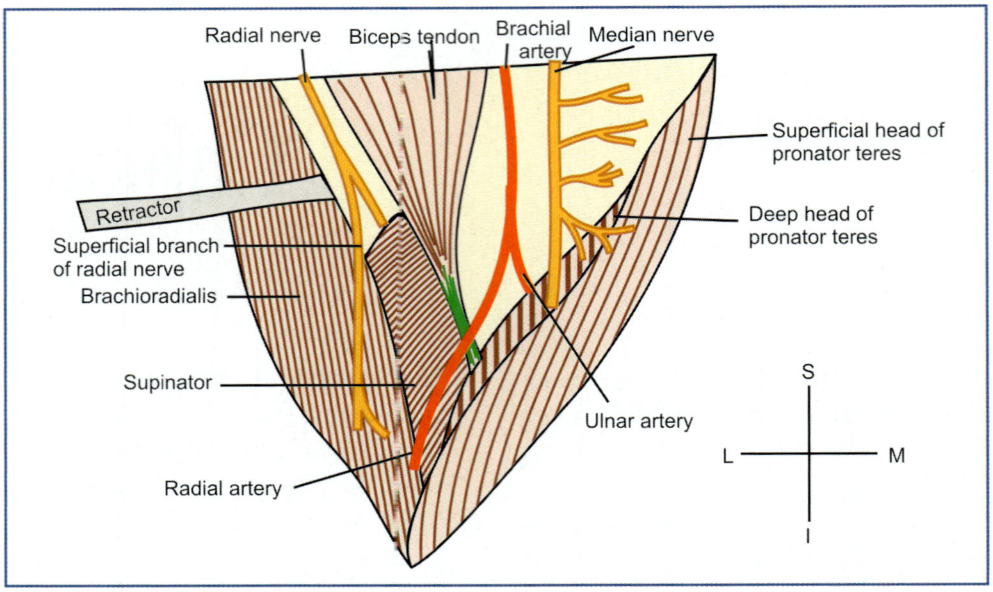

Fig. 16.2: Schematic diagram to show contents of cubital fossa

e. The radial nerve lies between the brachioradialis and brachialis muscles. At the level of lateral epicondyle it divides into superficial and deep branches. The deep branch gives a muscular twig to extensor carpi radialis brevis and supinator before entering the substance of supinator muscle (Many authors describe deep branch as posterior interosseous nerve). The superficial branch of radial nerve passes downwards under cover of the brachioradialis.

Anastomosis Around Elbow (Fig. 14.3)

The branches of the brachial, profunda brachii, ulnar and radial arteries take part in the anastomosis around the elbow. The branches from brachial and profunda brachii arteries are referred to as collateral and those of radial and ulnar arteries are referred to as recurrent. The collateral and recurrent arteries anastomose in front and behind the epicondyles of the humerus as follows.

a. On the medial side anteriorly, there is anastomosis between the anterior branch of inferior ulnar collateral (supratrochlear) artery and anterior ulnar recurrent artery.
b. On the medial side posteriorly, there is anastomosis between the superior ulnar collateral artery and the posterior ulnar recurrent artery.
c. On the lateral side anteriorly, there is anastomosis between the radial collateral artery and radial recurrent artery.
d. On the lateral side posteriorly, there is anastomosis between the middle collateral artery (supplemented by a twig from the supratrochlear) and interosseous recurrent artery.

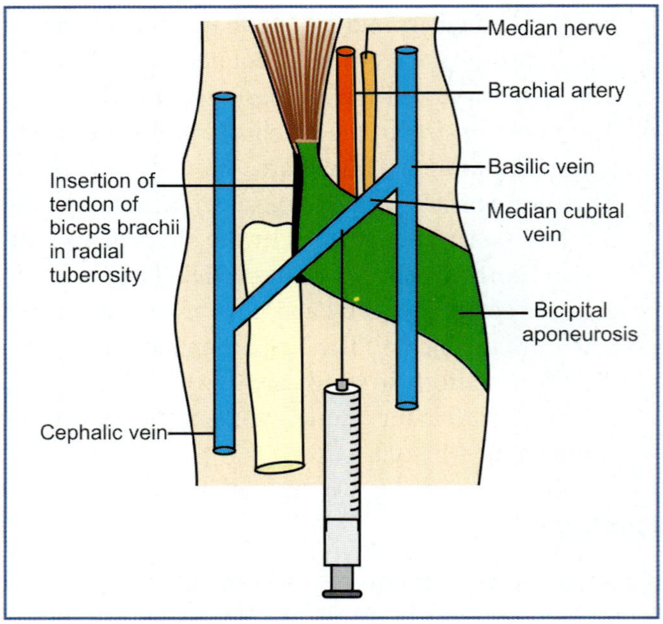

Fig. 16.3: Schematic diagram to show superficial veins at cubital fossa. Note that median cubital vein is preferred for venipuncture

Functional Importance

The arterial anastomosis ensures the normal circulation to forearm and hand when the elbow is flexed and when brachial artery is compressed temporarily.

17 Elbow Joint

The elbow joint is a hinge variety of synovial joint permitting movements of flexion and extension around a transverse axis. Three bones (humerus, ulna and radius) take part in this articulation hence it is described as a compound joint.

Articulating Surfaces (Fig. 17.1)

a. The lower end of humerus presents laterally placed capitulum and medially placed trochlea (pulley like in shape). These two structures are covered with articular cartilage. The capitulum articulates with the disc-shaped head of the radius to form humeroradial articulation. The trochlea articulates with the trochlear notch of the ulna (formed by articular areas of coronoid and olecranon processes) to form humero-ulnar articulation. Thus elbow joint consists of two articulations. The elbow joint and superior radioulnar joints share a common capsule hence the three joints together make up cubital articulation.

b. The articular surfaces of the humeroradial articulation are reciprocally curved. The closest contact between the head of radius and capitulum of humerus occurs in semi-flexed and mid-prone position of the forearm.

c. The articular surfaces of humeroulnar articulation are not reciprocally congruent because the trochlea of the humerus is not a simple uniform pulley as its medial flange projects downwards for a longer distance than its lateral counterpart. Moreover the trochlea is widest posteriorly, where its lateral edge is sharp. This is the reason why the humerus and the ulna are not in the same plane in extended and supinated position of forearm. The angulation between the arm and forearm is called carrying angle. However, in pronation of extended forearm they are in the same plane. This is for functional needs of human hand, as extended and semiprone forearm and hand are the necessary ingredients for optimum precision.

Fibrous Capsule (Fig. 17.1)

Being a hinge joint the articular capsule is lax and thin anteriorly and posteriorly but strengthened by collateral ligaments on either side.

a. Upper attachment of the capsule is as follows. Anteriorly, it is attached to the margins of articular surfaces covering capitulum and trochlea and to the margins of radial and coronoid fossae. Posteriorly, it is attached to the lateral trochlear margin and the edge of olecranon fossa extending slightly on the back of medial epicondyle close to the upper end of medial trochlear margin.

b. Lower attachment of the capsule to radius and ulna is as follows. Anteriorly, it is attached to the edges of coronoid process of the ulna and to the front of the annular ligament of radius. Posteriorly, it is attached to the superior and lateral margins of olecranon process and to the back of annular ligament.

Intra-articular Fossae

At the lower end of the humerus there are three fat filled intra-articular fossae. On the anterior aspect the coronoid fossa lies above the trochlea and the radial fossa above the capitulum. On the posterior aspect there is an olecranon fossa. During flexion of elbow, coronoid and radial fossae are occupied with upper border of coronoid process and head of radius respectively. During extension of elbow, the tip of the olecranon process of ulna occupies the olecranon fossa.

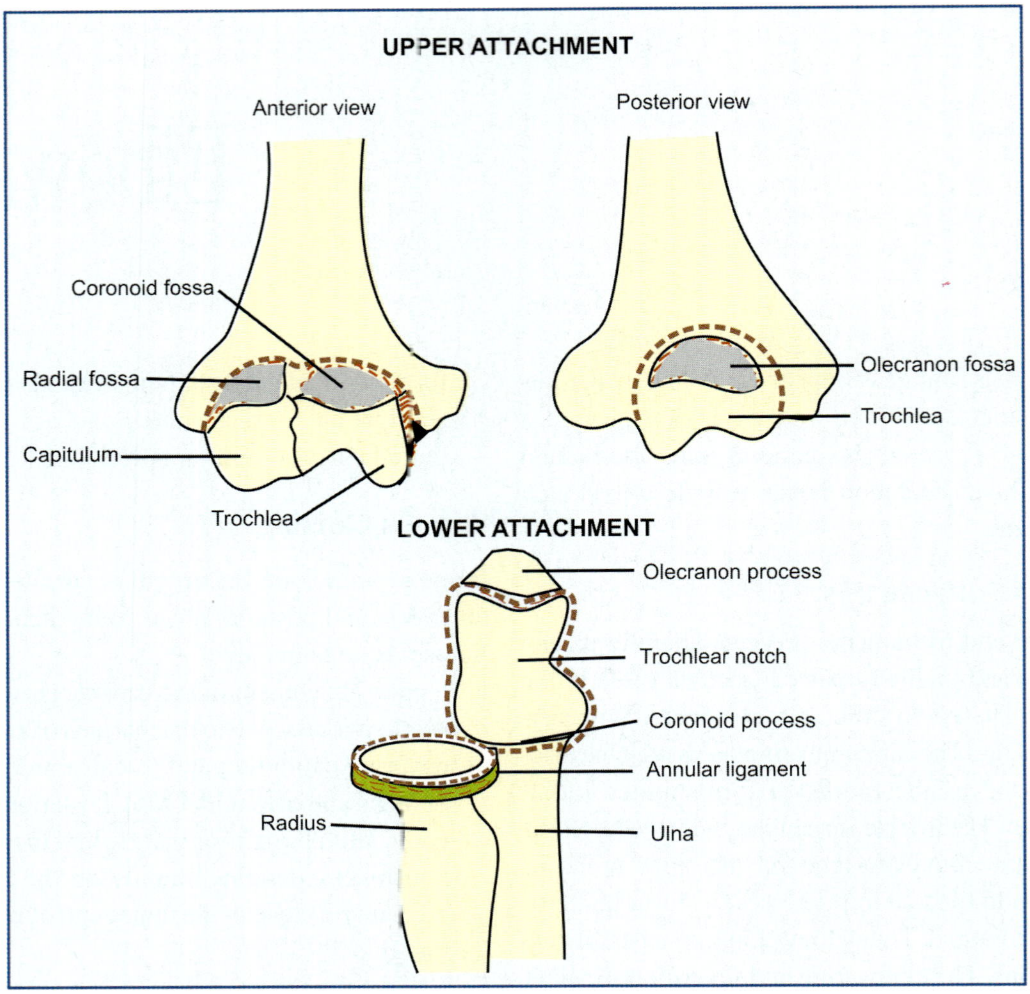

Fig. 17.1: Attachments of capsule of elbow joint (indicated by dotted line)

Synovial Membrane

It lines the fibrous capsule and all the intra-articular parts of the joint, which are not covered with articular cartilage. The fat pads in the fossae are intracapsular but extra-synovial. The synovial membrane projects under the annular ligament to surround the neck of the radius. Thus the elbow and superior radioulnar joints share a common synovial sheath.

Collateral Ligaments

a. The ulnar collateral ligament (Fig. 17.2) is triangular in shape and extends from medial epicondyle of humerus to the upper end of ulna. It consists of three parts, anterior, posterior and oblique (inferior), which enclose the thin area of the ligament. These parts share a common upper attachment to the medial epicondyle. However, their lower attachments are separate. The anterior thick band is attached to the medial border of the coronoid process and the posterior band to the medial border of olecranon process. The oblique band stretches between coronoid and olecranon processes connecting the lower ends of the two parts previously mentioned. The ulnar nerve lies on the medial surface the ligament, which gives origin to a few fibers of flexor carpi ulnaris muscle.

b. The radial collateral ligament extends from lateral epicondyle of humerus to the lateral part of the annular ligament surrounding the head of radius. Some of its posterior fibers cross the annular ligament to get attached to upper end of supinator crest of ulna. It gives origin to a few fibers of supinator.

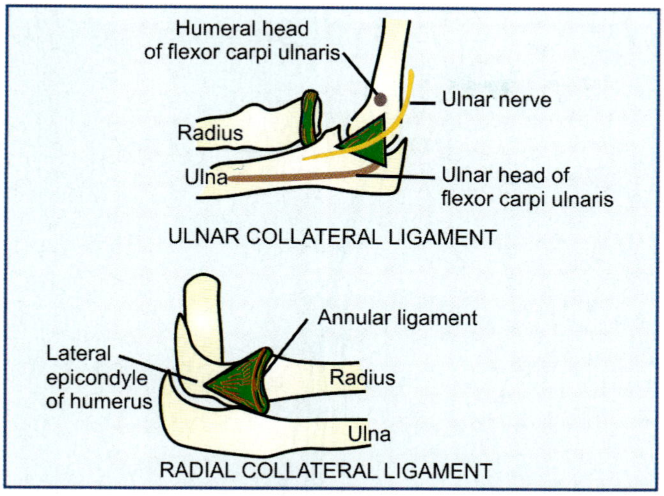

Fig. 17.2: Collateral ligaments of elbow joint. Note the ulnar nerve and origin of flexor carpi ulnaris in relation to ulnar collateral ligament

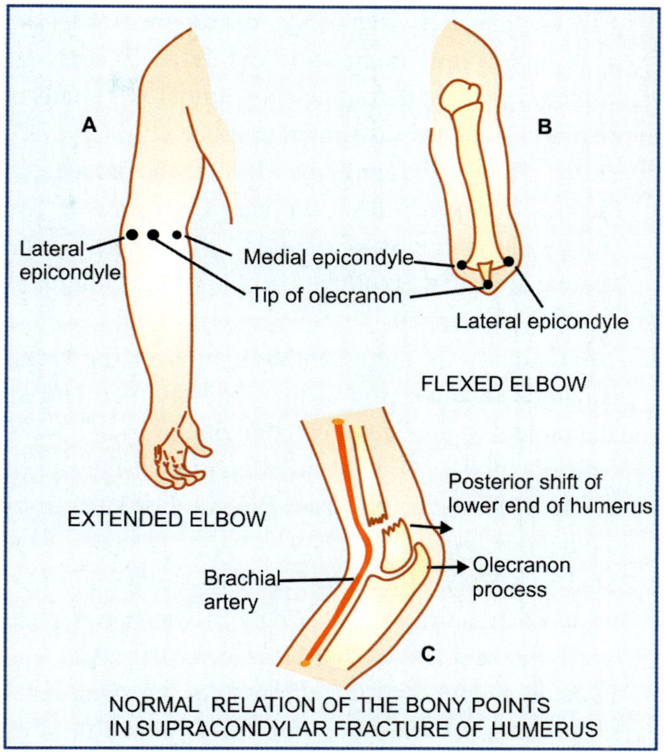

Fig. 17.3: Importance of bony points behind elbow

Relations of Joint

The anterior relations are the structures in the cubital fossa, namely, brachialis, biceps tendon, median nerve and brachial artery. Posteriorly, the joint is related to insertion of the triceps brachii with olecranon bursa between the tendon and joint capsule. Medially, the ulnar nerve is closely related to the posterior aspect of medial epicondyle and to the ulnar collateral ligament. In addition, it is related to the common origin of superficial flexor muscles of forearm. The common origin of the extensor muscles from the anterior aspect of the lateral epicondyle is related to the joint laterally.

Arterial Supply

Numerous articular branches from the arterial anastomosis around the elbow (Fig. 14.3) supply blood to the joint.

Nerve Supply

The articular branches of the radial nerve (through its branch to anconeus), of the musculocutaneous nerve (through a branch to brachialis) and of the ulnar and median nerves supply the joint.

Movements

a. Flexion is produced due to contraction of the brachialis, biceps brachii and brachioradialis muscles. The biceps brachii flexes the elbow in the supinated position of forearm and the brachioradialis in the midprone position.
b. Extension is produced by triceps brachii and anconeus assisted by gravity.

Clinical Highlights

a. At the back of the elbow there are three palpable bony points, medial and lateral epicondyles of humerus and the tip of olecranon process of ulna. In the extended elbow these points lie in a straight horizontal line. In flexed elbow they form an isosceles or equilateral triangle (Fig. 17.3A and B). Examination of these bony points is used in clinical practice to differentiate posterior dislocation of the elbow joint and the supracondylar fracture of humerus. In the former the olecranon process moves backwards from the lower end of humerus resulting in loss of the normal shape of the triangle. In the latter case the normal bony relation is retained since the olecranon shifts backward along with lower end of humerus.

b. The brachial artery is in danger of compression by the proximal fragment in supracondylar fracture of humerus proximal fragment of humerus, which is displaced forwards as shown in Figure 17.3C.
c. Pulled elbow is the condition in which the radial head escapes downward from the annular ligament. The children are more prone to pulled elbow because the annular ligament is tubular and the head of radius is not fully developed.
d. Tennis elbow is due to inflammation of the radial collateral ligament and of the periosteum around its attachment to the lateral epicondyle.
e. Golfer's elbow is due to inflammation at the site of common flexor origin from the anterior surface of medial epicondyle.
f. Student's elbow is due to inflammation of the subcutaneous olecranon bursa, caused by friction between the overlying skin and the hard surface of the desk.
g. In acute synovitis of the elbow joint the swelling is more conspicuous around the olecranon. For aspiration of fluid from the joint, the safest point is on either side of the olecranon.
h. The carrying angle (Fig.17.4) is the angulation between the long axis of arm and forearm, when the forearm is extended and supinated. The angle obliterates in pronated and extended forearm because in this position the human hand has optimum functional capacity. It also obliterates in flexed forearm. The carrying angle facilitates the movements of the forearm in relation to the hip and thigh. It is present mainly because the medial flange of trochlea projects downward 6 mm longer than its counterpart. Experts differ in interpreting the normal value of the carrying angle. If one defines carrying angle as angle of deviation of forearm from the axis of arm then its normal value ranges from 10-15° (slightly more in female). If one defines the carrying angle as the angulation (which is open laterally) between the long axis of the arm and that of the forearm then the normal value ranges from 160-170°. However, this definition is not consistent with the clinical terms-cubitus valgus and varus. In cubitus valgus deformity the forearm is deviated laterally more than normal due to increase in the carrying angle. The causes for this are, injury to the epiphysis of lateral epicondyle and supracondylar fracture. The cubitus valgus may gradually stretch the ulnar nerve behind the medial epicondyle resulting in its dysfunction. This may lead to a clinical condition called tardy ulnar palsy. In cubitus varus deformity the forearm is deviated medially due to reduction in the carrying angle as a consequence of which the ulnar side of the forearm touches the thigh. In cubitus rectus deformity the carrying angle is zero.

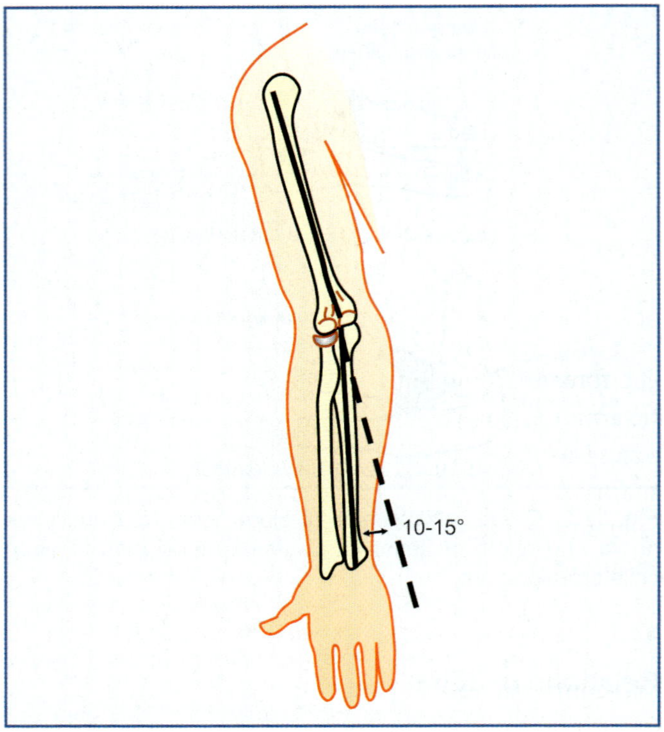

Fig. 17.4: Carrying angle (between arm and forearm)

18 Anterior Compartment of Forearm

The forearm extends from the elbow to the wrist. Like the arm it is enclosed in a sleeve of deep fascia. The two bones (radius and ulna) of the forearm and the intervening interosseous membrane divide the forearm into flexor compartment anteriorly and the extensor compartment posteriorly.

ANTERIOR COMPARTMENT (Fig. 18.1)

This compartment contains muscles, vessels and nerves. The superficial group of muscles consists of pronator teres, flexor carpi ulnaris, palmaris longus and flexor carpi radialis. These muscles have a common origin from the anterior aspect of medial epicondyle of humerus and are inserted into the carpus except the pronator teres, which is inserted into the middle of shaft of the radius. The intermediate group consists of flexor digitorum superficialis only. This muscle has common origin from medial epicondyle but is inserted into the digits. It acts on elbow, wrist, metacarpophalangeal (MCP) and proximal interphalangeal (PIP) joints. The deep group consists of flexor pollicis longus, flexor digitorum profundus and pronator quadratus. The flexor pollicis longus and flexor digitorum profundus are long muscles, which are inserted into the terminal phalanx of the digits. So, they act on wrist, metacarpophalangeal and interphalangeal (IP) joints.

Pronator Teres

This muscle is described in Chapter 20 along with muscles of pronation and supination.

Flexor Carpi Radialis

This muscle takes origin from the medial epicondyle. The muscle belly gives rises to a tendon about halfway down the middle of forearm. Near the wrist its tendon is related medially to the radial artery (Fig. 18.1). At the wrist the tendon passes deep to the flexor retinaculum in a separate osseofibrous canal, produced by the groove on the trapezium and the retinaculum. However, the tendon of flexor carpi radialis is located outside the carpal tunnel. It is inserted on the palmar surfaces of the bases of second and third metacarpal bones.

Nerve Supply

Flexor carpi radialis receives branches from the median nerve in the cubital fossa.

Actions

Acting alone it is the flexor of wrist joint. It acts synergistically with radial extensors of the carpus (ECRL and ECRB) to produce abduction of wrist (radial deviation).

Palmaris Longus

This muscle is not always present. It has a short belly and a long tendon. Since the median nerve lies just behind the thin palmaris longus tendon above the wrist, it may be mistaken for a tendon. The palmaris longus tendon is used as a graft in surgical repair of damaged flexor tendons in the hand.

Palmaris longus has a common origin from medial epicondyle of humerus. Distally, its tendon passes in front of the flexor retinaculum with which its fibers mingle and beyond this it becomes continuous with the apex of palmar aponeurosis.

Nerve Supply

The muscle receives nerve supply from the median nerve in the cubital fossa.

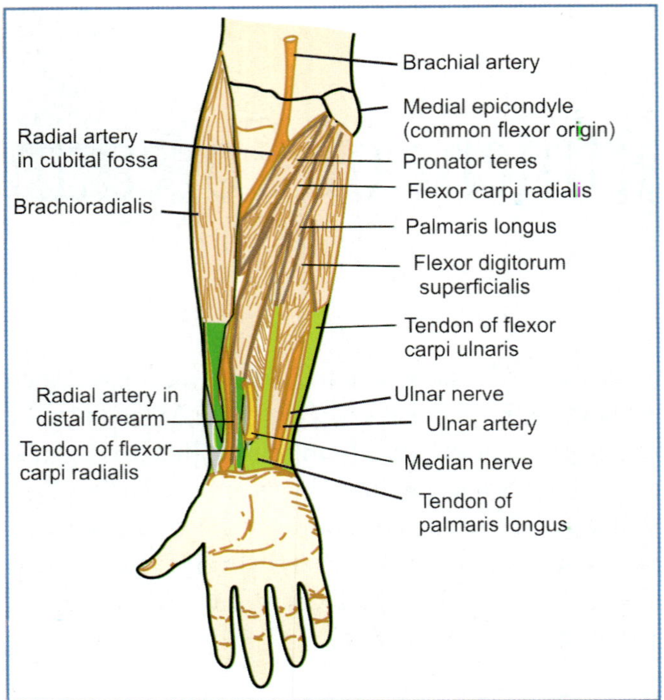

Fig. 18.1: Superficial structures in anterior compartment of forearm (Note that at wrist radial artery is lateral to tendon of flexor carpi radialis)

Action

It is a weak flexor of elbow joint.

Testing Muscle Function

The tendon of palmaris longus can be made prominent by asking the subject to bring together index finger and little finger and at the same time to flex the wrist.

Flexor Carpi Ulnaris

This muscle takes origin by two heads. The humeral head arises from common flexor origin of medial epicondyle and the ulnar head from the medial margin of olecranon process and the upper two-thirds of the posterior margin of ulna through a common aponeutrosis. The ulnar nerve enters the forearm between the two heads of this muscle. The compression of ulnar nerve in this location is known as cubital tunnel syndrome. At the wrist, the tendon of flexor carpi ulnaris lies medial to the ulnar nerve (Fig. 18.1). The muscle is inserted into pisiform bone, which is the sesamoid bone in its tendon. The insertion is prolonged through the pisohamate ligament to the hamate and through pisometacarpal ligament to base of fifth metacarpal bone.

Nerve Supply

The muscle receives branches from ulnar nerve (It is the only muscle of common flexor origin not supplied by median nerve).

Actions

Flexor carpi ulnaris is a flexor of wrist, when acting singly but in combination with extensor carpi ulnaris it produces adduction of wrist (ulnar deviation).

Flexor Digitorum Superficialis or Sublimis (FDS)

This is a broad muscle that lies deep to the four superficial flexor muscles. It takes origin by two heads, the humero-ulnar head from common flexor origin of medial epicondyle, ulnar collateral ligament and medial margin of olecranon process of ulna and the radial head from the anterior oblique line of radius. A fibrous band connects the two heads and the median nerve and ulnar artery pass underneath this band. The muscle ends in four tendons, which are bunched together, so that the tendons for middle and ring fingers lie anterior to those for index and little fingers. The tendons pass deep to the flexor retinaculum within the carpal tunnel. Here, they are enclosed in a common synovial sheath along with the flexor digitorum profundus tendons. On reaching the bases of proximal phalanges, each digital tendon enters the fibrous flexor sheath along with respective tendon of flexor digitorum profundus. The superficialis tendon splits in two slips, which pass posteriorly around the profundus tendon (Fig. 18.2). Behind the profundus tendon the two slips join to exchange some fibers (chiasma of Camper) and then insert in the palmar aspect of the sides of middle phalanx of the medial four digits.

Nerve Supply

The median nerve supplies branch to that part of flexor digitorum superficialis, which gives origin to the tendons for the medial three digits in the cubital fossa. It supplies the part of muscle giving origin to the tendon of index finger in the forearm.

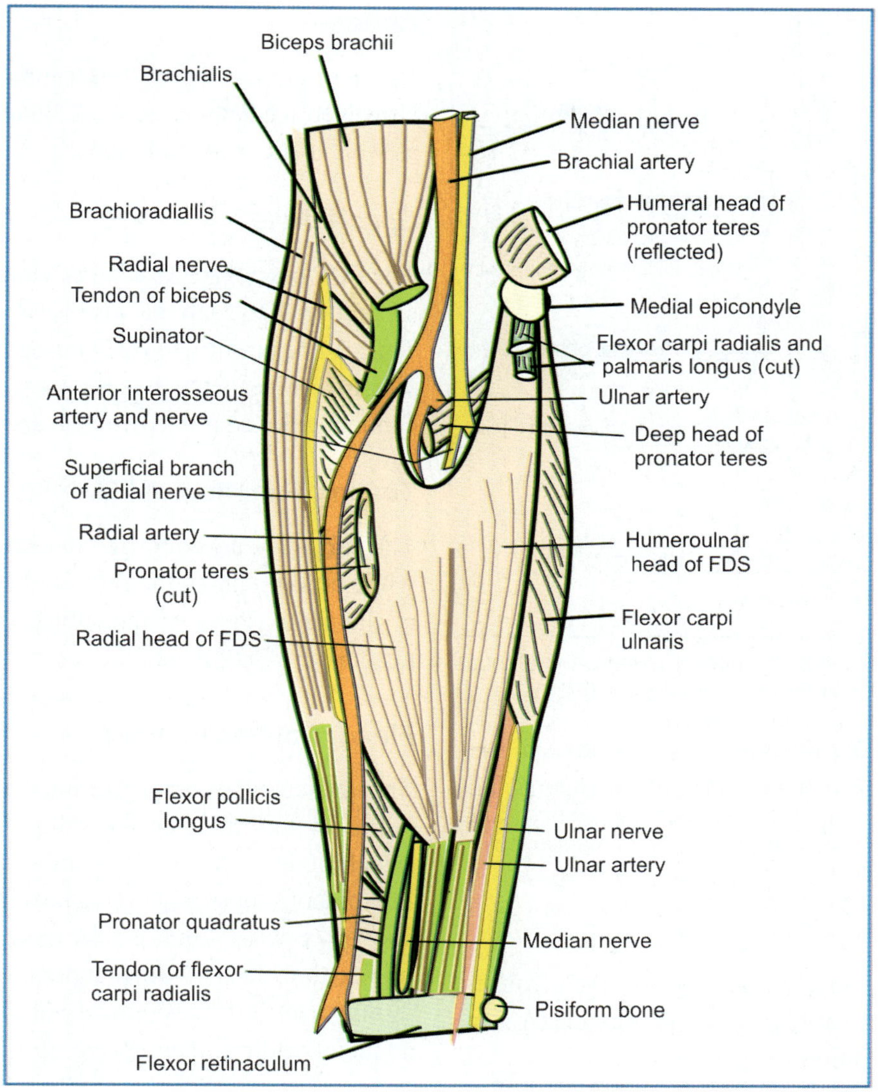

Fig. 18.2: Deeper structures in the anterior compartment of forearm. Note: The posterior relations of radial artery from above downwards

Actions

The FDS produces flexion of middle phalanx at the PIP joint and weak flexion of the proximal phalanx at the MCP joint. Each tendon can act independently of others.

Testing Function of FDS (Fig. 18.4)

The subject is asked to flex the middle phalanx of the finger (to be examined) while holding down the adjoining fingers in extension (to eliminate action of flexor digitorum profundus). If the subject is able to flex the middle phalanx the FDS is intact.

Flexor Digitorum Profundus (FDP)

This muscle takes origin from the anterior and medial surfaces of the upper three-fourth of the shaft of ulna, from adjacent interosseous membrane and upper three fourth of the posterior border of ulna by an aponeurosis. About halfway down the forearm four tendons are formed, though only the one to the index finger appears to be separate. The tendons pass deep to the flexor retinaculum and are enclosed in a common synovial sheath (ulnar bursa) with the tendons of flexor digitorum superficialis. After entering the palm, the tendons diverge towards respective digits. Each tendon gives origin to the lumbrical

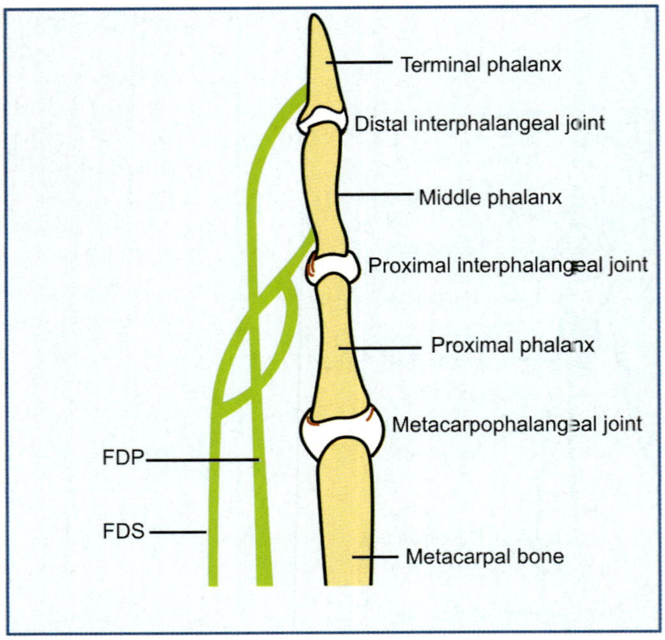

Fig. 18.3: Mode of insertion of flexor digitorum profundus (FDP) and flexor digitorum superficialis (FDS)

muscle and enters the fibrous flexor sheath, where it perforates the tendon of flexor digitorum superficialis. Finally each tendon is inserted in the base of respective terminal phalanx (Fig. 18.3).

Nerve Supply

The medial half of muscle receives branches from the ulnar nerve and the lateral half by the anterior interosseous branch of the median nerve.

Actions

Its main action is to flex the terminal phalanx of the digit. However, it can produce weak flexion of middle phalanx as well as the proximal phalanx.

Special Note

The FDP cannot act on a single finger due to insufficient separation of the part that gives origin to separate tendons. This can be confirmed by noticing that the terminal phalanx of a finger, (which is flexed at MCP and PIP joints), cannot be flexed if other fingers are in extended position.

Testing Function of FDP (Fig. 18.4)

The subject is asked to flex the finger (to be examined) while holding down the proximal and middle phalanges of the same finger. If the subject can flex the terminal phalanx the FDP is intact.

Flexor Pollicis Longus

This muscle takes origin from the anterior surface of the radius (below the anterior oblique line up to the upper attachment of pronator quadratus) and the adjacent interosseous membrane. The muscle ends in a tendon just above the wrist. The tendon passes deep to the flexor retinaculum in the carpal tunnel. In the palm it passes distally between the opponens pollicis and oblique head of adductor pollicis. It enters the fibrous flexor sheath at the

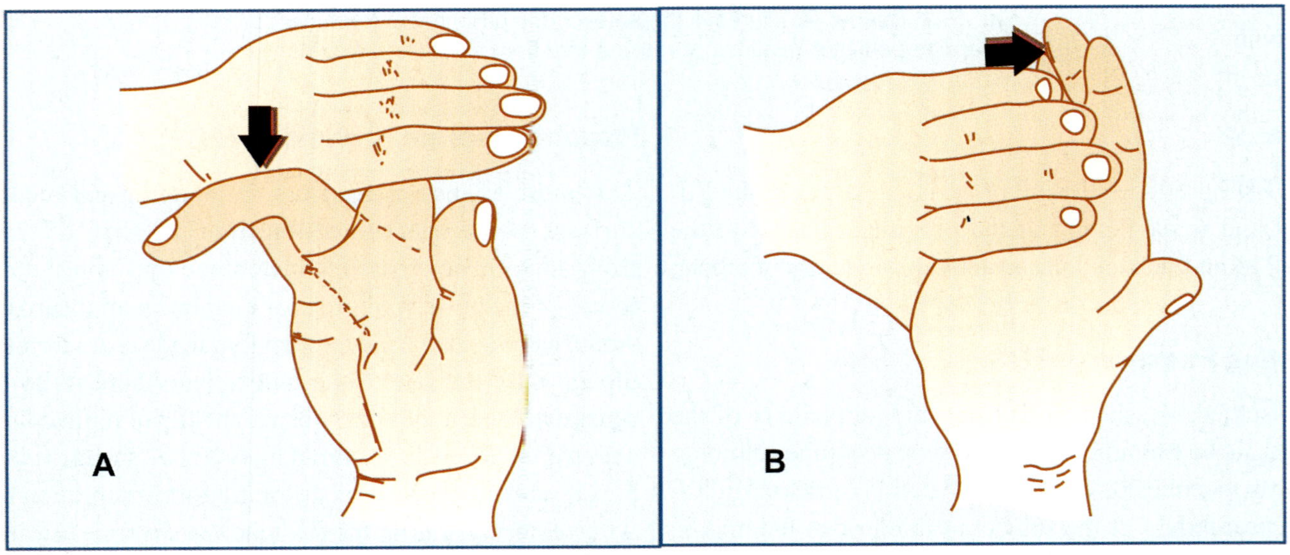

Fig. 18.4: Method of testing function of FDS (A) and of FDP (B)

base of the proximal phalanx and is inserted at the base of distal phalanx of thumb. The radial bursa covers the tendon from 2.5 cm proximal to the flexor retinaculum to its insertion.

Nerve Supply

The anterior interosseous branch of median nerve supplies the muscle in the forearm.

Action

Its action is to flex the phalanges of thumb.

Testing Function of FPL

The subject is asked to flex the distal phalanx of thumb against resistance, while the proximal phalanx is held stationary.

Clinical Highlights of Flexor Tendons

a. In traumatic injuries, the cut tendons are often repaired surgically. The tendon grafting can be done using the tendon of palmaris longus muscle.
b. Avascular necrosis of the tendon is a complication of suppurative tenosynovitis. When the pressure in the synovial sheath rises to a high level due to accumulation of the pus inside the tough fibrous sheath, it may compress the blood vessels thus interfering with the blood supply of the tendons. The arteries reach the tendons inside the digital synovial sheath via vincula tendinum, which are fibrous slips enclosed in synovial membrane. The vincula brevia are seen near the insertion of the tendon but vincula longa are closer to the base of the finger.

Pronator Quadratus

This muscle is described in Chapter 20 along with muscles of supination and pronation.

NERVES OF FOREARM

Superficial Branch of the Radial Nerve

The superficial branch of the radial nerve passes downward in the lateral part of the forearm under cover of the brachioradialis. It lies successively on the supinator, pronator teres, radial head of flexor digitorum superficialis and flexor pollicis longus muscles. The nerve is in close lateral relation to the radial artery in the middle third of its course. It leaves the artery about seven cm above the wrist, passes deep to the tendon of brachioradialis and curves round the lateral side of radius as it descends. On the dorsum of the hand the nerve gives 4-5 digital branches after piercing the deep fascia. The superficial branch of the radial nerve is purely sensory. It supplies a variable area of the dorsum and its digital branches supply the lateral three and half digits. Therefore, there will be sensory loss on the dorsum of the hand if the nerve is cut in the forearm.

Ulnar Nerve

The ulnar nerve enters the forearm from the back of the medial epicondyle passing between the humeral and ulnar heads of flexor carpi ulnaris lying in close contact with the ulnar collateral ligament. It descends along the medial side of forearm lying on flexor digitorum profundus and covered with flexor carpi ulnaris. In the lower part of forearm it becomes superficial, covered only by skin and fasciae. Superficial to flexor retinaculum it lies in a fascial canal called Guyon's canal lateral to the pisiform bone. The ulnar artery is separated from it in its upper third but in the distal two-third they form a single close neurovascular unit. The nerve terminates under cover of the palmaris brevis muscle into superficial and deep branches. The ulnar nerve and artery are vulnerable to injury at the superficial location in Guyon's canal on the flexor retinaculum.

Surface Marking

A line joining the back of the medial epicondyle of the humerus to the pisiform bone represents the ulnar nerve in the forearm.

Branches

In forearm, the ulnar nerve gives articular branch to the elbow joint. It gives muscular branches to the flexor carpi ulnaris and medial half of flexor digitorum profundus (part that sends tendons to little and ring fingers). Nearer the wrist it gives palmar cutaneous and dorsal cutaneous branches. It terminates on the flexor retinaculum in superficial and deep branches.

Median Nerve

The median nerve leaves the cubital fossa to enter the forearm between the humeral and ulnar heads of pronator teres muscle. It passes downward behind the tendinous bridge connecting the humeroulnar and radial heads of flexor digitorum superficialis and remains closely adherent to the deep surface of the same muscle. Its posterior relation is the flexor digitorum profundus muscle. About five cm proximal to the flexor retinaculum the nerve becomes superficial to the tendons of flexor digitorum superficialis. Here, it is very superficial in position being posterior to palmaris longus tendon (Fig.18.1) and enters the carpal tunnel along with the long flexor tendons of digits. The median nerve and median artery (which supplies blood to the nerve and is a branch of the anterior interosseous artery) form a neurovascular bundle in the middle part of forearm.

Branches in Cubital Fossa

i. Articular branches supply elbow and superior radio-ulnar joints.
ii. Muscular branches supply pronator teres, palmaris longus, flexor carpi radialis and flexor digitorum superficialis (FDS).

Branches in Forearm

i. The anterior interosseous nerve is the first branch to arise.
ii. A muscular branch to part of FDS giving origin to tendon of index finger.
iii. Just proximal to the flexor retinaculum, it gives off the palmar cutaneous branch, which crosses the flexor retinaculum and supplies the skin of the palm overlying the thenar eminence.

Anterior Interosseous Nerve

The anterior interosseous nerve (Fig.18.2) arises from the median nerve as it leaves the cubital fossa. It soon joins company with the anterior interosseous artery and the two descend on the anterior surface of the interosseous membrane. The nerve passes posterior to the pronator quadratus muscle to end in front of the wrist. The anterior interosseous nerve supplies lateral half of the flexor digitorum profundus (which sends tendons to index and middle fingers), flexor pollicis longus and pronator quadratus muscles. Its articular branches supply the distal radioulnar, radiocarpal (wrist) and intercarpal joints.

ARTERIES OF FOREARM

Radial Artery

The radial artery (Fig. 18.2) is one of the terminal branches of brachial artery. It extends from the level of the neck of the radius in the cubital fossa to the proximal end of the first intermetacarpal space on the dorsum of the hand. The artery then enters the palm between the heads of first dorsal interosseous muscle to continue as the deep palmar arch. The course of the radial artery can be divided into three parts, in the forearm, at the wrist and in the palm.

Relations in Forearm

Anteriorly in the proximal part the radial artery is related to the fleshy belly of brachioradialis and in the distal part to the skin and fasciae. So in the distal forearm the radial artery is quite superficial. Posteriorly it is related from above downwards (Fig. 18.2) to tendon of biceps brachii, supinator, pronator teres, flexor digitorum superficialis, flexor pollicis longus, pronator quadratus and the lower end of radius. Laterally it is related proximally to the fleshy belly of brachioradialis and distally to the tendon of brachioradialis. In its middle third radial nerve comes in close lateral relation of the artery. Its medial relations are different proximally and distally. The pronator teres muscle is a medial relation proximally and the tendon of flexor carpi radialis is the medial relation distally (where its pulse is felt lateral to this tendon).

Relations at Wrist

The radial artery takes a curve from the styloid process of radius backwards across the anatomical snuffbox. It first passes deep to the two tendons (abductor pollicis longus and extensor pollicis brevis), which form the anterior boundary of the snuffbox. Then the artery comes in relation to the carpal bones in the floor of the snuffbox, namely scaphoid and trapezium. The cephalic vein lies superficial to the artery in the snuffbox. Lastly, the artery passes deep to the extensor pollicis longus tendon, which forms the posterior boundary of the snuffbox and approaches the proximal end of the first intermetacarpal space.

Relations in Palm

The radial artery leaves the dorsum of the hand by passing between the two heads of the first dorsal interosseous muscle. After reaching the palm it takes a transverse course medially across the palm. It anastomoses with the deep branch of the ulnar artery to complete the deep palmar arch at the base of fifth metacarpal bone.

Surface Marking

In the forearm, a line drawn from a point one cm below the midpoint of the interepicondylar line at the elbow to the point of radial pulse (lateral to the tendon of flexor carpi radialis against the lateral aspect of lower radius) represents the radial artery. A curved line from the distal end of radius towards the lateral side of wrist reaching the proximal end of the first intermetacarpal space represents the artery at the wrist. A four cm long horizontal line across the palm at the level of the distal border of the hook of hamate represents the radial artery in the palm.

Branches of Radial Artery

i. In the cubital fossa, the radial artery gives the radial recurrent artery.
ii. In the forearm, its branches are, the muscular, anterior radial carpal or palmar carpal branches and superficial palmar branch.
iii. At the wrist, it gives the posterior radial carpal branches or dorsal carpal and the first dorsal metacarpal artery.
iv. In the palm, it gives radialis indicis, princeps pollicis and deep palmar arch.

Clinical Highlights

i. The point where the radial pulse is felt is anterior surface of the distal end of radius lateral to the tendon of flexor carpi radialis (Fig. 18.5).

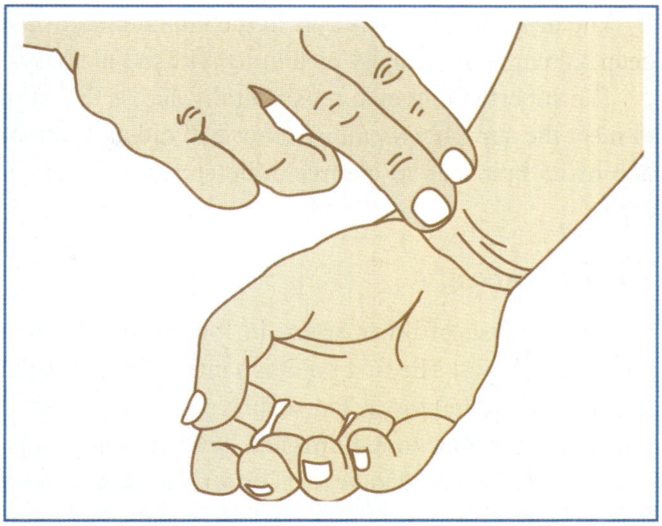

Fig. 18.5: Palpation of radial pulse

ii. For arterial puncture the radial artery is chosen since it is superficial in the distal forearm. In this procedure blood is withdrawn for the purpose of arterial blood examination, usually blood gas analysis.
iii. The radial artery is one of the limb arteries used as a homograft in coronary artery bypass surgery.
iv. Allen test is performed to find out the patency of the arteries of the forearm. For testing the radial artery, first the ulnar artery is compressed against the anterior surface of the ulna, while the patient clenches the fist tightly (this is to close off the superficial and deep palmar arches). Then the patient is asked to open the fist. The skin of the palm which is at first white, regains its color as blood flows into the palmar arches through the patent radial artery.

Ulnar Artery

The ulnar artery is the larger of the two terminal branches of the brachial artery. It begins at the level of neck of radius in the cubital fossa. It leaves the cubital fossa deep to the deep (ulnar) head of pronator teres, to enter the forearm. Its course in the forearm can be divided into two parts. In the upper third of the forearm the ulnar artery takes as oblique course to reach the medial margin of the forearm. In the lower two-thirds the artery passes vertically down along the medial margin of forearm to reach the wrist. Then it crosses the flexor retinaculum superficially (Fig. 18.2) and at the pisiform it divides into deep and superficial branches.

The deep branch takes part in the completion of the deep palmar arch medially by uniting with radial artery.

The superficial branch runs laterally across the palm to meet the superficial palmar branch of radial artery or one of its branches to complete the superficial palmar arch.

Surface Marking

To draw course of ulnar artery in forearm mark three points as follows. The first point is same as for the radial artery at the cubital fossa. The second point coincides the junction of the upper one-thirds and lower two-thirds of a line from medial epicondyle to pisiform. The third point is the pisiform bone. A line joining the first and second points represents the oblique part of the ulnar artery. A line joining the lower end of the above line to the third point represents the straight part of ulnar artery.

Relations

The oblique part is situated deeply compared to the vertical part of the artery. The anterior relations of the oblique part are the muscles that arise from medial epicondyle, namely, pronator teres, flexor carpi radialis, palmaris longus and flexor digitorum superficialis. The deep head of pronator teres intervenes between the ulnar artery and median nerve at the apex of cubital fossa. The anterior relations of the straight part are, the flexor carpi ulnaris in upper extent but towards the wrist it is covered with the skin and fasciae. Distally, it lies between flexor carpi ulnaris medially and flexor digitorum superficialis laterally before piercing the deep fascia along with the ulnar nerve. Thus, it passes in front of the flexor retinaculum. Posteriorly, it is related from above downward to brachialis, flexor digitorum profundus and flexor retinaculum. Medially, the ulnar nerve is in close relation in its lower two-third.

Relations at Wrist

The artery is covered by skin and superficial fascia. It lies superficial to flexor retinaculum along with the ulnar nerve. The ulnar nerve and pisiform bone are on its medial side. The artery and nerve are in a very exposed area at the wrist hence liable to injury.

Branches of Ulnar Artery

i. In the cubital fossa, the ulnar artery gives anterior and posterior ulnar recurrent arteries. The common interosseous artery is the main branch that takes origin from the lateral aspect of the ulnar artery in the cubital fossa.
ii. In the forearm, the branches of the ulnar artery are, the muscular and palmar and dorsal carpal branches.
iii. On the anterior surface of the flexor retinaculum, it divides in terminal branches, namely superficial and deep branches of ulnar artery.
iv. In the palm, the superficial branch takes main share in the formation superficial palmar arch and the deep branch helps in completion of the deep palmar arch.

Anterior Interosseous Artery

The anterior interosseous artery arises from the common interosseous branch of the ulnar artery at the superior border of the interosseous membrane (Fig. 18.2). It descends on the anterior aspect of the interosseous membrane along with the anterior interosseous nerve. As it reaches the upper margin of pronator quadratus, the artery passes through the interosseous membrane (Fig. 20.1) to enter the posterior compartment of the forearm. Here it runs down along with the posterior interosseous nerve to reach the back of the carpus in the fourth compartment deep to the extensor retinaculum.

Branches of Anterior Interosseous Artery

In the anterior compartment, the artery gives off a slender median artery, muscular branches, nutrient arteries to both radius and ulna and a descending branch to the anterior carpal arch. The median artery supplies the median nerve and sometimes accompanies it in to the palm, where it may take part in completion of superficial palmar arch on lateral aspect.

In the posterior compartment the artery gives muscular branches and the carpal branches, which take part in the dorsal carpal arch. It also supplies the extensor tendons.

19 Posterior Compartment of Forearm

The posterior compartment of the forearm contains extensor muscles, posterior interosseous nerve and both posterior and anterior interosseous arteries. A total of twelve muscles belong to the posterior compartment. They are divided into two sets (superficial and deep).

SUPERFICIAL MUSCLES

The superficial set contains the anconeus, brachioradialis, extensor carpi radialis longus, extensor carpi radialis brevis, extensor digitorum, extensor digiti minimi and extensor carpi ulnaris.

Anconeus (Fig. 19.1)

This is a triangular muscle with narrow origin and broad insertion. It takes origin from the posterior surface of lateral epicondyle of humerus and is inserted in olecranon process and posterior surface of upper fourth of ulna.

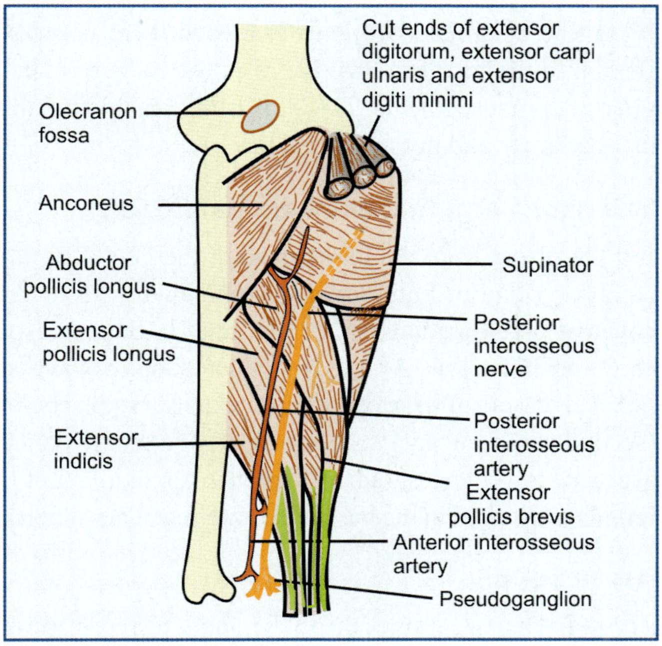

Fig. 19.1: Scheme to depict structures in posterior compartment of forearm

Nerve Supply

The nerve to anconeus is a branch of radial nerve in the spiral groove. It reaches the anconeus through the substance of the medial head of triceps brachii.

Action

The anconeus is an extensor of the elbow joint.

Brachioradialis (Fig. 18.1)

This muscle takes origin above the elbow and is inserted above the wrist. It is regarded as a borderline muscle since developmentally it is an extensor muscle but functionally and topographically it is the flexor muscle. It takes origin from the upper two-thirds of the lateral supracondylar ridge of humerus and is inserted in radius just above the styloid process (origin above elbow and insertion above wrist). The tendons of abductor pollicis longus and extensor pollicis brevis cross the tendon of brachioradialis above the wrist. The upper part of the muscle forms the lateral boundary of cubital fossa and here the radial nerve lies deep to it. At the wrist, the radial artery lies between the tendon of the brachioradialis laterally and of flexor carpi radialis medially.

Nerve Supply

The muscle receives branches from the radial nerve in the anterior compartment of arm.

Actions

Brachioradialis is the flexor of the elbow joint in midprone position of forearm. It is believed to bring the supinated forearm to midprone position and supinate the fully pronated forearm to midprone position.

Testing Muscle Function

The elbow of the subject is flexed to 90° and the forearm is kept in midprone position. Now the subject is instructed to flex the elbow against resistance. A normal muscle can be seen and felt.

Supinator Jerk Reflex

When the distal end of radius is tapped there is reflex flexion of the forearm. Positive response indicates integrity of spinal segments C7-C8. It is the brachioradialis that contracts and not the supinator.

Extensor Carpi Radialis Longus (ECRL)

It takes origin from the lower third of the lateral supracondylar ridge of humerus. It passes downward under cover of brachioradialis and superficial to the extensor carpi radialis brevis. At the wrist, the tendons of the two radial extensors of wrist pass deep to extensor retinaculum (second compartment) lodged in a groove on the dorsal aspect of lower end of radius. The extensor carpi radialis longus is inserted in the base of second metacarpal bone.

Nerve Supply

The radial nerve supplies the ECRL in the arm just above the elbow.

Extensor Carpi Radialis Brevis (ECRB)

It takes origin from common extensor origin on anterior aspect of lateral epicondyle of humerus. It passes downward deep to the corresponding longus muscle lying in direct contact with radial shaft. It is inserted in the bases of second and third metacarpal bones.

Nerve Supply

The deep branch of the radial nerve (posterior interosseous nerve) supplies the ECRB above the proximal margin of supinator.

Actions of the Radial Extensors of the Carpus

Both ECRL and ECRB along with extensor carpi ulnaris produce extension or dorsiflexion of the wrist. Both the carpal extensor muscles along with flexor carpi radialis act synergistically to produce abduction or radial deviation of wrist.

Testing Function of ECRL and ECRB

The subject clenches the fist and dorsiflexes the wrist in radial side against resistance. The ECRL and ECRB muscles can be palpated and their tendons can be felt near the insertion.

Extensor Digitorum

This muscle arises from the common extensor origin on anterior aspect of lateral epicondyle of humerus. The muscle gives rise to four tendons in mid-forearm. The tendons of extensor digitorum and the tendon of extensor indicis are lodged in the fourth compartment deep to the extensor retinaculum. On the dorsum of the hand the tendons are connected by tendinous interconnections, which restrict the independent actions on the fingers. Each tendon expands in to the extensor expansion over the proximal phalanx and is inserted through it to the base of the middle phalanx and that of terminal phalanx. The parts and attachments of the extensor expansion are described with the interossei and lumbrical muscles of the hand.

Nerve Supply

The posterior interosseous nerve supplies the muscle.

Actions

The extensor digitorum acts on the metacarpophalangeal joints to produce extension (the extension at interphalangeal joints takes place mainly by lumbricals and interossei muscles).

Testing Muscle Function

The subject is asked to keep the elbow and the anterior aspect of forearm and the palm on the table. After the examiner stabilizes the wrist of the subject with one hand, the subject extends the MCP joint of each finger against resistance.

Extensor Digiti Minimi

This is a separate extensor of the little finger. It arises from common extensor origin on the front of lateral epicondyle and passes downwards along the medial side of extensor digitorum. It passes deep to the extensor retinaculum in the fifth compartment. On the dorsum of the hand, it usually splits into two slips and is inserted in the extensor expansion of little finger.

Nerve Supply

The extensor digiti minimi receives twigs from posterior interosseous nerve.

Action

The extensor digiti minimi helps in extension of the metacarpophalangeal joint of the little finger.

Extensor Carpi Ulnaris

This muscle takes origin from the common extensor origin on the front of lateral epicondyle and from the posterior subcutaneous border of ulna in common with the origin of flexor carpi ulnaris. Its tendon passes deep to the extensor retinaculum in the sixth compartment, where it lies in a groove between head and styloid process of ulna. It is inserted in the base of the fifth metacarpal bone.

Nerve Supply

The posterior interosseous nerve supplies it.

Actions

Along with the two radial extensors of the carpus (ECRB and ECRL) it produces extension of wrist. The synergistic action with flexor carpi ulnaris produces adduction or ulnar deviation of wrist.

Testing Muscle Function

The subject is asked to keep the closed fist in position of ulnar deviation against resistance.

DEEP MUSCLES (Fig. 19.1)

The deep set contains from above downward, the supinator, abductor pollicis longus, extensor pollicis longus, extensor pollicis brevis and the extensor indicis.

Supinator

This muscle is described in Chapter 20 along with muscles of supination and pronation.

Abductor Pollicis Longus (APL)

The muscle takes origin from posterior surface of both radius and ulna and the interosseous membrane. Its long tendon spirals round the tendons of brachioradialis and the radial extensors of the carpus. The tendons of abductor pollicis longus and extensor pollicis brevis enclosed in common synovial sheath pass deep to the extensor retinaculum in the first compartment. The two tendons form the anterior margin of the anatomical snuffbox. The tendon of abductor pollicis longus is inserted in the radial side of the base of first metacarpal bone.

Nerve Supply

The posterior interosseous nerve supplies it.

Actions

The APL abducts and extends the thumb at the first carpometacarpal joint of thumb.

Testing Function of APL

The subject holds the forearm in midprone position and is then asked to abduct the thumb against resistance. The tendon of APL stands out in the margin of anatomical snuffbox.

Extensor Pollicis Brevis (EPB)

This muscle takes origin from the posterior surface of radius below the origin of abductor pollicis longus as well as from the adjacent interosseous membrane. Its tendon closely follows the tendon of abductor pollicis longus. The extensor pollicis brevis is inserted in the dorsal surface of proximal phalanx of thumb.

Nerve Supply

The posterior interosseous nerve supplies it.

Actions

It extends the proximal phalanx of the thumb and the first metacarpal bone.

Testing Function of EPB

Ask the subject to extend the proximal phalanx of thumb at the MCP joint against resistance (the forearm is resting on the table in prone position).

Clinical Highlights of Synovial Sheath Around APL and EPB

In de Quervain's tenosynovitis there is inflammation of the synovial sheath around the tendons of abductor pollicis longus and extensor pollicis brevis. This produces swelling and pain along the lateral aspect of the wrist. Symptoms usually subside after incising the tendon sheath.

Extensor Pollicis Longus (EPL)

This muscle takes origin from the posterior surface of ulna below the origin of abductor pollicis longus and from the interosseous membrane. Its long tendon hooks round the Lister's or dorsal tubercle of radius deep to the extensor retinaculum in the third compartment. It then passes along the posterior margin of the anatomical snuffbox. It is inserted in the base of the terminal phalanx of thumb. On the dorsum of the proximal phalanx, though there is no extensor expansion proper, the sides of the extensor pollicis longus tendon receive connections from the tendon of extensor pollicis brevis on the lateral side and from the insertion of adductor pollicis and first palmar interosseous muscles from the medial side.

Nerve Supply

The posterior interosseous nerve supplies the muscle.

Arterial Supply

The muscle belly receives arterial twigs from posterior interosseous artery but its tendon receives twigs from anterior interosseous artery, radial artery and first dorsal metacarpal artery amongst several other sources.

Actions

The EPL extends the thumb at the interphalangeal and first carpometacarpal joints.

Testing Function of EPL

The subject is asked to extend the distal phalanx of thumb against resistance.

Rupture of EPL Tendon

The spontaneous rupture of the tendon may occur due to ischemia, in case of injury to anterior interosseous artery. This artery or its branches may be injured in Colles fracture. The tendon ruptures, where it changes direction around the dorsal tubercle of radius. The patient feels that the thumb has "dropped" as the interphalangeal joint of the thumb cannot extend. This is also described as hammer thumb deformity.

Extensor Indicis

This takes origin from posterior surface of ulna below the origin of extensor pollicis longus. Its tendon passes along with the extensor tendons deep to the extensor retinaculum in the fourth compartment. It is inserted in the dorsal digital expansion of index finger.

Nerve Supply

The posterior interosseous nerve supplies it.

Action

It helps in extension of index finger.

POSTERIOR INTEROSSEOUS NERVE

This is the only nerve of the posterior compartment of forearm. It is a purely motor nerve.

The deep terminal branch of radial nerve continues as posterior interosseous nerve. It travels in the substance of the supinator muscle, which wraps round the proximal part of radius. As the nerve passes through the supinator it is closely related to the lateral aspect of neck of radius. Then it enters the back of forearm through the lower part of supinator (Fig.19.1).

Course

At first the nerve lies between the superficial and deep extensor muscles but at the distal border of extensor pollicis brevis it passes deep to extensor pollicis longus and directly rests on the interosseous membrane. In its upper part the posterior interosseous artery accompanies it but distally the anterior interosseous artery accompanies it. The posterior interosseous nerve and anterior interosseous artery reach the dorsum of the carpus, where they occupy the fourth compartment deep to the extensor retinaculum. Here, the nerve terminates in a pseudoganglion.

Branches (Fig. 19.2)

a. Before the posterior interosseous nerve enters the supinator it supplies extensor carpi radialis brevis and supinator in the cubital fossa.
b. While passing through the supinator it again supplies the supinator.
c. In its initial course at the back of forearm, it gives three short branches to the extensor digitorum, extensor digiti minimi and extensor carpi ulnaris. Then it gives longer branches to extensor pollicis longus, extensor indicis, abductor pollicis longus and extensor pollicis brevis. The branches from the pseudoganglion are given to the carpal ligaments and articulations.

Clinical Highlights

a. Posterior interosseous nerve (PIN) syndrome is due to compression of the nerve deep to the arcade of Frohse, which is a musculotendinous structure at the proximal edge of supinator muscle. In this syndrome, the extensor carpi ulnaris is usually affected first so that attempted wrist extension causes radial deviation due to overaction of radial extensors. There is weakness of extension and abduction of thumb (thumb drop) besides weak extension of fingers (finger drop).
b. The posterior interosseous nerve is of particular interest to the orthopedic surgeon because of its close relation to the neck of radius. The nerve is liable to injury in dislocation of the head of radius or during surgical exposure of upper part of radius. To locate the nerve, the orthopedic surgeons use Henry's method as follows. With elbow flexed at 90° and forearm supinated, the point of entry of nerve in the proximal edge of supinator lies three fingers below the radial head.

POSTERIOR INTEROSSEOUS ARTERY

It is one of the terminal branches of the common interosseous artery, which arises from the ulnar artery in cubital fossa. It enters the posterior compartment through the gap between the upper margin of interosseous membrane and the oblique cord. It passes downwards between the supinator and abductor pollicis longus. On the surface of the abductor pollicis longus muscle it accompanies the posterior interosseous nerve. It ends by anastomosing with the terminal part of anterior interosseous artery and dorsal carpal arch.

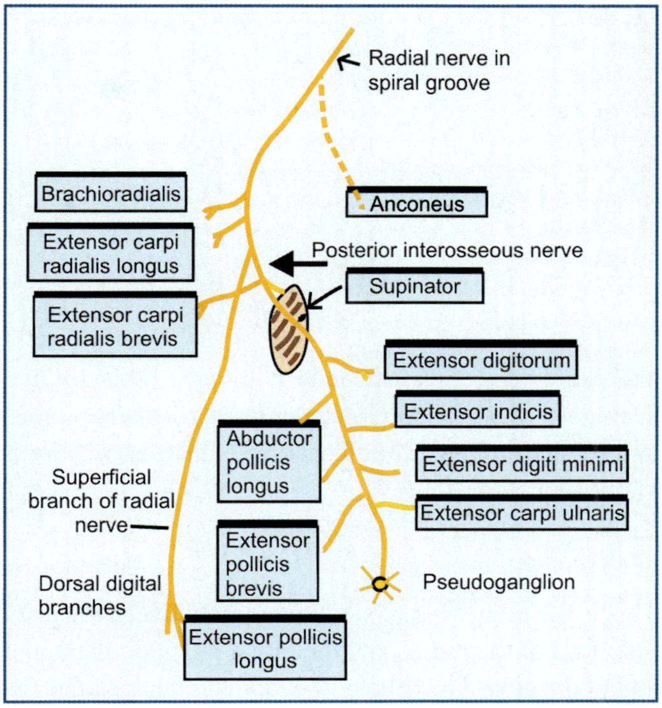

Fig. 19.2: Scheme to show nerve supply of muscles in extensor compartment of forearm

Branches

In cubital fossa, it gives the interosseous recurrent artery, which anastomoses with the radial collateral branch of profunda artery. In the posterior compartment it mainly gives muscular branches.

20 Radioulnar Joints

The radius and ulna articulate with each other by two synovial joints, the superior and inferior radioulnar joints, and by the middle radioulnar joint, which is of fibrous variety (Fig. 20.1).

SUPERIOR RADIOULNAR JOINT

This is the pivot type of synovial joint between the disc-like head of the radius and the radial notch on the upper end of the ulna. The head of the radius is held against the radial notch of ulna by a strong band called the annular ligament, which encircles the head of the radius and is attached to both the margins of the radial notch of ulna. The annular ligament and the radial notch together form an osseofibrous ring (Fig. 20.2) for the head of the radius to rotate during pronation and supination. The quadrate ligament is a weak bond between the neck of radius and lower margin of radial notch of ulna. The fibrous capsule of the elbow joint covers the joint. The synovial membrane lines the annular ligament and the fibrous capsule internally and is continuous with that of the elbow joint. Inferiorly, the joint is supported by the quadrate ligament, which spreads from the neck of radius to the radial notch of ulna. There is a difference in the shape of the annular ligament in adults and children, which is the basis of its clinical importance. In adults the cup shape of the ligament and its firm attachment to the neck of the radius prevent its downward displacement. On the contrary, in children the head tends to slip out of the ring due to the tubular shape of ligament and the smaller circumference of the head of radius resulting in a clinical condition called "pulled elbow".

INFERIOR RADIOULNAR JOINT (Fig. 22.1)

This is the pivot type of synovial joint between the head of ulna and the ulnar notch on the lower end of radius. The fibrous capsule surrounds the joint cavity and is attached to the margins of the articular surfaces. The capsule is thicker in front and behind but lax superiorly. The synovial membrane lines the capsule and projects in front of the interosseous membrane and behind the pronator quadratus as a narrow recess. The articular disc is attached medially to a pit between the styloid process and the head of the ulna and laterally to the inferior margin of the ulnar notch of the radius. Its peripheral part merges with the capsules of the radioulnar and wrist joints. The disc excludes the ulna from the wrist joint and provides the ulnar head a platform to rotate during movements of supination and pronation (Figs 20.1 and 22.1).

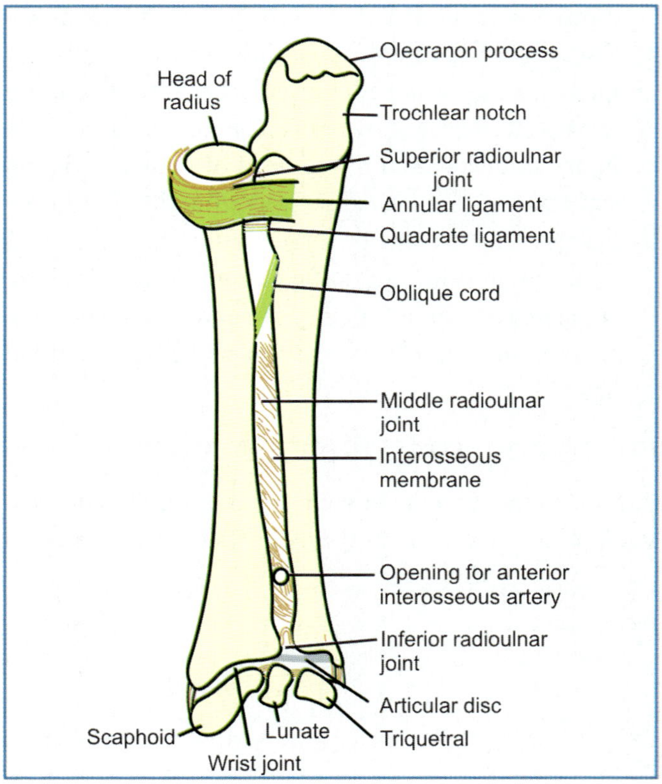

Fig. 20.1: Radioulnar joints

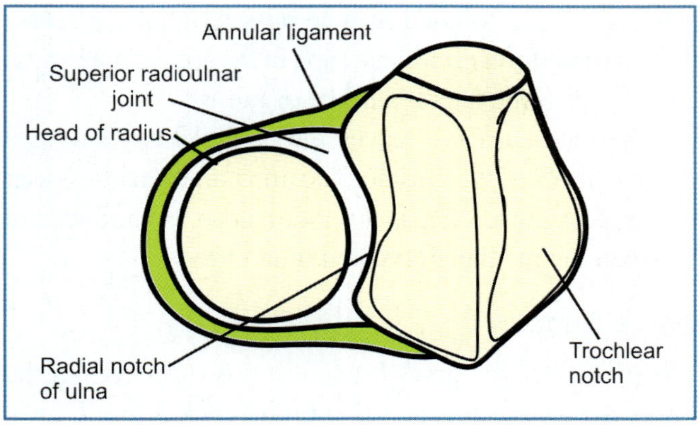

Fig. 20.2: Section of superior radioulnar joint showing attachment of annular ligament to radial notch of ulna

MIDDLE RADIOULNAR JOINT

This is a longitudinally oriented joint between the shafts of the radius and ulna. The oblique cord and the interosseous membrane are the connecting bonds between the two bones. This joint belongs to syndesmosis type of fibrous joint. The oblique cord extends from the lateral side of ulnar tuberosity to the lower limit of radial tuberosity.

INTEROSSEOUS MEMBRANE

This is a thick sheet of collagenous tissue between the interosseous borders of the two bones. The fibers in the membrane are directed downwards and medially from radius to ulna. Proximally the membrane starts about 2 to 3 cm below the radial tuberosity and distally it reaches upto the level of distal radioulnar joint, where it fuses with the capsule of this joint.

Relations of Anterior Surface

The three deep muscles of the front of the forearm, flexor digitorum profundus, flexor pollicis longus and pronator quadratus take origin from the anterior surface. The anterior interosseous nerve and vessels lie in close relation to this surface, At the upper margin of the pronator quadratus the anterior interosseous vessels pass through the interosseous membrane to enter the posterior compartment but the nerve descends up to the lower limit of the membrane.

Relations of Posterior Surface

The four deep muscles of the back of forearm, abductor pollicis longus, extensor pollicis brevis, extensor pollicis longus and extensor indicis take origin from the posterior surface. The lower part of the posterior surface is closely related to the posterior interosseous nerve and anterior intreosseous artery. The posterior interosseous vessels enter the posterior compartment through the gap between the upper margin of the membrane and the oblique cord.

Functions

The interosseous membrane transmits the compression forces from radius to ulna. The midprone position of the forearm, when the membrane is under tension is favorable for weight transmission. The other function of the membrane is that it increases the area of origin of deep flexor and extensor muscles of the forearm.

Supination and Pronation (Fig. 20.3)

The superior and inferior radioulnar joints permit the movements of supination and pronation. The movements take place around a mobile vertical axis passing through the center of the head of the radius and the lower end of ulna. The head of the radius rotates within the osseofibrous ring. In the movement of pronation, the radius carrying the hand with it turns anteromedially across the ulna with the result that the lower part of radius comes to lie medial to ulna and the palm faces posteriorly. During supination,

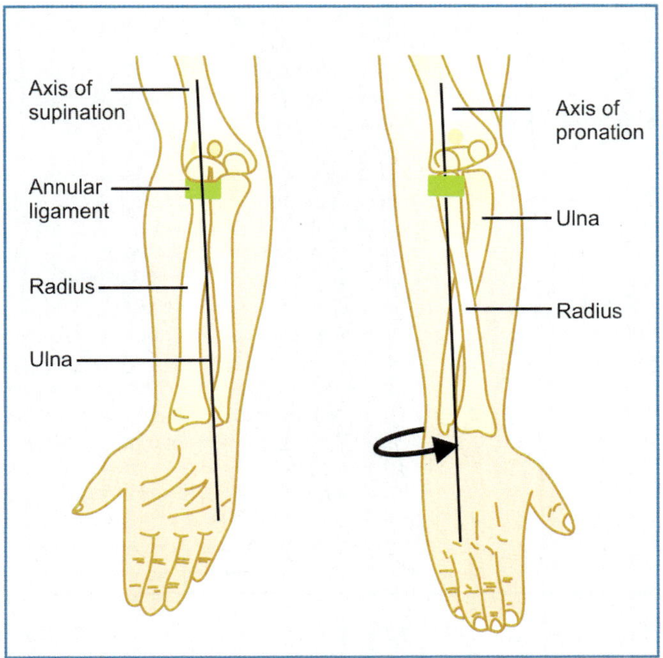

Fig. 20.3: Movements of pronation and supination

the radius comes back to its position lateral to ulna so that the palm faces anteriorly. The supination is a more powerful movement as is evident from the design of the screws. The supination is equated to the screwing movement while pronation to the unscrewing movement. The opening of a lock with the key in right hand is an example of supination while the action of locking with the key in right hand is an example of pronation.

MUSCLES OF PRONATION (Fig. 20.4)

Pronator Teres

This muscle takes origin by two heads. The humeral head is larger and more superficial than the ulnar head, which is deeper and smaller. The humeral head arises from the lower part of the medial supracondylar ridge of humerus and from the common flexor origin on the front of medial epicondyle. The ulnar head arises from the medial border of coronoid process of ulna. The two heads join each other and the combined muscle passes obliquely across the proximal forearm for insertion in the area of maximum convexity on the lateral surface of radius.

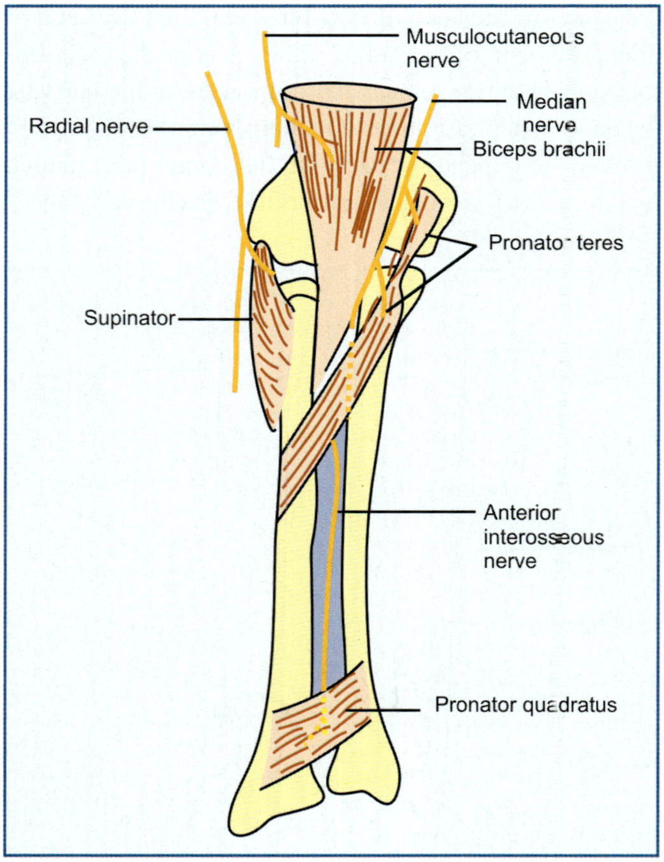

Fig. 20.4: Schematic representation of muscles of pronation and supination along with their nerve supply

The median nerve leaves the cubital fossa between the two heads of the muscle. The ulnar artery passes deep to the deep head. Thus, the ulnar head is sandwiched between the median nerve and ulnar artery.

Nerve Supply

The median nerve gives branch to pronator teres in the lower part of the arm and also in the cubital fossa.

Actions

The pronator teres rotates the radius in such a way that the palm is turned medially and hence faces posteriorly (in movement of pronation). It is also a weak flexor of elbow.

Testing Muscle Function

After flexing the elbow roughly to 20°, the subject is asked to supinate the forearm fully. After this the subject attempts to pronate the forearm against resistance. If normal, the contraction of the muscle is felt in upper part of forearm.

Pronator Quadratus

This is a quadrilateral and flat muscle, which is located deeply in the distal part of the forearm. It arises from the bony ridge on the anterior surface of the lower one fourth of the shaft of ulna. The fibers pass laterally and downward for insertion on the anterior surface of lower fourth of radius. The muscle lies in contact with the anterior surface of the lower part of the interosseous membrane. A synovial pouch called the sacciform recess, from the inferior radioulnar joint extends between pronator quadratus and interosseous membrane. The anterior interosseous nerve descends behind the posterior surface of the muscle. The space of Parona or deep forearm space lies between the long flexor tendons and the anterior surface of the pronator quadratus.

Nerve Supply

The anterior interosseous branch of the median nerve supplies the muscle.

Actions

It is the chief pronator of the forearm. It is assisted by the pronator teres only in rapid and forceful pronation.

MUSCLES OF SUPINATION (Fig. 20.4)

Biceps Brachii

This is a muscle of the anterior compartment of arm. It takes origin by two tendinous heads from the scapula. The short head takes origin from the tip of the coracoid process of scapula along with coracobrachialis. The long head takes origin from the supraglenoid tubercle of scapula. The tendon of the long head is intracapsular but extrasynovial in position. It leaves the shoulder joint by passing beneath the transverse humeral ligament to enter the intertubercular sulcus. The synovial sheath covers the tendon up to the level of surgical neck of humerus. The two heads of the biceps fuse to form a fusiform belly, which ends in a flat tendon about six to seven cm above the elbow. In the cubital fossa the tendon lies lateral to the brachial artery. It is inserted on the posterior part of radial tuberosity. The medial border of the tendon sends a fibrous expansion called the bicipital aponeurosis, which extends medially in front of the brachial artery and median nerve to get attached to the deep fascia of the forearm and through it to the subcutaneous posterior border of ulna.

Nerve Supply

The biceps brachii is supplied by musculocutaneous nerve.

Actions

The biceps brachii can act on three joints (shoulder, elbow and superior radioulnar) since it crosses all the three joints. On the radioulnar joint it acts as powerful supinator of the forearm. The biceps has its maximum supinating power, when the elbow is flexed at right angle. In this position of the elbow the insertion of the biceps is in line with the rest of the muscle. The action of the biceps on the elbow joint is flexion. Its action on shoulder joint is flexion. The long head of biceps helps in stabilizing the head of humerus during movements of the shoulder joint.

Testing Muscle Function

The subject flexes the elbow against resistance, when the forearm is supinated and extended.

Popeye Deformity

The rupture of the tendon of long head of biceps brachii (due to chronic tendonitis in elderly or in weight lifters or in swimmers) results in a sudden appearance of a swelling in the lower part of front of arm (Fig. 20.5). This is due to the detached muscle belly taking the shape of a ball. This appearance resembles the arm of a cartoon character named Popeye.

Supinator

This muscle belongs to the extensor compartment of forearm (Figs19.1 and 20.6) but is seen in the floor of cubital fossa anteriorly and also in the posterior compartment of forearm. It is attached to three bones, namely, humerus, ulna and radius and two ligaments and is disposed in two laminae (superficial and deep). The superficial lamina arises by tendinous fibers from the lateral aspect of lateral epicondyle of humerus, radial collateral ligament of elbow joint and annular ligament of superior radioulnar joint. The deep lamina arises by muscular fibers from the supinator crest of ulna and a small area in front

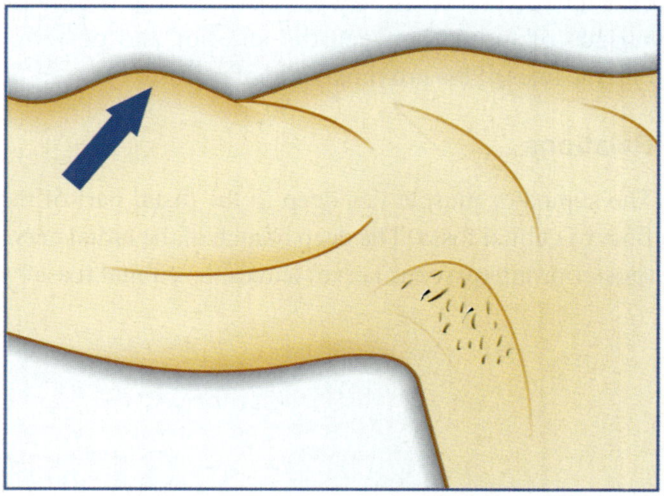

Fig. 20.5: Popeye deformity. The bulge in arm indicated by arrow is produced by biceps brachii consequent to the rupture of its long head

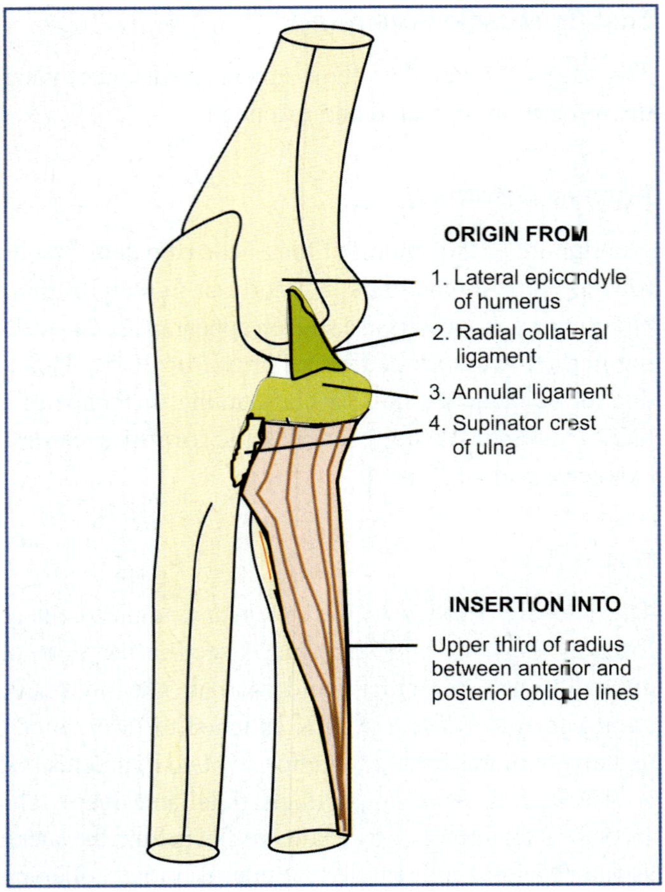

Fig. 20.6: Showing areas of origin and insertion of supinator muscle in posterolateral view

of it. The fibers of both laminae spiral round the upper one-third of radius, as they are inserted in to the lateral surface of radius between the anterior and posterior oblique lines of the proximal third of radius.

Relations

The supinator muscle lies deep in the distal part of the floor of cubital fossa. The deep branch of the radial nerve (posterior interosseous nerve) leaves the cubital fossa by entering the substance of the supinator at its proximal edge. The nerve travels between the two laminae and enters the posterior compartment just above the distal border of the supinator. The proximal edge of the superficial lamina of the supinator is fibro-tendinous (arcade of Frohse) in some percentage of population. This is a common site of compression of the nerve, producing posterior interosseous nerve (PIN) syndrome.

Nerve Supply

Posterior interosseous nerve supplies a branch usually before it enters the muscle and also as it passes through the muscle.

Actions

The action of the supinator is to rotate the shaft of the radius laterally and thereby bring about supination of the forearm. In the flexed forearm the role of supinator is to fix the radius (the prime supinator being biceps brachii) but in extended forearm the supinator is the prime supinator.

Testing Muscle Function

The subject is asked to supinate forearm against resistance in extended and fully pronated position.

Clinical Highlights

Fractures of the lower end of radius (Colles' fracture) and that of ulna are liable to produce distortion of the inferior radioulnar joint. Loss of pronation leads to interference with writing. The hand is almost handicapped if the capacity to pronate and to supinate is lost either due to joint disorder or muscle weakness. Pronation is lost in the lesion of median nerve at or above the level of the elbow. Supination is lost in injury to radial nerve at or above elbow and injury to the musculocutaneous nerve.

21 Retinacula at Wrist

The wrist is a junctional zone between the forearm and the hand. The tendons of the extensor muscles of the forearm cross the wrist from behind while the tendons of the flexor muscles cross in front. Since the tendons cross a series of joints at the carpus they are held tightly against the carpus to prevent their bow stringing. The deep fascia of the wrist is modified to form flexor and extensor retinacula to strap down these tendons.

FLEXOR RETINACULUM (Fig. 21.1)

The size of the flexor retinaculum is 2.5 × 2.5 cm. It is a square-shaped dense thickening of the deep fascia. The retinaculum is attached to the pisiform bone and hook of the hamate medially and to the scaphoid and the margins of the groove on trapezium laterally. Proximally, it is continuous with the deep fascia of forearm and distally with the palmar aponeurosis.

Surface Marking

Cup the palm of the hand by spreading the fingers (as though to grasp a large ball). The hollow between the proximal parts of the thenar and hypothenar eminences marks the position of flexor retinaculum distal to the distal flexure crease of the wrist. The retinaculum is quite deep from the skin because its anterior surface is covered with origin of thenar and hypothenar muscles. The surgeon operating on flexor retinaculum for the first time must be aware of this fact.

Relations

a. Anterior or superficial relations are, the ulnar nerve and vessels, the palmar cutaneous branch of ulnar nerve, the palmaris longus tendon and the palmar cutaneous branch of median nerve from medial to lateral side. The ulnar nerve and vessels are protected in Guyons canal inside the substance of the flexor retinaculum. The thenar and hypothenar muscles take origin from the anterior surface of the retinaculum.
b. Posterior or deep relations are the flexor tendons and the median nerve. The tendon of flexor carpi radialis passes through a separate tunnel in relation to the groove of trapezium. The median nerve along with four tendons of flexor digitorum superficialis, four tendons of flexor digitorum profundus and one of flexor pollicis longus passes through the carpal tunnel.

Clinical Highlights

The carpal tunnel syndrome (CTS) is produced as a result of compression of median nerve in the carpal tunnel. Some causes of CTS are chronic tenosynovitis or inflammation of the synovial sheaths surrounding the tendons in the carpal tunnel, myxoedema, pregnancy and anterior dislocation of the lunate bone. The effects of median nerve compression are as follows:

a. Numbness, tingling and burning pain in lateral three and half fingers are the early symptoms. The sensory loss develops in the same fingers in due course of time.

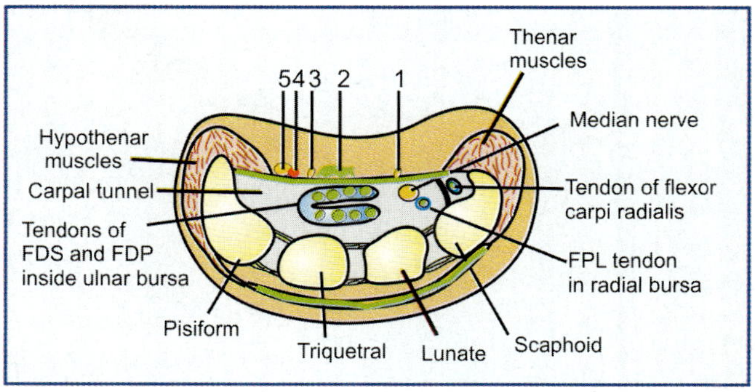

Fig. 21.1: To show relations of flexor retinaculum of hand. Note its anterior relations from lateral to medial: 1-Palmar cutaneous branch of median nerve, 2-Tendon of palmaris longus, 3-Palmar cutaneous branch of ulnar nerve, 4-Ulnar artery, 5- Ulnar nerve.

b. Weakness of thenar muscles and flattening of thenar eminence are the symptoms and signs of loss of motor function. Gradually, it will lead to ape thumb deformity if left untreated.

Surgical cutting of flexor retinaculum is one of the methods of relieving pressure on the median nerve.

EXTENSOR RETINACULUM

This is the rectangular shaped thickening of deep fascia (about 3.5 cm long) on the back of the wrist.

It is attached medially to pisiform and triquetral and laterally to the anterior border of lower end of radius. Proximally it is contienuous with the deep fascia at the back of forearm and distally with the deep fascia on the dorsum of hand.

Relations (Fig. 21.2)

a. The posterior or superficial relations are the superficial branch of the radial nerve and the dorsal cutaneous branch of the ulnar nerve.

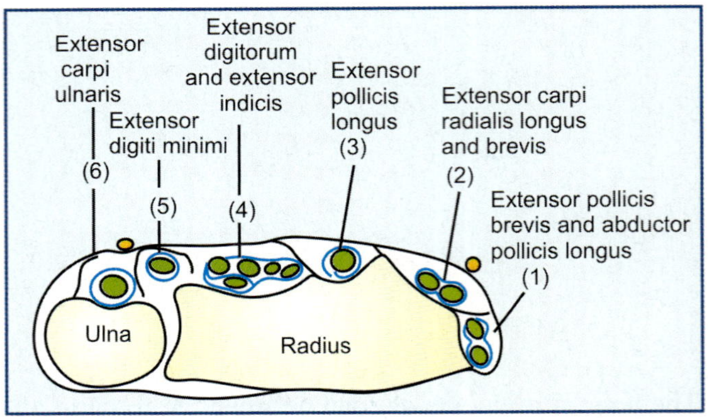

Fig. 21.2: Scheme to show relations of extensor retinaculum. Note the superficial branch of radial nerve and dorsal cutaneous branch of ulnar nerve in superficial relation to retinaculum

b. Anterior or deep aspect of the extensor retinaculum sends septa to the back of radius and ulna so that six osseofibrous compartments are formed for the passage of the extensor tendons. The compartments are numbered from lateral to medial side and their contents are shown in Figure 21.2.

22 Wrist Joint

The wrist joint is an ellipsoid type of synovial joint permitting movements along two axes. The anatomical name of the joint is radiocarpal joint, which is suggestive of the fact that of the forearm bones only the radius (and not the ulna) takes part in its formation. This is a functional necessity as the radius is able to carry the hand with it during pronation and supination.

Articular Surfaces (Fig. 22.1)

The proximal articular surface is concave in shape. The concavity is formed by the articular area on the inferior surface of the lower end of the radius along with the inferior surface of the articular disc of the inferior radioulnar joint. The distal articular surface is reciprocally convex. It is formed by proximal surfaces of scaphoid, lunate and triquetral bones from lateral to medial side.

Ligaments

The joint is surrounded by the fibrous capsule, which is strengthened by the palmar and dorsal radiocarpal ligaments and the carpal collateral ligaments.

Fibrous Capsule

The fibrous capsule is attached to the articular margins of the proximal and distal articular areas, including the articular disc. It is lined by synovial membrane. The anterior part of the capsule is thickened laterally to form palmar radiocarpal ligament, and medially to form palmar ulnocarpal ligament. Posteriorly, the capsule is strengthened to form dorsal radiocarpal ligament. These ligaments are attached distally mainly to the proximal row of carpal bones and also to the capitate (a bone of distal row).

Carpal Collateral Ligaments

The radial carpal collateral ligament extends from the styloid process of the radius to the scaphoid and trapezium. The ulnar carpal collateral ligament extends from the ulnar styloid process to the triquetral and pisiform.

Relations

Anteriorly, the joint is related to the tendons of the long flexors (flexor pollicis longus, flexor digitorum superficialis and profundus), carpal flexors (flexor carpi radialis and flexor carpi ulnaris) and the median and ulnar nerves. The posterior relations are the long extensor tendons of the digits (extensor digitorum, extensor indicis and extensor digiti minimi) and the carpal extensors (extensor carpi ulnaris, extensor carpi radialis longus and brevis) along with long and short extensors of the thumb (extensor pollicis longus and brevis) and the abductor pollicis longus. The radial artery in the anatomical snuffbox is related laterally.

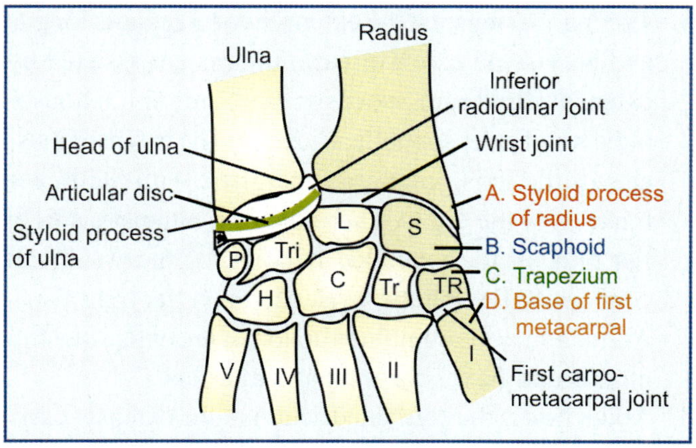

Fig. 22.1: Skeleton of wrist (P-Pisiform, Tri-Triquetral, L-Lunate, S-Scaphoid, TR-Trapezium, Tr-Trapezoid, C-Capitate, H-Hamate). Note that bones A, B, C, D are in the floor of anatomical snuffbox

Nerve Supply

The articular branches of anterior and posterior interosseous nerves supply the joint.

Arterial Supply

The palmar and dorsal carpal arches are the source of arterial supply. The carpal arches are the arterial anastomoses on the front and back of the wrist deep to the long tendons. The arteries that take part in the cruciate palmar arch are the palmar carpal branch of radial artery, palmar carpal branch of ulnar artery, descending branch of anterior interosseous artery and the recurrent branches of deep palmar arch. In the dorsal carpal arch the following four arteries tale part, the dorsal carpal branch of radial artery, dorsal carpal branch of ulnar artery and carpal branches of anterior and posterior interosseous arteries.

Movements

The flexion is described as palmar flexion and extension as dorsal flexion. The adduction is known as ulnar deviation and abduction as radial deviation. Circumduction is the sequential combination of the above movements. The movements of the wrist joint and of the intercarpal joints are inter-linked and therefore produced by the same set of muscles.

a. The main flexors, the flexor carpi radialis and flexor carpi ulnaris are assisted by the flexor digitorum superficialis, flexor digitorum profundus and flexor pollicis longus muscles.
b. The main extensors, the extensor carpi radialis longus and brevis and extensor carpi ulnaris are assisted by extensor digitorum, extensor digiti minimi, extensor indicis and extensor pollicis longus. The extensor muscles of the wrist joint are synergistic with the flexor muscles of the digits. Therefore one can make a tight fist only in the extended position of the wrist and conversely flexing the wrist can open the tight fist.
c. Adduction is the combined action of the extensor carpi ulnaris and flexor carpi ulnaris muscles.
d. Abduction is the combined action of the extensor carpi radialis longus and brevis and flexor carpi radialis muscles. The abductor pollicis longus and extensor pollicis brevis also contribute.

Clinical Highlights

a. The ganglion is a localized cystic swelling on the dorsum of the wrist arising from either the capsule of the joint or from the synovial sheath surrounding the extensor tendons or of the intercarpal joints. It usually presents as a painful lump and causes discomfort during the movements of wrist.
b. Colles' fracture (Fig. 22.3) is a common fracture of the distal part of the radius due to a fall on the outstretched hand. There is displacement of the lower radial fragment backwards and upwards and as a result the normal relationship of the tips of the ulnar and radial styloid processes is lost. The tip of the radial styloid process may be at the same level or higher than the tip of the ulnar styloid process. The wrist is swollen and its movements are limited and painful.

ANATOMICAL SNUFFBOX

This is a hollow space, which appears on the lateral side of the back of the wrist in the fully extended position of the thumb (Fig. 22.2).

Boundaries

This space is bounded on the ulnar side (posteriorly) by the extensor pollicis longus tendon and on the radial side (anteriorly) by the tendons of abductor pollicis longus and extensor pollicis brevis. The floor consists of four bony parts, in the proximal to distal order, styloid process of

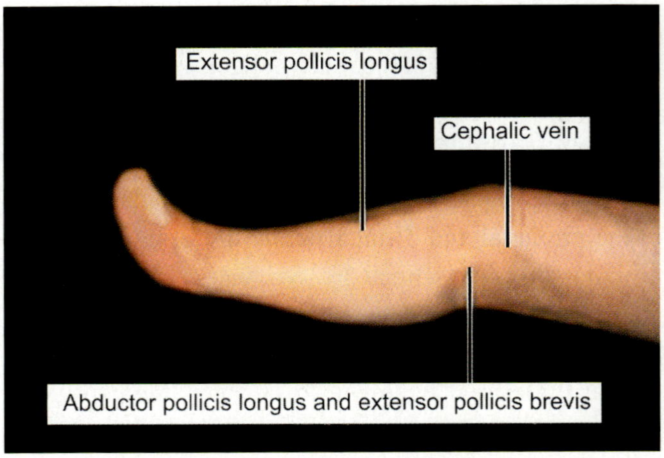

Fig. 22.2: Showing the tendons forming boundaries of anatomical snuffbox

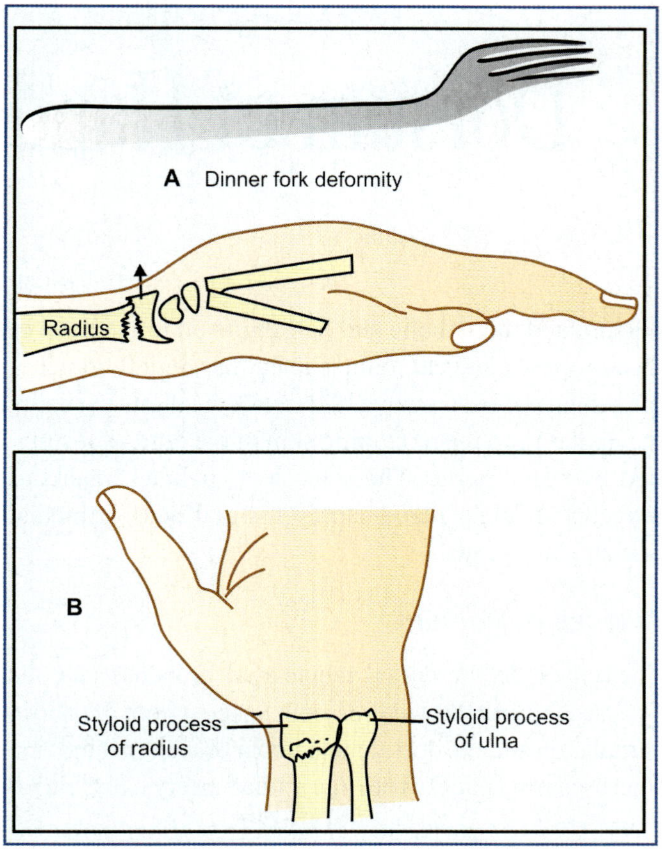

Fig. 22.3: Colles' fracture (at lower end of radius). In 'A' note the dorsal displacement of distal fragment of radius. In 'B' the styloid processes of radius and ulna are at the same level due to proximal displacement of distal fragment of radius

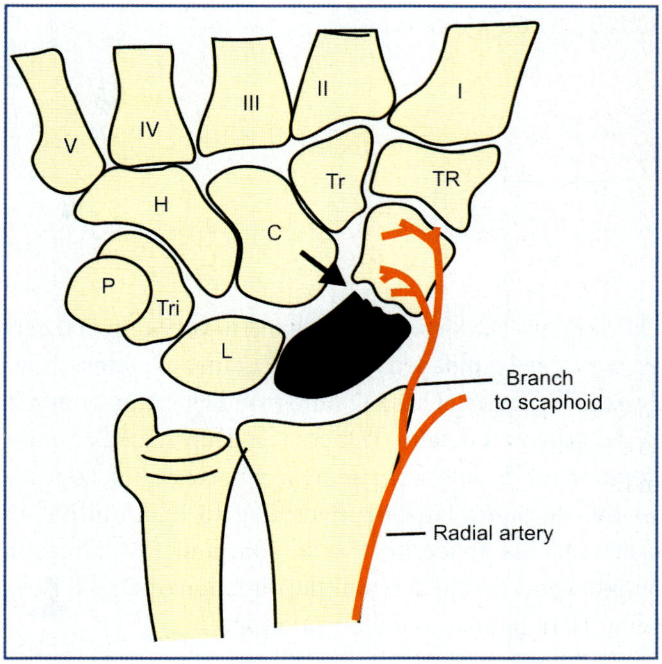

Fig. 22.4: Effect of fracture of scaphoid on its arterial supply. (Note that the arterial supply of the proximal segment is via distal segment which undergoes avascular necrosis in fracture, indicated by arrow)

radius, scaphoid, trapezium and base of the first metacarpal (Fig. 22.1). These bony parts can be felt through the roof. The fascial roof contains the cephalic vein and superficial branch of radial nerve. The radial artery passes via the anatomical snuffbox to the dorsum of the hand. On light pressure applied in the floor, pulsations of the radial artery can be felt.

Clinical Highlights

The scaphoid, which is in the floor of the anatomical snuffbox, is a frequently fractured carpal bone. The fracture is suspected if there is tenderness in the snuffbox. The scaphoid is more prone to fracture and necrosis due to following anatomical reasons. A narrow waist separates the proximal and distal parts of the scaphoid. Its nutrient artery (a branch of the radial artery) enters the distal part of the bone (Fig. 22.4). So, in fracture of the waist of the scaphoid, its proximal part is deprived of the blood supply and hence undergoes avascular necrosis.

23 Dorsum of Hand

The skin on the dorsum of the hand is very thin and can be very easily pinched. The subcutaneous veins show through it clearly. These features are in striking contrast to the skin on the palm. If there is a deep-seated abscess in the palm, its outer sign in the form of swelling appears on the dorsum. This happens due to availability of subcutaneous space on the dorsum and formation of lymphedema on the dorsum (the direction of lymph flow being from palmar to the dorsal aspect).

Structures on Dorsum

The dorsum has the dorsal venous network or arch, cutaneous nerves and vessels apart from the long extensor tendons of the digits. The deep fascia of the dorsum is extremely thin and is attached to the extensor tendons, which are devoid of the synovial sheaths here. An aponeurotic layer is formed under the skin by intertendinous connections. In this way, two fascial spaces, the dorsal subcutaneous space and the dorsal subaponeurotic space are seen on the dorsum. The infection of the subaponeurotic space usually results from laceration of the knuckles, as for example in tooth bite on the fist.

Nerves on Dorsum (Fig. 23.1)

As there are no intrinsic muscles on the dorsum, the nerves that are encountered here are purely sensory. The cutaneous nerves that supply the dorsum are, superficial branch of the radial nerve, the dorsal cutaneous branches of the ulnar nerve and the palmar digital branches of median and ulnar nerves. The superficial terminal branch of the radial nerve divides into four dorsal digital nerves, which supply the skin of the radial side of the hand as well as the lateral three and half digits up to the level of approximately the middle of middle phalanx. The dorsal cutaneous branches of ulnar nerve supply the remaining dorsum and medial one and half digits up to the level of distal interphalangeal joint. The palmar digital branches of median nerve come over the tips of the digits to supply the nailbed and the remaining skin of the digits not supplied by radial nerve. The same way, palmar cutaneous branches of ulnar nerve supply the nail beds of medial one and half digits.

Arteries of Dorsum

These include the dorsal metacarpal branches (for the first, second and third interosseous spaces) from the dorsal carpal arch and the dorsal metacarpal branch (for the first interosseous space) from the radial artery. The radial

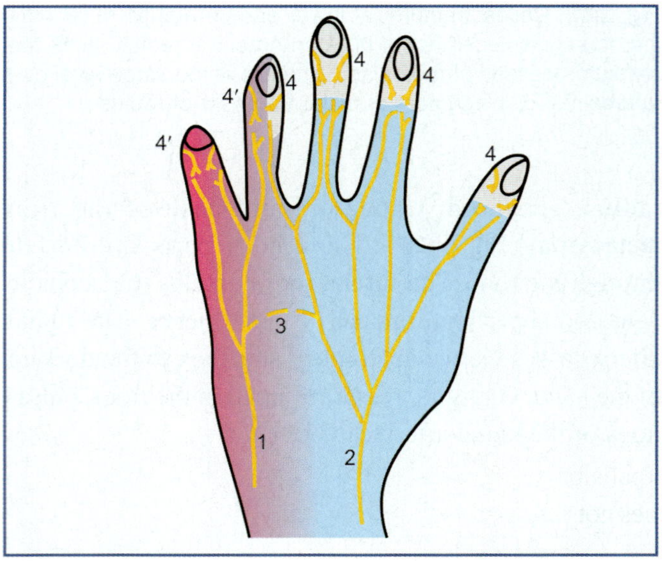

Fig. 23.1: Sensory nerves of dorsum of hand

1. Dorsal cutaneous branch of ulnar nerve
2. Superficial branch of radial nerve
3. Communication between digital branches of ulnar and radial nerves
4. Palmar digital branches of median nerve

4′. Palmar digital branches of ulnar nerve

artery enters the dorsum via the anatomical snuffbox. Here, it gives the first dorsal metacarpal artery before leaving the dorsum between the two heads of first dorsal interosseous muscle. The perforating branches (proximal perforating arteries) from the deep palmar arch reinforce the medial three metacarpal arteries. Distally the dorsal metacarpal arteries are connected to the common palmar digital arteries by the distal perforating branches. On reaching the bases of the digits the metacarpal arteries divide into dorsal digital arteries for the supply of the adjacent fingers.

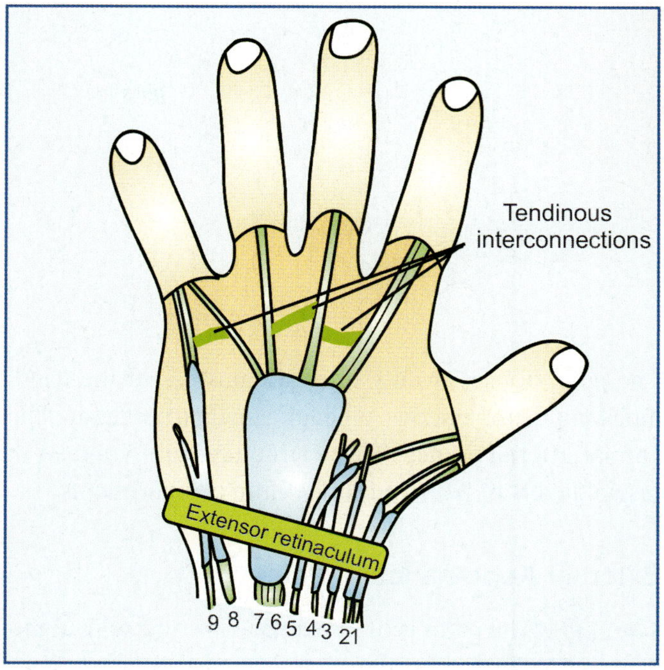

Fig. 23.2: Extensor tendons with their synovial sheaths (shown in blue) on dorsum of hand

1. Extensor pollicis brevis
2. Abductor pollicis longus
3. Extensor carpi radialis longus
4. Extensor carpi radialis brevis
5. Extensor pollicis longus
6. Extensor indicis
7. Extensor digitorum
8. Extensor digiti minimi
9. Extensor carpi ulnaris

Extensor Tendons on Dorsum (Fig. 23.2)

The tendons of the extensor muscles pass deep to the extensor retinaculum. All the tendons are covered with synovial sheath partially. Except for the three carpal extensors (ECRL, ECRB, ECU) the rest of the tendons cross the dorsum of the hand to reach the digits for insertion. The extensor tendons of the medial four digits are connected by tendinous interconnections (conexus intertendineus), which restrict the independent movements of the digits. The tendon of extensor digiti minimi usually splits in two on the dorsum. The extensor digiti minimi and extensor indicis tendons fuse with the respective tendon of the extensor digitorum distal to the conexus. Due to this the MCP joints of these fingers can be extended even if the MCP joints of the middle and ring fingers are flexed. Since the middle and ring fingers receive only one tendon it is not possible to extend their MCP joints, when the MCP joints of the index and ring fingers are flexed. The extensor tendons form a dorsal expansion over the metacarpophalangeal (MCP) joint and the proximal phalanx. The extensor expansion provides insertion not only to the extensor tendons but also to the interosseous and lumbrical muscles. In the case of thumb the extensor expansion is not present. The abductor pollicis longus does not reach the thumb phalanx. The tendon of extensor pollicis longus reaches the terminal phalanx. The tendon of extensor pollicis brevis sends a connection to the long extensor tendon on the proximal phalanx from the lateral aspect. A similar connection is present on the medial aspect from the insertion of first palmar inerosseous and the adductor pollicis. The details about the parts of the extensor expansion are described in Chapter 26 along with interossei and lumbricals.

24 Palm

The palm houses twenty intrinsic muscles of the hand, nine long flexor tendons, ulnar and median nerves and the palmar arterial arches. These structures are wrapped in fascial layers of palm in four definite compartments.

External Appearance of Palm

The skin of the palm is of thick glabrous type with abundant sweat glands. The skin shows characteristic papillary ridges, which are responsible for the fingerprints. Another peculiarity of palmar skin is its firm anchorage to the deep fascia at the skin creases (flexure lines) of palm. These lines are of importance in some diseases, like for example, Down syndrome (trisomy-21), where a single transverse crease on the palm (simian crease) is characteristic. Normally there are two transversely disposed palmar creases. The distal palmar crease (heart line) lies just proximal to the metacarpophalangeal joints (MCP joints). The proximal palmar crease is called the headline. The skin creases at the roots of the fingers are situated about 2-3 cm distal to the heart line. The middle skin crease of each finger lies at the level of PIP joint. The distal skin crease of the finger lies proximal to DIP joint. There is one longitudinally oriented crease laterally. On its lateral side, there is an elevated area called thenar eminence. A less well-marked area on the medial side is known as hypothenar eminence.

Superficial Fascia of Palm

The subcutaneous fat interspersed with dense fibrous tissue connects palmar aponeurosis to the skin. The superficial fascia is modified as superficial transverse metacarpal ligament at the web margins of the hand. The palmaris brevis muscle is located in the superficial fascia.

Palmaris Brevis (Fig. 24.1)

The palmaris brevis is present on the medial side across the base of hypothenar eminence. It arises from the flexor retinaculum and the palmar aponeurosis near its apex and is inserted in the dermis of medial margin of hand. It is subcutaneous in location, hence falls in the category of panniculus carnosus. The muscle receives nerve supply from superficial branch of ulnar nerve. Its contraction improves the grip of hand.

Palmar Aponeurosis (Fig. 24.1)

The palmar aponeurosis is a triangular thickening of the deep fascia in the central region of the palm. It is composed of longitudinally oriented fibers joined by transverse connections. The apex of the palmar aponeurosis is directed proximally, where it is continuous with flexor retinaculum and the tendon of palmaris longus. Its base extends distally to the level of distal palmar crease, where it splits into four digital slips for the medial four digits. Each slip divides in two parts to get attached at a deeper plane to the deep transverse metacarpal ligament, to the capsule of the corresponding MCP joint, base of proximal phalanx and to the fibrous flexor sheath of corresponding digit. Superficially, it is attached to the skin and the superficial transverse metacarpal ligament. The medial and lateral palmar septa arise from the respective margins of the palmar aponeurosis and incline in dorsal direction. The medial septum attaches to the fifth metacarpal while the lateral one to the first metacarpal. These septa are responsible for dividing the palm into fascial compartments. Near its apex, the palmaris brevis takes origin from its medial aspect. The palmar aponeurosis not only protects the nerves and vessels in the palm but also helps to improve the grip of the hand.

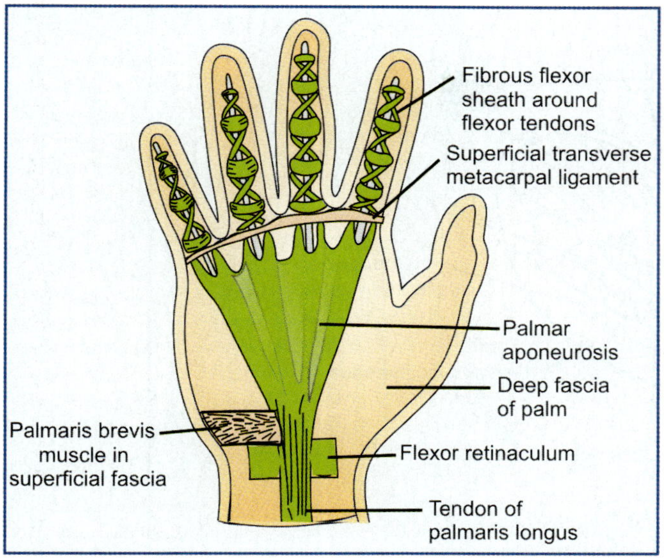

Fig. 24.1: Schematic diagram to depict modifications of deep fascia of palm

Dupuytren's Contracture

This is a condition in which the medial part of the palmar aponeurosis undergoes progressive shortening. This exerts pull on the little and ring fingers causing flexion deformity. Surgical division of the shortened part of the aponeurosis (fasciotomy) is done to straighten the bent fingers.

Fibrous Flexor Sheath (Fig. 24.1)

The fibrous flexor sheath is the thickened deep fascia on all five digits. The sheath extends from the level of head of metacarpal to the base of distal phalanx. It has a very thick and unique structure (consisting of five dense and stiff annular pulleys and three thin and lax cruciform pulleys). The sheath is attached to the margins of the phalanges. Thus, the phalanges and the sheath together form an osseofibrous tunnel in each digit. The tunnel for the thumb houses one tendon of flexor pollicis longus while the tunnels for the other digits house two tendons, one each of flexor digitorum superficialis and flexor digitorum profundus. The tunnel is closed distally by the attachment of the sheath to the phalanx beyond the insertion of flexor pollicis longus (thumb) and flexor digitorum profundus (other digits). The synovial sheath surrounds the tendons to allow frictionless movements of the tendons inside the tunnel. The arteries are carried to the tendon by the synovial folds, the vincula longa and brevia. The vincula longa are located near the roots of the fingers while the vincula brevia are found closer to the insertion of the tendons.

Fascial Compartments of Palm (Fig. 24.2)

The deep fascia of the palm is disposed in two layers, which wrap the intrinsic muscles, the long flexor tendons, the nerves and vessels of the palm. The deep fascia covering the thenar and the hypothenar areas turns posteriorly to become continuous with the deeper layer of fascia covering the anterior surfaces of the metacarpals, the interosseous muscles between them, and the adductor pollicis. These two fascial layers are connected to each other by means of the medial and the lateral palmar septa arising from medial and lateral margins respectively of the palmar aponeurosis. There are four fascial compartments, thenar, hypothenar, intermediate and adductor.

a. The thenar compartment contains abductor pollicis brevis, flexor pollicis brevis and opponens pollicis.
b. The hypothenar compartment contains abductor digiti minimi, flexor digiti minimi, and opponens digiti minimi.
c. The intermediate compartment contains the long flexor tendons surrounded by synovial sheaths, lumbricals, palmar arterial arches and the branches of the median and ulnar nerves.
d. The adductor compartment contains only the adductor pollicis muscle.

Palmar Spaces

The palmar spaces are known as the fascial spaces of palm. Under normal conditions there are no well-defined spaces inside the fascial compartments. However, the fascial spaces in the palm become apparent in the intermediate fascial compartment if there is collection of pus. A new septum called midpalmar septum (or intermediate palmar septum) develops in this compartment to divide it in the thenar and midpalmar spaces (Fig. 24.2).

The palmar spaces include midpalmar space, thenar space, web spaces, pulp spaces and forearm space of Parona.

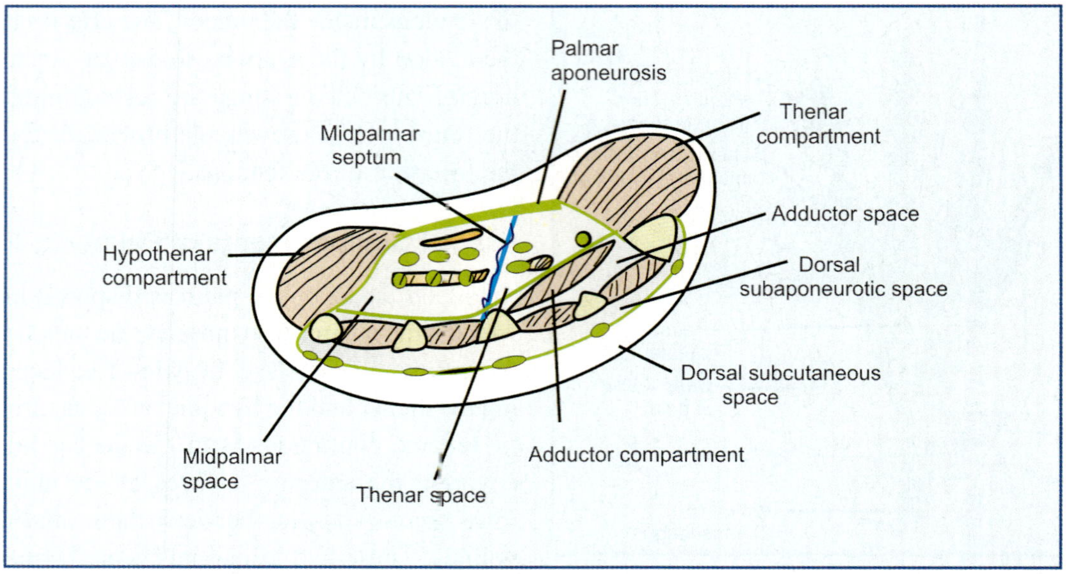

Fig. 24.2: Schematic transverse section of hand to show fascial compartments and fascial spaces

Boundaries of Midpalmar Space

a. Anteriorly (from superficial to deep), following structures are present, palmar aponeurosis, superficial palmar arch, flexor tendons of medial three digits covered in ulnar bursa and medial three lumbrical muscles.
b. Posteriorly, there is fascia covering the third and fourth interossei and the metacarpal bones.
c. The medial boundary is medial palmar septum.
d. The lateral boundary is midpalmar septum.
e. Proximally, the space extends upto the level of distal margin of flexor retinaculum, where normally it is closed, but sometimes may extend deep to the retinaculum.
f. Distally, the space extends upto the level of distal palmar crease beyond which it communicates with the medial two web spaces by corresponding lumbrical canals.

Boundaries of Thenar Space

a. Anteriorly, (from superficial to deep) following structures are present, palmar aponeurosis, superficial palmar arch and the flexor tendons of index finger covered with synovial sheath. The tendon of flexor pollicis longus may be present anteriorly or laterally.
b. Posteriorly, there is fascia covering the adductor pollicis muscle.
c. The lateral boundary is the lateral palmar septum.
d. The medial boundary is the midpalmar septum.
e. Proximally, the space extends to the level of distal margin of flexor retinaculum, where normally it is closed, but sometimes may extend deep to the retinaculum.
f. Distally, the space extends to the level of distal palmar crease beyond which it communicates with the first web space (and sometimes the second web space) by the corresponding lumbrical canal.

Palmar Spaces and Synovial Sheaths

a. The radial bursa is the synovial sheath surrounding the flexor pollicis longus tendon. It extends from the forearm (2 cm proximal to the proximal margin of flexor retinaculum) to the level of the base of terminal phalanx of thumb (Fig. 24.3). The radial bursa is in immediate anterior relation of thenar space.
b. The ulnar bursa is the common synovial sheath surrounding the tendons of flexor digitorum superficialis and profundus. It extends from the forearm (2 cm proximal to proximal margin of flexor retinaculum) to the midpalm level where the ulnar bursa

ends as a cul-de-sac but retains its continuity with the digital sheath around the flexor tendons of the little finger. The ulnar bursa and its distal extension in the little finger are in immediate anterior relation to midpalmar space. Beyond the common sheath the tendons of index, middle and ring fingers are devoid of synovial sheath until they enter the fibrous flexor sheath. The radial and ulnar bursae may communicate with each other.

Clinical Highlights

Tenosynovitis (inflammation of synovial sheath surrounding a tendon) of little finger can infect the ulnar bursa and that of thumb can infect the radial bursa. This in turn may infect the midpalmar and thenar spaces. With the current trend of liberal use of antibiotics in clinical practice to control infections, the occurrence of abscesses in palmar spaces is much reduced. However, if pus collects in these spaces it is drained through lumbrical canals. The midpalmar space communicates with third and fourth web spaces via corresponding lumbrical canals and the thenar space communicates with first web space by means of first lumbrical canal (Fig. 24.3). The web spaces are the ideal sites for opening the lumbrical canals to let out the pus in the palmar spaces (if midpalmar and thenar spaces are analogous to "pus tanks" then lumbrical canals are the "pus taps", which can be opened in web spaces to let out the pus).

Web Spaces

There are four subcutaneous spaces within the folds of skin connecting the bases of the proximal phalanges. From its free margin each web space extends up to the level of metacarpophalangeal joint. The contents of the web space are, the subcutaneous fat, superficial transverse metacarpal ligament (natatory ligament or a German name, Schwmmband ligament), interosseous and lumbrical tendons and digital nerves and vessels.

Pulp Spaces

The pulp space (Fig. 24.4) is a subcutaneous space between the distal phalanx and the skin of the terminal digit. It is closed proximally by the fusion of the fibrous flexor sheath (deep fascia) to the skin of the digit at the distal crease on the anterior aspect and by fusion of the deep fascia to the periosteum of terminal phalanx on the posterior aspect. The pulp space contains subcutaneous fatty tissue, which is loculated by tough fibrous septa extending from the skin to the phalanx, sensory nerves and the digital artery. Before entering the space the digital

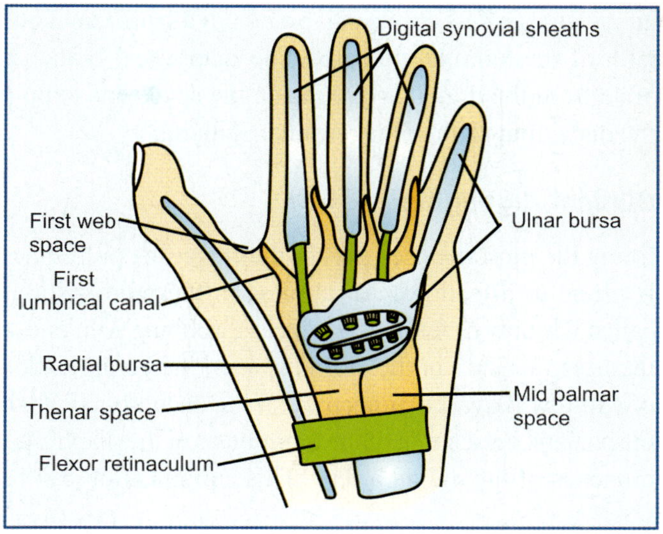

Fig. 24.3: Schematic depiction of synovial sheaths of flexor tendons (Note that common synovial sheath of FDS and FDP tendons has been removed partly to expose palmar spaces. Also note that lumbrical canals are the extensions of palmar spaces)

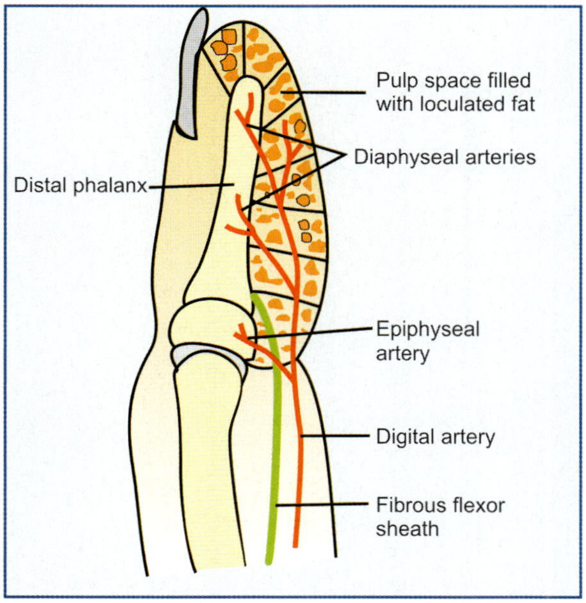

Fig. 24.4: Longitudinal section of digit to show pulp space and arterial supply of distal phalanx

artery gives off its epiphysial branch to the proximal one fifth of the terminal phalanx. The diaphyseal branches arise from the digital artery inside the space and supply the distal four-fifth of the terminal phalanx.

Clinical Highlights

Being the most exposed part of the finger the pulp space is prone to infections. An abscess in the pulp space is called whitlow or felon. It produces throbbing pain due to increased tension in the closed space. The complication of whitlow is avascular necrosis of the distal four-fifth of the phalanx on account of the thrombosis of the diaphyseal branches of the digital artery. This complication can be avoided if the abscess is drained at the right time by putting a small incision on the point of maximum tenderness.

Forearm Space or Space of Parona

Though it is located in the forearm, the space of Parona is included under palmar spaces because it is in continuity with the palmar spaces behind the flexor tendons through the carpal tunnel. The long flexor tendons wrapped in synovial sheaths form its anterior boundary. The pronator quadratus muscle is its posterior boundary. Very rarely this space gets filled with pus if the inflamed radial or ulnar bursa bursts here. For draining this space, incisions are placed on either side of the lower third of the forearm.

25 Arteries and Nerves of Palm

ARTERIAL ARCHES OF PALM

The hand is provided with abundant blood supply through branches of the radial and ulnar arteries, which form the superficial and deep arches.

SUPERFICIAL PALMAR ARCH (Fig. 25.1)

This arterial arch lies between the palmar aponeurosis and the long flexor tendons.

Modes of Completion of Arch

The superficial branch of the ulnar artery mainly contributes to the superficial palmar arch. The completion of the arch on the lateral side is variable. In the most usual mode, the superficial palmar branch of radial artery joins the superficial branch of the ulnar artery. Sometimes either the princeps pollicis or the radialis indicis (branches of radial artery) may complete the arch. Rarely it is the median artery, a branch of anterior interosseous artery, which completes the arch.

Branches

Three common palmar digital arteries and one proper digital artery arise from the convexity of the arch. These digital arteries receive more blood from the palmar metacarpal arteries (branches of deep palmar arch), which join them nearer the webs. The proper digital artery supplies the medial side of the little finger. Each common palmar digital artery divides into two proper digital arteries. The six proper digital arteries thus formed supply the adjacent sides of the medial four fingers.

Surface Marking

A distally convex line drawn from the distal border of fully extended thumb across the palm to meet the hook of the hamate represents the superficial arch.

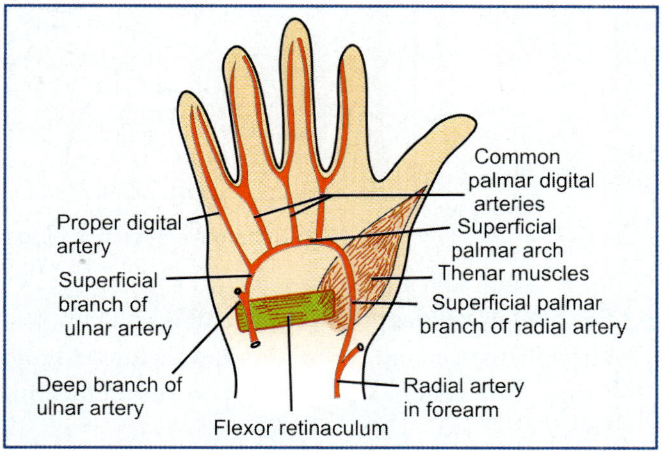

Fig. 25.1: Common mode of formation of superficial palmar arch

DEEP PALMAR ARCH (Fig. 25.2)

This arterial arch is located deep in the palm between the flexor tendons in front and the interossei muscles and the metacarpal bones behind.

Formation

The continuation of the radial artery in the palm mainly forms the deep palmar arch, which is completed on the medial side by the deep branch of ulnar artery. The radial artery at first passes behind the oblique head of adductor pollicis muscle and then between the two heads of the same muscle. It courses in the medial direction crossing the interossei muscles and the bases of the metacarpal bones. The deep branch of the ulnar nerve lies in the concavity of the arch.

Branches

a. Palmar metacarpal arteries are three in number and they join the common palmar digital arteries (the branches of superficial palmar arch).

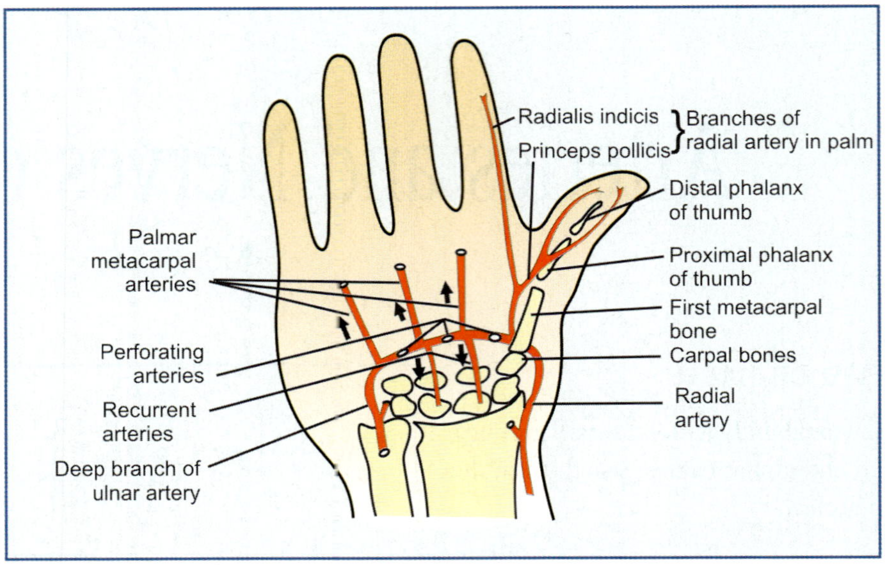

Fig. 25.2: Schematic depiction of formation and branches of deep palmar arch

b. Perforating arteries are three in number and they pass through the second, third and fourth interosseous spaces to anastomose with the dorsal metacarpal arteries.
c. Recurrent arteries turn proximally and pass in front of the carpus to take part in the formation of palmar carpal arch.

Surface Marking

A four cm long horizontal line drawn across the palm from a point just distal to the hook of the hamate represents the deep palmar arch. It is 1 to 1.5 cm proximal to the superficial palmar arch.

Bleeding Injury to Arterial Aches

Injury to arterial arches in the palm causes uncontrollable bleeding. The compression of the brachial artery against the humerus (Fig.14.5) is the most effective method to arrest bleeding in such cases. Tying or clamping the radial or ulnar or both radial and ulnar arteries proximal to the wrist fails to control the bleeding because of the connections between the palmar and dorsal carpal arches with the arterial arches.

MEDIAN NERVE IN PALM (Fig. 25.3)

The median nerve enters the palm under the distal margin of flexor retinaculum. It divides almost immediately into six branches (recurrent nerve, three proper palmar digital nerves and two common palmar digital nerves).

a. The short and thick recurrent branch is the lateral most. It turns proximally on the distal margin of the flexor retinaculum to enter the thenar muscles. This branch supplies abductor pollicis brevis, opponens pollicis and the superficial head of flexor pollicis brevis.
b. The lateral or first proper palmar digital nerve supplies the radial side of the thumb.
c. The second proper palmar digital nerve supplies the medial side of the thumb.
d. The third proper palmar digital nerve supplies the radial side of the index finger and also gives a motor branch to the first lumbrical muscle, which enters the muscle from its superficial aspect.
e. The lateral common palmar digital nerve gives a motor twig to the second lumbrical muscle, which enters the muscle from its superficial aspect. It then divides into two proper palmar digital nerves for the adjacent sides of index and middle fingers.
f. The medial common palmar digital nerve divides into two branches for the adjacent sides of middle and ring fingers.

All the proper palmar digital branches cross over the tips of the respective digits and supply the nailbed on the dorsum but the area may extend beyond the nail bed.

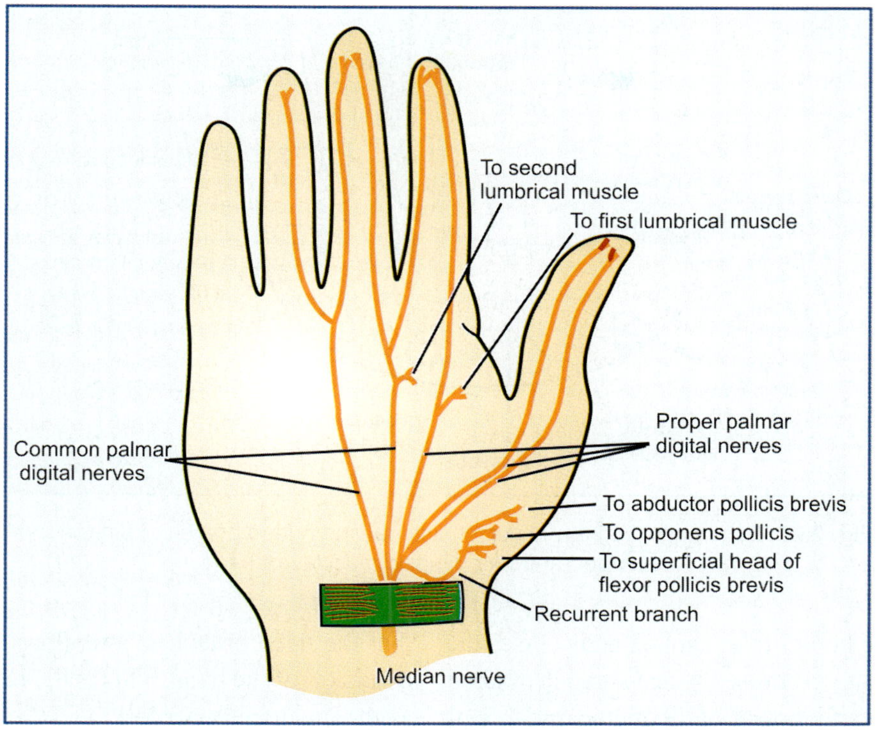

Fig. 25.3: Muscular and cutaneous branches of median nerve in hand

ULNAR NERVE IN PALM

The ulnar nerve terminates on the anterior surface of the flexor retinaculum in close relation to the pisiform bone into a smaller superficial and a larger deep branch.

Superficial Branch of Ulnar Nerve (Fig. 25.4)

The nerve enters the palm under cover of the palmaris brevis muscle, which it supplies and then divides, into one proper digital and one common digital branch. The proper digital branch supplies the skin on the palmar aspect of the ulnar side of the little finger. The common palmar digital runs toward the fourth interdigital cleft to divide into two proper digital nerves for the supply of adjacent sides of little and ring fingers. The digital nerves cross over the tips of the digits to supply the skin on the dorsal aspect of the digits. In some cases there may be a communication between the common palmar digital branches of ulnar and median nerves.

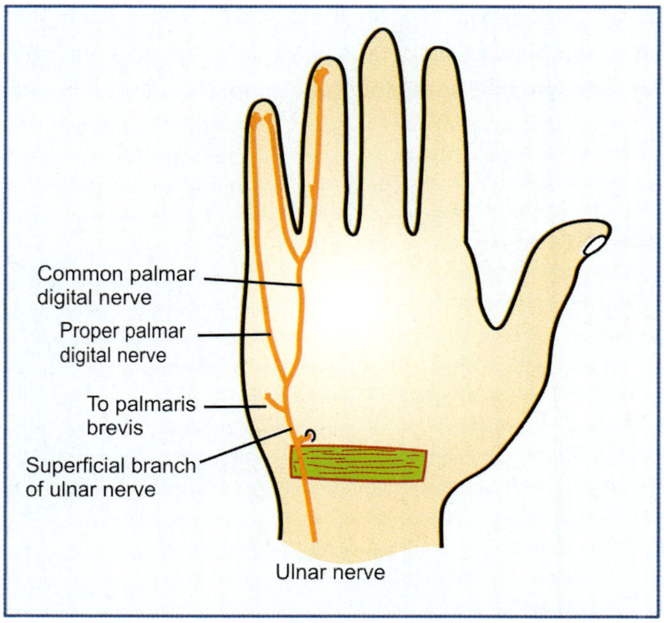

Fig. 25.4: Distribution of superficial branch of ulnar nerve in hand

Deep Branch of Ulnar Nerve in Palm (Fig. 25.5)

From its origin the deep branch of the ulnar nerve enters the hypothenar compartment of the palm, where it gives motor twigs to the abductor digiti minimi, flexor digiti minimi and opponens digiti minimi muscles. It turns deeply between the flexor and abductor digiti minimi muscles. Accompanied by the deep branch of ulnar artery the nerve

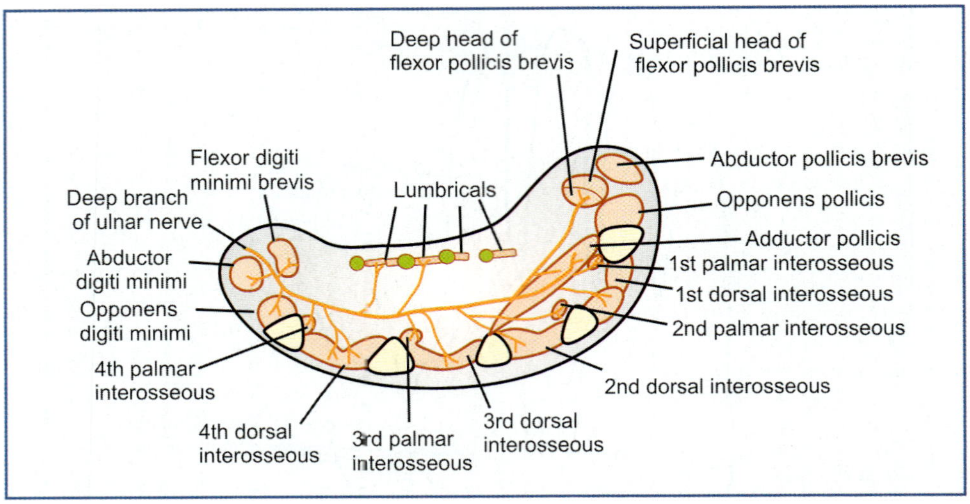

Fig. 25.5: Schematic diagram to depict distribution of deep branch of ulnar nerve to fourteen and half intrinsic muscles of hand

turns laterally on the hook of the hamate and crosses the palm. On its medio-lateral course the deep branch of ulnar nerve lies on the proximal parts of the metacarpal bones dorsal to the long flexor tendons. The deep branch supplies all the interossei and medial two lumbricals (the branches enter the deep aspect of the lumbrical muscles). It supplies the deep head of the flexor pollicis brevis also and ends by supplying the adductor pollicis muscle. Thus, it is clear that the deep branch of the ulnar nerve is essential for precision of the hand. This is the reason why it is known as the musician's nerve.

Clinical Highlights

The damage to this nerve causes ulnar claw hand, in which the medial two fingers show clawing (lateral two fingers do not show clawing due to functional lumbricals).

26 Intrinsic Muscles of Hand

There are twenty intrinsic muscles, which are located in the palm. They can be divided into four groups for descriptive purposes. The subcutaneous group contains palmaris brevis. The muscles acting on the little finger are called hypothenar muscles. The muscles acting on the thumb are thenar muscles and the adductor pollicis muscle. Those acting on the fingers are the interossei and lumbrical muscles.

HYPOTHENAR MUSCLES

The hypothenar muscles consist of three short muscles, the abductor digiti minimi medially and the flexor digiti minimi laterally, on a superficial plane. The opponens digiti minimi lies on a deeper plane. Their common action is deepening the cup of palm for proper grip.

a. Abductor Digiti Minimi

Abductor digiti minimi originates from the pisiform bone and piso-hamate ligament and the tendon of flexor carpi ulnaris. It is inserted in the ulnar side of the base of proximal phalanx of little finger. It abducts the little finger away from the fourth finger.

Abductor digiti minimi is the first muscle to show weakness in ulnar nerve lesion hence it is essential to know to test the function of the muscle.

Testing Function of Abductor Digiti Minimi

The subject is asked to place the back of the hand on the table and to abduct the little finger against resistance. It is interesting to note that for contraction of abductor digiti minimi it is necessary to fix its origin from flexor carpi ulnaris (FCU) tendon. This is achieved by active contraction of FCU muscle, which is indicated by a taut tendon of FCU at the wrist while testing the abductor digiti minimi.

b. Flexor Digiti Minimi

Flexor digiti minimi or flexor digiti minimi brevis takes origin from the hook of hamate and adjacent flexor retinaculum and is inserted along with abductor digiti minimi on the ulnar side of the base of proximal phalanx of little finger. It flexes the little finger at MCP joint.

This muscle is tested clinically in suspected cases of ulnar nerve lesion, since the loss of function of this muscle may be the only sign initially.

Testing Function of Flexor Digiti Minimi

The subject is asked to flex the MCP joint of little finger against resistance.

c. Opponens Digiti Minimi

Opponens digiti minimi muscle has a common origin with the flexor digiti minimi and is inserted in the ulnar side of the shaft of the fifth metacarpal bone.

It causes flexion of fifth metacarpal bone. It draws the bone anteriorly and laterally thus deepening the hollow of the palm.

Nerve Supply of Hypothenar Muscles

All the three muscles receive branches from the deep branch of the ulnar nerve.

THENAR MUSCLES

The thenar muscles consist of three short muscles, the abductor pollicis brevis laterally and flexor pollicis brevis medially, in the superficial plane and opponens pollicis on a deeper plane.

a. Abductor Pollicis Brevis

Abductor pollicis brevis takes origin from the tubercle of scaphoid, trapezium and the adjoining part of flexor retinaculum and is inserted in the lateral side of the base of proximal phalanx of thumb. The muscle abducts the thumb.

This muscle is tested clinically, in case of median nerve compression in the carpal tunnel. It is the first muscle to show weakness in carpal tunnel syndrome.

Testing Function of Abductor Pollicis Brevis

The subject is asked to abduct the thumb in a plane at right angles to the palmar aspect of index finger against the resistance of examiner's own thumb.

b. Flexor Pollicis Brevis

Flexor pollicis brevis has two heads. The superficial head takes origin from the tubercle of trapezium and the deep head takes origin from the capitate and trapezoid bones. The muscle is inserted in common with the abductor pollicis brevis on the lateral side of the base of the proximal phalanx of the thumb. There is usually a sesamoid bone at the site of insertion.

This muscle is a flexor of the thumb.

c. Opponens Pollicis

Opponens pollicis takes origin from the tubercle of the trapezium and the adjacent part of the flexor retinaculum. It is inserted in the lateral half of the palmar surface of first metacarpal bone.

It flexes and medially rotates the first metacarpal bone so as to help in opposition of the thumb.

Testing Function of Opponens Pollicis

This muscle is tested by asking the subject to touch the tip of little finger with the point of thumb or by asking the subject to make a circle with the thumb and index finger.

Nerve Supply of Thenar Muscles

The recurrent branch of median nerve supplies the abductor pollicis brevis, opponens pollicis and superficial head of flexor pollicis brevis. The deep branch of ulnar nerve supplies the deep head of flexor pollicis brevis.

ADDUCTOR POLLICIS (Fig. 26.1)

This muscle has two heads of origin. The oblique head arises form the capitate bone and bases of the second and third metacarpal bones. The transverse head takes origin from the palmar aspect of third metacarpal bone. The adductor pollicis is inserted in the medial side of the base of the proximal phalanx of thumb.

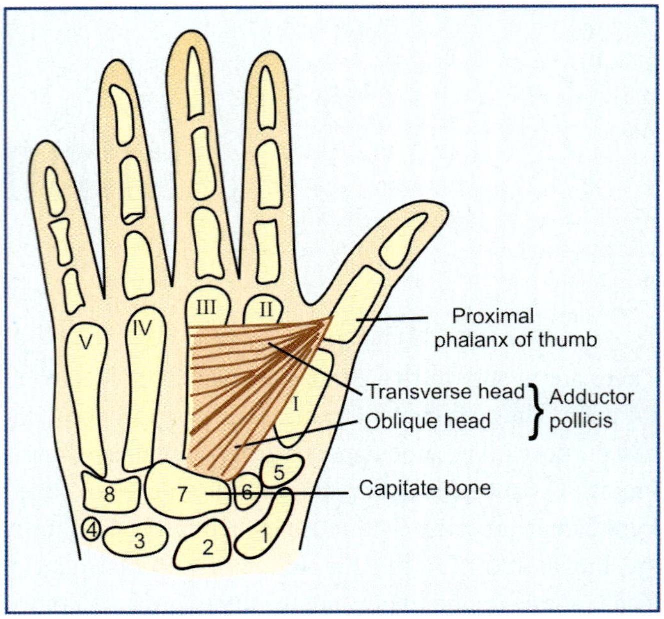

Fig. 26.1: Showing origin and insertion of adductor pollicis muscle

It adducts the thumb from the abducted position.

Nerve Supply

The deep branch of the ulnar nerve supplies it with its terminal branches.

Testing Function of Adductor Pollicis

Froment's test is performed to assess the strength of the adductor pollicis muscle. With both palms held together a card is kept between the thumbs and index fingers of the patient. Then the patient is asked to grip the card tightly. Thumb on the affected side flexes at the IP joint due to action of flexor pollicis longus, which compensates the action of adductor pollicis.

LUMBRICAL MUSCLES

Lumbrical is a Latin word, which means earthworm. The shape of the lumbrical muscle is like that of earthworm. The lumbricals are four tiny muscles, which take origin from flexor digitorum profundus tendons. Each lumbrical ends in a tendon, which enters the web space and turns dorsally along the lateral side of the metacarpophalangeal joint, to go for insertion into the corresponding extensor expansion. Therefore, lumbricals are the connecting link between the flexor and extensor tendons of the digits (Fig. 26.2). A connective tissue sheath called lumbrical canal surrounds each lumbrical tendon (for clinical importance of these canals read palmar spaces).

Comparison of Lateral and Medial Lumbricals

Feature	*Lateral*	*Medial*
Number	First and second	Third and fourth
Type	Unipennate	Bipennate
Nerve supply	Digital branches of median nerve	Deep branch of ulnar nerve
Point of nerve entry	From superficial surface	From deep surface

Actions of Lumbricals

The lumbricals flex the metacarpophalangeal joints and extend the interphalangeal joints.

Testing Function of Lumbricals

The subject is asked to flex the metacarpophalangeal joint of the extended finger to be tested against resistance.

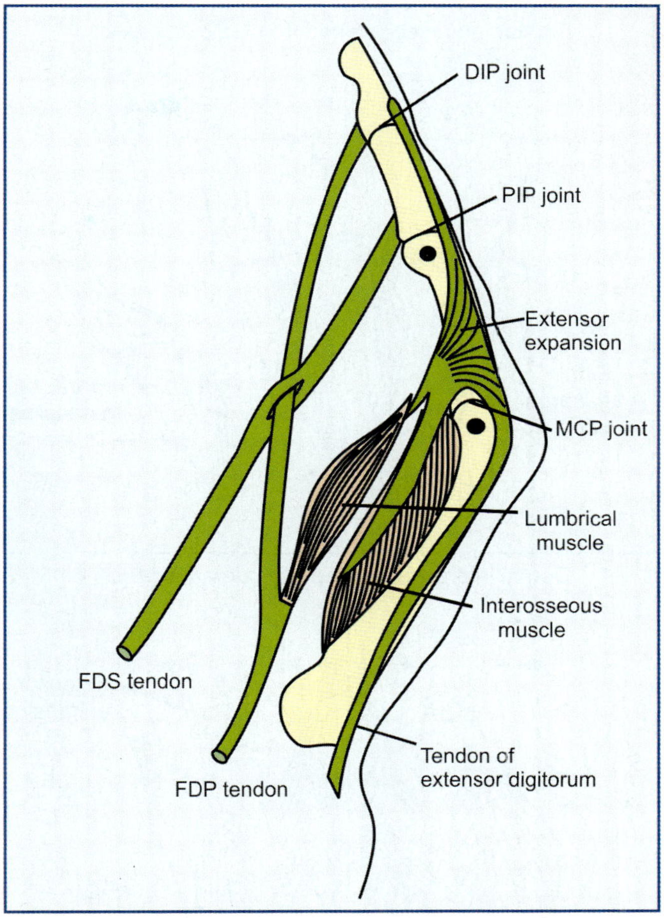

Fig. 26.2: Schematic diagram showing insertion of flexor and extensor tendons in the digit. (Note that interossei and lumbrical muscles pass anterior to MCP joint and posterior to PIP and DIP joints)

INTEROSSEI MUSCLES (Fig. 26.3)

There are two sets of interossei, palmar and dorsal. Each set consists of four muscles. The interossei are numbered one to four from lateral to medial side. Of the four palmar interossei the first one is not well developed and it works in unison with adductor pollicis. The palmar interossei are unipennate while the dorsal ones are bipennate muscles.

Nerve Supply

The deep branch of the ulnar nerve supplies all the interossei muscles.

Adduction of Fingers

The palmar interossei are adductors of the fingers from the central axis passing through the middle finger. The second palmar interosseous adducts the index finger, the third adducts the ring finger, and the fourth adducts the little finger. There is no adduction movement of the middle finger since no palmar interosseous is attached to it.

Abduction of Fingers

The dorsal interossei are abductors of the middle three fingers. The first dorsal interosseous abducts the index finger away from the middle finger, the second abducts the middle finger on the radial side, the third abducts the middle finger on the ulnar side and the ring finger is abducted away from the middle finger by the fourth muscle. This explains why there are two dorsal interossei for the middle finger. Since the little finger has its own abductor no dorsal interosseous muscle is attached to it.

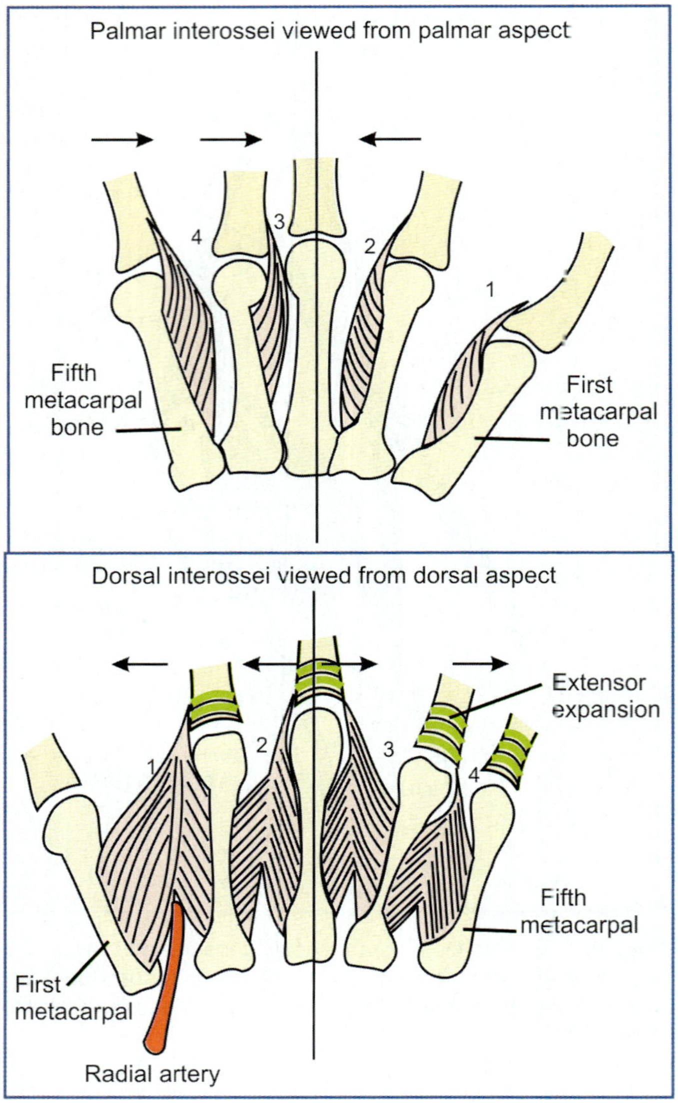

Fig. 26.3: Interossei muscles of right hand (Note that interossei adduct or abduct digits in relation to axis passing through third digit)

EXTENSOR EXPANSION (Fig. 26.4)

To understand the mode of insertion of the lumbricals and the interossei it is necessary to know the parts of the extensor expansion. Each extensor tendon flattens into the extensor expansion over the dorsal aspect of the MCP joint.

Parts of Extensor Expansion

The extensor expansion is triangular in shape. Its base encircles the MCP joint on all sides except the palmar aspect. Each basal angle is fixed to the deep palmar metacarpal ligament. Its thickened lateral margin receives the insertion of lumbricals and interossei. Its thick axial part carries the insertion of the extensor tendon or tendons. The axial part and the margins are interconnected by fibrous tissue nearer the base so as to ensure the firm anchorage of the expansion to the back of MCP joint. Closer to the PIP joint the axial slip splits in to three slips of which the central one is attached to the base of the middle phalanx. Each collateral slip joins the lateral margin of its side and then unites with the fellow of the other side on the dorsal aspect of the middle phalanx. The united collateral slips cross the DIP joint and gain attachment to the base of the terminal phalanx. The central and collateral slips function independently. The central slip carrying the insertion of the extensor tendon acts on the MCP joint while the collateral slips carrying the insertion of lumbricals and interossei act on MCP, PIP and DIP joints.

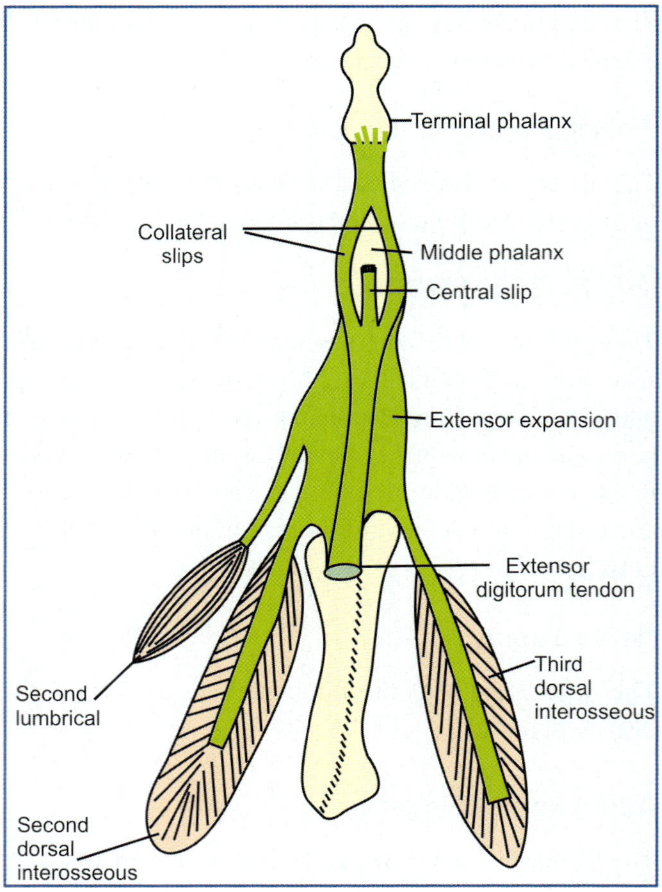

Fig. 26.4: Showing insertion of interossei and lumbrical muscles into extensor expansion of right middle digit

The slips of extensor expansion are closely applied to the dorsal aspects of the interphalangeal joints. In fact they replace the fibrous capsule of IP and MCP joints on the dorsal aspect.

Clinical Highlights

a. Mallet finger or baseball finger deformity (flexed terminal phalanx) results, when the extensor expansion is torn at its insertion in the base of terminal phalanx.
b. Boutonniere deformity results, when the insertion of extensor expansion in the middle digit is torn giving rise to flexed middle phalanx and extended terminal phalanx.

Muscles Attached to Extensor Expansion of Each Digit

Though it is not important clinically to know the attachments of the individual muscles to the extensor expansion of each finger, it is a good academic exercise (as it helps in understanding the actions of the muscles). Note that the lumbricals reach the lateral basal angle of the extensor expansion. One should practice to learn the specific attachments of the interossei muscles through the adduction and abduction actions of the fingers on one's own hand.

Combined Actions of Interossei and Lumbricals

The interossei and lumbricals together flex the metacarpophalangeal joints and simultaneously extend the interphalangeal joints. They can perform this unusual combination of actions due to their relations to the axes of movements of these joints (Fig. 26.2). These muscles cross the metacarpophalangeal joints on palmar aspect therefore they are able to flex the joints. Through the extensor expansion the muscles cross the interphalangeal joints on dorsal aspect. Accordingly the pull of the muscles is transferred to the dorsal side of the axes of the interphalangeal joints, which they extend.

Testing Function of Dorsal Interossei

The principle of testing the dorsal interossei is to assess the capacity of middle three fingers to abduct against resistance. To test the first muscle the index finger is abducted. To test the second muscle the extended middle finger is crossed dorsally over the extended index finger (good luck sign). To test the third muscle the middle finger is abducted towards the ring finger and for the fourth muscle ring finger is abducted.

Testing Function of Palmar Interossei

The principle of testing the palmar interossei is to assess the capacity of index, ring and little fingers to adduct against resistance. To test the second muscle the index finger is adducted towards the middle finger. To test the third muscle ring finger is adducted and for the fourth muscle little finger is adducted.

Clinical Highlights

Paralysis of all the interossei and lumbricals produces complete or true claw hand deformity (Fig 4.4) in which there is hyperextension of MCP and hyperflexion of PIP and DIP joints of all fingers.

27 Movements of Thumb and Fingers

The **thumb** enjoys free mobility compared to the other fingers hence functionally it is regarded as one half of the hand. An opposable thumb is a human character. It is designed for grasping objects. The anatomical peculiarity of the thumb is that it has two phalanges and one metacarpal bone. Moreover its metacarpal is at right angles to the plane of other metacarpals. The base of the first metacarpal articulates with the trapezium to form the first carpometacarpal joint. It is a saddle variety of synovial joint, which confers great mobility to the thumb (Fig. 27.1). Following movements take place in this joint:

a. The flexion-extension movements take place in the plane of the palm around an antero-posterior axis. In flexion the palmar surface of the thumb moves across the palm towards the ulnar border till the thumb comes in contact with the palm. Flexion is always accompanied by conjunct (automatic) medial rotation. In extension the thumb moves away from the palm so that its dorsal surface comes to face the dorsum of hand. Extension is necessarily accompanied by lateral rotation of thumb.
b. In abduction the thumb moves away from the index finger at right angles to the plane of the palm. In adduction the thumb is brought back to the resting position (in front of and in contact with the palmar surface of the index finger).
c. In opposition the tip of the thumb is brought in contact with the base or tip of any other finger. It is a composite movement consisting of abduction, flexion and medial rotation. It can be defined as the movement of flexion with medial rotation of abducted thumb. In reposition the opposed thumb is brought back to the resting position. In this movement there is extension, lateral rotation and adduction of abducted thumb.
d. Circumduction is an angular motion of the thumb consisting of flexion, abduction, extension and adduction.

First Carpometacarpal Joint (Fig. 22.1)

It is also called the trapezio-metacarpal joint. It is a saddle type of synovial joint. The articulating ends consist of, the distal articular surface of trapezium and the proximal articular surface of the base of first metacarpal bone. Both the articulating surfaces are reciprocally concavo-convex. The fibrous capsule lined with synovial membrane covers the joint. The carpometacarpal ligaments reinforce the joint.

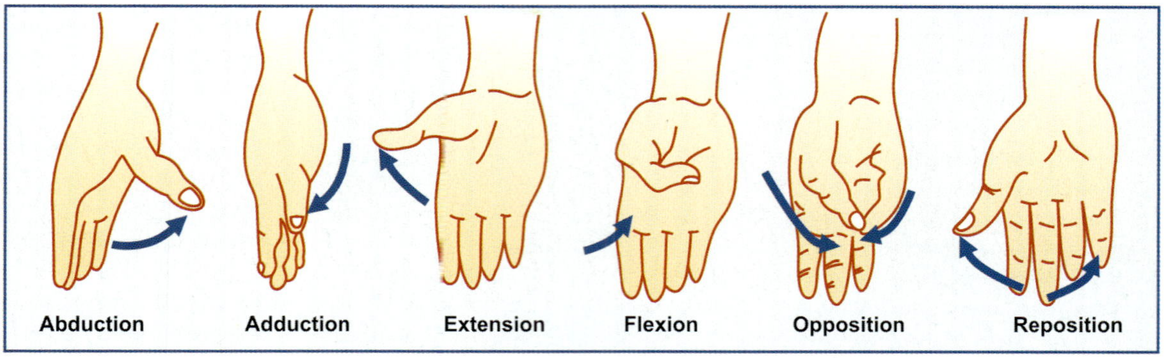

Fig. 27.1: Movements of the thumb

Muscles Acting on Thumb

A total of nine muscles act on the thumb. The long muscles are extensor pollicis longus and brevis, abductor pollicis longus and flexor pollicis longus. The short muscles are the three thenar muscles, adductor pollicis and the first palmar interosseous.

a. The flexion is produced by flexor pollicis longus and flexor pollicis brevis.
b. The extension is produced by extensor pollicis brevis, extensor pollicis longus and abductor pollicis longus.
c. The adduction is produced mainly by adductor pollicis assisted by first palmar interosseous muscle.
d. The abduction is produced mainly by abductor pollicis brevis, which is assisted by abductor pollicis longus.
e. The opposition movement is the synergistic actions of abductor pollicis longus and brevis, opponens pollicis and flexor pollicis brevis.
f. The reposition (reverse of opposition) is by synergistic actions of extensor pollicis brevis and longus, abductor pollicis longus and brevis (for extension and lateral rotation) and adductor pollicis muscles.

Metacarpophalangeal (MCP) Joints

The knuckles indicate the positions of the MCP joints. These joints are condyloid types of synovial joints. The articulating ends are the convex metacarpal head and the spherical fossa on the base of the proximal phalanx. The fibrous capsule covers the joint except dorsally where it is replaced by extensor expansion. The collateral ligaments support the joints on either side. The palmar ligament is very strong. It is in the form of a fibrous plate attached firmly to the base of proximal phalanx, but loosely to the neck of the metacarpal. This plate undergoes excursions relative to the movements of the joint. The margins of the palmar ligament give attachment to deep transverse ligament, fibrous flexor sheath, and slips of palmar aponeurosis, collateral ligaments and transverse fibers of extensor expansion.

Movements

The movements of flexion-extension and adduction-abduction take place at these joints. The flexor digitorum superficialis assisted by flexor digitorum profundus flex the joints in power grip. The interossei and lumbricals flex these joints in precision grip. Extension is produced by extensor digitorum. In the case of little finger extensor digiti minimi assists likewise, extensor indicis assists the extension of index finger. In the thumb, the range of movements is much less at the MCP joint.

Interphalangeal (IP) Joints

These joints consist of two rows, the proximal interphalangeal (PIP) joints and the distal interphalangeal (DIP) joints. The PIP and DIP joints are simple hinge types of synovial joints. The thumb has only one interphalangeal joint. On the dorsal aspect the capsule of these joints is replaced by the extensor expansion. Collateral ligaments, which are slack, support the joints, when the fingers are extended.

Movements

IP joints permit movements of flexion-extension. The flexor digitorum superficialis is the main flexor at the PIP joint. The flexor digitorum profundus alone causes flexion of DIP joint. The interossei and lumbricals produce the extension. In fully extended position of MCP joint the distal part of extensor digitorum is slackened, so that it becomes ineffective at IP joints. This can be understood from the claw hand deformity, in which MCP joints are hyperextended and IP joints are flexed in-spite of normal extensor digitorum. In other words the extensor digitorum can extend the MCP joints only.

Clinical Highlights

a. In swan neck finger there is hyperextension of PIP and flexion at DIP joints due to degeneration of the flexor digitorum superficialis tendon and of the insertion of extensor expansion in the terminal digit.
b. In buttonhole finger there is flexion at PIP and hyperextension at DIP joint due to rupture of the central slip of extensor expansion.
c. The mallet finger (baseball finger) is due to injury to the attachment of extensor expansion in distal phalanx so the terminal phalanx is flexed.

Grip Positions of Hand

a. In the precision grip (picking up a needle between tips of thumb and index finger) there is pad-to-pad opposition of index pulp and thumb pulp. The first metacarpal is flexed, abducted and opposed at trapezio-metacarpal or first carpometacarpal joint. The proximal phalanx of thumb is abducted and flexed at MCP joint. The index finger is flexed at MCP joint. The thenar muscles, interossei and lumbrical muscles of the first space are active during precision grip. Both median and ulnar nerve are necessary for this. The precision activities of the digits in a person using keyboards of a piano are dependent on the interossei muscles.

b. In the power grip the four fingers pulps are opposed to thenar eminence. The thumb base and the thenar pad provide fixed buttress. The MCP joints of other fingers are flexed by interossei and lumbricals. Both long flexor muscles flex the PIP joints but the DIP is flexed by flexor digitorum profundus alone. So the profundus is more powerful in power grip. In power grip ulnar nerve is more important.

c. In the key grip the thumb pulp is pressed against the side of the curled index finger. In this position the thumb is partially opposed and index finger is flexed. So for thumb opposition median nerve is responsible and for flexion of metacarpophalangeal joint of index finger first dorsal interosseous (ulnar nerve) is necessary.

d. In the hook grip (baggage grip) the middle phalanges are flexed at the PIP joints. In this grip the heavy objects like a bucket or suitcase are supported by the middle phalanges. The flexor digitorum superficialis is the main active muscle in this grip. Hence, median nerve is responsible for the hook grip.

28 Long Nerves of Upper Limb

MEDIAN NERVE

The median nerve originates from the brachial plexus by two roots. The lateral root arises from the lateral cord and carries (C5), C6, and C7 fibers in it. The medial root arises from the medial cord and carries C8 and T1 fibers in it. The medial root crosses the third part of the axillary artery and unites with the lateral root either in front of or on the lateral side of the artery in the axilla to form the median nerve. So, the root value of the median nerve is (C5), C6, C7, C8 and T1.

Course and Relations

a. In the axilla, the median nerve lies on the lateral side of the third part of the axillary artery. It enters the arm at the lower border of teres major muscle along with other nerves and the vessels in the axilla.
b. In the arm, initially, the median nerve lies in lateral relation to the brachial artery. It crosses in front of the brachial artery at the level of insertion of the coracobrachialis and travels downwards to the cubical fossa in medial relation to the artery. It gives sympathetic fibers to the brachial artery in the arm and a branch to the pronator teres just above the elbow.
c. In the cubital fossa, the median nerve is located medial to the brachial artery. The nerve and the artery are protected by the bicipital aponeurosis. Here it gives muscular branches from its medial side to pronator teres, flexor carpi radialis, palmaris longus and flexor digitorum superficialis. It also gives articular branches to elbow and superior radioulnar joints. The median nerve leaves the cubital fossa between the humeral (superficial) and ulnar (deep) heads of pronator teres. At this point the anterior interosseous branch arises from the median nerve.
d. In the forearm, the median nerve passes downwards behind the tendinous bridge between the humeroulnar and radial heads of flexor digitorum superficialis. During its descent in the forearm it remains adherent to the deep surface of flexor digitorum superficialis. About 5 cm proximal to the flexor retinaculum the median nerve becomes superficial (hence vulnerable to laceration injuries) lying along the lateral edge of FDS tendons and immediately posterior to the palmaris longus tendon as it approaches the flexor retinaculum. In the mid-forearm it gives muscular branch to part of FDS, which continues as the tendon for index finger. Before entering the carpal tunnel it gives off the palmar cutaneous branch, which supplies the skin overlying the thenar eminence and the lateral part of the palm.
e. In the carpal tunnel, the median nerve lies deep to flexor retinaculum. It is anterior to the tendons of FDS, FDP and of flexor pollicis longus. There is tight packing of nine tendons, their synovial sheaths and the median nerve in the carpal tunnel. Therefore, in case of narrowing of the carpal tunnel due to any cause median nerve is liable to compression.
f. In the palm, the median nerve flattens at the distal border of the flexor retinaculum and divides into six branches (Fig. 25.3). The most lateral branch, which is thick and short, is called the recurrent branch because it doubles back on the flexor retinaculum to gain entry into the thenar compartment. This branch supplies flexor pollicis brevis (superficial head), abductor pollicis brevis and opponens pollicis. The remaining five branches consist of lateral three proper digital branches and two common digital branches. The proper digital branches supply the sides of the thumb and radial side of index finger. The digital branch for the radial side of index finger also supplies the first lumbrical. The

lateral common digital branch after supplying second lumbrical divides into two proper digital branches for the adjacent sides of index and middle fingers. The medial common digital branch divides into two proper digital branches, which go to the adjacent sides of middle and ring fingers. The palmar digital branches supply the dorsal aspect of the distal 1½ to 2 digit of the same fingers via their dorsal branches. They give articular branches to the metacarpophalangeal and interphalangeal joints and are sensory to the fibrous flexor sheaths.

Special Note

Median nerve is called laborer's nerve because it supplies flexor muscles that are responsible for baggage or hook grip.

Clinical Highlights (Figs 28.1 and 28.2)

The effects of the lesion or injury of the median nerve depend on the level of lesion.

a. At the elbow the causes of nerve injury are, supracondylar fracture of humerus, application of tight tourniquet, during venipuncture in the cubital fossa and pronator syndrome (entrapment of nerve between two heads of pronator teres or under the fibrous arch connecting the two heads of flexor digitorum superficialis). This results in paralysis of pronator teres, flexor digitorum superficialis, flexor carpi radialis, palmaris longus, flexor pollicis longus, pronator quadratus and lateral half of flexor digitorum profundus. The motor effects are loss of pronation and hand of Benediction deformity, which is due to paralysis of both superficial and deep flexors of the middle and index fingers. The ring and little fingers can be kept in flexed position due to retention of the nerve supply of their FDP. Ape thumb or simian hand deformity is due to paralysis of thenar muscles. In this deformity, the thumb comes to lie in line with other fingers and there is thenar atrophy. There is loss of sensation over the central part and lateral half of the palm and lateral three and half digits (Fig. 28.2A).
b. Injury at mid-forearm results in pointing index deformity due to paralysis of part of FDS muscle that continues as the tendon of index finger. The other defects like ape thumb and sensory loss are similar to those seen at previous level of lesion.
c. Injury at carpal tunnel results in carpal tunnel syndrome. The causes are, myxoedema (deficiency of thyroxine), tenosynovitis of flexor tendons, pregnancy and rheumatoid arthritis of wrist. Initially the patient experiences symptoms like, numbness, tingling and pins and needles sensations in the lateral three and half digits. In due course, there may be total sensory loss in these digits. There is no sensory loss on the lateral part of palmar skin because of the sparing of palmar cutaneous branch in lesion at this level (Fig. 28.2B). If untreated 'ape thumb' deformity may set in due to paralysis of thenar muscles.
d. The superficial laceration at wrist, usually, due to cut injury and accidents may damage the palmar cutaneous branch only so that there is loss of sensation over the skin overlying the thenar eminence but no motor deficit. The deep laceration at the wrist due to knife cut or glass cut injures the median nerve and its palmar cutaneous branch. This produces ape thumb deformity, sensory loss on the lateral part of palm and in the lateral three and half digits.
e. Injury to recurrent branch of the median nerve produces paralysis of thenar muscles, causing ape thumb but no sensory loss.

ULNAR NERVE

The ulnar nerve arises in the axilla from the medial cord of brachial plexus. Its root value is C8 and T1. It may receive fibers from the C7 ventral ramus via the lateral cord or through a direct connection.

Course and Relations

a. In the axilla, the ulnar nerve lies medial to the third part of axillary artery between it and the axillary vein. It enters the arm as part of the main neurovascular bundle.
b. In the arm, the ulnar nerve is in the medial relation to the brachial artery upto the level of insertion of coracobrachialis, where it pierces the medial intermuscular septum to enter the posterior compartment of the arm. Here, it courses downward on the medial head of the triceps along with the superior ulnar

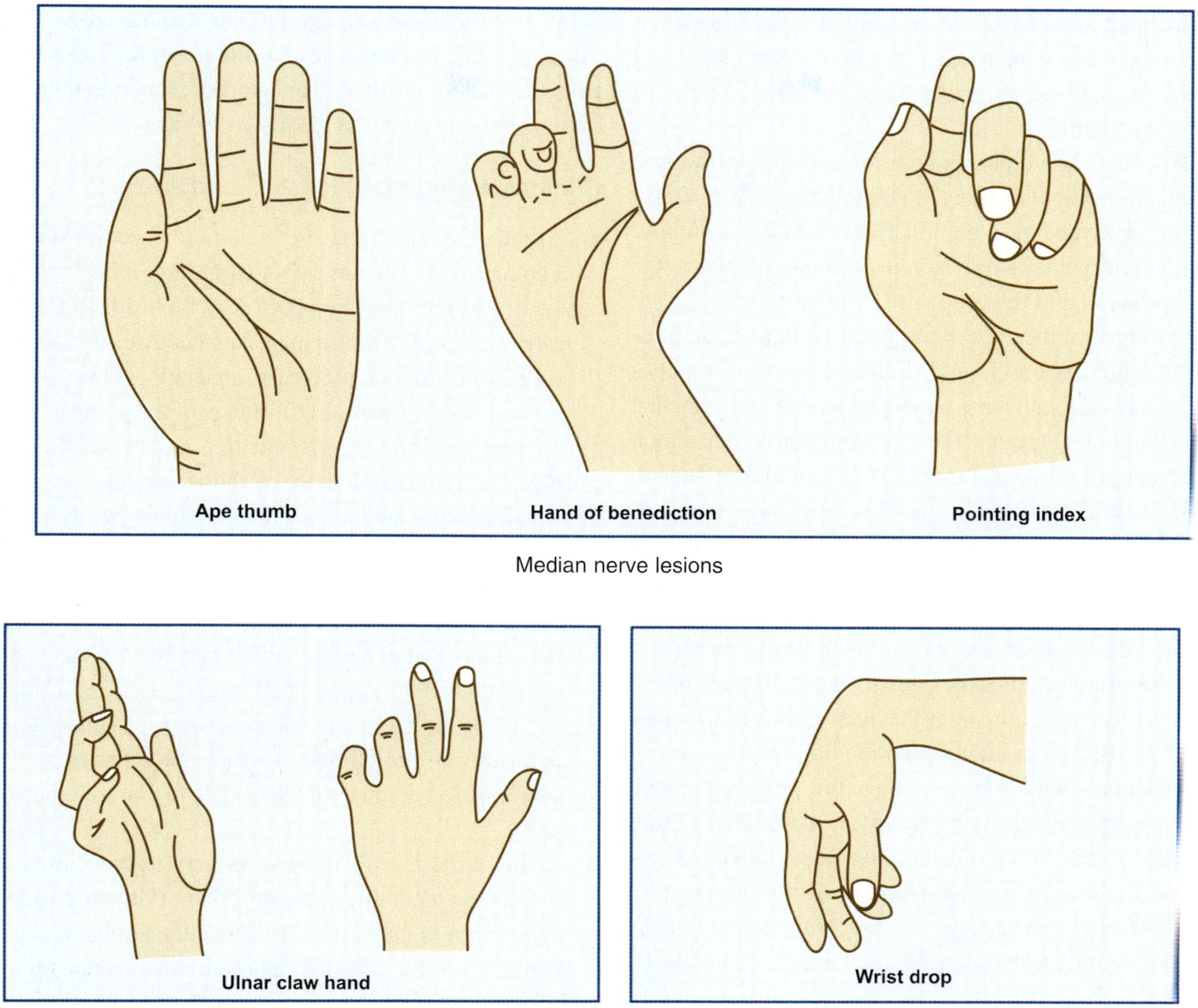

Fig. 28.1: Motor effects of lesions of long nerves of upper limb

collateral artery. At the back of the medial epicondyle the ulnar nerve is lodged in a groove. Pressure on the ulnar nerve at this site produces "funny bone" symptoms, with tingling along the hypothenar eminence and little finger. In leprosy the ulnar nerve is one of the peripheral nerves, which is thickened and hence is palpable at this site in the early stages of the disease.

c. The ulnar nerve enters the forearm between the humeral and ulnar heads of flexor carpi ulnaris, superficial to and in intimate contact with ulnar collateral ligament of the elbow joint. In its further course the ulnar nerve lies on the flexor digitorum profundus and is covered with flexor carpi ulnaris in the upper third of forearm. In this part of its course the ulnar nerve and artery are widely separated from each other. In the lower two thirds of the forearm the nerve becomes superficial and lies lateral to the flexor carpi ulnaris tendon. In this part of its course the ulnar nerve and the ulnar artery descend together (the artery being on the lateral side of the nerve). The ulnar nerve gives articular branch to the elbow joint and the muscular branches to the medial half of flexor digitorum profundus and to the flexor carpi ulnaris. The palmar cutaneous branch arises at the midforearm level and the dorsal branch arises 5 cm proximal to flexor retinaculum.

d. The ulnar nerve passes anterior to the flexor retinaculum (in Guyon's canal) on the lateral side of pisiform bone and medial to the ulnar artery. It divides under cover of palmaris brevis in its terminal branches, the superficial and the deep.

e. In the palm, the superficial terminal branch supplies the palmaris brevis and divides into two branches namely, one proper palmar digital branch for the medial side of little finger and the other common palmar digital branch for the adjacent sides of little and ring fingers. The dorsal branches cross over to the dorsal side to supply the nail bed of the medial one and half digits as well as variable area of skin of the digits. The deep terminal branch supplies the hypothenar muscles and turns deeply between the abductor digiti minimi and flexor digiti minimi muscles. The deep branch of the ulnar artery accompanies the deep branch of the ulnar nerve. Both turn laterally on the base of the hook of the hamate bone and cross the palm. The deep branch of ulnar nerve lies in the concavity of the deep palmar arch. It ends in the substance of the adductor pollicis muscle. It supplies the hypothenar muscles, palmar and dorsal interossei, medial two lumbricals, adductor pollicis and the deep head of the flexor pollicis brevis.

Special Note

The deep branch of the ulnar nerve is called 'musician's nerve' because it innervates all the small muscles of hand involved in fine movements of hand.

Surface Marking

To show the course of ulnar nerve in the arm one should join the following three points. The first point corresponds to the junction of the anterior two-thirds and posterior one-third of a line joining the lower ends of the anterior and posterior axillary folds in the abducted and laterally rotated position of the arm. The second point is marked at the middle of the medial margin of the arm. The third point is on the posterior aspect of the medial epicondyle. To mark the ulnar nerve in the forearm a line is drawn from the back of the medial epicondyle to a point in front of the wrist just lateral to the pisiform bone.

Clinical Highlights (Figs 28.1 and 28.2)

a. At the elbow the ulnar nerve is in exposed position. The causes of nerve injury at this site are, cubital tunnel syndrome (compression between two heads of flexor carpi ulnaris), fracture of medial epicondyle and cubitus valgus (due to increased carrying angle). This results in weakness of flexor digitorum profundus muscle to the ring and little fingers and consequent inability to flex the terminal phalanx of these fingers. There is clawing at the medial two fingers due to paralysis of interossei and medial two lumbricals. The atrophy of interossei results in guttering on the dorsum of hand. There is loss of adduction of thumb. There is sensory loss in the medial half of palmar and dorsal aspects of hand and medial one and half fingers (Fig. 28.2D and E). Tardy or late ulnar nerve palsy occurs in valgus deformity of the elbow, in which the ulnar nerve is subjected to a gradual stretch leading to a late or gradual palsy.

b. At the wrist the ulnar nerve is very superficial and therefore vulnerable to compression (Guyon's canal syndrome) or laceration. This usually results in claw hand deformity, which is more obvious compared to the lesion at elbow (ulnar nerve paradox). The reason for this is as follows. The lesion at the wrist spares the flexor digitorum profundus, which brings about powerful flexion at the interphalangeal joints causing marked clawing. Sensory loss is limited to medial one and half digits only because the palmar and dorsal cutaneous branches are spared.

c. In the palm the deep branch of ulnar nerve may be compressed against the hamate bone, when the hand is used as a mallet or if a vibrating tool rubs against it. This gives rise to ulnar clawing of the hand but no sensory loss.

d. Froment's sign is positive in ulnar nerve paralysis. When the patient pinches a piece of paper between thumb and index finger, the thumb on the affected

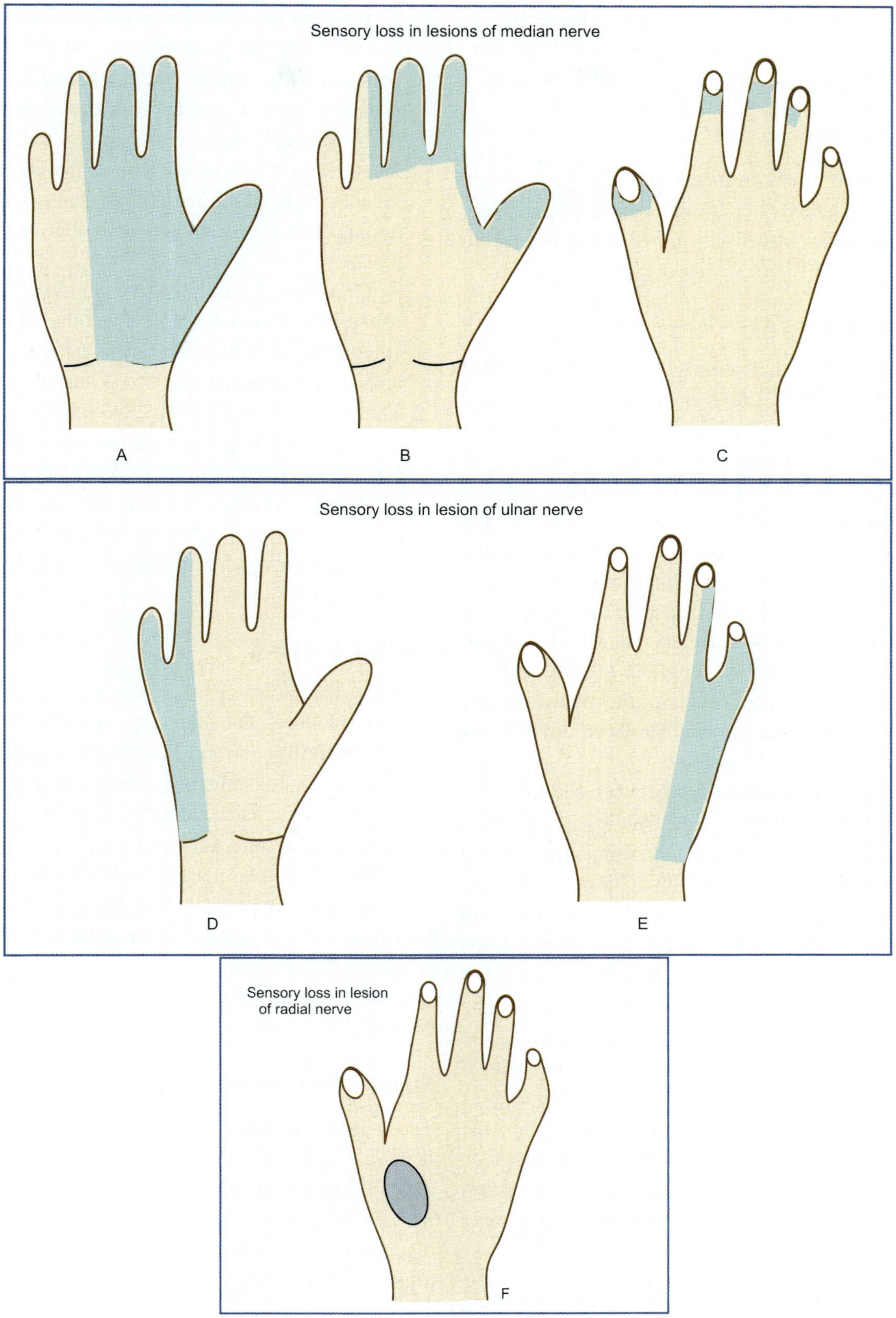

Fig. 28.2: Sensory effects due to lesions of long nerves of upper limb

side flexes. This is due to weakness of adductor pollicis muscle (supplied by ulnar nerve), which permits uncontrolled contraction of flexor pollicis longus.

RADIAL NERVE

The radial nerve arises from the posterior cord of the brachial plexus in the axilla. It is the largest branch of the brachial plexus. Theoretically, the nerve carries fibers from all the roots but T1 fibers are not constant.

Course and Relations

a. In the axilla, the radial nerve lies posterior to the third part of the axillary artery and anterior to the three muscles forming the posterior wall of the axilla (subscapularis, teres major and latissimus dorsi). The radial nerve gives off its posterior cutaneous nerve of arm in the axilla. It leaves the axilla as a part of the principal neurovascular bundle to enter the arm at the level of lower border of teres major muscle.
b. In the upper medial part of the arm, the radial nerve lies posterior to the brachial artery. Here it gives medial muscular branches to the long and medial heads of the triceps brachii. The branch for the medial head of triceps lies very close to the ulnar nerve and hence is called the ulnar collateral nerve.
c. The radial nerve soon passes between the long and medial heads of triceps to enter the lower triangular space, through which it reaches the spiral groove along with the profunda brachii vessels. This neurovascular bundle in the spiral groove lies in direct contact with the humerus, between the lateral and the medial heads of triceps. In the spiral grove the branches of the radial nerve are, posterior muscular and cutaneous. The posterior muscular branches supply the medial and lateral heads of triceps and the anconeus. The branch to anconeus lies in direct contact with the humerus as it passes downwards through the substance of the medial head (along with the middle collateral branch of profunda brachii artery). The cutaneous branches are, posterior cutaneous nerve of forearm and lower lateral cutaneous nerve of arm.
d. At the lower end of the spiral groove, the radial nerve is accompanied by radial collateral branch of the profunda artery. The two together pierce the lateral intermuscular septum of the arm and enter the anterior compartment, where they descend between the brachialis and brachioradialis and more distally between the brachialis and extensor carpi radialis longus muscles. In this location, the radial nerve supplies branches to brachioradialis and extensor carpi radialis longus. It also gives a few proprioceptive fibers to the brachialis.
e. At the elbow, the radial nerve is hidden under cover of the brachioradialis muscle. At the level of lateral epicondyle of humerus it terminates into superficial and deep branches in the lateral part of cubital fossa. The deep terminal branch (also otherwise described by authorities as posterior interosseous nerve) gives branches to supinator and ECRB before entering the substance of supinator to enter the posterior compartment. Further course of the posterior interosseous nerve is described in posterior compartment of the forearm.

Surface Marking

To draw the radial nerve in the arm three points are marked as follows. The first point coincides with the lower end of the axillary artery. For the second point, draw a line from the deltoid tuberosity (insertion of deltoid) to the lateral epicondyle. Then mark the second point at the junction of the upper one-third and lower two-thirds of this line. The third point is marked in front of the elbow about 1 cm lateral to the tendon of biceps brachii. A line joining the first two points represents the radial nerve in the spiral groove while the line joining the lower two points represents the radial nerve in the lateral side of the anterior compartment of arm.

Superficial Terminal Branch of Radial Nerve

The superficial branch of radial nerve is entirely sensory. It travels in the anterolateral part of the forearm under cover of brachioradialis. During its downward course the nerve lies successively on the pronator teres, flexor digitorum superficialis and flexor pollicis longus. The radial artery is on its medial side. About 7 cm above the wrist the nerve passes deep to the tendon of brachioradialis and turns dorsally in the direction of the anatomical snuffbox. In its further downward course the nerve can be rubbed against the tendon of extensor pollicis longus. In this relatively unprotected position the nerve is liable to be compressed by tight bracelets or watch- straps. Lying in the superficial fascia of the anatomical snuffbox the radial nerve divides into dorsal digital branches. It supplies a variable area of skin over the lateral side of the dorsum and lateral three and half digits. It may supply the proximal and middle phalanges or the proximal and half of the middle phalanges of the above digits.

Surface Marking of Superficial Terminal Branch

To mark the superficial terminal branch in the forearm three points are used. The first point is 1 cm lateral to the tendon of biceps brachii. The second point is at the junction of upper two-thirds and lower one-third of the lateral margin of the forearm. The third point is the anatomical snuffbox. A line joining the three points represents the radial nerve in the forearm.

Clinical Highlights (Figs 28.1 and 28.2)

a. In the axilla, the radial nerve is injured due to pressure of the crutch (crutch palsy). In this lesion all the muscles supplied by the radial nerve are paralysed. There is loss of extension at elbow (paralysis of triceps brachii), wrist drop (due to paralysis of wrist extensors), loss of extension at MCP joints of fingers (finger drop due to paralysis of extensor digitorum) and thumb drop due to paralysis of extensor pollicis longus and brevis. There is a variable sensory loss on the posterior aspect of the arm and forearm and on the dorsum of the hand. More often there is an isolated sensory loss on the dorsum of the hand at the base of the thumb (Fig. 28.2F).
b. In the arm, the radial nerve may be injured due to midhumeral fracture, inadvertent intramuscular injection in the triceps brachii or direct pressure as happens in saturday-night palsy. At this level the long head of the triceps is spared hence extension of the elbow is not totally lost. Otherwise the effects of injury are similar to those in the axilla.

29 Clinicoanatomical Problems and Solutions

CASE 1

An elderly man came to the hospital with the complaint of a pulsatile soft swelling in the left axilla of about two months duration. On examination it was found that abduction movement of his left arm was weak and restricted and there was sensory loss on the skin over lower half of deltoid muscle. There was slight edema (swelling) of the upper limb.

Questions

a. Which large blood vessel in the axilla is likely to give rise to a pulsatile swelling?
b. What is dilatation of a blood vessel called?
c. Give the extent and surface marking of this vessel in the axilla.
d. Name the muscle that crosses it anteriorly.
e. Describe with the help of diagrams the relations of this vessel.
f. Name the branches of this vessel in order.
g. Compression of which blood vessel will cause edema of the upper limb. Give the formation and termination of this vessel.
h. Explain sensory loss over the lower half of deltoid and restricted abduction in this case.

Solutions

a. Axillary artery
b. Aneurysm
c. The axillary artery extends from outer border of first rib to lower margin of teres major.
   For surface marking of axillary artery refer Chapter 5.
d. Pectoralis minor muscle
e. Refer to relations of axillary artery in Chapter 5
f. The superior thoracic artery is the branch of first part, acromiothoracic and lateral thoracic arteries are the branches of second part and subscapular, anterior and posterior circumflex humeral arteries arise from third part.
g. Compression of axillary vein results in edema of upper limb. This vein is formed at the lower margin of teres major muscle in the anterior compartment of arm by the union of basilic vein and venae comitantes of brachial artery (according to another view the basilic vein continues as axillary vein at the lower margin of teres major). The basilic vein becomes the subclavian vein at the outer margin of first rib.
h. The aneurysmal swelling compresses the axillary nerve, which is located posterior to the third part of axillary artery. The compression of motor fibers in the axillary nerve results in weakness of deltoid and restricted abduction. Similarly, compression of sensory fibers carried in upper lateral cutaneous nerve of arm (a branch of axillary nerve) gives rise to sensory loss in the skin over the lower half of deltoid (regimental badge anesthesia).

CASE 2

During difficult labor a baby was delivered in a hospital by applying forceps. After about two weeks the parents brought the baby to the pediatrician for check-up. The pediatrician observed that the baby's left arm was medially rotated and adducted while the forearm was pronated and extended.

Questions

a. Name the position of the upper limb seen in this newborn baby.
b. This position of the upper limb is characteristic of which clinical condition?
c. Injury to which part of brachial plexus is responsible for this condition.
d. Draw a simple labeled diagram of this part.
e. Paralysis of which muscles results in medial rotation of arm?
f. Paralysis of which muscles results in extended forearm?
g. Paralysis of which muscles results in adducted arm?
h. Enumerate the branches arising from the first two stages of brachial plexus.

Solutions

a. Porter's tip position
b. Erb's palsy
c. Upper trunk or Erb's point
d. Refer to Chapter 4 on Brachial Plexus.
e. Infraspinatus and teres minor
f. Biceps brachii, brachialis and brachioradialis
g. Supraspinatus and deltoid
h. From root stage-dorsal scapular nerve and long thoracic nerve and from trunk stage- suprascapular nerve and nerve to subclavius.

CASE 3

A 40-year-old woman came to the surgeon with the complaint of hard, painless lump in the upper, outer quadrant of the right breast. Examination revealed enlarged axillary lymph nodes on the right side and loss of mobility of the breast on the same side. X-ray of vertebral column showed irregular shadows in the bodies of L4 and L5 vertebrae.

Questions

a. Name the most probable clinical condition affecting the right breast.
b. Name the three muscles related to the base of the breast.
c. How is the fixity of the breast to the pectoralis major tested?
d. What is the reason of irregular shadows in the lumbar vertebrae in the above case? Explain the venous route of the spread of breast cancer with the help of diagram.
e. Which part of the breast is in contact with the pectoral group of lymph nodes and how does this part enter the axilla?
f. Describe lymphatic drainage of breast.
g. Draw diagram to show arterial supply of breast.

Solutions

a. Malignancy or cancer of breast
b. Pectoralis major, serratus anterior and aponeurosis of external oblique abdominis.
c. The patient with suspected malignancy of breast is subjected to this examination (Fig. 2.4). The patient is asked to press the hand on the hip forcibly to contract pectoralis major. After this the clinician moves the breast over the pectoral fascia in the direction of muscle fibers of pectoralis major. Free mobility indicates no infiltration of cancer cells in to the pectoral fascia and muscle.
d. Cancer cells deposit into vertebral bodies. For venous route of cancer spread refer to Figure 2.8.
e. Axillary tail of Spence enters the axilla by passing through foramen of Langer.
f. Refer Chapter 2 for lymphatic drainage of breast.
g. Refer to Figure 2.5. for arterial supply of breast.

CASE 4

A man involved in automobile accident was brought to the casualty. On examination it was found that his left shoulder was flattened and the head of humerus was palpable in the infraclavicular fossa. An A-P X-ray of the shoulder confirmed the diagnosis of anterior dislocation of shoulder joint. For the operation of reduction of the head of humerus, the orthopedic surgeon used the anterior approach for which skin incision was placed along the deltopectoral groove.

Questions

a. Which long blood vessel is located in the deltopectoral groove?
b. After retracting the deltoid and pectoralis major muscles from each other, which bony part of scapula is exposed?

c. Name the two muscles, which are attached to this bony part by a conjoint tendon.
d. Draw a diagram to show the relations of the shoulder joint.
e. Which nerve is in danger of injury in anterior dislocation of shoulder joint?
f. Describe the origin, course and distribution of this nerve.
g. Name the muscles in the rotator cuff and give nerve supply of each.
h. Of the four rotator cuff muscles, which muscle is not the rotator of arm?

Solutions

a. Cephalic vein
b. Coracoid process
c. Coracobrachialis and short head of biceps brachii
d. Refer to Figure 13.3
e. Axillary nerve
f. Refer to chapter 12
g. SITS muscles are supraspinatus, infraspinatus, teres minor and subscapularis.
h. Supraspinatus is not the rotator of arm. The infraspinatus and teres minor are lateral rotators and subscapularis is the medial rotator.

CASE 5

A man, whose work involved carrying heavy loads on the shoulder, experienced difficulty in raising the right arm vertically upwards. The examining physician asked the man to press his hands against the wall in front. It was found that the medial border and inferior angle of his right scapula became prominent.

Questions

a. Which muscle is tested in this man to detect the injury to which nerve?
b. Name the deformity of scapula caused by injury to this nerve.
c. Draw a diagram of brachial plexus to show the origin of this nerve.
d. How does this nerve enter the axilla?
e. Name the muscle in the medial wall of axilla to which this nerve is intimately related. Give the attachments of the muscle.
f. What is the action of this muscle in hyperabduction of arm? Does it act alone or in combination with other muscle?

Solutions

a. The serratus anterior is tested to detect injury to long thoracic nerve.
b. Winging of scapula or winged scapula
c. Refer to Chapter 4.
d. Through the apex of axilla
e. Serratus anterior (refer to Chapter 3)
f. It causes forward or lateral rotation of scapula along with upper and lower fibers of trapezius.

CASE 6

A gardener while digging soil cut his right ring finger by sharp edge of a broken glass. After about 3 to 4 days he developed fever and his entire ring finger was swollen and painful.

Questions

a. Name the structure in the ring finger that is likely to be inflamed.
b. What is the clinical condition called?
c. In what structure is the digital synovial sheath protected?
d. What is peculiar about the appearance of this structure?
e. Name the palmar spaces in the intermediate compartment of palm giving boundaries of each.
f. Name the channels that connect these spaces to the web spaces.
g. What is the surgical importance of these channels?

Solutions

a. Digital synovial sheath
b. Tenosynovitis
c. Fibrous flexor sheath
d. Fibrous flexor sheath is the modified deep fascia showing peculiar architecture of alternate annular pulleys and cruciform pulleys.
e. Midpalmar and thenar spaces (refer to Chapter 24)
f. Lumbrical canals

g. Lumbrical canals are opened up surgically in corresponding web spaces to drain the pus from palmar spaces.

CASE 7

An elderly woman with a history of fall on the outstretched hand developed localized pain and a swelling on the dorsal aspect of the wrist. When movements of wrist became painful she was brought to the hospital. X-ray findings confirmed the diagnosis of fracture of the lower end of radius.

Questions

a. What is the name of the fracture of the lower end of the radius and the typical deformity of the hand as a result of this fracture?
b. Why does the normal relationship of the styloid process of radius and ulna change consequent to this fracture?
c. Name the space in which the styloid process of radius is felt.
d. Which bones form the floor of this space?
e. Give the anterior and posterior boundaries of this space.
f. Which nerve crosses the roof of this space?
g. Draw a diagram to show the distribution of this nerve.

Solutions

a. Colles' fracture- dinner fork deformity.
b. Since the distal fragment of radius shifts posteriorly and upward its styloid process is also pulled up. Hence both ulnar and radial styloid processes are either at the same level or the ulnar becomes higher.
c. Anatomical snuffbox.
d. From proximal to distal—styloid process of radius, scaphoid, trapezium, base of first metacarpal bone.
e. Anterior—Abductor pollicis longus and extensor pollicis brevis, posterior-extensor pollicis longus.
f. Superficial branch of radial nerve.
g. Refer to Figure 23.1.

CASE 8

While attempting to collect a blood sample from the median cubital vein, the trainee nurse finds that blood in the syringe is bright red. She immediately withdraws the needle. When she reinserts the needle slightly medial to the previous puncture the patient experiences sharp pain, which radiates to the lateral three digits.

Questions

a. Name the superficial veins that are connected by the median cubital vein giving direction of blood flow in this vein.
b. Which fascial structure supports the median cubital vein?
c. What are the attachments of this fascial structure?
d. Which structures lie deep to the fascial structure?
e. Which structure, when pierced by needle gives rise to radiating pain in lateral three digits?
f. Name the muscles of the forearm and palm, which are paralysed if this structure is cut in the cubital fossa.

Solutions

a. Cephalic vein laterally and basilic vein medially are connected by median cubital vein, which carries blood from cephalic vein to basilic.
b. Bicipital aponeurosis
c. It extends from the main insertion of biceps brachii tendon in to posterior part of radial tuberosity to the deep fascia of forearm and to the posterior subcutaneous margin of ulna.
d. Median nerve and brachial artery
e. Median nerve
f. Four superficial muscles of forearm (pronator teres, FCR, palmaris longus and FDS), 21/2 muscles in the deep part of forearm via its anterior interosseous branch (flexor pollicis longus, pronator quadratus and lateral half of FDP), 41/2 muscles in palm (first and second lumbricals, abductor pollicis brevis, opponens pollicis and superficial head of flexor pollicis brevis)

CASE 9

An obese elderly woman with history of myxoedema (deficiency of thyroxine) complained of pins and needles sensation in the index and middle fingers of her right hand. On examination it was found that the thenar eminence of right hand was flattened and the patient was unable to bring the tips of the thumb and little finger together.

Questions

a. Name the clinical condition from the symptoms and signs.
b. Name the boundaries of the carpal tunnel and enumerate its contents.
c. Compression of which content is responsible for the above condition?
d. Inability to touch the thumb and little finger is suggestive of the weakness of which muscle?
e. Which structure is cut to relieve symptoms in this condition?
f. Mention the attachments and anterior relations of this structure
g. Anterior dislocation of which carpal bone may also produce similar syndrome?

Solutions

a. Carpal tunnel syndrome
b. Anteriorly flexor retinaculum and posteriorly carpal bones. The contents are, long flexor tendons of FDS, FDP and FPL covered with synovial sheaths and median nerve.
c. Median nerve
d. Opponens pollicis
e. Flexor retinaculum
f. Flexor retinaculum is attached medially to pisiform and hook of hamate and laterally to scaphoid and trapezium. Anteriorly it is crossed by from lateral to medial- palmar cutaneous branch of median nerve, palmaris longus tendon, palmar cutaneous branch of ulnar nerve, ulnar artery and ulnar nerve.
g. Lunate bone.

CASE 10

A patient suffering from Hansen's disease (leprosy) came to the hospital with complaint of weakness in the right hand. On examination it was found that there was sensory loss in medial one and half fingers and medial side of palmar and dorsal aspects of hand. In addition there was flattening of hypothenar eminence and difficulty in holding a card between thumb and index finger.

Questions

a. Name the nerve that is affected in this patient.
b. Describe the course and branches of this nerve in the palm.
c. Give reason for flattening of hypothenar eminence.
d. Explain the inability of the patient to hold the card between thumb and index finger.
e. Name the branches (giving the level of their origin) of this nerve that supply the skin of the dorsal and palmer aspects of the hand.
f. Name the deformity that will result if all muscles supplied by this nerve in the palm are paralyzed.

Solutions

a. Ulnar nerve
b. Refer to description of ulnar nerve in Chapter 28 and Figures 25.4 and 25.5 in Chapter 25.
c. Due to paralysis of hypothenar muscles (abductor digiti minimi, flexor digiti minimi and opponens digiti minimi).
d. To hold the card between thumb and index finger the adduction of thumb is necessary. The adduction of thumb is lost due to paralysis of adductor pollicis in this patient.
e. The palmar cutaneous branch takes origin from ulnar nerve in the middle of the forearm. It passes superficial to the flexor retinaculum to enter the palm. The dorsal cutaneous branch arises from the ulnar nerve a little above the wrist and enters the dorsum of hand to supply the skin of medial side.
f. Clawhand.

SINGLE BEST RESPONSE TYPE MCQs

1. Which of the following is a communicating bursa around the shoulder joint?
A. Supra-acromial **B.** Subacromial
C. Supracoracoid **D.** Subscapular

2. Which of the following is not attached to humerus?
A. Teres minor **B.** Brachialis
C. Biceps brachii **D.** Infraspinatus

3. Which part of brachial plexus is the continuation of ventral ramus of 7th cervical spinal nerve?
A. Medial cord **B.** Upper trunk
C. Middle trunk **D.** Lateral cord

4. **Regarding the long heads of biceps and triceps which of the following is true?**
   A. Both extracapsular
   B. Triceps extracapsular, biceps intracapsular
   C. Both intracapsular
   D. Triceps intracapsular, biceps extracapsular

5. **Subacromial bursa separates coracoacromial arch from the tendon of:**
   A. Subscapularis B. Teres minor
   C. Supraspinatus D. Infraspinatus

6. **Which one of the following has action similar to that of teres minor?**
   A. Supraspinatus
   B. Infraspinatus
   C. Subscapularis
   D. Teres major

7. **On which aspect are the interphalangeal joints in hand devoid of capsule?**
   A. Posterior B. Anterior
   C. Medial D. Lateral

8. **Which forms the anterior fold of axilla?**
   A. Pectoralis major
   B. Pectoarlis major and minor
   C. Pectoralis muscles and subclavius
   D. Clavipectoral fascia

9. **Epitrochlear lymph nodes lie along:**
   A. Median cubital vein
   B. Cephalic vein above elbow
   C. Basilic vein above elbow
   D. Brachial artery above elbow

10. **In the anterior compartment of arm the radial nerve does not supply:**
    A. Brachialis
    B. Brachioradialis
    C. Extensor carpi radialis longus
    D. Extensor carpi radialis brevis

11. **In climbing a tree the following two muscles contract together:**
    A. Teres major and teres minor
    B. Latissimus dorsi and teres major
    C. Pectoralis major and latissimus dorsi
    D. Teres major and pectoralis major

12. **Ligaments of Cooper are modifications of:**
    A. Axillary fascia
    B. Pectoral fascia
    C. Fatty tissue of breast
    D. Fibrous stroma of breast

13. **Which is not a branch of deep palmar arch:**
    A. Proximal perforating
    B. Recurrent
    C. Palmar metacarpal
    D. Common palmar digital

14. **Rotter's lymph nodes belong to which level of axillary nodes?**
    A. Level-I B. Level-II
    C. Level-III D. None

15. **Froment's test indicates the integrity of:**
    A. First and second palmar interossei
    B. First and second dorsal interossei
    C. Adductor pollicis
    D. First and second lumbricals

16. **First lumbrical canal is the extension of:**
    A. Ulnar bursa
    B. Thenar space
    C. Radial bursa
    D. Midpalmar space

17. **Which of the following does not connect radius and ulna?**
    A. Annular ligament
    B. Interosseous membrane
    C. Oblique cord
    D. Quadrate ligament

18. **Which of the following is not the modification of deep fascia?**
    A. Extensor retinaculum
    B. Palmar aponeurosis
    C. Extensor expansion
    D. Fibrous flexor sheath

19. **Hammer thumb deformity is due the rupture of the tendon of:**
    A. Flexor pollicis longus
    B. Abductor pollicis longus
    C. Extensor pollicis brevis
    D. Extensor pollicis longus

20. Abduction of the middle finger is brought about by:
- A. Third dorsal interosseous
- B. Third lumbrical
- C. Second and third dorsal interossei
- D. Second and third lumbricals

21. Ulnar collateral ligament of elbow joint is related to:
- A. Median nerve
- B. Basilic vein
- C. Ulnar nerve
- D. Ulnar artery

22. The artery supplying the scaphoid enters the bone at:
- A. Waist
- B. Distal half
- C. Proximal half
- D. Proximal end

23. Which dermatome overlies the little finger?
- A. T1
- B. C8
- C. C7
- D. C6

24. Which of the following pierces the interosseous membrane?
- A. Posterior interosseous artery
- B. Anterior interosseous artery
- C. Common interosseous artery
- D. Posterior interosseous nerve

25. The skin overlying the thenar eminence is supplied by:
- A. Recurrent branch of median nerve
- B. Palmar cutaneous branch of ulnar nerve
- C. Palmar cutaneous branch of median nerve
- D. Lateral proper digital branch of median nerve

Key to MCQs

1 D	2 C	3 C	4 B	5 C	6 B	7 A
8 A	9 C	10 D	11 C	12 D	13 D	14 B
15 C	16 B	17 A	18 C	19 D	20 C	21 C
22 B	23 B	24 B	25 C			

MULTIPLE RESPONSE TYPE MCQs

Write T *(True)* or F *(False)* Against Each Statement

1. The supinator muscle:
- a. belongs to anterior compartment of forearm
- b. is attached to humerus, ulna and radius
- c. is the only supinator of forearm
- d. is supplied by anterior interosseous nerve

2. Mammary gland:
- a. develops from surface ectoderm
- b. is a modified sebaceous gland
- c. rests on pectoralis minor muscle
- d. its superficial lymph vessels drain into Rotter's nodes

3. Superficial branch of radial nerve:
- a. is entirely sensory
- b. arises from radial nerve in spiral groove
- c. supplies skin over lateral half of dorsum of hand
- d. if damaged causes wrist drop

4. Middle trunk of brachial plexus:
- a. is present in axilla
- b. is formed by union of C6 and C7 roots
- c. dorsal scapular nerve is its only branch
- d. is the continuation of C7 root

5. The first part of axillary artery is related:
- a. anteriorly to pectoralis major
- b. posteriorly to serratus anterior
- c. laterally to axillary vein
- d. medially to medial cord of brachial plexus

6. Upper trunk of brachial plexus:
- a. is located in posterior triangle
- b. is formed by the union of C5 and C6 nerve roots
- c. gives origin to dorsal scapular nerve
- d. when injured causes clawhand

7. Regarding arteria profunda brachii:
- a. it is a branch of brachial artery
- b. it lies in spiral groove with radial nerve
- c. its radial collateral branch anastomosis with interosseous recurrent artery
- d. pierces lateral intermuscular septum of arm

8. The pulp space:
   a. is present in terminal phalanx of all digits
   b. contains loculated fat
   c. its infection is known as whitlow
   d. whitlow may cause thrombosis of epiphyseal artery

9. Regarding lumbricals of hand:
   a. look like earthworm
   b. all lumbricals are bipennate
   c. are inserted in to lateral side of extensor expansion
   d. all are supplied by deep branch of ulnar nerve

10. Extensor muscles attached to front of lateral epicondyle of humerus:
   a. anconeus
   b. extensor carpi radialis longus
   c. extensor carpi ulnaris
   d. extensor digiti minimi

Annexure: Radiographs of Upper Extremity

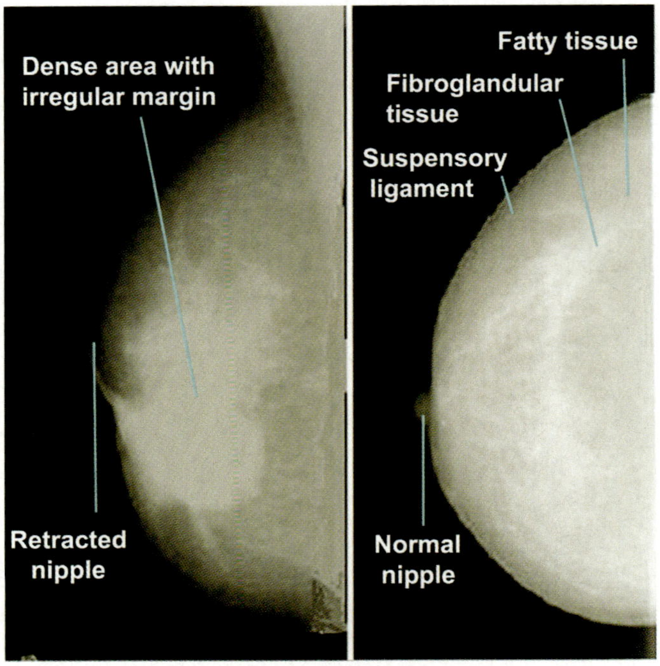

UL-R1. Mammograms showing malignancy and normal pattern of breast tissue

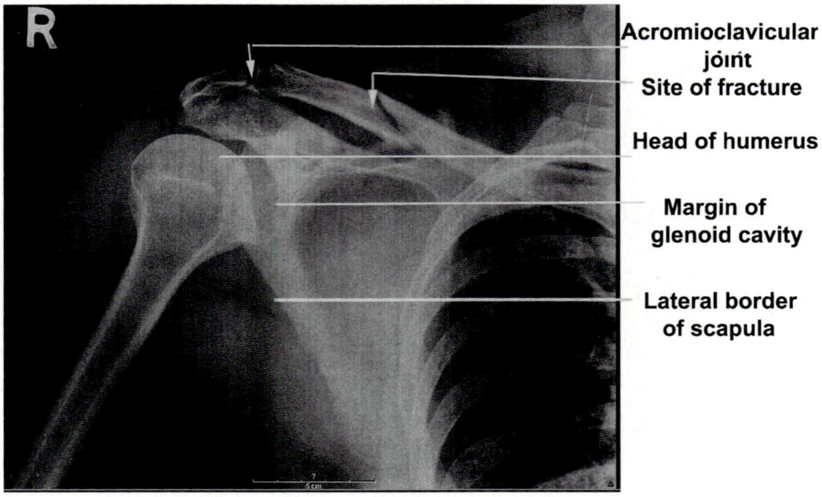

UL-R2. Radiograph of shoulder region with arm slightly abducted. Note the fracture of clavicle at the junction of lateral 1/3rd and medial 2/3rd

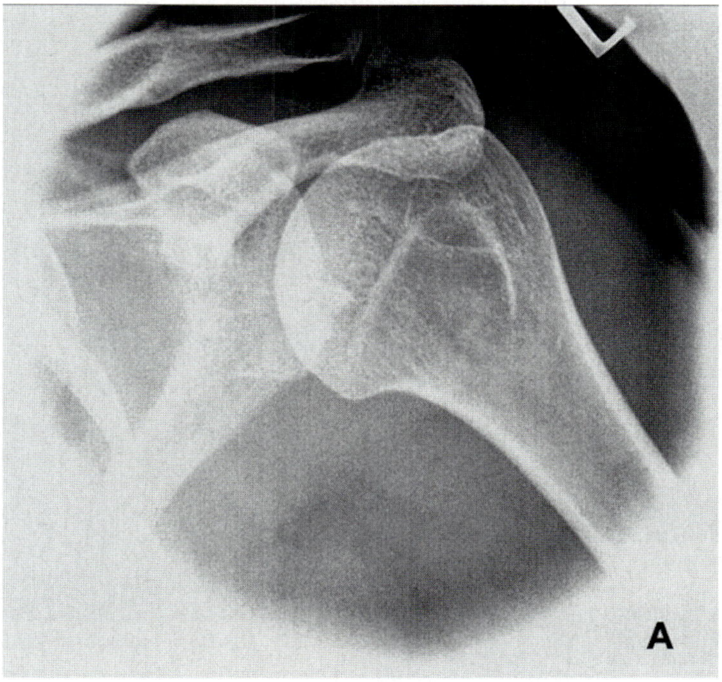

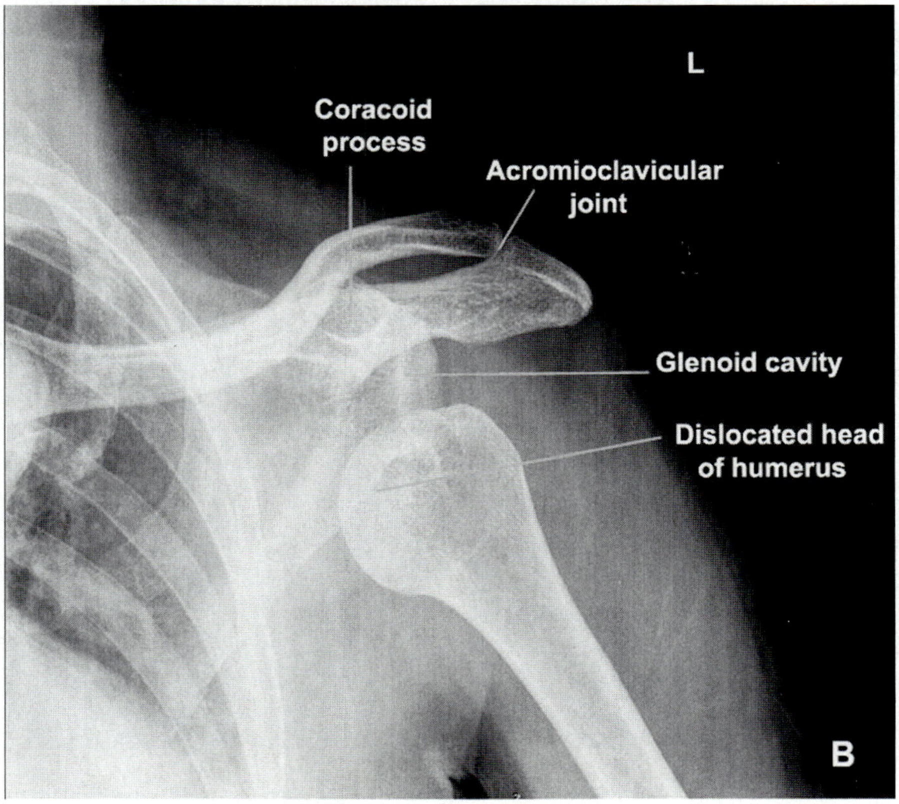

UL-R3. Radiographs of (A) Normal shoulder (glenohumeral) joint and (B) Anterior dislocation of shoulder

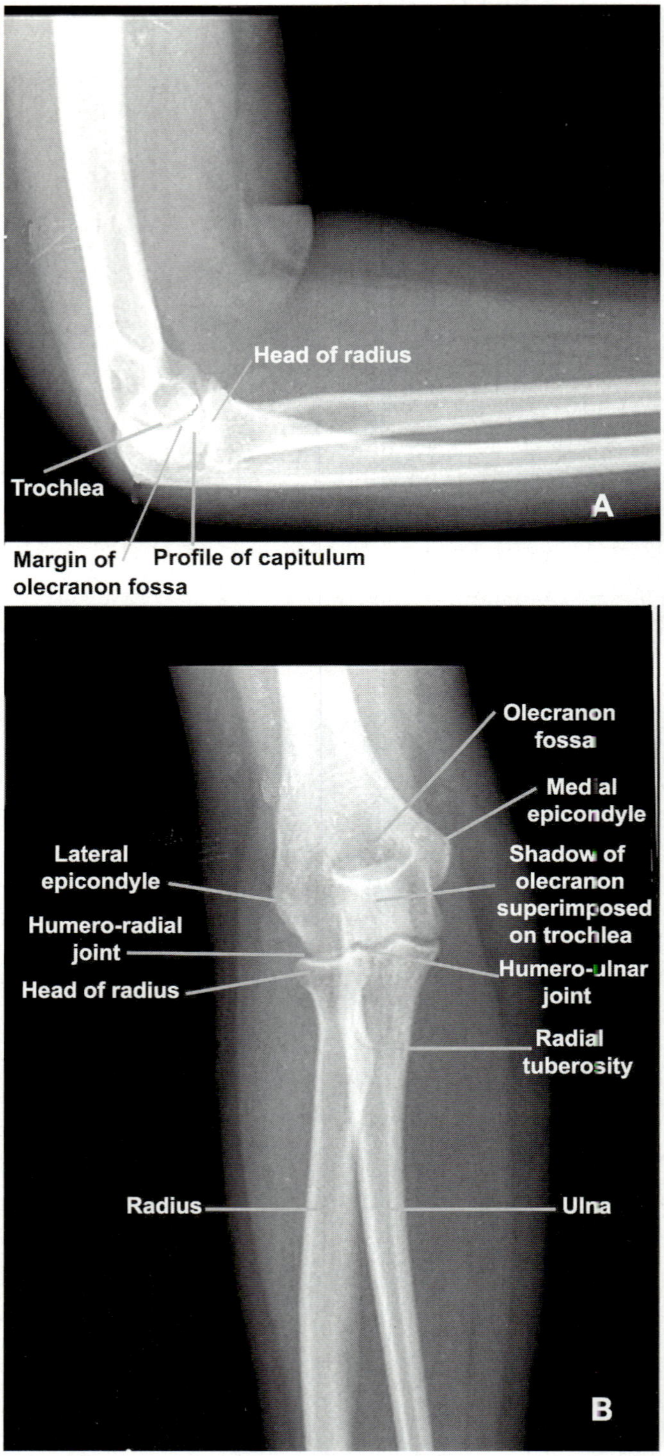

UL-R4. Radiographs of lateral view of flexed elbow joint (A) and anteroposterior view of extended elbow joint (B)

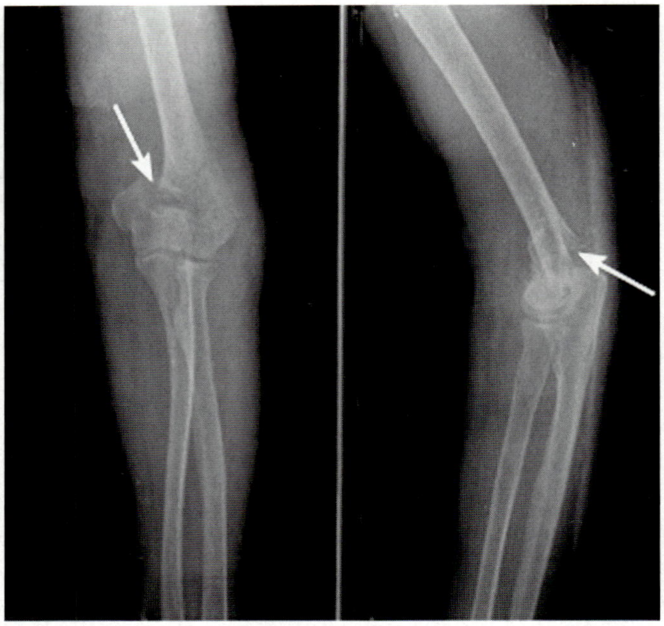

UL-R5. Suprocondylar fracture of left humerus

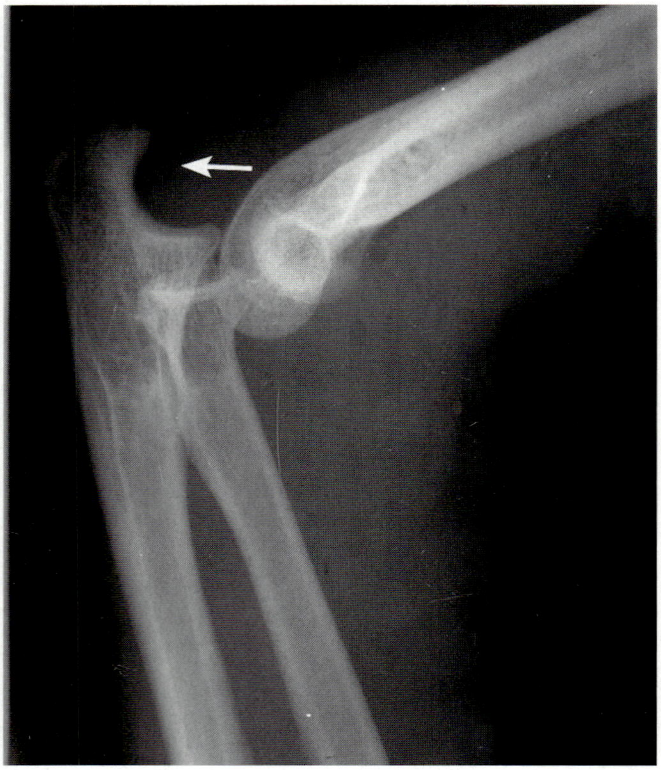

UL-R6. Posterior disc location of elbow joint

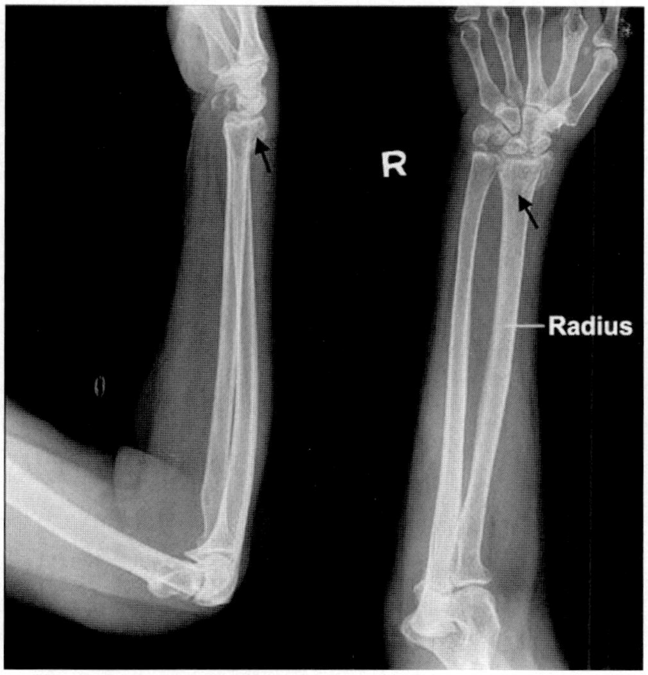

UL-R7. Colles' fracture of lower end of radius in anteroposterior and lateral views

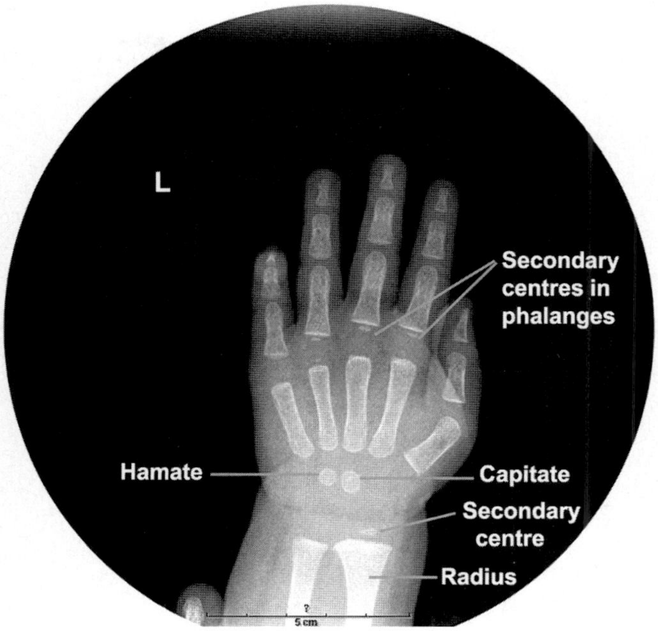

UL-R8. Radiograph of hand and wrist of one year old child

SECTION TWO

Thorax

30 Thorax

The thorax is the upper part of the trunk between the neck and the abdomen. It consists of thoracic wall and thoracic cavity, which protects the vital organs of respiration and circulation. In the lateral part of thoracic cavity on each side, the lung is enclosed in a serous sac called pleural cavity. The central part of the thoracic cavity between the two pleural cavities is called the mediastinum. The heart within the pericardial cavity is located in the mediastinum. The skeleton of the thorax is called thoracic cage or the rib cage. As the heart and the lungs are constantly moving, the thoracic cage necessarily has to be resilient. The thoracic wall or the chest wall (consisting of eleven intercostal spaces) is made of musculoskeletal elements (muscles, bones, cartilages and membranes).

BOUNDARIES OF THORACIC CAGE

The sternum and anterior parts of upper seven ribs and their costal cartilages form the anterior wall. The posterior thoracic wall is much longer. It is composed of twelve thoracic vertebrae with intervening discs and the posterior parts of the ribs. Twelve pairs of ribs form the lateral boundary on each side. The inlet of the thorax (upper opening) is kidney-shaped. It is nearly 10 cm in transverse diameter and 5 cm in anteroposterior diameter. Its boundaries are the body of first thoracic vertebra, the inner margins of the first ribs and their costal cartilages and the upper margin of manubrium sterni (Fig. 30.1). The first rib slopes downwards and forwards hence the first thoracic vertebral level is higher than that of the upper margin of the manubrium. Because of the inclination of the thoracic inlet, the apex of the lung with the overlying pleura appears to project into the base of the neck. The thoracic outlet is much wider than the inlet. The twelfth thoracic vertebra is its posterior boundary. The eleventh and the twelfth ribs lie on either side while the costal margins and the xiphoid process complete the outlet in front. The outlet is closed by a musculomembranous partition called the thoracic diaphragm. Because the diaphragm projects on either side as cupula in the thoracic cavity the upper abdominal organs are covered by lower part of thoracic cage.

Clinical Examination of Thoracic Wall

The pectoral region forms the front of the anterior chest wall and the scapular region forms part of the posterior chest wall. Deeper to these regions are the intercostal spaces, deeper to which are the contents of the thoracic cavity. For examination of the heart and great vessels of the thorax and for examination of the lungs and pleural cavities, the clinician examines the anterior and posterior chest walls. The methods of examination consist of inspection, palpation, percussion and auscultation, for which the familiarity with the skeletal and soft tissue landmarks is essential. Certain lines of orientation are

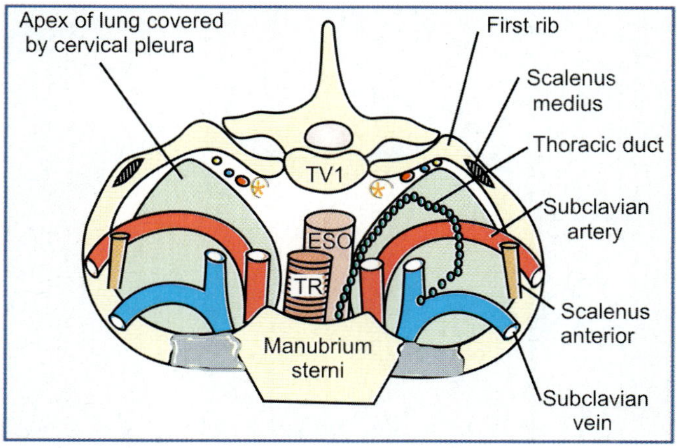

Fig. 30.1: Schematic diagram to illustrate structures passing through thoracic inlet. Anterior relations of neck of first rib: Sympathetic ganglion, superior intercostal artery, first posterior intercostal vein (highest intercostal vein), and ascending branch of T1 ventral ramus

necessary to delineate the internal structures as well as to identify safe sites for approaches to the internal organs.

Surface Landmarks

On the anterior aspect of the chest wall the suprasternal notch is a palpable. It is at the level of T2 vertebra. The trachea can be palpated in this notch. The sternal angle or angle of Louis is a palpable. It lies at the level of the disc between T4 and T5 vertebrae. The second rib articulates with it and hence is useful in counting ribs and intercostal spaces (the first rib is hidden behind the clavicle). The xiphisternal joint is at the level of disc between T8 and T9 vertebrae. The xiphoid process lies opposite T9 vertebrae. It can be palpated in the floor of epigastric fossa. The lowest part of costal margin corresponding to tenth rib in midaxillary line is at the level of L3 vertebra.

On the posterior aspect of the chest wall, the spines of the thoracic vertebrae are palpable in the midline. The scapula is located in the upper part of the back of thorax. Its superior angle lies opposite T2 vertebra. The spine of the scapula is subcutaneous and its root is at the level of T3 vertebra. The inferior angle of scapula corresponds to T7 vertebra and the seventh rib overlies it. Besides the bony landmarks, some reference lines are useful for the surface marking of the pleura, lungs and the apex of the heart. The midsternal line passes through the midline of sternum. The midclavicular line passes through the midpoint of the clavicle. The anterior axillary line corresponds to the anterior axillary fold and the posterior axillary line to the posterior axillary fold. The midaxillary line passes through the midpoint of the base of the axilla. The scapular line passes through the inferior angle of the scapula.

31 Inlet of Thorax

The thoracic inlet is the upper opening of the thoracic cavity by which it communicates with the neck and the upper extremity. It is kidney-shaped and is inclined downwards and forwards. Its boundaries (Fig. 30.1) are, the first thoracic vertebra posteriorly, upper margin of manubrium sterni anteriorly and the inner margin of the right and left first rib on either side. The structures that pass through the thoracic inlet can be subdivided into two groups. In the midline there are two strap muscles of the neck (sternothyroid and sternohyoid), inferior thyroid veins, trachea and the esophagus. On the right of the midline, the brachiocephalic artery and the right brachiocephalic vein are present. On the left of the midline, the left common carotid artery, left brachiocephalic vein, left recurrent laryngeal nerve and the thoracic duct are present. Laterally, on each, side the apex of the lung and the cervical pleura project upwards. The sympathetic chain, superior intercostal artery and the ventral ramus of the first thoracic nerve lie posterior to the lung apex but in front of the neck of the first rib. The internal thoracic artery, vagus nerve and phrenic nerve descend in relation to the medial aspect of lung apex. The subclavian vessels pass in front of the lung apex in lateral direction to cross the superior surface of the first rib. The scalenus anterior and medius muscles descend to gain insertion in the first rib. The Sibson's fascia is attached to the inner margin of first rib (Fig. 38.4).

The relations of the superior surface of the first rib are worthy of note. The subclavian vein lies in a groove on this surface in front of scalene tubercle (where scalenus anterior is inserted) and the subclavian artery and lower trunk of the brachial plexus are related just behind the tubercle (Fig. 31.1).

Scalene Triangle

The scalene triangle is a narrow triangular space bounded anteriorly by the scalenus anterior, posteriorly by scalenus medius and inferiorly by upper surface of the first rib. Its contents are, the lower trunk of the brachial plexus and the subclavian artery.

Clinical Highlights

In the presence of a cervical rib (Fig. 31.1) or a congenitally hypertrophied scalenus anterior muscle, the scalene triangle is unduly narrowed. As a consequence the subclavian artery and the lower trunk of the brachial plexus are liable to compression. This results in neuro-vascular symptoms, which are collectively called thoracic outlet syndrome (actually a misnomer) or cervical rib syndrome or scalenus anterior syndrome.

a. The compression of the subclavian artery results in pallor and coldness of the upper limb. There is reduction in the force or obliteration of the radial pulse on affected side. This is confirmed by Adson's test done as follows. The patient sits on the stool and is asked to take deep breath in and to turn the face to the affected side. There is reduction in radial pulse on the affected side in the presence of cervical rib or hypertrophied scalenus anterior muscle. Distal to the scalene triangle (site of compression) the subclavian artery may show dilatation (Fig. 31.1).
b. Though located outside the scalene triangle the subclavian vein is also liable for compression and it gives rise to distension of the superficial veins, edema and pain in the upper limb.

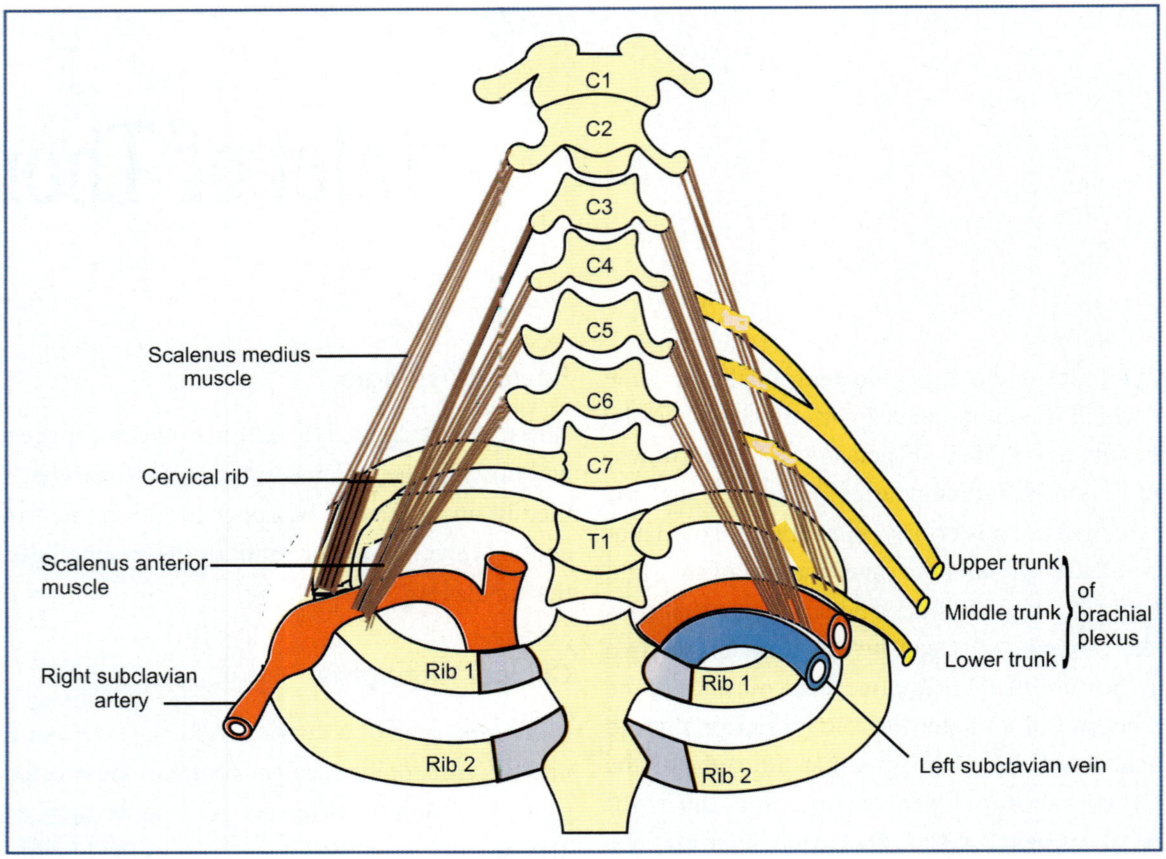

Fig. 31.1: Simplified scheme to show the effects of cervical rib on neurovascular structures related to superior surface of first rib. Note poststenotic dilatation of right subclavian artery due to cervical rib

c. The compression of lower trunk of brachial plexus results in symptoms like numbness, tingling and pain along the ulnar border of the hand and little finger. There may be weakness and wasting of small muscles of the hand. Advanced cases may show flattening of hypothenar eminence and guttering of the interosseous spaces on the dorsum of the hand.

Surgical Treatment

To alleviate symptoms due to cervical rib, the surgical treatment consists of removal of the rib. The periosteum of the rib must be removed in order to prevent regeneration of the rib. If hypertrophy of scalenus anterior muscle is the cause of symptoms then the operation of scalenotomy is performed.

Intercostal Spaces

The space between two adjacent ribs and their costal cartilages is called intercostal space. There are eleven intercostal spaces bounded by twelve ribs on each side. The upper nine spaces are close anteriorly but the short tenth and eleventh spaces have open anterior ends, which reach the level of mid-axillary line. Each intercostal space (Fig. 32.1) contains intercostal muscles, intercostal vessels and intercostal nerve. The intercostal nerve and vessels travel in the neurovascular plane, which lies between internal and innermost intercostal muscles.

Intercostal Muscles

The intercostal muscles lie in three layers. From the superficial to deeper plane they are, the external intercostal, internal intercostal and the innermost intercostal muscles.

a. External intercostal muscle takes origin from the lower margin of the rib above and is inserted in to the upper margin of the rib below, belonging to the particular intercostal space. It consists of fleshy interosseous part (between the ribs) and membranous interchondral part, which is known as anterior intercostal membrane

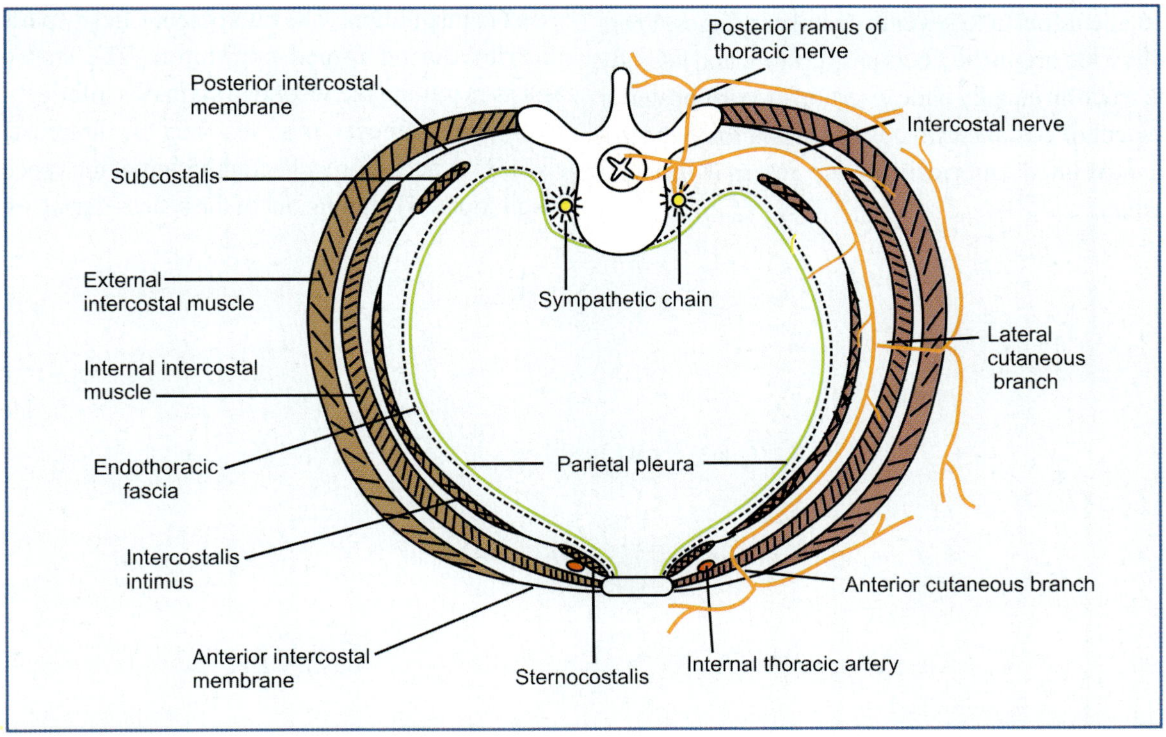

Fig. 32.1: Showing typical intercostal space on right side (Note that course, communications and branches of typical intercostal nerve are shown on the left side)

(between costal cartilages). The direction of the muscle fibers is downwards, forwards and medial.

b. Internal intercostal muscle takes origin from the costal groove of the rib above and is inserted in the upper margin of the rib below. It consists of fleshy and membranous parts. The longer fleshy part extends posteriorly up to the angle of the rib. It is subdivided into intercartilaginous and interosseous parts. The short membranous part (called posterior intercostal membrane) is located beyond the angle of the rib. The direction of the muscle fibers is downward, backward and lateral.

c. Innermost intercostal muscle is a discontinuous muscle layer, which is separated from costal pleura by endothoracic fascia. It is divided into sternocostalis, intercostalis intimus and subcostalis from before backwards.

   i. The sternocostalis (transversus thoracis) lies behind sternum and costal cartilages (Fig 34.3). It takes origin from the posterior aspects of lower part of body of sternum, xiphoid process and also from adjacent fourth to seventh costal cartilages. From this wide origin the fibers pass upward and laterally to reach an equally wide insertion in to the posterior aspect of costal cartilages of second to sixth ribs. It is related anteriorly to the internal thoracic artery.

   ii. The intercostalis intimus originates from the ridge above the costal groove of the upper rib and is inserted on the upper margin of the lower rib.

   iii. The subcostalis muscles are present in the posterior part of lower intercostal spaces only. The muscle arises from the inner surface of the rib near its angle and is inserted in inner surface of the lower ribs after crossing one or two spaces.

Nerve Supply

The intercostal muscles receive nerve supply from the corresponding intercostal nerves.

Actions

The external intercostal muscles elevate the ribs to increase the antero-posterior and transverse diameters of the thorax. The internal intercostal muscles have dual actions. Their intercartilaginous fleshy parts act synergistically with external intercostal muscles and hence assist in inspiration. The interosseous fleshy parts depress the ribs during forced expiration. The sternocostalis assists in pulling the second to sixth ribs inferiorly. Collectively the intercostal muscles keep the intercostal spaces rigid. This action prevents indrawing of the spaces during inspiration and bulging out of the spaces during expiration.

33 Intercostal Nerves

The intercostal nerves are the anterior primary rami of thoracic spinal nerves. They are eleven in number on each side, being equal to the number of intercostal spaces. The anterior primary ramus of twelfth thoracic spinal nerve, since it lies below the twelfth rib is called subcostal nerve. The unique feature of the intercostal nerves is that they retain their segmental character, unlike the anterior primary rami from the other regions of the spinal cord (which tend to form nerve plexuses).

Classification of Intercostal Nerves

a. Typical intercostal nerves are the ones that are confined to their own intercostal spaces in the thoracic wall. The third, fourth, fifth and sixth intercostal nerves are the typical nerves.
b. Atypical intercostal nerves extend beyond the thoracic wall for distribution partly or entirely. The first, second and seventh to eleventh intercostal nerves belong to this type. The ventral ramus of first thoracic spinal nerve contributes to the lower trunk of the brachial plexus hence the first intercostal nerve is very small. The lateral cutaneous branch of the second intercostal nerve (intercostobrachial nerve) supplies the skin of the floor of axilla and of medial side of adjacent arm. The seventh to eleventh intercostal nerves (thoraco-abdominal nerves) leave the thoracic wall at the costal margin to enter and supply the anterior abdominal wall.

Communications

Each intercostal nerve communicates with sympathetic ganglion by two branches. The white ramus communicans (WRC) carries preganglionic fibers from the intercostal nerve to the sympathetic ganglion and the gray ramus communicans (GRC) carries postganglionic fibers back to the intercostal nerve from the ganglion (Fig. 4.2). The postganglionic sympathetic fibers supply pilomotor fibers to the arrectores pilorum muscles, sudomotor fibers to the sweat glands and vasomotor for the smooth muscle of the blood vessels in the skin of the area of sensory supply of the intercostal nerve.

Functional Components

The intercostal nerve is composed of four functionally different types of nerve fibers. The general somatic efferent. (GSE) fibers supply the striated muscles. The general somatic afferent (GSA) fibers bring cutaneous sensations to the spinal cord. The general visceral efferent (GVE) fibers are the sympathetic fibers for the supply of the smooth muscle of the skin (arrectores pilorum), sweat glands and the blood vessels of the skin. The general visceral afferent (GVA) fibers bring visceral sensations to the spinal cord.

Typical Intercostal Nerve

The typical intercostal nerve (Fig. 32.1) enters the intercostal space posteriorly at the vertebral end. At first the nerve turns laterally behind the sympathetic trunk. It travels towards the intercostal space between the parietal pleura and the posterior intercostal membrane. The nerve enters the costal groove of the corresponding rib to course laterally and forwards in the neurovascular plane, lying below the intercostal artery. At the sternal (anterior) end of the intercostal space the nerve crosses in front of the internal thoracic artery and pierces the interchondral part of internal intercostal muscle, anterior intercostal membrane and sternocostal origin of pectoralis major muscle. It terminates as anterior cutaneous nerve.

Branches

a. The collateral branch arises from the posterior part of the intercostal nerve before it reaches the angle of the rib. This branch follows the inferior margin of the space in the neurovascular plane (Fig. 33.1) and may rejoin the main trunk. The collateral nerve and the main trunk supply muscular branches to the intercostal muscles and the serratus posterior superior muscle in the back.
b. The lateral cutaneous branch arises from the nerve along with the collateral branch and runs with the main trunk for a small distance and divides in anterior and posterior branches. The posterior branches supply the skin of back overlying the scapula and latissimus dorsi muscle and anterior branches supply the skin overlying the pectoralis major muscle.
c. The sensory branches are given to the parietal pleura and the periosteum of the ribs.
d. The anterior cutaneous nerve supplies the skin of the pectoral region.

Clinical Highlights

a. The intercostal nerve block is given to produce local anesthesia in one or more intercostal spaces by injecting the anesthetic solution around the intercostal nerve near its origin, just lateral to the vertebra.
b. The diseases of the thoracic vertebrae may irritate the intercostal nerves and thereby cause radiating pain in the area of cutaneous distribution of the affected nerves.
c. The pus from the tuberculous thoracic vertebrae may track along the neurovascular plane of the space and point at the sites of emergence of the anterior and lateral cutaneous nerves (lateral margin of sternum and midaxillary line).
d. In herpes zoster (shingles) of the thoracic spinal ganglion the cutaneous vesicles appear in the dermatomal area of the intercostal nerve.
e. Considering the positions of the intercostal and collateral neurovascular bundles in an intercostal space (Fig. 33.1) it is safe to insert a needle midway between the two ribs or a little lower.

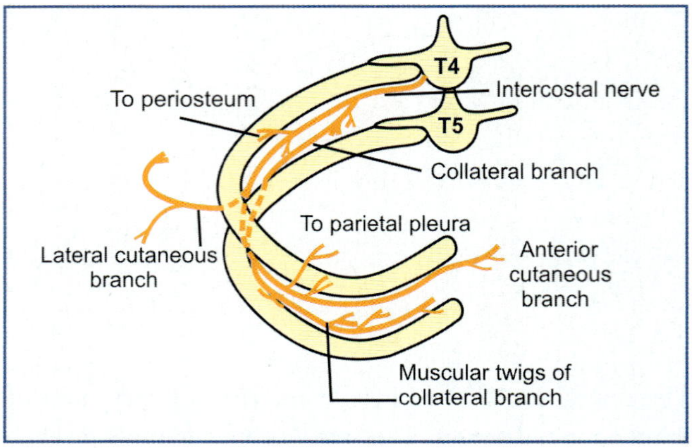

Fig. 33.1: Scheme to depict typical intercostal nerve in fourth intercostal space

Atypical Intercostal Nerves

a. The first intercostal nerve differs from the typical nerve in the following respects. It is the smallest intercostal nerve because a large part of the first thoracic ventral ramus is contributed to the brachial plexus (Fig. 33.2). It gives no collateral or cutaneous branches. It courses along the lower surface of the first rib. The neurovascular structures are arranged as nerve, artery and vein (NAV) from above downward (reverse of VAN arrangement). Due to absence of its cutaneous branches the T1 dermatome is absent on the front of

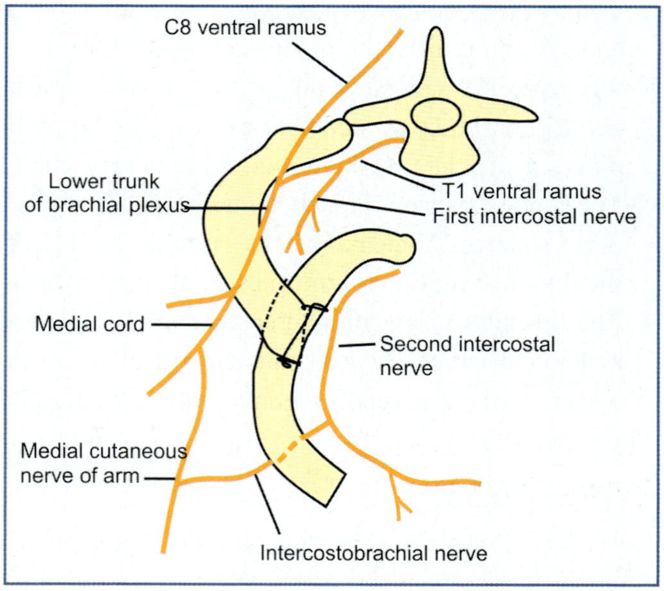

Fig. 33.2: Highly simplified scheme to depict atypical features of first and second intercostal nerves

the chest. Hence, T2 dermatome is placed adjacent to C4 dermatome at the level of sternal angle (Fig. 1.5).

b. The second intercostal nerve differs from the typical nerve in the following respects. Its lateral cutaneous branch enters the axilla as intercostobrachial nerve to join the medial cutaneous nerve of arm and supplies the skin of the floor of axilla and upper medial aspect of arm.

c. The thoracoabdominal nerves are described in Chapter 127 (anterior abdominal wall). During their thoracic course they supply the intercostal muscles of the respective spaces and also give sensory branches to the parietal (costal) pleura. Irritation of these nerves in pleurisy (inflammation of parietal pleura) may cause reflex spasm of anterior abdominal muscles and referred pain to the anterior abdominal wall. Therefore, when a patient complains of pain in the abdominal wall and examination reveals abdominal rigidity, radiograph of chest must be taken to rule out pathology in the pleura.

34 Blood Vessels of Thoracic Wall

The thoracic wall is richly supplied with blood by means of posterior and anterior intercostal arteries. The upper nine intercostal spaces contain three arteries, one posterior intercostal and two anterior intercostal arteries, per space. The lower two spaces being too short and with open anterior ends, contain a single posterior intercostal artery in each space.

Posterior Intercostal Arteries

a. In the upper two intercostal spaces the posterior intercostal arteries are the branches of superior intercostal artery (which in turn is a branch of the costocervical trunk of the subclavian artery).

b. In the lower nine spaces the posterior intercostal arteries arise from the descending thoracic aorta (Figs 34.1 and 51.1). The right posterior intercostal arteries are longer than the left arteries, because the descending aorta lies along the left of the vertebral column. Each posterior intercostal artery enters the posterior end of the intercostal space and travels forward in it lying above the nerve and below the vein (VAN) in the neurovascular plane. Near the angle of the rib it gives off a collateral branch. Towards the anterior end of the space the main arterial trunk anastomoses with the upper anterior intercostal artery, while its collateral branch anastomoses with the lower anterior intercostal artery.

Anterior Intercostal Arteries

a. In the upper six spaces the anterior intercostal arteries are the branches of internal thoracic artery on each side (Fig 34.3).

b. In the seventh to ninth spaces the anterior intercostal arteries are the branches of musculophrenic artery on each side.

c. The tenth and eleventh spaces do not have anterior intercostal arteries. The posterior intercostal arteries of these spaces enter the anterior abdominal wall because these short spaces are open anteriorly.

The upper and lower anterior intercostal arteries in each of the upper nine spaces pass laterally and backwards along the upper and lower margins of the respective spaces. At the junction of anterior one-third and posterior two-thirds of each space the main trunk of the posterior intercostal artery anastomoses with the upper anterior intercostal branch while the collateral artery anastomoses with the lower anterior intercostal branch. The free anastomoses between anterior and posterior intercostal arteries establish communications between the first part of subclavian artery and the descending thoracic aorta. In a condition of narrowing of the arch of aorta (coarctation) distal to the origin of left subclavian artery, the blood is filled in the descending aorta via these intercostal anastomoses.

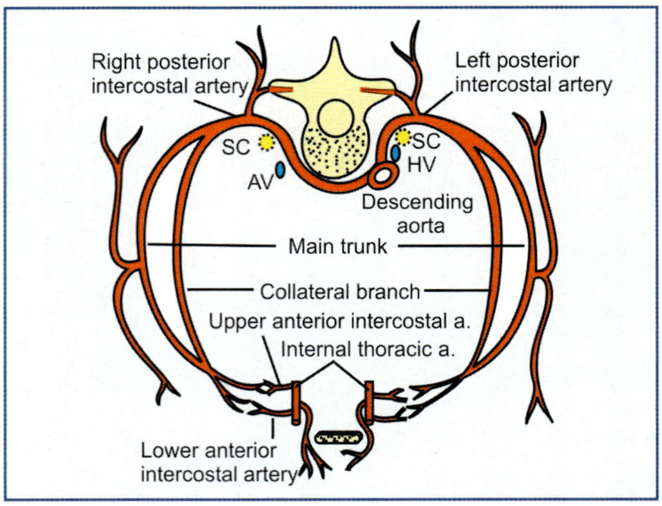

Fig. 34.1: Anastomoses of intercostal arteries in upper six intercostal spaces. SC-Sympathetic chain, AV-Azygos vein, HV-Hemiazygos vein

Intercostal Veins

a. The anterior intercostal veins of the upper six spaces drain into the internal thoracic vein, and those of succeeding three spaces into the musculophrenic vein.
b. The posterior intercostal veins reach the vertebral end of the intercostal spaces and receive intervertebral veins from the internal vertebral venous plexus. Their mode of termination on the two sides is different with the exception of highest intercostal vein (Fig. 34.2).
   i. The first or highest intercostal vein on the right side opens in right brachiocephalic vein and on the left it opens in the left brachiocephalic vein.
   ii. The veins of second and third spaces unite to form left superior intercostal vein, which opens in left brachiocephalic vein. The right superior intercostal vein is formed by the union of second, third and fourth posterior intercostal veins and it opens in arch of the azygos vein.
   iii. The veins of the remaining spaces open in vertical part of azygos vein on the right side. However, on the left side, the veins of the fourth to seventh spaces often into accessory hemiazygos vein (superior hemiazygos vein) and those from the eighth to eleventh spaces open into inferior hemiazygos vein.

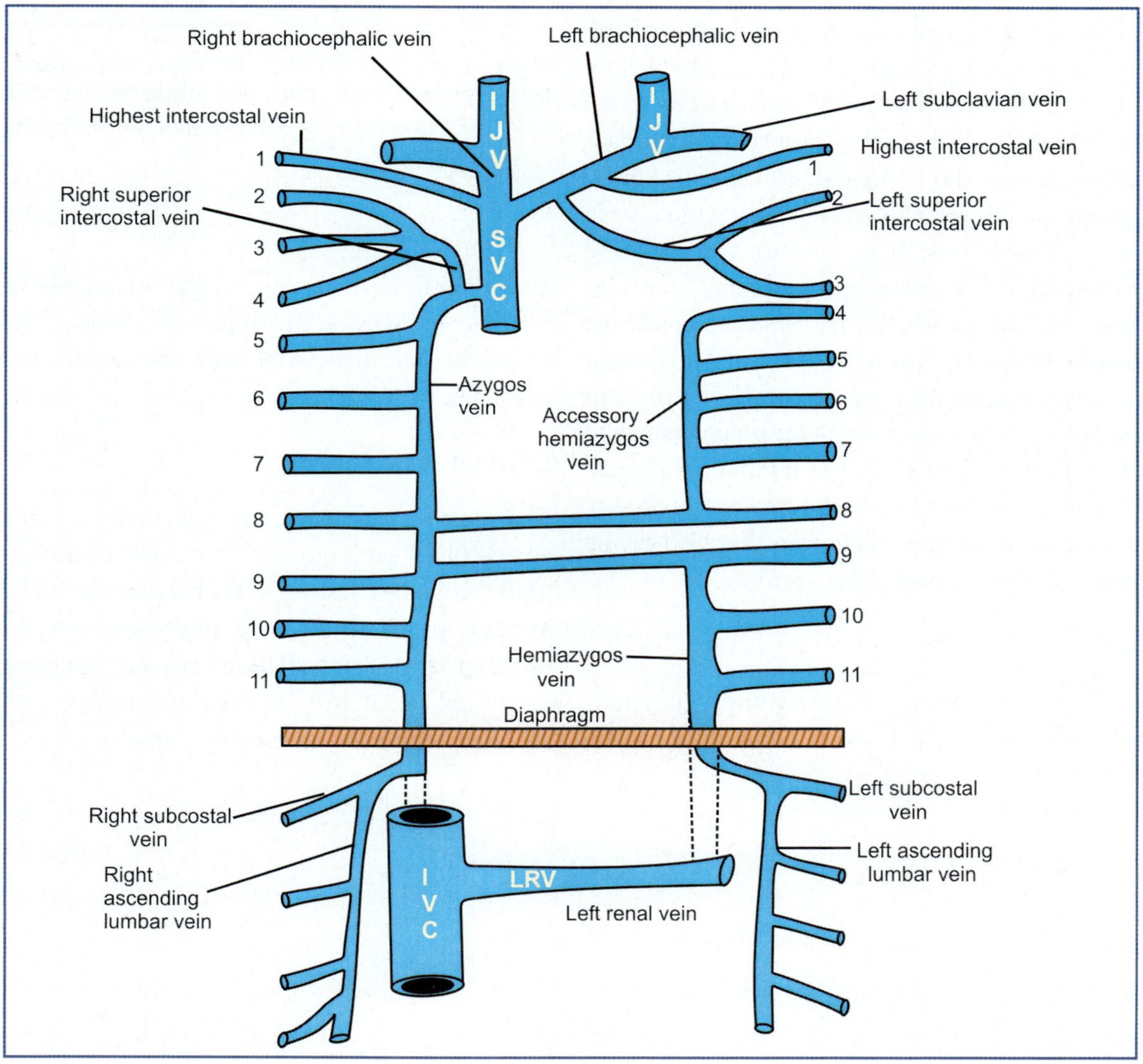

Fig. 34.2: Simplified scheme to depict veins of thoracic wall

Lymphatic Drainage of Intercostal Spaces

The intercostal and parasternal (internal mammary nodes) are the two groups of lymph nodes that drain the soft and hard tissues of the intercostal space. The intercostal nodes are located in the posterior part of the intercostal spaces near the heads of the ribs. The parasternal nodes form longitudinal chains along the course of internal mammary (thoracic) artery.

Internal Mammary or Internal Thoracic Artery

The internal mammary artery (Fig. 34.3) is a branch of the first part of the subclavian artery in the root of the neck. It descends behind the medial end of the clavicle and the upper six costal cartilages about one cm from the margin of the sternum. Upto the level of third cartilage the artery is closely related to the costal pleura but below this the sternocostalis muscle intervenes between it and the pleura. The artery is crossed anteriorly by the upper six intercostal nerves and is separated from the skin by internal intercostal muscle, external intercostal membrane and pectoralis major muscle. It ends in the sixth intercostal space by dividing into superior epigastric and musculophrenic arteries. The venae commitantes accompany the internal mammary artery up to the level of third costal cartilage. Above this level the venae comitantes unite to form a single vein, which opens in to the brachiocephalic vein of the corresponding side. The internal mammary artery in female, supplies the breast. It may be necessary to locate the artery for safe ligation in the third or the second intercostal space during mastectomy.

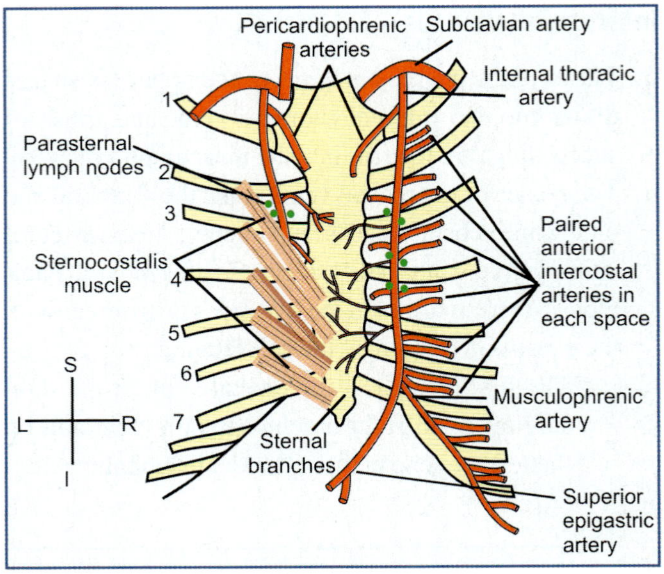

Fig. 34.3: Internal thoracic (mammary) artery viewed from inner aspect of anterior thoracic wall (Note that sternocostalis is shown only on left side and perforating cutaneous branches are not labeled)

Branches

The branches of the internal mammary artery are, pericardiacophrenic, pericardial, thymic, mediastinal, sternal and perforating. It also gives a pair of anterior intercostal arteries per space in the upper six spaces. The superior epigastric and musculophrenic arteries are its terminal branches.

Clinical Highlights

The internal mammary artery is favored over other vessels as a coronary graft (Fig. 46.3) because internal mammary grafts are longer lasting. It is observed that these arteries are less prone to develop atherosclerosis due to the histological peculiarity of their wall (containing elastic tissue only) and peculiarity of their endothelial cells, which secrete chemicals that prevent atherosclerosis.

35 Development of Respiratory System

The development of lungs is intimately associated with the development of the pleural cavities. The intraembryonic coelom divides to form the pleural, pericardial, and peritoneal cavities. It is a horseshoe-shaped space enclosed in splanchnopleuric and somatopleuric layers. Its midline part is the future pericardial cavity and the two tubular parts are the forerunners of the peritoneal cavity. The narrow connections between the above two parts are called the pericardioperitoneal canals (future pleural cavities).

Partition between Pericardial and Pleural Cavities

The lung bud invaginates the pericardio-peritoneal canal of its side and expands in all directions forming a double-layered pleural cavity. The splanchnopleuric layer forms the visceral pleura and the somatopleuric layer forms the parietal pleura. The right and left pleuro-pericardial membranes develop from the body wall mesoderm. The membranes elongate with the expansion of the lung buds and finally fuse with each other. This results in complete partitioning of the pericardial cavity from the right and left pleural cavities. The membranes give rise to the fibrous pericardium except its base, which develops from the septum transversum.

Partition between Pleural and Peritoneal Cavities

The communication between the pleural and peritoneal cavities is closed by the development of right and left pleuro-peritoneal folds from the body wall mesoderm. These folds extend medially and fuse with the septum transversum and the dorsal mesentery of the esophagus. In this way peritoneal cavity is separated from the pleural cavities.

Laryngotracheal Tube

A laryngotracheal groove appears in the floor of the caudal end of the pharynx (cranial end of foregut) at fourth week of intrauterine life (Fig.35.1). As this groove deepens and elongates in caudal direction, it is separated from the cranial end of the foregut by formation of a tracheo-esophageal septum. Thus, the laryngotracheal tube is formed from the endoderm of foregut. It gives rise to the epithelium of larynx, trachea, bronchi, bronchioles and alveoli of the lungs. The splanchnopleuric mesoderm forms the connective tissue, smooth muscle and cartilage of the respiratory passages. The cranial end of the tube forms the larynx, the succeeding part develops into trachea and the caudal end bifurcates to develop into bronchi and lungs.

Development of Bronchial Tree and Lungs

The caudal end of the laryngotracheal tube divides into right and left lung buds (Fig. 35.1). Each lung bud invaginates the medial wall of the pericardio-peritoneal canal (Fig. 35.2) of the respective side and undergoes repeated divisions. The development of the lung and bronchial tree takes place in three stages.

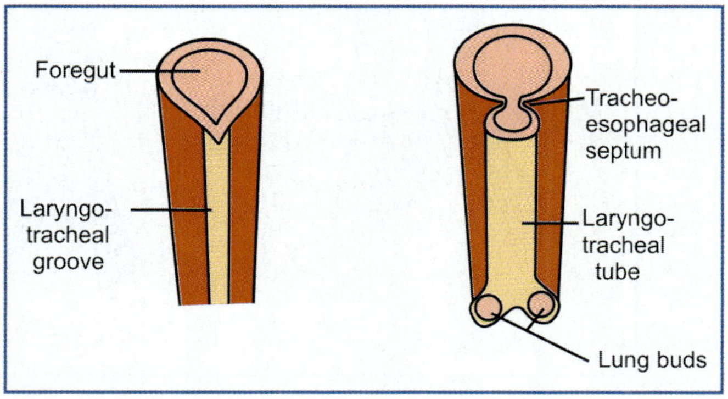

Fig. 35.1: Formation of laryngotracheal tube and lung buds

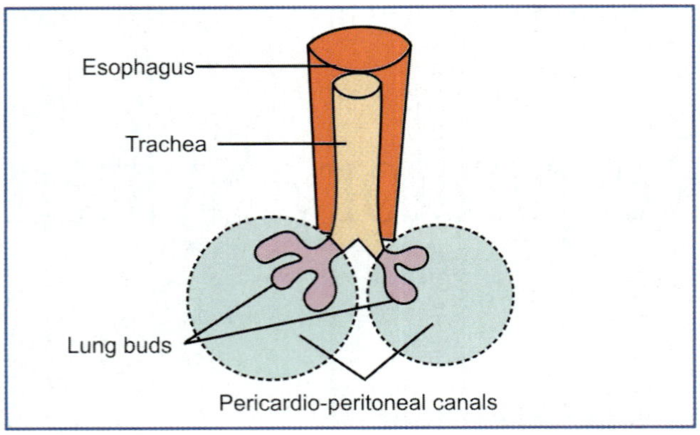

Fig. 35.2: Invagination of lung buds into pericardio-peritoneal canals

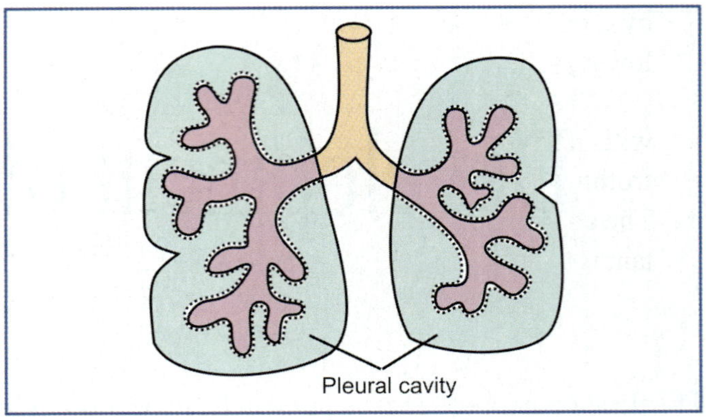

Fig. 35.3: Glandular phase of developing at 8 weeks of intrauterine life

a. The glandular phase (Fig. 35.3) lasting upto sixteen weeks is characterized by development of solid tubular outgrowths (resembling the ducts of a gland) of the lung bud.
b. The canalicular phase lasting from sixteen weeks to twenty-six weeks is characterized by rapid proliferation of the ducts, which gradually acquire lumina. The blood vessels proliferate and establish contacts with the canalized ducts.
c. The alveolar phase extends from twenty-six weeks to birth and continues postnatally until the age of eight years. From the seventh month of intrauterine life, the alveoli start differentiating. Many alveoli establish close contact with capillary endothelium. The alveolar cells become squamous type but a few retain their cuboidal shape and acquire secretory properties, an indication of surfactant production. With the onset of these structural and functional changes, the developing lungs are capable of normal function, thus increasing the chances of the fetus to survive, if born prematurely. Before birth, the alveoli are filled with amniotic fluid containing a small quantity of mucin and surfactant. Because of this the lungs sink in water. At the first breath after birth, the lung fluid is absorbed or expelled from respiratory passages and the lungs are filled with air. Hence, after the first breath the lungs float in water. The alveoli are prevented from collapse by the surfactant.

Congenital Anomalies

a. Tracheo-esophageal fistula (TEF) is a common anomaly, in which there is communication between trachea and esophagus. This is due to incomplete or defective tracheo-esophageal septation accompanied

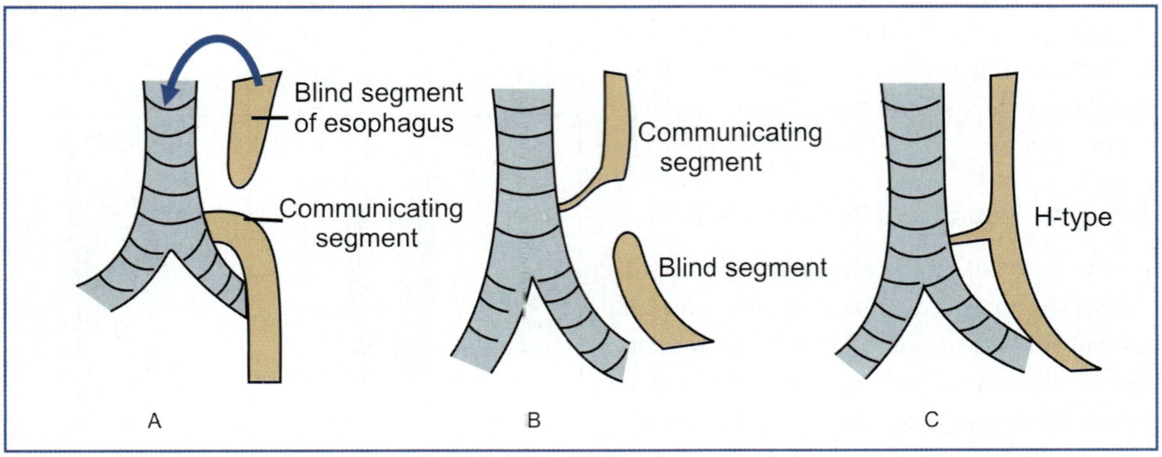

Fig. 35.4: Types of tracheo-esophageal fistulae (TEF). A is the most common type of TEF. It leads to chemical pneumonitis in newborn

by esophageal atresia. In about 90 percent of TEF the lower segment of esophagus opens into the trachea (Fig. 35.4) closer to its termination. A newborn baby with this type of TEF will present with excessive frothing and choking with first feed.

b. The absence of or inadequate secretion of the surfactant is the cause of collapse of alveoli after birth. This is one of the causes of death in neonatal period (respiratory distress syndrome).

c. The apex of right lung may be divided by the pleural fold carrying the azygos vein in its bottom. The medial part of the divided apex is called lobe of the azygos vein. This may cast a shadow in the lung apex in the radiograph, which may be mistaken for disease.

36 Mediastinum

The mediastinum is a midline, narrow and elongated space (containing many structures including heart and great vessels) between the right and left pleural cavities. Since it intervenes between the pleural cavities it is also described as a partition. Its boundaries are, anteriorly sternum, posteriorly thoracic vertebrae and on each side the mediastinal pleura (Fig. 36.1). The mediastinum extends from the inlet of thorax to the diaphragm (Fig. 36.2). It is connected to the lung on each side by the root of the lung.

Subdivisions (Fig. 36.2)

The mediastinum is broadly divided into superior and inferior parts by means of an imaginary line passing through the manubrio-sternal joint and the disc between T4 and T5 vertebrae. The inferior mediastinum is further subdivided into anterior, middle and posterior parts.

Superior Mediastinum

It is the space that lies behind the manubrium sterni and in front of the upper four thoracic vertebrae. Its upper limit is the thoracic inlet and lower limit is the plane passing through the disc between the fourth and fifth thoracic vertebrae. On each side it is bounded by mediastinal pleura.

Contents of Superior Mediastinum (Fig. 36.3)

a. The sternohyoid and sternothyroid muscles originate from the back of manubrium and the longus colli muscle is present on the front of upper thoracic vertebrae.
b. The arch of aorta and its branches (left subclavian, left common carotid and brachiocephalic).
c. The veins are, the superior vena cava, right and left brachiocephalic veins and the terminal part of azygos vein. The left superior intercostal vein courses upwards to open into the left brachiocephalic vein.

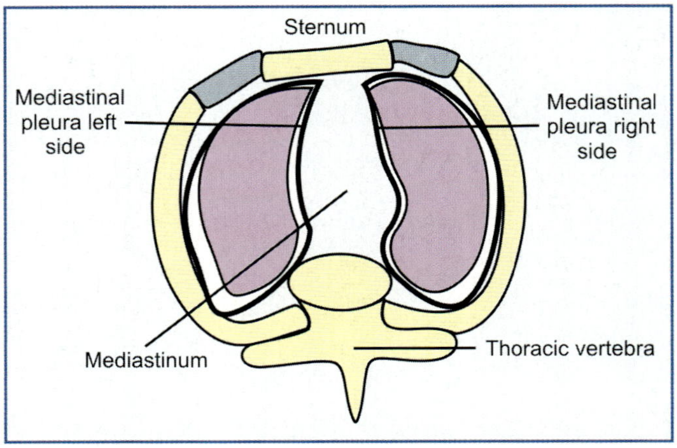

Fig. 36.1: Boundaries of mediastinum as seen in crosssection of thoracic cavity

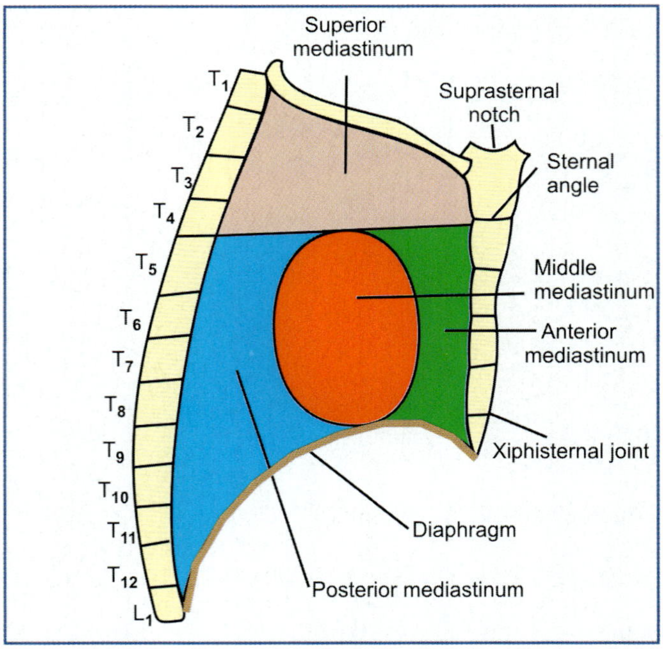

Fig. 36.2: Subdivisions of mediastinum

d. The remnant of the thymus is usually present.
e. The nerves on the right side are the right vagus and the right phrenic nerves and on the left side are the

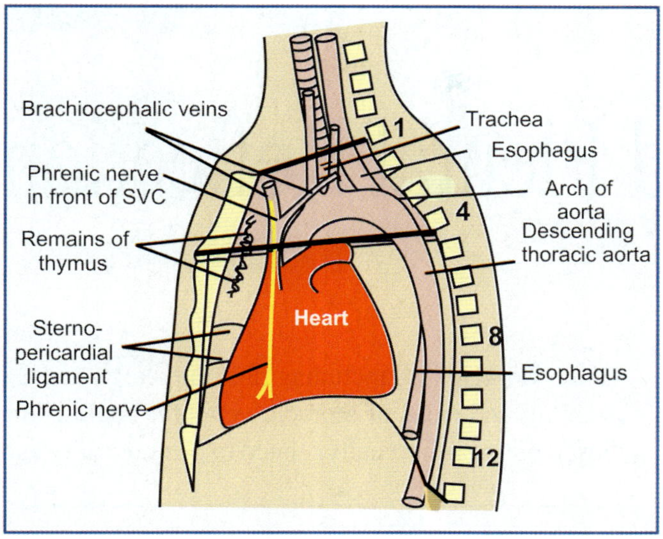

Fig. 36.3: Scheme to show a few contents of mediastinal subdivisions in lateral view

left vagus, left phrenic and left recurrent laryngeal nerves.

f. The esophagus and trachea enter from the neck and the thoracic duct passes through the posterior mediastinum and the superior mediastinum to the neck.
g. Lymph nodes.

Anterior Mediastinum

The anterior mediastinum is a narrow space that lies posterior to the body of sternum and in front of the fibrous pericardium. The diaphragm limits it below and its upper limit is upto the level of sternal angle, where it becomes continuous with superior mediastinum. Its contents are, the sternopericardial ligaments, remains of thymus, lymph nodes and areolar tissue.

Middle Mediastinum

The middle mediastinum lies between the anterior, superior and posterior mediastinal spaces. Inferiorly it is limited by the diaphragm and laterally by the mediastinal pleura and the root of the lung on each side. Its contents are, the pericardium, heart and the pulmonary vessels, tracheal bifurcation, terminal bronchi, phrenic nerves and the deep cardiac plexus.

Posterior Mediastinum

The anterior boundary is by the tracheal bifurcation, pulmonary vessels, and fibrous pericardium while the lower eight thoracic vertebrae lie posteriorly. On each side there is mediastinal pleura. The posterior mediastinum gives passage to the esophagus, descending thoracic aorta, azygos and hemiazygos veins, thoracic duct and the vagi. Lymph nodes are scattered along the esophagus. The splanchnic nerves from the sympathetic chain (which lies outside the limits of the mediastinum, behind the costal pleura) enter the posterior mediastinum.

Clinical Highlights

a. The mediastinal contents may be compressed due to a space-occupying lesion producing diverse signs and symptoms (mediastinal syndrome). For example, an enlarged lymph node in superior mediastinum may compress on the trachea, esophagus and the left recurrent laryngeal nerve resulting in symptoms like difficulty in breathing, difficulty in swallowing and hoarseness of voice respectively.
b. The mediastinal shift is an indication of lung pathology. The mediastinum shifts to the affected side due to appreciable reduction in lung volume and decrease in intrapleural pressure as happens in atelectesis or collapse of lung. On the contrary, in pneumothorax or hydrothorax, the mediastinum shifts towards the normal side (Fig. 37.4) because of the high pleural pressure on the affected side. Mediastinal shift is detected by palpating the trachea in the suprasternal fossa.
c. Mediastinitis is the inflammation of the loose connective tissue of the mediastinum. It usually occurs when deep infections of the neck spread downwards along the fascial continuity between the two regions (Fig. 39.2).
d. Mediastinoscopy is a diagnostic procedure used to obtain biopsy of lymph node in the superior mediastinum by introducing mediastinoscope through a small incision placed just above the suprasternal notch.
e. In the lateral or oblique radiographs of thorax, the heart shadow representing the middle mediastinum lies above the anterior part of the diaphragm. The retrosternal space representing the anterior mediastinum lies in front of the cardiac shadow. The retrocardiac space, which is equivalent to posterior mediastinum, is seen between the heart and the vertebral column. This space is occupied by the descending thoracic aorta and the esophagus.

Pleura and Pleural Reflection

37

The pleura is a smooth shining serous membrane that covers the lungs. It is divisible in two parts, visceral and parietal. The visceral pleura covers the lung surface and gives it a glistening appearance. The pleura that lines the internal surfaces of the thoracic walls, is called the parietal pleura. The visceral and the parietal layers of the pleura are continuous with each other along the root of the lung and at the pulmonary ligament, which extends downwards from the hilum as a double-layered pleural fold. The pleural cavity is a potential space enclosed between the visceral and parietal pleura and contains a small amount of serous fluid.

Visceral Pleura

The visceral pleura dips into the fissures of the lungs. It is inseparable from the lung tissue. It shares the blood supply and nerve supply (autonomic nerves) with that of the lungs and is insensitive to pain. It develops from splanchnopleuric mesoderm.

Parietal Pleura

The parietal pleura is more extensive than the visceral pleura. It is supported on its external surface by a thick layer of endothoracic fascia. The parietal pleura develops from somatopleuric mesoderm hence is supplied by somatic nerves and is pain sensitive

Subdivisions of Parietal Pleura (Fig. 37.1)

It is subdivided into four parts depending on the location, costal (costovertebral) pleura, mediastinal pleura, diaphragmatic pleura and cervical pleura or dome of pleura. These different parts are continuous with each other along the lines of pleural reflection.

a. The costal pleura covers the anterior, lateral and posterior aspects of the lung. It lines the inner aspect of the thoracic wall including ribs, intercostal spaces, sternum and sides of thoracic vertebral bodies. The costal pleura is internally related to pleural cavity and

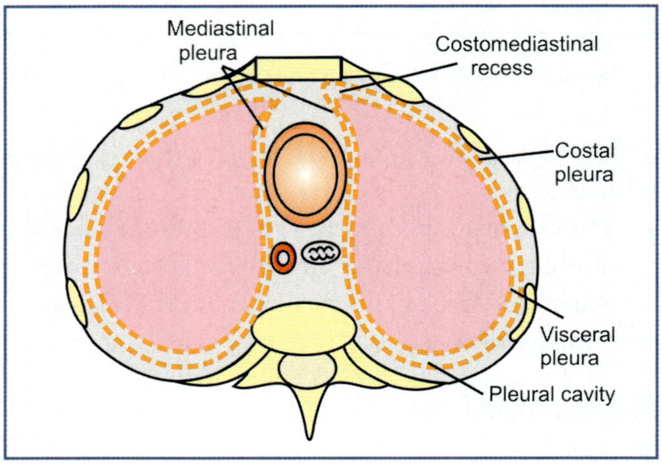

Fig. 37.1A: A scheme to show pleural cavity and costomediastinal recess in cross-section

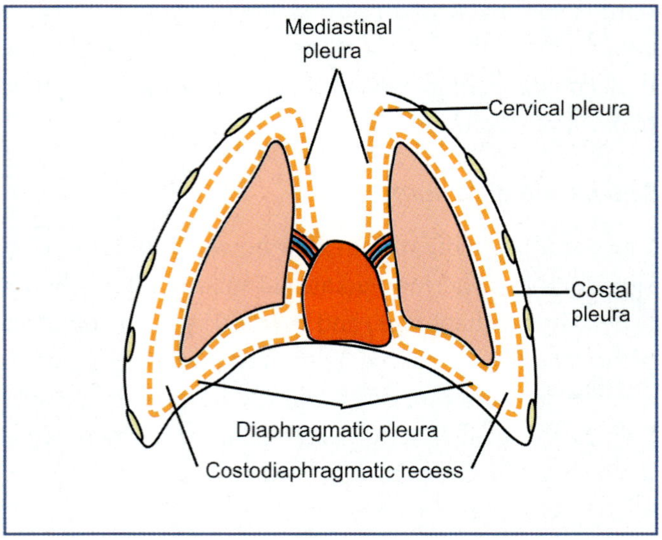

Fig. 37.1B: Pleural cavity and costodiaphragmatic recesses. (Note: The continuity of visceral and mediastinal pleura at hilum of lung)

visceral pleura. Its external surface is covered by endothoracic fascia. Anteriorly, the internal thoracic vessels directly rest on the pleura in the first intercostal space. Its other anterior relations are the sternum, costal cartilages, ribs and intercostal muscles. Posteriorly it is related to the sympathetic chain and its branches. At the posterior end of the intercostal space the intercostal nerve lies between the costal pleura and the posterior intercostal membrane.

b. The mediastinal pleura comes in contact with the structures in the corresponding side of the mediastinum since it covers the anterior part of the medial surface of the lung. It encloses the structures inside the lung root and becomes continuous with the visceral pleura at the hilum of lung. It extends below the lung hilum as pulmonary ligament, which is a connecting bond between the mediastinum and the medial surface of the lung below the hilum.
c. The diaphragmatic pleura covers the superior surface of diaphragm. It is related superiorly to the base of the lung, which is separated by the pleural cavity.
d. Above the level of inner margin of first rib, the costal pleura becomes the cervical pleura. It enters the root of the neck to cover the apex of the lung. It extends posteriorly up to the neck of first rib, which is at a higher level compared to the rest of the first rib. The cervical pleura is protected by suprapleural membrane or Sibson's fascia (Fig. 38.4), which extends from the tip of transverse process of seventh cervical vertebra to the inner margin of first rib. The subclavian vessels and the scalenus anterior muscle are related to it anteriorly. The sympathetic chain, superior intercostal artery and ventral ramus of first thoracic spinal nerve (Fig. 30.1) are its posterior relations (same as those of the apex of the lung).

Surface Marking of Lines of Pleural Reflections

Anteriorly, the costal pleura become continuous with the mediastinal pleura at the back of the sternum along the costo-mediastinal line of pleural reflection (Fig. 37.2). Inferiorly, the costal pleura is continuous with the diaphragmatic pleura along the costo-diaphragmatic line of pleural reflection (Fig. 37.3). Posteriorly, the costal pleura is continuous with the mediastinal pleura by the side of the vertebral column along the costo-vertebral line

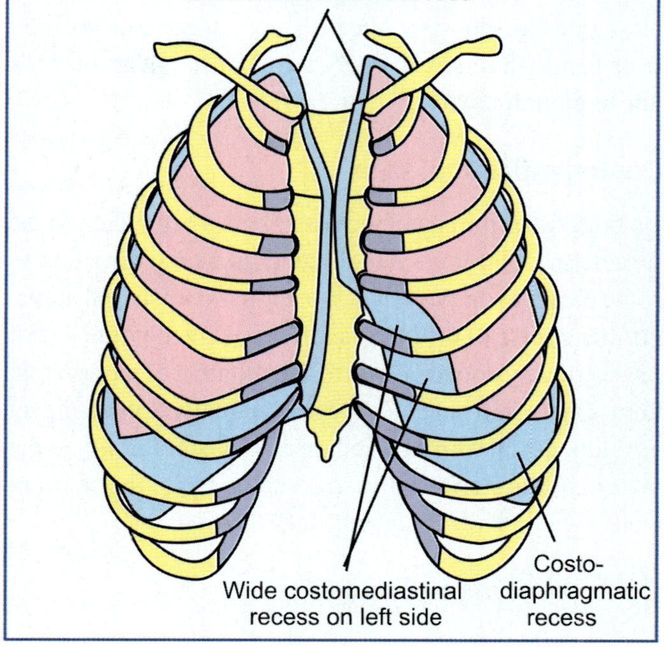

Fig. 37.2: Lines of pleural reflection in relation to thoracic cage as seen from anterior aspect (Note that pleura crosses right costoxiphoid angle but not the left)

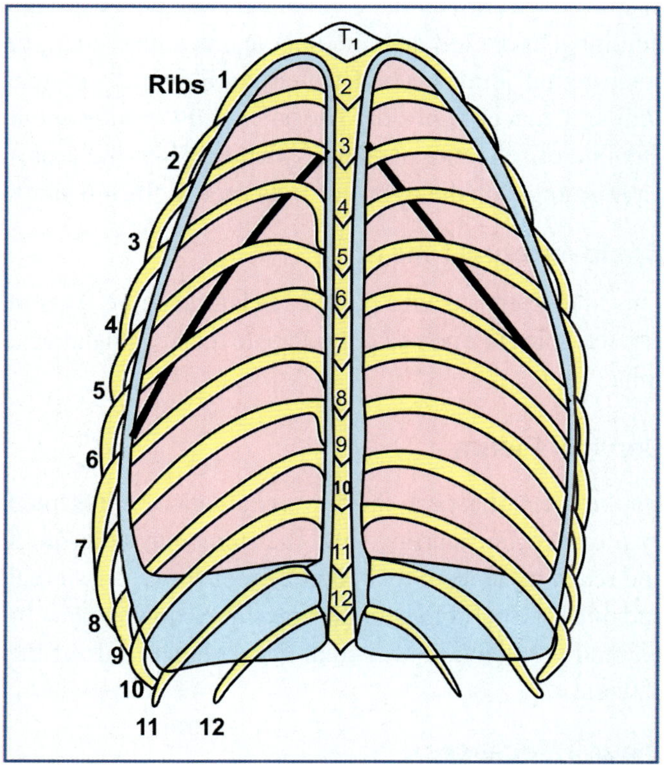

Fig. 37.3: Lines of pleural reflection in relation to thoracic cage as seen from posterior aspect

Section two

of pleural reflection (Fig. 37.3). The surface marking of these lines is important because any puncture or incision at or inside the lines is likely to result in pneumothorax (air in pleural cavity).

Costomediastinal Line

On both sides, the costomediastinal lines begin behind the sternoclavicular joint and descend in medial direction to come closer to each other at the midpoint of sternal angle. Further course of the lines is different. On the right side it runs vertically downward up to the midpoint of xiphisternal joint. On the left side it descends vertically upto the level of fourth costal cartilage and then deviates laterally to the margin of the sternum and descends close to the sternum up to the left sixth costal cartilage.

Costodiaphragmatic Line

On the right side the costodiaphragmatic line begins at the midpoint of xiphisternal joint and turns laterally along the seventh costal cartilage to reach the eighth rib in the midclavicular line, tenth rib in the midaxillary line, and twelfth rib in the scapular line to finally end at the level of spine of twelfth thoracic vertebra about 2 cm from the midline. On the left side the line begins at the left sixth costosternal joint, beyond which it follows the course similar to that of right side. The noteworthy feature about this line of reflection is that it extends below the costoxiphoid angle on the right side only (not on the left side).

Costovertebral Line

This line extends from a point 2 cm lateral to the seventh cervical spine to a point 2 cm. lateral to the twelfth thoracic spine.

Cervical Pleura

On the anterior aspect, the cervical pleura is represented by a curved line starting from the sternoclavicular joint and reaching upward to a point 2.5 cm above the sternal end of clavicle. From here the line curves down to meet a point at the junction of medial and middle thirds of the clavicle.

Pleural Recesses

The pleural recesses are the extensions of the pleural cavities along the lines of pleural reflections. These spaces are unoccupied by lung during quiet breathing. The recesses are present because the pleural cavities are larger than the lung volumes. They are present at two locations.

a. The costomediastinal recesses (Fig. 37.1A) are present along the costomediastinal lines of pleural reflection. Along this line the anterior margin of the lung does not coincide with the acute anterior margin of the pleural cavity. Thus, this recess is limited by junctional parts of the costal and mediastinal pleurae. The right recess is very narrow and of uniform size. The left recess, however, is wide at the level of fourth to sixth costal cartilages. The deviation of the anterior margin of the lung (due to the presence of cardiac notch) is much more compared to that of the pleural line, at this site. The left costomediastinal recess is responsible for the presence of the area of superficial cardiac dullness. Except for the wider part of the left recess the rest of the costomediastinal recesses are filled with lung during deep inspiration.
b. The costodiaphragmatic recesses (Fig. 37.1B) are present along the costodiaphragmatic lines of pleural reflection. Along this line the lower margin of the pleura is two-rib distance below the lower margin of the lung. This recess is limited by the costal and diaphragmatic pleurae and is unoccupied by the lung in quiet breathing. In deep inspiration, however the recesses of both sides are partially filled. The right recess is related to the liver and posterior surface of right kidney and the left recess to the fundus of the stomach, spleen and posterior surface of the left kidney. The costo-diaphragmatic recess being the most dependent part of the pleural cavity shows widening in the radiograph, when a small quantity of fluid accumulates in it. This may be the first indication of fluid in the pleural cavity. Therefore, these recesses are examined routinely in the radiographs of the chest. In posterior approach to the kidney while removing a section of the twelfth rib, care should be taken not to injure the inferior margin of pleura in relation to the twelfth rib.

Nerve Supply and Blood Supply of Pleura

The visceral pleura is insensitive to pain due to its autonomic nerve supply. It receives blood from the bronchial arteries. The parietal pleura, being supplied by somatic nerves is sensitive to painful stimuli. The pain is referred to the thoracic and abdominal walls or to the neck and shoulder. The costal pleura receives twigs from intercostal nerves. The peripheral part of diaphragmatic pleura receives branches from the intercostal nerves and its central part from the phrenic nerves. The mediastinal pleura is supplied by the phrenic nerve. The arterial supply is derived from the intercostal and internal mammary arteries.

Functional Importance of Pleural Cavity

When the lungs expand and contract during normal breathing, they slide back and forth within the pleural cavity. To facilitate this a thin film of fluid is present inside the pleural cavity. The mesothelial cells of the serous membrane secrete a small quantity of interstitial fluid continuously into the pleural space. The total amount of fluid is kept at the minimal level by a unique method of pumping out the excess fluid by lymphatic vessels. This mechanism of continuous turnover of the fluid is responsible for maintaining the cavity as a potential space and for maintaining the negative pressure in the pleural cavity, which is necessary to retain the visceral pleura in contact with the parietal pleura. If there is positive pressure in the pleural cavity (pneumothorax) the inherent elastic recoil of the lung tissue pulls the visceral pleura away from the parietal pleura causing collapse of the lung.

Clinical Highlights

a. Pleurisy (pleuritis) is inflammation of the parietal pleura. It gives rise to pain, which is aggravated by respiratory movements and is radiated to thoracic and abdominal walls. Inflammation of pleura by tuberculous bacilli is quite common in India.
b. Pneumothorax means air in the pleural space. Air may enter the pleural cavity as a result of penetrating injuries of thorax, tear of visceral or parietal pleura or inadvertent puncture of pleural cavity by the clinician while drawing fluid from the cavity. The primary effect of pneumothorax is the collapse of lung on the affected side. The collapsed lung is not able to oxygenate blood. Lowering of O_2 tension in blood gives rise to shortness of breath and cyanosis. The mediastium shifts to the normal side compressing the normal lung also.
c. Pleural effusion means excess fluid in pleural cavity. This condition gives rise to dullness on percussion and reduction in the intensity of the breath sounds. Due to the collapse of the lung on the affected side the mediastinum shifts to the normal side, which can be confirmed by shift of the trachea (Fig. 37.4). Fluid level can be confirmed by radiographic examination. If there is watery fluid in the pleural cavity it is called

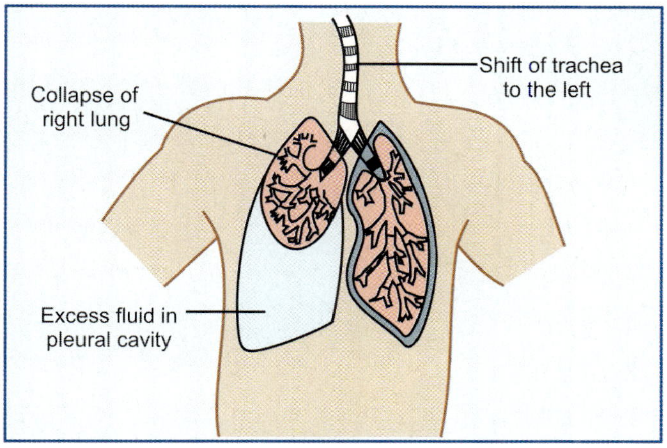

Fig. 37.4: Pleural effusion on right side

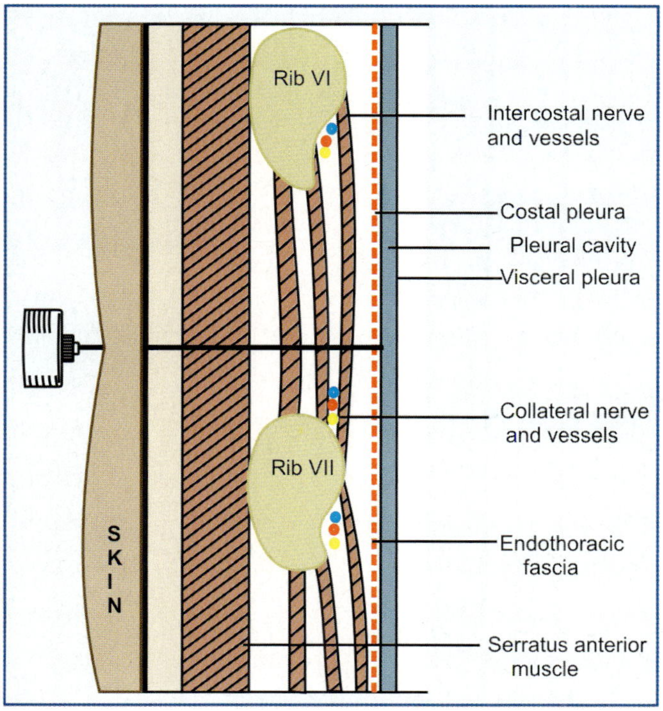

Fig. 37.5: Layers of thoracic wall pierced in succession by the needle during pleural tapping along posterior axillary line. Note VAN arrangement of neurovascular bundles in intercostal space

Section two

hydrothorax. Accumulation of pus is called pyothorax, of blood is known as hemothorax and of lymph is called chylothorax.

d. The thoracocentesis or pleural tap is done to remove excess fluid from the pleural cavity. This is performed with the patient in sitting position. Usually the needle is inserted in the posterior axillary line or the midaxillary line through the lower part of fifth or sixth intercostal space. The needle passes in succession the skin, fasciae, serratus anterior, intercostal muscles, endothoracic fascia and the costal pleura before entering the pleural cavity (Fig. 37.5).

38 Lungs

Each lung lies free in its own pleural cavity, attached to the mediastinum only by its root and the pulmonary ligament. The lungs of the children are pink in color unlike in the adult, where deposition of carbon particles (inhaled from atmospheric air) imparts grayish black color to the lungs. During life the lungs are soft, elastic and spongy. Being air-filled they float on water. The lungs of the new-born before the first breath sink in water.

Gross Features

Each lung is conical in shape with a rounded apex and a broad base (Fig. 38.1). It has costal and medial surfaces. The medial surface is subdivided into, anterior larger and concave mediastinal surface and posterior smaller vertebral surface. The mediastinal surface bears the hilum of the lung. The sharp anterior border separates the mediastinal and costal surfaces. The rounded posterior border separates the vertebral and costal surfaces and the inferior border intervenes between the base and other two surfaces.

External Features of Right and Left Lungs

a. The weight of the right lung is 600 gm and that of left lung is 550 gm. The right lung is broader and shorter than the left lung because the massive liver pushes the right dome of the diaphragm upwards.
b. The oblique and horizontal fissures divide the right lung in three lobes (upper, middle and lower) while the oblique fissure divides the left lung in two lobes (upper and lower).
c. The anterior margin of the right lung is sharp and straight. The anterior margin of left lung is sharp but not straight as it presents a cardiac notch and a projecting lingula below it.
d. The relations of the structures at the hilum on the two lungs are different (Fig. 38.2). The structures from above downwards in the right lung are, eparterial bronchus, pulmonary artery, hyparterial bronchus and inferior pulmonary vein and in the left lung, pulmonary artery, principal bronchus and inferior pulmonary vein.

However, none of these differences is reliable in assigning side to an isolated lung. For identification of the side of the lung it is held in anatomical position (as if it belongs to the holder's own body) with the help of apex and base, borders and surfaces.

Surface Markings of Fissures (Fig. 38.3)

a. The oblique fissure is marked by a line passing downward and forward, which starts at the posterior aspect about 2 cm lateral to the spine of third thoracic vertebra. The line crosses the fifth rib in the mid-axillary line and reaches the sixth costal cartilage 7-8 cm lateral to the mid-line (or at the sixth costochondral junction).

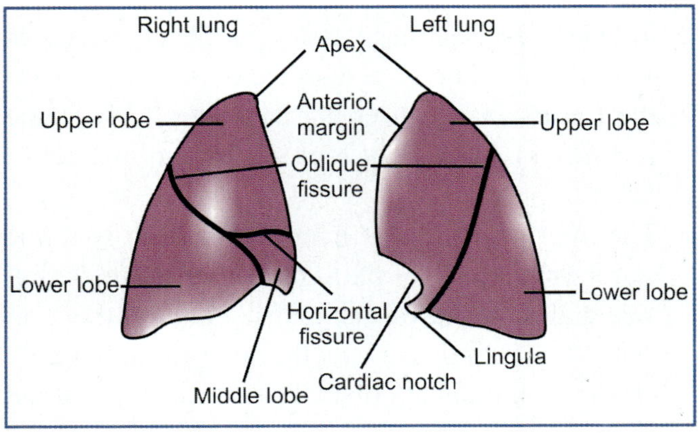

Fig. 38.1: Lobes and fissures of lungs viewed from anterior aspect. Note that lingula belongs to upper lobe of left lung

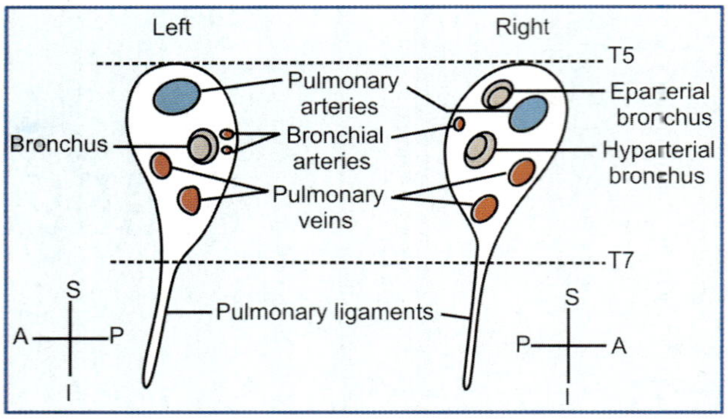

Fig. 38.2: Relationship of structures at hilum of right lung and left lung. Note the vertebral level of the hilum

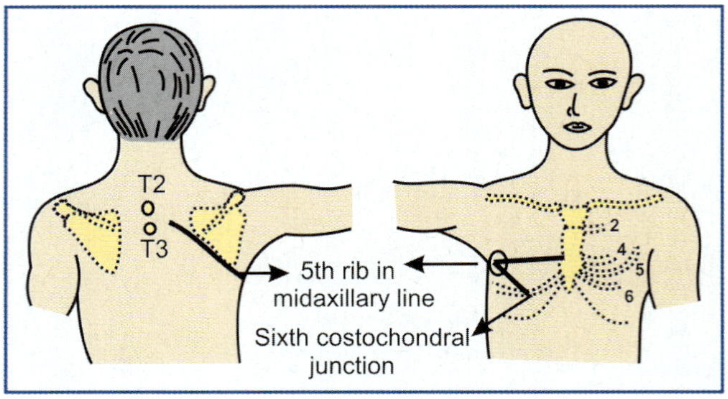

Fig. 38.3: Surface marking of fissures of right lung. Oblique fissure is drawn on both posterior and anterior aspects while horizontal fissure is drawn on anterior aspect alone. Note that the arm is abducted to 90°

Roughly, the oblique fissure corresponds to the medial border of the scapula in the fully abducted position of the arm.

b. The horizontal fissure runs along the level of the right fourth costal cartilage and rib to meet the oblique fissure in the midaxillary line.

Surface Marking of Lung

a. The summit of the apex of the lung is about 2 5 cm above the medial end of the clavicle. It is 3-4 cm above the sternal end of the first rib but does not extend above the neck of first rib.
b. The anterior margin of right lung coincides with the costo-mediastinal line of pleural reflection. The anterior margin of left lung coincides with the costo-mediastinal line of pleural reflection up to the level of fourth costal cartilage. Below this level, it deviates from the mid-line for a distance of 3.5 cm between the fourth and sixth costal cartilages (due to the presence of cardiac notch on the anterior margin of lung).
c. The inferior margin of lung is indicated by a line starting at the level of sixth costal cartilage on the left side and midpoint of the xiphisternum on the right side. Traced further it cuts the sixth rib in the mid-clavicular line, eighth rib in the mid-axillary line and tenth rib in the scapular line.
d. The posterior margin of lung extends vertically upwards from the transverse process of the tenth thoracic vertebra to a point lateral to the spine of the seventh cervical vertebra.

Auscultation Sites

In order to find out the disease or normalcy of the pleura or lung the clinician hears the breath sounds with the help of a stethoscope (auscultation). The knowledge of the surface marking of the lung is of use in delineating lung lobes on the surface of the chest wall.

a. The apex of the lung is auscultated above the medial third of the clavicle anteriorly and in the upper part of suprascapular region posteriorly.
b. The upper lobe of the right lung is best heard anteriorly in the area extending from the clavicle to the level of fourth costal cartilage while that of left lung is best heard in the area up to the level of sixth costal cartilage.
c. The middle lobe is heard anteriorly between the right fourth and sixth ribs in front of the midaxillary line.
d. The apical or superior segment of the lower lobe (on both sides) is heard posteriorly in the interval between the medial border of the scapula and the vertebral spines. The basal segments of the lower lobe (on both sides) are heard posteriorly in the infrascapular region up to the level of tenth rib.

Relations of Apex

The relations of the apex of the lung (Fig. 38.4) are clinically important. The apex is covered with the dome of the cervical pleura. The suprapleural membrane or Sibson's

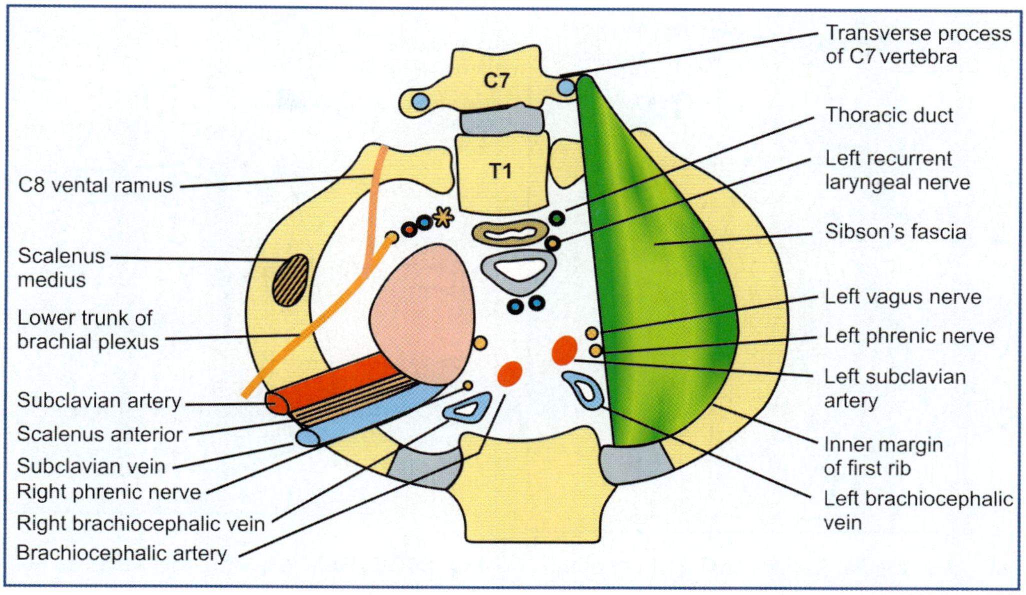

Fig. 38.4: Simplified scheme showing relations of apex of lung. [On the right side Sibson's fascia is removed to expose the relations. Observe the sequence of posterior relations (not labeled)]

fascia protects the apex and the covering pleura in the root of the neck. This fascia is derived partly from endothoracic fascia and partly from scalenus minimus or pleuralis muscle.

a. Anteriorly the apex is grooved by subclavian artery and vein. The scalenus anterior passes between the two vessels to reach its insertion on the scalene tubercle on the inner margin of first rib.
b. Posteriorly it is related to the sympathetic chain, highest intercostal vein, superior intercostal artery and ascending branch of the ventral ramus of the first thoracic nerve (from medial to lateral side). These structures are the anterior relations of the neck of the first rib.
c. Lateral relations of the apex are, the scalenus medius muscle and the lower trunk of brachial plexus.
d. Medial relations are different on the two sides. On the right side, from anterior to posterior the structures are right brachiocephalic vein, right phrenic nerve, brachiocephalic artery, right vagus and trachea. On the left side the order of structures is, left brachiocephalic vein, left subclavian artery, left recurrent laryngeal nerve, esophagus and thoracic duct.

Malignancy of Lung Apex

The malignancy of the apex of the lung may present as symptoms and signs produced due to spread of cancer to neighboring structures. Spread of cancer in subclavian or brachiocephalic vein produces venous engorgement and edema in the arm or neck and face. Pressure on the subclavian artery results in diminished pulse in the arm (brachial or radial, etc.) on the affected side. Infiltration in the phrenic nerve results in paralysis of hemi-diaphragm. Pancoast syndrome comprises of effects due to involvement of structures in posterior relation of the lung apex, erosion of the first and or second ribs, pain in ulnar distribution and wasting of small muscles of hand (due to injury to ventral ramus of T1 or lower trunk of brachial plexus) and Horner's syndrome (due to injury to sympathetic chain).

Medial Surface

The medial surface of the lung has a larger mediastinal surface, which is characterized by hilum of the lung and pulmonary ligament. This surface presents markings and grooves produced by the structures in the mediastinum. The smaller and convex vertebral surface is devoid of markings.

a. On the mediastinal surface of the right lung (Fig. 38.5A) there is a large cardiac impression in front and below the hilum. The right atrium and the right ventricle (mainly in the anterior part) are related here. The upper part of the cardiac impression is continuous with the

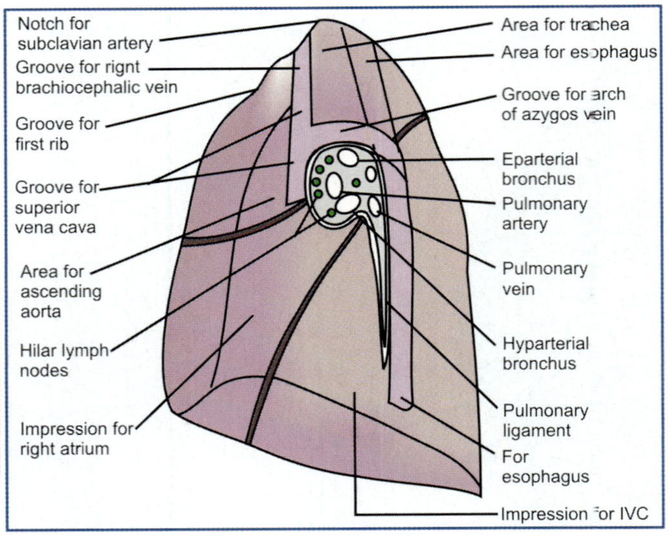

Fig. 38.5A: Relations of medial (mediastinal and vertebral) surface of right lung

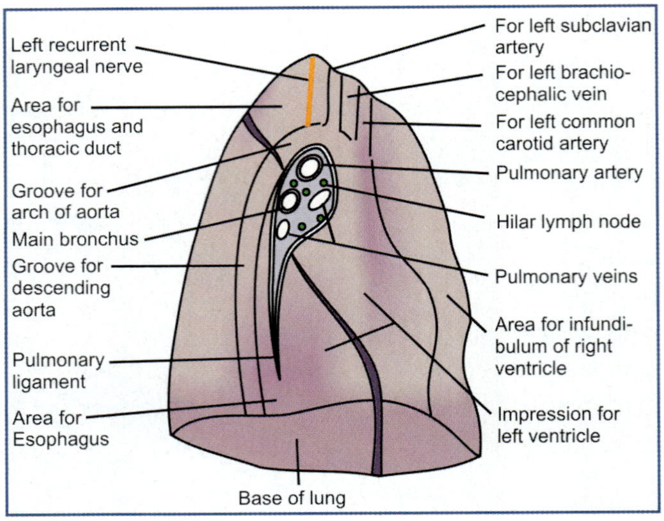

Fig. 38.5B: Relations of medial (mediastinal and vertebral) surface of left lung

groove for the superior vena cava, which is located in front of the hilum and is prolonged upwards as the groove for right brachiocephalic vein. A deep groove for the arch of azygos vein begins from the posterior margin of the groove for SVC and arches backwards over the hilum of the lung. Above the hilum the trachea and right vagus nerve are related posterior to the groove for SVC. The right phrenic nerve descends in front of the hilum and crosses the groove for SVC, cardiac impression and the groove for IVC. The esophagus makes a wide shallow groove behind the trachea, the hilum and the pulmonary ligament. However, this groove stops short of the lower margin of the lung. The inferior vena cava is related to the lung postero-inferior to the cardiac impression. A little below the apex, the right subclavian artery produces a notch on the anterior margin of the lung. The right first rib produces a notch on the anterior margin below that of right subclavian artery.

b. The vertebral surface of the right lung is in contact with the thoracic vertebrae and intervertebral discs. Besides this, it is related to posterior intercostal vessels and splanchnic nerves (branches of thoracic sympathetic chain).

c. On the mediastinal surface of the left lung (Fig. 38.5B) there is a large cardiac impression in front of and below the hilum. The left ventricle is mainly related to this area. The anterior part however is related to the infundibulum of right ventricle. The pulmonary trunk lies in front of the hilum in continuation of the area for infundibulum. The arch of aorta produces a deep and wide groove immediately above the hilum. This groove continues downwards behind the hilum and pulmonary ligament as the groove for descending thoracic aorta, which reaches the lower margin of the lung. The grooves for left subclavian artery and for left common carotid artery course upwards from the groove for arch of aorta. The left common carotid artery produces an anteriorly located short groove. The groove for left subclavian artery begins posterior to that of common carotid artery and runs upwards to cut the anterior margin just below the apex. The first rib comes in contact with this surface below that of left subclavian artery. The thoracic duct and esophagus are related behind the groove for left subclavian artery. The left brachiocephalic vein lies in a faint linear depression in front of the left subclavian artery. The left phrenic nerve descends in front of the hilum and crosses the cardiac impression. The lower esophageal impression lies in front of the groove for descending aorta and behind and below the lower end of the pulmonary ligament.

d. The convex vertebral surface of the left lung is related to the left aspects of thoracic vertebrae and intervening discs, posterior intercostal vessels and splanchnic nerves.

Root of Lung

The root of the lung connects the mediastinum to the lung. All the structures, which enter and leave the hilum of the lung, are enclosed in a tubular sheath of mediastinal pleura. This tubular sheath with its enclosed contents is called the root of the lung. The vertebral level of the lung root is T5 to T7. The contents of the root are, the bronchus (principal bronchus on the left side and the eparterial and hyparterial bronchi on the right side), pulmonary veins, pulmonary artery, bronchial vessels, lymph vessels, the hilar or bronchopulmonary lymph nodes and pulmonary nerve plexuses.

Pulmonary Ligament

It is a double fold of mediastinal pleura below the level of pulmonary hilum. It connects the mediastinal surface below the lung root to the side of posterior mediastinum. Therefore, the layers of the pulmonary ligament are continuous medially with mediastinal pleura, laterally with the visceral pleura and superiorly with the pleura covering the lung root. Its lower border is free. There is a potential space between the two layers of the pulmonary ligament, which provides a dead space for expansion of inferior pulmonary veins during increased venous return and for the descent of lung root during inspiration.

Bronchial Tree (Fig. 38.6)

The principal bronchus passes inferolaterally from the bifurcation of the trachea to the hilus of each lung. The bronchi divide in a tree-like manner within the lung. Each principal bronchus divides in to the secondary or lobar bronchi, which in turn divide into the segmental or tertiary bronchi.

Right Main Bronchus

This is wider, shorter and more vertical than the left bronchus. Therefore, an aspirated foreign body is more likely to enter the right lung than the left. The right main bronchus is 2.5 cm long. It gives its first branch, the superior lobar bronchus (eparterial bronchus) and then enters the hilum of the lung at the fifth thoracic vertebral level as the hyparterial bronchus.

a. The eparterial bronchus continues as the right superior lobar bronchus inside the lung and divides into three segmental bronchi namely, apical, anterior, and posterior.
b. The hyparterial bronchus divides into middle and right inferior lobar bronchi inside the lung. The middle lobar bronchus divides into two segmental bronchi called medial and lateral. The right inferior lobar bronchus divides into five segmental bronchi for the inferior lobe. The first branch to arise is the superior or apical segmental bronchus, which is given off from the posterior aspect and goes directly backwards to the superior segment of the inferior lobe. In the supine position of the body, this segmental bronchus projects directly posteriorly and since it is the first branch to arise, foreign body is inhaled into it. The superior bronchopulmonary segment of lower lobe is most dependent and hence secretions tend to collect in it (Fig. 38.7). The next branch to arise is called the medial basal bronchus to serve a small area below the hilum. The remaining bronchus divides into three segmental bronchi called anterior basal, posterior basal and lateral basal.

Left Main Bronchus

This bronchus is narrower, less vertical and longer than the right. It is 5 cm long. Passing to the left it lies in inferior relation to the aortic arch and crosses the esophagus anteriorly (producing esophageal constriction). It enters the hilum of the lung at the level of the sixth thoracic vertebra and divides into superior and inferior lobar bronchi.

a. The left superior lobar bronchus takes origin from the anterior aspect of the principal bronchus and curves laterally to divide into superior and inferior divisions. The superior division gives off an anterior segmental bronchus and is then called apicoposterior segmental bronchus, which soon divides into apical and posterior segmental bronchi. The inferior division descends towards the lingula and divides into superior and inferior lingular segmental bronchi.
b. The left inferior lobar bronchus gives off its first branch called the superior (apical) segmental bronchus for the upper part of the inferior lobe. Like on the right side this bronchus projects directly posteriorly and in the supine position tends to collect secretions. After a

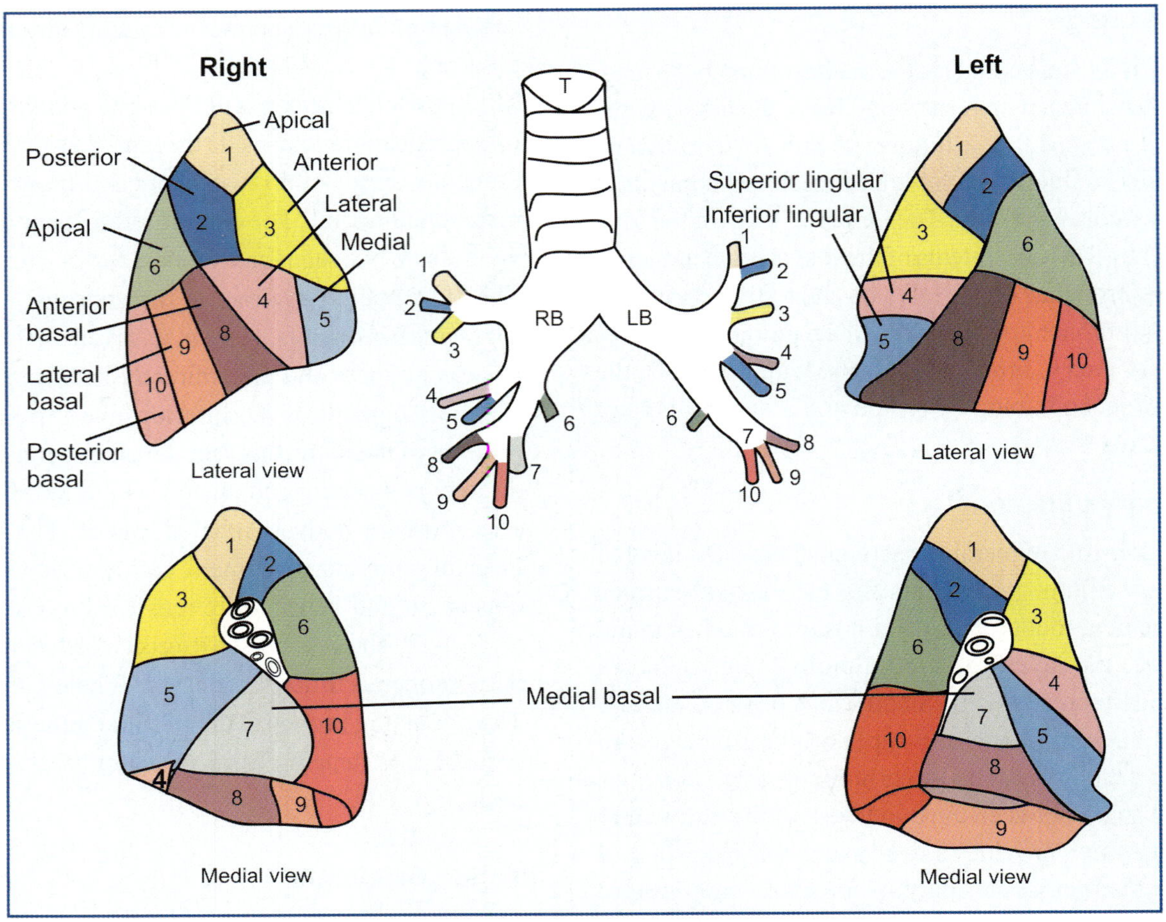

Fig. 38.6: Bronchopulmonary segments of lungs seen in lateral and medial views (Note: The difference in the division of bronchi as depicted in the bronchial tree)

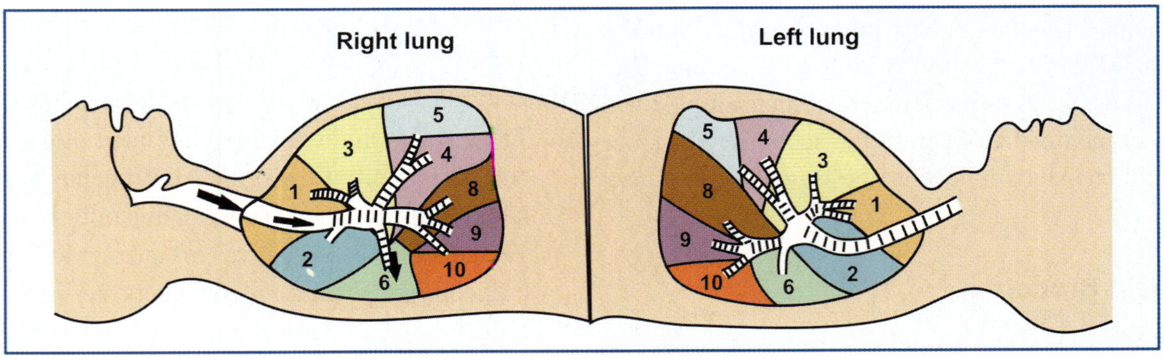

Fig. 38.7: Lateral view of bronchopulmonary segments and tracheobronchial tree in supine position of the body (Note that apical segment of lower lobe is most dependent in supine position. It is more prone to aspiration pneumonia on right side because right bronchus is in line with trachea compared to left bronchus)

further course of 1-2 cm the inferior lobar bronchus divides into anteromedial and posterolateral stems. The anteromedial stem divides into medial basal and anterior basal segmental bronchi while the posterolateral stem divides into lateral and posterior basal segmental bronchi. The areas of the inferior lobe to which these segmental bronchi go are essentially similar to that of the inferior lobe of right side.

Intrapulmonary Airways

Within each lung there are conducting airways (from lobar bronchi to terminal bronchioles) and respiratory areas (respiratory bronchioles, alveolar ducts, alveolar sacs and alveoli). The segmental bronchi branch until they become smaller and narrower progressively. Air passages less than 1 mm in diameter are termed bronchioles. They are devoid of cartilage and hence their wall consists of smooth muscle only. The bronchioles divide until they reach the stage of terminal bronchioles, which enter the lung lobule. The terminal bronchioles divide to give rise to respiratory bronchioles. A few alveoli sprout from the respiratory bronchioles, which divide to give rise to alveolar ducts. Each alveolar duct expands to form atrium, which expands in a number of alveolar sacs, which in turn are studded with alveoli. The alveoli are thin- walled pouches, which provide the respiratory surface for gaseous exchange. The alveoli are surrounded by pulmonary capillary bed. The alveolar epithelium is of simple squamous type. The type II cells are slightly larger and secrete surfactant. The blood-air barrier consists of alveolar epithelium, capillary endothelium and the basement membranes of the two in between.

Bronchopulmonary Segments

The bronchopulmonary segment is defined as a structural and functional unit of the lung parenchyma ventilated or aerated by a segmental or a tertiary bronchus.

Characteristic Features (Fig. 38.8)

The shape of the bronchopulmonary segment is pyramidal with apex pointing towards the hilum and the base towards the lung surface. Each segment has a covering of loose connective tissue. Each segment contains segmental structures, which are, the segmental bronchus and its further subdivisions, segmental branches of pulmonary artery and of bronchial artery. Air and impure blood pass in the center of each segment. The tributaries of pulmonary veins supported in loose connective tissue are located in the intersegmental planes. Thus, the pure blood passes along the periphery of each segment. Each segment can be delineated radiologically (bronchography). Segmental resection is surgical removal of a diseased bronchopulmonary segment. During surgery the segmental bronchus of the diseased segment is identified by dissection and it is clamped along with the blood vessels. This enables to delineate the segment, as the surface of that segment will darken due to loss of blood supply and air.

Names of Bronchopulmonary Segments (Fig. 38.6)

Lobes	*Right lung*	*Left lung*
Upper or superior	Apical Posterior Anterior	Apical Posterior Anterior Superior lingular Inferior lingular
Middle	Lateral Medial	
Lower or inferior	Apical or superior Medial basal Anterior basal Lateral basal Posterior basal	Apical or superior Medial basal Anterior basal Lateral basal Posterior basal

Blood Supply of Lungs

The pulmonary arteries take deoxygenated blood to the lungs. After entering the hilum it follows the pattern of division of the segmental bronchus. The arterioles accompanying the terminal and respiratory bronchioles are thin walled (without muscle fibers). These end up forming capillaries, which are in close proximity to the alveoli. The venous ends of the capillary beds join to form veins, which travel in the intersegmental plane. The intersegmental veins finally unite to form two pulmonary veins in each lung. Thus the pulmonary veins carry oxygenated blood from the lungs. The bronchial arteries provide nutrition to the bronchial tree upto the level of terminal bronchiole, which means to the non-respiratory portions of the lungs. The respiratory portions of the lungs are nourished from pulmonary capillary beds and directly from atmospheric air contained inside the alveoli.

Bronchial Vessels (Fig. 51.1)

The bronchial arteries supply the intrapulmonary bronchial tree and the connective tissue of lung parenchyma. The single right bronchial artery takes origin from either the left bronchial artery or the third right posterior intercostal artery or the descending aorta. On the left side there are

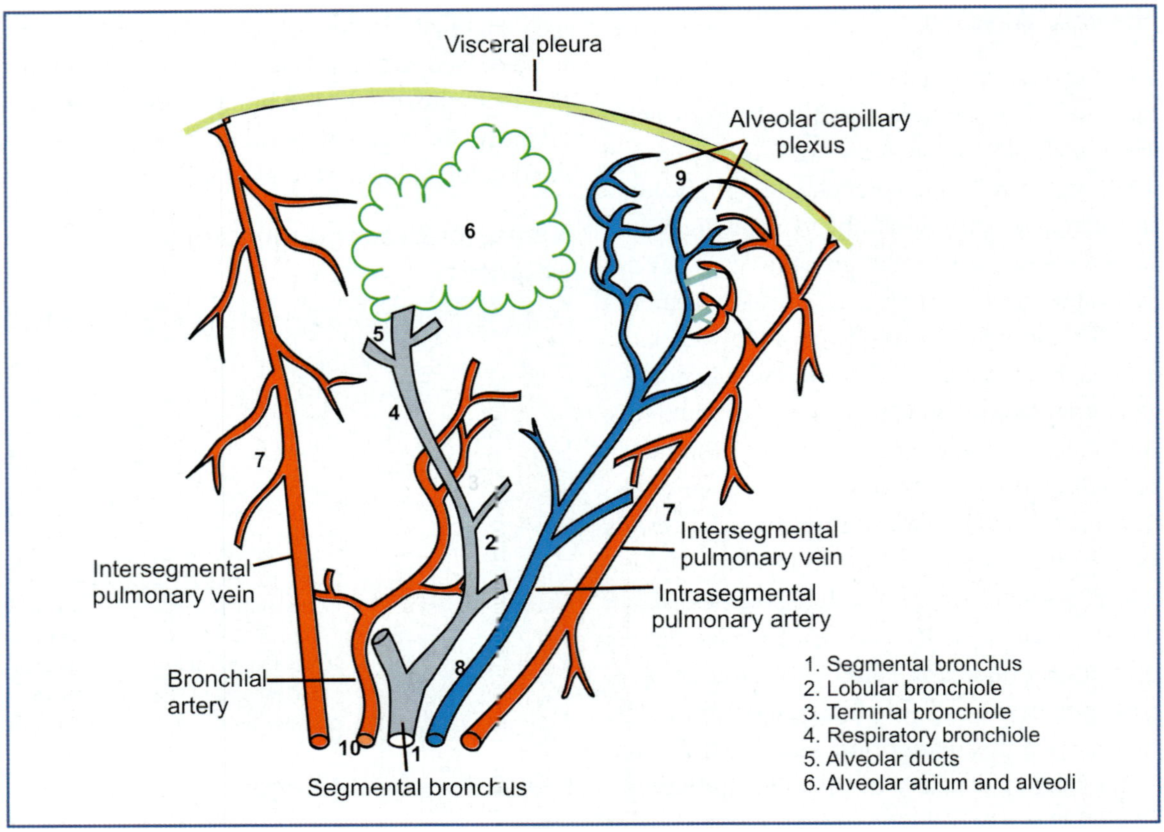

Fig. 38.8: Schematic diagram of a bronchopulmonary segment showing its blood vessels, ramifications of segmental bronchus and lung parenchyma

upper and lower bronchial arteries. Both are the branches of descending aorta at the level of tracheal bifurcation. The right bronchial vein opens into the azygos vein while the left bronchial vein opens into either the left superior intercostal vein or the accessory hemizygous vein.

Lymphatic Drainage (Fig. 38.9)

The lymphatic drainage of lung is important because lung cancer spreads by lymphatics paths. Two sets of lymphatic plexuses, superficial and deep, drain the lungs. The superficial plexus is subpleural in location and the deep plexus is seen along the bronchi and blood vessels. The two sets communicate with each other at the hilum and drain into the bronchopulmonary lymph nodes, which are also called hilar lymph nodes. These nodes are black in color due to the carbon particles drained from lungs. Efferent lymph vessels from the hilar nodes pass through tracheobronchial and paratracheal nodes. The tracheobronchial nodes communicate with the nodes in the base of the neck. These lymph nodes enlarge in pulmonary tuberculosis also. The enlarged nodes may sometimes obstruct a lobar bronchus causing collapse (atelectasis) of the entire lobe.

Nerve Supply

The lungs receive both sympathetic and parasympathetic nerves from the pulmonary plexuses. The afferent fibers from the lung originate in endings sensitive to stretch, which are involved in reflex control of respiration and coughing. The parasympathetic fibers are cholinergic while the sympathetic fibers are adrenergic. The parasympathetic stimulation causes bronchoconstriction and increased secretion of the glands. The sympathetic stimulation causes bronchodilatation, vasoconstriction and decreased secretion. The attack of bronchial asthma is produced due to spasm of the smooth muscles of the bronchioles.

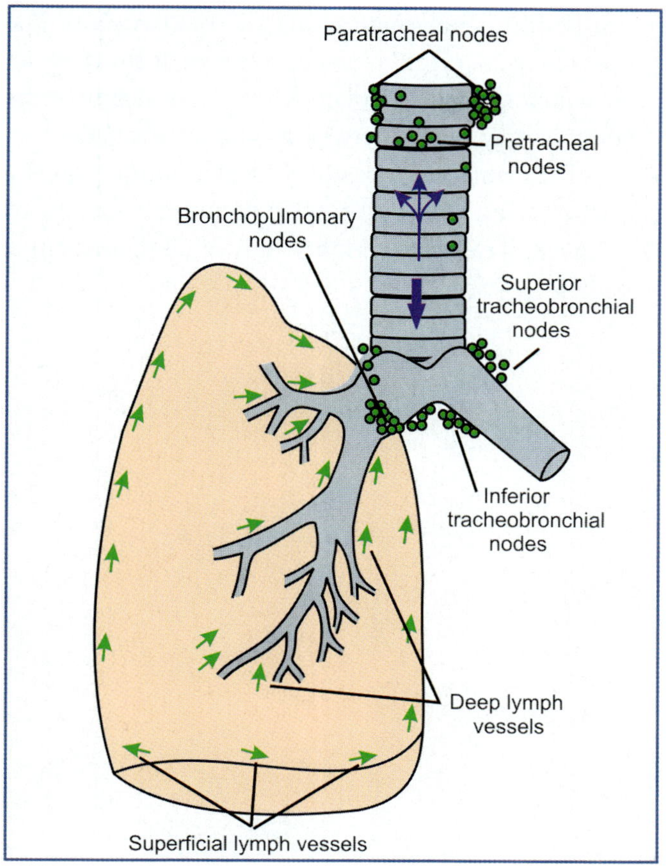

Fig. 38.9: Lymphatic drainage of lung and trachea

This may be precipitated by excessive vagal stimulation (due to exposure to cold air, dust, smoke, etc.). To counteract the spasm of the muscles either sympathomimetic or anticholinergic drugs are given. Sympathomimetic drugs like adrenaline mimic the action of sympathetic stimulation (bronchodilatation). Anticholinergic drugs like atropine nullify the bronchoconstriction action of cholinergic fibers, which results in dilatation of bronchii.

Radiological Anatomy

a. In a plain radiograph first the soft tissue shadows are examined. The trachea is identified in the midline in the superior mediastinum as a translucent air column. The lung fields are translucent, but the bronchovascular markings are seen as branching opacities throughout the lungs. The hilum is recognized as an opaque area because it contains large blood vessels and lymph nodes. The costodiaphragmatic recesses are visible and always examined for presence of fluid.

b. The CT scans and MRI of the thorax are also useful to study internal anatomy.

c. Bronchography is done to visualize the bronchial tree by injecting contrast medium. The preparation of the patient before the actual procedure is very important for obtaining the best results. To minimize the secretions in the bronchial tree the patient is encouraged to take out the sputum actively and is put under antibiotic cover. The patient is given nil by mouth five hours before the procedure. Premedication in the form of atropine is given intravenously thirty minutes prior to the procedure. Atropine is anticholinergic and hence reduces the secretion of bronchial glands. After spraying the nasal cavity, pharynx and larynx with 4% lignocaine a polythene catheter is passed through the nose or the mouth into the trachea and the contrast medium is injected through it. The patient is tilted into various positions necessary for filling the different bronchi. After this the radiographs are taken. Nowadays bronchography is replaced by CT scan.

Clinical Highlights

a. In bronchoscopy the interior of trachea and the bronchi is inspected using a bronchoscope. Carina is an important landmark visible through the bronchoscope. A flexible fiberoptic bronchoscope can be introduced under local anesthesia as a bedside procedure. Transbronchial biopsies can be obtained through this instrument.

b. Mendelson's syndrome is the aspiration pneumonia in the superior (apical) segment of the lower lobe (Fig. 38.7). The anatomical reason for this is that in the supine position of the body the superior segmental bronchus is the most dependent. Hence it tends to collect the secretions, which may obstruct the bronchus leading to collapse of the superior segment of the lower lobe (atelectasis) and pneumonia. This can be easily verified by percussive dullness in interscapular area and absence or diminished breath sounds in the same area.

c. The bronchiectasis is the condition in which bronchi and bronchioles are dilated. The segmental bronchi to the basal segments of the lower lobe are prone to this condition in which the smaller divisions of the bronchi become permanently dilated and filled with pus. Postural drainage is performed to remove pus by giving appropriate position to the patient.

d. The bronchogenic carcinoma originates from the epithelium of the bronchial wall. Cigarette smoke and automobile smoke increase the risk of this cancer. The presence of circular shadow (coin lesion) or an irregular shadow in a plain X-ray of chest may be the only finding in an otherwise asymptomatic patient.

The carcinoma spreads by local infiltration and by lymphatics. The surgical treatment consists of segmental resection or lobectomy or pulmonectomy.

39 Trachea

The trachea or windpipe is a tube that conducts air from the larynx to the principal bronchi. In the adult the trachea is about 12 cm long. It is situated partly in the neck and partly in the superior mediastinum (Fig. 39.1). The trachea lies in the midline in its cervical course but is deviated slightly to the right in its thoracic course. The trachea extends from the lower border of the cricoid cartilage (level with C6 vertebra) to the upper border of the fifth thoracic vertebra. Its upper end moves with larynx and the lower end moves with respiration. During deep inspiration, the tracheal bifurcation may descend to the level of the sixth thoracic vertebra. The walls of trachea are kept patent by 15 to 20 C-shaped cartilaginous rings. The posterior ends of the cartilaginous rings are held together by smooth muscle called trachealis, which flattens the posterior wall of the trachea. The soft posterior wall of the trachea allows for the expansion of the esophagus during swallowing. At its lower end, the trachea divides into right and left principal bronchi.

Importance of Carina

The lowest cartilaginous ring at the bifurcation of trachea is thick and broad in its central part. Its lower margin is called the carina, which is a hook-shaped or keel-shaped process curving downwards and backwards between the bronchi. The carina is visible as a sharp sagittal ridge at tracheal bifurcation during bronchoscopy. Hence it is a useful landmark. It is located about 25 cm from the incisor teeth and 30 cm from the external nares. The mucosa of trachea is most sensitive at carina. If the tracheobronchial lymph nodes in the angle between the principal bronchi enlarge (due to spread from bronchogenic cancer) the carina becomes distorted and flattened. Hence, morphological changes in the carina are looked for during bronchoscopy.

Comparative Features of Adult and Infant Trachea

a. The average diameter of adult tracheal lumen is 12 mm. In childhood the diameter in millimeters corresponds to the age in years. A four-year-old child will have tracheal diameter of 4 mm. Therefore, endotracheal tubes are graduated in mm.

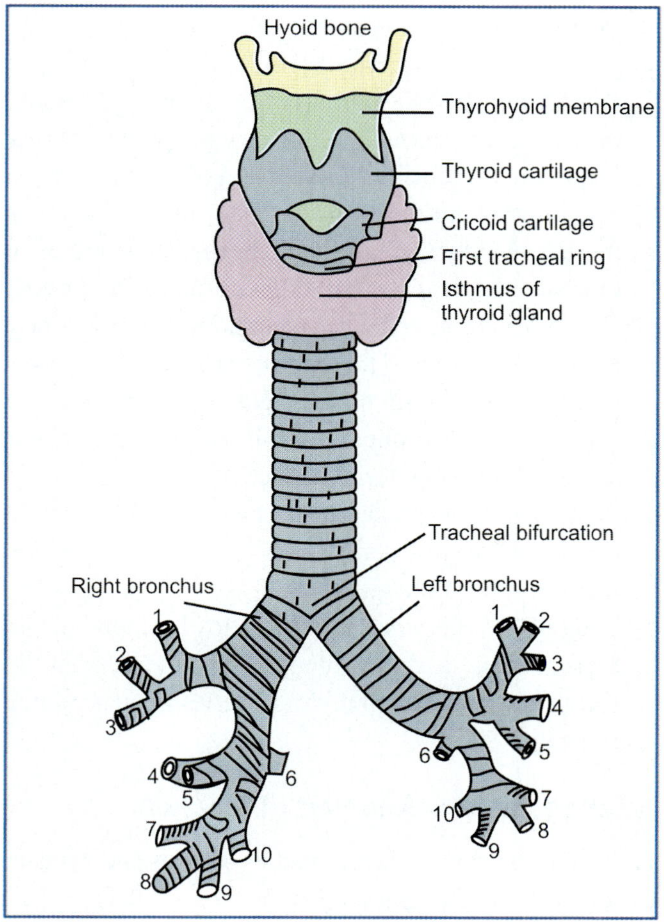

Fig. 39.1: Extent of trachea showing its continuity with larynx above and with bronchi below

b. The trachea is more deeply placed in children compared to the adult. Hence, tracheostomy is more difficult in child.
c. The left brachiocephalic vein may cross in front of the trachea in the suprasternal fossa in children. Similarly, the brachiocephalic artery may be related to the trachea on front just above the manubrium.
d. In children upto the age of two years the thymus is large hence it is in contact with the lower part of cervical trachea.

Relations of Cervical Part of Trachea (Figs 39.2 and 39.3A)

a. Anterior relations are very important as in the operation of tracheostomy these relations must be identified. Anteriorly following layers are seen from superficial to deep aspect, the skin, superficial fascia and the investing and pretracheal layers of deep fascia. The sternohyoid and sternothyroid muscles overlap it anterolaterally. The isthmus of the thyroid gland and the arterial anastomosis along its upper margin, cross the second to fourth or second to third tracheal rings. The inferior thyroid veins descend from the isthmus into the superior mediastinum. The jugular venous arch crosses the trachea in the suprasternal space. Thyroidea ima artery, when present is related anteriorly below the isthmus. The brachiocephalic artery forms a very close relation on the right side at the thoracic inlet. The pretracheal lymph nodes are present scattered on the anterior aspect.
b. Posteriorly, the trachea lies on the esophagus with recurrent laryngeal nerve in the groove between trachea and esophagus.
c. Laterally, the trachea is related to the lobes of the thyroid gland and the common carotid artery in the carotid sheath. Inferior thyroid arteries are also related laterally.

Relations of Thoracic Part of Trachea

The trachea is almost surrounded by arteries and veins in the superior mediastinum (Figs 39.3B and 39.4).

a. Anteriorly, the arch of aorta and its two branches, brachiocephalic and left common carotid arteries are in close relation to the trachea. The left brachiocephalic vein crosses the trachea from the left to right and receives the inferior thyroid veins, which descend in front of the trachea. Remains of thymus are related to the anterior surface. At the tracheal bifurcation, the deep cardiac plexus and tracheobronchial lymph nodes are seen.
b. Posteriorly, the trachea is in contact with the esophagus.
c. On the left side the trachea is related to the arch of aorta, left common carotid and left subclavian arteries. It is also related to the left recurrent laryngeal nerve.
d. On right side, it comes in contact with right lung and pleura between the groove for esophagus behind and the groove for superior vena cava in front (Fig. 39.3B). Its vascular relations on the right side are venous (right brachiocephalic vein, SVC and azygos arch). It is also related to the right vagus nerve.

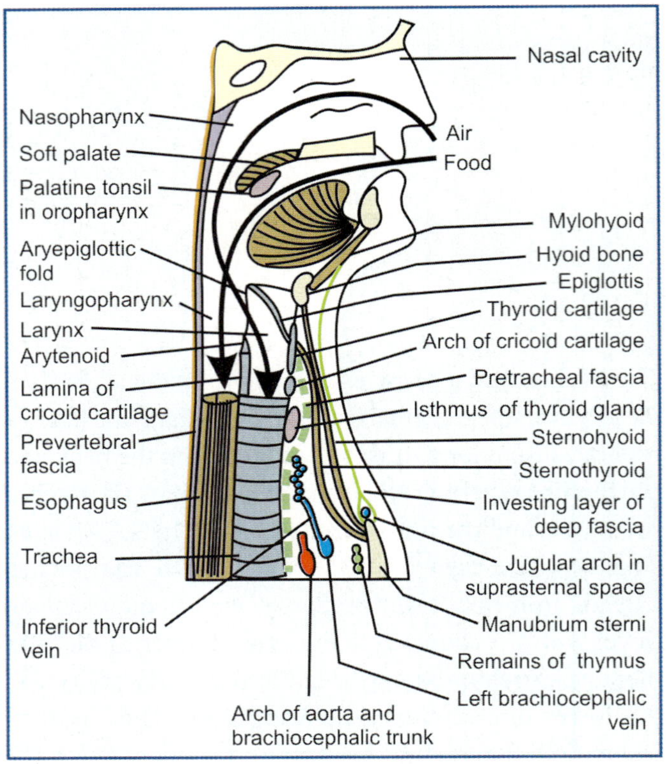

Fig. 39.2: Schematic median section showing some relations of trachea in the neck and in superior mediastinum. Note the crossing of air and foodpaths indicated by arrows

Surface Marking

The trachea is represented on the surface by a 2 cm wide midline band from the level of cricoid cartilage to the

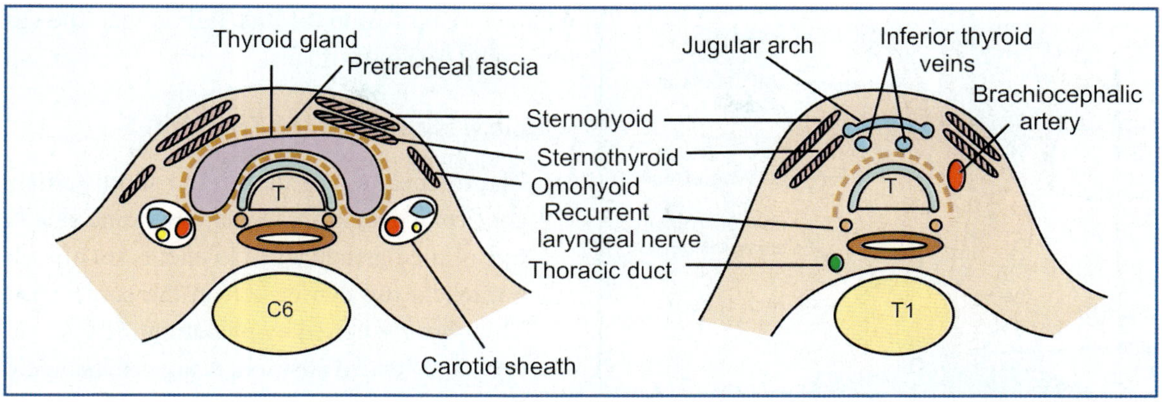

Fig. 39.3A: TS of neck at C6 and T1 vertebral levels showing relations of cervical part of trachea

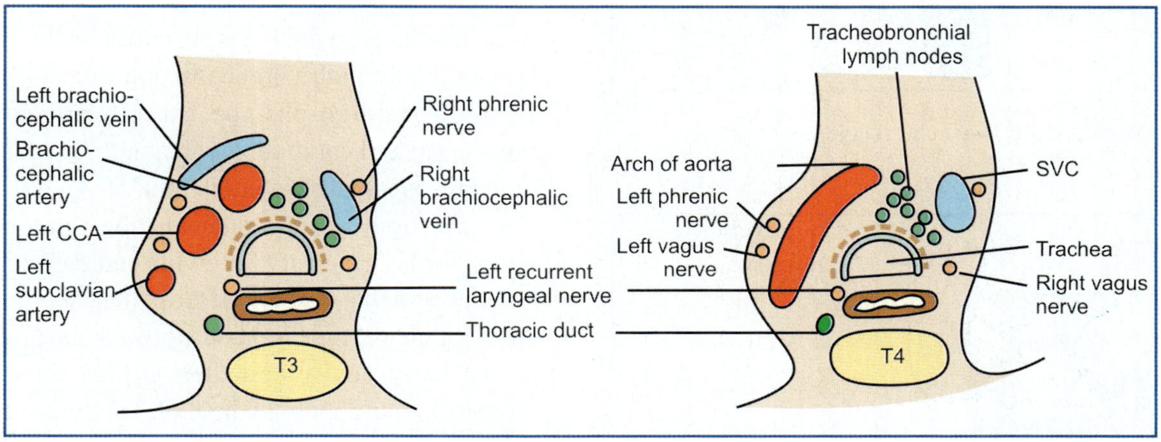

Fig. 39.3B: TS of superior mediastinum at T3 and T4 vertebral levels showing relations of trachea

sternal angle with a slight inclination to the right at the lower end.

Blood Supply (Fig. 39.5)

Inferior thyroid arteries are the main source of blood supply. The thoracic part of the trachea is supplied from the bronchial arteries. The descending and ascending branches of these sources anastomose on the surface of trachea. Tracheal veins drain into the inferior thyroid venous plexus.

Lymph Drainage

The lymph vessels drain into the pretracheal, paratracheal and tracheobronchial lymph nodes, which lie in close vicinity of the trachea from above downward (Fig. 38.9).

Nerve Supply

The nerve supply to the mucosa, tracheal glands and trachealis muscle is from the vagus nerves, recurrent laryngeal nerves and the sympathetic trunks.

Development

The trachea develops from the endodermal laryngotracheal groove. The groove forms the tube, which is separated from the developing esophagus by the tracheo-esophageal septum. If this process of separation is incomplete or if there is esophageal atresia, a communication is formed between the windpipe or trachea and food pipe or esophagus. This is known as tracheo-esophageal fistula or TEF (Fig. 35.2). In the common variety of TEF the upper segment of esophagus ends blindly but the lower segment is connected to the trachea at its bifurcation. It is a serious condition in the newborn, which needs immediate attention. The water or milk ingested by the infant gets accumulated in upper blind segment of esophagus. This is aspirated in the trachea. The gastric contents or bile may be regurgitated in the trachea through fistulous connection. Aspiration of fluid in lungs by both routes leads to aspiration or chemical pneumonia. The

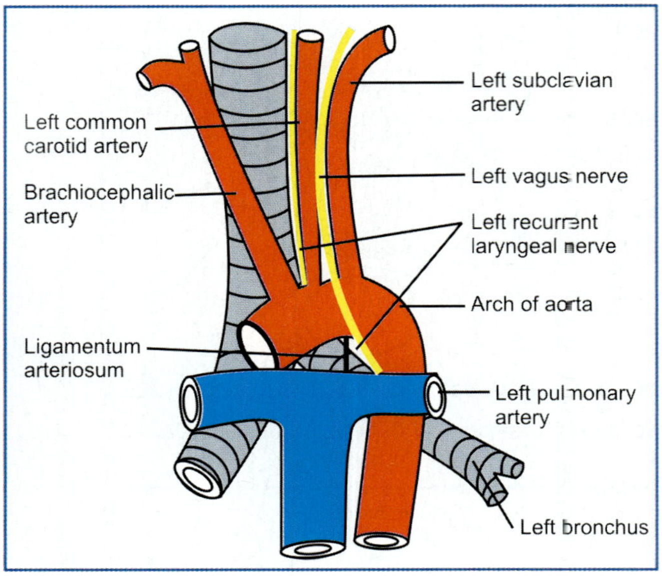

Fig. 39.4: Showing vascular relations of trachea

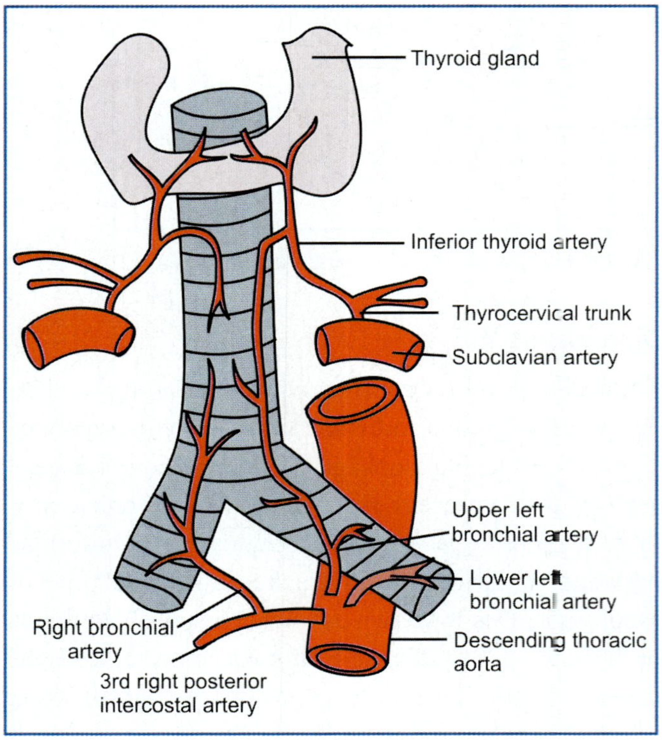

Fig. 39.5: Arterial supply of trachea

characteristic feature of this TEF is that, the stomach of the infant is filled with air.

Clinical Highlights of Trachea

a. The trachea is palpated in the suprasternal notch to confirm its position. Deviation to one side is suggestive of mediastinal shift. In aneurysm of arch of aorta a tracheal tug can be felt in the suprasternal notch. This sign is elicited by palpating the trachea with the neck in extended position. A tug is felt coinciding with the pulsation of the aorta.

b. The interior of the trachea is examined in the living with the bronchoscope. It is possible to take biopsies from tracheobronchial lymph nodes at the tracheal bifurcation through a bronchoscope.

c. In plain radiographs the trachea appears as a translucent and dark tubular area in the neck because of the presence of air column in it.

d. The insertion of endotracheal tube (endotracheal intubation) is necessary for giving general anesthesia. After positioning the head of the patient appropriately, an endotracheal tube is passed through the oral cavity or the nasal cavity and then guided through the laryngeal cavity with the help of a laryngoscope and pushed down till its tip reaches well above carina. The tube is guided keeping in mind the distance of the carina from the external nose or incisor teeth.

e. Tracheostomy is making an artificial opening in the trachea if there is airway obstruction at laryngeal level. The site for the opening is in the cervical part of the trachea. The steps of the procedure are described along with structures in the midline of the neck in Chapter 66.

f. Enlargement of structures in relation to trachea causes tracheal compression. Thyroid swellings are the most common cause of tracheal compression in the neck. The thoracic trachea may be compressed by enlarged lymph nodes or by aneurysm of arch of aorta in the superior mediastinum. Tracheal compression causes dyspnea or difficulty in breathing.

Section two

40 Diaphragm

The diaphragm is a movable partition between the thoracic and abdominal cavities. It is partly muscular and partly tendinous. It is the chief muscle of inspiration. The diaphragm descends during inspiration and ascends during expiration. During quiet breathing it descends for a distance of 1.5 cm. The movements of the diaphragm can be observed in the living by the fluoroscopic examination. The position of the diaphragm varies with posture. In supine posture the diaphragm is highest and shows maximum movements but reverse is the case in sitting position.

Parts and Relations

The superior surface of the diaphragm projects as two domes or cupola into the thoracic cavity. The domes are covered with diaphragmatic pleura. The base of each lung fits into the corresponding dome. In between the two domes there is a depressed area called the central tendon, with which the base of the fibrous pericardium fuses. The deeply concave inferior surface of the diaphragm forms the roof of the abdominal cavity. It is covered with peritoneum. The right side of this surface is moulded over the convexity of the right lobe of the liver, right kidney and right suprarenal gland while on left side the left lobe of the liver, fundus of stomach, spleen, left kidney and left suprarenal gland are in contact with the diaphragm.

Surface Marking

The right dome reaches a point as far as the upper border of the right fifth rib in the midclavicular line, but the left dome reaches as far as the lower border of the left fifth rib. On the posterior aspect the right dome is in level with a point 1.25 cm below the inferior angle of scapula, but the left dome is in level with a point 2.5 cm below the inferior angle of scapula. Thus, the right dome is at a higher level due to the presence of a large right lobe of the liver under it. The central tendon is at the level of a line joining the xiphisternal joint to the spine of eighth thoracic vertebra.

Attachments

The diaphragm has a circumferential origin from the margins of thoracic outlet (Fig. 40.1).

Origin

According to the site of origin the muscle fibers are divided in three parts.

a. Sternal fibers arise as two muscular slips from the back of the xiphoid process.
b. Costal fibers arise by six muscular slips from the inner surfaces of the costal cartilages and adjacent parts of the lower six ribs. The costal slips interdigitate with the origin of transversus abdominis muscle from the ribs.
c. Vertebral fibers arise by right and left crura and by arcuate ligaments on each side. The right crus is attached to the front of the bodies of the upper three lumbar vertebrae and the intervening intervertebral discs while the left crus is attached to the upper two lumbar vertebrae and the intervening discs. The median arcuate ligament is a poorly defined tendinous arch joining the two crura across the lower border of the twelfth thoracic vertebra. The right crus is larger in size because of the presence of heavy liver on the right side. A few fibers of the right crus deviate to the left of the midline to encircle the lower end of the esophagus. Some fibers of the right crus are attached to the duodeno-jejunal flexure as suspensory ligament of duodenum (muscle of Treitz). The medial and lateral arcuate ligaments or lumbocostal arches give origin to

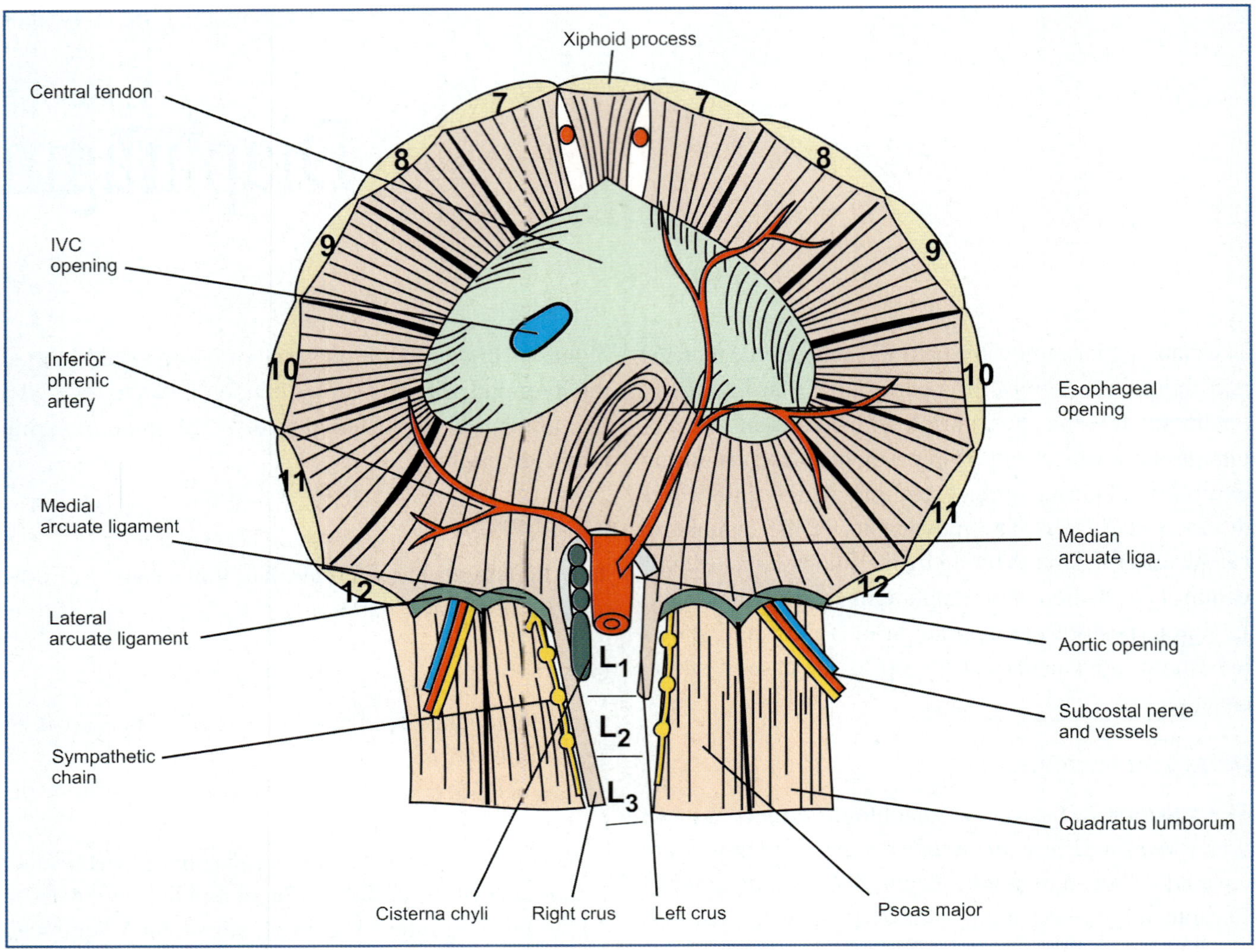

Fig. 40.1: Showing sternal, costal and vertebral origin of diaphragm from abdominal aspect

the diaphragmatic muscle. The medial arcuate ligaments are thickenings of fascia covering psoas major muscle stretching from the side of the body of the first lumbar vertebra to the middle of the front of the transverse process of the same vertebra. The lateral arcuate ligaments are the thickenings of upper margins of the anterior layer of thoracolumbar fascia in front of the quadratus lumborum muscle and stretch from the transverse process of first lumbar vertebra to the twelfth rib on each side.

Insertion

From this circumferential origin the muscle fibers converge towards the central tendon for insertion. The central tendon has no bony attachments. It is trifoliate in shape and is inseparably fused with the base of the fibrous pericardium.

Apertures in Diaphragm (Fig. 40.2)

There are three major apertures and a number of minor apertures in diaphragm for the passage of structures between thorax and abdomen.

Major Apertures

a. The quadrilateral vena caval aperture lies at the level of eighth thoracic vertebra. It is located in the central tendon to the right of the midline. The wall of the inferior vena cava is fused with the margins of the opening. The contraction of the diaphragm enlarges

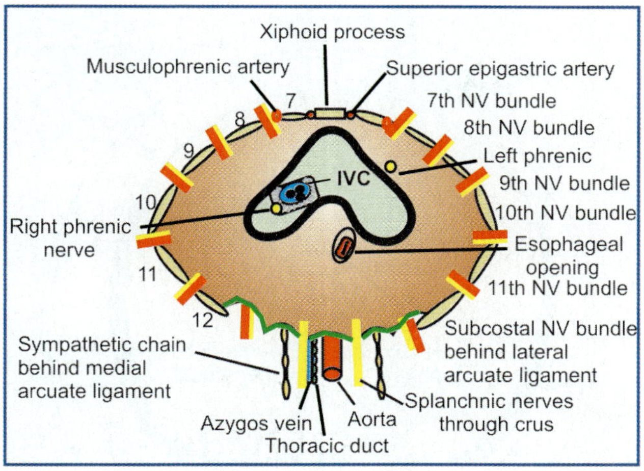

Fig. 40.2: Simplified diagram showing structures passing through diaphragm (NV bundle-intercostal neurovascular bundle)

the caval opening thereby dilating the vein and promoting the venous return. The branches of the right phrenic nerve pass through this opening along with IVC.

b. The elliptical esophageal hiatus is located in the muscular part of the diaphragm just posterior to the central tendon and to the left of the midline. The fibers of the right crus encircle it. It is at the level of the tenth thoracic vertebra. The contraction of the diaphragm has a sphincteric effect on the hiatus (pinchcock effect). The vagal trunks and the esophageal branches of left gastric vessels pass through the hiatus along with esophagus.

c. The rounded aortic opening lies posterior to the median arcuate ligament at the level of twelfth thoracic vertebra. The contraction of the diaphragm has no effect on this opening. The thoracic duct and vena azygos pass through the opening along with the aorta.

Minor Apertures

a. Superior epigastric vessels pass through a gap (space of Larry) between sternal origin and costal origin from seventh costal cartilage.

b. Musculophrenic vessels pass through the interval between slips of origin of diaphragm from the seventh and eighth ribs. The seventh intercostal nerve and vessels also pass through this interval.

c. The eighth to eleventh intercostal nerves and vessels pass through interval between the adjacent costal origins from subsequent ribs.

d. Subcostal nerves and vessels pass behind the lateral arcuate ligament.

e. Sympathetic chains pass behind the medial arcuate ligaments.

f. Greater, lesser and least splanchnic nerves pierce the crus of the corresponding side.

g. Hemiazygos vein pierces the left crus.

h. Right phrenic nerve passes usually through the IVC opening and the left phrenic nerve through the muscular part in front of the central tendon.

Nerve Supply

a. The phrenic nerves supply the muscle of the diaphragm. They pierce the diaphragm and ramify on its abdominal surface before entering the muscle (Fig. 41.1). The right phrenic nerve supplies the right half of the diaphragm upto the right margin of the esophageal opening. Left phrenic nerve supplies the left half of the diaphragm upto the left margin of the esophageal opening. Since the fibers of the right crus encircle the esophageal opening, it receives branches from both phrenic nerves.

b. The phrenic nerves give sensory fibers to the central part of diaphragm and the pleura and the peritoneum related to it. The lower intercostal nerves supply the peripheral parts of the diaphragm. Irritation of the pleura or the peritoneum of the central part of diaphragm gives rise to referred pain in front of and at the tip of the shoulder, which is the area of cutaneous supply of supraclavicular nerves (C3, C4).

Arterial Supply

a. Superior phrenic arteries (also called phrenic arteries), which are the last branches of thoracic aorta, are distributed to posterior part of the superior surface of the diaphragm. The musculophrenic and pericardiacophrenic branches of the internal thoracic artery supply anterior part of the superior surface of diaphragm.

b. Inferior phrenic arteries, which are the first branches of abdominal aorta, supply the inferior surface of the diaphragm.

Lymphatic Drainage

a. The thoracic surface drains as follows. Its anterior part drains into the anterior diaphragmatic nodes and parasternal nodes. The middle part drains in right and left lateral diaphragmatic nodes, parasternal nodes and posterior mediastinal nodes. The posterior part drains in posterior diaphragmatic nodes and posterior mediastinal nodes.

b. The abdominal surface drains as follows. The right half of diaphragm drains into lymph nodes lying along inferior phrenic artery and in the right lateral aortic nodes. The left half drains in preaortic nodes and in nodes around lower end of esophagus.

Actions

a. The diaphragm is a muscle of inspiration. When the diaphragm contracts the domes of the diaphragm along with the central tendon descend thereby increasing the vertical diameter of the thoracic cavity. Once the limit of the descent is reached the central tendon becomes a fixed point around which the diaphragm contracts. This contraction elevates the lower ribs thereby pushing forwards the sternum and the upper ribs, which increases the transverse and antero-posterior diameters of the thoracic cavity.
b. The contraction of the diaphragm raises the intra-abdominal pressure, which is useful in all expulsive activities like micturition, defecation and parturition. It also helps in weight lifting when the raised intra-abdominal pressure is kept sustained by closure of the glottis after taking a deep breath. This maintains the vertebral column in extended position, thus helping the trunk muscles in lifting heavy weights.
c. The contraction of the diaphragm facilitates venous and lymph return. The rise in the intra-abdominal pressure and decrease in the intra-thoracic pressure compress the blood in the inferior vena cava and lymph in the cisterna chyli. This results in upward movement of the blood towards the right atrium and of the lymph towards the thoracic duct.

Development (Fig. 40.3)

The diaphragm is entirely mesodermal and it develops in the neck of the embryo from four different sources, the septum transversum, right and left pleuroperitoneal membranes, dorsal mesentery of the esophagus and the body wall mesoderm. The muscle of the diaphragm develops from the third, fourth and fifth cervical myotomes and hence its motor innervation is from the phrenic nerve. When the diaphragm descends from the neck to its definitive position its nerve supply is also dragged down. This explains the long course of the phrenic nerves.

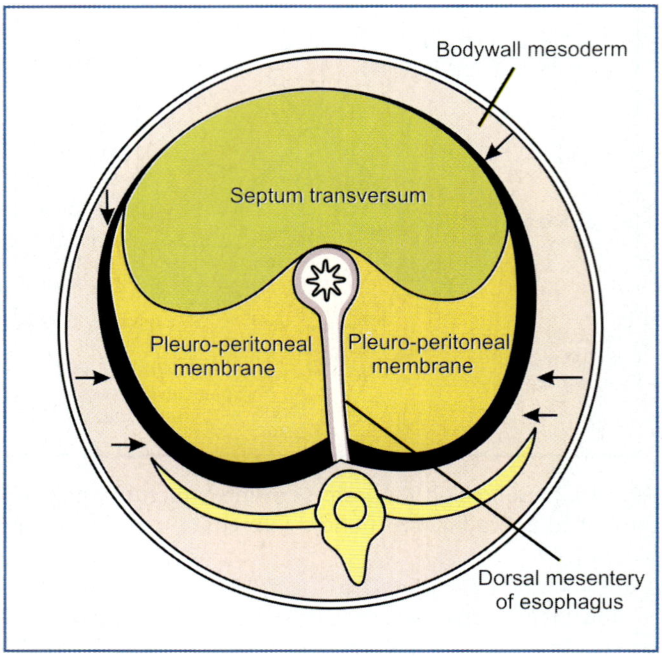

Fig. 40.3: Developmental sources of diaphragm

Congenital Diaphragmatic Hernia

a. Retrosternal hernia occurs through foramen of Morgagni, which is an enlarged space of Larry.
b. Posterolateral hernia occurs through the vertebrocostal triangle, which is also known as foramen of Bochdalek. It is a gap between the costal and vertebral origins of the diaphragm. The cause of this deficiency is assumed to be the failure of closure of the pleuroperitoneal canals due to non-development of pleuroperitoneal membrane. This occurs more commonly on the left side. The abdominal viscera may herniate through the defect into the thorax producing respiratory distress soon after birth. Immediate surgical correction is required to save the life of the newborn.

Clinical Highlights

a. The acquired diaphragmatic hernia (hiatus hernia) occurs through the esophageal opening (hiatus). It is of two types (Figs 40.4A and B).

i. In the sliding hernia the cardio-esophageal junction and the cardiac end of the stomach pass through the esophageal opening to enter the posterior mediastinum. This is caused due to weakness of the diaphragmatic muscle surrounding the esophageal opening and increased intra-abdominal pressure due to any cause. There is regurgitation or reflux of acid contents of the stomach into the esophagus causing peptic esophagitis (heartburn is the resulting symptom). The sliding hernia is usually associated with short esophagus.

ii. In the rolling hiatus hernia a part of the stomach passes through the esophageal opening into the posterior mediastinum. There is no reflux of gastric contents into the esophagus as the cardio-esophageal junction is in normal position.

b. Unilateral diaphragmatic paralysis is caused by damage to the phrenic nerve. The condition is diagnosed when an elevated hemidiaphragm is seen on fluoroscopy to move paradoxically. The bilateral diaphragmatic paralysis is a much more serious condition as it leads to respiratory failure.

c. Hiccups are the involuntary spasmodic contractions of diaphragm accompanied by the closure of the glottis. Hiccups are common in normal people and occur after eating or drinking as a result of gastric irritation. The other causes of hiccup include diaphragmatic irritation, phrenic nerve irritation, hysteria and uremia.

Mechanism of Respiration

The rhythmic movements of respiration produce alterations in the capacity of the thoracic cavity, which can be increased and then decreased in transverse, antero-posterior and vertical dimensions. The respiration rate in a healthy adult is 18-20/ minute. Each respiratory cycle consists of an inspiratory and an expiratory phase. Inspiration increases the thoracic volume with a simultaneous decrease in the intrapulmonary pressure. This ensures the inflow of air into the lungs until the pressures equalize. The expiration decreases thoracic volume with a simultaneous increase in the intrapulmonary pressure. This causes the air to flow out of the lungs until the pressures equalize.

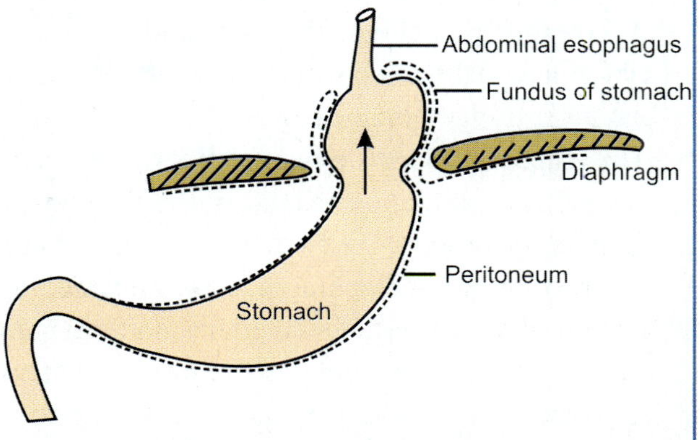

Fig. 40.4A: Sliding type of hiatus hernia

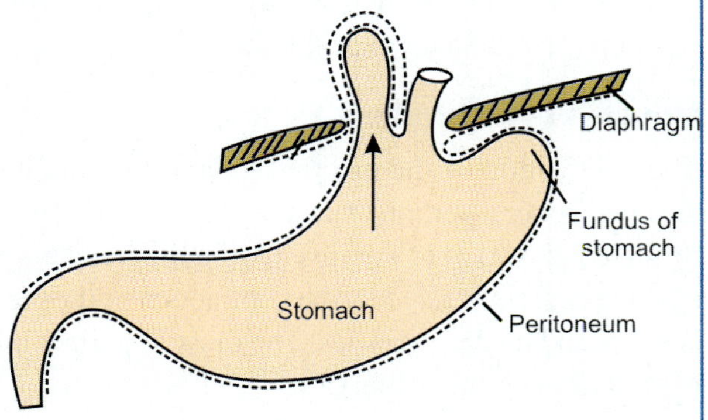

Fig. 40.4B: Para-esophageal/rolling type of hiatus hernia

Quiet Inspiration

a. The movements of the ribs take place at costo-vertebral and costo-transverse joints, which are the joints between the posterior ends of the ribs and the thoracic vertebrae.

In the pump-handle movement, the upper ribs (2-6) rotate around an axis, which passes through costo-vertebral and costo-transverse joints. This rotation results in upward and forward movements of the anterior ends of the ribs along with the sternum. The lower ribs (7-10) are elevated as a unit thereby lifting the lower end of the sternum upward and forward. The final effect is the increase in the antero-posterior diameter of the thoracic cavity.

In bucket-handle movement, the ribs are rotated along an axis, which passes through the tubercle of the rib and the middle of the sternum. The effect of this rotation is the elevation of the middle parts of the ribs in lateral direction so as to increase the transverse diameter of the thoracic cavity.

b. The diaphragm forms a mobile floor of the thoracic cavity. Its contraction results in the descent of the diaphragm by about 1-1.5 cm in quiet inspiration. The contraction of the diaphragm is accompanied by the reciprocal relaxation of the anterior abdominal muscles. The descent of the diaphragm results in increase in the vertical dimension of the thoracic cavity. The diaphragm can also act on the lower ribs at the end of its vertical descent. Keeping the central tendon as a fixed point the diaphragmatic contraction elevates the lower ribs thereby increasing the antero-posterior and transverse diameters of the thorax.

Muscles of Inspiration

The contraction of the external intercostal muscles and the interchondral portion of the internal intercostal muscles, results in elevation of the ribs. During movements of the ribs, the first rib is fixed by the contraction of the scalenus anterior and medius muscles. The most important muscle of inspiration is the diaphragm.

Forced Inspiration

Additional muscles are brought into play to increase the volume of the thoracic cavity. The first two ribs are elevated along with the manubrium sterni by active contraction of scaleni and sternomastoid muscles. The pectoral, levatores costarum and serratus anterior and posterior muscles elevate the ribs. The power of the diaphragmatic contraction is increased by fixing the twelfth rib with the help of active contraction of quadratus lumborum.

Quiet Expiration

Quiet expiration is largely a passive process. The elastic recoil of the lungs (intrinsic elastic recoil) and of the chest wall (extrinsic elastic recoil) accompanied by the relaxation of the diaphragm and external intercostal muscles is responsible for it. The relaxation of the diaphragm is accompanied by the reciprocal increase in the tone of anterior abdominal muscles. The extrinsic elastic recoil diminishes with age because the costal cartilages undergo calcification. Elderly people tend to breathe diaphragmatically. The diseases that reduce the intrinsic elastic recoil of the lungs, such as emphysema, affect the expiratory process and make it stressful.

Forced Expiration

Forced expiration is an active process brought about by the forcible contraction of the muscles of the anterior abdominal wall. In addition the quadratus lumborum contracts to pull the twelfth rib down. The interosseous parts of the internal intercostal muscles may also help in depressing the ribs. The serratus posterior inferior and latissimus dorsi muscles may also play a minor role.

41 Phrenic Nerves

The right and left phrenic nerves are the only motor supply to the muscle of the corresponding half of the diaphragm. The phrenic nerves originate from the cervical plexus in the neck. The phrenic nerve is a mixed nerve with 2:1 proportion of motor and sensory fibers. Its sensory fibers supply the diaphragmatic and mediastinal pleura, fibrous and parietal pericardium and diaphragmatic peritoneum of its side.

Origin

The phrenic nerve arises mainly from the ventral ramus of the fourth cervical nerve but receives contribution from the third and fifth cervical nerves also. Hence its root value is C3, C4, and C5 (Fig. 41.1). Accessory phrenic nerve, when present is a branch of nerve to subclavius (arising from Erb's point of brachial plexus). It carries C5 fibers and joins the phrenic nerve in the thorax (Fig. 41.2).

Course and Relations

The phrenic nerve has a long course, which can be divided into cervical and thoracic parts.

a. In its cervical course the phrenic nerve begins from the cervical plexus and descends on the anterior surface of the scalenus anterior muscle. The prevertebral layer of the deep cervical fascia plasters down the phrenic nerve to this muscle. During its descent, the nerve crosses the scalenus anterior muscle lateromedially. Anteriorly, the phrenic nerve is overlapped by internal jugular vein and sternomastoid. It is crossed by intermediate tendon of omohyoid, transverse cervical and suprascapular arteries, (and thoracic duct on the left side). Its posterior relation to the scalenus anterior muscle varies on two sides (Fig. 41.1). On the right side, it lies anterior to the muscle throughout its cervical course. However, on the left side its posterior relations are the scalenus anterior muscle and the first part of left subclavian artery. This is due to the fact that the left phrenic nerve leaves the scalenus anterior muscle from its medial margin near the root of the neck, unlike the right phrenic nerve, which retains its anterior relation to the muscle till the lower end of the muscle.
b. The right and left phrenic nerves pass through the thoracic inlet to enter the superior mediastinum. The left phrenic nerve enters the superior mediastinum between the left subclavian vein in front and the first part of the left subclavian artery behind. The right phrenic nerve enters the superior mediastinum by passing between the right subclavian vein in front and the right scalenus anterior muscle behind. Both the phrenic nerves cross the internal thoracic artery from lateral to medial side on its anterior aspect (Fig. 41.1).
c. The left phrenic nerve is longer than the right and the right phrenic nerve is shorter and more vertical in the thoracic course. Both the nerves at first pass through the superior mediastinum and then in front of the hilum of the respective lung to enter the middle mediastinum, where each descends in close relation of fibrous pericardium. The pericardiacophrenic vessels accompany the phrenic nerve in its thoracic course (Fig. 34.3). The relations of the thoracic part of right and left phrenic nerves are different.

The right phrenic nerve passes down along the right side of right brachiocephalic vein, superior vena cava, right atrium covered by right side of fibrous pericardium and lastly the thoracic part of inferior vena cava. In the middle mediastinum the nerve lies between the mediastinal pleura laterally and the fibrous pericardium medially. It leaves the thorax by passing through the vena

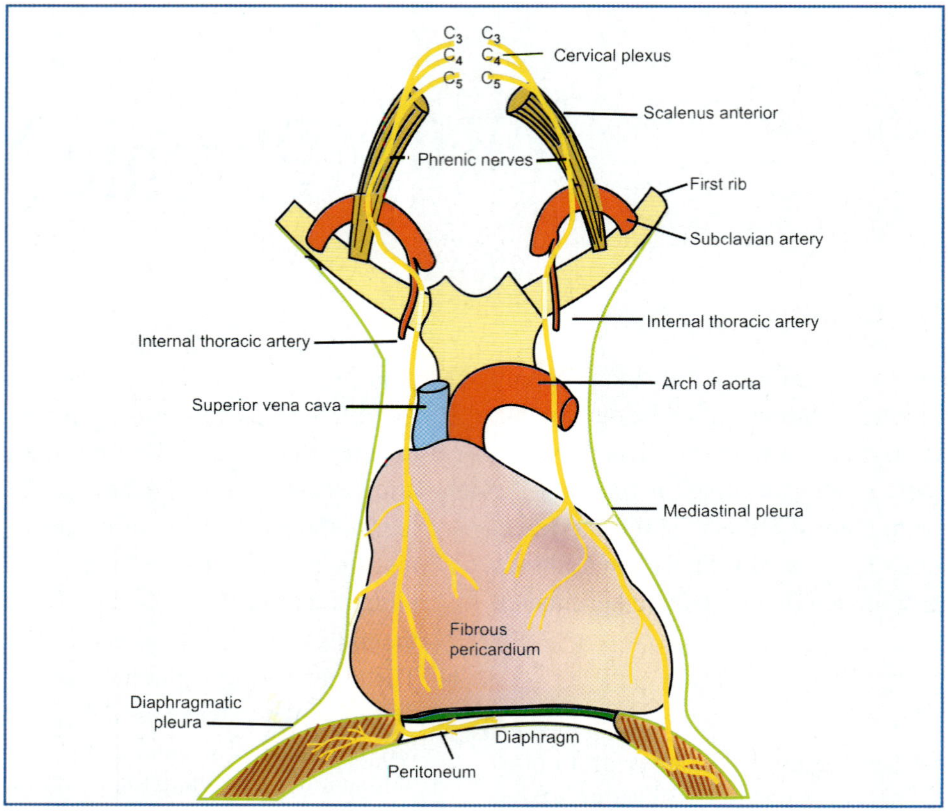

Fig. 41.1: Schematic diagram showing course and distribution of phrenic nerves (Note that the piece of rib between broken lines is assumed to be removed to expose the relation of phrenic nerve to internal thoracic artery)

caval opening or by piercing the central tendon in the vicinity of the opening.

The left phrenic nerve at first passes between left common carotid and left subclavian arteries and lies lateral to the left vagus nerve. Next, it crosses the left vagus nerve superficially and comes to lie medial to it. Both the nerves are crossed by left brachiocephalic vein. Then the phrenic nerve crosses the arch of aorta on its left and anterior aspect. After this the left phrenic nerve descends in front of the root of the left lung and in relation of the left ventricle covered by fibrous pericardium. In the middle mediastinum the nerve lies between the mediastinal pleura laterally and fibrous pericardium medially. It leaves the thorax by piercing the muscular part of diaphragm to the left of the anterior folium of the central tendon.

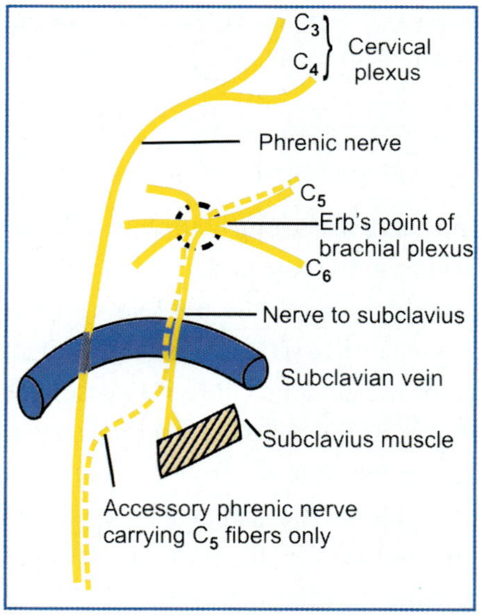

Fig. 41.2: Accessory phrenic nerve

Distribution

The phrenic nerves divide into branches, which ramify in the substance of the diaphragm or on its inferior surface and supply motor branches to anterior and posterior parts of muscle of the diaphragm. The sensory branches are given to the peritoneum lining the inferior surface of diaphragm, diaphragmatic pleura, mediastinal pleura and to the parietal and fibrous pericardium. In the inflammation of peritoneum or the pleura the pain is referred to the shoulder, which is the area of C4 dermatome.

Clinical Highlights

a. The phrenic nerve may be injured either in the neck or in the thorax. This results in paralysis of hemidiaphragm, which can be detected by X-ray screening. The paralyzed half of the diaphragm moves paradoxically during respiration and is pushed up in the thorax.

b. The avulsion of phrenic nerve is sometimes necessary in treating certain diseases. The nerve is approached via the base of the posterior triangle of the neck. It is freed from the prevertebral fascia in front of the scalenus anterior muscle and raised on a hook and then divided. The distal end of the nerve is grasped in a forceps and is twisted around the forceps and pulled upwards to tear out as much of the nerve as possible. In this way, the accessory phrenic nerve is also avulsed.

42 Development of Heart

The heart is the first organ to start function in the human embryo. During the third week of intrauterine life the angiogenic cells in the cardiogenic area at the cranial end of the embryonic disc form right and left endothelial cardiac tubes. Around 22nd day of development a single straight cardiac tube is formed by their fusion. Thus the cardiac tube is mesodermal in origin. It is located in the splanchnopleuric layer in the floor of the pericardial coelom. With the formation of the head fold of the embryonic disc, the pericardial coelom undergoes 180 degrees rotation. As a result of this, the cardiac tube and the splanchnopleuric layer come to lie on the dorsal aspect of the pericardial coelom. As the heart tube invaginates the splanchnopleuric mesoderm it gets encircled by it. The splanchnopleuric mesoderm forms the myoepicardial mantle around the cardiac tube. The endothe lium of the cardiac tube gives rise to the endocardium and the myoepicardial mantle to the myocardium and the epicardium (visceral layer of serous pericardium). The somatopleuric layer of pericardial coelom forms the parietal layer of serous pericardium. The cardiac tube is now suspended in the pericardial cavity by a dorsal mesocardium, which soon breaks down to form a communication between right and left halves of the pericardial cavity. This communication is the site of the transverse sinus of pericardium.

Subdivisions of Cardiac Tube

The cardiac tube is divisible into five chambers (Fig. 42.1). In cranio-caudal order the chambers are, truncus arteriosus, bulbus cordis, common ventricle, common atrium, and sinus venosus. A narrow atriventricular canal intervenes between the common ventricular and atrial chambers. The sinus venosus joins the atrial chamber by a midline sinu-atrial orifice. It is the venous end of the cardiac tube as it receives three pairs of veins on each side. Its two sides are drawn out as two horns. The truncus arteriosus is the arterial end of the cardiac tube and projects out as ventral aortic sac, which is connected by the arch arteries to the dorsal aortae on each side. By the end of 25 to 27 days the embryonic heart begins rhythmic beating.

Further Development of Cardiac Tube

The folding of the cardiac tube changes the tubular heart to a U-shaped bulbo-ventricular loop. Subsequently the sinus venosus moves upwards along with atrial chamber to lie behind and above the ventricle. The shape of the heart now changes to S-configuration (Fig. 42.2). At this

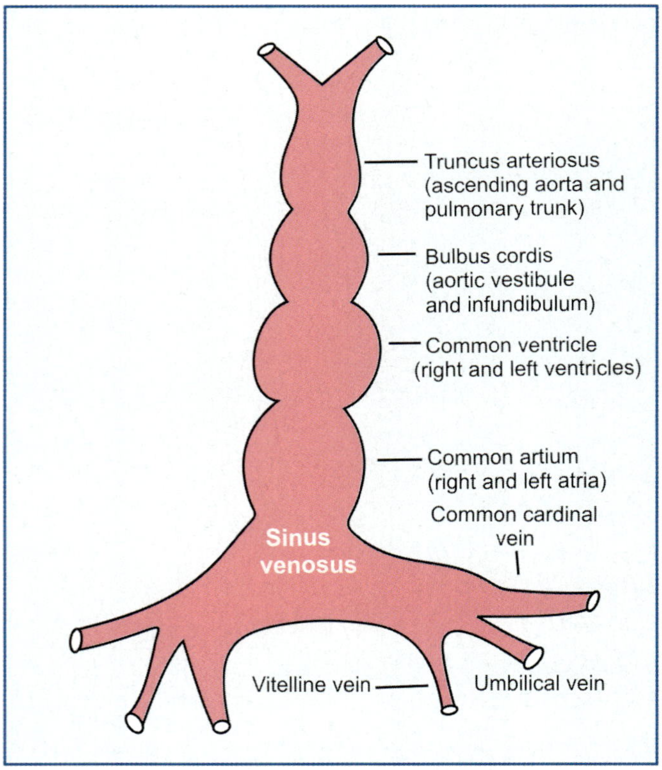

Fig. 42.1: Subdivisions of embryonic cardiac tube and their derivatives

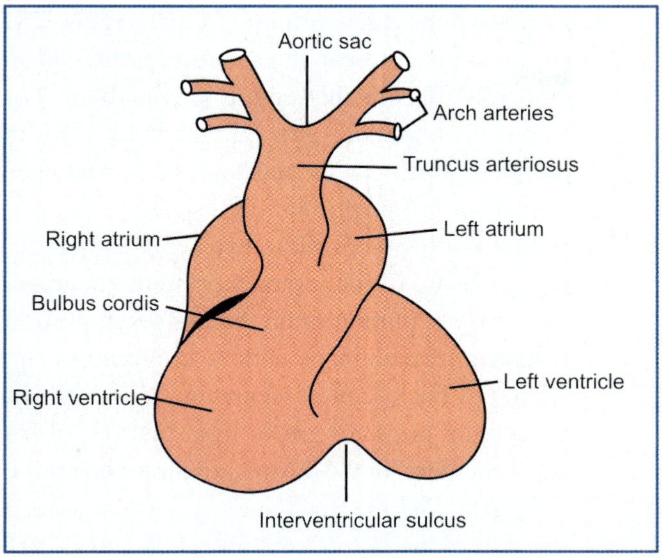

Fig. 42.2: S-shaped embryonic heart after folding of cardiac tube

stage the bulbus cordis and the ventricular chamber are separated by a deep bulbo-ventricular sulcus externally and a corresponding ridge internally. However, this sulcus becomes gradually shallower so that the bulbus cordis and the ventricle form a common chamber in continuation with truncus arteriosus. The sinus venosus is now posterior to the atrial chamber, which comes to lie behind the truncus arteriosus and the ventricle. The atrial chamber expands on either side of the truncus arteriosus. With these positional changes of the various parts, the contour of the embryonic heart resembles that of the adult heart.

Fate of Sinus Venosus (Fig. 42.3)

The sinus venosus is in communication with the atrial chamber by a mid-line sinuatrial orifice guarded by right and left venous valves. The left horn starts shrinking in size because of the diversion of blood from the left to the right side via transverse venous channels. The left horn is reduced to a tributary of the right horn, which grows proportionately very large in size. The position of the sinuatrial orifice is shifted to the right and its orientation becomes vertical. The cranial ends of the right and left venous valves fuse to form the septum spurium (Fig. 42.4). The right horn of sinus venosus is absorbed into the right half of the primitive atrial chamber to form the smooth sinus venarum of the right atrium. The left horn of the sinus venosus along with part of left common cardinal vein develops in to coronary sinus. The venous valves guarding the sinuatrial opening also undergo modifications. The superior and inferior limbic bands divide the right venous valve in to crista terminalis, valve of IVC opening and valve of coronary sinus opening. The sinus septum is a fold of inferior limbic band between the vena caval and coronary sinus openings. The sinus septum extends to gain attachment to the lower dorsal end of septum secundum. The left venous valve along with septum spurium fuses with the interatrial septum.

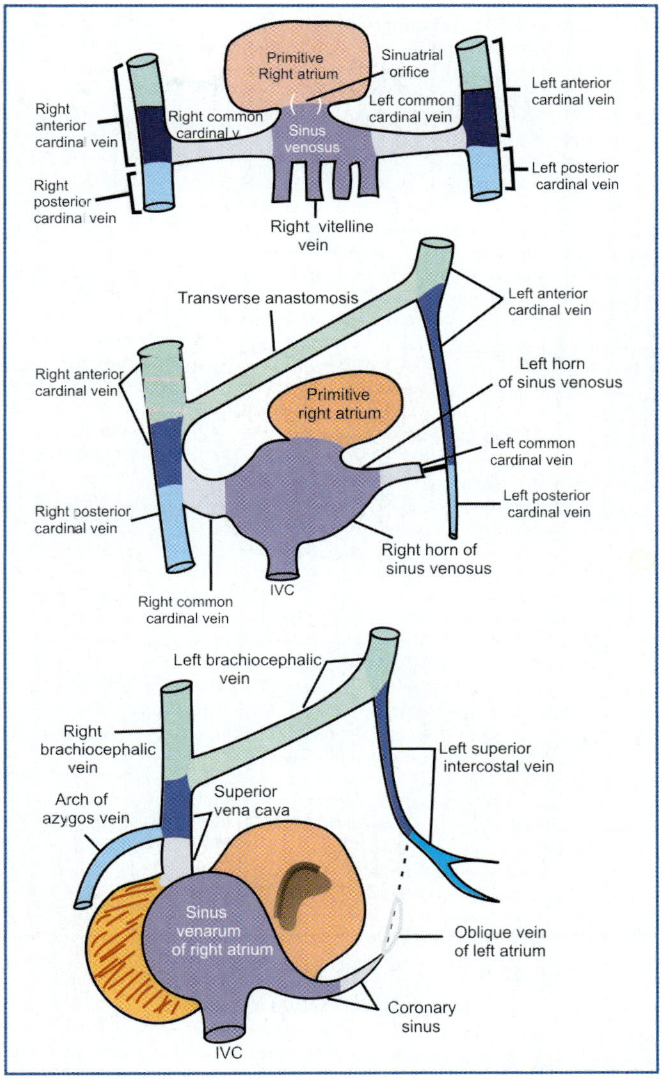

Fig. 42.3: Scheme to depict fate of sinus venosus. The figure also shows development of veins of thorax from cardinal veins

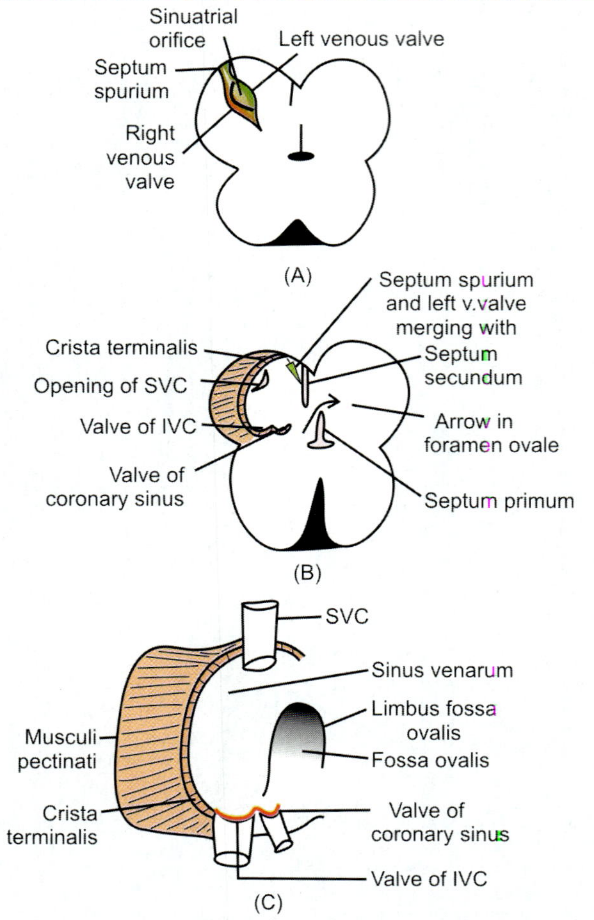

Fig. 42.4: Fate of right and left venous valves guarding sinuatrial orifice

Septation of Embryonic Heart

During 4-8 weeks of embryonic life septation simultaneously takes place in atrioventricular canal, atrium, ventricle, bulbus cordis and truncus arteriosus. The partition of a single heart tube in a four chambered pump, which contains four valves and gives rise to two blood vessels, is achieved by formation of seven septa, the septum intermedium, septum primum, septum secundum, aortico-pulmonary septum, proximal bulbar septum, distal bulbar septum and interventricular septum.

a. Septum intermedium divides the atrioventricular canal in to right and left halves. The dorsal and ventral walls of the atrioventricular canal develop endocardial cushions, which fuse with each other to form septum.
b. Interatrial septum is a valvular septum between the developing atria. This septum develops in stages because of its unique function during fetal life.
   i. At first a thin septum primum from the roof of the common atrium near the midline, grows down gradually towards the septum intermedium. The steadily narrowing gap between the septum primum and septum intermedium is called foramen primum or ostium primum (Fig. 42.5A).
   ii. Before the fusion of these two septa and consequent closure of the foramen primum, the upper part of the septum primum breaks down to form foramen secundum or ostium secundum (Fig. 42.5B). A thick septum secundum (to the right of the septum primum) grows from the roof of the atrial chamber, in the downward direction until it covers the foramen secundum on its right side.
   iii. The lower margin of septum secundum is free and concave (crista dividens). The oblique gap between the lower margin of septum secundum and the upper margin of septum primum is called foramen ovale (Fig. 42.5C). This foramen short-circuits the inferior vena caval blood to the left atrium. The flow of blood is unidirectional from the right to the left only. The septum primum acts as a flap valve since the pressure is greater in the right atrium than in the left in the fetal life. The foramen ovale closes after birth. This is accomplished as follows. The rise in the left atrial pressure soon after establishment of pulmonary circulation keeps the septum primum pressed against the septum secundum until they fuse. The septum primum becomes the floor of fossa ovalis and the lower margin of the septum secundum forms the limbus fossa ovalis. The functional closure of the foramen ovale occurs immediately after birth while the anatomical closure occurs 6 to 12 months after birth. In 15 to 20 percent of persons probe patency remains, which is symptom free.

Development of Pulmonary Veins (Fig. 42.5)

A single primary or common pulmonary vein develops from the dorsal wall of the left half of the common atrial chamber. This vein is believed to originate in the angiogenic cells in early dorsal mesocardium. These cells soon establish continuity with the endothelial cells of the cardiac tube. The single pulmonary vein divides into right and left pulmonary veins, which again divide and enter the lung

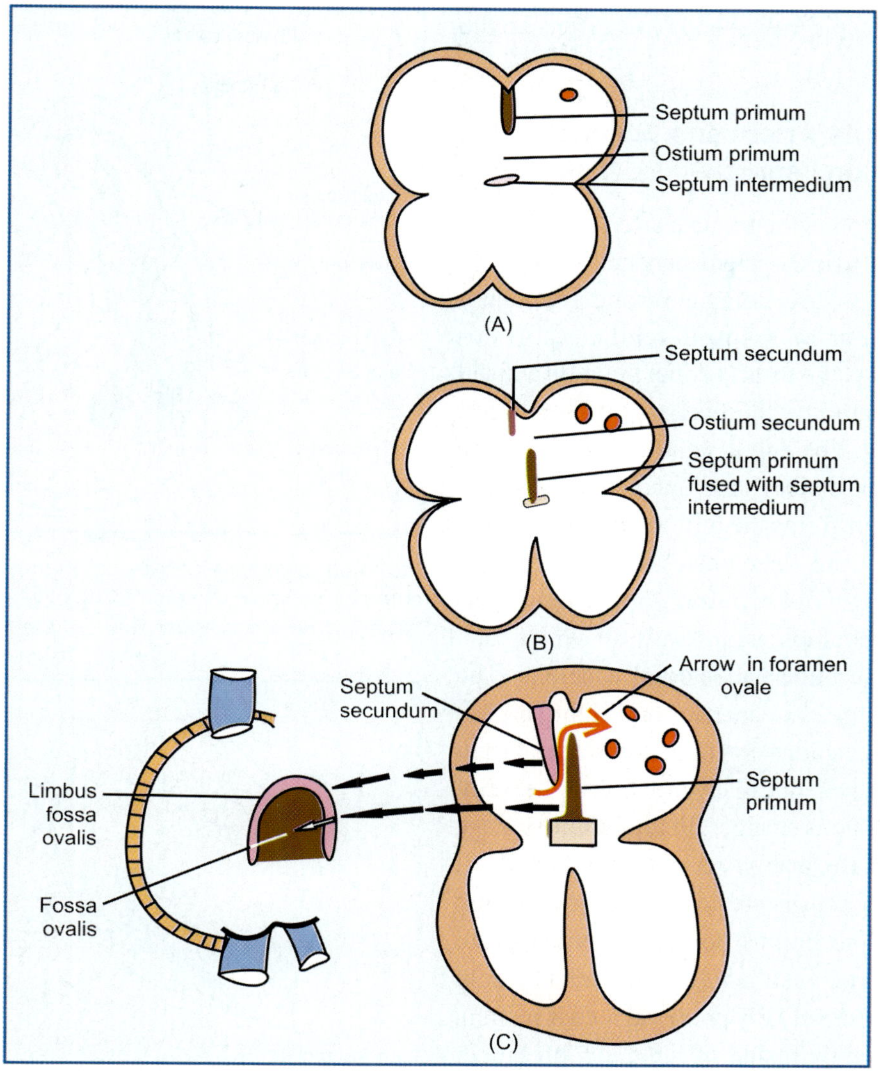

Fig. 42.5: Stages in development of interatrial septum. Figure also shows development of pulmonary veins in left atrium

bud. The common trunk of the original pulmonary vein with its right and left divisions until the bifurcation is absorbed in the common atrium on the left side. The result of this absorption is that four separate pulmonary veins establish communication with the left half of common atrium.

Developmental Sources of Atria

The right atrium develops from three sources, the rough part from the right half of common atrium, the smooth part or sinus venarum from the right horn of sinus venosus and the vestibule of the atrioventricular orifice from the right half of the A-V canal.

The left atrium develops from three sources, the rough part from the left half of common atrium, the smooth part from the absorbed parts of the pulmonary vein and the vestibule of the atrioventricular orifice from the left half of the A-V canal.

Atrioventricular Valves

The A-V valves are formed from the endocardial cushions in the right and left atrioventricular canals. The ventricular surface of the cushions is excavated to form the valves, which are attached to ventricular walls by trabecular cords modified later into chordae tendinae and papillary muscles. In this way, three leaflets are formed on the right side (tricuspid valve) and two leaflets on the left side (mitral valve).

Septation in Truncus Arteriosus, Bulbus Cordis and Common Ventricle (Fig. 42.6)

The process of septation in the truncus arteriosus, bulbus cordis and primitive ventricle is interdependent. The truncus arteriosus is divided into ascending aorta and pulmonary trunk by development of a spiral septum (aortico-pulmonary septum). At the trunco-conal junction a distal bulbar septum is formed by the fusion of right and left endocardial cushions. The spiral septum fuses with the distal bulbar septum and divides it into anterior and posterior parts. The anterior part forms the pulmonary valve at the origin of pulmonary trunk. The posterior part forms the aortic valve at the origin of ascending aorta. In each part one more cushion develops, as a result of which each orifice comes to have three endocardial cushions. The pulmonary cushions are, one anterior and right and left posterior. The aortic cushions are, one posterior and right and left anterior. However, due to levorotation of the heart, the position of the cushions changes. In the definitive stage the pulmonary cusps are, one posterior and right and left anterior and the aortic cusps are, one anterior and right and left posterior. The bulbus cordis is divided in to infundibulum and aortic vestibule (outflow tract of right and left ventricle respectively) by proximal bulbar septum. This septum is formed by fusion of right and left bulbar ridges.

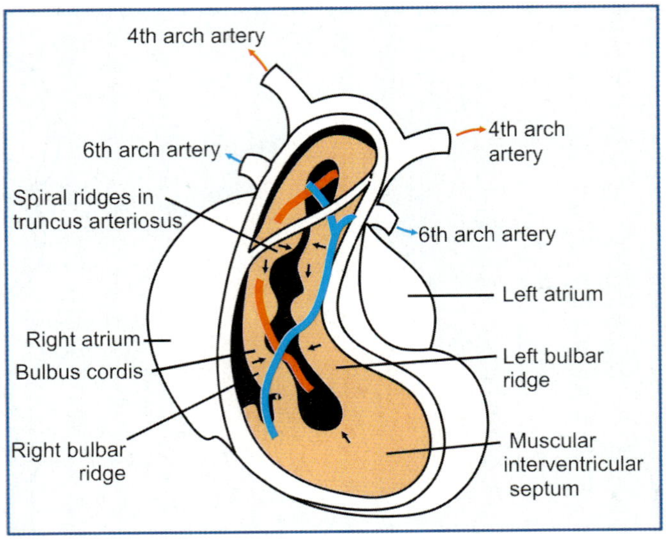

Fig. 42.6: Septation of truncus arteriosus, bulbus cordis and common ventricle. Note crossing of venous and arterial blood streams in truncus arteriosus

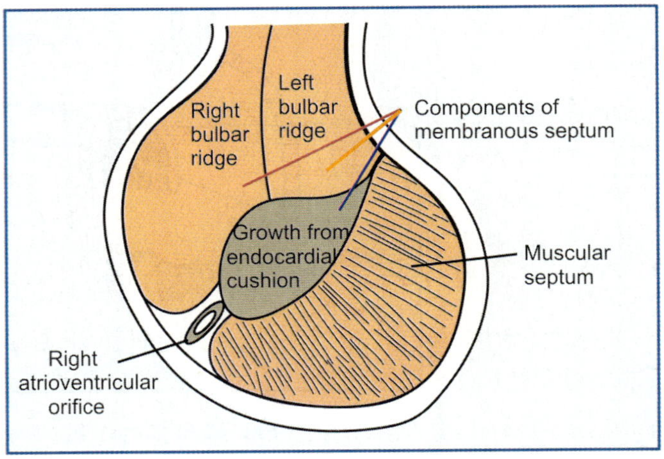

Fig. 42.7: Developmental sources of interventricular septum

Interventricular Septum (Fig. 42.7)

The interventricular septum is of composite origin because its muscular and membranous parts develop from separate sources. The muscular part is the first to develop from the floor of the bulbo-ventricular cavity. It divides the lower dilated part of the cavity into right and left halves. A large gap between the upper margin of the muscular septum and the bulboventricular ridge is called the interventricular foramen. The absorption of the ridge is essential for establishing the alignment between the bulbus and the ventricles. The interventricular foramen is closed to a certain extent by the right and left bulbar ridges of proximal bulbar septum, from above. The narrowed gap is completely filled by proliferation from the right end of endocardial cushion tissue of septum intermedium. Thus, the membranous part of septum develops from right bulbar ridge, left bulbar ridge and proliferation from endocardial cushion. The attachment of the septal cusp of the tricuspid valve divides the membranous septum in the fully developed state into an anterior interventricular part and a posterior atrioventricular part. The interventricular part develops from the proximal bulbar septum and the endocardial cushion proliferation, while the atrioventricular part is the right half of the endocardial cushion.

Developmental Sources of Ventricles

a. The right ventricle develops from two sources, the inflow part from the right half of common ventricle and the outflow part (infundibulum) from bulbus cordis.
b. The left ventricle develops from two sources, the inflow part from the left half of the common ventricle and the outflow part (aortic vestibule) develops from the bulbus cordis.

Development of Conducting Tissue

The nodal tissue develops from the sinus venosus close to the opening of the common cardinal vein. The right nodal tissue becomes the SA node around third month and is located near the opening of the superior vena cava in the upper part of the right atrium. The AV node develops from the left nodal tissue in the sinus venosus as well as in the endocardial cushions in the A-V canal around six-week stage of the embryo.

Congenital Anomalies

a. The heart may not be in the normal position. In dextrocardia the heart rotates to the right so that its apex is located in the right fifth intercostal space. In ectopia cordis the heart is exposed on the chest wall due to defective formation of anterior thoracic wall with cleft sternum.
b. Atrial septal defect (ASD) is the congenital anomaly, which becomes manifest in adult life. There are three types of ASD (Fig. 42.8) resulting in left to right shunt. The ostium secundum defect is one of the most common congenital heart defects. The persistence of the foramen secundum is due to excessive resorption in the septum primum or due to failure of development of septum secundum. The ostium primum defect is due to either to the failure of the septum primum to reach the endocardial cushions or due to defect in the endocardial cushions, so that foramen primum persists. Patent foramen ovale is due to failure of the septum primum and secundum to fuse after birth. This is extremely rare. In ASD there is increased load on the right side of the heart leading to progressive enlargement of right atrium, right ventricle and the pulmonary trunk. The disease manifests as effort intolerance (fatigue and breathlessness on exertion) in the third or fourth decade of life and thereafter. The atrial septal defects can be corrected by surgery.

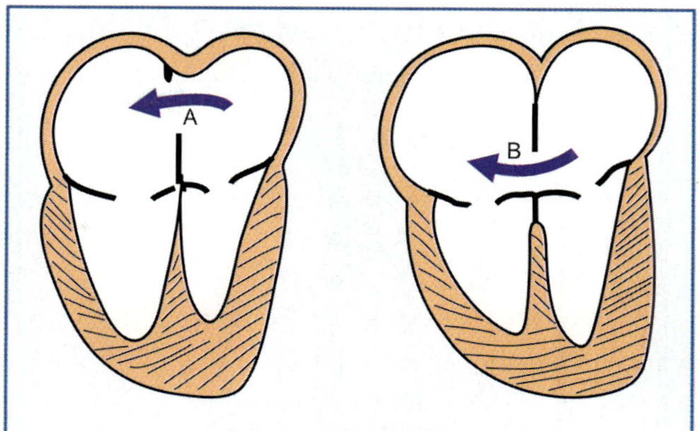

Fig. 42.8: Types of atrial septal defect (ASD). Note that both defects are in septum primum

c. Ventricular septal defects (VSD) involving the membranous part of the septum are very common. VSD may occur singly or in combination with other cardiac defects. The hemodynamic effects of VSD are quite serious. The blood flows from the left ventricle to the right ventricle and from here to the pulmonary circulation leading to enlargement of right ventricle, pulmonary trunk and pulmonary arteries. Large VSD may lead to pulmonary hypertension and congestive cardiac failure in infancy.
d. Tetralogy of Fallot (TOF) is a combination of four defects (Fig. 42.9), VSD, over-riding of aorta (ascending aorta having connection to both ventricles), pulmonary stenosis and right ventricular hypertrophy. The aorta carries mixed blood, which results in cyanosis. The effects of TOF are as follows. i. The right chambers of the heart are enlarged. ii. The pulmonary circulation does not receive much blood due to pulmonary stenosis. iii. The pulmonary artery is usually narrowed. iv. The child may have cyanotic spells especially during crying. v. There is shortness of breath or dyspnea on exertion, which is relieved by assuming squatting position for a few minutes. The reason for this is that squatting blocks the venous return and increases the peripheral resistance of the arteries so that more blood reaches the lungs. vi. The growth of the child is retarded due to hypoxia.

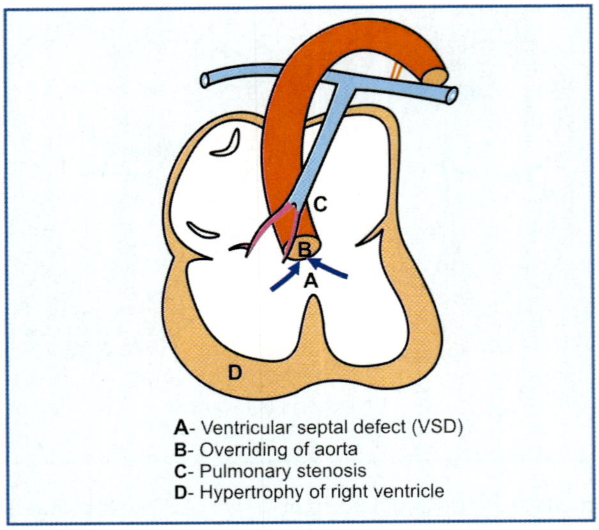

Fig. 42.9: Fallot's tetralogy

e. Pentalogy of Fallot (POF) is the name given to a condition in which the tetralogy is associated with the atrial septal defect (ASD).
f. Pink Fallot results if the pulmonary stenosis in TOF is not severe. In such cases there is bi-directional shunt across the VSD. Such patients do not have cyanosis and hence this TOF is called pink Fallot or acyanotic TOF.
g. Transposition of great vessels is associated with a large VSD. In this defect, the aorta originates from the right ventricle and the pulmonary trunk from the left ventricle. The left side of the heart is connected to pulmonary circulation only. The right side of the heart is connected to systemic circulation only. The two circulations are independent of each other. Life is sustained through mixing of blood via VSD.

Fetal Circulation (Fig. 42.10)

The circulation of blood in the prenatal life is different from that of postnatal life, primarily because the lungs of the fetus are not functional. The unique feature of fetal circulation is the presence of three shunts or bypass channels (ductus venosus, foramen ovale and ductus arteriosus) and three blood vessels connected to placenta (left umbilical vein and left and right umbilical arteries). The left umbilical vein carrying oxygenated blood originates in the placenta. It enters the fetus through the umbilical cord and umbilicus and reaches the liver, where it joins the left branch of the portal vein. Instead of circulating in the liver the blood is diverted from the left branch of portal vein to the inferior vena cava by the ductus venosus. The inferior vena cava brings this oxygenated blood to the right atrium, from where it is directed towards the foramen ovale by valve of the IVC. So the blood reaches the left atrium without passing through the pulmonary vessels and lungs. From the left atrium the blood reaches the left ventricle and to the aorta. The aorta receives the venous blood from the right ventricle through ductus arteriosus, which connects the aorta and the left pulmonary artery. Thus, the upper part of the body receives more oxygenated blood compared to the lower part because of mixing of venous blood in the aorta distal to the connection with the ductus arteriosus. The right and left umbilical arteries carry the deoxygenated blood from the lower end of abdominal aorta for purification in the placenta.

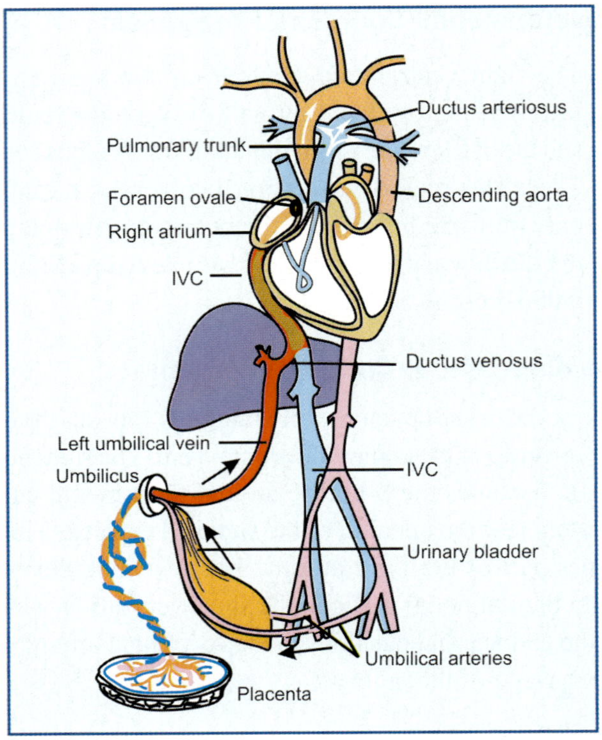

Fig. 42.10: Fetal circulation (Note: The short circuiting channels—ductus venosus, foramen ovale and ductus arteriosus)

Postnatal Changes in Fetal Circulation

The physiological closure of the three shunts and three blood vessels mentioned above occurs immediately after birth. The time of anatomical closure for the umbilical vessels and ductus venosus is two to three months after birth. The anatomical closure of ductus arteriosus occurs one to three months and that of foramen ovale six months after birth.

a. The left umbilical vein becomes the ligamentum teres of liver.
b. The ductus venosus becomes the ligamentum venosum.
c. The foramen ovale is replaced by the fossa ovalis and limbus fossa ovalis in the interatrial septum.
d. The ductus arteriosus becomes the ligamentum arteriosum.
e. The umbilical arteries undergo changes as follows. Their proximal patent parts form the superior vesical arteries and distal obliterated parts become the lateral umbilical ligaments.

Patent Ductus Arteriosus (PDA)

The patent ductus arteriosus (PDA) is a commonly seen in the rubella syndrome, which occurs in children whose mothers had German measles during the first two months of pregnancy. It may occur singly or in combination with other cardiac defects. In PDA the ductus arteriosus fails to obliterate postnatally. So a communication exists between the arch of aorta and left pulmonary artery (Fig. 42.11). Since the pulmonary arterial pressure is lower than that in the aorta, there is a continuous flow of blood from the aorta to the pulmonary artery. This is the reason for the presence of characteristic continuous murmur in PDA. The overloading of pulmonary circulation may result in enlargement of left atrium, left ventricle and ascending aorta. The symptoms of overload of pulmonary circulation are, recurrent respiratory infections, shortness of breath on exertion and palpitation. Surgical correction is feasible three to six months after birth.

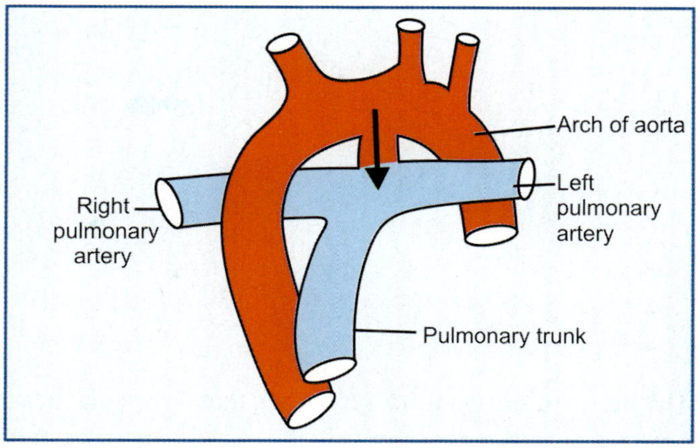

Fig. 42.11: Patent ductus arteriosus (PDA). Note the arrow in the patent ductus arteriosus

43 Pericardium

The pericardium is a fibroserous sac that covers the heart and the roots of great vessels in the middle mediastinum. It lies behind the body of the sternum and the second to sixth costal cartilages and in front of the fifth to eighth thoracic vertebrae. The pericardium is subdivided into the outer fibrous and inner serous pericardium. The pericardial cavity is enclosed between the parietal and visceral layers of serous pericardium and contains a small quantity of serous fluid. This facilitates the sliding of the two serous layers over each other during cardiac movements.

Development of Pericardium and Pericardial Sinuses

The pericardial cavity develops from the intraembryonic coelom. The cardiac tube invaginates the pericardial sac from the dorsal side. The splanchnopleuric mesoderm surrounds the cardiac tube. It gives rise to the myocardium and visceral pericardium. The somatopleuric mesoderm gives rise to the parietal pericardium. The visceral and parietal layers are continuous along a fold called dorsal mesocardium. With the degeneration of the dorsal mesocardium the visceral and parietal layers are in continuity only at the venous and arterial ends of the cardiac tube. After the folding of the cardiac tube its venous and arterial ends come close to each other and the space enclosed between them (space at the site of dorsal mesocardium) becomes the transverse sinus. In this way, in the definitive stage, the pulmonary trunk and ascending aorta representing the arterial end form the anterior boundary and the atria representing the venous end form the posterior boundary of the transverse sinus. The atria receive six veins, two in the right atrium and four in the left atrium. When these veins separate from each other (due to increase in size of the atria) the line of pericardial reflection becomes irregular. Along this irregular line a small recess of pericardial cavity is trapped. This recess is called the oblique sinus, which lies posterior to the left atrium. The lower part of the fibrous pericardium develops from septum transversum.

Fibrous Pericardium (Fig. 41.1)

It is a tough fibrous sac, which is shaped like a cone with an apex directed superiorly and a wide base inferiorly. The apex is continuous with the adventitia of great vessels at the level of sternal angle. The base blends with the central tendon of diaphragm. Inferior vena cava pierces the base posteriorly on the right side.

Anteriorly the fibrous pericardium is related to the structures in the anterior mediastinum. It is connected to body of sternum by upper and lower sternopericardial ligaments. The anterior margins of lungs and pleurae overlap this surface except over the bare area of the pericardium (opposite fourth and fifth costal cartilages on the left side), where the anterior margins of left lung and pleura deviate and the pericardium comes in direct contact with the thoracic wall. The part of the thymus in the anterior mediastinum is related to the upper part of pericardium in childhood.

Posteriorly the fibrous pericardium is related to the principal bronchi, the descending thoracic aorta and esophagus. This surface is pierced by four pulmonary veins.

Laterally it is related to the mediastinal pleura and through it to the mediastinal surface of respective lung. Phrenic nerve and pericardiacophrenic vessels descend on the left and right lateral surfaces of the fibrous pericardium. Incisions in the pericardium are always vertically placed to avoid injury to the phrenic nerves.

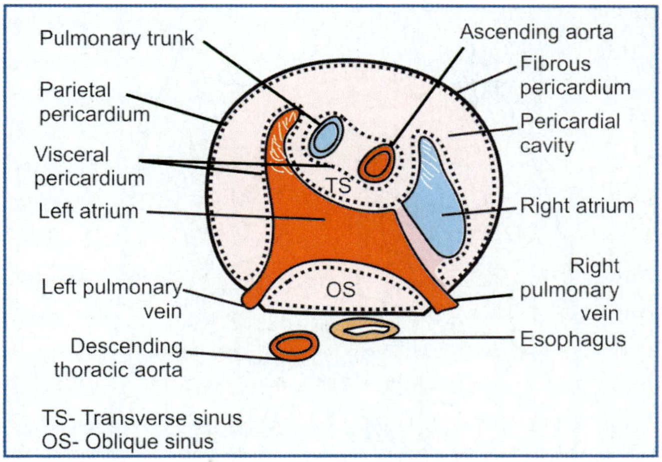

Fig. 43.1: Pericardial sinuses

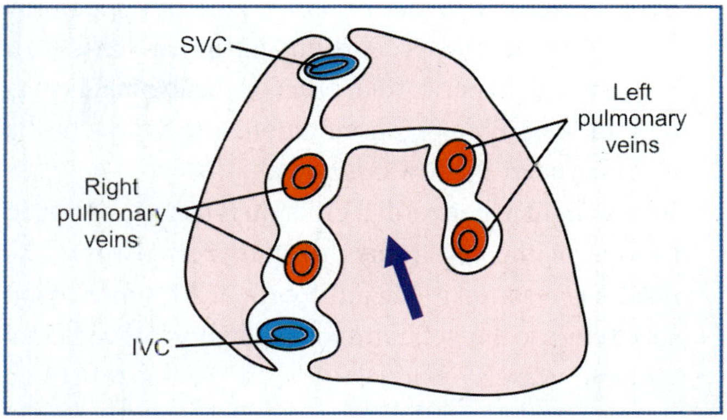

Fig. 43.2: Oblique sinus of pericardium (indicated by arrow)

Functions

The fibrous pericardium retains the heart in the middle mediastinum and prevents its over-distention. In the life-saving procedure, external cardiac massage the heart is squeezed inside the firm fibrous pericardium between the fixed vertebral column and somewhat resilient sternum and costal cartilages by applying rhythmic pressure to the lower sternum.

Blood Supply

The pericardial branches of the internal thoracic artery and of descending thoracic aorta provide arterial blood. The pericardial veins drain in the azygos and hemiazygos veins.

Nerve Supply

The phrenic nerves give sensory branches to the fibrous pericardium.

Serous Pericardium

The visceral layer (epicardium) covers the myocardium and the intrapericardial parts of the great vessels closely. It is reflected at the points, where the great vessels pierce the fibrous pericardium, on to the parietal layer, which lines the internal surface of the fibrous pericardium. Along the lines of pericardial reflection there are two pericardial sinuses, namely transverse and oblique.

Boundaries of Transverse Sinus (Fig. 43.1)

Anteriorly it is limited by the visceral pericardium covering the ascending aorta and pulmonary trunk and posteriorly by the visceral pericardium covering anterior surface of left atrium. The transverse sinus is open on either side and thus communicates the two halves of the pericardial cavity to each other. The transverse sinus provides space during cardiac surgery to clamp the ascending aorta and pulmonary trunk in order to insert tubes of heart lung machine in these vessels.

Boundaries of Oblique Sinus (Figs 43.1 and 43.2)

Anterior boundary is the visceral pericardium covering the posterior surface of left atrium. Its posterior boundary is the parietal pericardium lining the posterior surface of fibrous pericardium. On the right it is bounded by the pericardial reflection from IVC and right pulmonary veins. On the left it is limited by the pericardial reflection from left pulmonary veins. Superiorly there is pericardial reflection along the superior margins of the left atrium. The sinus is open inferiorly. The oblique sinus intervenes between the left atrium anteriorly and the esophagus posteriorly. It is believed to act as a bursa for the left atrium to expand during filling.

Blood Supply and Nerve Supply of Serous Pericardium

The parietal layer shares its blood supply and nerve supply with the fibrous pericardium. The visceral layer shares its blood supply and nerve supply with the heart.

Clinical Highlights

a. Inflammation of serous pericardium is called pericarditis, which may be due to bacterial or viral infections, rheumatic fever or uremia. Pain of pericarditis is referred to the precordium (front of chest) or epigastrium. In pericardial effusion, heart sounds may be faintly audible on auscultation. On X-ray chest a globular heart shadow is evident.

b. Excess fluid in pericardial effusion is usually removed by one of the two routes. In parasternal route the needle is inserted in the left fourth or fifth intercostal space close to the sternum avoiding injury to the internal thoracic vessels. Since the line of pleural reflection deviates in 4th and 5th intercostal spaces the needle does not pierce the pleura. This route is also preferred for giving intracardiac injections. In the subcostal (costoxiphoid) route (Fig. 43.3) the needle is introduced at the left costoxiphoid angle in an upward and backward direction to enter the pericardial cavity through the rectus sheath and the central tendon of diaphragm. Here too the pleura is saved because the pleural line of reflection does not extend below costal margin on the left side.

c. When there is rapid accumulation of fluid (blood or serous fluid) in the pericardial cavity it interferes with the atrial filling during diastole. This results in decreased cardiac output, increased heart rate and increased venous pressure. This is known as cardiac tamponade. Immediate tapping or aspiration of fluid is necessary to restore normal cardiac output.

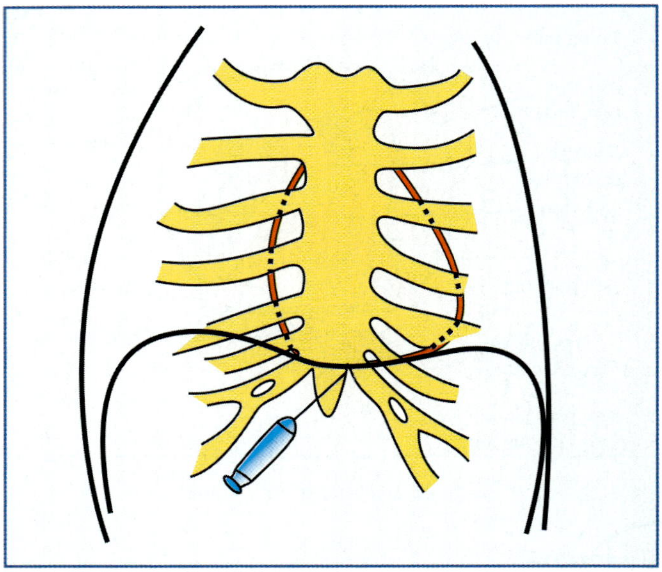

Fig. 43.3: Pericardiocentesis through left costoxiphoid angle

44 Gross Anatomy of Heart

The heart is a four- chambered muscular pump. The heart is covered with double-layered pericardium enclosing a potential pericardial cavity. Outermost covering of the heart and of the serous pericardium is called the fibrous pericardium. The muscle of the heart is known as myocardium, which contracts nonstop through out life. The right side of the heart consisting of right atrium and ventricle receives venous blood, which is pumped to the lungs for oxygenation by the pulmonary arteries. The left side of the heart consisting of left atrium and ventricle receives oxygenated blood, which is pumped to the entire body by the aorta and its branches. The interatrial septum and the interventricular septum are the partitions between atria and ventricles. There are four cardiac orifices, two atrioventricular orifices (mitral and tricuspid) and two semilunar orifices (pulmonary and aortic).

Orientation of Heart in Thorax

The heart is placed obliquely in the middle mediastinum of the thoracic cavity. Approximately two-thirds of it lies to the left and one-third to the right of the midline (Figs 44.1and 44.2). It makes an angle of 45° with the sagittal plane. Therefore, the terms right and left used in reference to relationship of cardiac chambers to each other are not strictly true. The correct perspective regarding the position and relations of the cardiac chambers is depicted in Figure 44.2, in which one can observe that the right part of the heart is in anterior location in respect to its left part due to the rotation of the heart to the left. The right atrium is anterior, inferior and to the right of the left atrium. The interatrial septum is inclined in a plane that is midway between the coronal and sagittal planes. The major part of right ventricle is anterior to the left ventricle. Hence if a knife is pushed into the chest by the side of the sternum in the left fifth or sixth intercostal space it will enter the right ventricle. However, the lower end of the right ventricle is to the right of the apical part of left ventricle and its superior extremity bearing pulmonary orifice is actually to the left, superior and anterior of the aortic orifice of the left ventricle. The left atrium forms the most posterior part of the heart. Therefore, it is very close to the esophagus located in the posterior mediastinum. The left ventricle is prominent inferiorly as it forms the left margin and the apex of the heart.

External Features

The average size of the heart is of that of a clenched fist of the person. The average weight of the adult heart is 280 gm. The atria are separated from the ventricles by an almost circular atrioventricular or coronary sulcus. This sulcus has an anterior part on the sternocostal surface (Fig. 44.3) and the posterior part between the base of the

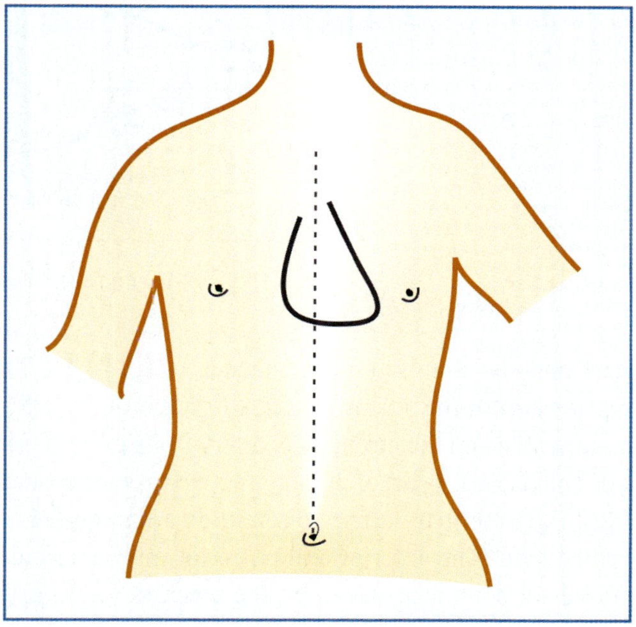

Fig. 44.1: Outline of normally positioned heart in relation to sagittal plane

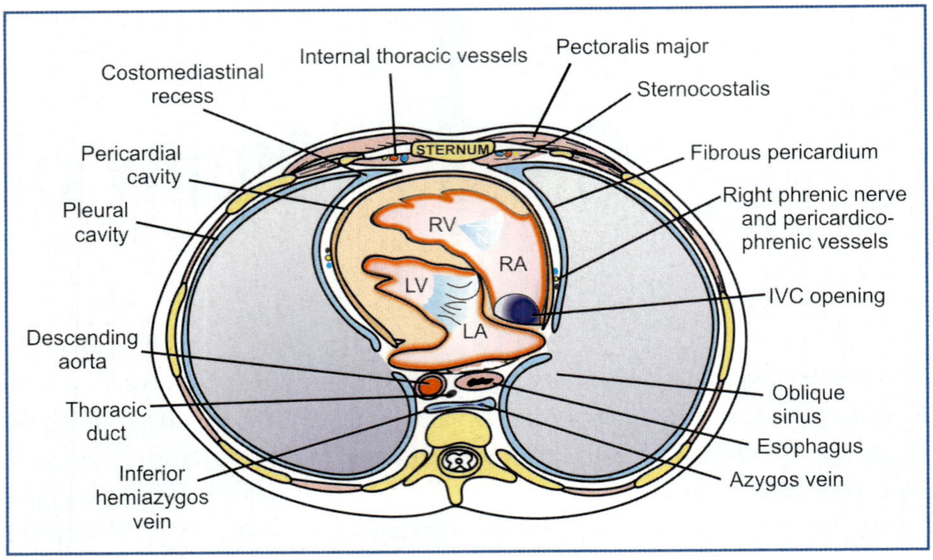

Fig. 44.2: Cross-section at T8 level to depict relations of heart and pericardium in thoracic cavity

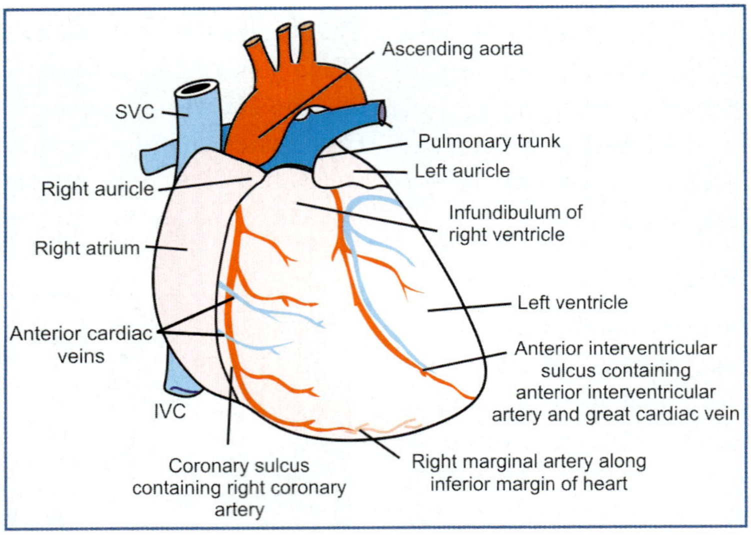

Fig. 44.3: Sternocostal surface of heart

heart and the diaphragmatic surface (Fig. 44.4). The anterior part of the sulcus contains right coronary artery on right side and the circumflex artery in its extreme left end. The posterior part of the sulcus contains the coronary sinus, right coronary artery, circumflex artery and small cardiac vein. The anterior and posterior interventricular grooves or sulci are located on the anterior and inferior surfaces respectively, indicating the line of attachment of the interventricular septum. Similarly there is an interatrial sulcus visible on the posterior aspect of the base of the heart. The point of junction of the atrio-ventricular, interatrial and posterior interventricular sulci is termed the crux of the heart. So, the crux (Fig. 44.5) is located in the posterior part of the atrioventricular sulcus.

Borders and Surfaces

The heart has a pointed apex directed inferiorly and a broad base directed posterosuperiorly. There are four

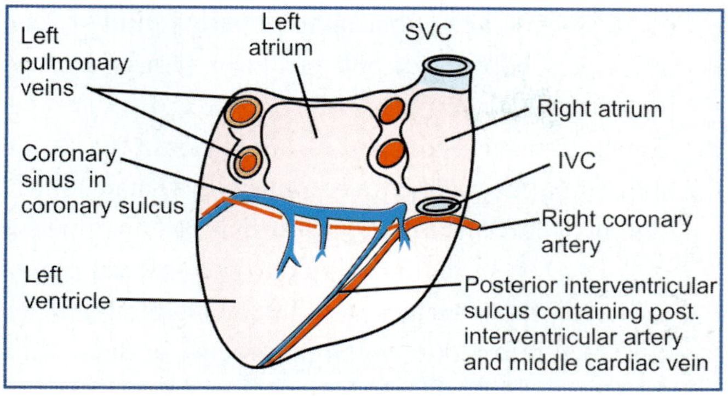

Fig. 44.4: Posterior (base) and diaphragmatic surfaces of heart

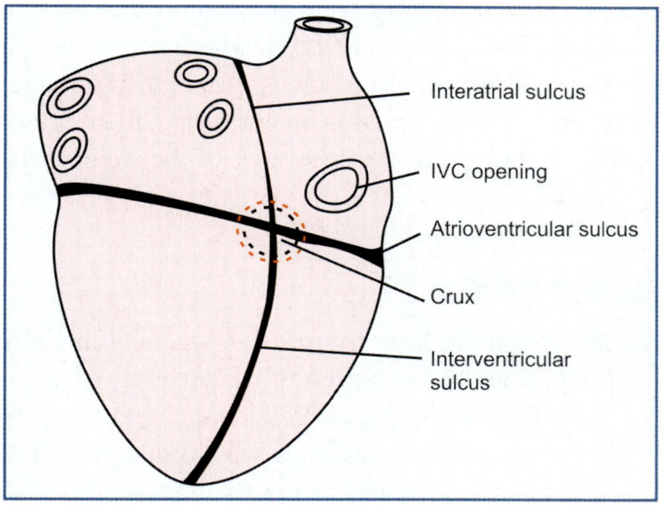

Fig. 44.5: Crux of the heart viewed from posterior aspect

margins limiting four surfaces. The margins are, superior, inferior (acute), right and left (obtuse). The surfaces are, anterior or sternocostal, inferior or diaphragmatic, left and right.

Apex of the Heart

The apex is the most mobile part of the heart. It is directed downward, forward and to the left and is formed by left ventricle only. The apex is located at the junction of inferior and left borders of the heart. It is separated from the anterior thoracic wall by left lung and pleura. Apex beat is the impulse produced by the apex when it impinges on the chest wall during systole. It may be visible in thin individuals. The character and position of the apex beat have clinical relevance. In enlargement or hypertrophy of left ventricle the apex shifts in downward and lateral direction. The common causes of the downward and lateral shift of the apex are, mitral regurgitation, aortic regurgitation and systemic hypertension. In right ventricular hypertrophy as happens in pulmonary stenosis, the apex shifts in lateral direction only.

Margins of Heart

a. The right margin is entirely formed by the right atrium and is almost vertical.
b. The inferior or acute margin is formed by right ventricle mainly with a very small contribution by the left ventricle. The right marginal branch of right coronary artery and the accompanying vein course along this margin. The anterior and posterior interventricular grooves cut this margin a little to the right of the cardiac apex, at a point called apical incisure or notch. The anterior and posterior interventricular arteries meet each other at this point.
c. The left or obtuse margin is formed by left ventricle mainly with a small contribution by left auricle superiorly. The left end of coronary sulcus and its contents, namely, circumflex artery and great cardiac vein cross the left margin. The marginal branch of circumflex artery runs along the left margin
d. The superior margin is formed by the upper margins of the atria and is hidden from the sternocostal surface by the ascending aorta and pulmonary trunk. The bifurcation of the pulmonary trunk coincides with this margin.

Surfaces of Heart

a. The sternocostal surface (Fig. 44.3) faces upwards, forwards and to the left. The right ventricle, right atrium, right auricle and a small strip of left ventricle and the left auricle contribute to it. The roots of the great vessels interrupt the anterior part of the atrioventricular sulcus. The part of the sulcus to the right of roots of the great vessels appears on the sternocostal surface between the right ventricle and atrium and extends up to the junction of right and inferior margins. The anterior part of the sulcus contains the right coronary artery embedded in the fat. The anterior cardiac veins cross over the sulcus to reach the right atrium. The ventricular part of the sternocostal surface lies to the left of the coronary sulcus. The anterior interventricular groove (sulcus) demarcates the two ventricles on this surface. It contains anterior interventricular branch of left coronary artery and the great cardiac vein embedded in fat. Superiorly and to the left, the right ventricle is prolonged as the infundibulum, which continues as the pulmonary trunk at the pulmonary orifice. Inferiorly and to the left, the left ventricle forms the apex of the heart. A finger -shaped left auricle projects on the sternocostal surface to overlap the left aspect of the pulmonary trunk. Anteriorly this surface is related (from within outwards) to the pericardium, anterior mediastinum, anterior margins of the lungs and pleura (including the left costo-mediastinal recess), the body of sternum and the third to sixth costal cartilages. The part related to the left costomediastinal pleural recess gives a dull note on light percussion (an area of superficial cardiac dullness).

b. The diaphragmatic surface is flat and rests on the central tendon of diaphragm. The left ventricle (left two-thirds) and the right ventricle (right one-third) contribute to this surface. The demarcating line between the two ventricles is the posterior interventricular groove, which contains posterior interventricular branch of right coronary artery and middle cardiac vein.

c. The base (Fig. 44.4) is also referred to as the posterior surface. It is the most fixed part of the heart. It is quadrilateral in outline and faces backwards and to the right. The left atrium forms the left two-thirds of the base and the right atrium forms the right one-third. A faint interatrial groove marks the demarcation between the two atria. The base lies at the level of fifth to eighth thoracic vertebrae in supine position. In standing position it descends by one vertebra. Six large veins open into the base of the heart. The four pulmonary veins (one pair on each side) open in the left atrium, the left pair being close to the left margin of the base and the right pair just to the left of interatrial groove. The two great veins open in the right atrial part of the base, the SVC at the right superior angle and the IVC at the right inferior angle of the base. The relations of the base (Fig. 43.1) are important. It is related anteriorly to the transverse sinus of pericardium and the roots of the great vessels and posteriorly to the oblique sinus of pericardium, which intervenes between it and posterior part of fibrous pericardium.

d. The left surface consists of almost entirely of the obtuse margin of the left ventricle with a small contri–bution of left atrium and its auricle at the superior end. The left surface is related to mediastinal pleura and mediastinal surface of left lung and pleura hence it is often referred to as left pulmonary surface. This surface is widest above, where it is crossed by the left part of the atrioventricular sulcus, which contains the circumflex artery, the great cardiac vein and the beginning of coronary sinus.

e. The rounded right surface is also described as the right pulmonary surface since it comes in contact with right lung and pleura. The sulcus terminalis (terminal groove), which is present on this surface, demarcates this surface from the atrial part of the sternocostal surface.

Surface Marking (Fig. 45.5)

a. The apex of the heart is marked by a point 9 cm away from the midline in the left fifth intercostal space.

b. The right margin is drawn by joining a point on the lower part of the second right intercostal space close to the sternum to a point on the right sixth costal cartilage 1-2 cm from the sternal margin.

c. The inferior margin is drawn by joining a point on the right sixth costal cartilage 1-2 cm from the margin of the sternum to a point representing the apex of the heart.

d. The left margin is drawn by a line joining the point representing the apex of the heart to a point on the second left intercostal space 1-2 cm from the sternal margin.

e. The superior margin is indicated by a line from a point on the upper part on the left second intercostal space 1-2 cm lateral to the sternal margin to a point close to the margin of the sternum in the lower part of right second intercostal space.

f. The anterior part of the atrioventricular sulcus is indicated by an oblique line extending from the sternal end of the left third costal cartilage to the sternal end of right sixth costal cartilage.

45 Chambers of Heart

RIGHT ATRIUM

The right atrium receives the venous blood from the entire body via SVC and IVC and from the heart via the coronary sinus. It lies anterior as well as to the right of the left atrium. Among the cardiac chambers the right atrium has the thinnest wall. The right atrium forms part of the sternocostal surface of the heart. The right auricle projects from it to overlap the right side of the base of the pulmonary trunk. The sulcus terminalis is a visible groove that extends from the right side of the SVC opening to the right side of the IVC opening.

Interior of Right Atrium (Fig. 45.1)

The cavity of the right atrium is divisible into three parts.

a. The sinus venarum is the smooth posterior part, which receives venous blood from following sources:
   i. The superior vena cava brings blood from upper half of the body. Its opening is located at the roof of the right atrium. An intervenous tubercle located below this opening, directs the superior vena caval blood to the tricuspid orifice in fetal life.
   ii. The inferior vena cava brings blood from the lower half of the body. Its opening (guarded by a small Eustachian valve) is at the lowest and posterior part of the atrium near the interatrial septum.
   iii. The coronary sinus, which is the vein of the heart brings blood from the myocardium. Its opening (guarded by a thin Thebesian valve) is located between the opening of IVC and the tricuspid orifice.
   iv. There are multiple small openings of venae cordis minimae scattered all over the atrial walls.
b. The right atrium proper and the auricle form the rough anterior part of the right atrium. This part presents important features.
   i. The crista terminalis is a C-shaped muscular ridge. It starts on the upper part of the interatrial septum, passes in front of the SVC opening and then turns along its lateral margin downward to reach the opening of the IVC. It demarcates the rough and smooth parts of the right atrium and coincides with the sulcus terminalis on the outer aspect of the atrium.
   ii. The musculi pectinati (so called because of resemblance to comb) are the parallel muscular ridges extending from the crista into the right auricle. The dense trabeculations of musculi pectinati inside the right auricle makes it a potential site for thrombi formation. The thrombi dislodged from the right atrium enter the pulmonary circulation and may produce pulmonary embolism.
   iii. The SA node is located in the right atrial wall in subepicardial position at the upper end of the

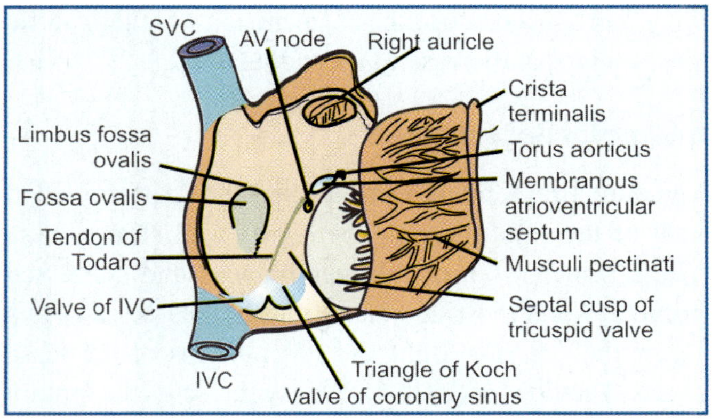

Fig. 45.1: Right lateral view of opened right atrium to depict its internal features

sulcus terminalis close to the opening of the superior vena cava.
  iv. The anterior cardiac veins open in the anterior aspect (rough part) of the atrium.

c. The vestibule of the tricuspid valve (Fig. 45.1) is the anteroinferior part (floor) of the right atrium, which leads into the tricuspid orifice. It shows three features:
  i. The Koch's triangle is an identifiable landmark in the right atrium during surgery. Its three boundaries are, the valve of coronary sinus (posteriorly), tendon of Todaro (superiorly), and the attached margin of the septal cusp of tricuspid valve (anteriorly). The tendon of Todaro is a subendocardial fibrous thickening from the point of confluence of valve of IVC and the limbus fossa ovalis to the most anterior point of the septal cusp of tricuspid valve. The AV node lies at the apex of Koch's triangle, which is a feature of the floor of the right atrium near the lower end of the interatrial septum. This description is according to " cardiac anatomy by Anderson and Backer", which is based on dissection and histological study of human hearts. However, the majority of texts (including Cunningham's manual of practical anatomy) describe its location in the lower part of interatrial septum.
  ii. The atrioventricular membranous septum is located antero-superior to the tendon of Todaro. It intervenes between the right atrium and the left ventricle.
  iii. The torus aorticus is the bulge in the atrial wall above the atrioventricular membranous septum, produced due to the adjacent non-coronary aortic sinus at the base of ascending aorta.

Interatrial Septum (Fig. 45.1)

The interatrial septum forms the septal or posteromedial wall of the right atrium. The septal wall shows fossa ovalis, which is an ovoid, membranous and depressed portion. A curved ridge called the limbus fossa ovalis forms the superior, right and left margins of the fossa ovalis. The floor of the fossa ovalis represents the septum primum and the limbus fossa ovalis is the remnant of the lower margin of the septum secundum of the fetal heart (Fig. 42.5). So the fossa ovalis with its limbus indicates the site of the valvular foramen ovale of fetal circulation. This foramen is normally completely obliterated after birth. A small slit (probe patency) may be found along the upper margin of the fossa ovalis in one-third of normal heart. The part of the septal surface above the limbus fossa ovalis is muscular and embryologically it is derived from the septum secundum.

Right Ventricle

The right ventricle receives blood from the right atrium through the tricuspid orifice and pumps it through the pulmonary orifice into the pulmonary trunk. The right ventricle takes large share in the formation of sternocostal surface of the heart and a small share in the diaphragmatic surface. The thickness of the ventricular wall is proportionate to its workload. In fetal stage the right ventricle pumps blood in the aorta through the ductus arteriosus, hence its wall is thicker than that of left ventricle. In postnatal stage the right ventricle pumps blood in pulmonary circulation, where systolic arterial pressure is 25-35 mm Hg. Hence the thickness of its walls is much less compared to that of left ventricle. Though the shape of the cavity of the right ventricle is classically described as crescentic, in the living the right ventricle has the shape of the bellows.

Interior of Right Ventricle (Fig. 45.2)

The cavity of the right ventricle is divisible in three parts. The inlet part containing the tricuspid valve, the trabecular body (ventricle proper) is the rough part. The outlet part (infundibulum or conus arteriosus) is the smooth part that leads into pulmonary valve. The inlet and outlet parts are present in the roof of the ventricle. The supraventricular crest, which is the largest muscular ridge in the right ventricle, separates the outflow and inflow parts. This crest is an arched structure consisting of a parietal limb and a septal limb. The parietal limb is part of the anterior wall of the ventricle and provides attachment to the anterior cusp of the tricuspid valve. The septal limb meets the interventricular septum, where it merges with the septomarginal trabecula. The supraventricular crest forms the posterior and the lateral aspects of the infundibulum.

a. Ventricular cavity proper (trabecular body) is characterized by presence of the muscular projections, which are collectively called the trabeculae carnae. There

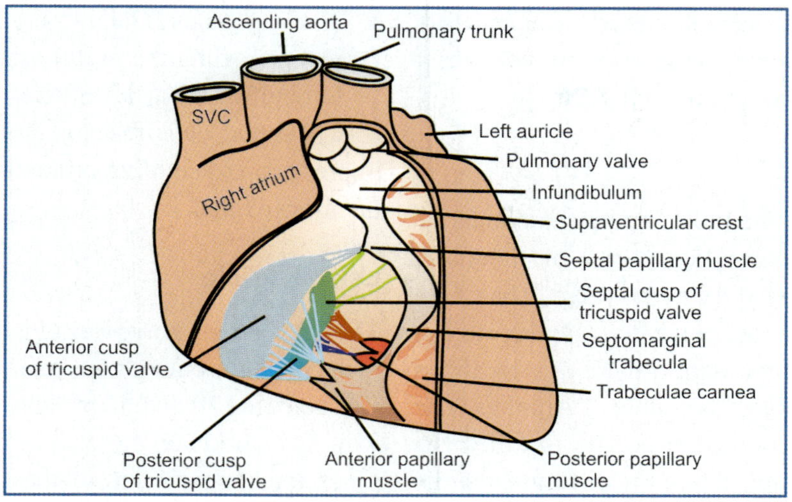

Fig. 45.2: Anterior view of opened right ventricle to depict its internal features

are three types of trabeculae in the right ventricle, namely, ridges, bridges and the papillary muscles.

i. The ridges are found all over the cavity in large numbers.
ii. The bridges are the elevations, which are fixed at the two ends but remain free in between. The septomarginal trabecula (moderator band) is the best example of this type. This trabecula passes from the interventricular septum to the base of the anterior papillary muscle. The important feature of this trabecula is that it carries the right branch of atrioventricular bundle (RBB) in its substance. This ensures early contraction of papillary muscles so that chordae tendineae are already taut before the ventricular contraction begins.
iii. The papillary muscles are conical muscular projections. Depending on their attachment to the ventricular wall, the papillary muscles are described as anterior, posterior and septal. The large anterior papillary muscle is attached to the right anterolateral wall, where it blends with the right end of the septomarginal trabecula. The posterior papillary muscle is attached to the inferior wall. The septal papillary muscles, when present are several small muscles attached to the septal limb of the septomarginal trabecula.

b. The inlet of the right ventricle shows the tricuspid valve. The orifice of the tricuspid valve accommodates the tips of three fingers. The annulus of this valve is a ring of collagenous tissue, which gives attachment to the cusps of the valve. The three cusps of the valve are termed anterior, posterior and septal (Fig. 45.2). The anterior cusp is attached to the supraventricular crest, the posterior to the posterior wall and the septal to the membranous interventricular septum. Each cusp has two surfaces (atrial and ventricular). The chordae tendineae arising from the anterior papillary muscle are attached to the anterior and posterior cusps; those from posterior papillary muscle to the posterior and septal cusps; and those from the septal muscles or directly from the septum to the anterior and septal cusps. During ventricular diastole when the intraventricular pressure is low the papillary muscles are relaxed and the chordae tendineae are slack. At this stage valves open and the apices of the cusps project into the ventricle. The blood flows freely from the right atrium to the right ventricle. During ventricular systole when the intraventricular pressure is increased the cusps are driven upward. The papillary muscles contract and tighten the chordae tendineae. This action is responsible for the closure of the valve by apposition of the atrial or smooth surfaces of the cusps. On the whole, the tricuspid valve is described as indeterminate, which means it is not very rigid structurally and hence functionally it is a very compliant valve.

c. The outlet part or infundibulum is funnel shaped. It supports the pulmonary orifice. Unlike the rest of ventricular cavity the infundibulum is smooth. The supraventricular crest constitutes its posterior and right lateral walls and the membranous septum separates it from the aortic vestibule of the left ventricle.

Pulmonary Valve

The pulmonary valve is the most superior and anterior valve. In normal individuals it lies anterior by about half its diameter, and to the left of the aortic valve. It has three semilunar cusps, right anterior, left anterior and posterior. In the midpoint of the free margin there is a localized thickening of fibrous tissue, the nodule of Arantius. The thin margin on either side of the nodule is called the lunule. The pulmonary sinuses are the dilatations in the wall of the pulmonary trunk just above the cusps. At the end of systole, when the intraventricular pressure falls, there is a tendency for blood to return to the ventricle. This blood fills the pulmonary sinuses thereby approximating the cusps to each other. At the beginning of ventricular systole the rise in pressure forces the cusps to open and project into the pulmonary trunk.

Left Atrium

The left atrium is cubical in shape. It is positioned behind and to the left of the right atrium. The pulmonary trunk and the ascending aorta conceal its anterior surface. The left atrium forms the left two-thirds of the base of the heart. The left auricle projects anterosuperiorly from it to overlap the left aspect of the pulmonary trunk. This chamber receives the oxygenated blood from two pairs of pulmonary veins and sends the same to the left ventricle through mitral orifice (For relations of the left atrium refer to base of the heart in Chapter 44).

Interior of Left Atrium

The left atrium is a relatively featureless cavity. Its interior can be divided into three parts:

a. The smooth part has the openings of the pulmonary veins, two on either side on its posterior wall. This part is developed from absorbed part of the embryonic pulmonary vein and its divisions.
b. The rough part is confined to the left auricle, which has musculi pectinati and develops from primitive atrium. The left auricle is a potential site for the formation of thrombi, which if dislodged, can result in embolism in systemic circulation.
c. The vestibule of the mitral valve is a narrow passage just preceding the mitral orifice and is derived from left half of the atrioventricular canal.

The septal wall of the left atrium may present a lunate impression (resembling a thumbprint) corresponding to the fossa ovalis.

Left Ventricle

The left ventricle is a powerful pump, which propels blood in the systemic circulation against the peripheral vascular resistance at 120/80 mm of Hg in normal state. In keeping with this workload, the wall of the left ventricle is three times thicker than that of the right ventricle. The left ventricle forms the cardiac apex, one-third of the sternocostal surface, two-thirds of the inferior surface and part of the left surface of the heart. The left ventricle receives the blood from the left atrium and pumps the same into the ascending aorta via the aortic orifice.

Interior of Left Ventricle

The cavity of the left ventricle is circular on cross section. The left ventricle is divisible in three parts, the inflow or inlet part containing the mitral valve, the trabeculated body or ventricle proper and the outflow part or vestibule. The interventricular septum forms the anterolateral wall of the ventricle.

a. The ventricle proper has rough walls with muscular projections called trabeculae carnae, which form a fine meshwork. The trabeculae are especially rich at the apex and on the inferior wall. The septum and the upper part of the anterior wall are relatively smooth. There are two papillary muscles. The anterior papillary muscle originates from the anterior wall and its chordae tendineae are attached to both the cusps of the mitral valve. The posterior papillary muscle originates from the inferior wall and its chordae tendineae are attached to both the cusps of the mitral valve.
b. The inflow part contains mitral valve, which is the most posterior valve of the heart. This valve lies superior, posterior and to the left of the tricuspid valve and posteroinferior and slightly to the left of the aortic valve. The mitral orifice can admit the tips of two fingers and its shape is like a horseshoe. The valve has two cusps hence the name bicuspid valve. The mitral cusps resemble in shape the Bishop's miter (crown). The

anterior cusp is attached to upper and right part of the margin of the orifice and is considerably longer. The posterior or mural cusp is attached to the lower and left part of the margin. The anterior cusp forms the only partition between left ventricular inflow and outflow orifices. The chordae tendineae are attached to the free margin of anterior cusp but to the free margin and ventricular surface of the posterior cusp. At the onset of diastole the mitral valve opens passively due to the lower pressure in the left ventricle. With the onset of atrial systole there is active opening of valve cusps and maximum filling takes place. During ventricular systole papillary muscles contract, which increases the tension in the chordae tendineae. This results in effective valve closure.

c. The outflow part or aortic vestibule is a smooth part of the left ventricle situated a little in front and to the right of the mitral valve. It develops from the left half of bulbus cordis. The aortic vestibule is virtually non-existent. The anterior cusp of the mitral valve and the adjacent part of fibrous skeleton of the heart (subaortic curtain) form its posterior wall. The membranous part of the interventricular septum forms its anterior and right walls and separates it from right ventricle and right atrium. The aortic valve is the upper limit of this so-called passage.

Aortic Valve

The aortic valve is made of three cusps or leaflets and is stronger in structure than the pulmonary valve. The free margins of the cusps project into the ascending aorta. Like the pulmonary valve the free margins of the cusps present nodule and lunules on either side of nodule. The cusps are supported within three aortic sinuses of Valsalva. According to the position of the cusps the sinuses are described as anterior, right posterior and left posterior. The anterior aortic sinus gives origin to right coronary artery and left posterior aortic sinus gives origin to left coronary artery. The right posterior aortic sinus is called the noncoronary sinus, which projects in the right atrium to produce torus aorticus. During diastole, the closed aortic valve supports an aortic column of blood. The three nodules are apposed and the valve is tightly closed. As the ventricular systole begins the pressure in the ventricle exceeds that of the aorta and the valve opens passively. The free margins of the cusps become almost straight lines making the orifice triangular when fully open. During ejection, a small amount of blood enters the sinuses, which helps to maintain the position of the valves during systole and initiate their approximation at the end of systole.

Interventricular Septum

The interventricular septum is a partition between the two ventricles. The septum is oriented in three different planes. Its attachment to the anterior wall is indicated by the anterior interventricular groove on the sternocostal surface and to the inferior surface by the posterior interventricular groove. The right surface of the septum faces forwards and bulges into the right ventricle, while the left surface looks backwards and is concave towards the left ventricle.

Parts of Interventricular Septum

a. The muscular part of the septum is larger and thicker.
b. The membranous part of the septum lies postero-superior to the muscular septum. It appears as a small oval transparent area, which is in continuity with the central fibrous body. The attachment of the septal cusp of the tricuspid valve divides the membranous part into the anterior interventricular part and a posterior atrioventricular part (Fig. 45.3). Thus, the interventricular part separates the aortic vestibule of the left ventricle from the infundibulum of the right ventricle and the atrioventricular part separates the aortic vestibule from the floor of the right atrium.

Conducting Tissue in Interventricular Septum

The membranous septum is pierced by the left branch of the atrioventricular bundle near its junction with the muscular part. The left surface of the muscular septum carries the left branch of atrioventricular bundle in the sub-endocardial position. The right branch of the atrioventricular bundle passes along the right surface of the septum in the subendocardial position. The septomarginal trabecula attached to this surface of the septum carries the right bundle to the anterior papillary muscle.

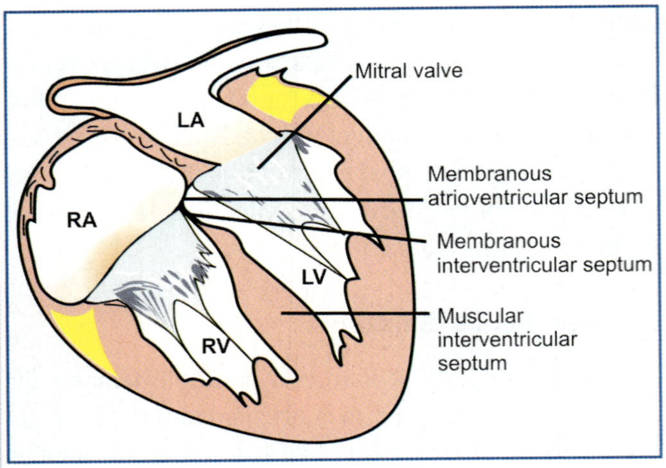

Fig. 45.3: Interventricular septum. Note that large part of septum is muscular. Its membranous part is continuous with atrioventricular septum

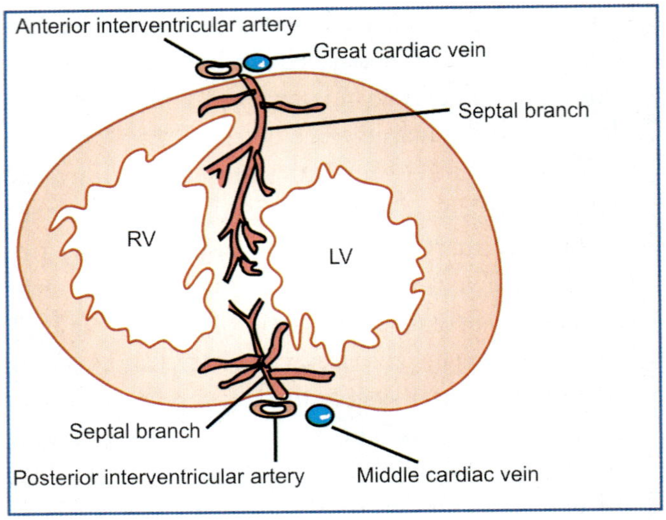

Fig. 45.4: Schematic diagram to show arterial supply of interventricular septum

Arterial Supply of Interventricular Septum (Fig. 45.4)

a. The anterior two-third of the septum receives anterior septal branches of anterior interventricular artery (a branch of left coronary artery).
b. Small posterior septal branches of the anterior interventricular and short septal branches of posterior interventricular artery (a branch of right coronary artery) supply the posterior one-third of the septum.

So, the left coronary artery takes a larger share in the arterial supply of the interventricular septum in the "right dominance." But in the case of the "left dominance" the entire supply is derived from the left coronary artery. The thrombosis of the septal branches will result in septal infarction and heart block.

Surface Markings of Cardiac Valves (Fig. 45.5)

a. The pulmonary orifice is indicated by a 2.5 cm long transverse line partly behind the left third costal cartilage and partly behind the adjacent left half of sternum.
b. The aortic orifice is denoted by an oblique line 2.5 cm long behind the left half of the body of sternum at the level of third left intercostal space.
c. A 3 cm long oblique line behind the left half of the sternum opposite the fourth left costal cartilage marks the mitral orifice.
d. A 4 cm long line placed vertically behind the right half of the sternum opposite the fourth intercostal space.

Surface Markings of Cardiac Auscultation Areas (Fig. 45.5)

a. Pulmonary valve—second intercostal space to the left of sternum.
b. Aortic valve—second intercostal space to the right of sternum.

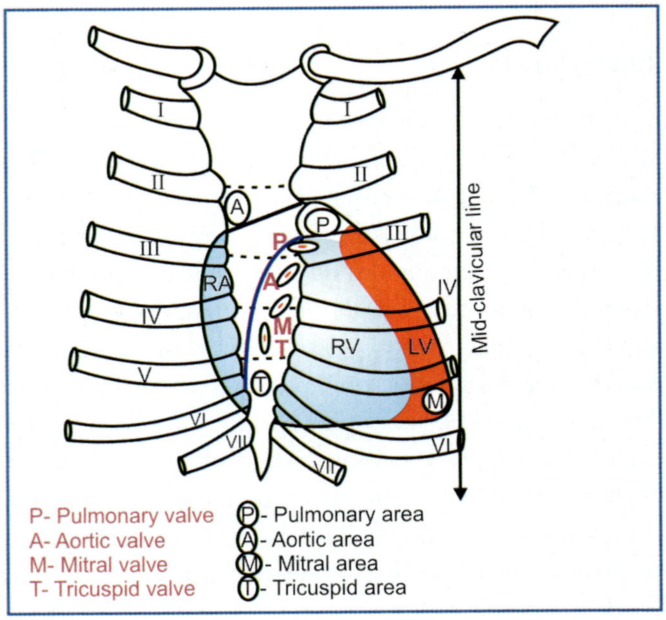

Fig. 45.5: Surface markings of cardiac borders, valves and auscultation areas

c. Tricuspid valve—fifth intercostal space over the center of the body of sternum.
d. Mitral valve—near the cardiac apex.

Radiological Anatomy of Heart

a. In the posteroanterior (PA) X-ray of chest the transverse diameter of the cardiac shadow of normal sized heart is equal to half the diameter of the chest. When it exceeds this ratio (1:2) it is suggestive of cardiac enlargement. The margins of the cardiac shadow are identifiable in the PA, RAO (right anterior oblique) and LAO (left anterior oblique) views of chest X-rays. The right margin of the cardiac shadow is formed by the SVC, right atrium and IVC from above downward. The aortic knuckle (prominence due to arch of aorta), pulmonary bay containing pulmonary trunk, left auricle and left ventricle, form the left margin from above downward. The inferior margin of the cardiac shadow merges with the shadow of the diaphragm and the liver.
b. In the right oblique anterior (ROA) view of chest X-ray the heart shadow shows all the four chambers. The posterior border of heart shadow is formed by left atrium. This view is used to assess the size of the left atrium in mitral stenosis with the help of Ba-swallow.
c. In the left oblique anterior (LOA) view of the chest X-ray the heart shadow is largely made up of right ventricle anteriorly and left ventricle posteriorly.
d. The serial CT scans of the thorax is the best way to study the anatomical relations of the heart and the surrounding structures to each other.
e. In cardiac catheterization and angiography the cardiac chambers are delineated with the help of the contrast medium. A special cardiac catheter is passed through the femoral vein to reach the right side of heart, while the left side of the heart is approached through the brachial or femoral artery.
f. Echocardiography (ECHO) is a modified ultrasound imaging of the heart. It is a simple and non-invasive procedure, which gives the details of internal anatomical features of the heart. The usual approach of this procedure is transthoracic. One drawback of this route is that it is not possible to properly see the structures at the base of the heart. This drawback is overcome by the transesophageal echography, which improves the imaging of the base considerably because the esophagus is separated from the base of the heart by at most 0.5 cm of tissue.

Clinical Highlights

Diseases of the valves of the heart are very common. Usually there is history of rheumatic fever in the childhood in such cases. Depending on the extent of the damage to the valve components the orifice may be narrowed causing stenosis or the valves may become incompetent causing regurgitation. These defects produce structural as well as functional effects.

a. The mitral stenosis (narrowing of mitral orifice) is most common in young age. There is obstruction to the left atrial blood during ventricular filling. This leads to rise in left atrial pressure followed by pulmonary venous hypertension, which is the cause of respiratory symptoms like, shortness of breath (dyspnea), cough and hemoptysis (blood in sputum). There is enlargement of left atrium, which may press on the esophagus causing dysphagia and on left recurrent laryngeal nerve causing hoarseness of voice (Ortner's syndrome). The stasis of blood in left auricle encourages clot formation. The detached clots form emboli, which enter the left ventricle, ascending aorta and the systemic circulation. The complications like gangrene of lower limb (due to occlusion of femoral artery), myocardial infarction (due to occlusion of coronary artery), stroke (due to occlusion of cerebral artery) or renal infarct (due to occlusion of segmental branch of renal artery) may occur once the emboli enter the systemic arterial tree. There are various options available for treating mitral stenosis. Mitral valvotomy means dilatation of the stenosed mitral orifice. In balloon valvotomy, a special balloon is introduced inside the left atrium through the arterial route. In the surgical treatment, the mitral valve is dilated by closed mitral valvotomy or open mitral valvotomy. In some cases the diseased mitral valve is replaced by artificial (prosthetic) valve.
b. In mitral regurgitation the mitral valve fails to close during systole. The hemodynamic effects are as follows. The blood from left ventricle regurgitates in to the left atrium during systole. So during diastole

there is overfilling of the left ventricle. In this process a part of blood shuttles between left atrium and left ventricle. This increases the workload of the left ventricle. Eventually gross dilatation and hypertrophy of left ventricle may culminate in left ventricular failure.

c. In aortic stenosis the blood accumulates inside the left ventricle causing its hypertrophy and dilatation. There is low cardiac output, which may manifest as angina pectoris and syncope (fainting) on exertion. The disease may culminate in left ventricular failure.

d. In aortic regurgitation incompetent aortic valve fails to close the aortic orifice completely during diastole. There is overfilling of left ventricle during diastole because it receives blood from left atrium as well as ascending aorta. The left ventricle undergoes dilatation and hypertrophy. Gradually this leads to left ventricular failure.

e. In tricuspid stenosis the tricuspid orifice is narrowed. The blood flow from right atrium to right ventricle is reduced, which results in reduction of blood in the pulmonary circulation. The net result is decreased cardiac output and elevation of right atrial pressure leading to systemic venous congestion and right heart failure.

f. Tricuspid regurgitation is a common clinical condition. The tricuspid orifice undergoes stretching as a result of right ventricular dilatation or infarction. The pressure in the right atrium increases due to regurgitation of blood into it during systole. Ultimately the right side of the heart dilates and gives rise to systemic venous congestion and right heart failure.

g. Pulmonary stenosis is almost always congenital, either isolated or as part of Fallot's tetralogy. The stenosis of the pulmonary orifice results in hypertrophy of the right ventricle and reduction in cardiac output.

46 Blood Supply and Nerve Supply of Heart

The myocardium beats nonstop throughout life and is capable of working harder during times of increased physical activities. Therefore, the oxygen demand of the myocardium is very high. The right and left coronary arteries supply blood to the heart. The stems of the two arteries and their major anastomosing branches (located in the sub-pericardial fat) encircle the heart like an obliquely inverted crown.

Unique Features of Coronary Arteries

a. The coronary arteries are the biggest vasa vasora (pleural of vasa vasorum) in the body because the heart is considered to be a modified blood vessel.
b. The coronary arteries are functionally end arteries but anatomically they are not. The branches of the two coronary arteries anastomose at arteriolar level, but the caliber of the anastomosing arteries is not sufficient to maintain normal circulation, if one of the arteries is suddenly blocked.
c. Unlike other arteries of the body, the coronary arteries fill mainly during diastole of the ventricles. Duration of the systole in a cardiac cycle is constant irrespective of the rate of heart. Therefore, in response to increase in heart rate (tachycardia) diastole will be shortened, thus reducing the coronary filling. So, in patients with coronary artery disease increase in heart rater due to any cause may precipitate ischemia (reduction in arterial supply).
d. The coronary arteries are more prone to athero-sclerosis (subendothelial deposition of fatty material) compared to other arteries hence ischemic heart diseases are very common.

Origin and Course of Right Coronary Artery (Figs 46.1A and B)

The right coronary artery takes origin from the anterior aortic sinus at the root of the ascending aorta. Its course can be divided into three segments.

a. The first segment extends from the aortic root to the coronary sulcus on the sternocostal surface. This segment of the artery courses between the pulmonary trunk and the right auricle in anterior direction to reach the left end of the coronary sulcus.
b. The second segment lies in the coronary sulcus on the sternocostal surface, where it runs almost vertically downward to reach the lower end of the right margin of heart. This segment is covered by sub-pericardial fat and is crossed by anterior cardiac veins.

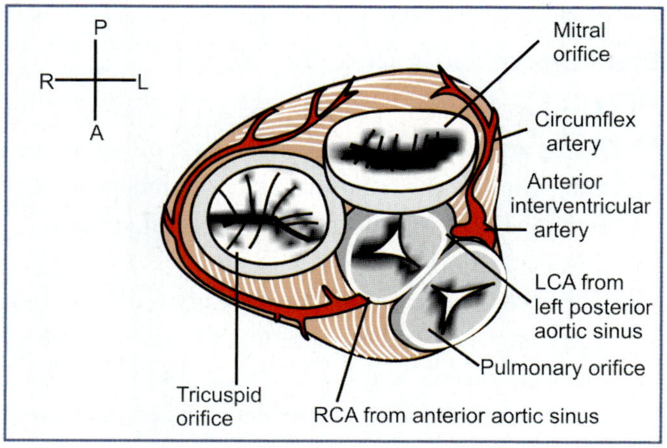

Fig. 46.1A: Cross-section through the plane of cardiac orifices showing origin of coronary arteries from sinuses at the base of ascending aorta

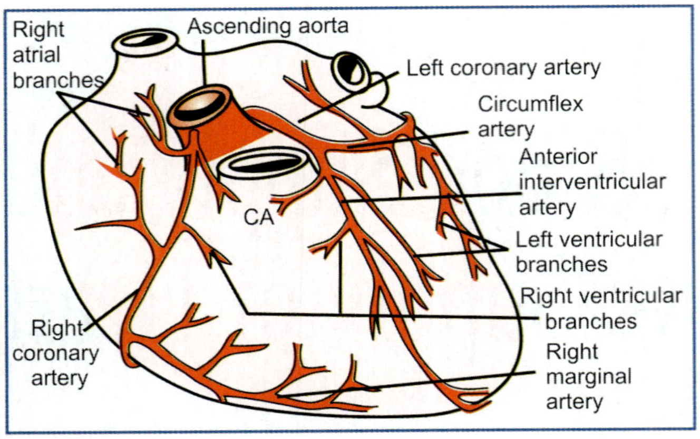

Fig. 46.1B: Course and branches of coronary arteries on sternocostal surface. Note the anastomosis of conus arteries (CA) on the surface of pulmonary trunk

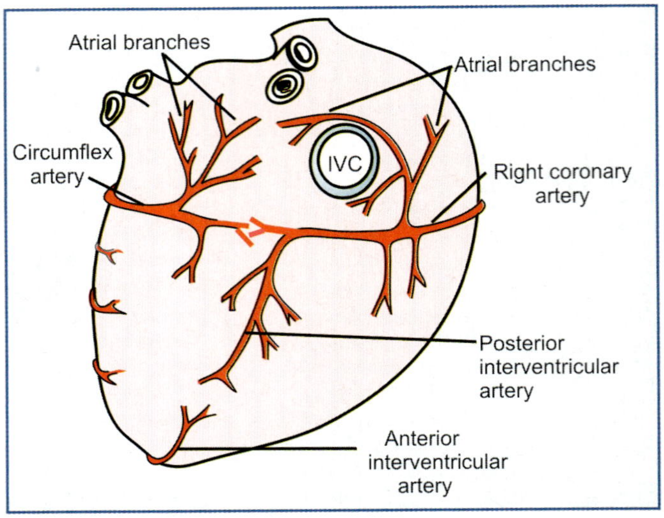

Fig. 46.2: Branches of right coronary artery and of circumflex branch of left coronary artery on posterior and inferior surfaces

c. The third segment of the artery occupies the right portion of coronary sulcus on the posterior aspect (Fig. 46.2) and runs upwards and to the left from the lower end of the right margin along with small cardiac vein.

Termination of Right Coronary Artery

The right coronary artery terminates by different modes in the posterior part of the coronary sulcus. In 60 percent of subjects it ends a little to the left of the crux by anastomosing with circumflex branch of the left coronary artery. In 10 percent of subjects, it terminates at the lower end of the right margin, while in another 10 percent it terminates between the right border and the crux. In the remaining 20 percent it reaches the left border by coursing the entire coronary sulcus, thus replacing a part of circumflex artery.

Branches of Right Coronary Artery

i. The first segment of the artery gives origin to right conus artery, which supplies the base of the pulmonary trunk. If the conus artery arises independently from the anterior aortic sinus, it is called the third coronary artery.
ii. The second segment of the artery gives off the right anterior atrial branch (supplying the anterior part of the right atrium and the SA node through a nodal branch), right anterior ventricular branches (supplying the anterior part of the right ventricle) and the right marginal artery, which travels along the inferior margin of the heart, supplying both the ventricles, on its way.
iii. The third segment of the artery gives off the right posterior ventricular branches (supplying the diaphragmatic surface of right ventricle), right posterior atrial branches and AV nodal branches. Lastly, it gives off a large posterior interventricular artery (termed as posterior descending artery in clinical texts), which travels in the posterior interventricular groove along with middle cardiac vein and supplies the diaphragmatic surface of both ventricles and the posterior one-third of the interventricular septum.

Area of Supply

The area of supply of the right coronary artery consists of right atrium, right ventricle except some part on the anterior wall closer to the anterior interventricular groove, posterior one-third of the interventricular septum, most of the conducting tissue and variable area of left atrium and ventricle.

Origin and Course of Left Coronary Artery (Figs 46.1A and B)

The left coronary artery takes origin from the left posterior aortic sinus at the root of the ascending aorta. It is larger in size and shorter compared to the right artery and supplies a greater volume of myocardium. Its short-stem courses anteriorly between pulmonary trunk and left auricle to emerge on the sternocostal surface, where it divides into terminal branches of equal size namely, anterior interventricular and circumflex arteries.

Branches of Left Coronary Artery

a. The anterior interventricular artery (termed as left anterior descending or LAD artery in clinical texts) descends in the anterior interventricular groove on the sternocostal surface accompanied by great cardiac vein. It terminates by meeting the end of the posterior interventricular artery either at the apex of the heart or in the posterior interventricular groove after winding round the apex. Its branches are, right and left ventricular, left conus and anterior septal. One of the left anterior ventricular branches is especially large and is called diagonal artery. The left conus artery anastomoses with the corresponding branch of the right coronary artery (Fig. 46.1B). The anterior septal branches supply the anterior two-thirds of the interventricular septum. Thus, it is evident that the anterior interventricular (LAD) artery supplies a large area of left ventricle and of the interventricular septum. Moreover, it is very much prone to atherosclerosis and narrowing in men. Hence, its block may cause massive and fatal infarction. On account of this, LAD has been named the " widow maker".
b. The circumflex artery continues in the left part of the coronary sulcus and curves round the left margin of the heart to appear in the left portion of the coronary sulcus on the posterior aspect (Fig. 46.2). Usually it terminates to the left of the crux by anastomosing with the right coronary artery but at times, it continues as the posterior interventricular artery. The circumflex artery gives rise to left marginal artery, ventricular branches to inferior surface of left ventricle and left atrial branches. It supplies the SA node and AV node in some percent of cases.

Area of Supply

The left coronary artery supplies most of the left ventricle, a narrow strip of right ventricle, anterior two-thirds of the interventricular septum and the left atrium.

Coronary Dominance

In the right dominance, the posterior interventricular artery arises from the right coronary artery, while in the left dominance the posterior interventricular artery is a branch of the left coronary artery. In balanced pattern, both the coronary arteries give origin to these branches, which run parallel in the posterior interventricular sulcus.

Coronary Anastomosis

In normal healthy heart, the coronary arteries are the true end arteries as these anastomoses are inadequate to maintain circulation in the event of sudden occlusion of a major branch of coronary artery. However, with slow onset occlusion in coronary arteries like in atherosclerosis, there is time for newer anastomoses to develop so that the normal nutrition of the myocardium is not affected.

Clinical Highlights

a. Coronary angiography is a radiological procedure by which coronary arteries are visualized after injecting a contrast medium into them. Angiography is useful in localizing the sites of the blocks in the coronary arteries or their branches. In this procedure, a special catheter is passed usually through the femoral artery up into the aorta till the base of the ascending aorta. The contrast material is injected in the coronary ostia located at this site and then the radiographs are taken.
b. In angina pectoris due to narrowing of coronary artery or arteries there is reduction in blood supply to the myocardium. This results in lack of sufficient oxygen to the myocardium (ischemia). As a consequence, on physical exertion the patient experiences pain in the chest. The typical anginal pain is of gripping or constricting type of retrosternal pain, which radiates to the inner side of left arm or shoulder or to the neck. Weakness, dizziness and perspiration accompany the pain, which is relieved after rest.
c. In myocardial infarction (MI), there is a complete block in the coronary artery or its major branch either due to thrombus or embolus formation on the atheromatous patch in the vessel. This results in complete loss of blood supply to the myocardium with consequent infarction. Massive myocardial infarction usually is fatal.
d. There are two methods by which the blood supply to the myocardium can be restored if the coronary artery or its branches are blocked. In one method, the narrowed segment of the artery is mechanically dilated

and in another method the diseased segment is bypassed by a segment of the patient's own healthy blood vessel from another site.

i. Percutaneous transluminal coronary angioplasty (PTCA) is the technique used for increasing the inside diameter of the narrowed coronary artery. In this method, a balloon catheter is passed into the coronary artery and the balloon is inflated at the site of the block so as to squash the raised atheromatous plaque against the wall of the artery.
ii. Coronary artery bypass graft (CABG) is a major surgical procedure. The patient's own vessels are used for the graft. The commonly used vessels are the great saphenous vein, the internal mammary artery and the radial artery. Amongst these, internal mammary artery graft is the most favored. This graft has greatest success rate because the wall of the internal mammary artery has elastic tissue in it and chances of re-stenosis are far less. In patients with multiple blocks (three or four), all the three blood vessels can be used. Figure 46.3 shows the internal mammary artery graft for blocked LAD and saphenous vein graft for right coronary block. A segment of saphenous vein in the thigh, is taken out and anastomosed with the ascending aorta on one hand and to the patent part of the affected artery beyond the block. The segment of vein is reversed during grafting so that its valves do not hamper the blood flow. While taking the radial artery graft, the patency of the ulnar artery is always ensured by Allen's test beforehand.

Veins of Heart (Fig. 46.4)

There are three major veins, which drain blood from the myocardium.

a. The coronary sinus is the chief vein of the heart. It collects venous blood from the myocardium and empties it into the right atrium.
b. There are three or four anterior cardiac veins, which directly open in the anterior part of the right atrium.
c. The venae cordis minimae (Thebesian veins) are scattered all over the myocardium and open directly in all the cardiac chambers.

Coronary Sinus

This is a short (2.5 cm long) and wide venous channel located in the posterior part of coronary sulcus between the left atrium and left ventricle. The myocardial fibers from the atrium often cover it superficially.

Development

The coronary sinus develops from the left horn of the sinus venosus and part of left common cardinal vein (Fig. 42.3). Some authors consider coronary sinus to develop from only the left horn of the sinus venosus.

Origin and Termination

The coronary sinus begins as the continuation of the great cardiac vein at the left end of the coronary sulcus. From here it courses downward and to the right lying between the left atrium and ventricle and opens in the smooth part of the right atrium. The opening of the coronary sinus is guarded by a small valve (called Thebesian valve) and is located between the IVC opening and the right A-V orifice.

Tributaries

a. Great cardiac vein begins at the cardiac apex. It ascends in the anterior interventricular groove to enter the coronary sulcus and follows this to reach the left border of the heart, where it joins the left end of the coronary sinus.

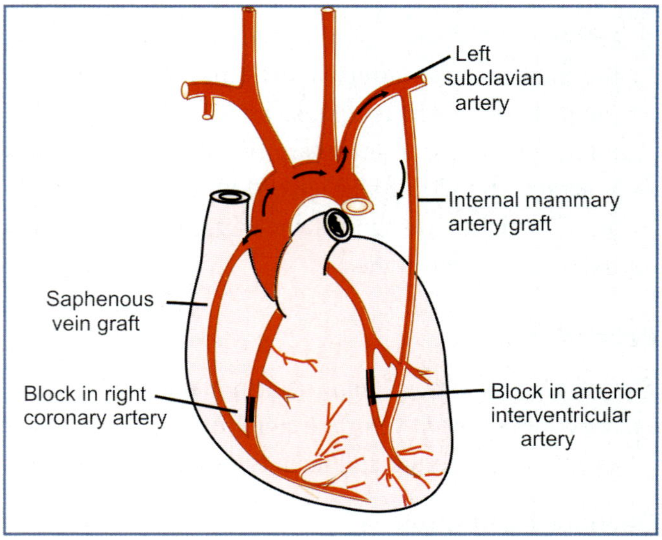

Fig. 46.3: Coronary artery bypass graft (CABG) using arterial and venous grafts

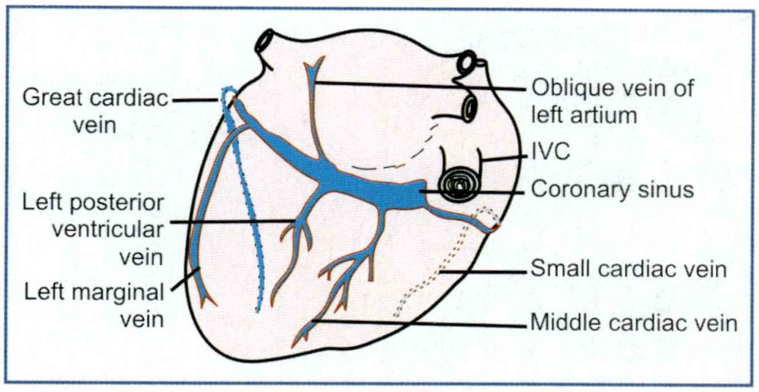

Fig. 46.4: Posteroinferior view showing veins of heart

b. Middle cardiac vein begins at the cardiac apex, ascends in the posterior interventricular groove and joins the coronary sinus at its right end.

c. Small cardiac vein has a variable course. It may follow the course of the right coronary artery in the anterior as well as in the posterior parts of the coronary sulcus and open in the right end of the sinus. In the majority of subjects it lies in the posterior part of the coronary sulcus along with right coronary artery. In such situations, the right marginal vein may open in it or independently in the right atrium. The small cardiac vein may take the place of right marginal vein so that it accompanies the right marginal artery as well as the right coronary artery in its posterior course. In a small percentage of cases, small cardiac vein opens in the right atrium directly.

d. Posterior vein of left ventricle lies parallel to the middle cardiac vein and opens in the coronary sinus somewhere in its middle.

e. Oblique vein of left atrium or oblique vein of Marshall opens near the left end of the coronary sinus. It is connected to the left superior intercostal vein by ligament of left vena cava (Fig. 42.3). The oblique vein and the ligament are the remnants of the left common cardinal vein.

Fibrous Skeleton of Heart

The fibrous skeleton (Fig. 46.5) of the heart gives support to the cardiac valves and the myocardium. It is described as a dynamically deformable tissue. The fibrous skeleton gives origin to the myocardium of atria and the ventricles and ensures electrophysiological discontinuity between the atria and ventricle except where the bundle of His penetrates the central fibrous body.

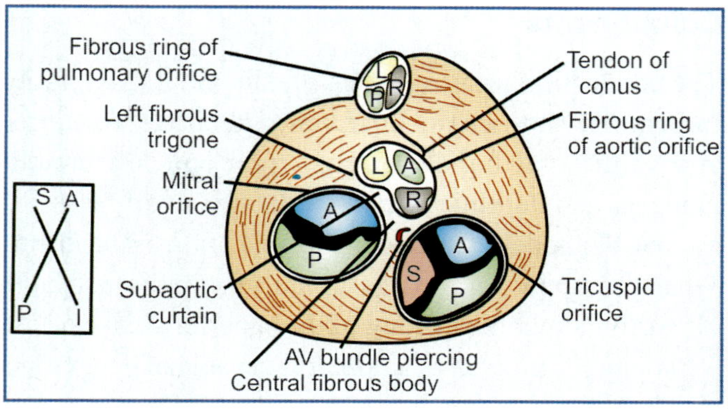

Fig. 46.5: Fibrous skeleton of heart viewed from above after removal of atria

Component Parts

The atrioventricular valves and the aortic valve are located close to each other and share a common fibrous ring (annulus) while the pulmonary valve has a separate fibrous ring, being a little away from the other three valves. At the aortic orifice the fibrous ring is the strongest. The pulmonary annulus is connected to the aortic annulus by the tendon of conus or infundibulum. The common fibrous tissue between the annulus of A-V valves behind and the aortic orifice in front is divisible into:

a. Left fibrous trigone, where the aortic and mitral valves meet.

b. Subaortic curtain between the aortic valve and the gap in the mitral valve annulus.

c. Right fibrous trigone, where the aortic, mitral and tricuspid rings meet and which is continuous with the membranous part of the interventricular septum.

The central fibrous body is the combination of right fibrous trigone and the membranous part of interventricular septum. The bundle of His penetrates this important structure. The tendon of Todaro is the collagenous connection between the central fibrous body and the valve of the inferior vena cava. The atrioventricular dehiscence is a serious condition resulting from the injury to the central fibrous body.

Conducting Tissue of Heart

The conducting tissue (Fig. 46.6) consists of excitable tissue, which consists of modified myofibers. This specialized tissue is responsible for maintaining the heart rate at 70-90 per minute in the adult.

Components

The conducting tissue consists of, sinuatrial (SA) node, internodal pathways, atrioventricular (AV) node, atrioventricular bundle of His, right and left bundle branches and Purkinje fibers (conduction myofibers).

a. The SA node is situated in the wall of the right atrium at the upper end of the crista terminalis partially surrounding the opening of the superior vena cava. It is subepicardial in position. It is capable of generating electrical impulses, hence, it is called the pacemaker of the heart. The SA node is a very vascular area of the heart.
b. It is believed that three internodal pathways exist across the atrial wall and they connect the SA node to the AV node. Similarly a path (Bachmann's bundle) connecting right and left atria is also believed to exist. But for want of histological evidence of these paths it is assumed that the internodal and interatrial conduction occurs through ordinary working myocardium.
c. The AV node is located in the triangle of Koch in the lower part of the right atrium to the left of the coronary sinus opening. It extends downwards upto the junction of interatrial septum and the central fibrous trigone. In this way the AV node is related to, both the AV valves, interatrial septum, membranous part of interventricular septum and the aortic valve. The AV node initiates the ventricular systole. The impulse is carried in the atrioventricular bundle to the ventricles. If the SA node is damaged the AV node can take over the function of the pacemaker.
d. The atrioventricular bundle of His is the only muscular connection between the myocardium of atria and ventricles. It passes through the central fibrous body and along the posterior margin of the membranous interventricular septum to the junction of the muscular and membranous parts of the septum. At this level it divides into two bundle branches, one for each ventricle. The right bundle branch (RBB) passes down on the right side of the interventricular septum. A part of this bundle enters the septomarginal trabecula, which carries it to the anterior papillary muscle, and the remainder breaks up into fine fibers, which supply the, rest of the right ventricle. The left bundle branch (LBB) pierces the septum and passes down in a superficial position on the left aspect of the septum. It divides into fibers that enter the ventricular musculature. The fibers of the bundle of His are in continuity with Purkinje fibers in the ventricular wall.

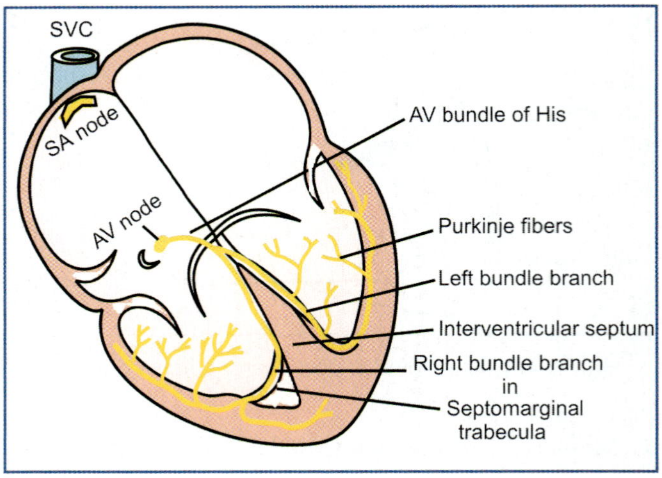

Fig. 46.6: Schematic diagram showing parts of conducting system of heart

Blood Supply of Conducting Tissue

Usually the SA node is supplied by the right coronary artery. In 35 percent- circumflex branch of left coronary may supply it. Usually the AV node and AV bundle are supplied by the right coronary artery but in 20 percent the circumflex branch of left coronary artery supplies. The right bundle branch receives blood from both right and left coronary arteries and the left bundle branch from the left coronary artery. In left coronary dominance entire septum receives branches from left coronary artery.

Nerve Supply of Heart

Both sympathetic and parasympathetic nerves control the action of heart through the cardiac plexuses and the coronary plexuses.

Efferent Nerve Supply

a. Parasympathetic efferent supply is via the cervical cardiac branches of vagus and cardiac branches of recurrent laryngeal nerves. The parasympathetic is cardioinhibitory in function.
b. The sympathetic supply is via the three cervical cardiac branches and a few thoracic cardiac branches of the sympathetic chain. The sympathetic is cardioaccelerator in function.

Afferent Nerve Supply

The heart is insensitive to touch, cutting; cold or heat but ischemia and resultant accumulation of metabolic products stimulate pain nerve endings in the myocardium. The pain sensation is carried in the middle and inferior cervical cardiac branches and thoracic cardiac branches of the sympathetic chain to the thoracic ganglia of the sympathetic chain (Fig. 46.7). From here, the impulse passes via the white rami to the thoracic spinal nerves (T1-T5) and to the dorsal root ganglia. The central processes of the neurons in the dorsal root ganglia carry the impulses to the posterior horns of T1 to T5 spinal segments (mostly of the left side). The afferent fibers in the vagus nerves reach the medulla oblongata and are concerned with reflexes controlling the cardiovascular activity.

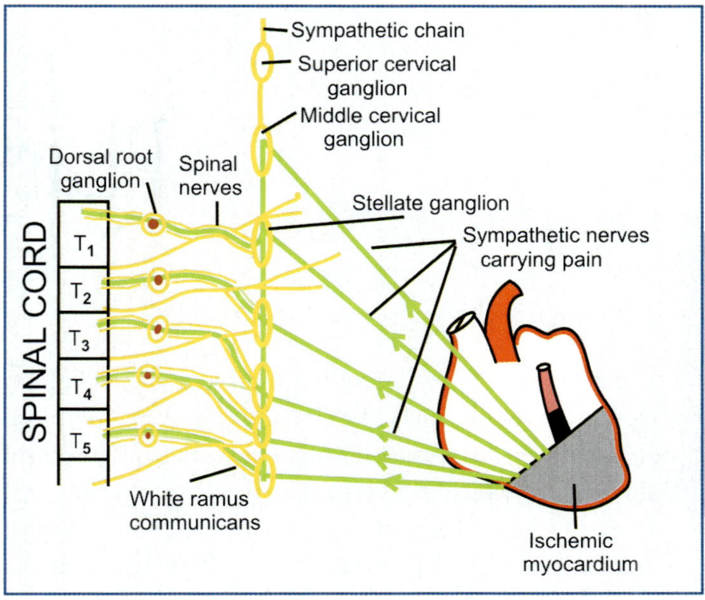

Fig. 46.7: Highly schematic diagram showing path of pain from ischemic myocardium to spinal cord

Referred Pain in Angina Pectoris

When the pain impulses from ischemic myocardium reach the spinal cord, they stimulate the somatic sensory neurons of the corresponding segments of the spinal cord, usually on the left side.

Thus, pain is felt in the cutaneous area of T1 and T2 segments, along the inner border of the left upper limb. The pain may also be felt in the precordium and back, which are supplied by T2 to T5 spinal nerves. It is worthy of note that individuals with transplanted heart do not experience anginal pain. This is so because transplanted heart is a denervated donor heart, in which regeneration of the nerves is not possible in the host.

47 Pharyngeal Arch Arteries

The basic arterial pattern of the embryo at the end of 4th week of development is like that of fishes. A pair of dorsal aortae is seen on the dorsal wall of the embryo. The dorsal aortae fuse below the level of the seventh inter-segmental arteries to form a single dorsal aorta. On the ventral aspect there is an aortic sac, which is the dilated part of the truncus arteriosus. As the neck elongates the aortic sac is drawn out cranially as right and left horns (limbs). These horns are equivalent to the ventral aortae of fishes. They are connected to dorsal aortae through a series of six aortic arch arteries that pass through the pharyngeal arches. The cranial arch arteries degenerate as the caudal ones make their appearance. Therefore at any given time all of the six arch arteries are never present. The fifth arch artery is rudimentary. The third, fourth and sixth arch arteries along with the aortic sac and dorsal aortae give rise to the definitive arteries of the thorax and neck.

Transformation of Arch Arteries (Fig. 47.1)

The symmetrical pattern of arch arteries and dorsal aortae undergoes following changes during 6th to 8th weeks.

a. The ductus caroticus, which is a segment of dorsal aorta between the third and fourth arch arteries

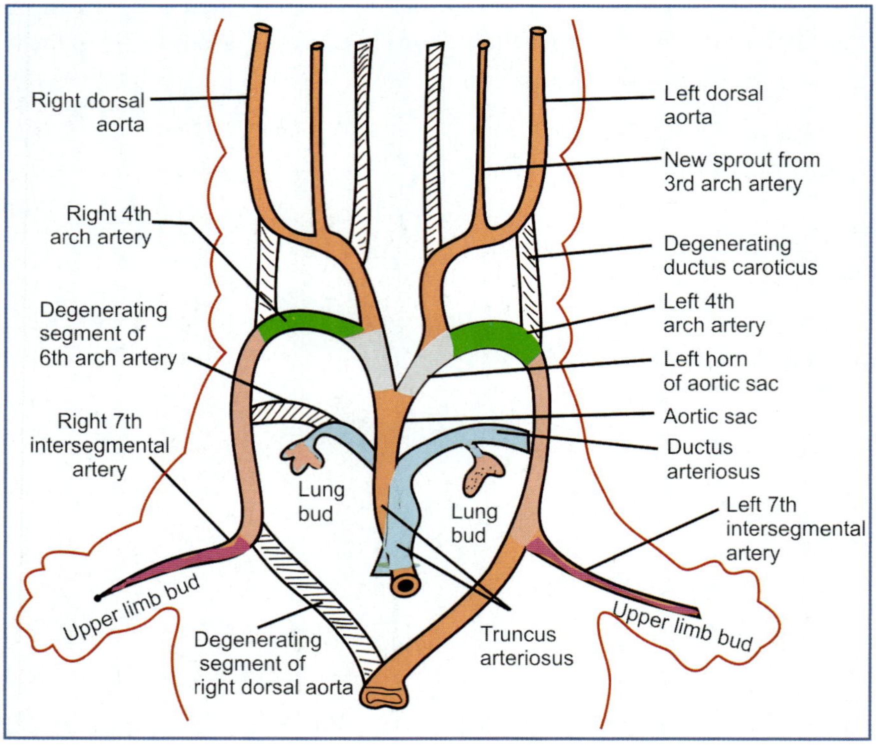

Fig. 47.1: Derivatives of pharyngeal arch arteries. Note the difference in developmental sources of right and left subclavian arteries

involutes on both sides. This creates a break in the dorsal aorta of each side.

b. The sixth arch arteries are divided in dorsal and ventral segments due to the appearance of a connection to the lung bud.
c. The dorsal segment of the sixth arch artery on the right side involutes.
d. The right dorsal aorta disintegrates between the origin of left seventh intersegmental artery and the point of its fusion with left dorsal aorta. This breaks the connection between right and left dorsal aortae.

Derivatives of Arch Arteries

a. The ventral segment of right sixth arch artery develops in to the right pulmonary artery.
b. The ventral segment of left sixth arch artery develops in to left pulmonary artery.
c. The dorsal segment of left sixth arch artery becomes the ductus arteriosus.
d. The arch of aorta develops from four sources as follows, aortic sac, left horn of aortic sac between sixth and fourth arch arteries, left fourth arch artery and part of left dorsal aorta (Fig. 50.5). (Some texts mention three developmental sources of the arch. This is probably because the aortic sac and its left horn are counted as one source).
e. The brachiocephalic artery develops from right horn of aortic sac between sixth and fourth arch arteries.
f. The common carotid artery develops from the right horn of aortic sac between fourth and third arch arteries plus a small contribution from the proximal part of third arch artery of its side.
g. The internal carotid artery develops from the distal part of third arch artery and the dorsal aorta above ductus caroticus.
h. The external carotid artery is a new sprout from the proximal part of third arch artery.
i. The left subclavian artery develops from the left seventh intersegmental artery.
j. The right subclavian artery develops from three sources, right fourth arch artery, part of right dorsal aorta and right seventh intersegmental artery.
l. The descending thoracic aorta and abdominal aorta are derived from the fused dorsal aortae.

Relationship of Arch Arteries to Recurrent Laryngeal Nerves

The recurrent laryngeal nerves are related to the dorsal segments of the sixth arch arteries. When the heart and the arch arteries descend from the neck to the thorax, the nerves are pulled down. Since the recurrent laryngeal nerves supply the larynx they retrace their course upwards. In this process, the nerves hook round the sixth arch arteries on both sides. On the right side, the dorsal segment of the sixth arch artery involutes and the fifth arch artery is rudimentary. Therefore, the right recurrent laryngeal nerve recurs around the lowest persisting arch artery on the right side, namely, the right subclavian artery. On the left side the dorsal segment of the sixth arch artery becomes the ductus arteriosus, which in postnatal life modifies into the ligamentum arteriosum. Therefore, the left recurrent laryngeal nerve hooks round the lowest persisting arch artery on the left side, namely, ligamentum arteriosum.

ANOMALIES OF ARCH ARTERIES

a. Patent ductus arteriosus (PDA) is the result of non-closure of ductus arteriosus after birth (Fig. 42.9). It may occur as an isolated anomaly or in combination with other cardiac defects. It is usually found in Rubella syndrome, which occurs in infants whose mothers had German measles during first two months of gestation. In PDA the blood shunts from the arch of the aorta to left pulmonary artery. This overloads the pulmonary circulation leading to progressive damage in the pulmonary vascular bed. The treatment consists of ligation and division of the ductus arteriosus.
b. Coarctation of aorta means narrowing of the lumen of the arch of aorta. There are two types of coarctation (Fig. 47.2). In preductal type the narrowing is proximal to the attachment of ductus arteriosus while in postductal type it is distal to the attachment of the ductus. In preductal type, the ductus is invariably patent while in the postductal type it is obliterated. The method of filling of the descending aorta distal to the narrowing is different in the two types. In the preductal type the aorta receives deoxygenated blood through the patent ductus arteriosus. In the postductal

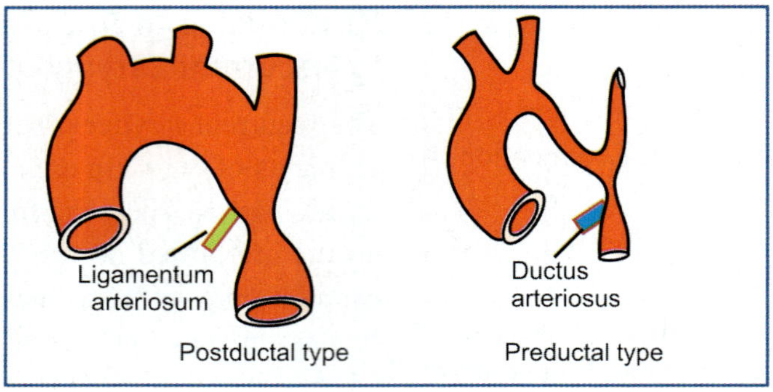

Fig. 47.2: Types of coarctation of aorta. Note that postductal type is seen in childhood and in adults while preductal type is seen in infants

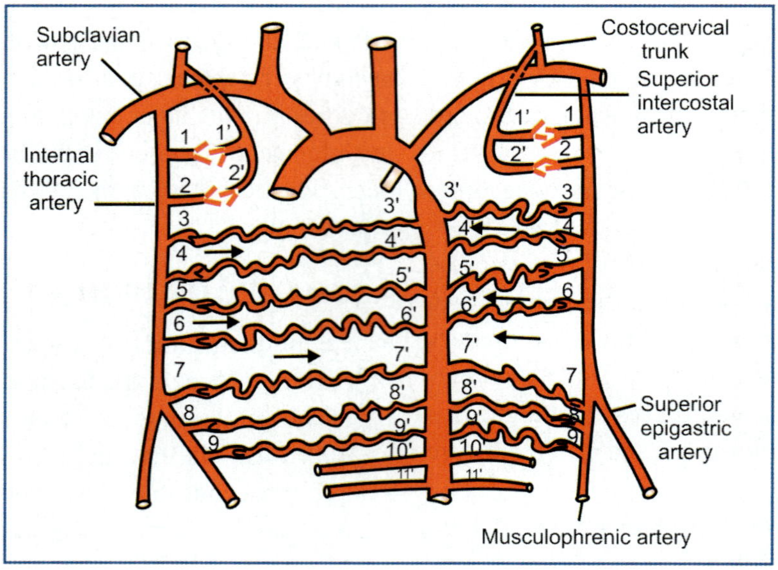

Fig. 47.3: Scheme depicting collateral circulation in postductal type of coarctation of aorta. Note that no. 1 to 9 are anterior intercostal arteries and 1' to 9' are posterior intercostal arteries. Note that 3rd to 9th posterior intercostal arteries are tortuous and show reversal of blood flow

type the aorta is filled with blood through collateral circulation (Fig. 47.3). The postductal coarctation is more common. Its characteristic signs are the radio-femoral delay and difference in the BP in the upper and lower extremities. Radiological sign of rib notching may be present. Rib notching is due to erosion of the lower borders of the ribs by the enlarged and tortuous posterior intercostal arteries. These arteries carry blood from the anterior intercostal arteries to fill the descending aorta. Thus, there is reversal of blood flow in the posterior intercostal arteries.

c. Aberrant right subclavian artery (Fig. 47.4) takes origin from the arch of the aorta beyond the left subclavian artery. It crosses behind the esophagus to reach the right side. The cause of this anomaly is the involution of the right fourth arch artery and the persistence of the normally disintegrating segment of right dorsal aorta. The anomaly can be confirmed radiologically since the aberrant artery indents the barium filled esophagus at the level of the fourth thoracic vertebra. Often, dysphagia is the main complaint. The aberrant right subclavian artery is responsible for the occur-

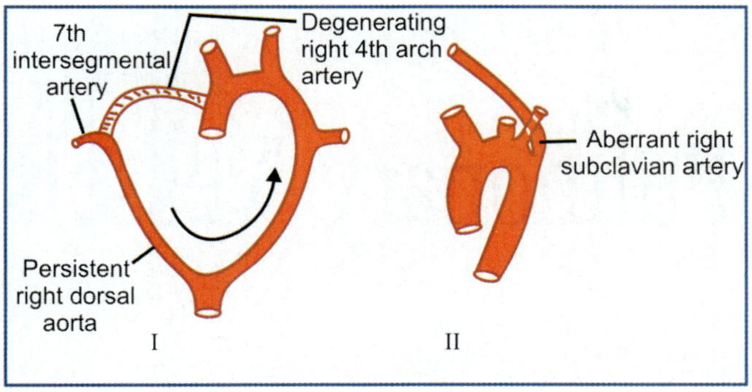

Fig. 47.4: Embryological basis of aberrant right subclavian artery. The arrow indicates the direction of upward migration and shortening of persistent right dorsal aorta to become fourth branch of aortic arch

rence of nonrecurrent right recurrent laryngeal nerve. This nerve fails to recur since the right subclavian artery does not develop from the right 4th arch artery. The nerve arises from the vertical part of vagus in the neck (Fig. 47.5).

d. The double aortic arch results if the part of right dorsal aorta beyond the seventh intersegmental artery fails to involute. This anomaly gives rise to a vascular ring in the thorax around the trachea and esophagus. The symptoms depend upon the tightness of the ring. There may be difficulty in deglutition and respiration due to compression of esophagus and trachea respectively.

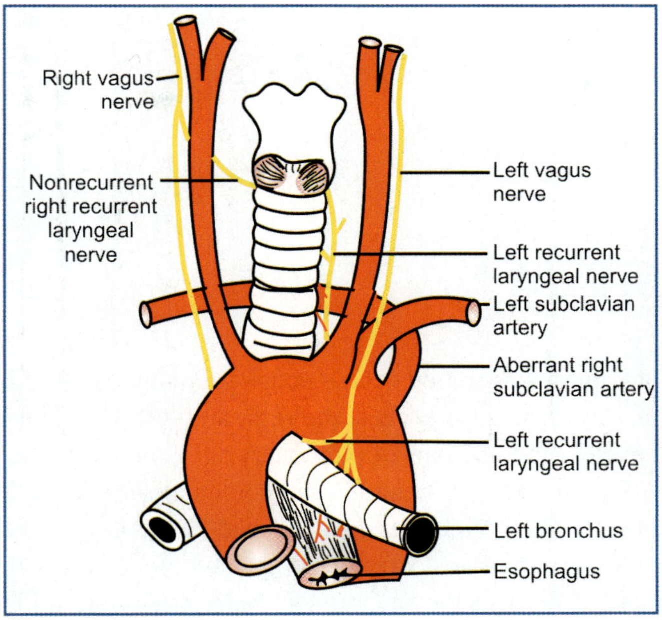

Fig. 47.5: Aberrant right subclavian artery. Note this anomaly is associated with nonrecurrence of right recurrent laryngeal nerve

48 Pulmonary Vessels

The pulmonary blood vessels consist of pulmonary trunk and its terminal branches, the right and left pulmonary arteries, and one pair of pulmonary veins on each side. The pulmonary arteries and veins communicate with each other at the pulmonary capillary bed in the lungs. The pulmonary arteries carry deoxygenated blood from the right ventricle to the lungs and the pulmonary veins bring oxygenated blood back to the left atrium.

Pulmonary Trunk

This vessel begins as the continuation of infundibulum of the right ventricle at the pulmonary valve (Fig. 48.1). It is 5 cm long and 3 cm wide. It systolic pressure is 15-25 mm of Hg. The pulmonary trunk bifurcates into right and left pulmonary arteries inside the fibrous pericardium. Its bifurcation is at the level of the superior margin of the atria (level with fifth thoracic vertebra).

Surface Marking

A 2.5 cm broad horizontal line is drawn at the level of left third costal cartilage, extending partly behind the sternum. This line represents the pulmonary valve. From either end of this line two parallel lines are drawn upward till the level of the upper margin of second costal cartilage.

Relations

The relation of pulmonary trunk to the ascending aorta is important. Both the vessels are covered in a common sleeve of visceral pericardium due to their common development from the truncus arteriosus. The pulmonary trunk is in front of the ascending aorta at its beginning but soon it comes to lie on the left of the ascending aorta. Both vessels form the anterior boundary of transverse sinus of pericardium hence lie in front of the left atrium. At its origin the pulmonary trunk is flanked by the corresponding coronary artery and auricle.

Pulmonary Arteries

The surface marking of the upper margin of the heart indicates the position of the pulmonary arteries. This line extends from a point 1.25 cm away from the right margin of sternum at the upper margin of third costal cartilage to a point 1.25 cm away from the left margin of sternum at the lower margin of left second costal cartilage. The right two-thirds of this line indicates the right pulmonary artery and the left one-third indicates the left artery.

Course and Distribution

a. The right pulmonary artery has a longer intrapericardial course than the left pulmonary artery. During its intrapericardial course it is related anteriorly (in succession) to the ascending aorta, SVC and the upper right pulmonary vein. Posterior to it but outside the fibrous pericardium, are the esophagus and the right main bronchus. After piercing the fibrous pericardium the artery enters the hilum of right lung, where it lies slightly below and in front of the eparterial bronchus. The upper

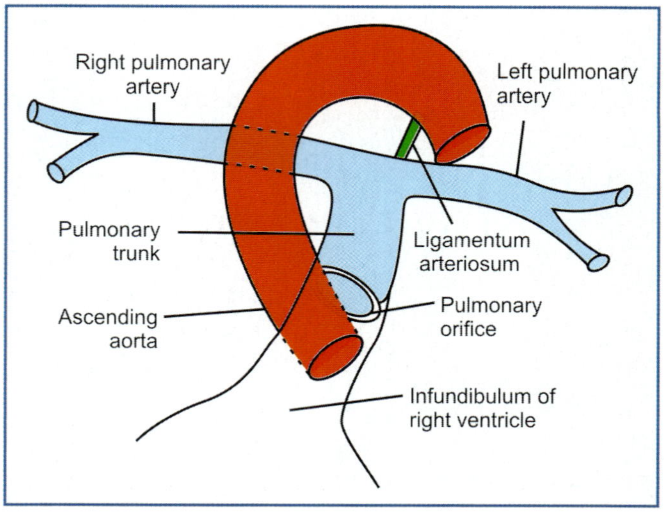

Fig. 48.1: Pulmonary trunk and its branches

right pulmonary vein is in front of the pulmonary artery while the hyparterial bronchus lies below and on a posterior plane. The inferior pulmonary vein is lowest in position. At the hilum of the lung the right pulmonary artery divides into two unequal branches. The smaller branch enters the upper lobe of the lung while the larger branch soon divides into lobar branches for the middle and the lower lobes. The lobar branches divide into segmental branches for individual bronchopulmonary segments of a particular lobe. Thus, the arterial divisions follow the pattern of bronchial tree.

b. The left pulmonary artery has a very short intrapericardial course. After it pierces the fibrous pericardium it is related anteriorly to left lung and pleura and posteriorly to the left main bronchus, descending aorta and left vagus nerve. Superiorly the ligamentum arteriosum connects it to arch of aorta. At the hilum of the left lung the left pulmonary artery is highest in location. The left main bronchus lies below and behind while left superior pulmonary vein lies in front and below the artery. The inferior pulmonary vein is the lowest structure at the hilum. The artery divides into two equal branches for the two lobes of the left lung. Each lobar branch gives off segmental branches corresponding to the number of bronchopulmonary segments. The segmental arteries repeatedly subdivide till they join the capillary bed surrounding the alveoli. The branching pattern of the left pulmonary artery shows frequent variations.

Pulmonary Veins (Fig. 48.2)

The pulmonary veins originate as small venous tributaries from the pulmonary capillaries. The veins lie in the planes separating the adjacent bronchopulmonary segments so that they are able to pick up oxygen from more than one segment. The intersegmental veins unite to form lobar veins. There are three lobar veins on the right side while there are two lobar veins on the left side. Of the three lobar veins on the right side those from the middle and lower lobes unite to form right inferior pulmonary vein. The lobar vein of the upper lobe continues as the right superior pulmonary vein. On the left side the lobar vein of upper lobe continues as left superior pulmonary vein while the one from the lower lobe is called the left inferior pulmonary vein. After emerging from the lung, the pair of veins on each side proceeds transversely to pierce the fibrous pericardium to open in the posterior wall of the left atrium. The walls of the pulmonary veins contain cardiac muscle fibers instead of the smooth muscle fibers. They are valveless veins.

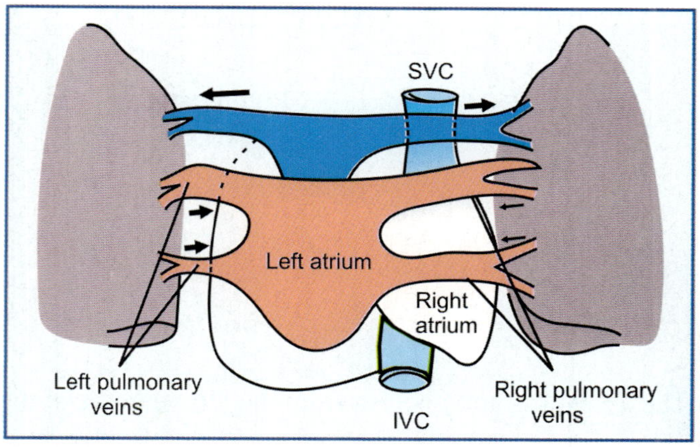

Fig. 48.2: Pulmonary vessels viewed from posterior aspect

Clinical Highlights

a The pulmonary edema means accumulation of serous fluid in the lung alveoli as a result of rise in the hydrostatic pressure of pulmonary capillaries. This happens when there is rise in pulmonary arterial pressure or if capillary permeability increases as for example in inflammation of lung tissue due to any cause. The common cause of pulmonary edema is left ventricular failure due to acute myocardial infarction, mitral stenosis, mitral regurgitation or systemic hypertension. It can also occur in pneumonia. In pulmonary edema the patient experiences intense dyspnea (breathlessness), sweating, frothy sputum and cyanosis.

b. The pulmonary embolism means occlusion of pulmonary artery or its branches by emboli. The emboli usually originate from thrombosis in distant peripheral veins like calf or pelvic veins or from the right auricle. Massive pulmonary embolism is a cause of sudden death. Predisposing factors for peripheral vein thrombosis are, prolonged immobilization, thrombophlebitis and postoperative period. Symptoms of pulmonary embolism include sudden dyspnea, anginal pain, hemoptysis (blood in sputum) and cyanosis.

49 Ascending Aorta

The ascending aorta begins from the left ventricle at the level of aortic valve. It continues as the arch of aorta at the level of sternal angle. Its length is 5 cm and diameter is 3 cm. It is entirely intrapericardial.

Surface Marking

The aortic valve is drawn on the left half of the body of sternum at the level of 3rd intercostal space by a line 2.5 cm broad. From the ends of this line two parallel lines are drawn in upward direction to reach the right half of sternum at the sternal angle. The upper end of the ascending aorta is represented by a line on the right half of the sternum at this level.

Sinuses of Valsalva

Just above the aortic valves the wall of the ascending aorta shows three dilatations, called aortic sinuses of Valsalva. Their positions are anterior, right posterior and left posterior. The anterior aortic sinus is called the right coronary sinus because it gives origin to right coronary artery. The left posterior sinus is called the left coronary sinus because it gives origin to left coronary artery. The right posterior sinus is called the non-coronary sinus.

Bulb of Ascending Aorta

It is a dilatation on the right side of the ascending aorta, which is subjected to constant thrust of the forceful blood current ejected from the left ventricle. This site is prone to aneurysm.

Relations

The ascending aorta pierces the apex of fibrous pericardium at the level of sternal angle. It is enclosed with the pulmonary trunk in a common sleeve of visceral pericardium. Its anterior relations can be subdivided in three levels. The lowest part is related to the infundibulum of right ventricle and the auricle of right atrium. Its middle part is in relation to the pulmonary trunk. Above this, it is related to the pericardium. The transverse sinus of pericardium is the posterior relation and it separates the ascending aorta from the left atrium. The SVC and the right atrium form close relation on the right side while the pulmonary trunk is related on the left side. Thus, The pulmonary trunk is at first in anterior relation and then comes on the left side.

Branches

The right and left coronary arteries are its two branches. The left coronary artery provides circumferential branches to the ascending aorta at its base.

Development

The ascending aorta develops from the truncus arteriosus after its partitioning by the spiral septum.

Aneurysm of Ascending Aorta

The aneurysm occurs at the bulb of the aorta. It may compress the pulmonary trunk, SVC, right atrium or right main bronchus (through the pericardium). It may cause anginal pain. Its serious complication is rupture, which results in rapid accumulation of blood in the pericardial cavity (hemopericardium).

50 Arch of Aorta

The arch of aorta (aortic arch) is located in the superior mediastinum. It is the continuation of ascending aorta and it continues as the descending thoracic aorta, both events take place at the level of sternal angle (Fig. 50.1). At its beginning the arch of aorta is anteriorly located while its termination is located posteriorly (very close to the left side of the fourth thoracic vertebra). The arch reaches the level of mid-manubrium, as it spans the distance between its two ends.

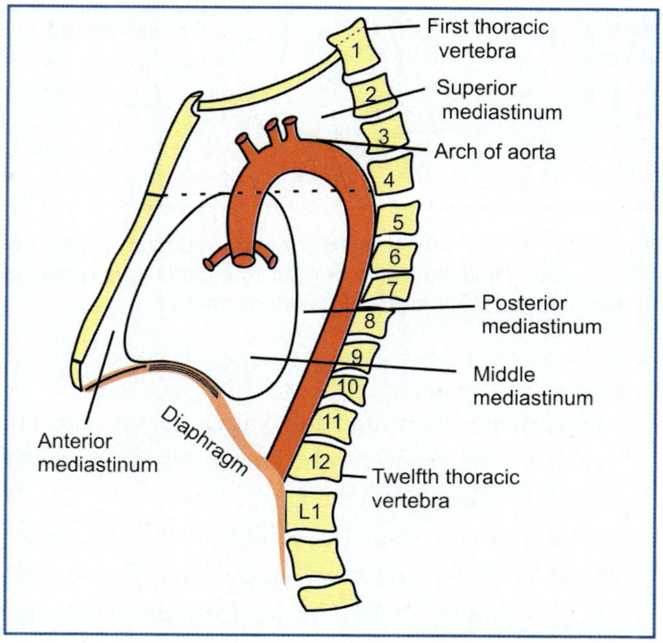

Fig. 50.1: Overall layout of aorta in mediastinum (Note that arch of aorta is the continuation of ascending aorta and it continues as descending aorta)

Course

The arch of aorta begins at the level of right second costal cartilage and turns backwards, upwards and to the left in front of the trachea. Having reached the middle of the back of manubrium, it turns backwards and downwards along the left side of the trachea upto the level of lower border of fourth thoracic vertebra, where it becomes the descending aorta. During its course it describes two convexities (first upward and second to the left). The aortic arch produces a deep groove on the left lung through the mediastinal pleura, above the hilum.

Surface Marking (Fig. 50.2)

The arch of aorta is represented by a curved and wide (2.5 cm) band, which connects the right second costal cartilage close to the sternum to the left second costo-sternal junction. The most convex point of this band reaches the midpoint of the manubrium sterni.

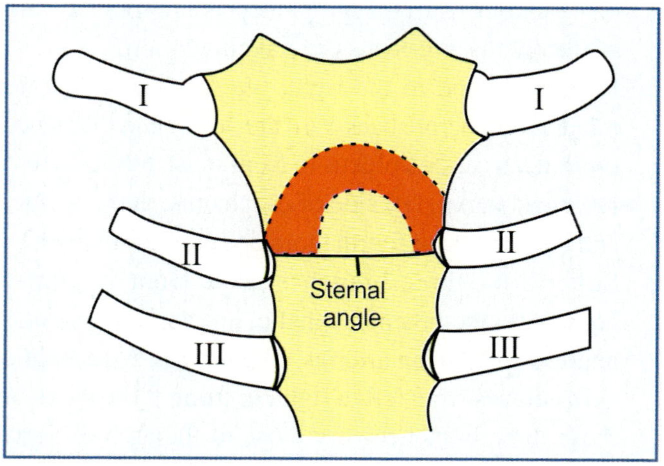

Fig. 50.2: Surface marking of arch of aorta

Relations

a. Anteriorly (Fig. 50.3) and to the left, the structures that cross the arch from anterior to posterior are, left phrenic nerve, inferior cervical cardiac branch of left vagus nerve, superior cervical cardiac branch of left

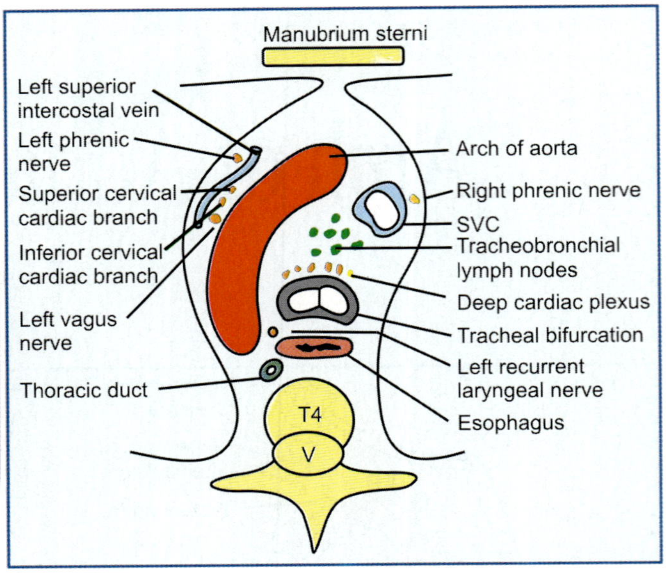

Fig. 50.3: TS at the level of T4 vertebra to depict relations of arch of aorta. (Note that left recurrent laryngeal nerve is related to right and posterior surface of arch of aorta)

sympathetic chain and left vagus nerve. The left superior intercostal vein also crosses the arch between the phrenic nerve and the vagus nerve.

b. Inferiorly, it is in relation to the bifurcation of pulmonary trunk, left pulmonary artery and the left main bronchus (Fig. 50.4 and 39.4). The ligamentum arteriosum connects the arch of aorta (distal to the origin of left subclavian artery) to the beginning of the left pulmonary artery. The left recurrent laryngeal nerve winds round the ligamentum and the superficial cardiac plexus lies on its anterior aspect. This ligament is a fibrous remnant of the ductus arteriosus of fetal circulation.

c. Posteriorly and to the right, the structures that are related from before backward are, lower end of trachea (with deep cardiac plexus in front of it), left recurrent laryngeal nerve, left side of esophagus, thoracic duct and the left side of fourth thoracic vertebra (Fig. 50.3).

d. Superiorly, three branches arise from its upper convexity, the brachiocephalic, left common carotid and left subclavian arteries. The left brachiocephalic vein courses from left to right, in front of the bases of these three branches very close to the arch of aorta (Fig. 50.4).

Branches

The brachiocephalic (innominate) artery arises from the summit of the arch. Beyond this the arch gives origin to left common carotid and left subclavian arteries. Occasionally, a fourth branch called thyroidea ima may arise from the arch. Some variations in the branches are, the left vertebral artery or inferior thyroid artery may arise from the arch.

Arterial Supply

Small twigs arise from the branches of the aortic arch and enter its wall from outside. These twigs (vasa vasora) supply blood to the outer part of the wall. The inner part of the tunica media is nourished from the blood in the lumen of the arch.

Development

The arch develops from four sources, aortic sac, left horn of aortic sac, left fourth arch artery and the left dorsal aorta (Figs 50.5 and 47.1). The congenital anomalies associated with the arch are, patent ductus arteriosus (Fig. 42.11), coarctation of aorta (Figs 47.2 and 47.3), aberrant right subclavian artery (Figs 47.4 and 47.5) and double aortic arch. For details of the development and anomalies of the arch refer to Chapter 47 on pharyngeal arches.

Aneurysm of Aortic Arch

The aneurysm of aortic arch is a localized dilatation of the vessel. A characteristic clinical sign of this condition

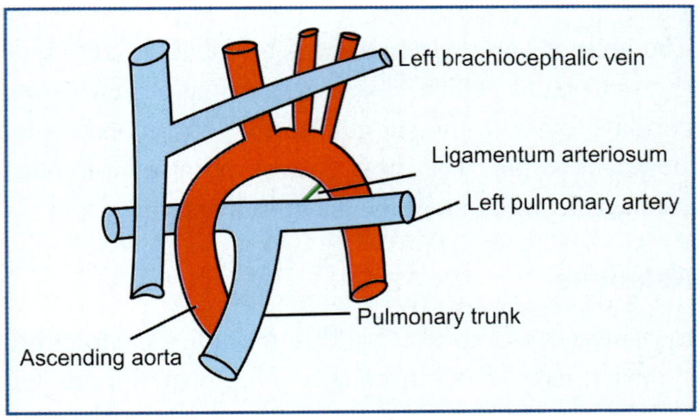

Fig. 50.4: Superior and inferior relations of arch of aorta

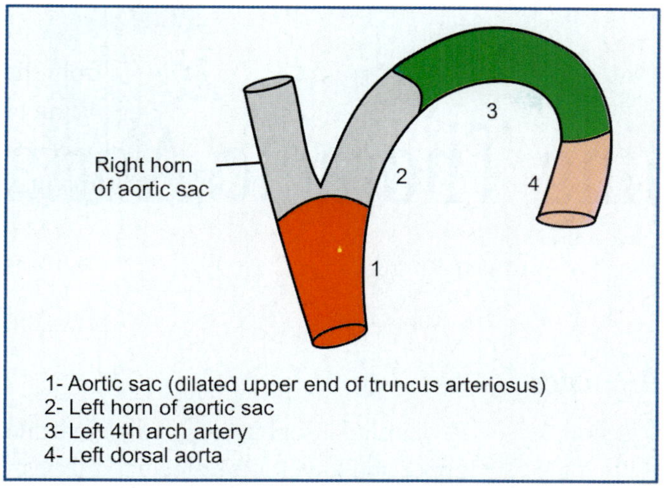

Fig. 50.5: Scheme to depict developmental sources of aortic arch

is the tracheal tug, which is a tugging sensation felt in the suprasternal notch, where trachea is palpated in extended position of the neck. The aneurysm usually causes compression of neighboring structures in the superior mediastinum producing diverse symptoms and signs (mediastinal syndrome). Pressure on esophagus will cause dysphagia, on trachea, stridor and dry cough, on left recurrent laryngeal nerve, hoarseness of voice and on sympathetic chain, Horner's syndrome. Compression of veins in superior mediastinum will cause venous congestion in the neck and upper limb. The aneurysm may rupture into bronchus, pleural cavity, pericardial cavity or esophagus leading to fatal hemorrhage.

Radiological Appearance

In the P-A view of X-ray chest the arch of aorta appears as a small projection at the upper end of the left margin of the cardiac shadow. It is called aortic knuckle. In LAO (left anterior oblique) view of X-ray chest a translucent space enclosed by the arch is identifiable. It is called aortic window in which faint shadows of pulmonary arteries may be seen.

Descending Thoracic Aorta 51

The descending thoracic aorta is located in posterior mediastinum. It extends from the left side of the lower border of fourth thoracic vertebra to the lower border of the front of the twelfth thoracic vertebra. At its upper end it is continuous with the arch of aorta. At its lower end it passes through the aortic opening of the diaphragm to become continuous with the abdominal aorta. At its commencement the aorta is to the left of the vertebral column. During its descent it gradually inclines towards the midline till it lies directly anterior to the vertebral column at its termination.

Surface Marking

A 2.5 cm broad line is drawn on the left part of the sternal angle and the adjoining part of second left costal cartilage. Another line of same breadth is drawn on the anterior abdominal wall about 2 to 2.5 cm above the transpyloric plane in the median plane. The ends of the broad lines are connected by two parallel lines to mark the aorta on the surface.

Relations (Fig. 51.1)

Anteriorly the descending aorta is related to, from above downwards, the left lung root, pericardium (with left atrium inside it), esophagus and the diaphragm. Posteriorly it is related to the vertebral column and hemiazygos veins. The upper part is related on the right side to the esophagus. The other relations on the right side are the thoracic duct and vena azygos. Its lower part comes in contact with the right lung and pleura. On the left side the descending aorta produces a deep vertical groove on the medial surface of the left lung (posterior to the hilum and extending upto the lower end of the medial surface).

Branches

Visceral	Pericardial, esophageal, mediastinal and upper and lower left bronchial arteries
Parietal	3rd to 11th posterior intercostal arteries Subcostal arteries Superior phrenic or phrenic arteries

Dissecting Aneurysm

The aortic dissection (dissecting aneurysm) is a condition that mostly affects the thoracic aorta. The blood from

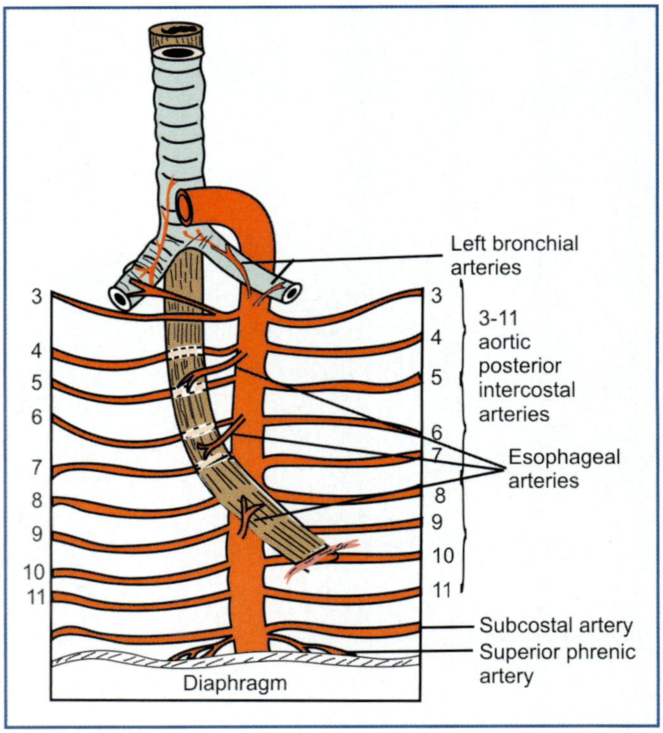

Fig. 51.1: Scheme to show branches of descending thoracic aorta

aortic lumen enters its wall through a tear in the intima. A channel of blood is created in the tunica media. This causes dilatation of the aorta. The patient usually experiences pain in the back due to compression of intercostal nerves. Occasionally, the aorta may rupture into the left pleural cavity. Surgical treatment consists of transection of diseased segment followed by end-to-end anastomosis or replacement with prosthetic vascular graft.

Veins of Thorax

52

Superior Vena Cava (SVC)

The superior vena cava (SVC) drains blood from the head and neck, upper limb, walls of thorax and upper abdomen into the right atrium of the heart. It is 7 cm long and is subdivided in two parts, extrapericardial in the superior mediastinum and intrapericardial in the middle mediastinum. The superior vena cava is without valves since gravity facilitates the flow inside. It is formed by the union of right and left brachiocephalic veins behind the lower border of right first costal cartilage close to the sternum (Fig. 52.1). It passes vertically downwards behind the first and second right intercostal spaces and pierces the fibrous pericardium to open in the upper posterior part of the right atrium at the level of the third costal cartilage. The arch of the azygos vein opens just before the superior vena cava pierces the fibrous pericardium. The intrapericardial part is closely related to the ascending aorta and the right pulmonary artery.

Surface Marking of SVC

This vein is represented by two parallel and vertical lines 2 cm apart starting from the lower border of the first costal cartilage to the upper border of the third costal cartilage close to the right side of sternum.

Brachiocephalic Veins

There are two brachiocephalic veins (Fig. 52.1). Each is formed behind the sternoclavicular joint by the union of the internal jugular and subclavian veins. The right and left brachiocephalic veins unite to form the SVC at the lower margin of right first costal cartilage close to the sternum. Both veins are devoid of valves. The right brachiocephalic vein is short (2.5 cm) and extends from the right sternoclavicular joint to the lower margin of first costal cartilage. Its tributaries are, the right vertebral vein, right internal thoracic vein, right inferior thyroid vein and the first right posterior intercostal vein. The left brachiocephalic vein is about twice as long as the right vein (6 cm). It runs obliquely across the superior mediastinum from the left sternoclavicular joint to the lower margin of first right costal cartilage, where it unites with the right vein. It is closely related to the posterior surface of the manubrium sterni. This relation should be kept in mind while performing sternal puncture. Posteriorly it is related to the three branches of the arch

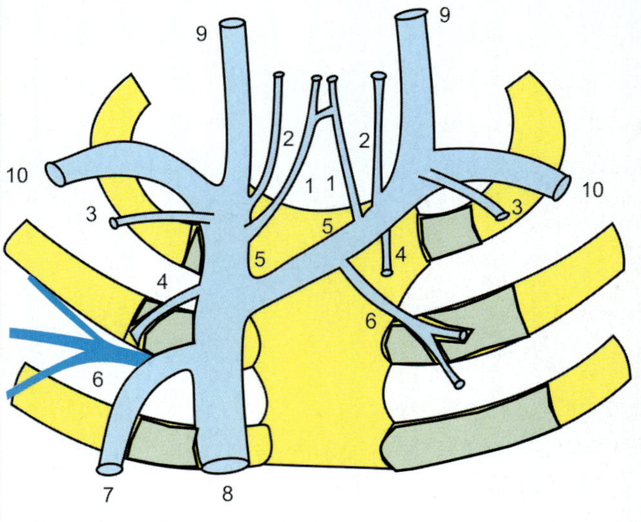

1- Rt. and Lt. inferior thyroid veins
2- Rt. and Lt. vertebral veins
3- Rt. and Lt. first posterior intercostal veins
4- Rt. and Lt. internal mammary veins
5- Rt. and Lt. brachiocephalic veins
6- Rt. and Lt. superior intercostal veins
7- Azygos vein
8- Superior vena cava
9- Rt. and Lt. internal jugular veins
10- Rt. and Lt. subclavian veins

Fig. 52.1: Formation, tributaries and termination of brachiocephalic veins (viewed from internal aspect)

of aorta and two nerves (left vagus and left phrenic). This vein receives the left vertebral vein, left internal thoracic vein, left inferior thyroid vein (sometimes both inferior thyroid veins drain into it), first left posterior intercostal vein, left superior intercostal vein, thymic veins and pericardial veins.

Azygos Vein (Fig. 34.2)

The name azygos means single or without a companion. The azygos vein is present on the right side only. It is provided with valves. It presents a tortuous appearance. The azygos vein begins in the abdomen usually as a continuation of lumbar azygos vein (which arises from posterior part of IVC) or is formed by the union of right ascending lumbar and right subcostal veins (Fig. 53.1). It leaves the abdomen through the aortic opening of diaphragm and enters the posterior mediastinum. Here it ascends vertically upwards lying in front of the vertebral column upto the level of the fourth thoracic vertebra, where it arches forwards superior to the hilum of the right lung (which it grooves) to open in the SVC just before the latter pierces the fibrous pericardium. The azygos vein receives a number of tributaries, right superior intercostal vein, right posterior intercostal veins from the fourth space onwards, right subcostal vein, ascending lumbar vein, hemiazygos vein, accessory hemiazygos vein, right bronchial vein, esophageal, pericardial and mediastinal veins.

Hemiazygos Vein (Inferior Hemiazygos Vein)

This vein is present on the left side. It is formed like the azygos vein in the abdomen from either the continuation of left lumbar azygos vein that arises from the posterior surface of the left renal vein or by the union of left ascending lumbar and the left subcostal veins. The hemiazygos vein pierces the left crus of the diaphragm and enters the posterior mediastinum. It passes vertically upward lying on the front of the vertebral bodies and crosses over to the right side in front of the eighth thoracic vertebra to open in the azygos vein. This vein receives, left ascending lumbar vein, left subcostal vein and the left posterior intercostal veins of the ninth to eleventh intercostal spaces.

Accessory Hemiazygos Vein (Superior Azygos Vein)

This vein begins as the continuation of usually the fifth posterior intercostal vein and descends on the left side of the vertebral column. At the level of the seventh thoracic vertebra it crosses over to the right side behind the descending aorta and the thoracic duct to open in the azygos vein. This vein receives the fifth to seventh left posterior intercostal veins and the left bronchial vein.

Posterior Intercostal Veins (Fig. 34.2)

There are eleven pairs of posterior intercostal veins. Each posterior intercostal vein drains its intercostal space. The vein of the first space (the highest intercostal vein) ascends in front of the neck of the first rib and then arches over the cervical pleura in anterior direction to open in the corresponding brachiocephalic vein.

The right superior intercostal vein begins by the union of right posterior intercostal veins of the second, third and often the fourth spaces. It opens in the arch of the azygos vein.

The left superior intercostal vein begins by the union of left posterior intercostal veins of the second, third and often the fourth spaces. It descends to the level of the vertebral end of the aortic arch and then crosses the left and anterior surfaces of the arch of aorta. It terminates in the left brachiocephalic vein. Its tributaries are the left bronchial vein, and sometimes the left pericardiacophrenic vein.

The posterior intercostal veins of the remaining spaces on the right side drain in the vertical part of azygos vein. The corresponding veins on the left side drain into hemiazygos veins.

The posterior intercostal veins communicate with anterior intercostal veins, which are the tributaries of internal thoracic veins. They communicate with the vertebral venous plexuses. This communication has clinical significance in venous spread of the cancer in the vertebrae and skull bones from primary cancer in the breast, prostate or thyroid gland.

Collateral Venous Circulation

The superior vena cava may be compressed at two sites, in the superior mediastinum or in the middle mediastinum.

Depending on the site of obstruction the different collateral pathways are developed. If the SVC is obstructed above the entry of the azygos vein the following routes drain the blood from the upper part of the body. The blood from the internal thoracic vein reaches the azygos vein via the anastomoses between the anterior and posterior intercostals veins. The internal thoracic vein communicates with the superior and inferior epigastric veins (of the anterior abdominal wall). So the veins of the anterior abdominal wall form another route to carry blood from the internal thoracic veins to the IVC. If the obstruction is below the entry of the azygos vein, venous blood from the upper part of the body reaches the right atrium via the IVC, which receives blood from the azygos vein. There is reversal of blood flow in the azygos vein, which pours blood in IVC through lumbar azygos or ascending lumbar veins. As a result, the superficial venous collateral channels are dilated along the lateral thoracic and abdominal walls.

Development of Veins of Thorax

During the fourth week of embryonic life there is a symmetrical pattern of venous channels (Fig. 42.3). The cardinal veins consists of anterior cardinal veins draining the cephalic half of the embryo, posterior cardinal veins draining the caudal half of the embryo and the common cardinal veins or the ducts of Cuvier formed by the union of anterior and posterior cardinal veins, which enter the respective horns of the sinus venosus. During the fifth to seventh weeks the symmetry of the venous pattern is lost because of the development of a transverse anastomotic intercardinal channel between the right and left anterior cardinal veins. This channel diverts the venous blood from the left to the right side, consequent to which the veins on the left side become smaller in size.

a. The right brachiocephalic vein develops from upper part of right anterior cardinal vein, which is cranial to the transverse anastomosis.
b. The left brachiocephalic vein develops from left anterior cardinal vein cranial to the transverse anastomosis and the transverse anastomosis itself.
c. The extrapericardial part of SVC develops from the right anterior cardinal vein caudal to the transverse anastomosis and its intrapericardial part develops from the right common cardinal vein.
d. The left superior intercostal vein develops from left anterior cardinal vein caudal to the transverse anastomosis and the terminal part of left posterior cardinal vein.
e. The oblique vein of Marshall is a remnant of left common cardinal vein. It is connected to the left superior intercostal vein by means of a ligament (ligament of left vena cava), which is also a remnant of left common cardinal vein.
f. The arch of azygos vein develops from the terminal part of right posterior cardinal vein.

53 Lymphatic Organs of Thorax

The lymphatic organs in thorax consist of thymus, thoracic lymph nodes and the thoracic duct.

THYMUS

The thymus is a complex lymphoid organ. It is the only lymphoid organ that is responsible for the differentiation of T-lymphocytes. The thymic secretory products are indispensable for the development and maintenance of an immunologically competent T-lymphocyte pool for the entire body. The thymus mainly lies in superior mediastinum with extension in anterior mediastinum in front of the pericardium. It is roughly pyramidal with base pointed inferiorly. The thymus is often bi-lobed but the two lobes are joined in the midline by connective tissue.

Age Changes

At birth, the thymus is well-developed and weighs about 30 g. At puberty, it reaches maximum size and weighs about 40 g. During adulthood, there is a gradual reduction in the weight as the lymphatic tissue is replaced by fatty tissue. In old age, it is much reduced in size and turns into a fibro-fatty mass. Therefore the number of lymphocytes inside the thymus is greatly reduced. However, lymphocyte production and differentiation persist throughout life.

Relations

In the superior mediastinum, anteriorly the thymus is related to the manubrium sterni, sternohyoid and sternothyroid muscles and posteriorly to left brachiocephalic vein, the arch of aorta and its three branches and trachea. In the anterior mediastinum, anterior relations are, the body of sternum and upper four costal cartilages and posterior relation is the fibrous pericardium.

Blood Supply

The branches of internal thoracic and inferior thyroid arteries supply the thymus. The thymic veins usually drain into the left brachiocephalic vein, though drainage into internal thoracic and inferior thyroid veins is also possible.

Lymphatic Drainage

The efferent lymphatic vessels drain into the brachiocephalic, tracheobronchial and parasternal lymph nodes. The thymus receives no afferent lymphatics.

Development

The endoderm of the third pharyngeal pouches of both sides gives rise to thymic epitheliocytes. The embryonic mesenchyme gives rise to the lymphocytes, connective tissue and blood vessels.

Function

Undifferentiated lymphocytes from the bone marrow enter the thymus from circulating blood. The lymphocyte-processing takes place within the thymus. The T-cells committed to the production of cell-bound or cell-mediated immunity are released into the circulation. Only when the T-cells start circulating through the lymph nodes and spleen, the lymphocytes within these structures become B-lymphocytes, which are committed to the production of a particular antibody.

Clinical Highlights

a. Patients with thymic aplasia, agenesis or hypoplasia, as occurs in DiGeorge syndrome and Nezelof's syndrome (refer to Chapter 72 on Branchial Apparatus) have lymphopenia, decreased immunity and die early from infection. DiGeroge syndrome presents with severest form of deficient T cell immunity.

b. The causes of thymic atrophy in young age are ionizing radiation, severe malnutrition, prolonged administration of glucocorticoids and cytotoxic drugs.
c. In hyperplasia of thymus there are lymphatic follicles in the thymic lobules. The patient may develop myasthenia gravis. The epithelial cell tumor of thymus called thymoma may present as myasthenia gravis. When the thymoma is large in size it may compress on trachea, esophagus and large veins in the superior mediastinum.
d. Myasthenia gravis is a chronic autoimmune disease of adults, in which there is reduction in the power of certain voluntary muscles for repetitive contractions. The cause is the destruction of acetylcholine receptor proteins of neuromuscular junction by autoimmune antibodies produced by T-lymphocytes. The muscles commonly involved are the levator palpebrae superioris (causing bilateral ptosis) and extraocular muscles (causing diplopia).

LYMPH NODES OF THORAX

The lymph nodes that drain the thoracic walls are arranged in two groups.
a. The parasternal nodes are located along each internal thoracic artery. They receive lymph vessels from mammary gland, deeper structures of supra-umbilical anterior abdominal wall, superior hepatic surface and the deeper parts of anterior thoracic wall. The efferents from the parasternal nodes unite with the efferents from tracheobronchial and brachiocephalic nodes to form the bronchomediastinal trunk.
b. The intercostal nodes are placed at the posterior end of the intercostal spaces. They receive deep lymph vessels from mammary gland and the posterolateral aspect of thoracic wall. Efferents from the nodes in lower 4 to 7 spaces on both sides unite to form the descending thoracic lymph trunk which descends to the abdomen through aortic orifice and may join the thoracic duct. Efferents from the nodes in the upper left spaces form the upper intercostal lymph trunk, which ends in the thoracic duct, and the corresponding ones on the right side join the right lymph trunk. The posterior nodes lie on the back of the crura of the diaphragm and are connected to the lateral aortic nodes in the abdomen and the posterior mediastinal nodes.

The lymph nodes that drain the thoracic contents consist of three groups.
a. The brachiocephalic nodes lie in the superior mediastinum anterior to the brachiocephalic veins. They receive lymph from thymus, thyroid, pericardium, heart and the lateral diaphragmatic nodes. Their efferents unite with those from tracheobronchial nodes to form right and left bronchomediastinal trunks.
b. Posterior mediastinal nodes lie vertically in the posterior mediastinum along the descending aorta and the esophagus. They receive lymph from the contents of posterior mediastinum, diaphragm including the lateral and posterior diaphragmatic nodes. Their efferents join the thoracic duct.
c. The tracheobronchial nodes (Fig. 38.9) consist of five subgroups. The paratracheal nodes are seen on the front and sides of the trachea. The superior tracheobronchial nodes lie in the angles between trachea and bronchi. The inferior tracheobronchial nodes are present in the angle between bronchi. The bronchopulmonary or hilar nodes are present in the hilum of the lung and the pulmonary nodes are inside the lung substance. These nodes drain lungs and bronchi, thoracic trachea, heart and receive lymph from posterior mediastinal nodes. Their efferents join the efferents of parasternal and brachiocephalic nodes to form right and left bronchomediastinal trunks. The right bronchomediastinal trunk opens independently at right jugulosubclavian junction. The left bronchomediastinal trunk opens into thoracic duct.

THORACIC DUCT

The thoracic duct is a thin-walled elongated lymph vessel about 45 cm long. It conveys the lymph from the body into the venous stream. The lymph in the thoracic duct has milky white appearance because it carries products of fat digestion from the intestine. The duct extends from the upper end of cisterna chyli on the posterior abdominal wall to the junction of left internal jugular and left subclavian veins, at the base of the neck. It is beaded in appearance due to the presence of numerous valves throughout its course. A constant valve guards the opening of the duct in the jugulosubclavian junction to prevent regurgitation of blood in the duct. The duct carries lymph from the entire body except the right half of thorax, right half of head and neck and the right upper limb.

Course and Relations (Fig. 53.1)

Its course can be divided into three parts, abdominal, thoracic and cervical.

a. The abdominal part of the thoracic duct begins at the lower border of the twelfth thoracic vertebra as a continuation of cisterna chyli (a receptacle of lymph on the posterior abdominal wall) and enters the thorax through the aortic opening of the diaphragm. At the aortic opening it is related anteriorly to the median arcuate ligament and posteriorly to the twelfth thoracic vertebra. The azygos vein is on its right and the aorta on its left.
b. In the posterior mediastinum, the thoracic duct ascends to the right of the midline lying on the vertebral bodies. On reaching the level of the fifth thoracic vertebra it gradually inclines to the left and enters the superior mediastinum at the left side of the sternal angle. The esophagus is related to it anteriorly. The azygos vein is on its right and thoracic aorta is on its left.
c. In the superior mediastinum, the thoracic duct ascends along the left margin of esophagus to the thoracic inlet. Anteriorly it is related to the arch of aorta and the left subclavian artery above it. Posteriorly it lies on the bodies of upper four thoracic vertebrae. On its right it is related to the esophagus and on its left it is related to the left lung and pleura.
c. The cervical part of the thoracic duct (Fig. 53.2) arches laterally at the level of transverse process of the seventh cervical vertebra. The summit of the arch is 3 to 4 cm above the clavicle. Anteriorly the arch is related to the carotid sheath and its contents. Its posterior relations are important. The ascending limb of its arch is related to left vertebral artery and vein, left stellate ganglion and left thyrocervical trunk and its three branches. The descending limb of the arch is related to the medial margin of scalenus anterior muscle, the left phrenic nerve and the first part of left subclavian artery.

Termination

In the usual mode of termination, the thoracic duct opens at the union of left subclavian and left internal jugular veins. However, either it may open in subclavian vein or IJV near their union or it may divide into a number of smaller vessels before termination.

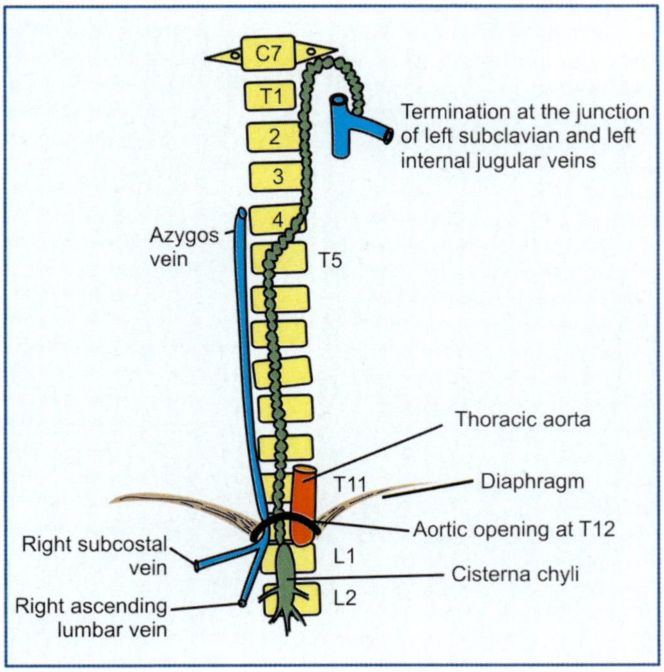

Fig. 53.1: Origin, course and termination of thoracic duct

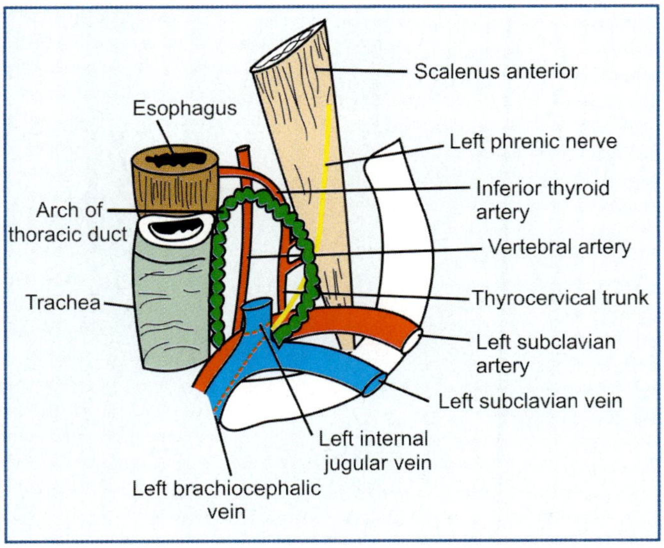

Fig. 53.2: Relations of cervical part of thoracic duct

Tributaries

A large number of tributaries join the thoracic duct throughout its course.

a. Descending thoracic lymph trunks (from lymph nodes of lower intercostal spaces)
b. Ascending lumbar lymph trunks (in abdomen)
c. Upper intercostal trunk of left side
d. Mediastinal trunks (from mediastinum, diaphragm and diaphragmatic surface of liver)
e. Left bronchomediastinal trunk (from lungs and mediastinum)
f. Left jugular trunk (from head and neck)
g. Left subclavian trunk (from upper limb).

Clinical Highlights

a. Injury to the thoracic part of the duct may cause chylothorax (lymph in the pleural cavity).
b. Thoracic duct may be obstructed by microfilarial parasites in which case it produces widespread effects like, chylothorax, chyloperitoneum and even the accumulation of lymph in the tunica vaginalis testis (hydrocele).
c. The cervical part of thoracic duct may be injured during removal of the supraclavicular lymph nodes. If the injury is not detected at the time of operation, postoperatively the patient may lose as much as 1 to 1.5 liters of lymph in 24 hours. Immediate ligation of the duct is necessary to stop the leakage.

Right Lymphovenous Portal

On the right side there are three lymph trunks that converge at the jugulosubclavian junction, the right jugular trunk draining the right half of head and neck, the right subclavian trunk draining the right upper limb and the right bronchomediastinal trunk from the right half of thorax. The termination of the three lymph trunks of right side is subject to variation. Usually the lymph trunks open independently in the jugulosubclavian junction. Occasionally, the three trunks unite to form the right lymphatic duct, which has a similar course in the neck like that of thoracic duct.

54 Autonomic Nerves of Thorax

The autonomic nervous system has sympathetic and parasympathetic components. The cervical and thoracic branches of vagus nerve (parasympathetic) and of the sympathetic chains form autonomic plexuses in thorax, which supply the visceral musculature and secretory glands through postganglionic branches. The visceral afferent fibers are carried from the viscera via the plexuses to the spinal cord and brainstem.

Vagus Nerve

The vagus nerve (tenth cranial nerve) originates in the medulla oblongata and carries the preganglionic parasympathetic fibers from the dorsal nucleus of vagus. These fibers leave the vagus nerve through its cervical and thoracic branches (superior and inferior cervical cardiac branches of vagus nerve). These take part in the formation of superficial and deep cardiac plexuses. The right recurrent laryngeal nerve is given off at the root of the neck from the right vagus. This nerve gives rise to thoracic cardiac branches.

Course and Branches in Thorax

In the superior mediastinum, the right vagus nerve lies on the right side of trachea. It is posteromedial to the SVC and then passes deep to azygos arch to reach the posterior side of the root of the right lung. The left vagus nerve is positioned between left common carotid and left subclavian arteries. Then it crosses the left side of the arch of aorta to reach the posterior side of the root of left lung. At the root of the lung each vagus nerve divides into a number of branches, losing its identity as individual nerve. Here the branches of the vagus join the sympathetic branches to form pulmonary plexuses. Below the lung root the vagal branches on both sides come in relation to the esophagus. The right vagus is located on the posterior side and the left vagus on the anterior side of the esophagus. Having taken part in the esophageal plexuses along with sympathetic branches the vagus nerves leave the thorax through the esophageal opening as posterior vagal trunk (right vagus) and anterior vagal trunk (left vagus). The branches of the vagus in the thorax are, thoracic cardiac branches, pulmonary branches and esophageal branches. As the left vagus nerve crosses in front of the left surface of the arch of aorta it gives off the left recurrent laryngeal branch, which winds round the ligamentum arteriosum and then passes upwards and medially deep to the arch of aorta. Like on the right side the left recurrent laryngeal nerve gives thoracic cardiac branches.

Visceral Afferent Fibers

There are visceral afferent fibers in these cervical and thoracic cardiac branches, which terminate in the sensory ganglia of the vagus nerve. The central processes of these ganglia carry the impulses to the medulla oblongata. In this way the vagus nerves carry sensations from the heart, great blood vessels and respiratory system, which are involved in maintaining the reflex activity of these organs.

Sympathetic Chains

Each sympathetic chain extends from the base of the cranium to the coccyx. It passes through the cervical, thoracic, lumbar and sacral (pelvic) regions. It bears a number of ganglia along its length, where majority of preganglionic fibers synapse. The sympathetic chain gives cervical cardiac and thoracic branches for the supply of the thoracic viscera. The cervical cardiac branches are three on each side and are named as superior, middle and inferior cervical cardiac branches according to the ganglion from which they originate.

Thoracic Branches of Sympathetic Chain

The sympathetic chain enters the thorax through the thoracic inlet. The thoracic part of the chain consists of eleven ganglia. The first thoracic ganglion is fused with inferior cervical ganglion to form cervicothoracic or stellate ganglion, which lies in front of the neck of the first rib. The thoracic sympathetic chain lies on the heads of the succeeding ribs, posterior to the costal pleura. It leaves the thorax behind the medial arcuate ligament to become continuous with lumbar part of the sympathetic trunk. The upper five ganglia supply the thoracic aorta and its branches. The pulmonary branches arise from second to sixth ganglia. The cardiac branches arise from second to fifth ganglia. The branches to the esophagus and trachea reach either directly or indirectly from plexuses. The greater, lesser and least splanchnic nerves leave the thorax to supply the abdominal organs and carry preganglionic sympathetic fibers for relay in the celiac ganglion in the abdomen. The greater splanchnic nerve arises from fifth to ninth ganglia and perforates the crus of diaphragm to enter the abdomen and end in the celiac and aorticorenal ganglia. The lesser splanchnic nerve arises from ninth to tenth ganglia and pierces the diaphragm along with greater splanchnic nerve and terminates in aorticorenal ganglion. The least splanchnic nerve from the lowest ganglion enters the abdomen with the sympathetic chain and ends in renal plexus.

Visceral Afferent Fibers

The visceral afferent fibers (from thoracic viscera) accompany the preganglionic and postganglionic sympathetic fibers and terminate in the dorsal root ganglia of the thoracic spinal nerves. They mediate pain and other nociceptive impulses to the spinal cord.

Autonomic Plexuses in Thorax

The autonomic plexuses are composed of the postganglionic sympathetic fibers, preganglionic parasympathetic fibers and small parasympathetic ganglia. The preganglionic parasympathetic fibers either synapse in these ganglia or synapse in the ganglia, which are located in the wall of the viscera. Besides these, the plexuses carry the visceral afferent fibers.

Superficial Cardiac Plexus

This plexus is located on the ligamentum arteriosum below the arch of aorta. The superior cervical cardiac branch of left sympathetic chain and inferior cervical cardiac branch of left vagus nerve take part in its formation. This plexus is in communication with the deep cardiac plexus, right coronary plexus and left anterior pulmonary plexus.

Deep Cardiac Plexus

This plexus is located in front of the bifurcation of trachea. The following nerves take part in its formation:

a. The cervical sympathetic branches inlcude middle and inferior cardiac branches of left sympathetic chain and the superior, middle and inferior cardiac branches of right sympathetic chain.
b. The thoracic sympathetic branches include cardiac branches of upper five thoracic sympathetic ganglia from both sides.
c. The cervical parasympathetic branches include superior cardiac branch of left vagus nerve and superior and inferior cardiac branch of right vagus nerve.
d. The thoracic parasympathetic branches include cardiac branches of the right and left recurrent laryngeal nerves in addition to direct branches of vagus nerves. The afferent fibers in the deep cardiac plexus carry pain sensation from the heart in the cardiac branches of middle and inferior cervical sympathetic ganglia and in the cardiac branches of thoracic sympathetic ganglia.

Coronary Plexuses

The right half of the deep plexus directly supplies branches to the right atrium and is in communication with right coronary plexus. The left half of the deep plexus is connected with superficial cardiac plexus and gives direct branches to the left atrium. It continues as the left coronary plexus. Thus, the right half of deep plexus and superficial cardiac plexus form the right coronary plexus, while the left coronary plexus is derived from the right and left halves of deep cardiac plexus.

Pulmonary Plexuses

There are two pulmonary plexuses, anterior and posterior in relation to the hilum of the lungs. Thoracic branches of vagus and sympathetic trunk (upper four or five ganglia) form them. The anterior pulmonary plexus on right side is in communication with right half of deep cardiac plexus while the plexus on the left side is in communication with left half of the deep cardiac plexus and with the superficial cardiac plexus. The two plexuses are interconnected. The network of nerves arising from the plexuses enters the lung along the bronchi, pulmonary and bronchial vessels. There are small ganglia in tracheobronchial tree, in which preganglionic vagal fibers synapse.

Esophageal Plexus

This plexus around the esophagus is composed of esophageal branches of fifth to ninth sympathetic ganglia, esophageal branches of both vagi and branches from the recurrent laryngeal nerves. The nerve cells in muscular and submucous layers of the esophagus are the relay stations for parasympathetic fibers. Congenital absence of these neurons results in achalasia or cardiospasm.

55 Esophagus

The esophagus is a muscular tube about 25 cm long. It is continuous above with laryngopharynx at the lower border of cricoid cartilage and below with the cardiac orifice of stomach. Its vertebral extent is from the sixth cervical to the eleventh thoracic vertebra. The main function of the esophagus is to transport food from the pharynx to the stomach.

Course (Fig. 55.1)

The esophagus passes through three regions of the body namely, neck, thorax and abdomen. Its thoracic part is the longest while the abdominal part is the smallest. The course of the esophagus is not straight as it shows three curves. The esophagus follows the concavity of the thoracic vertebral column. At the root of the neck, it inclines to the left by 0.5-1 cm from the midline. It comes back in the midline at the level of fifth thoracic vertebra. Again, it deviates to the left below the seventh thoracic vertebra and inclines anteriorly to pass through the muscular part of diaphragm at the level of tenth thoracic vertebra.

Surface Marking

The upper end of the esophagus is marked at the lower border of cricoid cartilage, which is palpable in the midline 5 cm above the suprasternal notch. From this level esophagus can be drawn as a 2.5 cm wide band passing down to the level of the left seventh costal cartilage 2.5 cm from its junction with the sternum.

Constrictions (Fig. 55.1)

There are four sites of constrictions or narrowing in the esophagus. The distance of each constriction is measured from the upper incisor teeth.

a. The first constriction at the pharyngoesophageal junction is at a distance of 15 cm.
b. The second constriction at a distance of 22.5 cm is produced by the arch of aorta as it crosses the anterior and lateral aspects of esophagus.
c. The third constriction at a distance of 27.5 cm is produced by left bronchus as it crosses the esophagus.
d. The fourth constriction at the esophageal opening in diaphragm is at a distance of 40 cm.

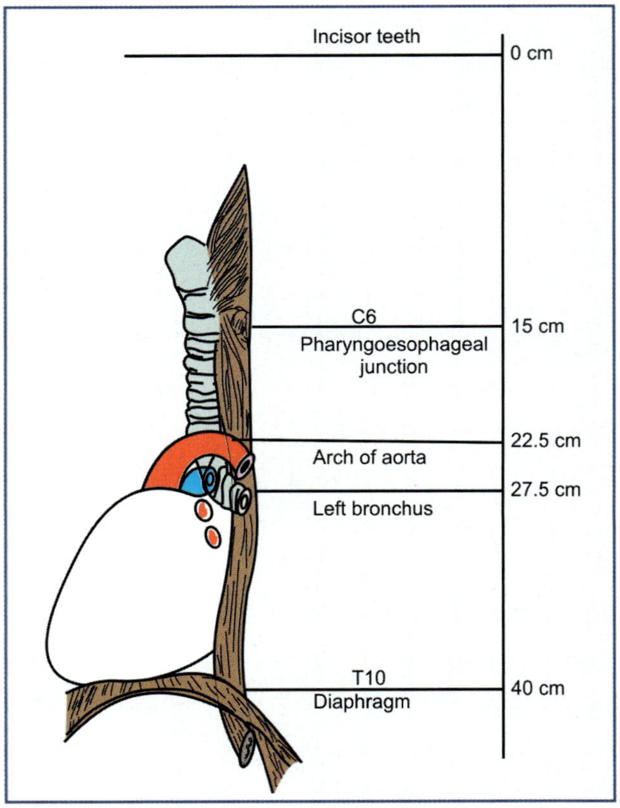

Fig. 55.1: Distances of esophageal constrictions from incisor teeth

The constrictions are the sites, where swallowed foreign bodies are stuck. These are the sites, where strictures develop after ingestion of caustic substances. Moreover, these sites have predilection for carcinoma of esophagus.

Relations of Cervical Esophagus

In the neck the esophagus is related anteriorly to the trachea and to recurrent laryngeal nerves in tracheoesophageal groove. Posteriorly it is related to the prevertebral fascia and vertebral column. The common carotid artery and lateral lobe of thyroid are its lateral relations. In addition, on the left side it is in relation to the thoracic duct at the root of the neck.

Relations of Thoracic Esophagus (Fig. 55.2)

Anterior relations (from above downwards) are trachea, arch of aorta, right pulmonary artery, left principal bronchus, fibrous pericardium and oblique sinus (separating it from left atrium) and diaphragm. Therefore, anteriorly the esophagus is very close to the left atrium of heart. In transesophageal ECHO, the instrument is passed through the esophagus to examine the base of the heart.

Posteriorly, it is in relation to the thoracic vertebrae in the superior mediastinum. In the posterior mediastinum the right posterior intercostal arteries cross the vertebral column behind the esophagus. In addition, the transverse parts of hemiazygos veins, thoracic duct, azygos vein and descending thoracic aorta are related posteriorly.

Left Lateral Relations

In the upper part of the superior mediastinum, it is related to left subclavian artery, thoracic duct, left recurrent laryngeal nerve and the left pleura and upper lobe of left lung are related on the left side. In the lower part of the superior mediastinum, its left edge is related to the arch

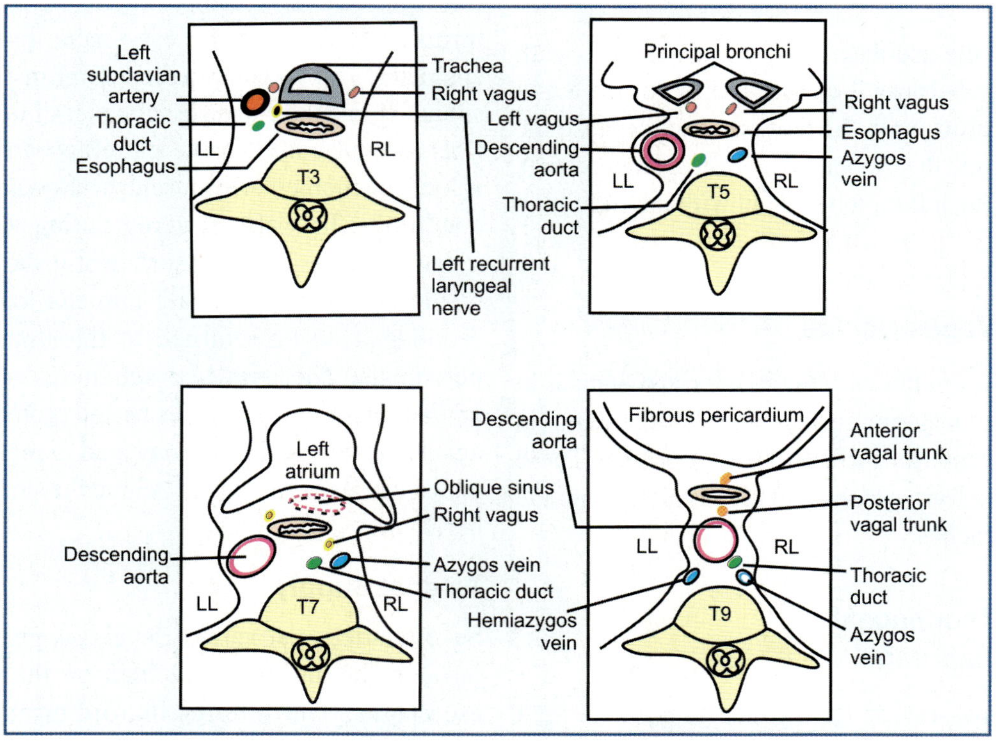

Fig. 55.2: Relations of thoracic part of esophagus from T3 to T9 vertebral levels. Note: The changing relations of descending aorta from above downward and of thoracic duct from below upward (LL—left lung, RL—right lung)

of aorta. In the posterior mediastinum, the descending aorta is on the left side in the upper part. The esophagus is also related to the left lung and pleura, where it makes an impression on the mediastinal surface of left lung behind the lower end of pulmonary ligament.

Right Lateral Relations

The esophagus produces a shallow vertical groove behind the hilum and pulmonary ligament of right lung. The arch of azygos vein is related at the level of sternal angle and the descending thoracic aorta is on the right side below the level of the crossing of the esophagus in front of the aorta.

Posterior Relations

In the superior mediastinum, the thoracic vertebrae are its posterior relations. In the posterior mediastinum at the level of fifth thoracic vertebra, the thoracic duct crosses behind the esophagus. Lower down, the descending aorta, thoracic duct and the azygos vein are posterior to the esophagus.

To sum up, the esophagus has triple relations with descending aorta because it crosses in front of the aorta. It has triple relations with the thoracic duct because the duct crosses behind the esophagus. The esophagus comes in contact with the left lung twice but with the right lung only once.

Relations to Vagus Nerves

Below the level of pulmonary hilum the right vagus is in contact with the posterior surface and the left vagus in contact with the anterior surface of the esophagus. These branches unite to form esophageal plexus along with the sympathetic branches.

Relations at Esophageal Aperture in Diaphragm

The esophagus passes through the muscular part of right crus of diaphragm at the level of tenth thoracic vertebra. The left vagus (now called anterior gastric nerve) is related anteriorly and the right vagus (now called posterior gastric nerve) is related posteriorly to it. The esophagus is also related to the esophageal branches of left gastric vessels.

Abdominal Part of Esophagus

This part is about 1 to 2 cm long and is the only part of the esophagus covered with serous membrane (peritoneum). It is related to the posterior surface of left lobe of liver and posteriorly to the left crus of diaphragm. The right and left vagus nerves enter the abdomen lying along the posterior and anterior surfaces respectively.

Lower Esophageal Sphincter

There is no anatomical sphincter at the gastroesophageal junction. Two mechanisms are believed to operate for preventing the gastroesophageal reflux. The lower esophageal sphincter shows a specialized area of circular smooth muscle, which possesses the physiological properties of the sphincter. The muscle in this area is maintained under tonic contractions by the intramural plexuses of enteric nervous system. The muscle fibers of the right crus of the diaphragm, which surround the terminal portion of the esophagus provide external sphincter. Thus, a combination of intrinsic physiological sphincter and the extrinsic sphincter of the crural muscle fibers provides an adequate antireflux barrier. This barrier is lowered momentarily during swallowing under normal conditions. It is also lowered during vomiting. If the intragastric pressure rises sufficiently, the acidic contents of the stomach regurgitate into the lower end of the esophagus, to be returned to the stomach by reflex peristalsis. The stratified squamous nonkeratinizing epithelium of the esophagus has no protective properties against gastric acid. This may lead to reflux esophagitis, which causes burning pain behind the sternum, known as heartburn.

Arterial Supply

Several arteries at various levels supply the esophagus through the anastomotic chain on the surface of the esophagus. The inferior thyroid artery supplies the cervical part of esophagus. The descending thoracic aorta and bronchial arteries give branches to the thoracic part of the esophagus. The left gastric and left inferior phrenic arteries supply the abdominal esophagus.

Venous Drainage

The cervical part of esophagus drains into inferior thyroid veins. The thoracic part drains into the azygos and hemiazygos veins. The drainage of the abdominal part is by left gastric vein, which is a tributary of portal vein. The veins of the middle part (systemic) anastomose with the veins of the lower part (portal). The portosystemic venous anastomosis is located in the submucous layer of the lower part of esophagus. In patients with portal hypertension, the submucous venous plexuses become enlarged. Such dilated venous plexuses covered with mucosa protrude in the lumen of lower esophagus. They are asymptomatic until they rupture causing a large bout of blood vomiting (hematemesis).

Lymphatic Drainage

From cervical part lymph drains in deep cervical nodes. From thoracic part lymph drains in posterior mediastinal nodes and from abdominal part and adjacent thoracic parts lymph drains in left gastric nodes.

Nerve Supply

The sympathetic efferent fibers are vasoconstrictors. Parasympathetic efferent fibers are motor to the musculature of esophagus as well as to the esophageal glands. The striated muscle in the upper two thirds receives nerve supply from vagus while the smooth muscle in the lower part receives nerve supply through the esophageal plexus. The sympathetic afferent fibers carry pain sensations. Pain fibers travel in the sympathetic nerves. Most painful sensation from the esophagus originates from lower thoracic and abdominal parts, since these parts are vulnerable to acid peptic esophagitis. The pain impulses reach the T4 and T5 segments of the spinal cord along the afferent sympathetic paths. Therefore, the pain is referred to the lower thoracic region and epigastric region of abdomen. At times, it is difficult to distinguish the esophageal pain from anginal pain.

Development

The esophagus develops from the endoderm of the foregut. The crucial step in the development of the esophagus is its luminal separation from the laryngotracheal tube by formation of a laryngotracheal septum. At this early stage of development the esophagus is very short but with the descent of heart it elongates. At the same time due to proliferation of lining endodermal cells, the lumen of the esophagus is obliterated. At the end of the embryonic phase, the lumen is recanalized. The muscle of the upper third of esophagus is striated like the pharynx, the muscle of the middle third is the mixture of both striated and non-striated and that of the lower third is non-striated only.

Anomalies

a. Esophageal atresia is due to failure of recanalization of the esophagus. It is associated with hydramnios because the fetus is unable to swallow the amniotic fluid.
b. Tracheoesophageal fistula or TEF (Fig. 35.3) is due to maldevelopment of the septum between the esophagus and the trachea. They are invariably associated with localized atresia of esophagus and hence hydramnios is a constant feature. The most feared complication is aspiration pneumonia in the neonate. A few types of tracheoesophageal fistulae are shown in Figure 35.3. In one type of fistula, the upper segment of the esophagus is blind but the lower segment communicates with the trachea just above the bifurcation by a narrow channel. This type occurs in 90% of cases. This fistula is characterized by cyanotic coughing attacks in neonate. The infant may cough up bile and the stomach is distended with air. In another type, the upper segment of esophagus communicates with the trachea and the lower segment ends blindly. In rare cases, a very narrow and oblique connection exists between the esophagus and trachea.
c. Anomalous blood vessels (duplication of aortic arch or aberrant right subclavian artery) may cause esophageal symptoms (dysphagia) in the first few days after birth but may remain symptomless.

Clinical Highlights

a. Radiological examination of esophagus by barium swallow is used for detection of the enlargement of left atrium in mitral stenosis.

b. Esophagoscopy is performed to directly inspect the interior of the esophagus. The mucosa in normal state is pale pink in color and thrown into vertical folds. The clinician undertaking this procedure must pass the esophagoscope carefully at the sites of constriction in the esophagus.

c. Dysphagia means difficulty in swallowing. Extrinsic causes of dysphagia are, pressure from aneurysm of aortic arch, enlarged lymph nodes, aberrant right subclavian artery (passing posterior to the esophagus), retrosternal goiter or enlarged left atrium. Intrinsic causes are strictures and carcinoma of esophagus.

d. Carcinoma of esophagus usually spreads by lymphatics and involves posterior mediastinal nodes. The direct spread through the wall of the esophagus can lead to involvement of lung, bronchi and aorta. The cancer from lower third of esophagus spreads to the gastric and celiac nodes in the abdomen.

e. The hiatus, hernia (Fig. 40.4) is an acquired condition in which the stomach herniates in the posterior mediastinum through the esophageal hiatus in the diaphragm. The sliding variety of hernia is due to short esophagus. In this condition the abdominal part of esophagus, cardioesophageal junction and part of fundus of the stomach enter the thorax. This may produce symptoms and the regurgitation of the acid contents in the esophagus results in peptic esophagitis. In rolling or paraesophageal hiatus hernia a part of the stomach enters the thorax but the cardioesophageal junction is normal in position. This type is usually symptomless.

56 Clinicoanatomical Problems and Solutions

CASE 1

A 35-year-old man came to the hospital with complaints of severe pain in the front of the right side of chest. The pain radiated down to the anterior abdominal wall. Auscultation of chest revealed absent breath sounds over the inferior lobe of the right lung and X-ray chest confirmed the presence of fluid in the pleural cavity on the right side.

Questions

a. Name the condition in which there is accumulation of fluid in the pleural cavity.
b. Give the boundaries of the pleural cavity and its normal content.
c. Name the various parts of parietal pleura giving nerve supply of each.
d. Enumerate the differences in parietal and visceral pleura.
e. Give explanation for radiation of pain to the anterior abdominal wall in this case.
f. Describe the pleural recesses.
g. Name the layers (from outer to inner direction), which a needle will encounter in the midaxillary line in 6th intercostal space to aspirate fluid from pleural cavity.

Solutions

a. Pleural effusion
b. The pleural cavity is a potential space that is bounded by visceral and parietal layers of pleura. Normally it contains very small quantity of serous fluid.
c. The parietal pleura is subdivided into four parts, costal (costovertebral), mediastinal, diaphragmatic and cervical. The costal pleura is supplied by intercostal nerves, mediastinal by phrenic nerves and diaphragmatic by both intercostal and phrenic nerves.
d. The visceral pleura is adherent to the lung surface and dips into the fissures of the lung. It develops from splanchnopleuric mesoderm, hence, it is supplied by autonomic nerves. It is pain insensitive. It shares its arterial supply and lymph drainage with lung. The extensive parietal pleura lines the internal surface of thoracic wall, mediastinum and upper surface of diaphragm. It develops from somatopleuric mesoderm hence, it is supplied by somatic nerves (intercostal and phrenic nerves). It is pain sensitive. It shares its arterial supply and lymph drainage with body wall.
e. The parietal pleura lining the lower part of the thoracic cavity is supplied by lower five intercostal nerves, which also supply the anterior abdominal wall. In this case the presence of fluid in the pleural cavity causes irritation of parietal pleura. Therefore, the pain from the chest is referred to the anterior abdominal wall.
f. There are two pleural recesses, costomediastinal and costodiaphragmatic, which are described in Chapter 37.
g. The layers pierced by the needle are skin, superficial and deep fasciae, serratus anterior muscle, intercostal muscles, endothoracic fascia and costal pleura (Fig. 37.5).

CASE 2

A 50-year-old male with a history of chronic smoking consulted the doctor because he had complaints of weight loss, persistent cough and blood in the sputum. He also noticed absence of sweating on the right side of face. On examination, partial ptosis and constriction of pupil were noted in the right eye. PA view of chest X-ray showed a lesion in the apex of right lung.

Questions

a. What is the probable clinical condition?
b. Name the posterior relations of the apex of the lung in medial to lateral order.
c. Involvement of which structure will produce partial ptosis and loss of sweating on the face?
d. Draw a diagram to show the lymphatic drainage of the lungs.
e. Write briefly on the bronchopulmonary segments of right lung.
f. Which bronchopulmonary segment is most dependent in supine position?
g. Give the origin of bronchial arteries on right and left sides.

Solutions

a. Malignancy of apex of right lung.
b. Sympathetic chain, highest intercostal vein, superior intercostal artery and ascending branch of T1 ventral ramus.
c. Sympathetic chain (producing Horner's syndrome)
d. Refer to Fig. 38.9
e. The bronchopulmonary segments of the lung correspond to the tertiary or segmental bronchi. The right principal bronchus divides into epiarterial and hyparterial bronchi before entering the lung. Inside the lung the epiarterial bronchus divides into anterior, posterior and apical tertiary bronchi of upper lobe. Hence in the upper lobe there are corresponding three segments. The hyparterial bronchus divides into middle lobar and inferior lobar bronchi inside the lung. The middle lobar bronchus divides into medial and lateral segmental bronchi for the corresponding bronchopulmonary segments of the middle lobe. The inferior lobar bronchus divides into five segmental bronchi, apical, superior basal, inferior basal, lateral basal and medial basal, corresponding to the five bronchopulmonary segments.
f. Apical (superior) bronchopulmonary segment of the lower lobe.
g. On the right side, a single bronchial artery takes origin from right third posterior intercostal artery. On the left side, two bronchial arteries take origin from descending thoracic aorta.

CASE 3

A 38-year-old man was brought to the casualty because of sudden onset of severe chest pain. On examination, his respiration and pulse were rapid. On auscultation, the heart sounds were faintly audible. X-ray chest showed a globular enlarged shadow suggestive of fluid around heart.

Questions

a. What is the site of fluid accumulation in this case?
b. Name the three layers of pericardium.
c. Give the nerve supply and arterial supply of fibrous pericardium.
d. Describe the pericardial sinuses.
e. Describe costoxiphoid approach to aspirate the fluid.
f. Write short note on the bare area of pericardium.

Solutions

a. Pericardial cavity
b. The outer layer is known as fibrous pericardium. Inner to this tough layer, there are two layers of serous pericardium, parietal layer and visceral layer (epicardium). The parietal layer lines the fibrous pericardium. The visceral layer covers the heart and intrapericardial parts of the great vessels.
c. The phrenic nerve supplies the fibrous pericardium. The pericardiophrenic branches of internal thoracic artery and pericardial branches of descending aorta provide arterial supply.
d. There are two pericardial sinuses, transverse and oblique, which appear during development of cardiac tube. The transverse sinus is present between the ascending aorta and pulmonary trunk in front and left atrium behind (Fig. 43.1). It is a passage connecting the right and left halves of pericardial cavity hence lined by visceral pericardium only. It develops between the arterial and venous ends of the cardiac tube, when the dorsal mesocardium of embryonic heart breaks

down. It provides a space to the cardiac surgeon during ligation of ascending aorta and pulmonary trunk in the operation of coronary artery bypass grafting.

The oblique sinus is a blind recess behind the left atrium enclosed by right and left pulmonary veins. It develops along the venous end of the cardiac tube, when the six veins separate and give rise to an irregular line of pericardial reflection (Fig. 43.3). This sinus is lined by visceral pericardium covering the posterior surface of left atrium and the parietal pericardium lining the posterior part of fibrous pericardium.

e. In costoxiphoid approach, the needle inserted through the left costoxiphoid angle in upward and backward direction, passes through the rectus sheath and the central tendon of diaphragm to enter the pericardial cavity. The advantage of this approach is that it avoids pleura since the line of pleural reflection does not cross the costoxiphoid angle on left side (Fig. 37.2).
f. The bare area of pericardium is the area, which is to the left of the sternal margin from 4th to 6th costal cartilages. This area is not covered by lung due to the presence of cardiac notch in the anterior margin of left lung (Fig. 37.2). The bare area is dull on percussion hence it is also known as area of cardiac dullness.

CASE 4

A 30-year-old woman with a history of rheumatic fever in childhood came to the hospital with complaints of dyspnea (shortness of breath) and weakness of 3 months duration. On auscultation, a prominent mid-diastolic murmur was heard. Echocardiography confirmed the narrowing of mitral orifice. Since the patient also had complaint of dysphagia (difficulty in swallowing). Ba swallow radiograph was taken.

Questions

a. What is the probable clinical condition affecting the mitral valve?
b. Give the surface marking of the mitral valve.
c. Which cardiac chamber is likely to enlarge in this condition?
d. What is the reason for dysphagia in this case?
e. What is the purpose of the Ba swallow radiograph?
f. Explain how a thrombus dislodged from left atrium can block the renal artery.
g. Draw a diagram to show the relationship of the pericardial sinuses to left atrium.
h. Give the developmental sources of left atrium.

Solutions

a. Mitral stenosis
b. The mitral valve is marked on the left half of sternum at the level of 4th costal cartilage.
c. Left atrium
d. Enlarged left atrium compresses the esophagus, which lies posterior to the left atrium.
e. In Ba swallow radiograph, the impression of left atrium on the esophagus can be visualized.
f. A thrombus dislodged from the left atrium will first enter the left ventricle and then the systemic circulation via the ascending aorta. The clot can reach renal artery, which is a branch of abdominal aorta.
g. Refer to Figure 43.1
h. The left atrium develops from left half of primitive atrium, absorbed parts of pulmonary veins and left half of atrioventricular canal.

CASE 5

A middle-aged obese man with a family history of coronary artery disease complained of tightness in the chest accompanied by profuse sweating and pain along the inner side of left upper limb. The patient had characteristic ECG changes and hence was admitted in the intensive care unit.

Questions

a. What is the probable clinical condition?
b. Trace the path of pain impulse from the heart to the spinal cord.
c. Name the arteries that supply blood to the heart and give their peculiarities.
d. Describe the origin, course and branches of each artery.
e. What is the difference between angina pectoris and myocardial infarction?
f. Name three blood vessels of the body that can be used for coronary artery graft.
g. To perform coronary angiography the cardiologist chooses the right femoral artery. Trace the path of catheter to the coronary ostia, where dye is injected.

Solutions

a. Myocardial infarction
b. For path of pain impulse from ischemic myocardium refer to Figure 46.7.
c. Right and left coronary arteries (for peculiarities refer Chapter 46).
d. Refer Chapter 46.
e. In angina pectoris there is mismatch between demand and supply. It means due to temporary narrowing of coronary arteries the myocardium does not receive sufficient blood, hence, pain is felt. In myocardial infarction the arterial supply to myocardium is totally cut off, which results in infarction (necrosis).
f. Saphenous vein, internal thoracic artery, radial artery.
g. Right femoral artery—right external iliac artery—right common iliac artery—abdominal aorta—descending thoracic aorta arch of aorta—ascending aorta and its sinuses.

CASE 6

An elderly patient presented with a pulsating swelling protruding from the upper margin of the sternum. On examination the sign of tracheal tug was positive. The CT scan of chest and aortic angiography showed localized dilatation of aortic arch.

Questions

a. Name the clinical condition.
b. In which part of mediastinum, is the arch of aorta located?
c. Give the boundaries and contents of this mediastinum.
d. Name the structures, which are likely to be compressed by the dilated aortic arch.
e. Describe the relations of the arch of aorta with the help of diagrams.
f. Give the developmental sources of the arch of aorta.
g. Name the connection between the arch of aorta and the left pulmonary artery in the fetus and in the adult.

Solutions

a. Aneurysm of arch of aorta
b. Superior mediastinum
c. Refer to Chapter 36.
d. The structures likely to be compressed are SVC, trachea, esophagus, phrenic nerves, left recurrent laryngeal nerve.
e. For relations of arch of aorta refer to Chapter 50.
f. The arch of aorta develops from aortic sac, left horn of aortic sac, left 4th arch artery and left dorsal aorta.
g. In the fetus the arch of aorta is connected to left pulmonary artery by means of ductus arteriosus and in the adult the two are connected by ligamentum arteriosum, which is a remnant of the ductus arteriosus.

CASE 7

A 58-year-old woman complained of dysphagia (difficulty in swallowing) for the duration of one month. Ba swallow and esophagoscopy were performed. A biopsy taken from the lesion in the lower third of esophagus confirmed the diagnosis of malignancy.

Questions

a. What is the vertebral extent of esophagus?
b. Name the structures that produce constrictions in the esophagus.
c. Give the lymphatic drainage of the esophagus.
d. Name the congenital vascular anomalies, which give rise to dysphagia.
e. Describe the arterial supply of esophagus.
f. What is the length of abdominal esophagus?
g. Write short note on hiatus hernia.

Solutions

a. Vertebral extent is from C6 to T11
b. First constriction located at upper end of esophagus by cricopharyngeus muscle, second by arch of aorta, third by left bronchus and lowest at esophageal hiatus in diaphragm.
c. Refer to Chapter 55
d. Double aortic arch, aberrant right subclavian artery.
e. The cervical part of esophagus receives branches from inferior thyroid arteries and the thoracic esophagus receives branches from bronchial arteries and from descending aorta. The lower part of esophagus receives branches from left gastric artery.
f. Two cm.
g. For hiatus hernia refer Chapters 40 and 55.

CASE 8

A 15-year-old girl came to the hospital with complaints of reduced exercise tolerance (feeling weak after slight exertion), leg cramps on walking and shortness of breath. On examination, radiofemoral delay was noted and BP in upper limb was—120/70 mm of Hg and in lower limb—90/60 mm of Hg. Chest X-ray showed rib notching. Echocardiography showed narrowing of arch of aorta beyond attachment of ligamentum arteriosum.

Questions

a. Name the condition in which there is localized narrowing in the arch of aorta.
b. Explain how the descending aorta is filled with blood in this condition
c. In which arteries there is reversal of blood in this case?
d. Give reason for notching of ribs.
e. Give the origin of anterior and posterior intercostal arteries in eleven intercostal spaces.
f. Name an important visceral branch of right third posterior intercostal artery.

Solutions

a. Coarctation of aorta
b. In postductal type of coarctation the descending aorta receives blood from enlarged and tortuous posterior intercostal arteries of 3rd to 9th spaces. These arteries receive blood from the anastomoses with anterior intercostal arteries from internal thoracic and its musculophrenic branch (refer Fig. 47.2).
c. Posterior intercostal arteries
d. The dilated and tortuous posterior intercostal arteries erode the ribs in the costal groove.
e. The upper six spaces are supplied with a pair of anterior intercostal arteries from internal thoracic artery (branches of internal thoracic artery 7th, 8th and 9th spaces receive anterior intercostal arteries) from superior intercostal artery (branch of costocervical trunk of subclavian artery). In 3rd to 11th spaces the posterior intercostal arteries are the direct branches of descending aorta.
f. Right bronchial artery.

MCQs—SINGLE BEST RESPONSE TYPE

1. **Which of the following is a typical intercostal nerve:**
   A. First B. Second
   C. Third D. Seventh

2. **The right bundle branch (RBB) travels in:**
   A. Triangle of Koch
   B. Moderator band
   C. Membranous interventricular septum
   D. Supraventricular crest

3. **Crista terminalis is a feature of:**
   A. Right ventricle B. Left ventricle
   C. Right atrium D. Left atrium

4. **The phrenic nerve supplies all, *except:***
   A. Fibrous pericardium
   B. Parietal layer of pericardium
   C. Pulmonary pleura
   D. Mediastinal pleura

5. **The most anterior valve of the heart is:**
   A. Mitral B. Tricuspid
   C. Pulmonary D. Aortic

6. **Conducting tissue of the heart is a modification of:**
   A. Epicardium B. Myocardium
   C. Endocardium D. Neural tissue

7. **Which of the following is related to the arch of aorta on its right side?**
   A. Left phrenic nerve
   B. Right phrenic nerve
   C. Left recurrent laryngeal nerve
   D. Right recurrent laryngeal nerve

8. **The lower margin of the lung cuts the following rib in midaxillary line:**
   A. 6th B. 8th
   C. 10th D. 12th

9. **The horizontal fissure runs along:**
   A. Right 4th rib anteriorly
   B. Left 4th rib anteriorly
   C. Right 4th rib posteriorly
   D. Left 4th rib posteriorly

10. Compared to right principal bronchus the left bronchus is:
A. Shorter, narrower, more vertical
B. Longer, wider, more horizontal
C. Longer, narrower, more horizontal
D. Shorter, wider, more vertical

11. Right venous valve develops into all, *except:*
A. Crista terminalis
B. Torus aorticus
C. Valve of IVC
D. Valve of coronary sinus

12. What is not true regarding the carina?
A. Mucosa most sensitive
B. Located at tracheal bifurcation
C. Located at a distance of 40 cm from incisor teeth
D. Visible in bronchoscopy

13. Which of the following is not related to superior surface of first rib?
A. Ventral ramus of T1
B. Lower trunk of brachial plexus
C. Subclavian artery
D. Subclavian vein

14. Foramen secundum is present in:
A. Septum secundum B. Septum primum
C. Septum intermedium D. Septum spurium

15. The nonrecurrent right recurrent laryngeal nerve is associated with:
A. Double aortic arch
B. Aberrant right subclavian artery
C. Transposition of great vessels
D. Coarctation of aorta

16. The diaphragmatic hernia can occur in the following sites, *except:*
A. Esophageal opening B. Bochdalek triangle
C. Foramen of Morgagni D. IVC opening

17. The following meet at the crux of the heart, *except:*
A. Interatrial groove
B. Posterior interventricular groove
C. Posterior atrioventricular groove
D. Sulcus terminalis

18. Which is located along the periphery of the bronchopulmonary segment?
A. Bronchial artery
B. Bronchial vein
C. Pulmonary vein tributary
D. Pulmonary artery branch

19. The acute margin of heart is:
A. Inferior B. Superior
C. Left D. Right

20. The diaphragm develops from all, *except:*
A. Septum transversum
B. Mesoderm of body wall
C. Ventral mesentery of esophagus
D. Pleuroperitoneal membranes

Key to MCQs

1 C	2 B	3 C	4 C	5 C	6 B	7 C
8 B	9 A	10 C	11 B	12 C	13 A	14 B
15 B	16 D	17 D	18 C	19 A	20 C	

MULTIPLE RESPONSE MCQs

Write T for true and F for false against each statement.

1. The boundary of the triangle of Koch:
A. Eustachian valve B. Tendon of Todaro
C. Thebesian valve D. Torus aorticus

2. Veins that opens directly in the cavity of heart:
A. Oblique vein of Marshal
B. Coronary sinus
C. Anterior cardiac vein
D. Venae cordae minimae

3. The interventricular septum:
A. Membranous part is prone to defects
B. Distal bulbar septum
C. Growth from endocardial cushions
D. Growth from floor of bulboventricular cavity

4. The thymus:
A. Receives afferent lymphatic vessels
B. Located in middle mediastinum only
C. Develops along with superior parathyroid glands
D. The primary lymphatic organ

5. **The thoracic duct drains lymph from:**
   A. Right upper limb
   B. Right lower limb
   C. Liver
   D. Right half of supraumbilical abdominal wall
6. **The thoracic part of esophagus is related to thoracic duct:**
   A. On the right side at T3 vertebral level
   B. Posteriorly at T5 vertebral level
   C. On the left at T7 vertebral level
   D. On the right at T9 vertebral level
7. **The right atrium develops from:**
   A. Right half of common atrial chamber
   B. Entire sinus venosus
   C. Right half of atrioventricular canal
   D. Truncus arteriosus
8. **The sixth arch arteries develop into:**
   A. Right pulmonary artery
   B. Left pulmonary artery
   C. Ductus arteriosus
   D. Ductus venosus
9. **The mediastinal surface of left lung shows impressions for:**
   A. Arch of aorta
   B. Brachiocephalic trunk
   C. Infundibulum of right ventricle
   D. Left ventricle
10. **The greater splanchnic nerve:**
   A. Carries preganglionic sympathetic fibers
   B. Carries preganglionic parasympathetic fibers
   C. The content of middle mediastinum
   D. Pierces central tendon of diaphragm

Annexure: Radiographs of Thorax

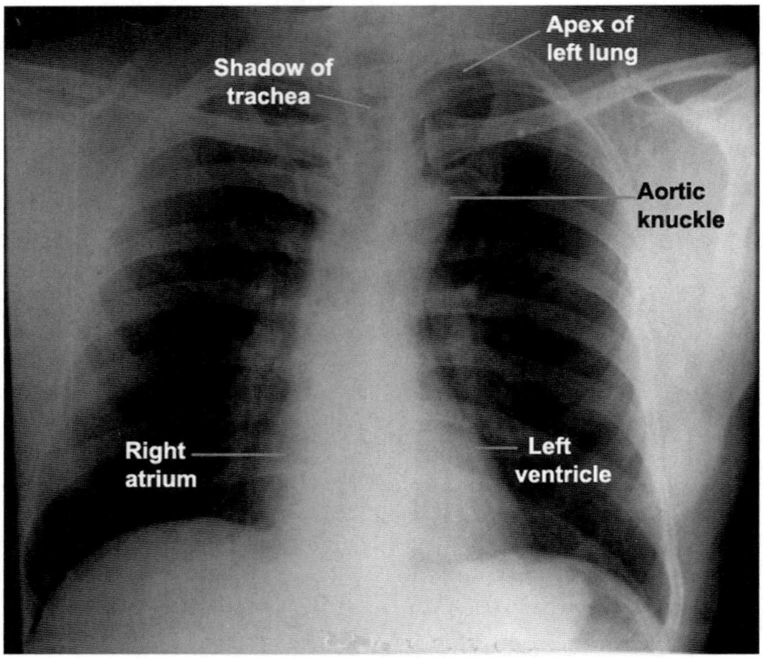

TH-R1. Posterior view of plain radiograph of chest

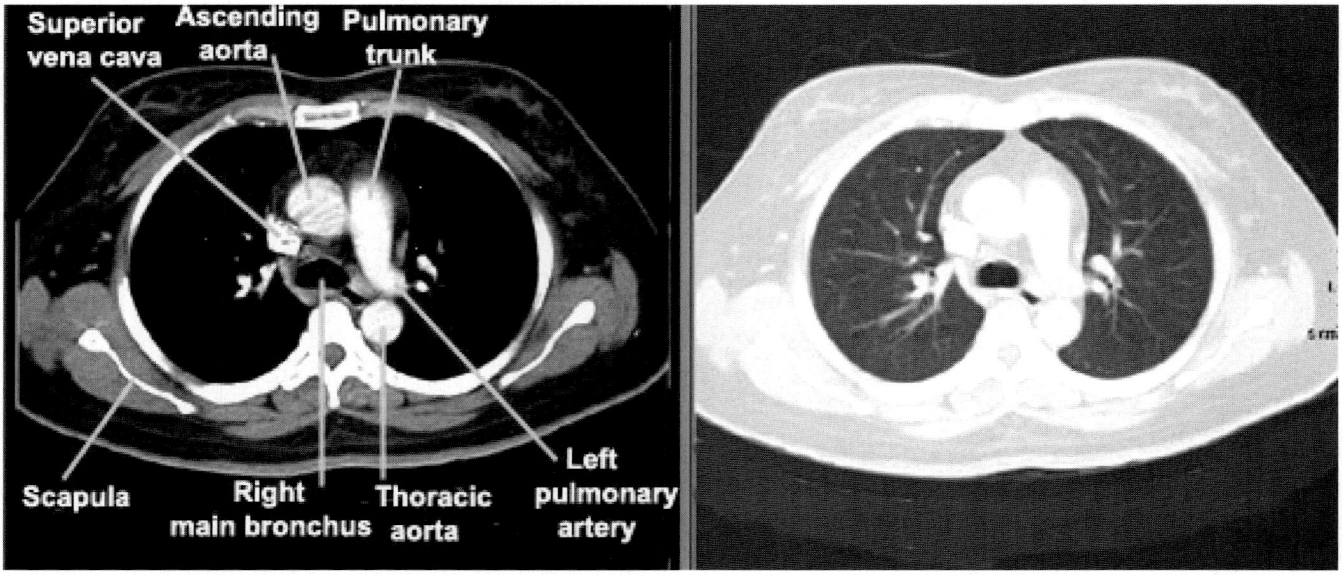

TH-R2. Cross-section of thorax at T5 level obtained by CT scan

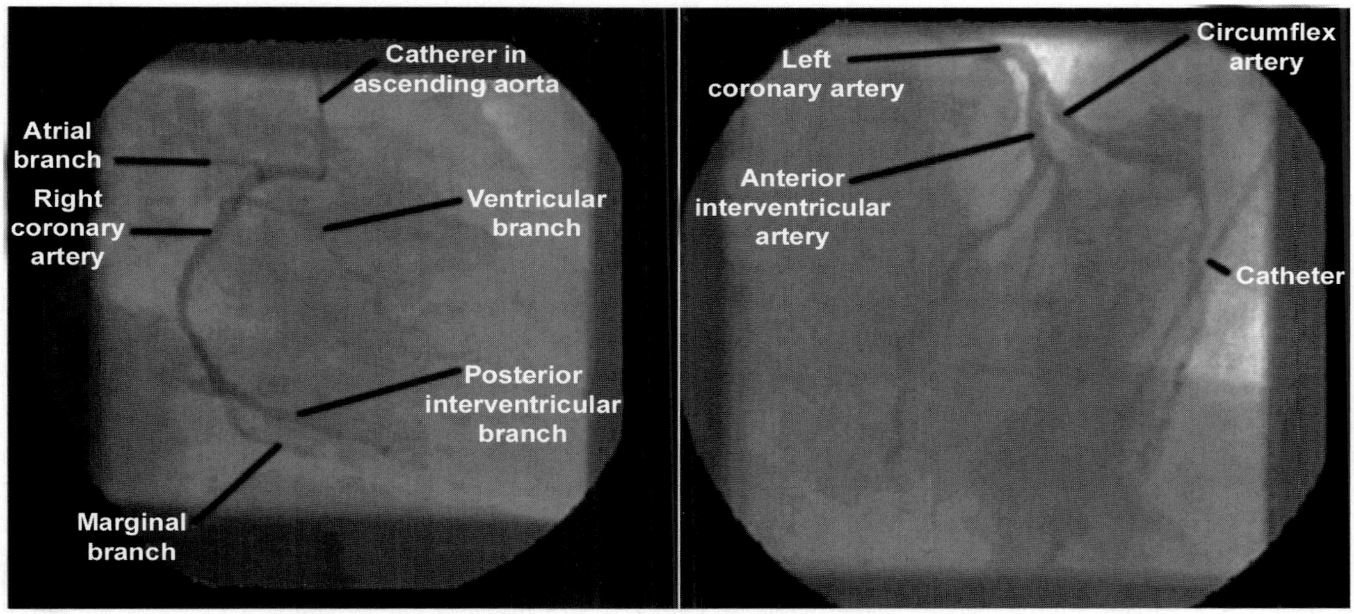

TH-R3. Coronary angiogram showing right and left coronary arteries

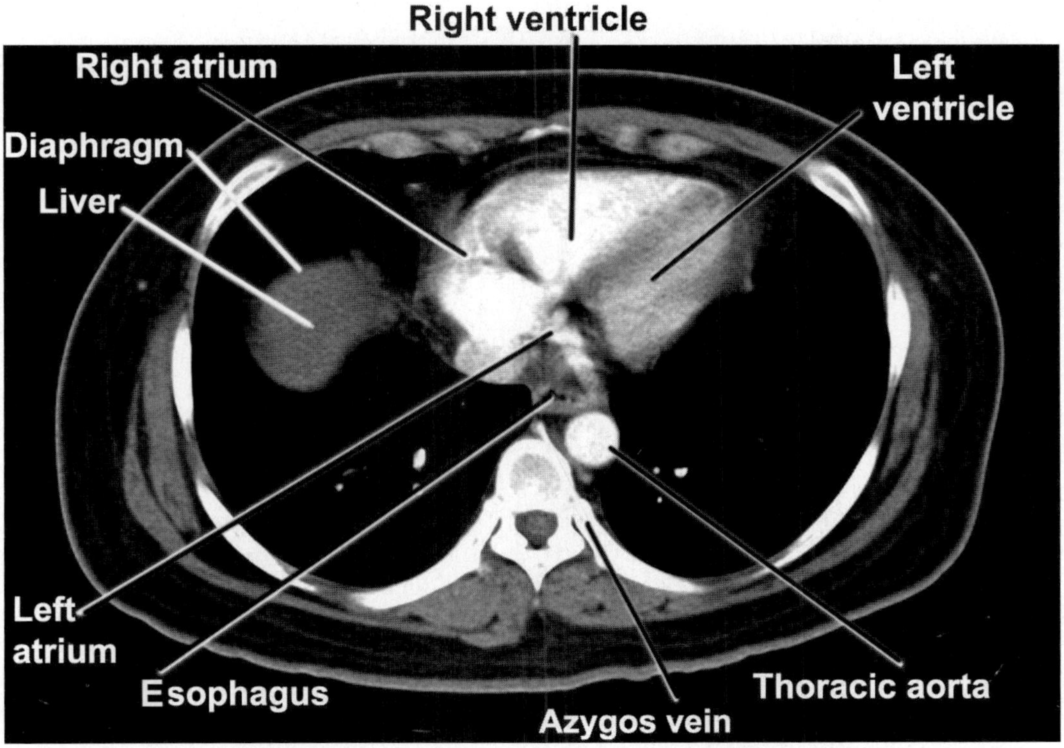

TH-R4. Cross-section of thorax at T7 T8 level obtained by CT scan with contrast

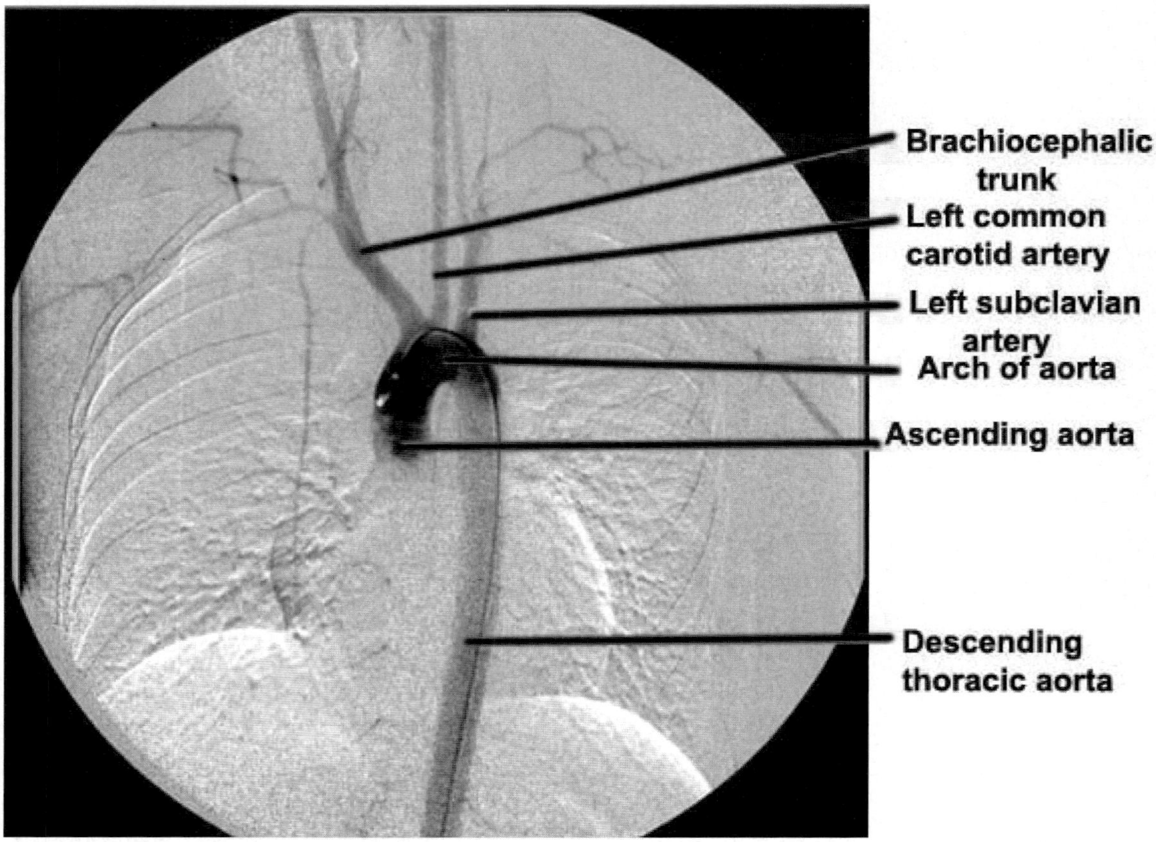

TH-R5. Digital subtraction angiogram showing different parts of aorta in thorax

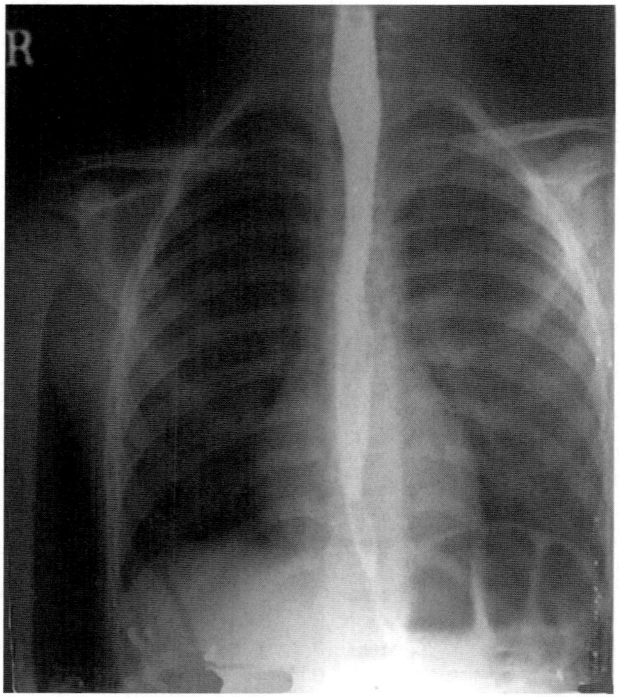

TH-R6. Barium swallow radiograph of 8-year-old boy showing cervical and thoracic parts of esophagus

SECTION THREE

Head and Neck

57 Scalp

The scalp is the soft tissue covering the cranial vault. It is limited anteriorly by the eyebrows and posteriorly by the superior nuchal lines and the external occipital protuberance. The superior temporal lines limit the scalp laterally on each side. The forehead, though not covered with hair is included in the scalp. A line extending from the auricle to the vertex on each side divides the corresponding half of scalp into anterior and posterior quadrants.

Layers (Fig. 57.1)

The scalp consists of five layers, skin, superficial fascia, musculoaponeurotic layer, subaponeurotic layer and pericranium from outer to inner side.

a. The skin of scalp is characterized by plenty of hair follicles, sebaceous and sweat glands. The sebaceous cysts of the scalp are quite common.
b. The superficial fascia is characterized by dense connective tissue. It contains the blood vessels and the nerves of the scalp. The fibrous strands in the superficial fascia are fixed to the walls of the blood vessels and this factor prevents retraction of the blood vessels, when injured. Hence scalp wounds bleed profusely. The bleeding in the scalp is controlled by application of direct pressure of the digit or by placing the surgical sutures.
c. The musculoaponeurotic layer consists of the epicranial aponeurosis (galea aponeurotica) and the frontal and occipital bellies of the occipitofrontalis muscle.

   The frontal belly has no bony attachments. Posteriorly, it is attached to the galea aponeurotica and anteriorly its fibers merge with those of superficial muscles of the forehead and the orbicularis oculi. It is inserted into the superficial fascia of the region of the eyebrow. The action of the frontal bellies is to produce horizontal wrinkles on the forehead and to raise the eyebrows.

   The occipital belly of each side takes origin from the highest nuchal line and the mastoid part of the temporal bone and is inserted into the galea aponeurotica.

   The first, second and third layers of the scalp are fused with each other and move as a single unit. The alternate contraction of occipital and frontal bellies moves the scalp forwards and backwards.

   The galea aponeurotica covers the vault like a helmet. Posteriorly between the occipital bellies it is attached to the occiput and the superior nuchal line. Anteriorly it merges with the superficial muscles between the two frontal bellies. Laterally it is attached partially to the superior temporal line and fuses with the temporal fascia in the temporal region via small extensions.
d. The subaponeurotic layer (fourth layer) forms a potential space filled with loose areolar tissue beneath the aponeurotic layer. The emissary veins, which communicate the veins of the scalp with the intracranial venous sinuses, pass through this space. This space is

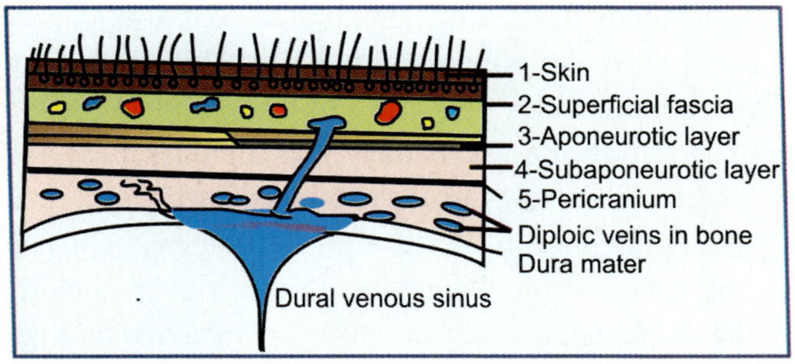

Fig. 57.1: Layers of scalp (Note that nerves and blood vessels are seen in superficial fascia. The emissary vein connects intracranial venous sinus to extracranial vein)

closed on all sides except anteriorly, where it extends in the upper eyelid (Fig. 57.2). It is known as the dangerous area of scalp due to following reasons:

i. Fluid that collects in this space tends to gravitate in the eyelid. In this way black eye is produced if there is bleeding in this space due to scalp injury on direct blow on the skull.
ii. The infection in this space readily enters the cranium through the emissary veins causing thrombosis of the venous sinuses or osteomyelitis of the cranial bones.
iii. In newborn children there is slow accumulation of blood in this space, when there is intracranial hemorrhage due to fracture of the bone of vault and associated dural tear. The leakage of blood outside the cranium in the potentially large subaponeurotic space delays the symptoms of cerebral compression. Hence the slow accumulation of blood in the fourth layer is known as safety valve hematoma.

e. Pericranium is the outer periosteum of the bones of the vault. It forms a loose covering for the bones except at the sutures, where it is continuous with the endocranium. Cephalhematoma is the collection of blood underneath the pericranium in fracture of the bones of the vault. Cephalhydrocele is accumulation of CSF beneath the pericranium due to tear of dura mater and arachnoid mater. Such swellings are restricted to the bones of the vault and are of the shape of the related bone.

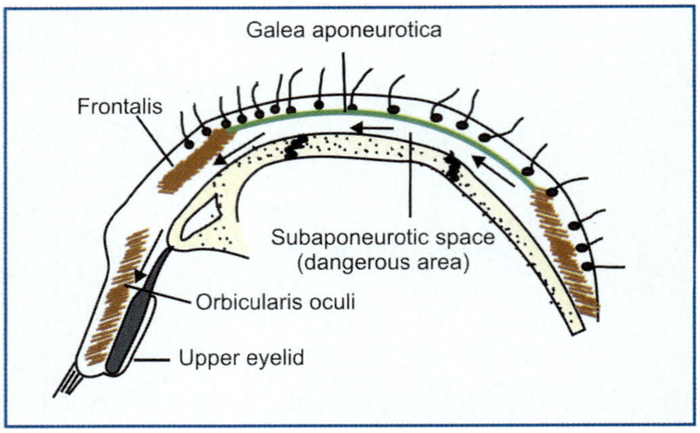

Fig. 57.2: Sagittal section of cranial vault showing continuity (indicated by arrows),of dangerous area of scalp with upper eyelid

Nerves of Anterior Quadrant (Fig. 57.3)

One motor and four sensory nerves are present in the anterior quadrant of the scalp.

a. The motor nerve is the temporal branch of the facial nerve for the supply of the frontal belly of the occipitofrontalis.
b. The sensory nerves, namely, the supratrochlear and supraorbital nerves are the terminal branches of frontal nerve (a branch of the ophthalmic nerve). The zygomaticotemporal nerve, a branch of zygomatic nerve (from maxillary nerve) enters the scalp through the foramen of same name in the zygomatic bone. The auriculotemporal nerve is a branch of mandibular nerve and enters the scalp via the temporal region.

Nerves of Posterior Quadrant (Fig. 57.3)

One motor and four sensory nerves are present in the posterior quadrant of the scalp.

a. The motor nerve is the posterior auricular branch of the facial nerve for the supply of the occipital belly of occipitofrontalis.
b. The sensory nerves are, the great auricular nerve (C2, C3) and the lesser occipital nerve (C2), which are the branches of the cervical plexus and enter the scalp behind the ear. The greater occipital nerve is a branch of dorsal ramus of C2. It is the thickest cutaneous nerve in the body and supplies the skin as far forward as the vertex. The third occipital nerve is a branch of dorsal ramus of C3. It lies medial to and lower than the greater occipital nerve and supplies the skin covering the external occipital protuberance.

Arterial Supply (Fig. 57.3)

The scalp is richly supplied with blood through the extensive anastomoses between the branches of the internal and external carotid arteries. The advantage of the profuse blood supply is that the wounds of scalp heal faster. However, if the lacerations of the scalp include galea aponeurotica the wound gapes because the occipito-frontalis muscles exert pull on the aponeurosis. Such wounds are always treated by surgical suturing to control bleeding and facilitate healing.

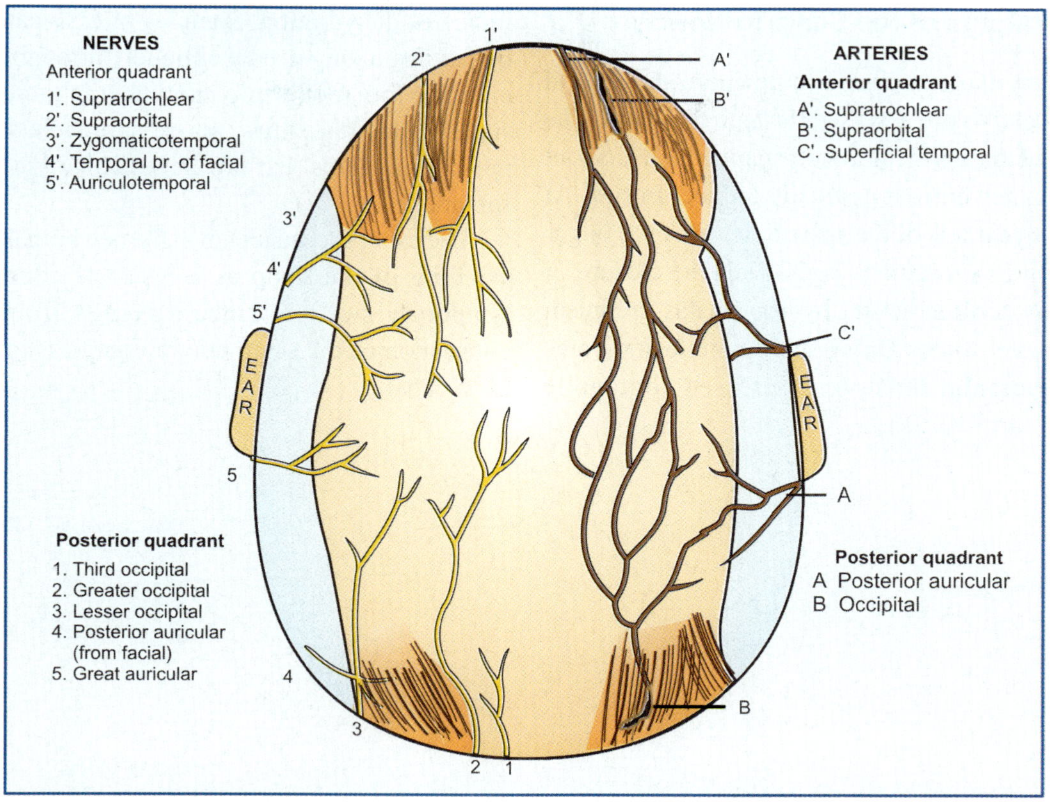

Fig.57.3: Nerves and arteries of scalp seen from above

a. The arteries in the anterior quadrant are, supratrochlear, supraorbital and the superficial temporal arteries. First two arteries are the branches of the ophthalmic artery (a branch of internal carotid artery). The superficial temporal artery is the terminal branch of the external carotid artery. The anterior branch of superficial temporal artery appears wavy particularly in the elderly. The superficial temporal artery pulse can be felt against the zygomatic process of the temporal bone in front of the tragus of the ear.
b. The arteries in the posterior quadrant are, the posterior auricular artery and the occipital artery (branches of external carotid artery).

Venous Drainage

The veins of scalp begin in the venous network. The supratrochlear and supraorbital veins unite to form the facial vein near the medial angle of eye. The supraorbital vein communicates with the superior ophthalmic vein by a communicating vein. The superficial temporal vein receives middle temporal and transverse temporal veins and then enters the substance of the parotid gland, where it unites with the maxillary vein to form the retromandibular vein. The posterior auricular vein joins the posterior division of retromandibular vein to form the external jugular vein. The occipital veins draining the posterior part of the scalp turn in the suboccipital triangle to join the vertebral and deep cervical veins. The parietal and mastoid emissary veins connect the venous network of scalp to the venous sinuses in side the cranium. The scalp veins can be used for intravenous infusion in early childhood, since these veins are constant in location. The preferred veins are superficial temporal, posterior auricular, supraorbital and supratrochlear veins.

Lymphatic Drainage

The lymph vessels of the anterior quadrant drain in the superficial parotid lymph nodes and those from the posterior quadrant drain in the occipital and retro-auricular lymph nodes. In infections and infestations (for example by lice) these lymph nodes are enlarged.

Clinical Highlights of the Scalp in Newborn

When a pediatrician examines the newborn the sutural lines and fontanelles are assessed through the scalp. The anterior fontanelle is a membranous gap, which is about 2.5 × 2.5 cm in newborn. It gradually reduces in size. At the end of first year it is of the size of the tip of the finger and by 18 months it becomes bony. Delayed closure of fontanelles may occur in rickets, hydrocephalus, cretinism and Down's syndrome. Bulging fontanelle indicates increase intracranial tension. Depressed fontanelle indicates dehydration. Samples of CSF can be obtained by passing a long needle obliquely through the scalp and anterior fontanelle into the subarachnoid space. The superior sagittal sinus can be approached (in case the peripheral veins are not accessible) via the anterior fontanelle.

The caput succedaneum in the newborn is the localized swelling of the scalp as a result of edema. This is a temporary swelling since it results from the venous congestion of the scalp due to compression through the birth canal.

58 Development of Face

The face develops from five facial prominences or processes, which surround the stomodeum of the embryo during the fifth week of intrauterine life. These facial processes are composed of mesenchymal proliferations covered by ectoderm. Each facial process has its own sensory nerve, ophthalmic nerve for frontonasal process, maxillary nerve for maxillary process and mandibular nerve for mandibular process. The final derivatives of the processes are innervated by the sensory branches of the respective nerves.

Facial Processes (Fig. 58.1A)

The frontonasal process forms the cranial boundary of the stomodeum. The bilateral mandibular processes form the caudal boundary of the stomodeum and bilateral maxillary processes (arising from the mandibular processes) are seen laterally. The olfactory pits appear on each side of the midline in the frontonasal process. As a result the frontonasal process is divided in median nasal process and lateral nasal processes (Fig. 58.1B). The median nasal process grows caudally much longer than the lateral nasal processes. The projecting part of the median nasal process forms a globular process (Fig. 58.1C), which is also described as intermaxillary segment. It has a labial component, upper jaw component and the palatal component.

Derivatives of Frontonasal Process

a. The cranial most undivided part of frontonasal process gives rise to forehead and upper eyelids.
b. The globular process (of the median nasal process) gives rise to philtrum of the upper lip and the premaxilla. The rest of the median nasal process intervening between the two olfactory pits gives rise to the nasal septum and the crest and tip of the nose.
c. The lateral nasal process gives rise to alae of the nose.

Derivatives of Maxillary Processes

Each maxillary process grows in medial direction below the developing eye to meet and fuse with lateral nasal process. At the line of fusion the deeper cells of the ectoderm form a solid cellular cord, which canalizes later to form nasolacrimal duct. The lower eyelid develops from the maxillary process and the lateral nasal process. Below the level of olfactory pit the maxillary process on each side grows toward the globular process to fuse with it to form the upper lip.

Developmental Sources of Upper Lip

The philtrum develops from the globular process and the right and left sides of the lip develop from the respective maxillary processes (Fig. 58.1D). The labial branches of infraorbital nerve alone supply the skin of the entire upper lip. This can be explained by the fact that the ectoderm of the maxillary process grows over the globular process and thus carries its nerve supply to the philtrum. The muscles of the upper lip are derived from the mesoderm of the second arch and hence are supplied by facial nerve.

Derivatives of Mandibular Processes

The lower lip is formed from the fusion of the two mandibular processes. The lower part of the cheek is also formed from this process. The muscles of the lower lip

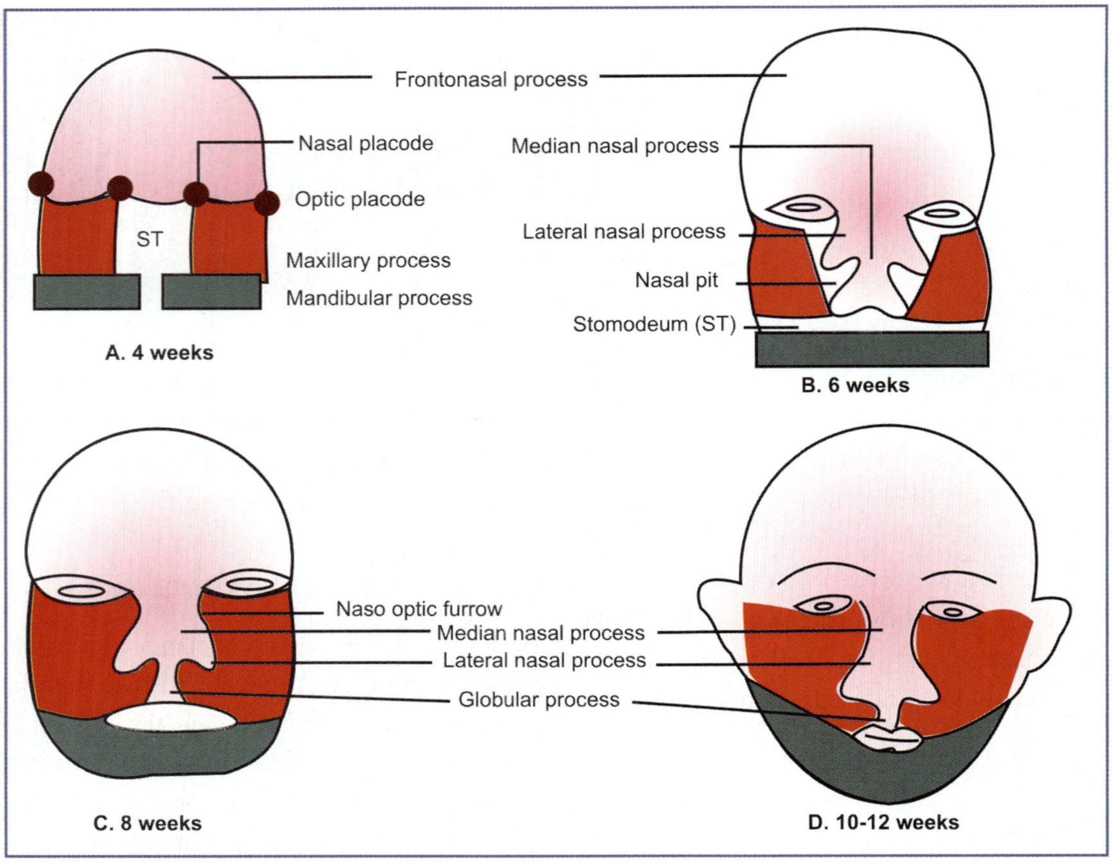

Fig. 58.1: Stages in development of face

develop from the mesoderm of second arch and hence supplied by seventh nerve. The angles of the mouth are originally placed laterally close to the developing auricle. Subsequently with fusion of the maxillary and mandibular processes the angle of the mouth shifts its position medially. Failure of fusion or arrest of fusion of these two processes results in macrostoma or large mouth. The excessive fusion between these two processes results in a very small mouth called microstoma.

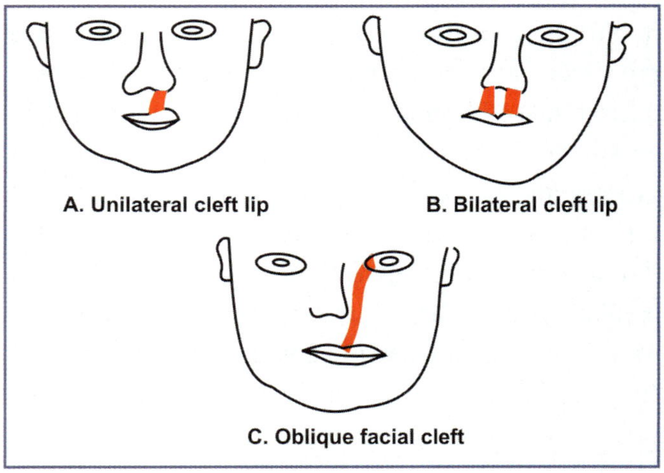

Fig. 58.2: Congenital anomalies of face

Congenital Anomalies

a. The harelip or cleft lip is more common in upper lip. The name harelip is used for the defects of upper lip because the upper lip of hare normally shows a cleft. The cleft lip may be an isolated defect or in combination with cleft palate (Fig. 58.3). In isolated cleft lip the defect may be in the central part or it may be on one side or both sides of the lip. Accordingly three types of defects are recognized. The central harelip is due to failure of fusion of the globular swellings to each

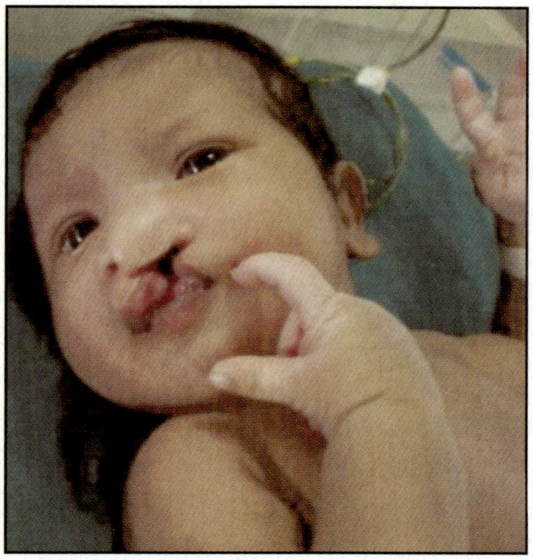

Fig. 58.3: One-month-old infant with left sided complete cleft lip (Note: The divided orbicularis oris muscle (Photo *courtesy* Department of Pediatric Surgery, Dr SMCSI Medical College, Karakonam)

other. Unilateral harelip is due to failure of fusion of maxillary process of one side with the corresponding globular swelling (Fig. 58.2A). The bilateral harelip is caused due to failure of fusion of the maxillary and globular processes on both sides (Fig. 58.2B). In the lower lip the defect is always central and occurs due to nonfusion of the two mandibular processes to each other. Apart from cosmetic effect, the infant has difficulty in sucking. In later stages there may be defective dentition and speech. Surgical repair is usually done by the age of three to six months.

b. The oblique facial cleft occurs, when the maxillary process fails to fuse with the lateral nasal process and the globular process. In this defect there is unilateral cleft lip and there is failure of formation of nasolacrimal duct.

59 Nerves and Blood Vessels of Face

The face extends from the hairline to the base of the mandible. The forehead is common to both the face and the scalp. The muscles of facial expression are important not only in emoting but also in the closure of the mouth and the eyes. They are inserted in the skin of face as there is no deep fascia in the face.

Sensory Nerves of Face (Fig. 59.1)

The skin of the face mainly receives branches from the three divisions of trigeminal nerve. Only a small area of skin covering the angle of mandible and the parotid gland is supplied by great auricular nerve (C2, C3). Thus, the C2 dermatome lies adjacent to the trigeminal area in the lower part of the face (Fig. 1.5). These nerves carry general sensations (touch, pain and temperature) from the facial skin and the proprioceptive sensations from the muscles of facial expression. There are free anastomoses between the sensory nerves of the face and the motor branches of facial nerve.

Branches of Ophthalmic Nerve

a. Supraorbital nerve is one of the terminal branches of frontal nerve. It ascends through the notch on the supraorbital ridge. It is the longer and larger nerve supplying the skin of the forehead, upper eyelid and the scalp as far back as the vertex.

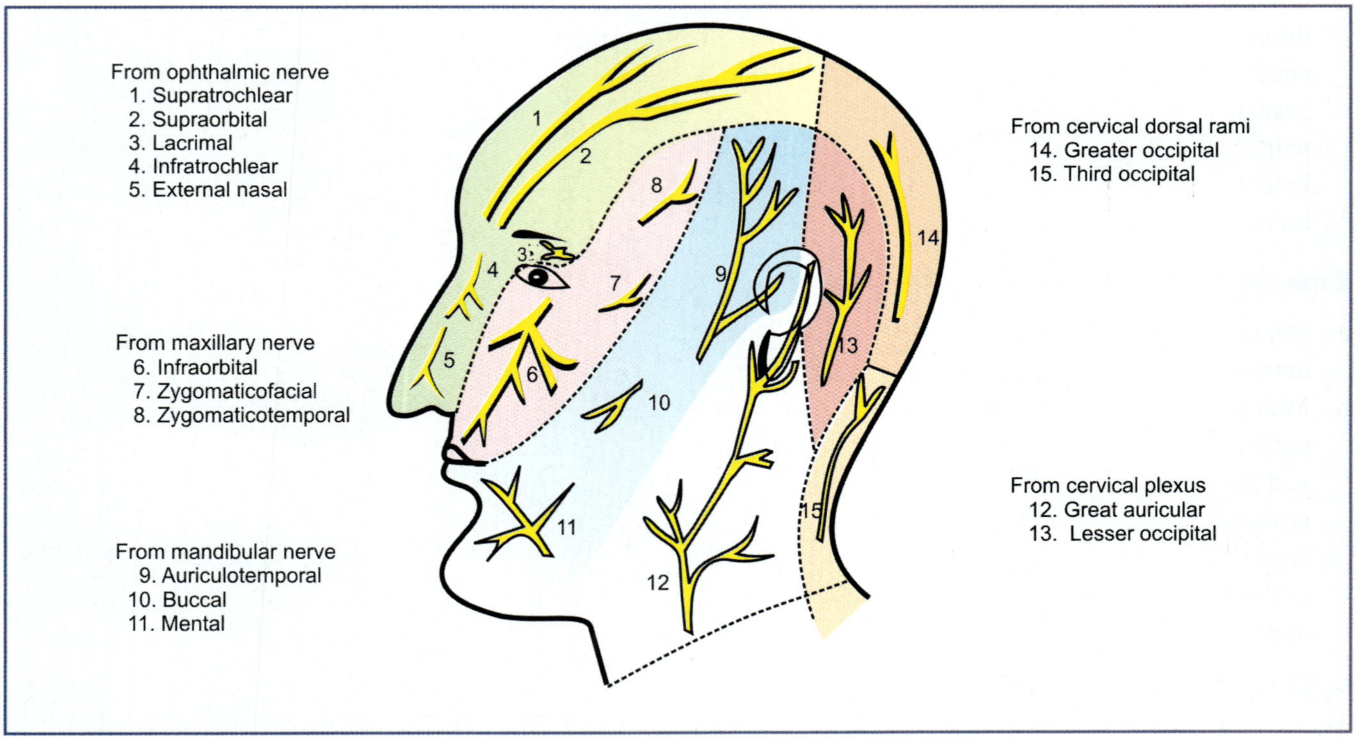

Fig. 59.1: Sensory nerves of face, scalp and auricle
(Note that great auricular nerve supplies the skin covering angle of mandible and parotid)

b. Supratrochlear nerve is the other terminal branch of the frontal nerve. It lies medial to the supraorbital nerve and supplies the medial part of the forehead and the upper eyelid.
c. Palpebral branch of lacrimal nerve supplies the lateral part of upper eyelid.
d. Infratrochlear branch of the nasociliary nerve supplies the medial part of upper eyelid and the root of the nose.
e. External nasal branch of the anterior ethmoidal nerve (from nasociliary nerve) supplies the midline of the nose including its tip.

Branches of Maxillary Nerve

a. Zygomaticofacial nerve, a branch of the zygomatic nerve, appears on the face through the zygomaticofacial foramen and supplies the skin of the prominence of cheek.
b. Zygomaticotemporal nerve, a branch of zygomatic nerve enters the temporal region through the foramen of the same name to supply the skin of the temple just lateral to the lateral angle of eye.
c. The infraorbital nerve enters the face by emerging through the infraorbital foramen, which lies between the origin of levator labii superioris above and levator anguli oris below. It immediately divides in three branches, which diverge in three directions. The palpebral branches supply the lower eyelid, the nasal branches supply the side of the nose and the labial branches supply the upper lip.

Branches of Mandibular Nerve

a. Buccal branch of mandibular supplies the cheek covering the buccinator.
b. Mental nerve arising from the inferior alveolar nerve comes out through the mental foramen of mandible and supplies the skin of the lower lip, chin and that covering the base of the mandible.
c. Auriculotemporal nerve enters the temple at the side of the face and supplies the area in front of the auricle and the temple.

Infiltration of Anesthetic Solution

The position of supraorbital nerve can be found out by palpation of supraorbital notch. If pressure is applied here it is very painful. To inject the supraorbital nerve the needle passes through the skin and the frontalis muscle at this point. As the supraorbital, infraorbital and mental foramina lie in the same vertical plane it is easy to locate the position of the other two foramina. The infraorbital nerve is infiltrated with anesthetic solution by passing the needle through the skin and the levator labii superioris at the position of infraorbital foramen. Similarly, the mental nerve can be approached at its point of emergence at the mental foramen.

The facial nerve is the motor nerve of the face and is described with muscles of facial expression in Chapter 60.

Blood Supply of the Face

The face is richly supplied mainly through branches of facial artery and superficial temporal artery. In addition branches of internal carotid artery (supratrochlear and supraorbital) and other arteries accompanying the sensory nerves of the face. There are extensive anastomoses between the arteries of the two sides. Therefore wounds of the face bleed profusely but heal rapidly.

Facial Artery (Figs 59.2 and 59.3)

This is the anterior branch of the external carotid artery, given off in the carotid triangle in the neck. The course

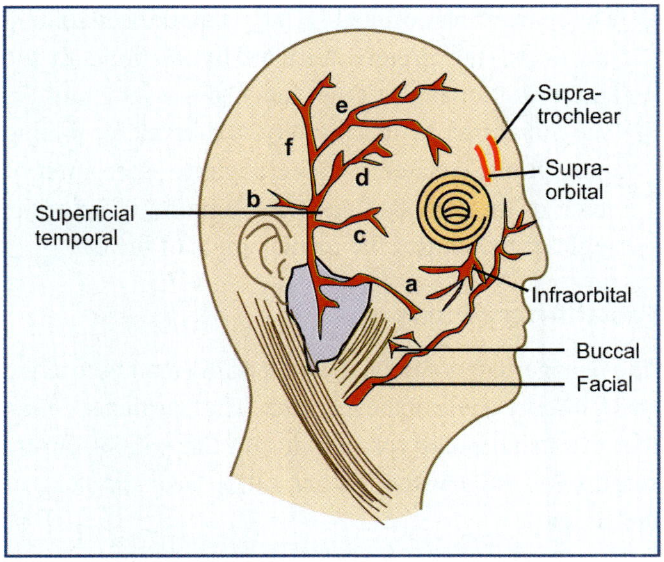

Fig. 59.2: Arterial supply of face

(Note: The numerous branches of superficial temporal and facial arteries. The other sources are: branches of ophthalmic (supratrochlear and supraorbital) and branches of maxillary (intraorbital and buccal). Branches of superficial temporal artery: a—transverse facial, b—anterior auricular, c—zygomatico-orbital, d—middle temporal, e—frontal, f—parietal)

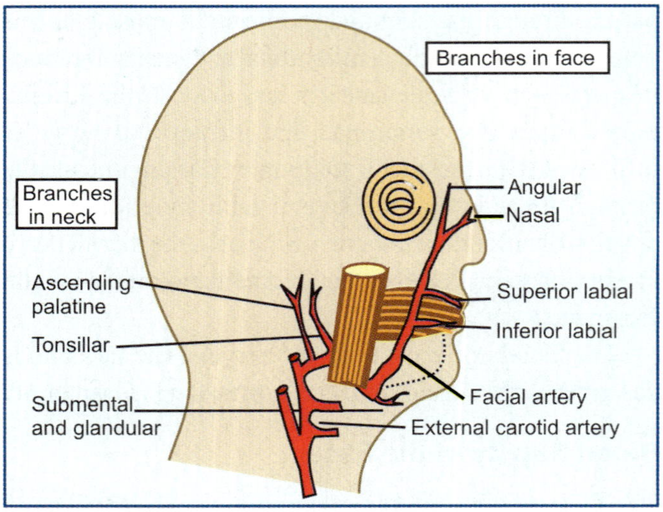

Fig. 59.3: Course and branches of cervical and facial parts of facial artery

of the facial artery is divided in two parts, the cervical and the facial. The facial artery is tortuous throughout its extent. The cervical part is tortuous to adapt to the movements of pharynx during deglutition. The facial part is tortuous to adapt to the movements of mandible, lips and cheek.

Surface Marking

a. The cervical part of facial artery is marked by joining the tip of the greater horn of hyoid bone to the anteroinferior angle of the clenched masseter muscle.
b. The facial part of facial artery is marked by joining three points (related to three angles), anteroinferior angle of the clenched masseter, a point, close to the angle of mouth and the medial angle of the eye.

Facial Artery Pulse

The facial artery is felt on the base of the mandible at the anteroinferior angle of the masseter. The anesthetists often feel the facial pulse for monitoring the patient during surgery (as the anesthetists are sitting near the head of the patient).

Course and Relations

a. The cervical part is of the facial artery is intimately related to the submandibular salivary gland. Occasionally its loop may extend upwards to come in lateral relation of the oropharynx. There are four branches in the neck, ascending palatine artery, tonsillar artery, glandular branches to submandibular gland and the submental artery, which is the largest and the last branch.
b. The facial part of the facial artery is quite long. The facial artery enters the face by piercing the deep fascia of the neck and crossing the base of the mandible at the anteroinferior angle of the masseter. It ascends in the superficial fascia of the face and lies on the superficial aspect of the buccinator and the levator anguli oris. Then the artery lies superficial or passes through the levator labii superioris to ascend embedded in the levator labii superioris alaeque nasi. The facial vein is posterior to the facial artery. There are four branches of facial artery in the face, namely, inferior labial, superior labial, lateral nasal and the angular artery, which is the continuation of the facial artery after the origin of its last branch (Fig. 59.3).

Arterial Anastomoses

a. The anastomoses between the right and left superior labial and right and left inferior labial arteries are clinically important. These anastomoses are by main trunks and hence deep wounds of the lips and incisions on the lips bleed freely from either end.
b. The facial artery anastomoses with the transverse facial artery (of superficial temporal artery) in the cheek.
c. Superior labial artery gives off a septal branch, which anastomoses with septal branches of nasopalatine and anterior ethmoid arteries inside the nasal cavity.
d. At the medial angle of eye the facial artery anastomoses with the dorsal nasal branch of ophthalmic artery.

Superficial Temporal Artery (Fig. 59.2)

This artery is one of the terminal branches of the external carotid artery, given off in the substance of the parotid gland at the level of neck of the mandible. It emerges from the base of the parotid gland along with the auriculotemporal nerve. It enters the anterior quadrant of the scalp and divides into its terminal branches, frontal and parietal.

In the substance of the parotid gland it gives transverse temporal artery, which leaves the gland from its anterior margin. It travels medially above the parotid duct to supply facial tissue. Other branches of this artery are, orbito-zygomatic, anterior auricular and middle temporal.

Superficial Temporal Pulse

This artery is felt anterior to the tragus of the ear against the zygomatic process of the temporal bone. The anesthetist, who sits near the head of the patient during the operation usually feels the superficial temporal pulse.

Venous Drainage of Face

The veins of the face correspond to the arteries. Of the various veins the facial vein is clinically important because of its connections with the cavernous venous sinus.

Facial Vein (Fig. 59.4)

The facial vein is formed by the union of supratrochlear and supraorbital veins at the medial angle of the eye. It lies posterior to the facial artery and is less tortuous than it. The vein runs downwards and laterally on the surface of levator labii superioris alaeque nasi and then on the buccinator muscle and the body of mandible. At the anteroinferior angle of masseter it enters the neck and pierces the deep fascia of the neck. It crosses the submandibular gland, the posterior belly of digastric muscle and stylohyoid muscle. It joins the anterior division of retromandibular vein to form the common facial vein a little anteroinferior to the angle of mandible. The common facial vein opens in the internal jugular vein.

Tributaries

The facial vein has a number of tributaries. It receives the supratrochlear and supraorbital veins at the medial angle of the eye. It collects blood from the ala of nose. The superior and inferior labial veins drain into the facial vein. The deep facial vein from pterygoid venous plexus opens on its posterior aspect. In the neck it receives submental and submandibular veins. The external palatine or paratonsillar vein is its tributary from the tonsil.

Communications

The facial vein and its communicating veins do not possess valves. Therefore, blood flows in them in both directions. The facial vein communicates with the cavernous sinus by two routes, namely, the superior ophthalmic vein and the pterygoid venous plexus (Fig. 59.4A and B). The deep facial vein connects the facial vein to the pterygoid venous plexus, which lies in the infratemporal fossa. This plexus communicates with the cavernous sinus via the emissary vein. The infective thrombus from a boil on the dangerous area of the face usually spreads via the deep facial vein,

Section three

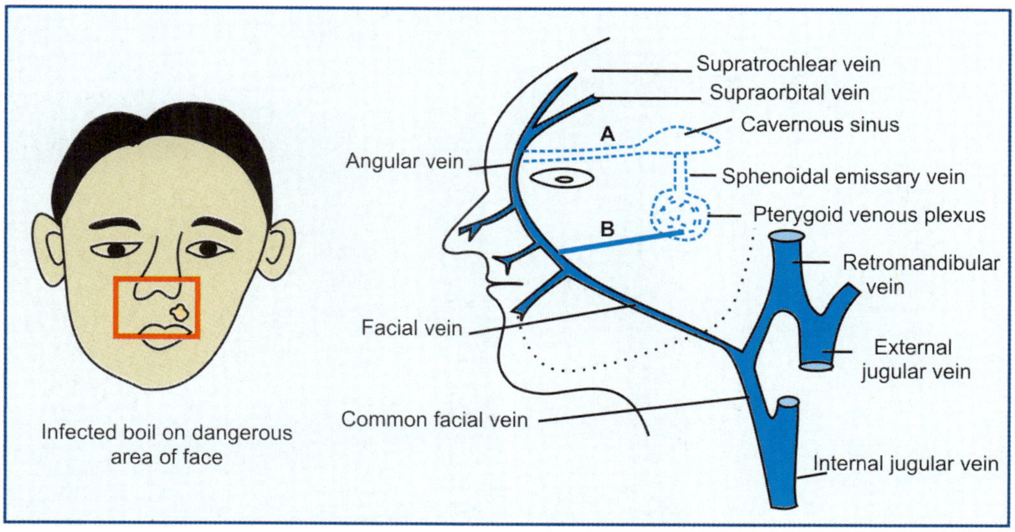

Fig. 59.4: Scheme to show dangerous area of face and its venous communications to cavernous sinus via superior ophthalmic vein (A) and deep facial vein, (B) pterygoid plexus—emissary vein route (The figure also shows formation, tributaries and termination of facial vein)

pterygoid plexus and the emissary vein. This spreads the infection to the sinus producing cavernous sinus thrombosis. The dangerous area of face (also known as mask area) includes the upper lip, lower part of nose and the adjoining cheek (Fig. 59.4).

Lymphatic Drainage

The face is divided in three zones from which the lymphatic vessels reach three different nodes. The upper area consisting of greater part of forehead, temple, lateral half of eyelid and lateral half of cheek drain to the preauricular or superficial parotid lymph nodes. The intermediate zone consisting of lower medial forehead, medial half of eyelid, nose, upper lip, lateral part of lower lip and medial part of cheek drain in the submandibular nodes. Some vessels first reach the buccal nodes and from there drain in submandibular nodes. The lower zone consisting of the central part of the lower lip and chin drains into the submental nodes.

60 Muscles of Facial Expressions

The muscles of the face arise from the facial bones and are inserted in the skin of the face. They are placed in the superficial fascia of the face. There is no deep fascia on the face except for the parotido-masseteric fascia, which is the deep fascia of neck extending in the face. The muscles of the face are able to express the various emotions through their contractions. They are arranged around the eyes, mouth and nose. The muscles around the mouth are arranged in the most complex manner and give rise to a variety of facial expressions. The facial muscles develop from the mesoderm of the second branchial arch hence are supplied by the facial nerve. Since the muscles are present in the superficial fascia they morphologically belong to the panniculus carnosus.

Classification (Fig. 60.1)

a. Muscles attached to the eyelids or orbital musculature
b. Muscles attached to the nose or nasal musculature
c. Buccolabial muscles, which include oral muscles and buccinator.

Orbicularis Oculi

This muscle is the sphincter of the eyelid. So it has protective function. Its shape is elliptical and is divided in orbital, palpebral and lacrimal parts.

a. The orbital part arises from the medial palpebral ligament and adjoining part of frontal bone. The fibers pass laterally in a series of concentric loops around

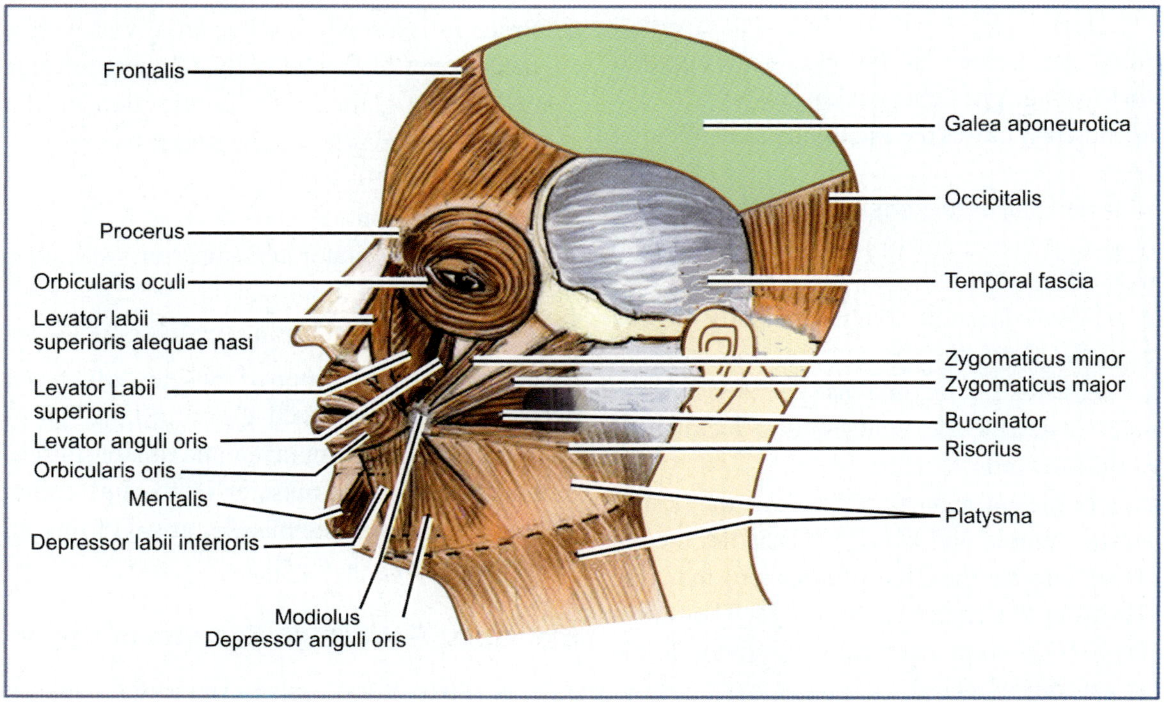

Fig. 60.1: Muscles of facial expression
(Note that parotid fascia and masseteric *fascia are not labeled in the figure)

the orbital margin. They turn down medially to go along the inferior orbital margin to come back for attachment to the medial palpebral ligament and the frontal process of maxilla below it. There is no bony attachment on the lateral side. The upper orbital fibers blend with the fibers of frontal belly of occipitofrontalis and with corrugator supercilii. Some fibers are inserted in the skin of the eyebrow. The lower orbital fibers blend with or overlap the attachments of levator labii superioris alequae nasi and levator labii superioris.

b. The palpebral part is present in both the eyelids. It takes origin from the medial palpebral ligament. The fibers pass through the eyelids and interlace laterally to give rise to lateral palpebral raphe. A small group of fine fibers close to the margin of each eyelid is called the ciliary bundle (Fig. 61.1).

c. The lacrimal part (Horner's muscle) takes origin from the lacrimal fascia, lacrimal crest and lateral surface of lacrimal bone. It passes laterally behind the lacrimal sac and divides in upper and lower slips, which enter the corresponding eyelids. Some fibers are inserted in the tarsus of the lid near the lacrimal canaliculi while others interlace with palpebral part.

Actions

a. The orbital part screws up the eye to give partial protection from bright light (winking).
b. The palpebral part closes the eye lightly as in blinking or in sleep.
c. The orbital and palpebral parts together close the eye forcibly as in protecting it from a blow or in strong expiratory effort.
d. The lacrimal part draws the eyelids medially thereby increasing the flow of tears towards the lacrimal puncta. It expands the lacrimal sac thereby creating the vacuum inside the sac, which aids in sucking the lacrimal fluid towards it.
e. The action of the entire muscle is to draw the skin of the eyebrow, temple and cheek towards the medial angle of eye. This has the effect of producing radiating skin folds from the lateral angle of eye. These skin folds may become permanent in old age giving rise to 'crow's feet appearance.

Nerve Supply

Temporal and zygomatic branches of facial nerve supply the orbicularis oculi muscle.

Paralysis of Orbicularis Oculi

The paralysis of orbicularis oculi in facial nerve injury, results in inability to close the eye. The lower eyelid sags down from the eyeball (called ectropion), which results in epiphora or spilling of tears on the cheek.

Blepharospasm

Blepharospasm is the involuntary and forcible contraction of orbicularis oculi resulting in closure of eyelids. It presents as brief and involuntary eye closure affecting one or both eyes. One method of treating this condition is by cutting the branches of facial nerve supplying orbicularis oculi. Another method consists of local injection of botulinus toxin, which blocks the release of acetylcholine at neuromuscular junction and thus prevents the contraction of the muscle.

Nasal Muscles

The nasal muscle group consists of the following small muscles.

a. Procerus is a small muscle partially blended with the medial end of frontal belly of occipitofrontalis and covers the glabella. Its contraction produces the transverse wrinkles on the bridge of nose.
b. Nasalis
c. Depressor septi
d. Nasal part of levator labii superioris alaeque nasi.

Buccolabial Group

This is an important group of muscles, which acts on the oral orifice and alters the shape of the lips. This muscular complex consists of sphincter and dilator muscles of the mouth. The intrinsic muscles of the lips comprise the sphincter. The extrinsic muscles arising from other sites come for insertion in the lips.

Elevators, Retractors, Evertors of Upper Lip

a. Labial part of levator labii superioris alaeque nasi

b. Levator labii superioris (raises and everts the upper lip)
c. Zygomaticus minor (elevator of upper lip)
d. Zygomaticus major (draws the angle of mouth upwards and laterally)
e. Levator anguli oris (raises the angle of mouth)
f. Risorius
g. Malaris (if present).

Depressors, Retractors, Evertors of Lower Lip

a. Depressor labii inferioris (draws the lower lip downwards)
b. Depressor anguli oris (draws the angle of mouth downwards and laterally)
c. Mentalis (the only muscle, which is not directly inserted in the lower lip or modiolus but acts on lower lip by raising the base of the lower lip so as to protrude or evert it).
d. Platysma (draws down the lower lip and angle of mouth).

Compound Sphincter of the Mouth

a. Orbicularis oris
b. Incisivus labii superioris
c. Incisivus labii inferioris.

Modiolus

The modiolus is a common point of insertion of as many as nine or ten muscles. It lies about 10 to 12 mm lateral to the angle of mouth. It is a fibromuscular condensation, where the extrinsic and intrinsic muscles converge. It can be palpated between the opposed thumb compressing the skin at the angle of mouth and index finger simultaneously compressing the oral mucosa at the same point. The shape of the modiolus is like that of the hub of a cart-wheel, but the muscles radiating from it lie in different planes. The complex integrated movements of modiolar muscles help in biting, chewing, drinking, sucking, swallowing and speaking apart from the facial expressions.

Orbicularis Oris

This is a sphincter muscle of the oral orifice. It is located within the upper and lower lips and is attached to both right and left modioli. In the upper lip its fibers intermingle with incisivus superioris (taking origin from incisive fossa of maxilla) and with maxillary and lower pterygomandibular fibers of buccinator in addition to depressor anguli oris fibers, which decussate in the upper lip. In the lower lip its fibers intermingle with incisivus inferioris (taking origin from the incisive fossa of the mandible) and with mandibular and upper pterygomandibular fibers of buccinator in addition to levator anguli oris fibers, which decussate in the lower lip. The muscle fibers are attached to the skin as well as to the mucosa of the lip. The main action of the muscle is to close the mouth.

Nerve Supply

Lower buccal and marginal mandibular branches of facial nerve supply the muscle.

Buccinator (Figs 60.2 and 62.1)

The meaning of the word buccinator is trumpeter. So this muscle is active in blowing through the mouth. It is grouped along with muscles of facial expression since it shares its development and nerve supply with them. It is actually an accessory muscle of mastication because it helps in chewing food. It is a deeply placed muscle of the cheek lying in the interval between the maxilla and mandible.

Attachments

a. The origin is from a C-shaped line from the outer surfaces of maxilla opposite the molar teeth, a tendinous band between the pterygoid hamulus and the maxillary tuberosity, anterior border of pterygomandibular raphe and outer surface of mandible opposite third molar tooth.
b. The insertion into the lips is rather complicated (Fig. 116.2). The fibers converge towards the modiolus. The maxillary fibers pass in the upper lip while the mandibular fibers pass in the lower lip. The pterygomandibular fibers cross at the modiolus. The upper fibers travel in the lower lip to join the similar fibers of the opposite side. The lower fibers pass through the upper lip to join the similar fibers of the opposite side.

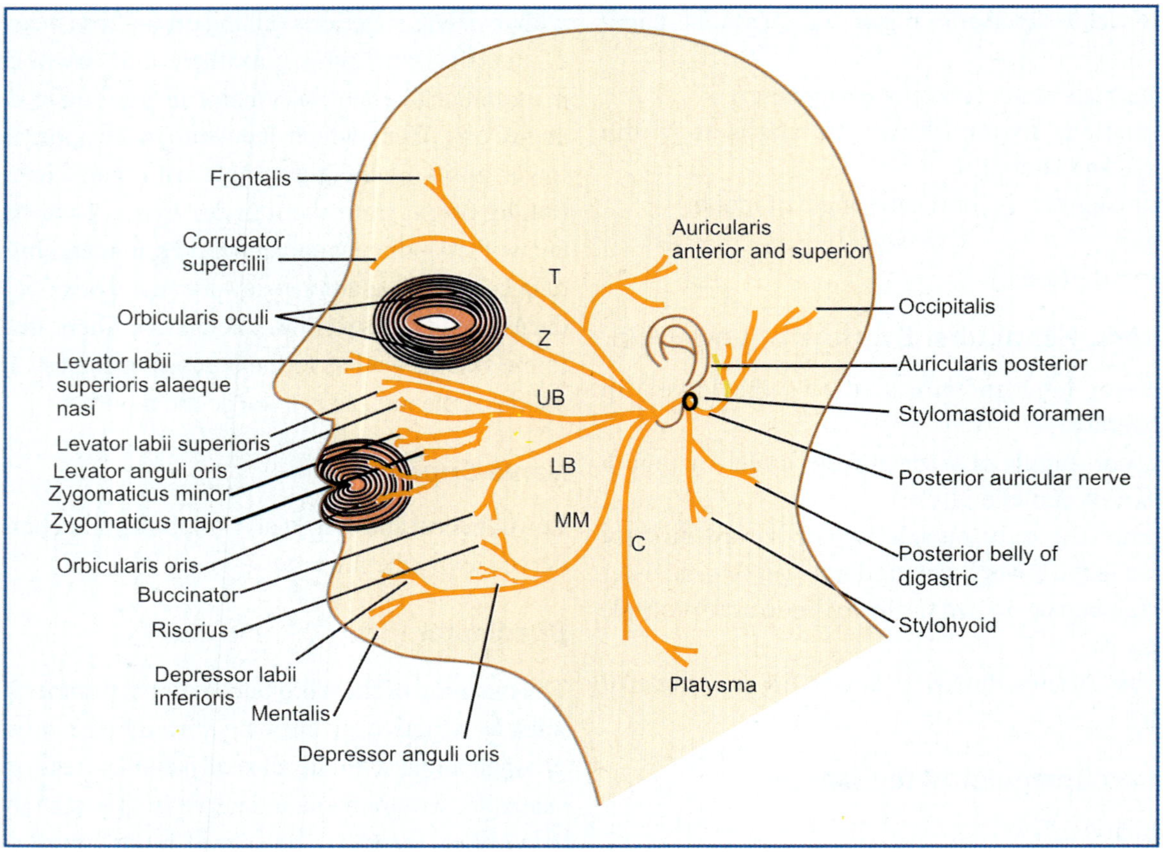

Fig. 60.2: Extracranial course and distribution of facial nerve. The branches of facial nerve in the face are: T—temporal, Z—zygomatic, UB—upper buccal, LB—lower buccal, MM—marginal mandibular, C—cervical

Relations (Fig. 166.2)

Posteriorly it is related to the anterior margin of superior constrictor muscle of pharynx, which also takes origin from the pterygomandibular raphe. Its deep surface is covered with mucosa of the vestibule of oral cavity. Superficially it is covered with buccopharyngeal fascia and buccal pad of fat. The facial vessels and branches of facial nerve and buccal branch of mandibular nerve lie superficial to it. The parotid duct and the buccal branch of mandibular nerve pierce the muscle. The tendon of tensor palati passes through the narrow gap behind the tendinous band (extending between the pterygoid hamulus and the maxillary tuberosity).

Nerve Supply

The lower buccal branches of facial nerve supply the buccinator.

Actions

The buccinator compresses the cheeks against teeth and gums. This action is helpful in mastication as it prevents food from collecting in the vestibule. It compresses the blown out cheeks and raises the intraoral pressure. This action is helpful in playing wind instruments and in whistling.

Paralysis of Buccinator

In paralysis of buccinator food tends to collect between the teeth and cheek (in vestibule of mouth) on the affected side. When the patient attempts to hold water in the mouth, the water escapes from the affected side quite unexpectedly. In many cases of facial palsy this is the presenting complaint.

Facial Muscles and Expressions

Contraction of individual muscles produces specific facial expression as shown below.

No	Muscle	Facial expression
1	Frontalis	Surprise
2	Procerus	Concentration
3	Zygomaticus major and levator anguli oris	Smiling and laughing
4	Zygomaticus minor, levator labii superioris alaeque nasi and levator labii superioris	Disdain and contempt
5	Depressor labii inferioris and depressor anguli oris	Sadness and sorrow
6	Risorius	Grinning
7	Mentalis	Doubt
8	Platysma	Horror and terror
9	Corrugator supercilii	Frowning

Testing Function of Facial Muscles

The various muscles of facial expression are individually tested in suspected facial nerve palsy.

a. To test the frontal belly of occipitofrontalis (frontalis) ask the subject to raise the eyebrows. Normally horizontal wrinkles are seen on the forehead.
b. To test orbicularis oculi ask the subject to close the eyelids tightly against resistance.
c. To test levator anguli oris ask the subject to show the teeth so that angles on both sides move equally.
d. To test orbicularis oris ask the subject to purse the lips tightly against resistance.
e. To test the buccinator ask the subject to blow out the cheeks keeping the mouth shut. Then tap on the cheek to see if air escapes from closed mouth.
f. To test the platysma ask the subject to clench teeth and simultaneously depress the angles of mouth. Normally longitudinal folds of skin become obvious in the neck, when platysma contracts.

Extracranial Course of Facial Nerve (Fig. 60.2)

The facial nerve leaves the cranium through the stylomastoid foramen. Immediately after the exit it gives three branches, posterior auricular branch for the supply of the occipital belly of occipitofrontalis and posterior auricular muscles, digastric branch for the posterior belly of digastric and a branch to the stylohyoid muscle. To reach the parotid gland the facial nerve courses forwards in lateral relation to the styloid process. This part of the trunk of the facial nerve can be exposed surgically between the mastoid process and the external acoustic meatus. The facial nerve enters the posteromedial surface of the parotid gland. Within the gland it runs forwards for a short distance superficial to the retromandibular vein and external carotid artery and then divides in temporofacial and cervicofacial trunks. The temporofacial trunk divides in temporal and zygomatic branches while the cervicofacial trunk divides in buccal, marginal mandibular and cervical branches. The five terminal branches radiate like a goose's foot (pes anserinus) from the anterior border of the parotid gland.

Branches in the Face

The motor branches for the facial muscles lie in the superficial fascia hence they are vulnerable to damage in facial lacerations.

a. The temporal branch leaves the gland through its upper surface and passes upwards and forwards in front of the auricle across the zygomatic arch to reach the temple. It supplies the anterior and superior auricular muscles, orbicularis oculi, frontalis and corrugator supercilii.
b. The zygomatic branch runs along the zygomatic arch and supplies the orbicularis oculi.
c. The buccal branches are two in number. The upper buccal branch passes above the parotid duct and supplies the procerus, zygomaticus major and minor, levator anguli oris, levator labii superioris, levator labii superioris alaeque nasi and nasal muscles. The lower buccal branch passes below the parotid duct and supplies the buccinator and orbicularis oris.
d. The marginal mandibular branch has unusual course. It first descends to the digastric triangle under the platysma and then curves upwards and forwards across the base of mandible at the anteroinferior angle of masseter and reaches the face after crossing the facial vessels. It supplies the risorius, depressor anguli oris, depressor labii inferioris and mentalis. The marginal mandibular branch is in danger of injury while placing incision for removal of submandibular gland.
e. The cervical branch enters the anterior part of the neck through the apex of the gland and supplies the platysma.

Communications

The branches of the facial nerve supplying the muscles of facial expression make plenty of anastomoses with the sensory branches of trigeminal nerve, which carries the proprioceptive sensations through these communications to the CNS.

a. The temporal branches communicate with auriculotemporal and zygomaticotemporal nerves.
b. The zygomatic branches communicate with zygomaticofacial and lacrimal nerves.
c. The upper buccal branches communicate with infraorbital and infratrochlear nerves.
d. The lower buccal branches communicate with buccal branch of mandibular nerve.
e. The marginal mandibular branch communicates with mental nerve.
f. The cervical branch communicates with transverse cutaneous nerve on neck.

61 Eyelids and Lacrimal Apparatus

The Latin equivalent of eyelid is palpebrae while the Greek equivalent is blepharon. The clinical conditions related to the eyelid are referred in terms of its Greek equivalent, for example, the inflammation of the margins of the eyelid is called blepharitis or congenital absence of the eyelid is called ablepharon. The eyelids protect the eyeball from direct and bright sunlight and injury. The upper eyelid is larger and more mobile than the lower. The eyelids are separated from the eyeball by the conjunctival sac.

External Features of Eyelids

Each eyelid has a free or palpebral margin from which cilia or eyelashes project. The space between the free margins of the two eyelids is called palpebral fissure. The meeting points of the two eyelids are called lateral and medial canthi or angles. At the margin of the eyelid the skin and the conjunctiva are continuous with each other. The lateral five-sixth of the margin of the eyelid bears cilia and hence is called the ciliary part. The medial one-sixth is devoid of cilia but contains the lacrimal canaliculus and hence is called the lacrimal part. At the junction of the two parts the lacrimal punctum is located. The lacrimal canaliculus begins at the punctum, is embedded in the medial one-sixth of the margin and ends medially in the lacrimal sac. The triangular area at the wide medial angle of eye is called the lacus lacrimalis. It contains a reddish body called the lacrimal caruncle (which is considered to be detached part of the eyelid). The plica seminularis is a fold of conjunctiva that is situated lateral to the caruncle.

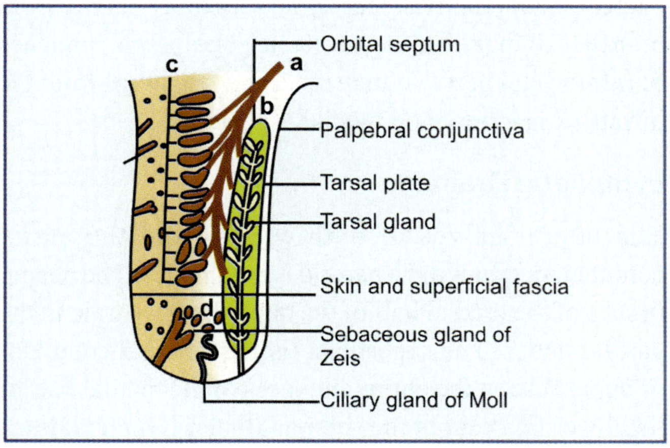

Fig. 61.1: Vertical section through upper eyelid
(Note: The muscles inside the upper eyelid: a—Levator palpebrae superioris, b—Müller's muscle, c—Orbicularis oculi, d—Ciliary bundle of muscle fibers)

Structure of Eyelids (Fig. 61.1)

The eyelids are made of five layers from without inward.

a. Skin of the eyelid is extremely thin and loosely attached to the dermis. It is composed of sweat and sebaceous glands. The large sized sebaceous glands at the lid margin are called Zeis's glands and the large-sized sweat glands near the lid margin are called Moll's glands. The ducts of the Moll's glands open in the hair follicles or in the ducts of the sebaceous glands. The inflammation of Zeis's gland is called stye, in which the gland becomes swollen, hard and painful.
b. Superficial fascia of the eyelid is devoid of fat and is composed of loose tissue. Hence edema of the eyelids is very common.
c. Muscular layer is composed of both striated and non-striated muscle fibers. The upper eyelid consists of palpebral part of orbicularis oculi, (supplied by facial nerve), ciliaris bundle, which is an isolated part of orbicularis oculi near the lid margin (supplied by facial nerve), levator palpebrae superioris (supplied by oculomotor nerve) and Müller's muscle or superior tarsal muscle, which is the non-striated muscle

(sympathetic innervation). The lower eyelid consists of palpebral part of orbicularis oculi, ciliaris bundle and the inferior tarsal muscle (involuntary muscle). The space beneath the muscular layer in the upper eyelid is called submuscular space. It is filled with loose areolar tissue and is continuous with the subaponeurotic space of scalp. This continuity is responsible for the appearance of black eye in bleeding injury to the skull vault. The submuscular layer contains the sensory nerves of the eyelid hence local anesthetic solutions are injected deep to the palpebral part of orbicularis oculi.

d. The tarsus and palpebral fascia together form the fourth layer. The tarsal plate consists of dense fibrous tissue and gives support to the eyelid. The tarsal plate of the upper lid is bigger and of almond shape while that of lower lid is smaller and of rod shape. The medial ends of the two tarsal plates are connected by medial palpebral ligament to the lacrimal crest of maxilla in front of the lacrimal sac. The lateral ends of the two tarsi are connected by the lateral palpebral ligament to the tubercle on the zygomatic bone (Whitnall's tubercle) within the orbital margin laterally. The superior tarsus gives attachment to the levator palpebrae superioris. The tarsi are connected to the orbital margin by the palpebral fascia or the orbital septum. The tarsal glands are embedded in the deep surface of the tarsus. These glands are called Meibomian glands. They are modified sebaceous glands. Their ducts open on lid margins by minute openings. The tarsal glands secrete oily fluid, which forms a thin film on the conjunctiva. This reduces the evaporation of tears. The inflammation of tarsal glands is called hordeolum internum. The chalazion is the cystic swelling of the tarsal gland.

e. Palpebral conjunctiva forms the innermost layer of the eyelids.

Conjunctiva

The conjunctiva is a transparent mucous membrane, which lines the inner surface of the eyelids and the front of the sclera of the eyeball. The part lining the lids is called palpebral conjunctiva and that lining the sclera is called the ocular or bulbar conjunctiva. The space between the palpebral and bulbar conjunctiva is called the conjunctival sac. At the sclerocorneal junction the epithelium of conjunctiva becomes continuous with the corneal epithelium. The palpebral conjunctiva is highly vascular. It is closely adherent to the tarsi. The tarsal glands are visible through it if the lid is retracted. The superior and inferior fornices of the conjunctival sac are located at the line of reflection of the conjunctiva from the lid to the eyeball. The superior fornix receives the ducts of the lacrimal gland. The conjunctival epithelium is in continuity with the skin and with the epithelium of ducts of tarsal glands at the palpebral margin and with the epithelium of lacrimal canaliculi at the lacrimal puncta.

Blood Supply of Eyelids

The eyelid receives the arterial supply from the lateral palpebral branches of lacrimal and medial palpebral branches of the ophthalmic arteries. The conjunctiva receives arterial supply from the palpebral arteries as well as the anterior ciliary arteries. The veins from the lids and palpebral conjunctiva drain in the facial vein while those from the bulbar conjunctiva drain in ophthalmic veins.

Nerve Supply

The upper eyelid including its palpebral conjunctiva receives nerve supply from the branches of ophthalmic nerve, namely, supratrochlear, supraorbital, infratrochlear and the lacrimal branches. The lower eyelid including its palpebral conjunctiva receives nerve supply mainly from branches of maxillary nerve, namely, palpebral branches of infraorbital nerve. It may receive a few twigs from the infratrochlear nerve on medial aspect.

Lymphatic Drainage

The lateral halves of both eyelids and the entire conjunctiva drain in the parotid lymph nodes. The deeper tissues of the medial half of the upper lid also drain in the parotid nodes. The superficial tissues of the medial half of upper lid and the entire thickness of the medial half of the lower lid drain in the submandibular lymph nodes.

Clinical Highlights of Eyelids

a. The word ptosis means drooping of the upper eyelid. The drooping is due to paralysis of levator palpebrae superioris. The oculomotor palsy is one of the causes of ptosis. Partial ptosis is due to paralysis of Müller's muscle as happens in Horner's syndrome. Bilateral ptosis is usually seen in myasthenia gravis.

b. The sagging or eversion of the lower eyelid (ectropion) is due to paralysis of orbicularis oculi due to facial palsy. This results in spilling of the tears.

Lacrimal Apparatus

The lacrimal apparatus consists of the lacrimal glands that secrete the lacrimal fluid (tears) and the lacrimal passages that drain the lacrimal fluid into the nasal cavity. A film of fluid is continuously distributed on the surface of conjunctiva and cornea by periodic blinking of the eyelids. The lacrimal fluid plays a role in protecting and nourishing the cornea.

Components of Lacrimal Apparatus (Fig. 61.2)

The lacrimal apparatus consists of, lacrimal gland, lacrimal ducts, conjunctival sac and lacus lacrimalis, lacrimal puncta, lacrimal canaliculi, lacrimal sac and nasolacrimal duct.

Lacrimal Gland

The lacrimal gland is a serous gland and hence the tears are watery in consistency. It has two parts, larger orbital and smaller palpebral. The orbital part is situated above the eyeball and is lodged in the lacrimal fossa on the inferior aspect of the orbital plate of frontal bone or the medial aspect of the zygomatic process of frontal bone. The palpebral part is located in the lateral part of the upper eyelid. The orbital and palpebral parts are continuous with each other around the lateral margin of levator palpebrae superioris. Thus, the orbital part lies above the levator palpebrae superioris and the palpebral part lies below it. The orbital part lies behind the orbital septum and the palpebral part lies in front of it. The ducts of the lacrimal gland are about a dozen in number. Some ducts drain the orbital part and others drain the palpebral part but all ducts traverse through the palpebral part. The ducts open in the lateral part of superior conjunctival fornix. When the palpebral part of the gland is surgically removed all the ducts are also removed, resulting in a condition, where production of lacrimal fluid takes place but its drainage is hampered. Accessory lacrimal glands are minute glands that lie near the fornices in both eyelids. If the lacrimal gland is surgically removed the accessory lacrimal glands are able to carry out its functions.

Secretomotor Nerve Supply (Fig. 61.3)

The preganglionic fibers originate in the lacrimatory nucleus in the pons. They are carried through the nervus intermedius of the facial nerve and leave in the greater petrosal branch of the facial nerve. The union of greater petrosal and the deep petrosal nerves form the nerve of pterygoid canal or Vidian nerve. This nerve carries the preganglionic fibers to the sphenopalatine ganglion for synapse. The postganglionic secretomotor fibers are

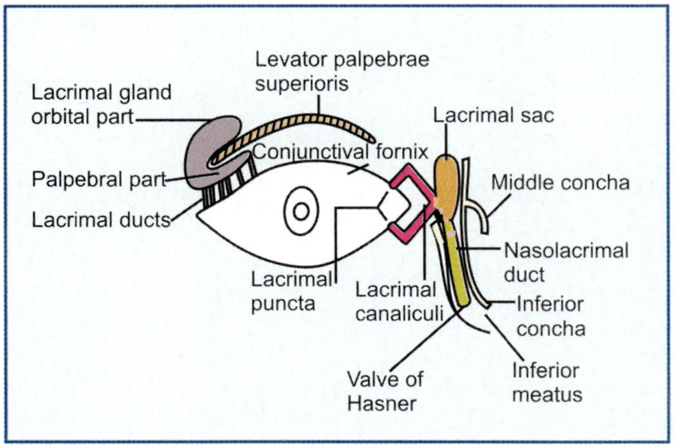

Fig. 61.2: Scheme to show components of lacrimal apparatus

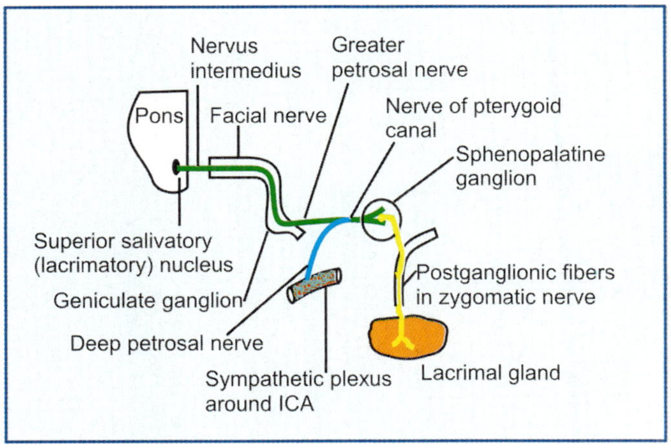

Fig. 61.3: Pathway of secretomotor nerve supply of lacrimal gland

Section three

carried in the zygomatic nerve to the lacrimal gland via a communication with the lacrimal nerve.

Conjunctival Sac

This receives the lacrimal fluid at its superior fornix and the fluid is transferred to the conjunctival sac for spreading evenly to form a thin film over the cornea and conjunctiva. As the new fluid is formed the older fluid is gradually drifted toward the lacus lacrimalis.

Lacrimal Canaliculi

The superior and inferior lacrimal canaliculus begins at the lacrimal punctum, which is located at a slightly raised papilla projecting toward the lacus lacrimalis. The lacrimal puncta lie on the lid margins about six mm lateral to the medial angle of the eye. Each canaliculus runs medially in the respective lid margin to open in the lacrimal sac. The course of the canaliculus is not straight but at first it turns downward or upward (depending on the eyelid) and then turns medially.

Lacrimal Sac

The lacrimal sac is located in the lacrimal groove just posterior to the medial margin of the orbit. The lacrimal sac is one cm long and half a cm wide. Its upper end is blind and its lower end is continuous with the nasolacrimal duct. Nearer its upper end it receives the lacrimal canaliculi laterally. The sac is closely coved with lacrimal fascia except on medial aspect. A few fibers of lacrimal part of orbicularis oculi take origin from the lacrimal fascia. So the contraction of this muscle exerts a pull on the fascia causing the expansion of sac thereby helping to suck the lacrimal fluid in the sac. It is related to the medial palpebral ligament anteriorly in front of lacrimal fascia. Posteriorly it is in relation to the lacrimal part of orbicularis oculi with lacrimal fascia and a minute plexus of veins between them. The lacrimal groove lies medially and separates the sac from anterior ethmoidal cells and middle meatus of nasal cavity. Dacryocystitis is the inflammation of lacrimal sac. The main symptom in this common condition is epiphora (spilling of tears) because of block in the sac or the nasolacrimal duct.

Nasolacrimal Duct

This duct begins at the lower end of the lacrimal sac. It is narrowest at its upper end. It passes through an osseous canal in the lateral, posterior and downward direction to open in the inferior meatus of the nasal cavity. Its lower opening is guarded by a mucosal fold (called a lacrimal fold or valve of Hesner), which prevents air and nasal secretions from being carried upwards in the reverse direction during raised intranasal pressure.

62 Parotid Gland

The word parotid is derived from pars and otis (near the ear). The parotid gland is the largest among the salivary glands.

General Features

The parotid gland weighs about 25 gm and resembles in shape an inverted pyramid. It is a compound tubulo-alveolar type of gland consisting mainly of serous acini. The parotid duct carries the watery secretion of the gland to the vestibule of the mouth. The secretion forms the saliva and helps in moistening the mouth and in the formation of the bolus of the food.

Location (Fig. 62.1)

The parotid gland is located below, in front and behind the ear lobule. It fills the hollow between the ramus of mandible and the mastoid process. It extends between the external acoustic meatus above to just posteroinferior to the angle of mandible. Posteriorly it overlaps the sternocleidomastoid and anteriorly it crosses the masseter.

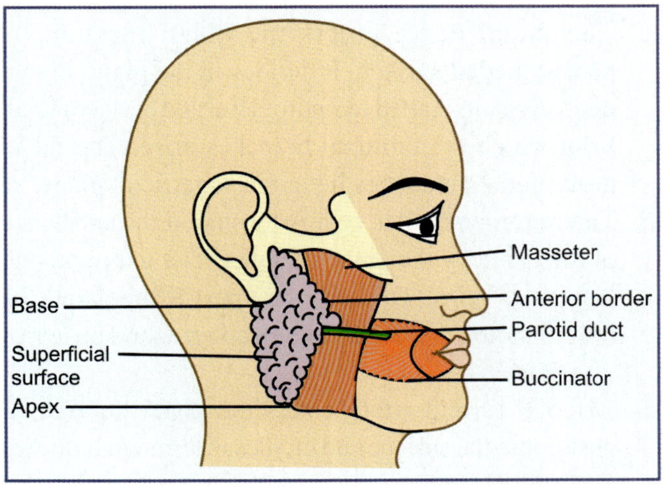

Fig. 62.1: Location and parts of parotid gland (Note: The accessory parotid gland above the parotid duct)

Parts, Surfaces and Borders

The parotid gland has a narrow base and a rounded apex that points inferiorly. It has three borders (medial, anterior and posterior) and four surfaces, namely, superficial or lateral, anteromedial, posteromedial and superior or base. The medial border separates the anteromedial and postero-medial surfaces. The anterior border separates the superficial and anteromedial surfaces. The posterior border intervenes between the superficial and posteromedial surfaces.

Processes

a. The glenoid process is the part of the base or superior surface of the gland lodged between the external acoustic meatus and the capsule of temporomandibular joint. Swelling and inflammation of glenoid process, for example in mumps, give rise to pain during eating.
b. The pterygoid process is the extension of the deep part of the gland between the medial pterygoid muscle and the ramus of mandible.
c. The facial process is the part that extends on the face along the duct. A part of it becomes separate above the duct as accessory parotid gland.

Surface Marking (Fig. 62.2)

To draw the curved anterior border three points are marked as follows. The first point coinciding with the head of the mandible is in front of the tragus of ear. The second point is marked on the center of the masseter muscle. Third point lies just posteroinferior to the angle of mandible. The posterior border is drawn by joining the third point to the fourth point, which is marked at the upper end of the anterior margin of mastoid process. A line joining

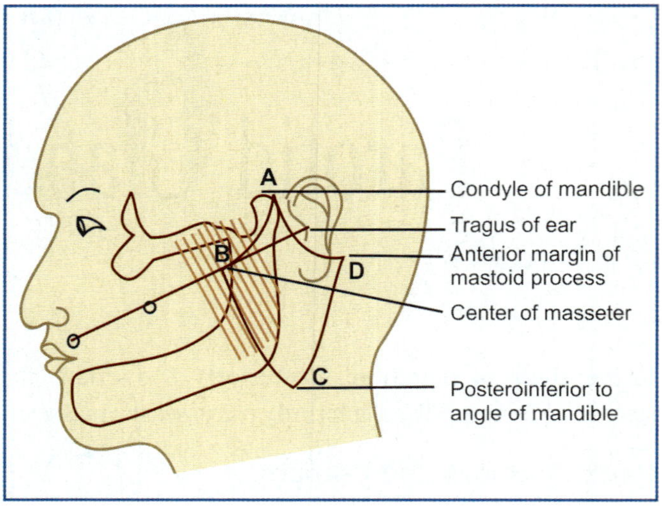

Fig. 62.2: Surface marking of parotid gland and parotid duct. Line A-B-C—represents anterior margin, line C-D—posterior margin and line D-A—superior margin. Parotid duct is represented by middle-third of a line from tragus to a point midway between ala of nose and red margin of upper lip

the first and fourth points represents the upper border of the parotid. This line is concave upwards and may be drawn either across the lobule of the ear or by lifting the lobule of the ear.

Fascial Capsule

The parotid gland is enclosed in a fascial capsule derived from the investing layer of deep cervical fascia. At the lower end of the parotid the fascia splits in superficial and deep layers. Extremely dense superficial layer is attached to the lower border of zygomatic arch. The inflammatory swellings of the parotid gland are very painful because of the unyielding nature of this dense fascia. This layer blends with the epimysium of masseter to form parotidomasseteric fascia. The deep layer of the fascial capsule is relatively thin and is attached to the styloid process, tympanic plate and the mandible. The fascial layer extending between the styloid process and the angle of mandible is called stylomandibular ligament, which intervenes between the parotid and the submandibular salivary glands.

Relations (Fig. 62.3)

a. The superficial or lateral surface is covered by skin, superficial fascia including the posterior fibers of platysma and the dense capsule of the gland. The superficial parotid lymph nodes and the cutaneous twigs of the great auricular nerve lie in the superficial fascia.
b. The anteromedial surface is closely related to the ramus of the mandible and the masseter attached to its lateral surface and medial pterygoid attached to its medial surface.
c. The posteromedial surface is very large and hence comes in contact with many structures. It is related to the mastoid process and the two muscles attached to it, namely, sternocleidomastoid and posterior belly of digastric. It is also related to the styloid process and the three muscles attached to it, namely, stylohyoid, styloglossus and stylopharyngeus. The internal carotid artery and internal jugular vein are separated from the parotid gland by the styloid apparatus. Last four cranial nerves are also located near these vessels. The external carotid artery grooves this surface before entering the gland.
d. The medial border of the gland may project medially so much that it touches the lateral wall of the oropharynx. Hence the medial border is also known as the pharyngeal border.
e. The narrow superior surface is related to the external acoustic meatus and the temporomandibular joint. The auriculotemporal nerve is embedded in the capsule near the superior surface.
f. The apex lies between the sternocleidomastoid and the angle of mandible and it overlaps the posterior belly of digastric.

Contents (Fig. 62.3)

a. The facial nerve enters the gland through its posteromedial surface. It divides in the gland in two main divisions called temporofacial and cervicofacial, from which the terminal branches arise. The facial nerve and its branches lie in the superficial plane.
b. The retromandibular vein is formed in the substance of the gland by the union of superficial temporal and maxillary veins. Towards the apex of the gland the retromandibular vein divides in anterior and posterior divisions.
c. External carotid artery enters the gland through its posteromedial surface and divides in terminal branches (superficial temporal and maxillary) at the level of and posterior to the neck of the mandible.

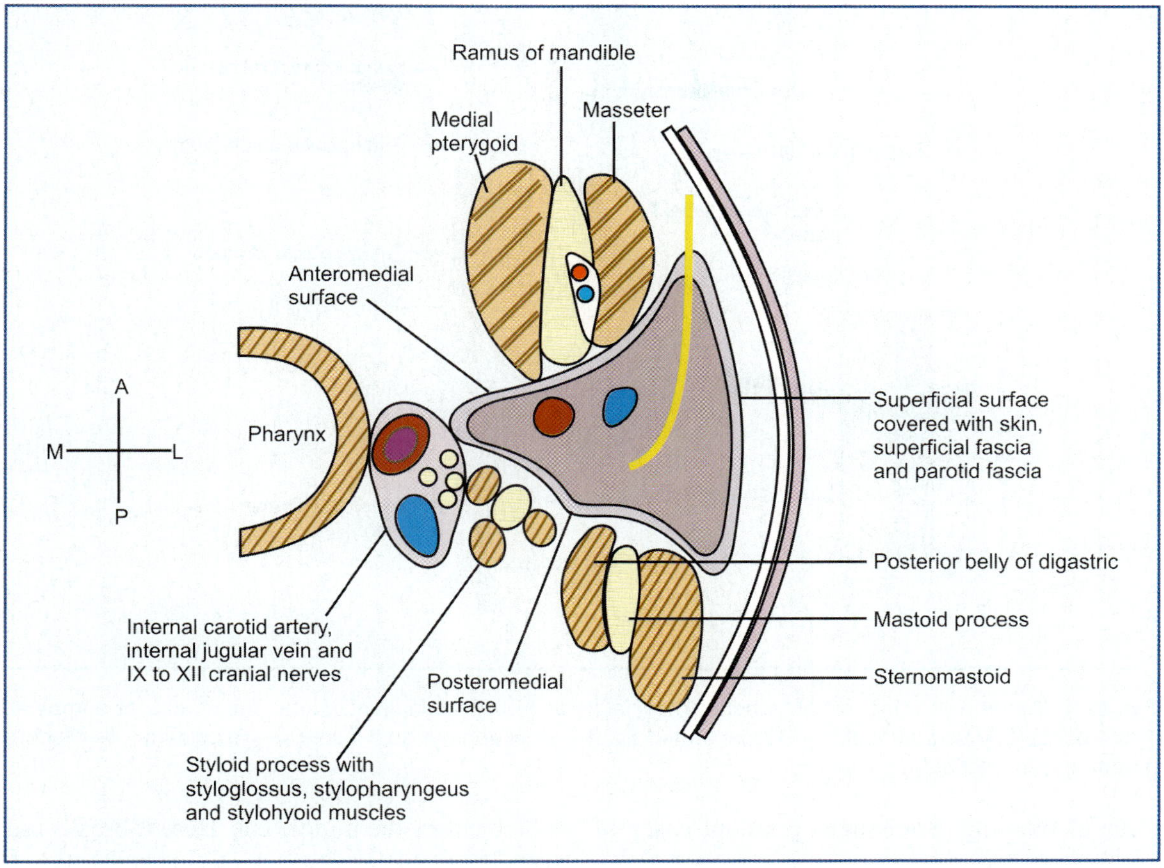

Fig. 62.3: Schematic horizontal section to show relations of right parotid gland
(Note: The contents of gland (from superficial to deep): facial nerve, retromandibular vein and external carotid artery)

The facial nerve is the most superficial structure inside the gland. The retromandibular vein is deeper to the facial nerve and the external carotid artery is the deepest. The nerve and the vein constitute a plane called faciovenous plane, which divides the gland in superficial and deep parts.

Apart from these three major structures the parotid also contains deep group of parotid lymph nodes and a part of the auriculotemporal nerve.

Exit of Structures from the Gland (Fig. 62.4)

a. The structures that leave the anterior border are the zygomatic branch of facial nerve, transverse facial vessels, upper buccal branch of facial nerve, parotid duct, lower buccal branch of facial nerve and marginal mandibular branch of facial nerve.
b. The base or superior surface gives passage to the temporal branch of facial nerve, auriculotemporal nerve and superficial temporal vessels.
c. The apex gives passage to the cervical branch of facial nerve and the retromandibular vein or its two divisions.
d. The maxillary artery leaves through the anteromedial surface (maxillary vein enters the gland via the same surface).

Parotid Duct or Stensen's Duct

The parotid duct is five cm long. It drains the secretions of the gland to the vestibule of the mouth. It emerges from the anterior border of the parotid along with branches of facial nerve and crosses the masseter. At the anterior margin of this muscle it turns sharply medially to pierce the buccal pad of fat, buccopharyngeal fascia, buccinator muscle and the buccal mucosa (Figs 62.1 and 62.4). It opens in the vestibule of mouth at the level of the crown of the upper second molar tooth. The oblique course of the duct between the buccinator and the oral mucosa acts as a valve, which prevents distension of the parotid duct

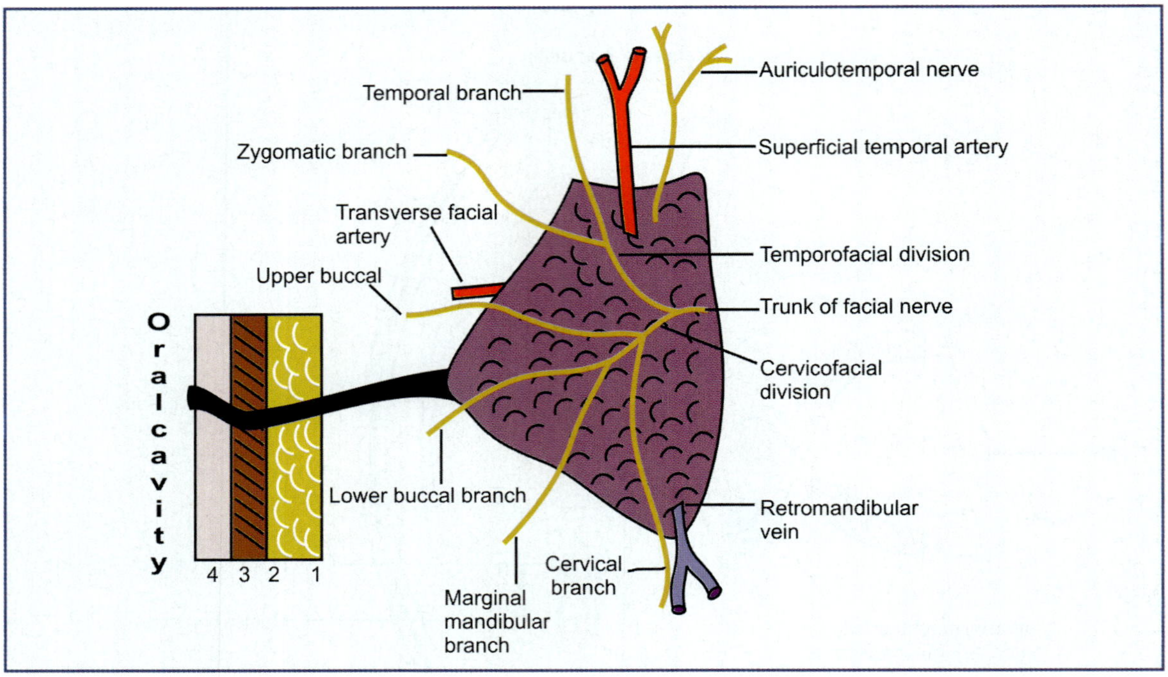

Fig. 62.4: Scheme showing exit of branches of facial nerve from parotid gland (Note: The structures numbered 1 to 4 pierced by parotid duct. 1—Buccal pad of fat, 2— Buccopharyngeal fascia, 3—Buccinator, 4—Mucous membrane of vestibule)

during forceful blowing. Sometimes resistant cases of chronic recurrent parotitis are treated by injecting antibiotic through the oral aperture of the duct.

Surface Marking of Parotid Duct

The middle third of the line starting from the lower border of tragus to the point between the ala of the nose and the red margin of the lip represents the parotid duct.

Parotid Sialography

This is a radiological procedure for visualizing the parotid duct and its branching pattern. It is performed in cases where narrowing or obstruction of the main duct or its intraglandular branches is suspected. The contrast medium is injected into a small cannula passed through the oral aperture of the duct and the radiograph is taken.

Secretomotor Nerve Supply (Fig. 62.5)

The preganglionic parasympathetic fibers taking origin in the inferior salivary nucleus in the medulla oblongata are carried in the glossopharyngeal nerve. These fibers leave the ninth nerve in its tympanic branch (Jacobson's nerve), which enters the middle ear. Here it breaks in tympanic plexus, which gives rise to lesser petrosal nerve. This nerve enters the middle cranial fossa, from where it enters the infratemporal fossa to terminate in the otic ganglion. The postganglionic fibers from the ganglion join the auriculotemporal nerve, which supplies the secretomotor fibers to the gland.

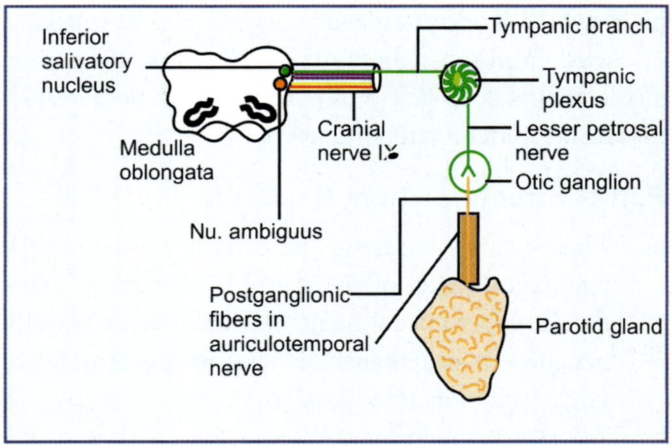

Fig. 62.5: Pathway of secretomotor nerve supply of parotid gland

Lymphatic Drainage

The parotid gland drains in deep and superficial group of parotid lymph nodes. The deep nodes are within the substance of the gland while the superficial nodes lie in the superficial fascia covering the lateral surface of the gland. The parotid lymph nodes drain in the deep cervical nodes.

Development

The parotid gland is ectodermal in origin. It arises from the buccal ectoderm as an outgrowth, which gives rise to the parotid duct and the gland. The site of origin of the outgrowth is retained as the oral orifice of the duct.

Clinical Highlights

a. The parotid swellings may be due to inflammation of the gland or due to tumors (benign or malignant). Since the gland is positioned below, behind and in front of the lobule of the ear its swellings obliterate the normal hollow just below the lobule of the ear, which is invariably lifted in the parotid swellings.
b. The parotid abscess presents as a slight swelling with redness on the surface of the swelling accompanied by acute excruciating pain. It results from bacterial parotitis (the infection due to bad oral hygiene traveling from the mouth via the duct). The parotid abscess does not show fluctuation, when ripe due to its unyielding capsule. While draining the abscess the surgical incision on the parotid fascia is placed transversely in the direction of the branches of the facial nerve.
c. Mumps is a non-suppurative viral infection of the parotid gland, in which there is painless enlargement of the gland.
d. Tumors of parotid gland are very common. A painless slow growing tumor is benign in nature. It does not damage facial nerve. On the contrary, the malignant growth is characterized by rapidly growing painful swelling, which involves the facial nerve producing facial palsy. Therefore, it is very essential to examine the function of facial nerve by testing the muscles of facial expression in parotid tumors. The palpation of the deep group of cervical lymph nodes for finding out the spread of cancer is also essential. Occasionally cancer may spread to the temporomandibular joint. This results in painful and restricted movements of the jaw.
e. During surgical excision of benign tumors of parotid gland the facial nerve is preserved either by following the facial nerve (nerve is exposed in the interval between the bony external meatus and the mastoid process and then traced into the gland till its divisions are identified) or by following the faciovenous plane, which consists of facial nerve and retromandibular vein. Identification of this plane during surgery is done by following the external jugular vein towards the gland upto the posterior division of retromandibular vein in the substance of the gland. The facial nerve is not injured if the excision of parotid is done along the faciovenous plane.
f. Auriculotemporal syndrome or Frey's syndrome is sometimes encountered during the healing process after surgery on the parotid gland. Two sensory nerves (auriculotemporal and great auricular) in close relation to the gland may be cut during surgery. During the process of regeneration secretomotor fibers in the auriculotemporal nerve, accidentally join the great auricular nerve. As a result of this mix up, while eating, instead of production of saliva there is perspiration over the skin over the parotid gland (supplied by great auricular nerve) due to reflex stimulation of the sweat glands.

63 Triangles of Neck

The sternomastoid muscle is a prominent landmark, which serves to divide the neck in the anterior and posterior triangles (Fig. 63.1).

Boundaries of Posterior Triangle

The intermediate third of clavicle, the anterior border of trapezius and the posterior border of sternomastoid bound the posterior triangle. The muscles forming the floor of the triangle are the semispinalis capitis, splenius capitis, levator scapulae and scalenus medius, from above downward. The inferior belly of omohyoid divides the posterior triangle in upper larger occipital triangle and lower smaller subclavian triangles.

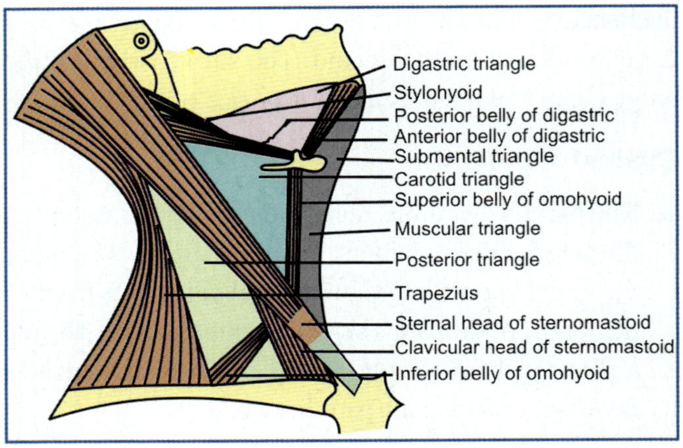

Fig. 63.1: Lateral view of neck depicting boundaries of triangles of neck (Note that inferior belly of omohyoid divides the posterior triangle into upper occipital and lower supraclavicular [subclavian] triangles)

Boundaries of Anterior Triangle

The boundaries of the anterior triangle are as follows, body of the mandible above, anterior midline of the neck and the anterior margin of sternomastoid muscle. The superior belly of omohyoid and the digastric muscle divide the common anterior triangle in four smaller triangles.

a. The submental triangle is a space between the anterior bellies of right and left digastric muscles on each side and body of the hyoid bone. It is a single midline triangle in the suprahyoid region.
b. The anterior and posterior belly of digastric muscle and the base of the mandible bound the digastric triangle.
c. The anterior border of sternomastoid, posterior belly of digastric and superior belly of omohyoid bound the carotid triangle.
d. The muscular triangle is bounded by the anterior midline of the neck, superior belly of omohyoid and the sternomastoid muscle.

64 Cervical Fascia

Superficial Fascia

The superficial fascia of the neck contains the platysma muscle in the front besides the cutaneous nerves and the anterior jugular and external jugular veins.

Platysma

The platysma takes origin from the fascia covering the pectoralis major and the deltoid muscles (Fig. 1.3). Passing in front of the clavicle the platysma spreads out as a thin sheet in the superficial fascia of the neck. The muscles of the two sides meet in the midline. The anterior fibers insert in the lower margin of the body of mandible. The posterior fibers cross in front of the mandible and get attached to the modiolus at the angle of mouth and to the lower lip.

Nerve Supply

The cervical branch of facial nerve supplies the platysma.

Actions

The platysma depresses the mandible and draws the angle of mouth in the inferior direction.

Clinical Highlights

a. While suturing the skin incision in the neck the platysma also must be sutured, otherwise the skin scar will be stretched and healing will be delayed.
b. This muscle is often tested in suspected Bell's palsy by asking the patient to clench the teeth and simultaneously depress the angles of mouth. This should produce visible contraction of the normal muscle in the neck.

Deep Fascia of Neck

The deep fascia of the neck or fascia colli is arranged in three layers (Fig. 64.1).

a. The outer layer is called the investing layer of deep fascia because it invests the neck like a collar.
b. The middle layer is called the pretracheal fascia because it lies in front of the trachea. It is confined to the anterior aspect of the neck.
c. The deepest layer is called the prevertebral layer because it lies in front of the bodies of cervical vertebrae. It spreads laterally on both sides across the floor of the posterior triangles.

Attachments of Investing Layer

This layer roofs anterior and posterior triangles of the neck and splits to enclose two muscles, namely, sternomastoid and trapezius. It is attached posteriorly to the ligamentum nuchae and the spine of the seventh cervical vertebra. It passes forwards on each side and splits to enclose the trapezius muscle. The two layers unite at the anterior margin of the trapezius to form a single layer, which roofs the posterior triangle. At the posterior margin of sternomastoid the fascia splits again to enclose the same muscle. The spinal part of the accessory nerve lies just beneath the investing layer of deep fascia in the roof of the posterior triangle. At the anterior margin of the sternomastoid the two layers reunite to form a single layer, which roofs the anterior triangle. The fascial layers of the two sides are continuous with each other in the midline anteriorly. The upper attachments of the fascia are very wide so for descriptive purposes, they are subdivided in anterior and posterior attachments.

Upper attachment on anterior aspect is as follows:

a. In the midline, the fascia is attached to the hyoid bone and the symphysis menti.
b. Laterally the fascia is attached to the base of the mandible but it splits in the submandibular region to enclose the submandibular gland. The superficial layer

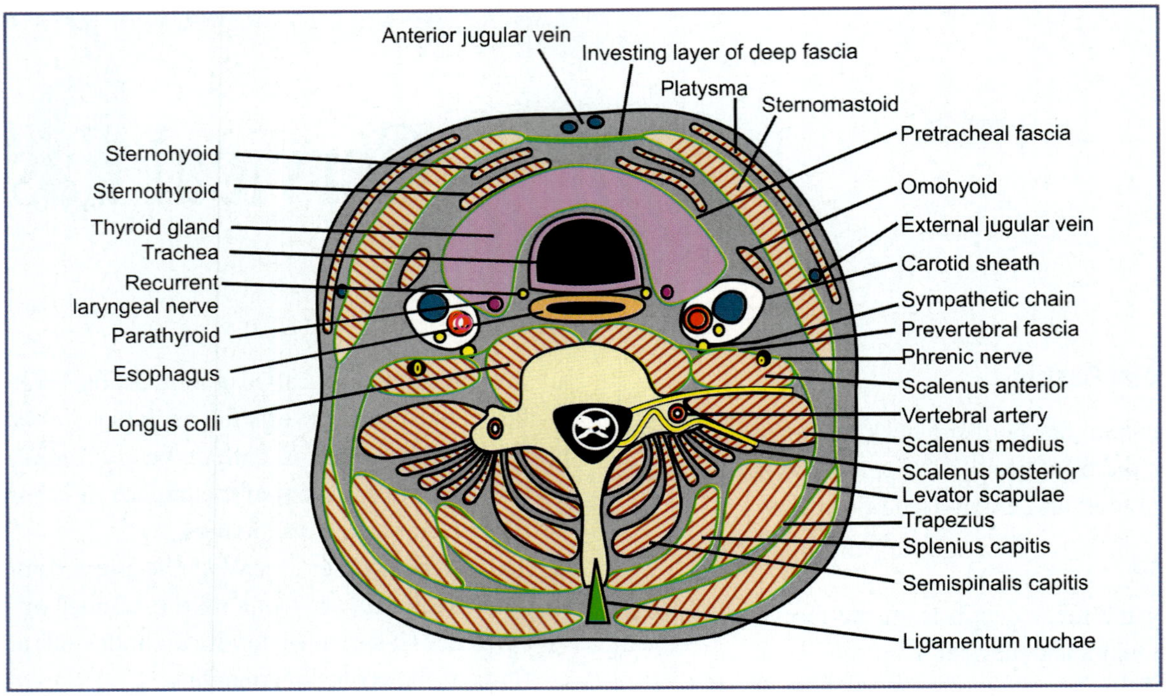

Fig. 64.1: Cross-section at the lower part of neck depicting disposition of layers of cervical fascia (Note: The ventral ramus of spinal nerve between scalenus anterior and medius on right side)

is attached to the base of the mandible and the deep layer is attached to the mylohyoid line of the mandible.

c. At the apex (lower end) of the parotid gland the fascia again splits in two layers to enclose the parotid gland. The superficial layer is very strong and is called parotidomasseteric fascia, which is attached to the zygomatic arch. The deep layer is attached to the styloid process and the lower surface of tympanic plate at the base of the skull. The part of the deep layer between the styloid process and the angle of the mandible is called the stylomandibular ligament and it separates the parotid from the submandibular gland. The upper attachment on the posterior aspect is linear, beginning at the external occipital protuberance and going laterally along the superior nuchal line to the mastoid process and the cartilaginous part of external acoustic meatus.

Lower attachment of the fascia is to the suprasternal notch of the manubrium sterni (Fig. 39.2), upper surface of clavicle and the acromion and spine of scapula. At its lower attachment the deep fascia splits twice to enclose two spaces, suprasternal and supraclavicular.

Suprasternal Space of Burns

This space is enclosed between the two layers of the investing fascia after it splits above the manubrium sterni. Its superficial layer is attached to the anterior border of suprasternal notch and the deep layer to the posterior margin. The space contains the sternal head of sternomastoid, the jugular venous arch connecting the anterior jugular veins, interclavicular ligament and occasional lymph node.

Supraclavicular Space

Above the middle third of the clavicle the fascia splits to form two layers, which attach to the anterior and posterior margins of the superior surface of the clavicle and enclose the supraclavicular space in the lower part of the roof of posterior triangle. The space contains the terminal part of external jugular vein and the supraclavicular nerves.

Attachments of Pretracheal Layer

a. Superiorly the pretracheal fascia is attached to the hyoid bone in the midline and to the oblique line of thyroid cartilage on each side.

b. Inferiorly (Fig. 39.2) it passes in front of the trachea and inferior thyroid veins and enters the superior mediastinum behind the suprasternal notch. Its lower end blends with the apex of the fibrous pericardium.
c. Laterally it covers the strap muscles and then forms the anterior wall of the carotid sheath, beyond which it merges with the loose fascia under the sternomastoid muscle.

Relation of Pretracheal Fascia to Thyroid Gland (Fig. 73.3)

The pretracheal fascia forms the false capsule for the thyroid gland. The ligament of Berry is the part of the fascia extending from the back of the thyroid lobe to the cricoid cartilage. The attachment of the pretracheal fascia to the cricoid and thyroid cartilages and the hyoid bone is responsible for movement of thyroid gland with deglutition.

Attachments of Prevertebral Fascia

This layer lies behind the pharynx and esophagus and in front of the prevertebral muscles.

a. Superiorly it is attached to the base of the cranium.
b. Inferiorly it enters the thorax through thoracic inlet and blends with the anterior longitudinal ligament on the front of the bodies of the upper three thoracic vertebrae.
c. Laterally it forms the posterior wall of the carotid sheath and passes in front of the scalenus anterior, scalenus medius and levator scapulae, splenius capitis and semispinalis capitis muscles. It then passes over the deep muscles of the back to reach the ligamentum nuchae (according to other view it merges with the fascia under the trapezius).

Relations of Prevertebral Fascia

The prevertebral fascia forms the fascial floor of the posterior triangle of the neck. Its relations are surgically important. The cervical plexus, phrenic nerve, brachial plexus, long thoracic nerve and dorsal scapular nerve, subclavian artery and scalene muscles lie behind the fascia. The sympathetic chain, carotid sheath and the subclavian vein are located in front of the fascia. The retropharyngeal space, pharynx and esophagus are in front

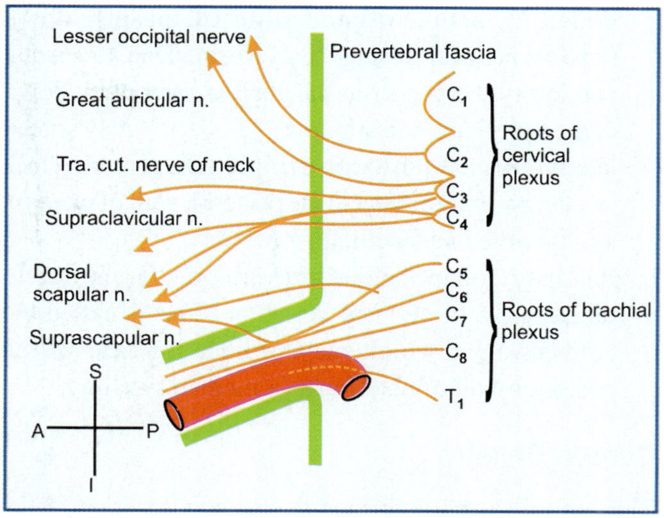

Fig. 64.2: Scheme to show some branches of cervical and brachial plexuses piercing prevertebral fascia (Note: The prolongation of prevertebral fascia around brachial plexus and subclavian artery as cervicoaxillary fascia)

of the fascia in the midline of the neck. In the interval between the scalenus anterior and medius the prevertebral fascia forms a tubular cervicoaxillary sheath around the brachial plexus and the subclavian artery. This sheath is carried into the axilla (Fig. 64.2).

Structures that Pierce Prevertebral Fascia (Figs 64.2 and 76.1)

a. The cutaneous branches of the cervical plexus (supraclavicular nerves, great auricular nerve, lesser occipital nerve and transverse cutaneous nerve of neck)
b. Suprascapular nerve and nerve to subclavius (from Erb's point)
c. Grey rami communicans from the sympathetic chain to the cervical spinal nerves.

Spaces in Relation to Prevertebral Fascia

a. Retropharyngeal space filled with loose areolar tissue lies in front of the prevertebral fascia and behind the pharynx and esophagus. It acts as a bursa for the pharynx to move. This extends inferiorly to the mediastinum. This space is divided in right and left parts by a midline fibrous septum that joins the prevertebral fascia to the buccopharyngeal fascia covering the pharynx. Each half of the space contains a few lymph nodes. In acute inflammation of these nodes a retropharyngeal abscess may form. Due to fascial continuity the pus from the abscess may track down in the superior mediastinum (Fig. 39.2). It may spread laterally in the posterior triangle and give rise to a swelling or may project in the posterior wall of pharynx as a paramedian swelling.

b. Pus may collect behind prevertebral fascia due to tuberculosis of cervical vertebrae. This is called the cold abscess, which may project forward in the posterior wall of pharynx as a median swelling.

Carotid Sheath

The carotid sheath is formed due to condensation of the deep cervical fascia. It encloses the carotid arteries, internal jugular vein and the vagus nerve and extends from the base of skull to the root of the neck. The lateral wall of the sheath is relatively thinner compared to the medial to allow for the expansion of the internal jugular vein. The pretracheal fascia fuses with its anterior wall and the prevertebral fascia lies in its posterior wall. The ansa cervicalis (C1, C2, C3) lies embedded in its anterior wall. The sympathetic trunk is closely related to its posterior wall. The deep cervical lymph nodes are embedded in the sheath. Therefore, during block dissection of the neck the carotid sheath is exposed for removal of the deep lymph nodes and the internal jugular vein.

Contents of Carotid Sheath (Fig. 66.3)

The carotid sheath contains the common carotid artery up to the upper border of thyroid cartilage and the internal carotid artery above this level. The internal jugular vein is present in the entire extent of the sheath in lateral relation to the arteries. The vagus nerve is present in the entire extent in posterior relation to the arteries and the vein. The superior and inferior cervical cardiac branches and the pharyngeal and superior laryngeal branches of vagus originate inside the sheath.

65 Posterior Triangle

The posterior triangle is an important region of the neck as it contains the supraclavicular part of the brachial plexus. It is in communication with the axilla via cervicoaxillary canal, which gives passage to the neurovascular structures from the posterior triangle to the axilla for onward transmission to the upper limb.

Boundaries (Fig. 65.1)

The posterior triangle of neck has anterior and posterior boundaries, base, fascial roof and muscular floor. The posterior margin of sternomastoid muscle forms its anterior boundary and the anterior margin of the trapezius muscle forms its posterior boundary. Middle third of the clavicle forms the base. The apex lies at the superior nuchal line of the occipital bone between the attachments of the trapezius and sternomastoid. The fascial roof of the triangle is the investing layer of deep fascia of neck.

Subdivisions

The inferior belly of omohyoid muscle divides the posterior triangle in a larger upper occipital triangle and a smaller lower subclavian or supraclavicular triangle. The inferior belly of omohyoid, sternomastoid and trapezius muscles bound the occipital triangle. The supraclavicular triangle is bounded by inferior belly of omohyoid, sternomastoid and middle third of clavicle. The surface anatomy of this triangle is the lower part of the hollow above the clavicle known as greater supraclavicular fossa (which is also known by a fancy name—the saltcellar).

Muscular Floor

For general purposes it is accepted that the muscular floor consists mainly of three muscles, from above downward, splenius capitis, levator scapulae and scalenus medius.

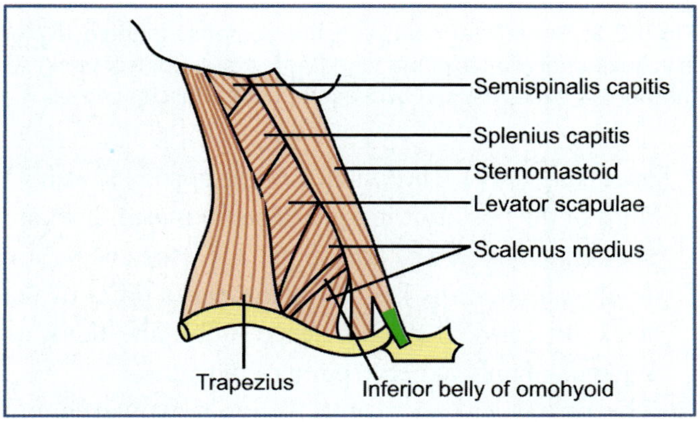

Fig. 65.1: Boundaries of posterior triangle of neck and muscles in its floor

Occasionally above the splenius capitis vertically oriented semispinalis capitis is also seen (Fig. 65.1). Alternate way to describe the floor is to divide it according to the two triangles. In the occipital triangle floor consists of, from above downward, splenius capitis (occasionally preceded by semispinalis capitis), levator scapulae and scalenus medius muscles. In the supraclavicular triangle, besides scalenus medius, the first rib and first digitation of serratus anterior muscle are included in the floor. The prevertebral layer of deep cervical fascia covers the muscular floor like a carpet. The first rib and the first digitation of the serratus anterior are not covered with prevertebral fascia.

Superficial Contents (Fig. 65.2)

a. The cutaneous branches of the cervical plexus enter the posterior triangle by piercing the prevertebral fascia around the midpoint of the posterior border of the sternomastoid. The cutaneous nerves are, great auricular, lesser occipital, transverse cervical nerve and medial, intermediate and lateral supraclavicular nerves. The lesser occipital nerve hooks the spinal

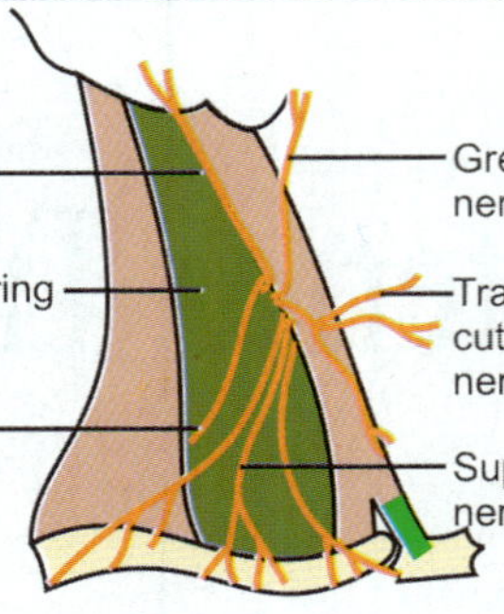

Fig. 65.2: Superficial nerves inside posterior triangle (Note: The seven nerves bunching together at nerve point of neck. All the nerves except spinal accessory, pierce fascial carpet)

accessory nerve. The junction of the upper and middle third of the posterior margin of sternomastoid, where six cutaneous nerves and spinal accessory nerve are in close relation is known as the nerve point of the neck. In cervical plexus nerve block anesthetic is injected mainly at nerve point of the neck.

b. The spinal accessory nerve runs downwards and laterally lying in intimate relation to the fascial roof but between the roof and floor. It leaves the triangle by entering the anterior margin of trapezius 5 cm above the clavicle. The spinal accessory nerve takes origin by rootlets from the anterior horn cells of the C1 to C5 segments of the spinal cord. The rootlets join in the cervical vertebral canal to form the nerve trunk, which enters the cranium through the foramen magnum. The spinal part joins the cranial part of the accessory nerve in the posterior cranial fossa to form the accessory or the eleventh cranial nerve. This nerve leaves the cranium via the jugular foramen. Immediately after the exit it divides in cranial and spinal parts. The spinal part crosses in front of the tip of the transverse process of the atlas and descends laterally deep to the posterior belly of digastric to enter the carotid triangle and then into the substance of the sternomastoid muscle. As it enters the posterior triangle, it is hooked by the lesser occipital nerve. Since, it is superficially placed in the triangle, it is vulnerable to injury. It supplies the sternomastoid and the trapezius muscles.

The surface marking of the accessory nerve is as follows. Draw a line from a point in front of the tragus of ear to a point midway between mastoid process and the angle of the mandible (this point coincides with transverse process of atlas). From here carry the line to the midpoint of the posterior margin of the sternomastoid muscle and further downward to a point on the anterior margin of the trapezius about 5 cm above the clavicle.

c. Branches of C3 and C4 ventral rami cross the triangle along with spinal accessory to supply proprioceptive fibers to the trapezius muscle.

Deeper Contents (Fig. 65.3)

a. The supraclavicular part of brachial plexus trunk stage of the plexus and few branches of the supraclavicular plexus) is located in the supraclavicular triangle. The upper trunk gives off suprascapular nerve and the nerve to subclavius. The accessory phrenic nerve (carrying C5 fibers from nerve to subclavius to the phrenic nerve) may be present occasionally. The branches from the root stage of brachial plexus (long thoracic nerve and dorsal scapular nerve) enter the posterior triangle. The dorsal scapular nerve (from C5 root) pierces the scalenus medius to appear at its lateral margin and then it descends lying in front of the levator scapulae muscle. It leaves the occipital triangle behind the anterior margin of the trapezius. The upper two roots of the long thoracic nerve pierce the scalenus medius and unite on its surface to form the long thoracic nerve, which descends on the anterior surface of the scalenus medius. The nerve enters the axilla through the cervicoaxillary canal. Its lowest root from C7 joins the long thoracic nerve in the axilla.

The trunks of the brachial plexus are close to the surface in the supraclavicular triangle as the skin, platysma and the investing layer of deep fascia only cover them. The structures crossing in front of the trunks are, inferior belly of omohyoid, the external jugular vein, transverse cervical artery and the supraclavicular nerves. The upper and middle trunks lie above the subclavian artery but the lower trunk lies posterior to it. The brachial plexus and the subclavian artery are enclosed in the cervicoaxillary fascia, which is the extension of the prevertebral fascia. The subclavian vein is outside the fascial sheath.

b. The suprascapular and transverse cervical arteries are the branches of the thyrocervical trunk from the first

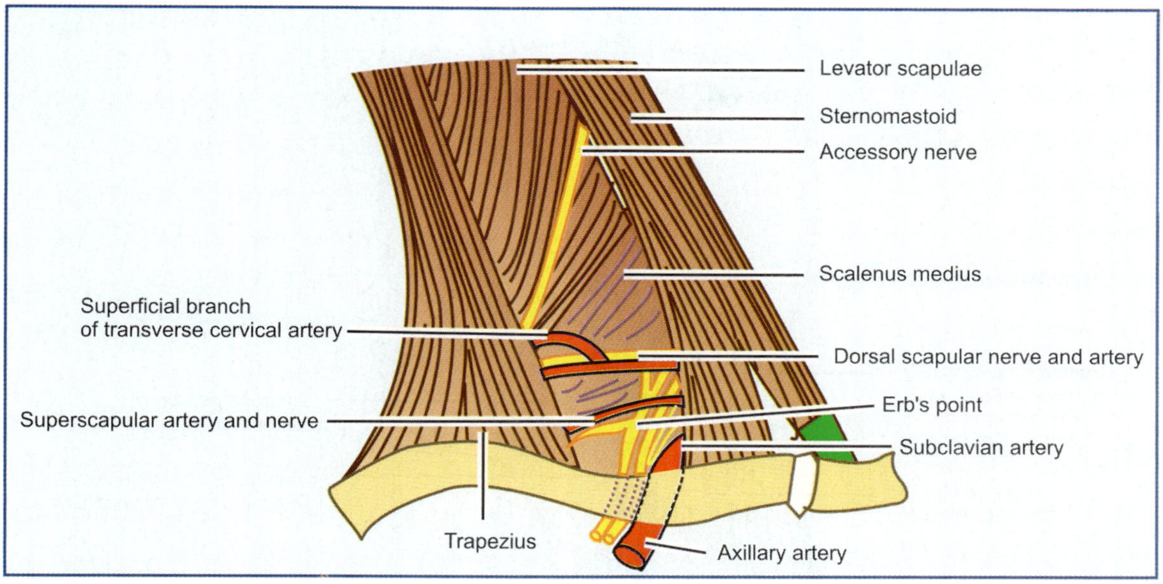

Fig. 65.3: Deeper contents of lower part of posterior triangle. The external jugular vein with its tributaries and inferior belly of omohyoid have been removed for better exposure of the contents (Note: The trunks of the brachial plexus and branches of subclavian artery. The origin of suprascapular nerve and nerve to subclavius from Erb's point. Long thoracic nerve is not shown)

part of subclavian artery. They turn in lateral direction to enter the posterior triangle, where the suprascapular artery accompanies the suprascapular nerve. The superficial branch of the transverse cervical artery accompanies the spinal accessory nerve and the deep branch of the same artery accompanies the dorsal scapular nerve (sometimes the dorsal scapular branch of the third part of subclavian artery replaces the deep branch of transverse cervical artery).

c. The third part of the subclavian artery and the subclavian vein are the contents of lowest part of the triangle.
d. The terminal part of the external jugular vein after piercing the fascial roof enters the supraclavicular triangle to open into the subclavian vein.
e. Occipital artery, which is a branch of external carotid artery, runs a part of its course near the apex of the posterior triangle.
f. A few cervical lymph nodes, belonging to superficial group, lie close to the accessory nerve along the posterior margin of the sternomastoid. The supraclavicular lymph nodes belonging to the inferior deep cervical group lie in the supraclavicular triangle in close relation to the posterior margin of the sternomastoid muscle.

External Jugular Vein (Fig. 65.4)

The external jugular vein is formed just behind the angle of the mandible by the union of the posterior auricular vein and the posterior division of the retromandibular vein. It runs in the superficial fascia on the surface of the sternomastoid muscle and so it is a very visible vein. It crosses the sternomastoid muscle from medial to lateral side to reach its posterior margin and enters the superficial fascia of the roof of the posterior triangle. It travels downwards to the supraclavicular triangle, where it pierces the fascial roof about 2 to 3 cm above the clavicle at the posterior margin of sternomastoid. One noteworthy feature is that the wall of the vein is adherent to the fascia, where it pierces the deep fascia. If the vein is cut at this point, it cannot close due to the traction exerted by the attached fascia. So the vein is exposed to the atmosphere, which may cause fatal venous air embolism unless the cut end is occluded immediately. The vein runs for a short distance in the supraclavicular triangle before opening in the subclavian vein behind the clavicle along the margin of the sternomastoid. There are valves at its termination and at about 4 cm above the clavicle. Though the external jugular vein can easily serve as a venous manometer to assess pressure in right side of the heart yet in clinical

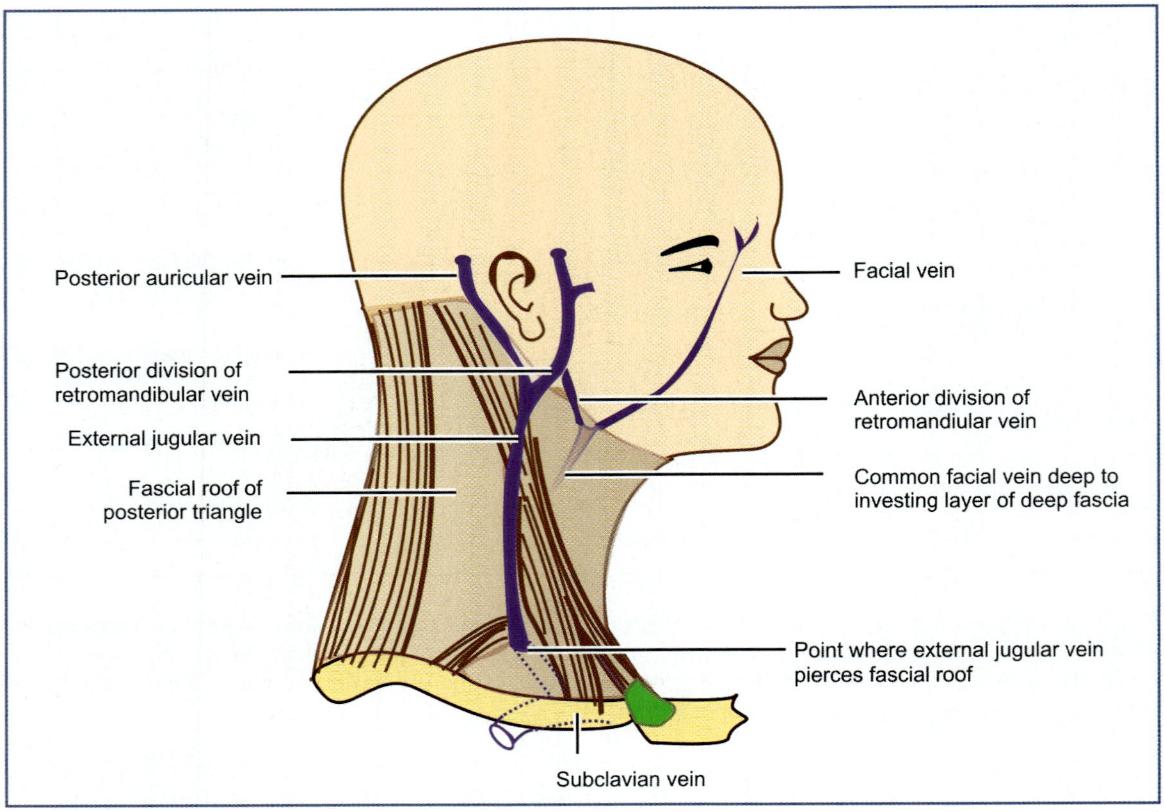

Fig. 65.4: Formation and termination of external jugular vein
(Note that EJV enters the supraclavicular triangle to terminate into subclavian vein)

practice it is the internal jugular vein that is used for this purpose. There are two reasons for not using the external jugular vein, it has valves at two places and it passes through the deep fascia, which makes it liable to external compression.

Tributaries

Apart from its formative tributaries, the external jugular vein receives, transverse cervical vein, suprascapular vein, anterior jugular vein and the veins that drain the posterior part of the scalp and neck. Sometimes a communicating vein (running across the clavicle) from the cephalic vein joins the external jugular vein. To sum up, the external jugular vein drains blood from wide areas, which include scalp, parts of face, neck and back, and some deeper parts as well.

Surface Marking

The external jugular vein is often visible in the living. It can be made more visible by blowing through the mouth against resistance or by applying digital pressure in the supraclavicular triangle gently. However a line joining two points corresponding to its upper and lower ends represents the vein. The upper point is just below and behind the angle of mandible and the lower point is deep to the clavicle just behind the margin of the sternomastoid.

Clinical Highlights of Supraclavicular Triangle

The supraclavicular triangle is important in the clinical examination of a patient. This region is inspected from the front but palpated from behind.

a. The trunks of the brachial plexus can be felt on deep palpation behind and just above the middle third of the clavicle. For brachial plexus block the anesthetic agent is injected around the trunks just above the midpoint of clavicle. Injuries to the trunks of the brachial plexus are commonly due to trauma at birth or due to motorcycle accidents or stab wounds. Injury to the upper trunk causes Erb's palsy and injury to the lower trunk results in Klumpke's palsy.

b. The supraclavicular lymph nodes are palpated here (Fig. 65.5). The left supraclavicular nodes are enlarged in cancer of the stomach colon and testis. These nodes are called Virchow's nodes. If the left supraclavicular lymph nodes are enlarged in cancer of stomach it is called Troisier's sign. The cancer of the lung or breast spreads to the supraclavicular nodes of the side of the lesion.

c. The subclavian vein at this site is often used for central venous access. Through the central venous catheter it is safe to give powerful drugs and it can also be used for long-term feeding in a serious patient (specially when all the peripheral veins are thrombosed or collapsed).

d. The pulsations of the subclavian artery can be felt on deep pressure behind the middle third of the clavicle. The bleeding due to severe lacerations of the brachial or axillary artery can be controlled by compressing the third part of the subclavian artery downward and backward against upper surface of the first rib.

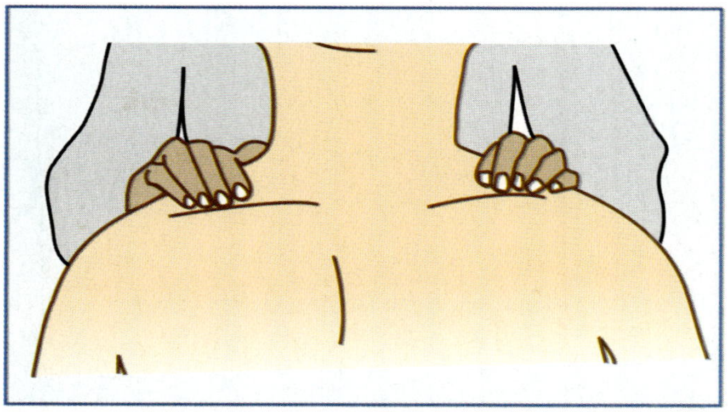

Fig. 65.5: Palpation of supraclavicular lymph nodes from behind

66 Midline Region of Neck

The median region of the front of neck extends from the chin to the suprasternal notch. It is divided in suprahyoid and infrahyoid regions. The suprahyoid region contains the submental triangle (Fig. 66.1). The infrahyoid region contains the bilateral muscular triangles and the midline structures. The identification of the midline structures is essential during the operation of tracheostomy. It is also useful in clinical examination of the midline swellings in the neck.

Suprahyoid Region

a. The superficial fascia in the suprahyoid region contains the submental lymph nodes. The anterior jugular veins begin here by the union of several small superficial veins. The anterior jugular veins run down close to the midline and enter the suprasternal space, where they unite with each other by a transverse connection called the jugular arch. Each vein turns laterally and passes deep to the sternomastoid muscle

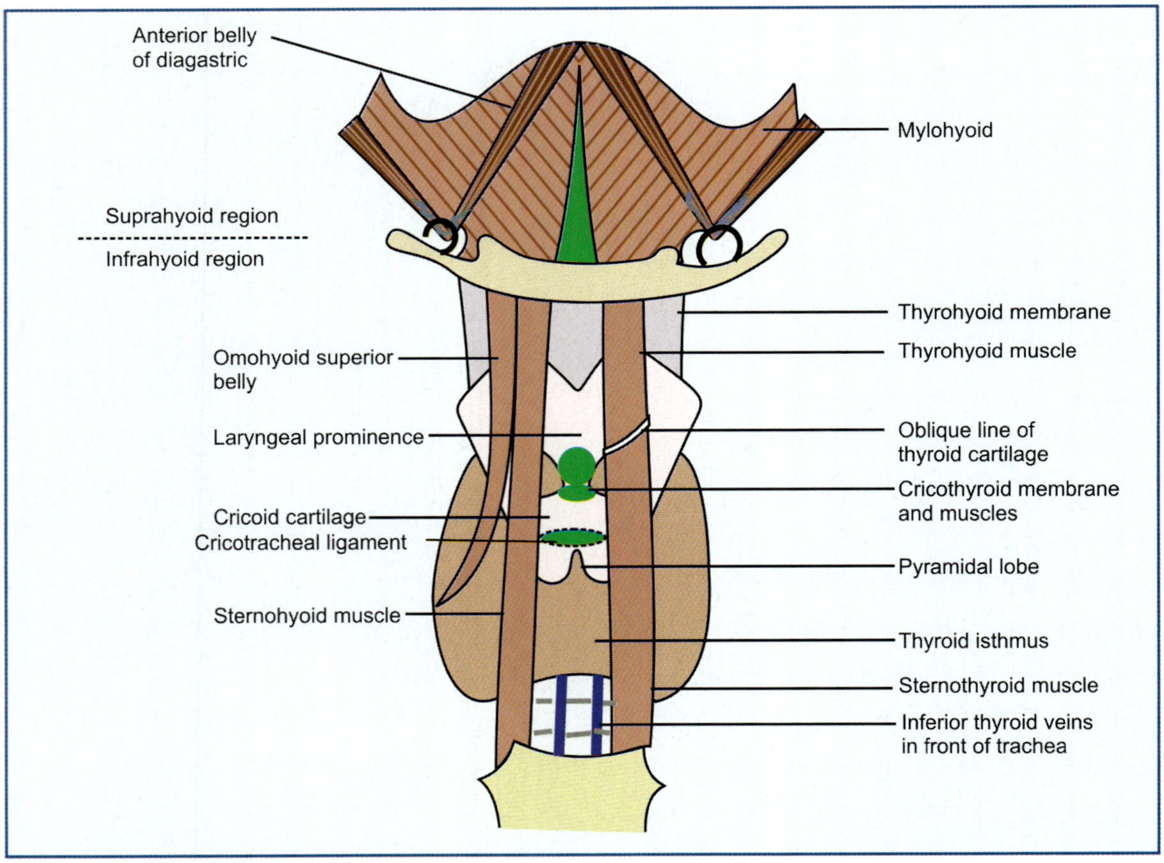

Fig. 66.1: Structures in the median region in anterior part of neck
(Note that left sternohyoid has been removed to expose the attachments of sternothyroid and thyrohyoid muscles)

to reach the base of the posterior triangle, where it opens in the external jugular vein.

b. The anterior bellies of the digastric muscles and the hyoid bone bound the submental triangle in the suprahyoid region. The floor of the triangle is formed by mylohyoid muscle of both sides. The right and left mylohyoid muscles together form the oral diaphragm by joining at the midline raphe.

Infrahyoid Region

The following structures are found in this region from above downwards (Fig. 66.2):

a. The body of the hyoid bone is palpable despite the fact that the hyoid bone gives attachment to a number of muscles and ligaments. The hyoid is located 1 cm below and six cm behind the chin and is highly mobile. Its vertebral level is C3.
b. The thyrohyoid membrane extends from the upper margin of the thyroid cartilage and passes deep to the body of hyoid bone to get attached to its upper margin. Its median part is called median thyrohyoid ligament, which is separated from the hyoid by a bursa. Internal laryngeal nerve and superior laryngeal vessels pierce the thyrohyoid membrane.
c. Laryngeal prominence (Adam's apple in male) can be palpated and seen in the midline. The upper border of thyroid cartilage corresponds to C4 vertebra and the lower border to C5 vertebra.
d. The cricoid cartilage is at the level of sixth cervical vertebra. Its anterior arch is palpable in the midline. Cricothyroid membrane or ligament extends between the arch of the cricoid and the thyroid cartilage. The cricothyroid branch of the superior thyroid artery runs across this membrane to anastomose with its counterpart. The cricothyroid muscle lies on the cricothyroid membrane on each side. This muscle is exceptional in that it is the only intrinsic muscle of the larynx, which lies on the external aspect of the larynx. At the lower end of cricoid cartilage the larynx continues as the trachea.
e. The first tracheal ring is palpable below the lower margin of cricoid arch.
f. The isthmus of the thyroid gland lies in front of the second to fourth (or second to third) tracheal rings. At times a small pyramidal lobe projects up from the isthmus and it may give rise to a slender slip of muscle called lavator glandulae thyroidae or a fibrous band, which attaches the isthmus to the hyoid bone. The

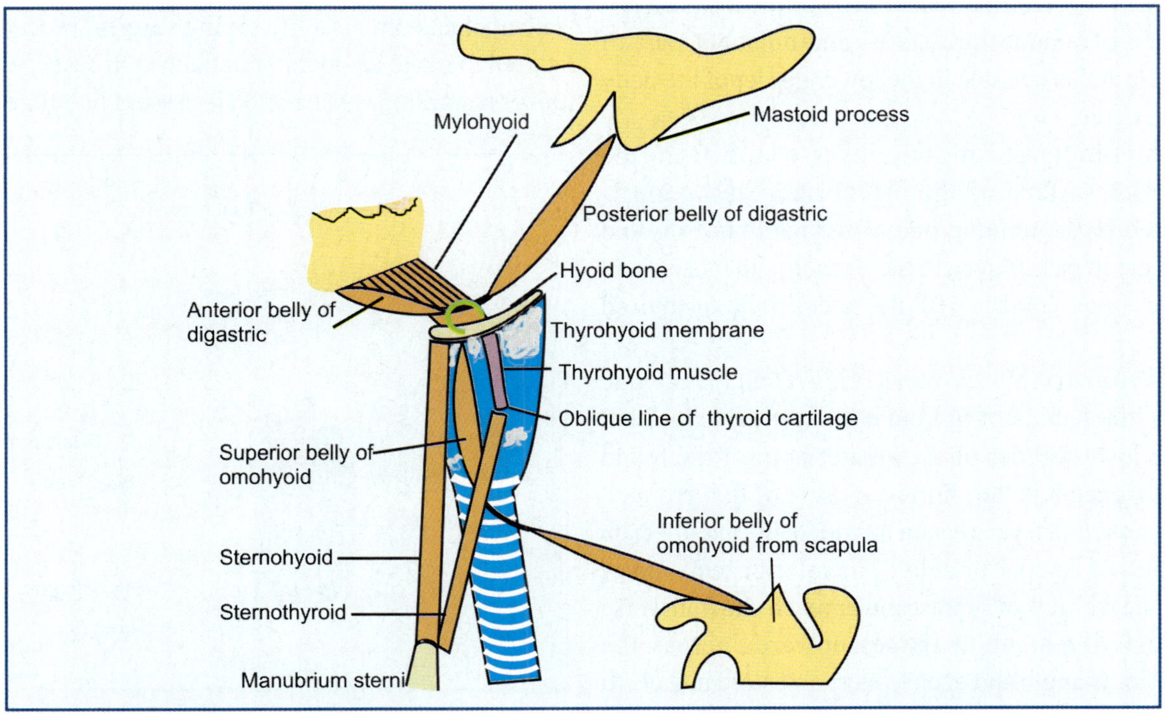

Fig. 66.2: Scheme to depict bony attachments of suprahyoid and infrahyoid muscles

pyramidal lobe and the levator glandulae thyroidae are remnants of the embryological thyroglossal duct. Along the superior margin of the isthmus there is a rich anastomosis between the terminal parts of the anterior branches of superior thyroid arteries.

g. The lateral lobes of the thyroid gland lie on the lateral aspects of trachea. Below the isthmus the anterior aspect of trachea is related to the inferior thyroid veins and thyroidea ima artery (if present). The trachea is deeply placed below the level of isthmus.

h. The suprasternal space of Burns with its contents (jugular venous arch, sternal head of sternomastoid, occasional lymph nodes and interclavicular ligament) is the lowest among the midline structures.

Infrahyoid or Strap Muscles (Fig. 66.2)

These muscles are called the ribbon muscles due to their shape. They are also called pretracheal muscles because of their position in front of the trachea. There are four muscles in this group. The sternohyoid, sternothyroid and thyrohyoid muscles form the floor of the muscular triangle and they cover the trachea, larynx, thyroid gland and thyrohyoid membrane. The superior belly of the omohyoid forms the lateral margin of the muscular triangle.

a. The sternohyoid muscle takes origin from the posterior surface of manubrium sterni and adjacent part of clavicle and is inserted in the lower border of the body of the hyoid.

b. The sternothyroid muscle takes origin from the posterior surface of the manubrium sterni and is inserted in the oblique line of the lamina of thyroid cartilage. It passes deep to the sternohyoid muscle and lies in direct contact with the lateral lobe of thyroid gland.

c. The thyrohyoid muscle takes origin from the oblique line of the lamina of thyroid cartilage and is inserted in the lower border of the greater horn of the hyoid bone. Hence it is the shortest muscle of this group.

d. The omohyoid muscle has an inferior belly, intermediate tendon and a superior belly. The inferior belly arises from the margins of suprascapular notch and transverse scapular ligament. It passes upwards across the posterior triangle and deep to sternomastoid muscle to terminate in a tendon, which is strapped down to the clavicle by the deep fascia. The superior belly takes origin from the intermediate tendon and passes vertically across the anterior triangle for insertion in the lower border of the body of the hyoid bone.

Nerve Supply of Strap Muscles (Fig. 66.3)

The ansa cervicalis is a loop-shaped nerve plexus with the root value of C1, C2 and C3. The C1 fibers from the hypoglossal nerve form the superior limb or descendes hypoglossi. The C2 and C3 fibers from the cervical plexus form the inferior root or descendes cervicalis. The two roots are joined by a loop called ansa. The loop is plastered to the anterior wall of the carotid sheath. The branches to sternohyoid, sternothyroid and inferior belly of omohyoid muscles arise from the loop. The branch from the superior limb of the ansa supplies the superior belly of omohyoid. The thyrohyoid nerve, a direct branch of the hypoglossal nerve carrying C1 fibers, supplies the thyrohyoid muscle.

Actions

The strap muscles move the larynx and hyoid during speech and swallowing. They depress the hyoid bone or fix it when acting with suprahyoid muscles.

Clinical Highlights

The tracheostomy is a life saving surgical procedure that is used to make an opening in trachea in cases, where the upper respiratory obstruction is present like for example,

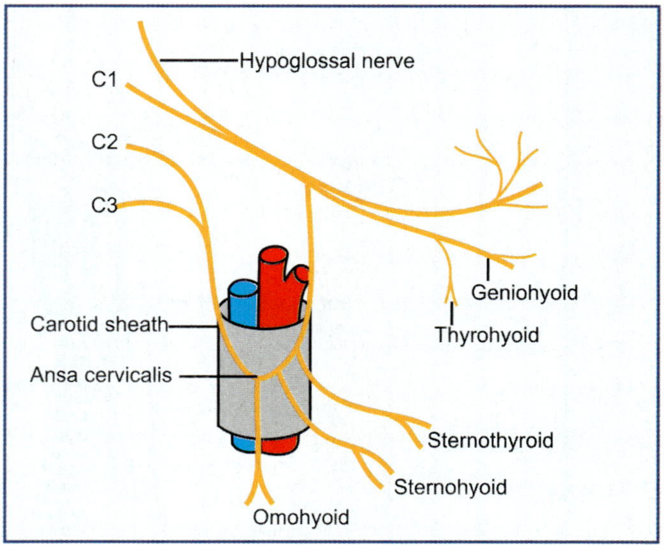

Fig. 66.3: Nerve supply of strap muscles (Note that ansa cervicalis is plastered to anterior wall of carotid sheath)

in impaction of foreign body in the larynx or laryngeal edema. Sound knowledge of the anatomy of the midline structures is essential to perform this operation. Depending on the level of the opening in relation to isthmus of thyroid gland the tracheostomy is either high or low. In high tracheostomy the incision is placed above the isthmus in the first tracheal ring. This is relatively dangerous procedure as one is likely to enter laryngeal cavity due to injury to adjacent cricoid cartilage with subsequent stenosis or narrowing of lower end of larynx. Hence low tracheostomy through second to fourth tracheal rings is preferred.

Steps in Low Tracheostomy

a. The head of the patient is kept in the extended position by keeping a pillow under the shoulders. This position brings the trachea forwards. The skin incision can either be vertical or transverse. The vertical incision is placed from the level of cricoid cartilage for 2.5 to 3.5 cm downward exactly in the midline. A 5 cm long transverse incision is placed 2 fingers breadth above the sternal notch.
b. The incision is deepened to cut in succession the superficial fascia with platysma, investing layer of deep fascia and the pretracheal fascia.
c. The interval between the right and left sternohyoid muscles is opened up and the sternothyroid muscles are retracted.
d. Isthmus of the thyroid gland is identified and retracted upward (and not cut so as to avoid bleeding from the highly vascular isthmus).
e. A vertical incision is placed in the second to fourth tracheal rings and an endotracheal tube is inserted through the opening in the trachea.

67 Carotid Triangle

The carotid triangle is so called because all the three carotid arteries (common, external and internal) are present inside it and moreover the carotid arteries are very superficial here. In the living person the triangle is visible as small depression anterior to sternomastoid muscle and behind the hyoid bone.

Boundaries of Carotid Triangle (Fig. 67.1)

The carotid triangle presents three boundaries (anterosuperior, anteroinferior and posterior), floor and roof.

The anterosuperior boundary is formed by posterior belly of digastric and the stylohyoid muscles. The anteroinferior boundary is formed by superior belly of omohyoid muscle. The posterior boundary is formed by anterior margin of the sternomastoid muscle. The floor consists of parts of four muscles, hyoglossus and thyrohyoid anteriorly and middle and inferior constrictors of the pharynx posteriorly. The roof consists of the skin, superficial fascia with platysma and the investing layer of deep fascia of neck. The hyoid bone is located at its anterior angle.

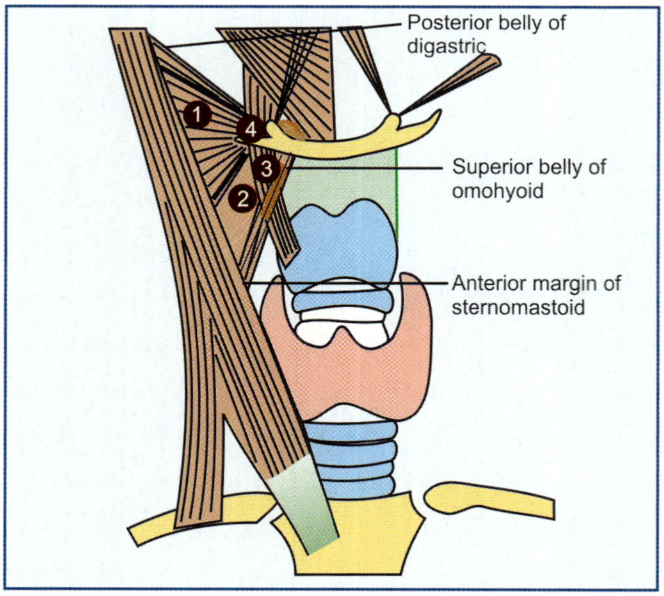

Fig. 67.1: Schematic diagram depicting boundaries of carotid triangle (Note: The muscles in the floor 1. Middle constrictor, 2. Inferior constrictor, 3. Thyrohyoid, 4. Hyoglossus)

Contents (Fig. 67.2)

a. The bifurcation of the common carotid artery into internal and external carotid arteries takes place at the level of upper margin of thyroid cartilage. The

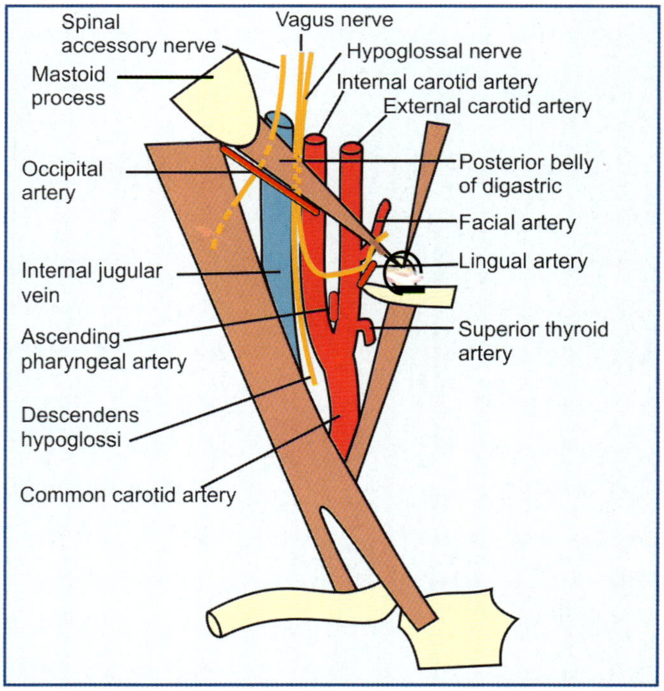

Fig. 67.2: Contents of carotid triangle (Note: Bifurcation of common carotid artery and 5 branches of external carotid artery)

internal carotid artery is posterolateral to the external carotid artery in the triangle. The external carotid artery gives five of its branches here (see below). At the bifurcation the common carotid artery including the adjacent internal carotid artery show a small dilatation called carotid sinus, which is supplied by the sinus branch of glossopharyngeal nerve. It is a baroreceptor for controlling intracranial blood pressure. The carotid body is a small neurovascular structure situated close to posterior wall of the carotid sinus. It acts as a chemoreceptor controlling the oxygen tension within the artery.

b. The internal jugular vein passes through the carotid sheath lying in lateral position compared to the common carotid and the internal carotid arteries. It receives tributaries corresponding to the branches of the external carotid artery.
c. The vagus nerve passes vertically downward in posterior position inside the carotid sheath. It gives superior laryngeal nerve, which divides in internal and external laryngeal nerves here. The spinal accessory nerve crosses the superolateral angle to enter the sternomastoid muscle. The hypoglossal nerve enters the triangle deep to the posterior belly of digastric between the internal jugular vein and internal carotid artery. It crosses superficial to internal and external carotid arteries and the loop of the lingual artery from lateral to medial side. Inside the triangle the hypoglossal nerve gives off superior root of ansa cervicalis and a branch to thyrohyoid. The ansa cervicalis is formed in the anterior wall of the carotid sheath. The cervical sympathetic chain extends vertically posterior to the carotid sheath and in front of the prevertebral fascia.
d. The jugulo-digastric and jugulo-omohyoid lymph nodes are located in the vicinity of the internal jugular vein.

Carotid Pulse

The carotid triangle contains a large number of arteries (three carotid arteries and five branches of external carotid artery) because of which a massive arterial pulsation is felt here to a palpating finger and hence is the preferred site for taking carotid pulse (Fig. 67.3). The carotid pulse is palpable just lateral to the upper margin of thyroid cartilage.

Branches of External Carotid Artery (Fig. 67.2)

a. The ascending pharyngeal artery is the first branch of external carotid artery. It ascends between the internal carotid artery and the wall of the pharynx
b. The superior thyroid artery is the first anterior branch of the external carotid artery. It gives infrahyoid, superior laryngeal and sternomastoid branches in the triangle. The superior laryngeal artery accompanied by internal laryngeal nerve enters the larynx by piercing the thyrohyoid membrane. The superior thyroid artery leaves the triangle by descending deep to the superior belly of omohyoid towards thyroid gland.
c. The lingual artery arises from the anterior aspect behind the tip of the greater horn of the hyoid. It forms a loop around the greater horn of the hyoid. The loop of the lingual artery is crossed by the hypoglossal nerve. The lingual artery passes deep to the hyoglossus.
d. The facial artery arises from the anterior aspect just above the origin of lingual artery. It leaves the triangle by passing deep to the posterior belly of digastric to enter the digastric triangle.
e. The occipital artery takes origin at the level of facial artery. It passes backward and upward under cover of the posterior belly of digastric. It gives off upper and lower sternomastoid branches.

Internal Jugular Vein

This vein is located lateral to the carotid arteries in the carotid sheath. In the carotid triangle it receives superior thyroid vein, common facial and lingual veins.

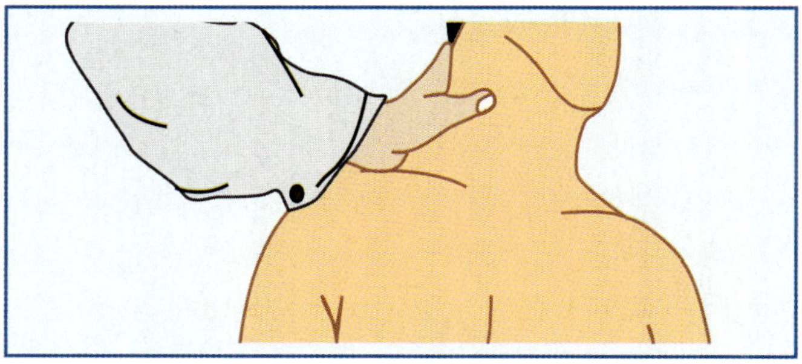

Fig. 67.3: Site of palpation of carotid pulse

Nerves in the Triangle

a. The spinal part of the accessory nerve crosses the posterosuperior angle of the carotid triangle to enter the sternomastoid muscle.

b. The hypoglossal nerve descends at first lying between the internal carotid artery and internal jugular vein. Then it crosses the internal and external carotid arteries and the loop of the lingual artery superficially to disappear under the intermediate tendon of digastric muscle. In the carotid triangle the hypoglossal nerve gives two branches, superior root of the ansa cervicalis and the thyrohyoid branch, both of which carry the C1 fibers.

c. The ansa cervicalis is formed by the union of the superior and inferior limbs or roots in the anterior wall of the carotid sheath (Fig. 66.3) in the triangle. The inferior root of the ansa cervicalis from the C2 and C3 ventral rami descends along the lateral surface of the internal jugular vein.

d. The vagus nerve runs down inside the carotid sheath lying on a posterior plane in between the internal jugular vein laterally and carotid arteries (either the common or internal carotid artery) medially. In the carotid triangle it gives rise to pharyngeal and superior laryngeal branches. The superior laryngeal branch divides into the internal and external laryngeal nerves.

e. The cervical sympathetic trunk lies embedded in the posterior wall of the carotid sheath.

Deep Cervical Lymph Nodes

A chain of deep cervical lymph nodes lies in intimate relation to the internal jugular vein. The jugulo-digastric nodes lie above the posterior belly of digastric and jugulo-omohyoid below it. Painless enlargement of these nodes due to tuberculosis is quite common. Some times the affected lymph nodes liquefy due to degeneration and form a cold abscess. The pus remains confined deep to the investing layer of deep fascia. But eventually the deep fascia is eroded at one point and the pus flows in the superficial fascia-giving rise to collar-stud abscess.

68 Digastric Triangle

The digastric triangle is the superficial part of the submandibular region.

Boundaries (Fig. 68.1)

The anterior belly of digastric muscle forms its anteroinferior boundary and the posterior belly of digastric muscle and stylohyoid muscle form the posteroinferior boundary. Superior boundary is the base of the mandible and an imaginary line from the angle of mandible to the tip of mastoid process. The mylohyoid and hyoglossus muscles and anterior part of the middle constrictor are in the roof (referred to as floor by many authors). The skin, superficial fascia (including platysma) and the deep fascia form the floor (referred to as roof by many authors). The superficial fascia contains the cervical branch of facial nerve and cutaneous branches of transverse cervical nerve.

Subdivisions of Triangle

The digastric triangle is subdivided in anterior and posterior parts, which have different contents.

Contents of Anterior Part

The superficial lobe of submandibular salivary gland completely fills the triangle. The submandibular lymph

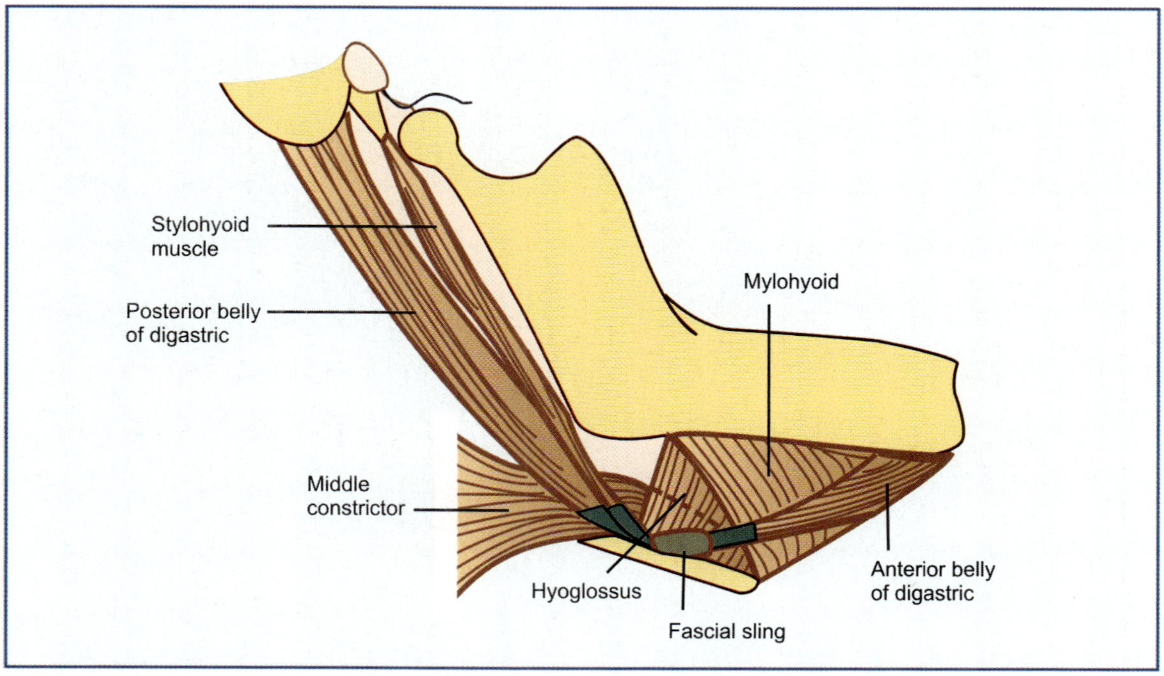

Fig. 68.1: Simplified scheme to depict the boundaries of digastric triangle (Note: The muscles in the floor)

nodes are embedded in the superficial surface of the salivary gland. The facial artery and its cervical branches are intimately related to the salivary gland. The formation of common facial vein takes place in the triangle. The mylohyoid nerve enters the triangle and supplies the anterior belly of digastric and mylohyoid muscles. The hypoglossal nerve accompanied by lingual veins passes superficial to the hyoglossus to reach the tongue.

Contents of Posterior Part

The posterior part of the digastric triangle lies behind the ramus of the mandible. It contains the lower part of the parotid gland, external carotid artery and the carotid sheath with its contents, glossopharyngeal nerve and the three muscles attached to the styloid process (stylohyoid, styloglossus and stylopharyngeus).

69 Submandibular Region

The submandibular region is located between the body of mandible and the hyoid bone. Its superficial parts include submental and digastric triangles and their contents. Its deeper part includes the deep part of the submandibular gland, the submandibular duct, sublingual gland with its ducts and the hypoglossal nerve and lingual artery. The lingual nerve enters the region from the infratemporal fossa while the glossopharyngeal nerve enters the posterior end from the posterior part of the digastric triangle. The hypoglossal nerve, glossopharyngeal nerve, lingual nerve and lingual artery pass through the submandibular region to reach the root of the tongue. The hyoglossus is the key muscle of this region.

Digastric Muscle (Fig. 69.1)

The digastric muscle consists of two bellies joined by an intermediate tendon giving it a V-shape. The anterior belly takes origin from the digastric fossa of the mandible and the posterior belly originates from the digastric groove on the medial aspect of the mastoid process. The intermediate tendon is attached to the junction of body and greater horn of hyoid bone by a fibrous sling.

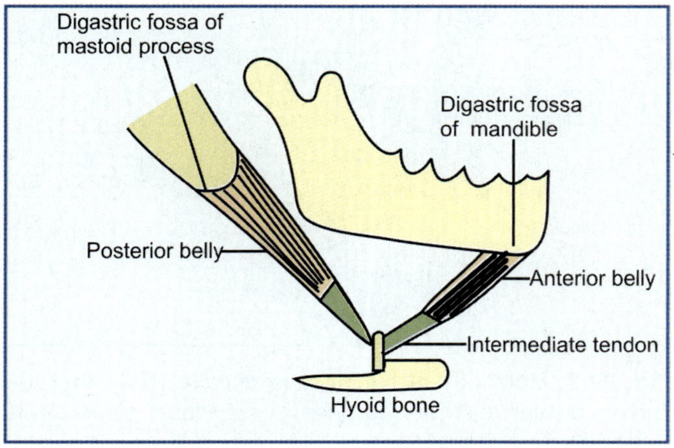

Fig. 69.1: Attachments of digastric muscle

Development and Nerve Supply

a. The posterior belly of digastric muscle develops from the mesoderm of second branchial arch hence it is supplied by the facial nerve.
b. The anterior belly develops from the mesoderm of first branchial arch and hence is supplied by the nerve to mylohyoid, which is a branch of inferior alveolar nerve (from mandibular).

Actions

The digastric muscle causes the depression and retraction of the mandible (assists in opening the mouth). It causes elevation of hyoid (assists in deglutition).

Relations of the Posterior Belly

The digastric muscle has numerous relations since it forms the boundary of both the digastric and carotid triangles of the neck.

a. The superficial structures that come in relation to the muscle are, retromandibular vein, common facial vein, great auricular nerve and cervical and marginal mandibular branches of facial nerve. The mastoid process and parotid salivary gland are its superficial relations posteriorly. The sternomastoid covers it and the submandibular salivary gland lies superficial to it in the anterior part.
b. Its deep relations (Fig. 67.2) are the three great vessels of the neck, internal jugular vein, internal and external carotid arteries. The hypoglossal, vagus and spinal accessory nerves pass deep to it high up in the neck. The hypoglossal nerve passes deep to the posterior belly at the level of angle of the mandible to enter the carotid triangle. But it again passes deep to the intermediate tendon to enter the digastric triangle.

c. The stylohyoid muscle is closely related to the upper border of the posterior belly near the base of skull. The facial nerve lies between the stylohyoid and the posterior belly at its exit from the stylomastoid foramen.
d. The occipital artery leaves the carotid triangle by passing upwards along the lower margin of the posterior belly.

Relations of Anterior Belly

This muscle forms the boundary of the submental and submandibular triangles. In the suprahyoid region it is related to the mylohyoid muscle.

Stylohyoid Muscle

This is a small muscle, which arises from the styloid process of the temporal bone and passes along the upper border of the posterior belly of digastric to reach its insertion at the hyoid bone. It receives its nerve supply from the facial nerve as soon as the exit of the nerve from the stylomastoid foramen. Its action is to draw the hyoid bone upward and backward.

Hyoglossus Muscle (Fig. 69. 2)

This is the extrinsic muscle of the tongue but forms a key muscle of the submandibular region due to its numerous relations. It is a quadrate muscle taking origin from the upper surface of the greater horn and body of the hyoid bone. It passes upwards partially covered with the mylohyoid on the superficial aspect and partially covering the genioglossus on the deep aspect, for insertion in the side of the root of the tongue.

Relations

a. The superficial or lateral surface is related to the mylohyoid muscle in its anterosuperior part. The rest of the superficial surface is related to the following important structures from above downward, the lingual nerve, submandibular ganglion, deep part of submandibular gland with the submandibular duct and the hypoglossal nerve with accompanying veins. These structures and the hyoglossus are related to the medial surface of the submandibular gland.
b. The deep or medial surface is related to middle constrictor and genioglossus muscles. The lingual artery courses in anteriorly along this surface lying on the middle constrictor. The second part of the lingual artery courses in a forward direction lying on the deep surface. The glossopharyngeal nerve and stylohyoid ligament also pass deep to the muscle.
c. Structures passing deep to the posterior margin are, the lingual artery, glossopharyngeal nerve and stylohyoid ligament.
d. Structures passing deep to the anterior margin are, the lingual artery and genioglossus muscle.

Thus, it is clear that the first part of the lingual artery is related to the posterior margin of the hyoglossus, the second part to its deep surface and the third part to its anterior border.

Nerve Supply

The hyoglossus receives branches from the hypoglossal nerve along with other lingual muscles.

Actions

The hyoglossus depresses the side of the tongue.

Mylohyoid Muscle

This muscle is positioned in the suprahyoid region in such a way that it forms the floor of the submental triangle but

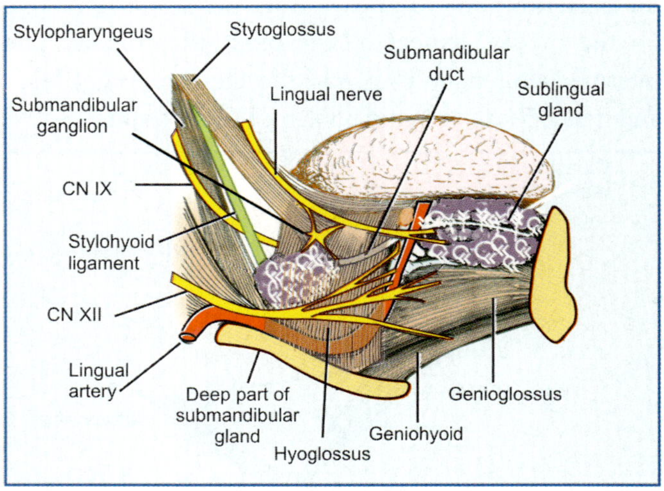

Fig. 69.2: Relations of hyoglossus muscle (Note that the submandibular duct passes deep to sublingual gland on its way to the floor of oral cavity)

its posterior fibers form the anterior part of the roof of the digastric triangle.

Attachments (Fig. 69.3)

The mylohyoid muscle is triangular in shape with wide origin and narrow insertion. It takes origin from the entire mylohyoid line of the mandible. It goes backwards to insert in the central part of the body of the hyoid bone. The muscles of the two sides meet and fuse in the midline at the median fibrous raphe to form a continuous muscular sheet in the floor of the mouth. Hence the mylohyoid muscles together constitute the oral diaphragm. The submandibular salivary gland is related to the muscle at three sites. The superficial and deep parts of the submandibular salivary gland are continuous with each other around the free posterior margin. The superficial part of the gland is in contact with the inferior surface and the deep part is in contact with the superior surface of the muscle. Thus the mylohyoid gives the submandibular gland a U-shape.

Relations of Inferior or External Surface

The inferior surface of the muscle is in part related to the structures in the submental triangle and in part to those in the digastric triangle. Thus it is related to platysma, anterior belly of digastric muscle, submental vessels and mylohyoid nerve and vessels. The medial surface of the superficial part of submandibular gland contained in the digastric triangle is also related to this surface.

Relations of Superior or Internal Surface (Fig. 69. 4)

The geniohyoid muscle lies very close to the median fibrous raphe. The posterior part of mylohyoid is in relation to hyoglossus. There are certain structures separating the two muscles namely, lingual nerve with submandibular ganglion hanging from it and the deep part of the submandibular gland with the submandibular duct. The lowest structure is the hypoglossal nerve with accompanying lingual veins. The anterior part of mylohyoid is related to genioglossus. Between these two muscles lies the sublingual gland. The third part of the lingual artery lies above the sublingual gland.

Nerve Supply

The mylohyoid nerve (a branch of inferior alveolar) supplies the mylohyoid and the anterior belly of digastric.

Actions

The muscle elevates the floor of the mouth in the first stage of deglutition. Acting from below it can depress the mandible.

Ludwig's Angina

Due to the proximity of the oral cavity and submandibular region, the intraoral infections like for example cellulitis

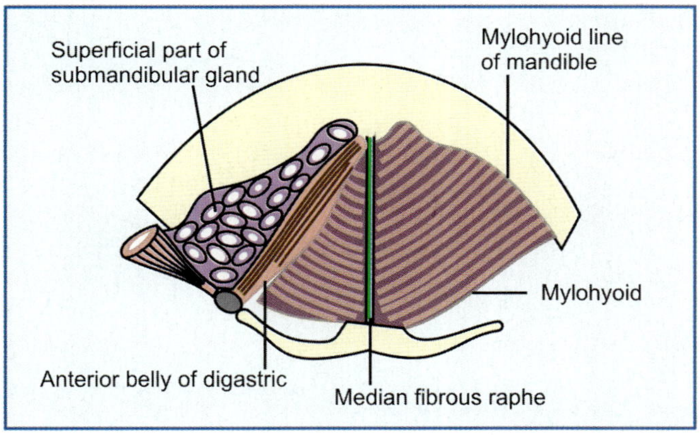

Fig. 69.3: To show mylohyoid muscle and some relations of its inferior surface (Note: Wide origin from mandible and narrow insertion in hyoid bone)

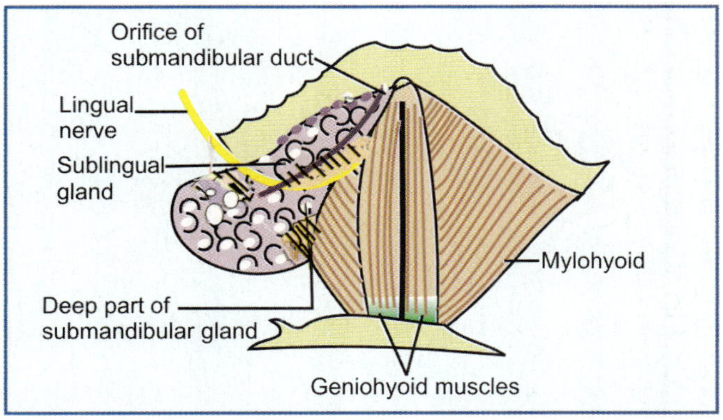

Fig. 69.4: To show superior surface of mylohyoid and its relations after removal of hyoglossus (Note that sublingual gland drains by multiple ducts in the floor of oral cavity)

spread rapidly to the submandibular region through the mylohyoid cleft. This cleft is present between the mylohyoid and hyoglossus muscles, which is more on a posterior plane than the mylohyoid. The cellulites causes swelling in the submandibular region due to rapid collection of pus, which remains confined within the rigid fascial barriers. This condition is called Ludwig's angina. It is characterized by putrid halitosis (bad smell of breath). To drain the fluid mylohyoid muscles are divided by surgical incisions.

Geniohyoid Muscle (Fig. 69.4)

This is a small muscle, which is located above the mylohyoid muscle but very close to the midline. It arises from the inferior mental spine or genial tubercle on the back of symphysis menti and is inserted in the anterior surface of the body of hyoid bone. The muscles of the two sides may fuse with each other. It receives twigs from the C1 fibers brought to it in the branch from the hypoglossal nerve. The geniohyoid elevates the hyoid and draws it forwards.

70 Submandibular and Sublingual Salivary Glands

The submandibular salivary gland is a mixed type of compound racemose gland. It pours its relatively viscous secretion by the submandibular duct against gravity in the floor of the oral cavity.

Parts (Fig. 70.1)

The gland consists of a larger superficial part, which fills the digastric triangle and a smaller deep part, which lies above the mylohyoid muscle. The two parts are continuous with each other around the free posterior margin of the mylohyoid muscle.

Fascial Capsule (Fig. 70.2)

The investing layer of deep fascia splits to enclose the submandibular salivary gland. The superficial layer covers the superficial surface of the gland and is attached to the lower border of the mandible. The deep layer covers the medial surface and is attached to the mylohyoid line of the mandible. The submandibular lymph nodes are almost embedded in the gland within the fascial capsule. If the lymph nodes are secondarily involved in cancer of the tongue or lip or primarily involved in tuberculosis, the excision of the lymph nodes along with submandibular gland is mandatory due to their close proximity.

Bi-digital Palpation of the Gland

The submandibular gland is palpated by the index finger placed in the floor of the mouth and the thumb placed below the floor, anteromedial to the angle of mandible. This is possible because the deep part is palpable from oral cavity and superficial part by the thumb below the mylohyoid.

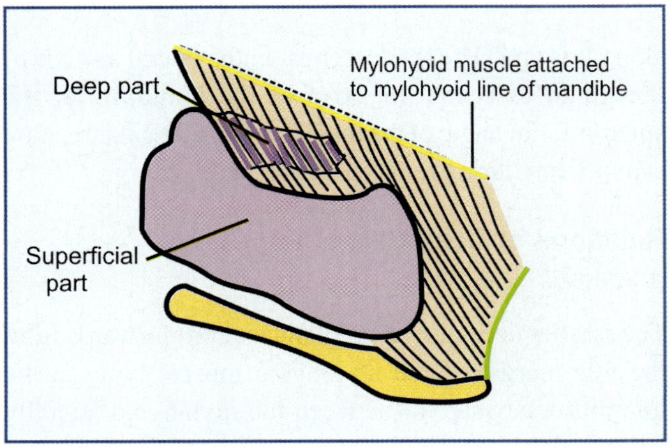

Fig. 70.1: Schematic diagram depicting continuity of two parts of submandibular gland around the posterior margin of mylohyoid muscle

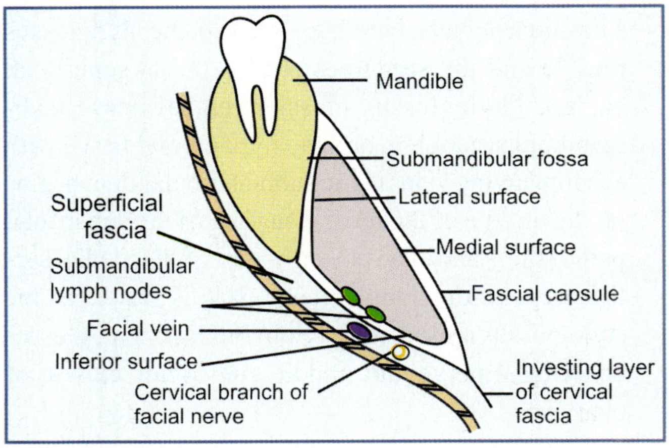

Fig. 70.2: To show fascial capsule and surfaces of submandibular salivary gland

Surface Marking

The upper convex margin of the gland is drawn by joining the point at the angle of mandible to a point on the middle of the base of the mandible. The lower margin is convex downwards. It is marked by a line joining the two ends of the upper margin and extending below the level of the greater horn of the hyoid bone.

Relations of Superficial Part of Gland

The superficial part has three surfaces. The superficial or inferior surface faces towards the skin. The lateral surface is in contact with the submandibular fossa of the mandible while the medial surface is the most extensive. The posterior end of the gland is in contact with the stylomandibular ligament, which separates it from the parotid gland.

a. The superficial surface is covered with the skin, superficial fascia with platysma, facial vein, cervical and marginal mandibular branches of facial nerve and investing layer of deep fascia. The submandibular lymph nodes are embedded in this surface (Fig. 70.2).
b. The lateral surface is in contact with the submandibular fossa on the inner surface of mandible. The posterior part of this surface is in contact with medial pterygoid muscle. Between the medial pterygoid and this surface the facial artery passes forwards and inferiorly.
c. The relations of the medial surface (Fig. 70.3) are different in its anterior, intermediate and posterior parts. The anterior part is related to the mylohyoid muscle, mylohyoid nerve and vessels and submental vessels. The intermediate part is related to the hyoglossus muscle and the structures resting on its superficial surface (styloglossus muscle, lingual nerve, submandibular ganglion and the hypoglossal nerve with accompanying veins). The submandibular duct begins on the middle of the medial surface of the superficial part of the gland. The posterior part of the medial surface beyond the hyoglossus muscle is related to the styloglossus muscle and stylohyoid ligament, glossopharyngeal nerve and middle constrictor muscle of pharynx.

Relationship to Facial Artery (Fig. 70.4)

The facial artery is related to the gland twice. The artery grooves the posterior end of the gland as it runs upwards along this end. Then it descends on the lateral surface of the gland to reach the base of the mandible at the anteroinferior angle of the masseter. This vascular relation is important during removal of the gland.

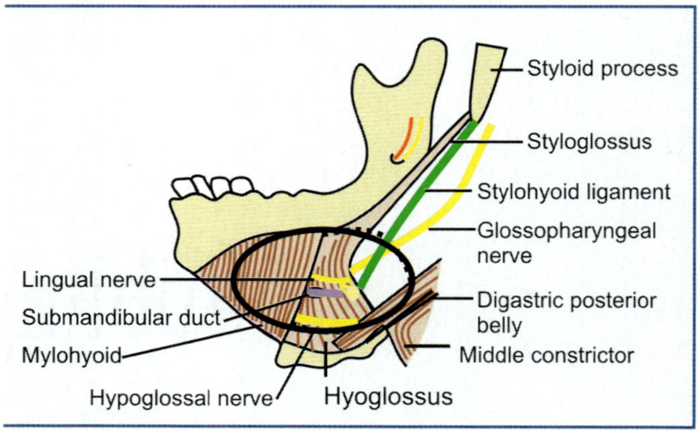

Fig. 70.3: Relations of medial surface of superficial part of submandibular gland (Note that outline of medial surface of gland is shown in foreground for reference)

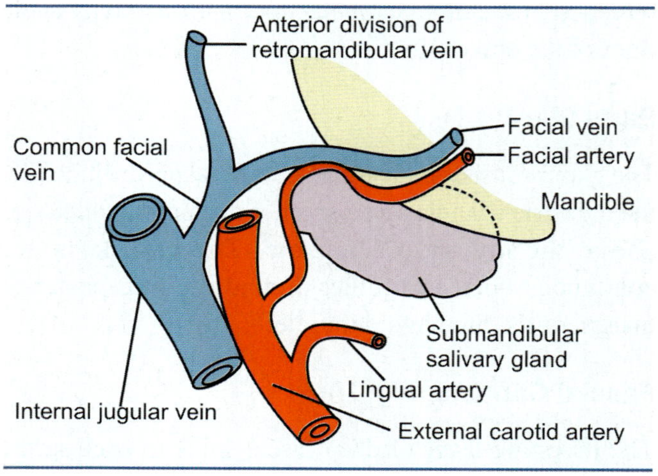

Fig. 70.4: Relation of facial vessels to submandibular salivary gland

Relations of Deep Part of the Gland (Figs 69.1 and 70.5)

The smaller deep part of the gland extends forwards from the free margin of the mylohyoid muscle lying in the intermuscular interval between the mylohyoid laterally and hyoglossus medially. It is situated between the lingual nerve and the submandibular ganglion above and the hypoglossal nerve below. The submandibular duct passes through the deep part.

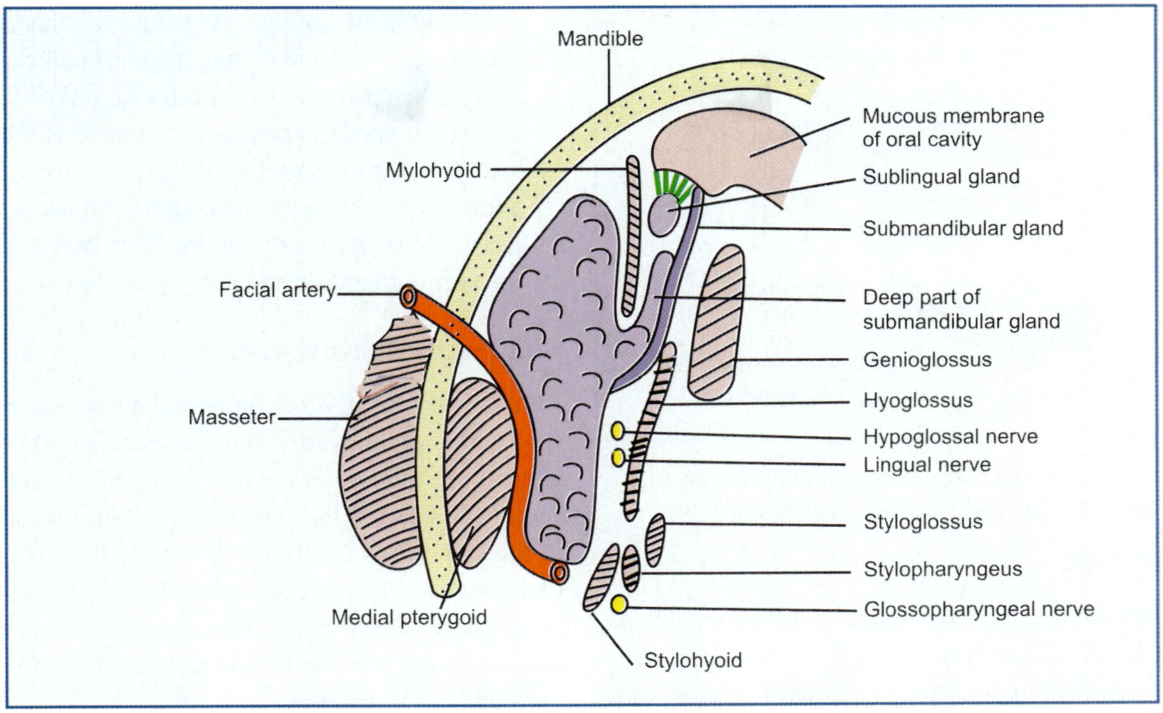

Fig. 70.5: To show origin and termination of submandibular duct and relations of the gland in schematic horizontal section of submandibular region

Submandibular or Wharton's Duct

The submandibular duct is about five cm long and begins on the medial surface of the superficial part of the gland (Fig. 70.5) near the posterior margin of the mylohyoid, where it enters the deep part of the gland. The duct emerges from the anterior end of the deep part and runs forwards and upwards between the sublingual gland and the genioglossus muscle to open in the floor of the mouth at the summit of the sublingual papilla by the side of the frenulum of tongue. As it traverses the deep part of the gland it receives small ducts from it. The submandibular duct has triple relation with the lingual nerve (Fig. 70.6). The lingual nerve is at first above the duct. At the anterior border of the hyoglossus the nerve crosses the duct from lateral to medial side to reach the tongue. Thus the nerve is related to its lateral, inferior and medial aspects. The duct can be palpated in the floor of the mouth. Its narrowest part is the orifice by which it opens in the oral cavity.

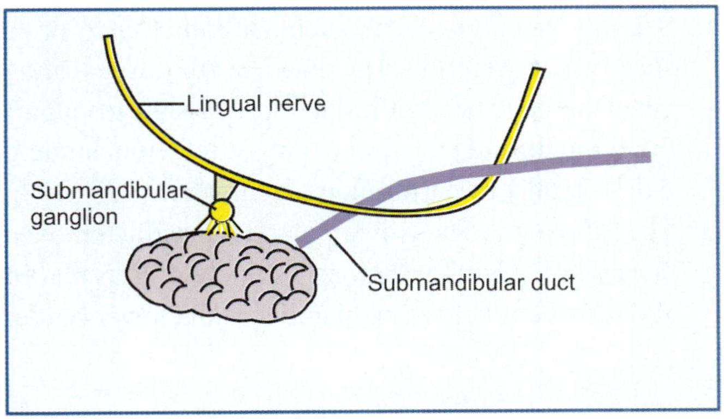

Fig. 70.6: Showing triple relation of lingual nerve to submandibular duct

Secretomotor Nerve Supply (Fig. 70.7)

The preganglionic parasympathetic fibers originate from the superior salivatory nucleus in the pons. These fibers join the facial nerve and leave it through its chorda tympani branch, which joins the lingual nerve in the infratemporal fossa. The lingual nerve brings the preganglionic fibers the submandibular ganglion, which is a peripheral parasympathetic ganglion. The postganglionic fibers directly enter the gland.

Lymphatic Drainage

The gland drains in the submandibular lymph nodes.

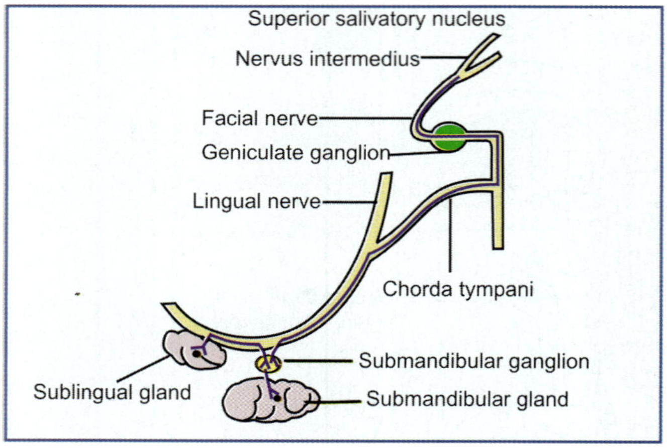

Fig. 70.7: Pathway of secretomotor nerve supply of submandibular and sublingual salivary glands

Section three

Development

The submandibular and sublingual salivary glands are believed to develop as outgrowths from the endoderm of the linguogingival sulcus during sixth week of embryonic life.

Clinical Highlights

a. Salivary calculi occur in submandibular duct due to stasis of the secretion. The gland swells during eating when the stone blocks the duct. It is possible to palpate the stone through the oral cavity or to demonstrate it radiologically by performing sialography.
b. The submandibular salivary gland is usually removed because of calculi or tumor. A skin incision is placed about five cm below and parallel to the lower border of mandible, beginning at the angle of mandible. This is necessary to avoid cutting the marginal mandibular and cervical branches of the facial nerve. The facial artery is ligated in two places so that a segment of the artery is removed with the excised gland. While cutting the duct care is taken not to injure the lingual nerve. After dissecting out the deep part of the gland the entire gland is removed.

Sublingual Salivary Gland

This salivary gland is of compound racemose and mixed type with predominantly mucous secretion. It is situated beneath the mucosa of the oral cavity in contact with the sublingual fossa on the inner surface of the mandible close to the symphysis menti. Occasionally the right and left glands are fused with each other. Each sublingual gland has eight to twenty ducts. The smaller ducts open in the summit of the sublingual fold separately. A few open in the submandibular duct.

Relations

Superiorly the sublingual gland is related to the mucosa of floor of the mouth and inferiorly to the mylohyoid muscle. Posterior to it lies the deep part of submandibular gland. The sublingual fossa of mandible is its lateral relation and the submandibular duct and lingual nerve are related medially. The secretomotor supply reaches the gland through the branches of lingual nerve, which receives postganglionic fibers from the submandibular ganglion.

71 Sternomastoid Muscle

The sternomastoid or sternocleidomastoid is a key muscle in the neck. It is useful in dividing the neck into anterior and posterior triangles. It is enclosed in a fascial sheath of the investing layer of deep cervical fascia. The sternomastoid muscle becomes visible on turning the head to the opposite side.

Attachments (Fig. 71.1)

The muscle takes origin from the two bones of the shoulder girdle and is inserted into the two bones of the cranium. It takes origin by sternal and clavicular heads, which fuse to form a single belly. The sternal head arises by a tendon from the upper part of the anterior surface of the manubrium sterni. The clavicular head arises by fleshy fibers from the upper surface of the medial one-third of the clavicle. The triangular gap called lesser supraclavicular fossa between the two heads, is occupied by the terminal part of internal jugular vein. The insertion of the muscle is on the lateral surface of the mastoid process and on the lateral half of the superior nuchal line.

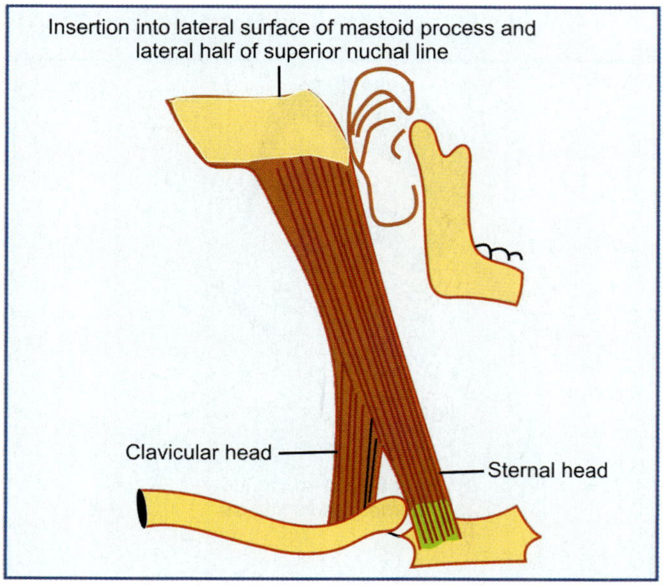

Fig. 71.1: Attachments of sternomastoid muscle [Note: Lesser supraclavicular triangle (fossa) between clavicular and sternal heads]

Actions

a. The contraction of sternomastoid muscle of one side causes downward movement of the head towards the shoulder of same side and rotation of the head to the opposite side (so that the face faces to the opposite side).
b. The contraction of both muscles causes the flexion of the cervical part of vertebral column.
c. The two muscles acting together elevate the thoracic cage through attachment to the sternum and thus help in forced inspiration.

Nerve Supply

The sternomastoid receives motor supply from spinal part of the accessory nerve. The proprioceptive sensation from the muscle is carried in C2 and C3 ventral rami.

Testing Muscle Function

a. To test the right muscle place your hand on the subject's chin on the left side and ask the subject to turn the head towards the left shoulder against resistance. The right sternomastoid becomes prominent and taut if its nerve supply is intact. The left muscle can be tested likewise.
b. To test both muscles simultaneously place your hand on the point of the subject's chin and ask him to press down against resistance. If active both muscles stand out.

Relations

For descriptive purposes the sternomastoid muscle is divided in different parts namely, superficial and deep surfaces and anterior and posterior margins.

a. The superficial surface is related to the external jugular vein, which descends on this surface. The great auricular nerve and transverse cutaneous nerve cross this surface.
b. The deep surface is related to structures in the anterior and posterior triangles of the neck. This surface is divided in three regions by superior belly of omohyoid and posterior belly of digastric muscles, which cross on the deep aspect of the muscle. The part below the omohyoid is related to sternoclavicular joint, sternothyroid and sternohyoid muscles and the anterior jugular vein. The part between the omohyoid and posterior belly of digastric has following relations. The anterior part of the deep surface is related to the carotid arteries, internal jugular, facial and lingual veins and the vagus nerve, ansa cervicalis and the deep cervical lymph nodes. The posterior part of the deep surface is related to the splenius, levator scapulae and scalene muscles, cervical plexus and upper part of brachial plexus, phrenic nerve and suprascapular and transverse cervical arteries. The occipital artery crosses the muscle just below the lower border of the posterior belly of digastric. At this point the accessory nerve passes deep to the muscle and pierces its deep surface to enter its substance. Near its insertion the sternomastoid is related to the mastoid process and the muscles inserted in it, namely, splenius, longissimus capitis and posterior belly of digastric.
c. The anterior margin of the sternomastoid bounds the carotid triangle above and the muscular triangle below. The clinical importance of the anterior margin is as follows. The branchial cysts and branchial fistulae (congenital anomalies of cervical sinus as described in Chapter 72) appear as swellings in relation to this margin. The branchial cyst appears at the junction of upper and middle one-third while the branchial fistula opens at the junction of lower and middle third of the anterior margin.
d. The midpoint of the posterior margin is called the nerve point because the following nerves emerge from this point (Fig. 65.2), cutaneous branches of cervical plexus (great auricular, lesser occipital, transverse cervical, and three supraclavicular nerves) and the spinal accessory nerve. The lesser occipital nerve hooks round the accessory nerve and runs along the posterior margin above the nerve point. The superficial lymph nodes are located around the nerves at this point. Enlargement of these nodes may be the cause of compression of the nerves.

Section three

Clinical Highlights

a. Torticollis or wryneck (Fig. 71.2) is the deformity in which head is bent to the affected side while the face (or chin) turns to the opposite side. There are several causes of this condition. Congenital torticollis occurs due to development of fibrous tissue tumor in the muscle before birth. The sternomastoid tumor is the swelling in the muscle as a result of birth injury. It subsides gradually in majority of cases but in a few instances it may cause shortening of the muscle, which results in muscular torticollis.
b. Bezold abscess is the complication of acute mastoiditis. Because the muscle is inserted in the mastoid process, pus in the mastoid process breaks through its tip and enters the sheath of the muscle. The Bezold abscess appears as a swelling in the upper part of the neck.

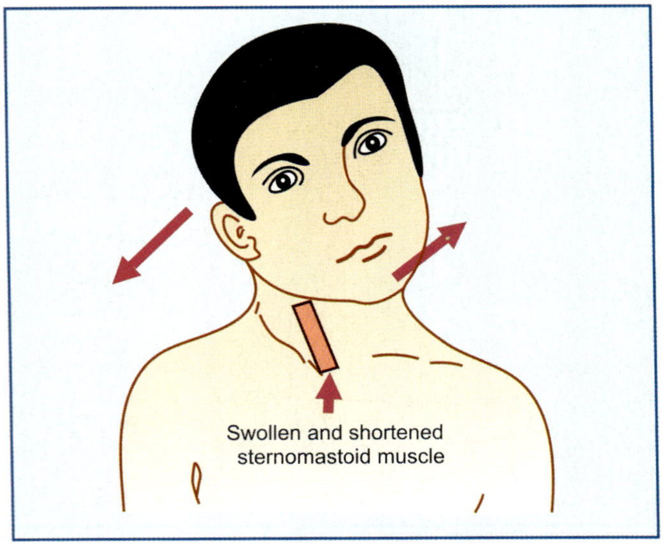

Fig. 71.2: Torticollis (wryneck)
(Note that head is tilted towards affected side and face towards normal side)

72 Branchial Arches (Pharyngeal Arches)

In the four-weak-old human embryo the neck is not recognizable. Subsequently, the neck develops with the appearance of a series of branchial or pharyngeal arches in the lateral wall of developing pharynx (at the end of the fourth week and during the fifth week) in the region between the stomodeum and the pericardium. The pharyngeal arches appear in craniocaudal order as thickenings of the mesoderm in the pharyngeal wall. A total of six pharyngeal arches develop in human embryo but the fifth arch is transient in existence.

Each arch consists of a mesodermal core (forerunner of skeletal muscles and cartilage) containing the artery and the nerve (Fig. 72.1). Each arch has an ectodermal cleft, endodermal pouch and the cleft membrane separating the two (as described below).

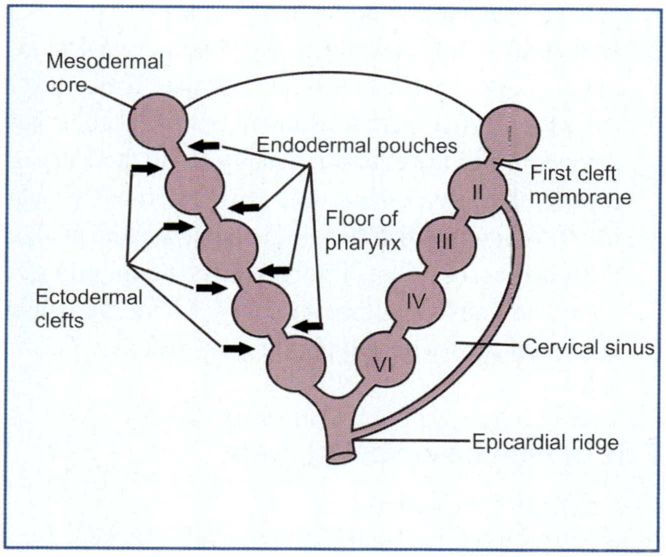

Fig. 72.1: Pharyngeal arches (I through IV and VI) (Note that Vth arch being rudimentary is not shown. Cervical sinus is enclosed by the ectoderm of the arches and ectoderm of overhanging second arch)

Ectodermal Clefts

The ectoderm covering the pharyngeal arches dips as pharyngeal clefts in between the adjoining arches.

Endodermal Pouches

The endoderm lining the pharyngeal arches grows out as pharyngeal pouches in between the adjoining arches.

Cleft Membranes

The ectoderm of the clefts and the endoderm of the pouches meet each other to form a bi-germinal cleft membrane. Only the first cleft membrane is tri-germinal because mesoderm enters in between the endoderm and ectoderm. This is the reason why the first cleft membrane alone persists. The others disintegrate.

Nerves of Arches

a. Only the first arch has two nerves. The mandibular nerve is the nerve of the first arch. It is also described as post-trematic nerve of first arch. The chorda tympani nerve (a branch of facial nerve) is the pretrematic nerve of first arch.
b. The facial nerve belongs to second arch.
c. The glossopharyngeal nerve belongs to third arch.
d. The vago-accessory complex belongs to the fourth arch.
e. The recurrent laryngeal nerve belongs to the sixth arch.

Development of Cervical Sinus

During the development of pharyngeal arches, the neck of the embryo presents an uneven appearance. The second arch grows faster inferiorly to overlap the succeeding arches. The ectoderm- lined space between the overhanging second arch and the succeeding arches is called the cervical sinus. The lower end of the growing second arch fuses with the epipericardial ridge so that the cervical sinus becomes a closed space. Soon, the cervical sinus undergoes obliteration, after which the smooth contour of the neck is restored.

Anomalies of Cervical Sinus (Fig. 72.2)

a. Branchial cyst develops if a part of the sinus persists along the anterior margin of the sternomastoid muscle just below the angle of mandible. It presents as a painless fluctuant swelling in the neck.
b. Branchial fistula develops when the cervical sinus remains open at its caudal end. The fistula may be of three types. An external fistula or branchial sinus has an opening on the exterior, usually along the anterior margin of the sternomastoid above the sternoclavicular joint. An internal fistula has an opening in the wall of the tonsillar fossa just in front of its posterior pillar. A complete fistula is a rare anomaly, where the fistula communicates with the pharynx as well as with the skin.

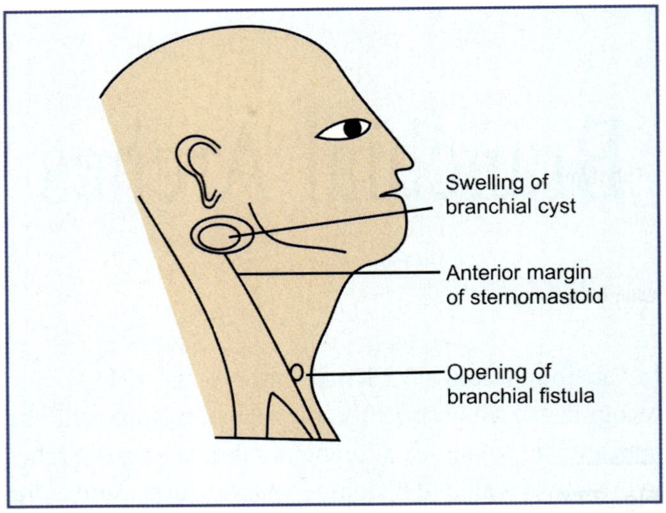

Fig. 72.2: Anomalies of cervical sinus along anterior margin of sternomastoid

Fate of First (Mandibular) Arch

Ectodermal Derivatives

The dorsal part of the first cleft forms the external acoustic meatus.

Endodermal Derivatives

The dorsal part of the first pouch unites with the dorsal part of the second pouch to form tubotympanic recess, which gives rise to the auditory tube, middle ear and tympanic (mastoid) antrum.

First Cleft Membrane

The first cleft membrane is unique in that it is composed of three germ layers. It develops into the tympanic membrane.

Mesodermal Derivatives

a. The skeletal derivatives of the first arch cartilage (Meckel's cartilage) gives rise to malleus, incus, anterior ligament of malleus, sphenomandibular ligament and the mandible (Fig. 72.3).
b. The muscles developed from the first arch mesoderm are the four muscles of mastication, tensor tympani, tensor palati, mylohyoid and anterior belly of digastric. The mandibular nerve supplies all the eight muscles.

Fate of Second (Hyoid) Arch

Endodermal Derivatives

The ventral part of the second pouch forms the tonsil.

Mesodermal Derivatives

a. The second arch cartilage (Reichert's cartilage) gives rise to the stapes, and styloid process of temporal bone,

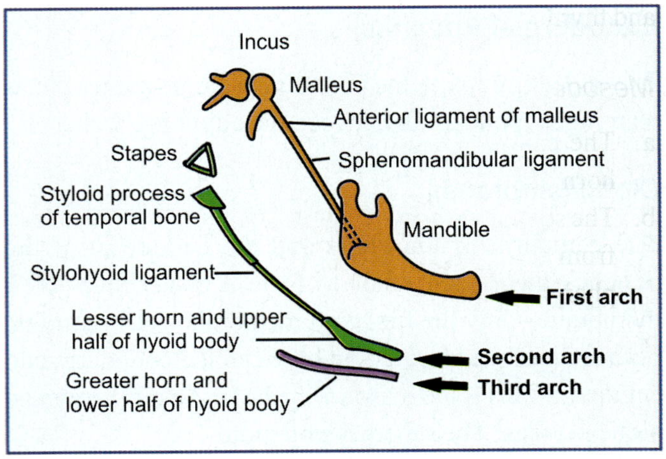

Fig. 72.3: Schematic illustration of skeletal derivatives of I, II, and III branchial arches

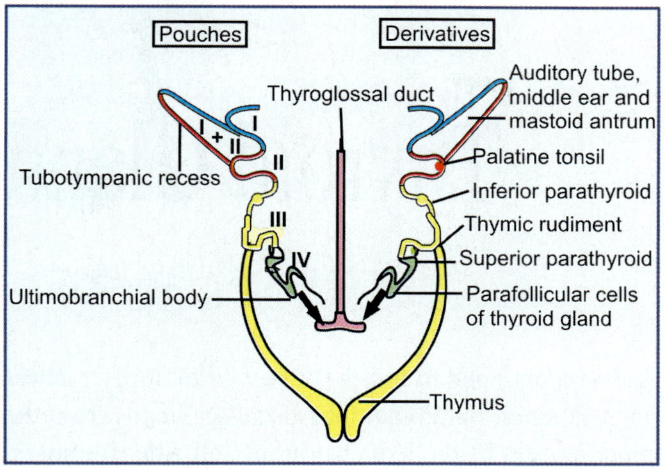

Fig. 72.4: Derivatives of pharyngeal pouches (Note: The contribution of ultimobranchial body in formation of parafollicular cells of thyroid gland)

stylohyoid ligament, lesser horn of hyoid bone and the upper part of the body of hyoid bone (Fig. 72.4).

b. The muscles developed from the second arch are, the occipitofrontalis, muscles of facial expression including platysma, auricular muscles, stapedius, buccinator, posterior belly of digastric and the stylohyoid. The facial nerve supplies all these muscles.

Fate of Third Arch

Endodermal Derivatives

The third pouch gives rise to the inferior parathyroid gland and thymus.

Mesodermal Derivatives

a. The cartilage of the third arch gives rise to greater horn of the hyoid bone and the lower part of its body.

b. The stylopharyngeus muscle is the only one developed from the third arch and is supplied by the glossopharyngeal nerve.

Fate of Fourth and Sixth Arches

Endodermal Derivatives

The fourth pouch gives rise to the superior parathyroid gland.

Ultimobranchial Body

Lower part of fourth pouch (along with rudimentary fifth pouch) forms the caudal pharyngeal complex or ultimobranchial body, which grows downwards to meet the lower end of the thyroglossal duct. It gives rise to C-cells of thyroid gland.

Mesodermal Derivatives

The cartilages of the larynx are derived from the fourth and sixth arches. The muscles developed from the fourth and sixth arches are the muscles of the pharynx (except stylopharyngeus), muscles of soft palate (except tensor palati) and the muscles of larynx.

Anomalies of Pharyngeal Pouches

a. DiGeorge syndrome (third and fourth pharyngeal pouch syndrome) results from failure of development of third and fourth pouches. This syndrome is characterized by thymic hypoplasia (resulting in selective T cell deficiency and greatly reduced cell-mediated immunity) and absence of parathyroid glands (resulting in hypocalcemia and tetany). When the above deficits are accompanied by cardiac defects, abnormalities of face and cleft palate, CATCH 22 spectrum results. Deletion of long arm of chromosome 22 is the reason of the multiple anomalies.

b. Nezelof's syndrome results due to failure of development of only the third pharyngeal pouch. Here, superior parathyroid glands are present but inferior parathyroid glands and thymus are absent. Therefore, there is normal function of parathyroid glands.

73 Thyroid Gland

The thyroid gland is a highly vascular endocrine gland situated in the lower part of the front of the neck in close relation to larynx and trachea (Fig. 39.1). The follicular cells of the thyroid gland secrete triiodothyronine (T3) and tetraiodothyronine (T4) hormones, which raise the rate of metabolism. The hormones are stored in the follicles of the gland as thyroglobulin. The parafollicular cells secrete calcitonin, which is a hypocalcemic hormone.

General Features (Fig. 73.1)

The thyroid gland weighs approximately 25 gm in adult being slightly heavier in female. It consists of right and left lobes, which are connected by an isthmus. Each lobe is around 5 cm in length, 3 cm in breadth and 2 cm in thickness. The lobes extend from the oblique line of the thyroid cartilage to the level of fifth or sixth tracheal ring and correspond to C5-T1 vertebrae. The isthmus lies against the second to fourth (or second to third) tracheal rings. A small pyramidal lobe usually extends from the upper margin of the isthmus on the left side. It may be attached to the hyoid bone by a slip of a muscle called levator glandulae thyroidae. The upward shift of thyroid is arrested by the attachment of sternothyroid muscle to the oblique line of thyroid cartilage. On the contrary, the short neck and strong strap muscles push the lower pole of a normally located but enlarged gland downward in the superior mediastinum and give rise to the retrosternal goiter.

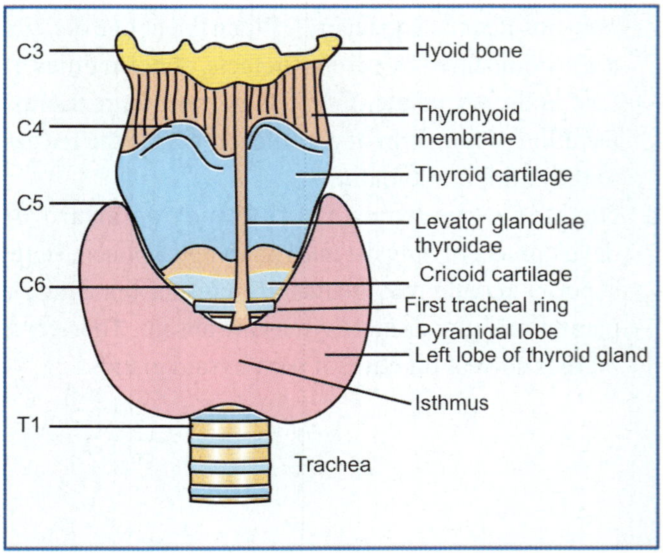

Fig. 73.1: Location and parts of thyroid gland Vertebral level (C5 to T1) of thyroid lobe is shown on right side

Development (Figs 72.1 and 73.2)

The thyroid gland develops from the endoderm of the floor of the embryonic pharynx at the foramen caecum, which lies at the junction of the anterior two-thirds and posterior one-third of the developing tongue. The cells of the thyroid rudiment pass through the substance of the tongue to form the thyroglossal duct, which courses downwards in the midline anterior to the hyoid bone. The duct usually recurs posterior to the hyoid bone before proceeding down in front of thyroid and cricoid cartilages. The bi-lobed lower end of the thyroglossal duct gives origin to the follicular cells of the thyroid gland. The caudal pharyngeal complex (ultimobranchial body) joins each side of the lower end of thyroglossal duct to give origin to parafollicular cells. The thyroid gland starts functioning from the fourth month of intrauterine life.

Remnants of Thyroglossal Duct

The cranial end of the thyroglossal duct is indicated by the foramen caecum of the tongue. The caudal end of the duct may persist as pyramidal lobe (extending from the isthmus and the occasional levator thyroidae glandulae

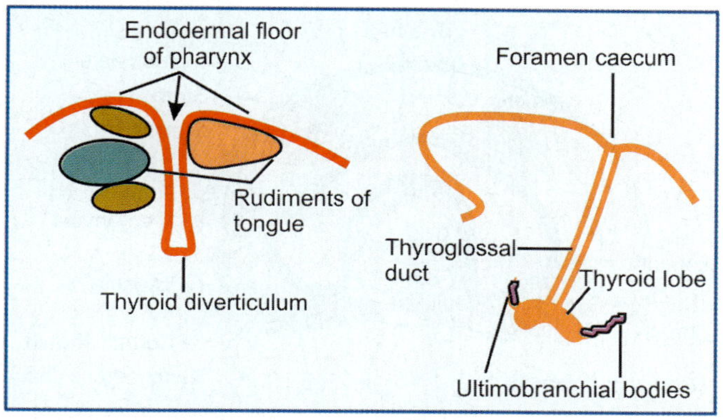

Fig. 73.2: Simplified diagram showing relationship of developing tongue and developing thyroid gland

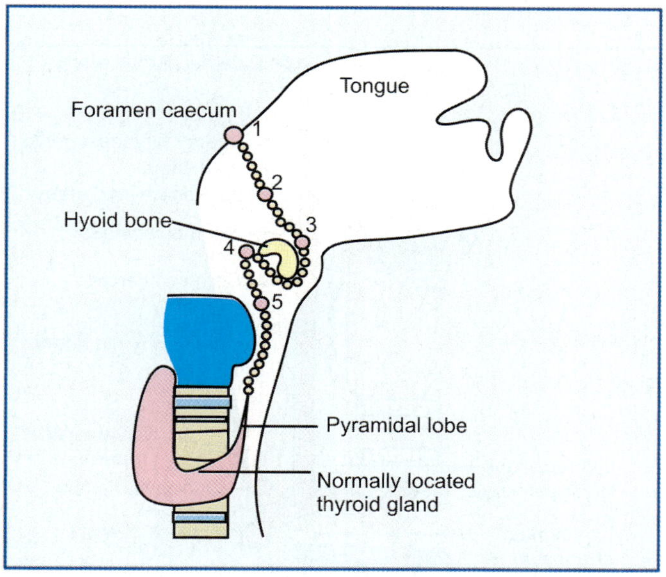

Fig. 73.3: Course of thyroglossal duct and sites 1 through 5 of ectopic thyroid tissue and sites 3, 4 and 5 of thyroglossal cysts. (1) Lingual, (2) Intralingual, (3) Suprahyoid, (4) Retrohyoid, (5) Infrahyoid

(a fibromuscular slip attaching the pyramidal lobe to the hyoid bone). The rest of the thyroglossal duct disappears.

Congenital Anomalies (Fig. 73.3)

a. If the thyroglossal duct fails to descend, the thyroid gland may remain in the oral cavity on the dorsum of the tongue. Such an anomaly is called lingual thyroid.
b. Other ectopic sites of the thyroid gland are along the course of the thyroglossal duct, intralingual, suprahyoid, retrohyoid or infrahyoid.

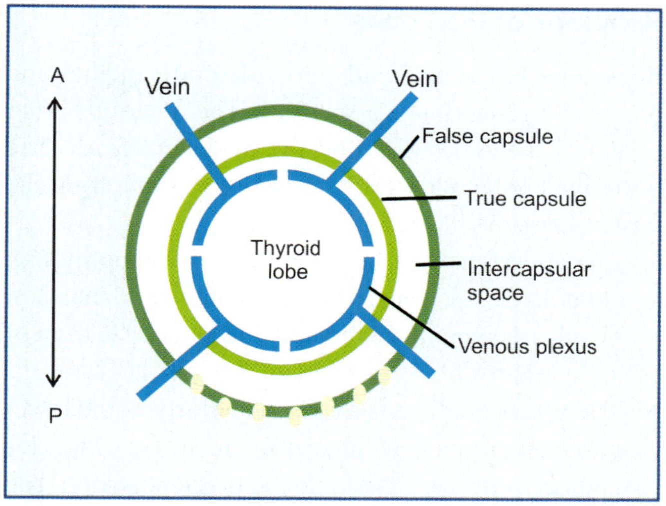

Fig. 73.4: Scheme to depict capsules of thyroid gland and relation of venous plexus to true capsule (Note that false capsule is weak posteriorly)

c. The duct may persist as thyroglossal cyst, which usually presents as midline swelling in the neck. Usually it is found in the vicinity of the hyoid bone. During surgical removal of the cyst the body of hyoid bone is also removed to prevent recurrence.
d. A thyroglossal fistula is formed when the cyst breaks through the skin.

Capsules of Thyroid Gland (Fig. 73.4)

The thyroid gland has a true capsule (fibrous) and a false capsule (fascial). The true capsule is the condensation of the connective tissue at the periphery of the gland. The venous plexus lies deep to the true capsule. The false capsule is derived from the pretracheal layer of deep cervical fascia. The pretracheal fascia is attached above to the oblique line of thyroid cartilage. On the posteromedial aspect of the lobe the fascial capsule is thickened to form the suspensory ligament of Berry, which is attached to the arch of cricoid cartilage. This ligament holds the gland firmly in contact with the larynx and thus prevent it from sliding down, when enlarged. During surgical removal of the gland, the ligament of Berry must be identified and cut. The attachments of the pretracheal fascia to the thyroid and cricoid cartilages and also to the hyoid bone are responsible for the movements of the thyroid during swallowing (deglutition) and speech.

Relations of the Lobes

Each lobe has superficial (anterolateral), medial and posterior (posterolateral) surfaces. The anterior border separates the superficial and the medial surfaces. The posterior border separates the medial surface from the posterolateral surface (Fig. 73. 5).

a. The superficial surface is related to sternothyroid, sternohyoid and superior belly of omohyoid muscles, which are laterally covered by the anterior margin of sternomastoid.
b. The medial surface is related superiorly to the lower parts of larynx and pharynx and to two muscles namely, inferior constrictor and cricothyroid. The external laryngeal nerve lies between these two muscles. The inferior part of the medial surface is related to the trachea and esophagus. The recurrent laryngeal nerve lies between these two tubes. This nerve is related to the inferior thyroid artery. The nerve passes upwards in the groove between the trachea and esophagus to lie immediately behind the cricothyroid joint and the ligament of Berry.
c. The posterolateral surface is related to the carotid sheath (with its contents), sympathetic chain behind the carotid sheath and to the prevertebral fascia and longus colli directly behind. On the left side the lower pole may be closely related to the arch of the thoracic duct.
d. The anterior border is related to the anterior branch of superior thyroid artery.
e. The posterior border is related to the parathyroid glands and the anastomosis between the superior and inferior thyroid arteries.

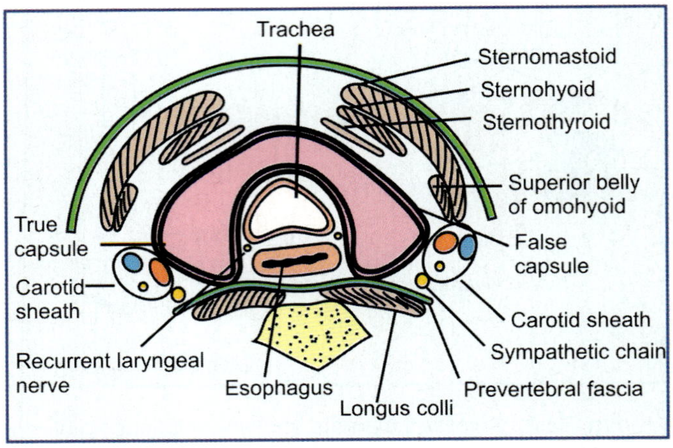

Fig. 73.5: Scheme to show relations of lobe of thyroid gland

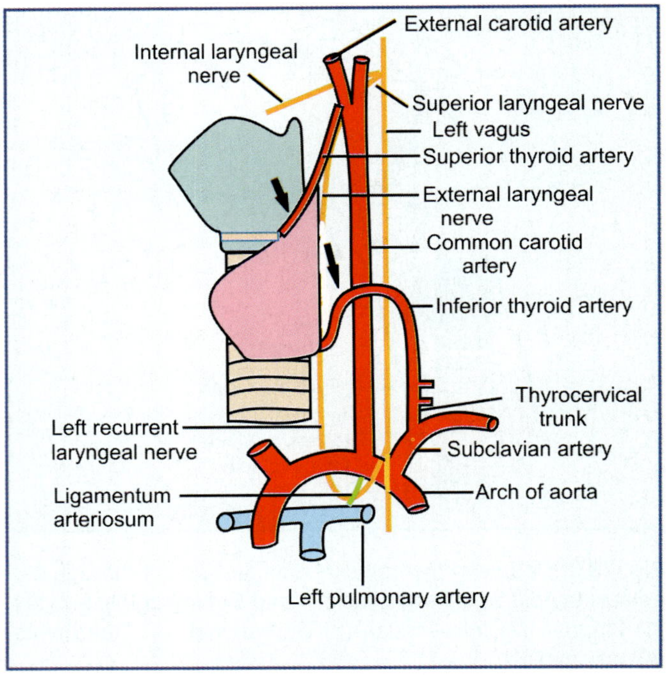

Fig. 73.6: Showing relations of thyroid arteries and accompanying nerves on left side (Note that upper arrow indicates safe site to ligate superior thyroid artery and lower arrow to ligate inferior thyroid artery)

Relations of Isthmus

a. Anteriorly it is covered from within outwards by pretracheal fascia, strap muscles, investing layer of deep fascia, superficial fascia with anterior jugular veins and the skin.
b. Posteriorly it rests on second to third or second to fourth tracheal rings.
c. Along its upper margin the terminal parts of anterior branches of both superior thyroid arteries take part in a rich anastomosis, which supply twigs to the anterior surface of the isthmus also.
d. Along its lower margin the inferior thyroid veins emerge and the thyroidea ima enters at the same level. The vascular relations of the isthmus are to be kept in mind during tracheostomy.

Arterial Supply (Fig. 73.7)

The superior and inferior thyroid arteries and an occasional arteria thyroidea ima (ima means single or unpaired)

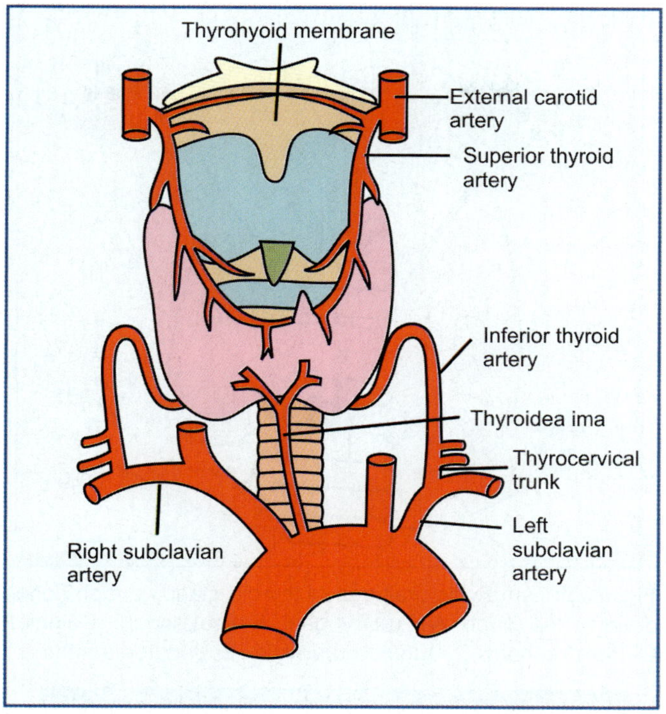

Fig. 73.7: Arterial supply of thyroid gland

provide rich blood supply to the gland. The thyroid arteries are large-sized and show arterial loops so as to accommodate upward and downward movements of the thyroid gland.

a. The superior thyroid artery is a branch of external carotid artery in the carotid triangle. It descends to the superior pole of the lateral lobe of the thyroid gland in company with external laryngeal nerve. At the upper pole the artery enters the gland but the nerve goes deep. Hence the lower pole is the safest site for tying the superior thyroid artery.
b. The inferior thyroid artery arises from the thyrocervical trunk of the first part of subclavian artery. It forms a loop with upward convexity to reach the level of sixth cervical vertebra and then descends to reach the base of the lateral lobe of the gland. It pierces the prevertebral fascia and then enters the lower part of the gland, where it is very close to the recurrent laryngeal nerve. Hence it is safer to tie the inferior thyroid artery or its branches as away from the lower pole of the gland as possible. On the left side it is advisable to be more careful because of the danger of injuring the arch of the thoracic duct. The inferior thyroid artery and the thoracic duct may lie very close to each other at the root of the neck. Ascending branch of the inferior thyroid artery anastomoses with the descending branch of the superior thyroid artery along the posterior margin of the gland. While tying the branches of inferior thyroid artery, its ascending branch supplying the parathyroid glands is always preserved (being the main supply of these glands).
c. Thyroidea ima is a branch of arch of aorta or brachiocephalic trunk. It ascends in front of the trachea and enters the isthmus. It is not always present.
d. There are accessory thyroid arteries from the esophageal and tracheal branches of inferior thyroid arteries that give additional supply to the gland.

Venous Drainage (Fig. 73.8)

The thyroid veins do not accompany the arteries. The veins arise from venous plexus that lies deep to the true capsule. The superior thyroid vein emerges from the upper pole and terminates in the internal jugular vein. A very short middle thyroid vein emerges from the lobe and terminates in internal jugular vein. The inferior thyroid veins emerge from the lower margin of isthmus and descend on the anterior surface of trachea to open in the left brachiocephalic vein (though occasionally they open in respective brachiocephalic veins). The right and left veins frequently communicate with each other in front of the trachea. On injury these veins are a source of bleeding

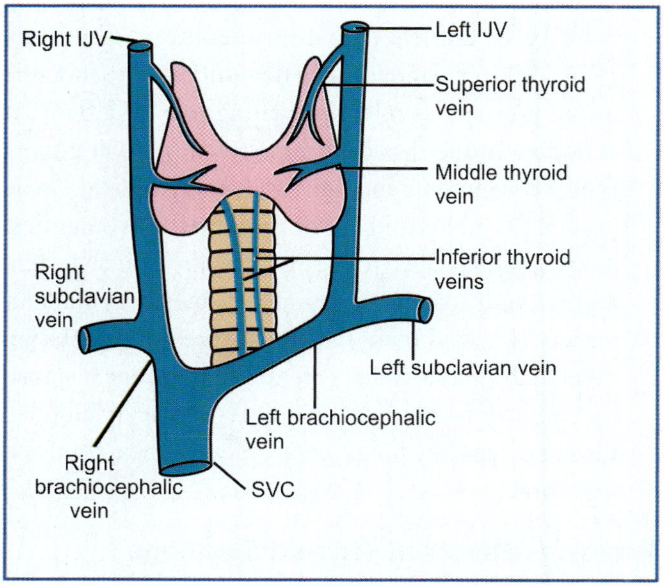

Fig. 73.8: Venous drainage of thyroid gland

during tracheostomy. A fourth vein (Kocher's) is occasionally met with between inferior and middle veins. It opens in the internal jugular vein.

Lymphatic Drainage (Fig. 73.9)

The lymph from the upper part of the gland reaches the upper deep cervical nodes (jugulodigastric) either directly or through the prelaryngeal nodes. The lymph from the lower part of the gland reaches the lower deep cervical group (jugulo-omohyoid) either directly or through the pretracheal (Delphic) and paratracheal nodes. Some lymph vessels may drain in brachiocephalic nodes in the superior mediastinum while others may directly reach the thoracic duct. The lymphatic spread of papillary carcinoma of the thyroid gland manifests in an interesting way. The thyroid gland looks normal but the deep cervical lymph node of the jugular chain is enlarged and contains thyroid tissue.

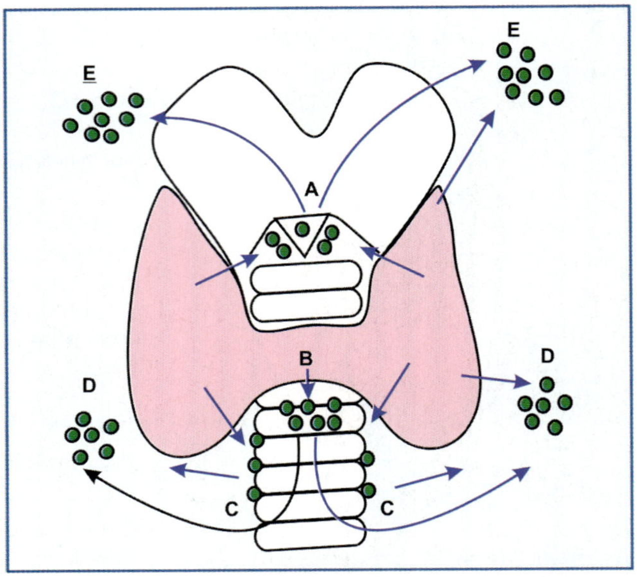

Fig. 73.9: Lymphatic drainage of thyroid gland. Lymph nodes draining the gland: A–Prelaryngeal, B–Pretracheal (Delphic), C–Paratracheal, D–Jugulo-omohyoid, E–Jugulodigastric

Clinical Highlights

a. Hypofunction of thyroid gland in infants and children is called cretinism and in adult, is called myxedema. Cretinism is the leading cause of mental retardation in children.
b. Hyperfunction of thyroid gland is called thyrotoxicosis or toxic goiter.
c. The term goitre means enlargement of thyroid gland due to any cause. The goiter may present as a smooth swelling or a nodular swelling. The thyroid swelling usually is confined to the midline in the neck (Fig. 73.10) and moves with deglutition. The endemic goitre presents as a large swelling due to deficiency of iodine in the diet or drinking water. Such goiters produce symptoms and signs of hypothyroidism. Toxic goiters (hyperthyroidism or thyrotoxicosis) manifest as symptoms related to the eye, cardiovascular system and nervous system. They are of diffuse or nodular variety. Thyroid malignancy may present as enlargement of the gland. Some types of thyroid cancer spread by lymph vessels while other types spread by blood to distant places like lungs, ends of long bones, skull and vertebrae.

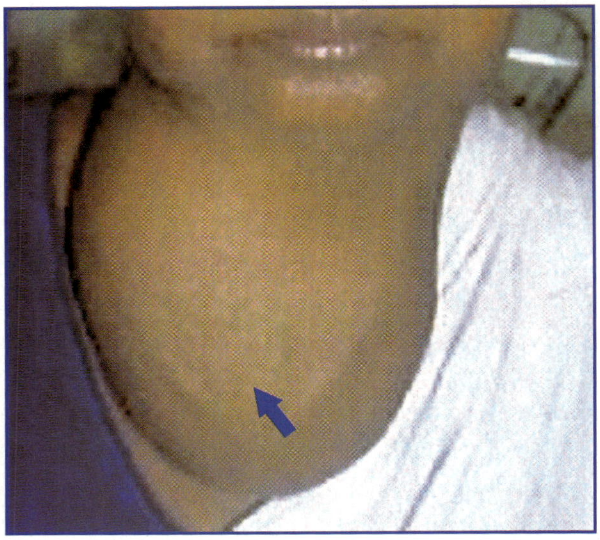

Fig. 73.10: Photo of a patient with enlarged thyroid gland (*Courtesy:* Department of Medicine, Dr SMCSI Medical College, Karakonam)

Pressure Effects of Thyroid Swellings

The enlarged thyroid gland tends to compress the structures that are its anatomical relations. The pressure effects may be varied, depending on the structure or structures compressed as shown below.

No.	*Structure*	*Effect of compressed*
1	Trachea	Dyspnea or shortness of breath
2	Esophagus	Dysphagia or difficulty in swallowing
3	Recurrent laryngeal nerve	Hoarseness of voice
4	Carotid sheath	Posterior displacement
5	Sympathetic chain	Horner's syndrome

Operations on Thyroid Gland

a. Isthmusectomy means removal of the thyroid isthmus. It is done if the thyroid swelling arises from the isthmus and to relieve tracheal obstruction due to compression by the isthmus.
b. Thyroid lobectomy consists of removal of the lobe along with the isthmus.
c. Near-total thyroidectomy consists of total thyroid lobectomy on the affected side with conservation of small thyroid tissue (between the esophagus and trachea) on the normal side.
d. Total thyroidectomy includes removal of the entire gland.

Complications of Thyroid Surgery

Injury to the recurrent laryngeal nerve while tying the inferior thyroid artery or its branches is the most feared complication. In 1 percent of cases the right recurrent laryngeal nerve may be non-recurrent arising from the right vagus higher up in the neck. The reason for this anomaly is that the right subclavian artery is aberrant (Fig. 47.5). Therefore, if the surgeon does not locate the nerve in its normal position on the right side he or she must keep in mind the possibility of nonrecurrent right recurrent laryngeal nerve. Inadvertent removal of parathyroid glands along with thyroid results in parathyroid insufficiency (tetany). This can also result due to injury to the artery supplying the parathyroid glands.

PARATHYROID GLANDS

The parathyroid glands are small (6 × 3 × 2 mm) endocrine glands along the posterior margin of the lobe of thyroid gland. They are inside the fascial capsule of the thyroid gland. There are two pairs of parathyroid glands consisting of right and left superior and right and left inferior glands. The secretion of parathyroid glands is called parathyroid hormone or parathormone. It maintains the blood calcium level by mobilizing the stored calcium from the bones. Its action is opposite to that of thyrocalcitonin.

Location (Fig. 73.11)

The superior parathyroid gland of each side is usually on a level with the junction of upper and middle thirds of lateral lobe of thyroid gland. The inferior gland lies behind the lower end of the thyroid gland on each side near the angle between the inferior thyroid artery and recurrent laryngeal nerve.

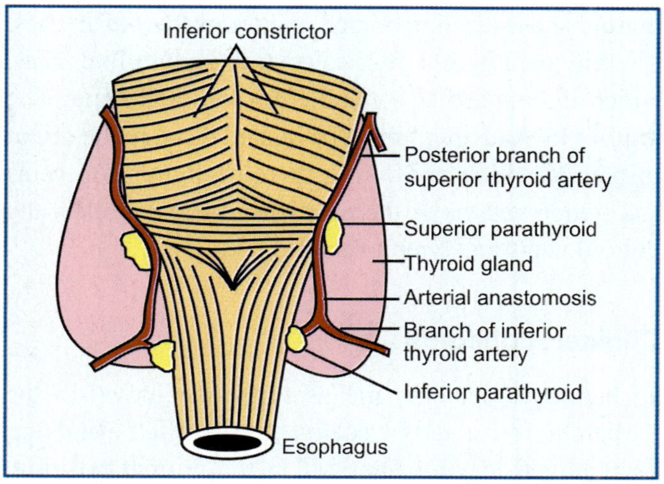

Fig. 73.11: Posterior view of lower pharynx and upper esophagus to show location of parathyroid glands

The parathyroid glands appear as small yellowish brown bodies. They are identified during surgery by isolating a small arterial branch that runs from the inferior thyroid artery to each parathyroid gland. Sometimes histological demonstration by taking frozen section is the only way to identify the gland during surgery.

Development (Fig. 72.3)

The superior parathyroid glands develop from the endoderm of the fourth pharyngeal pouch on each side. The inferior parathyroid glands develop along with thymus from the endoderm of third pharyngeal pouch. Both descend to reach their definitive positions. At times the inferior parathyroid may descend in superior mediastinum. In DiGeorge syndrome both thymus and all four parathyroid glands are congenitally absent but in Nezelof's syndrome thymus and inferior parathyroid glands are absent but superior parathyroid glands are present.

Blood Supply

Both the superior and inferior parathyroid glands receive mainly small branches from the inferior thyroid arteries. The superior pair also receives branches from the anastomosis between the posterior branch of superior thyroid and ascending branch of inferior thyroid arteries. The tiny parathyroid arteries enter the hilum-like areas, which distinguish the gland from the fat lobule. The inferior thyroid artery must be ligated distal to the origin of parathyroid artery during thyroidectomy. The veins and lymph vessels of the parathyroid glands follow the thyroid veins and lymph vessels.

Clinical Highlights

a. Parathyroidectomy means surgical removal of the parathyroid glands. Usually, three and half glands are removed leaving one half in the normal position. Alternatively, all the four glands are removed and a few pieces of one gland are implanted in the muscle of the forearm on one side (nondominant) or in sternomastoid where they grow and produce required hormone.
b. Parathyroid insufficiency results in tetany, which is characterized by low serum Ca, convulsions and carpopedal spasms due to increased neuromuscular excitability, and sensory symptoms like, numbness and tingling in hands and feet.
c. Excess of parathormone leads to rise in blood calcium level due to excessive absorption from bones. This leads to fragility of bones and proneness to fractures.

Blood Vessels of Neck 74

The carotid arteries (common, internal and external) and the subclavian arteries pass through the neck. The external carotid and the subclavian arteries give branches in the neck. The jugular veins (anterior, external and internal) and the subclavian veins are the major venous channels of the neck.

COMMON CAROTID ARTERIES (CCA)

Due to the difference in the origin of the common carotid arteries, the left artery is longer than the right. The left common carotid artery is a direct branch of the arch of aorta in the superior mediastinum. The right common carotid artery is one of the terminal branches of the brachiocephalic trunk behind the right sternoclavicular joint. Each common carotid artery terminates by dividing in the external and internal carotid arteries at the level of upper margin of thyroid cartilage in the carotid triangle. The cervical course of the right and left arteries is similar.

Surface Marking

a. The left common carotid artery is marked by drawing two parallel lines about 8 to 10 mm apart joining the three points as follows. The lowest point lies just to the left of the center of manubrium sterni. The second point corresponds to the left sternoclavicular joint. The third point is marked on the anterior margin of the left sternomastoid at the level of upper margin of the thyroid cartilage.
b. The right common carotid artery is drawn on similar lines by joining the point on the right sternoclavicular joint and the point at the level of upper margin of thyroid cartilage on the anterior margin of the right sternomastoid.

Cervical Course of Common Carotid Artery (CCA)

Each common carotid artery is enclosed in the carotid sheath along with the internal jugular vein and the vagus nerve. It runs up along the anterior margin of the sternomastoid but on a deeper plane. It is related posteriorly to the sympathetic chain. It lies successively on the subclavian artery, vertebral artery and at the level of the carotid tubercle on the inferior thyroid artery. The thoracic duct crosses behind the lower part of the left artery and the right recurrent laryngeal nerve crosses behind the right artery. The artery is crossed by the superior belly of omohyoid at the level of cricoid cartilage. Below this level it is deeply placed because the sternomastoid and the infrahyoid muscles overlap it. But, above the level of omohyoid the artery is closer to the surface. Medially the common carotid artery is related to larynx and pharynx upto the lower margin of cricoid cartilage, below which it is related to the trachea and esophagus. The thyroid gland, recurrent laryngeal nerve and inferior thyroid artery are its medial relations. The internal jugular vein is the immediate lateral relation inside the carotid sheath.

Carotid Sinus and Body

The carotid sinus is a slight dilatation at the bifurcation of common carotid artery and the commencement of internal carotid artery. It is a baroreceptor and hence richly innervated by carotid sinus branch of the glossopharyngeal nerve and branches of vagus and sympathetic chain. Carotid sinus hypersensitivity or digital pressure on one or both carotid sinuses may cause excessive slowing of heart rate, fall in BP and fainting (cardinal features of carotid sinus syndrome). The carotid body is a small reddish structure behind the common carotid bifurcation. These bodies function as respiratory chemoreceptors to monitor blood oxygen and carbon dioxide levels. The glomus cells and ganglion cells in them receive nerve supply from the same sources as the carotid sinus.

The carotid bodies show enlargement in people, who live in high altitudes and in patients with hypoxia due to chronic lung diseases. The carotid body tumor or potato tumor of neck is a benign growth of carotid body usually adherent to all the three carotid arteries. It is a pulsatile swelling that moves transversely (vertical movement being prevented by the fork of the bifurcation of common carotid artery). When sufficiently enlarged it compresses the adjacent carotid sinus thereby precipitating an attack of carotid sinus syndrome.

INTERNAL CAROTID ARTERY (ICA)

The internal carotid artery supplies the large part of the cerebral hemisphere, pituitary, the eye and orbit, forehead and part of nasal cavity. It begins at the bifurcation of common carotid artery and ascends in the carotid sheath to reach the base of the skull. It enters the petrous part of the temporal bone by entering the carotid canal, in which it travels to reach the foramen lacerum, through the upper opening of which it enters the middle cranial fossa.

Relations (Fig. 74.1)

a. The anterior relations at the carotid triangle and above the triangle are different. The ICA is fairly superficial in the carotid triangle. Its anterior relations are, the skin, superficial fascia, deep fascia and anterior border of sternomastoid. It is crossed by occipital artery and hypoglossal nerve. The external carotid artery is anteromedial to the internal carotid artery. Above the carotid triangle the anterior relations are as follows. The posterior belly of digastric and stylohyoid muscles cross it. The posterior auricular artery, styloid process and stylopharyngeus muscle, glossopharyngeal nerve and pharyngeal branch of vagus are the other structures that cross it. The parotid gland and its contents (external carotid artery and its bifurcation, facial nerve, retromandibular vein) lie in front of the artery. In the posterior part of the digastric triangle the external carotid artery lies superficial and lateral to the internal carotid artery. However, the styloid process, stylopharyngeus muscle, glossopharyngeal nerve, pharyngeal branch of vagus and the deep part of parotid gland separate the two arteries.

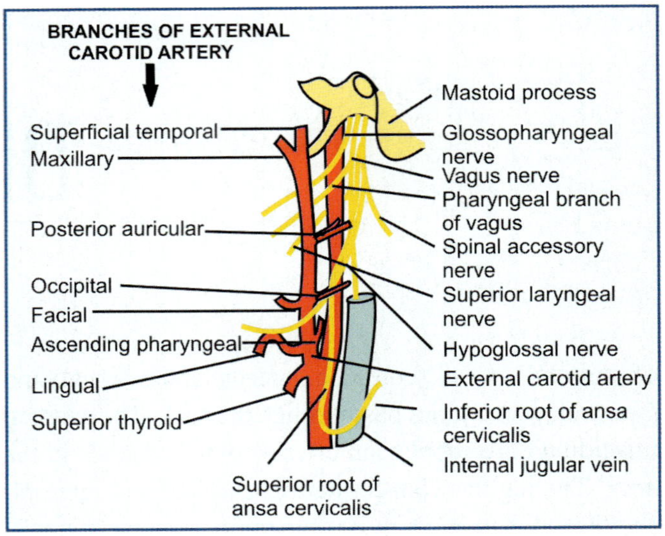

Fig. 74.1: Neurovascular bundle of neck (Note that CN XII crosses superficial to internal carotid, external carotid and lingual arteries but deep to occipital artery)

b. Behind the carotid sheath the ICA is related to the longus capitis muscle and the sympathetic chain. The superior laryngeal branch of the vagus passes posterior to the artery.
c. The internal carotid artery is closely related to lateral wall of oropharynx in the region of tonsillar fossa. Therefore, tonsil is its medial relation.
d. The internal jugular vein is on its lateral aspect and the vagus nerve is on the posterolateral aspect inside the carotid sheath.

Atherosclerosis

If the cervical part of internal carotid artery is narrowed due to atherosclerosis it may lead to impairment of vision or blindness and cerebral ischemia. The visual effects are produced because the ophthalmic artery is an intracranial branch of the ICA.

EXTERNAL CAROTID ARTERY (ECA)

This artery takes origin from the common carotid artery in the carotid triangle at the upper border of thyroid cartilage. It terminates in the substance of the parotid gland by dividing in superficial temporal and maxillary arteries at the back of the neck of mandible.

Relations in Carotid Triangle

The external carotid artery is anteromedial to the internal carotid artery in the carotid triangle. It gives rise to branches in the carotid triangle and lies closer to the surface, having the same superficial relations as the internal carotid artery. Medial relations of the artery in the triangle are the pharyngeal wall, superior laryngeal nerve and ascending pharyngeal artery. The hypoglossal nerve, the lingual vein, common facial vein and superior thyroid vein cross the artery in the triangle. As it leaves the carotid triangle it is crossed by posterior belly of digastric and the stylohyoid muscles.

Relations in the Posterior Part of Digastric Triangle

Here the artery lies in the narrow gap between the parotid and the pharynx. It changes its relation to the internal carotid by coming in lateral relation from the anteromedial relation. Medially it is separated from the internal carotid artery by the styloid process and the muscles attached to it. The ninth cranial nerve and pharyngeal branch of vagus cross the artery before it enters the substance of the parotid gland through the posteromedial surface of the gland.

Branches in Carotid Triangle (Fig. 67.2)

a. Ascending pharyngeal artery is the first branch in the carotid triangle. It is a long slender branch that runs close to the pharyngeal wall. It is distributed to the pharynx, auditory tube, tonsil, palate, middle ear and meninges.
b. Superior thyroid artery arises from anterior aspect. It runs downward and medially towards the superior pole of thyroid gland. Its named branches, from above downwards are, infrahyoid, superior laryngeal, sternomastoid, cricothyroid and glandular (anterior and posterior). The superior laryngeal branch is accompanied by internal laryngeal nerve while the superior thyroid itself is accompanied by external laryngeal nerve.
c. Lingual artery is the chief supply of the tongue. It arises from the anterior aspect opposite the tip of the greater horn of hyoid. It is divided in three parts by the hyoglossus muscle. The first part of the lingual artery lies in the carotid triangle. It forms a characteristic upward loop, which is crossed by the hypoglossal nerve. The second part passes deep to the hyoglossus muscle. The third part is known as arteria profunda linguae or deep lingual artery. It ascends along the anterior border of the hyoglossus lying on the medial aspect of genioglossus. On reaching the undersurface of the tongue it runs forwards beneath the mucous membrane on the side of the frenulum linguae. It ends at the tip of the tongue by anastomosing with the artery of opposite side. It gives a few named branches (suprahyoid from the first part, dorsal lingual from the second part, and the sublingual from the third part). The first part of the lingual artery is the preferred site for applying ligature.
d. Facial artery is a big artery that has a cervical and facial course. Like the lingual artery it forms a loop in its cervical course. Its relation to the submandibular gland is very important. Details of the artery are given along with blood supply of face.
e. Occipital artery arises from the posterior aspect of the external carotid artery at the level of facial artery. It leaves the carotid triangle by following the lower margin of posterior belly of digastric muscle. At first it crosses the anterior aspect of the transverse process of atlas and then traverses the vascular groove on the medial aspect of mastoid process. Here it lies deep to the digastric and other muscles attached to the mastoid process. In its further course the occipital artery enters the roof of the suboccipital triangle, where it lies on the semispinalis capitis (which is in the floor of the apical part of the posterior triangle of the neck). It pierces the insertion of trapezius two to three cm from the midline to enter the superficial fascia of the posterior quadrant of the scalp in company with the greater occipital nerve. The occipital artery has a wide area of distribution. It gives two sternomastoid branches in the carotid triangle. Deep to the mastoid process it gives stylomastoid (in two-thirds of subjects), mastoid and auricular branches. In the suboccipital region, there are the muscular and the descending branches, which anastomose with the transverse cervical artery. The occipital artery may injure in the fracture of the base of skull near the mastoid process. This may result in bleeding and formation of a

hematoma behind the ear, which may displace the pinna forwards (Battle's sign).

Branches of ECA Outside Carotid Triangle

f. Posterior auricular artery arises just above the digastric and stylohyoid muscles. Its named branches are, stylomastoid (in one-third of subjects), auricular and occipital arteries.

g. Superficial temporal artery is the smaller terminal branch of the external carotid artery given off in the substance of the parotid gland. This artery leaves the parotid gland through its base and crosses the root of the zygomatic arch to enter the anterior quadrant of the scalp. About five cm above the root of the zygoma the superficial temporal artery divides in its anterior (frontal) and posterior (parietal) branches. Apart from branches to parotid gland the named branches of the artery are, transverse facial, anterior auricular, zygomatico-orbital, middle temporal (which perforates the temporal fascia and grooves the squamous temporal bone) and the terminal branches. The arterial pulse can be felt at the root of the zygomatic arch in front of the auricle. The temporal arteritis is the connective tissue disease of the elderly (over 60 years), in which the temporal arteries become palpable, thickened and painful. Tortuosity of the arteries in the elderly is a common feature.

h. Maxillary artery is the other terminal branch of the external carotid artery. It leaves the parotid gland to enter the infratemporal fossa. The details of the artery are dealt along with the infratemporal and pterygopalatine fossae.

Subclavian Artery (Fig. 74.2)

The subclavian arteries have a wide area of distribution as they supply the upper limb, part of neck and part of thoracic and abdominal walls, the contents of posterior cranial fossa and the spinal cord.

Origin and Termination

The right subclavian artery is a branch of brachiocephalic artery hence it begins behind the right sternoclavicular joint. The left subclavian artery is the direct branch of the arch of aorta hence it begins in the superior mediastinum. Thus, the left subclavian artery is longer than the right. Each subclavian artery continues at the outer border of the first rib as the axillary artery.

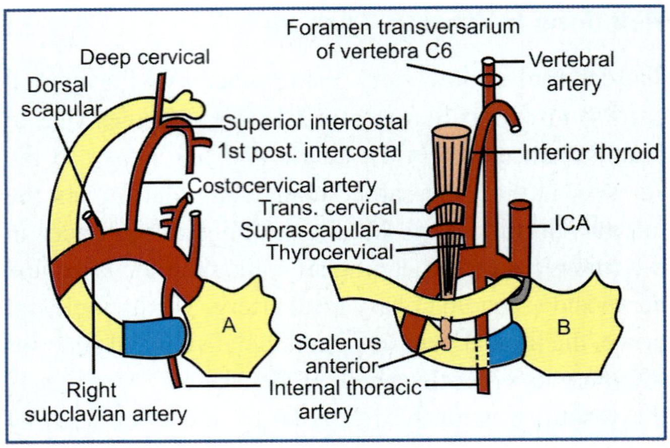

Fig. 74.2: Simplified scheme to show branches of right subclavian artery. Fig. A shows branches of costocervical trunk and Fig. B of thyrocervical trunk

Surface Marking

a. The left subclavian artery is marked by 8 mm wide line, which starts at the left margin of the manubrium sterni at the level of the center of manubrium. This line is extended to the left sternoclavicular joint and then to the midclavicular point with upward convexity.

b. The right subclavian artery is marked by a similar line, which starts at the right sternoclavicular joint and extends laterally to the midclavicular point with an upward convexity.

Parts of Subclavian Artery

The scalenus anterior muscle crosses in front of the artery to reach the first rib for insertion. The muscle divides the subclavian artery in three parts. There are differences in the relations of the first part on the two sides but the second and third parts are identical on the two sides. The third part of the artery is the content of the posterior triangle.

First Part of Right Subclavian Artery

This part extends from the right sternoclavicular joint to the medial margin of right scalenus anterior. It ascends about two cm above the clavicle to take an arched course. The first part of the subclavian artery forms the base of the scalenovertebral triangle.

Relations

a. Anteriorly the first part is covered by several structures hence it is deeply placed. The sternomastoid, sternohyoid and sternothyroid muscles cross in front of it. The union of right internal jugular and right subclavian veins to form right brachiocephalic vein takes place in front of the first part. The right vertebral vein crosses it. The nerves that cross the artery in front are, right vagus and its cervical cardiac branches, cervical cardiac branches of right sympathetic chain and ansa subclavia (a connection between the middle and inferior sympathetic ganglia).

b. Two nerves loop round the inferior aspect (ansa subclavia and right recurrent laryngeal nerve).

c. The posterior relations are the apex of the right lung, cervical pleura and suprapleural membrane. The same two nerves come in posterior relations after hooking round the inferior aspect.

First Part of Left Subclavian Artery

a. The thoracic part of the first part of the left subclavian artery is related to the structures in the superior mediastinum. Anteriorly it is in relation to the left common carotid artery, left vagus, left phrenic nerve and left brachiocephalic vein. Its posterior relations are the left side of esophagus and thoracic duct. Medially it is related to trachea, left recurrent laryngeal nerve, esophagus and thoracic duct and laterally it is in contact with the mediastinal surface of the left lung and pleura.

b. The relations of the cervical part of the first part of the left subclavian artery are similar to those on the right side except for the following differences. The thoracic duct and left phrenic nerve cross the artery in front. The left recurrent laryngeal nerve does not hook round the artery and hence is not related to its inferior and posterior aspects.

Second Part of Subclavian Arteries

Anteriorly the artery is related to the scalenus anterior muscle and the subclavian vein in front of the muscle. Posteriorly there are lung and pleura, Sibson's fascia and lower trunk of brachial plexus. Superiorly it is related to the upper and middle trunks of brachial plexus.

Third Part of Subclavian Arteries

The third part extends from the lateral margin of the scalenus anterior to the outer margin of the first rib. It lies in the subclavian triangle of the neck. This is the most superficial part of the subclavian artery and hence it can be approached just lateral to the posterior margin of the sternomastoid muscle and can be compressed against the first rib with shoulder depressed and the pressure being directed in downward, backward and medial direction.

Relations of Third Part

The third part is related anteriorly to the external jugular vein and its tributaries and nerve to subclavius. The clavicle lies in front of it. The subclavian vein is present anteroinferiorly while the lower trunk of brachial plexus lies posteroinferiorly. The left lung and pleura form the posterior relations. The middle and superior trunks of the brachial plexus lie superiorly. The artery is in direct contact with the superior surface of first rib inferiorly. The subclavian artery and the lower trunk of the brachial, plexus lie in a narrow scalene triangle bounded by the superior surface of the first rib and the scalenus anterior and medius muscles. The cervical rib may further narrow the triangle producing symptoms of arterial and neural compression giving rise to the cervical rib or thoracic outlet syndrome (Fig. 31.1).

Branches of First Part (Fig. 74.2)

There are three branches from the first part, vertebral, thyrocervical, and the internal mammary arteries. The costocervical trunk is the branch of the first part on the left side only.

a. The vertebral artery (refer to the suboccipital triangle in Chapter 80).

b. Thyrocervical trunk at once breaks up in three branches, inferior thyroid, suprascapular and transverse cervical.

i. The inferior thyroid artery forms a loop to reach the inferior pole of the thyroid gland. First it runs up along the medial margin of scalenus anterior then turns medially just below the transverse process of the sixth cervical vertebra and finally it descends on the longus colli to reach the inferior pole of the thyroid gland. As the inferior thyroid artery nears the thyroid gland it is closely related to the recurrent laryngeal nerve. The branches of the inferior thyroid artery are, ascending cervical, inferior laryngeal, pharyngeal, tracheal, esophageal and glandular to thyroid and parathyroid glands. The inferior thyroid artery is clinically important since it may be injured in surgery on thyroid gland).

ii. The suprascapular artery turns laterally across the scalenus anterior muscle to reach the posterior triangle. Here it crosses anterior to the third part of the subclavian artery and the brachial plexus. The suprascapular artery and the nerve leave the posterior triangle along with the inferior belly of omohyoid and reach the scapular region. Further course of the artery is described along with muscles of the back.

iii. The transverse cervical artery divides in superficial and deep branches in the posterior triangle. Frequently the deep branch takes origin directly from the third part of the subclavian artery. In that case it is called the dorsal scapular artery, which accompanies the dorsal scapular nerve to the back. In such cases the superficial branch represents the transverse cervical artery and travels along the accessory nerve to the deep surface of the trapezius muscle.

c. The internal mammary artery (internal thoracic) takes origin from the inferior aspect of the subclavian artery. Its further course is described in Chapter 34 on blood vessels of the thoracic wall.

Branches of Second Part

The costocervical trunk takes origin from the posterior aspect of the second part of the subclavian artery on the right side and from the first part of the subclavian artery on the left side. Sometimes it takes origin from the first part on both sides. It divides in the superior or highest intercostal and deep cervical branches at the neck of the first rib (Fig. 74.3). The superior intercostal artery descends in front of the neck of the first rib and gives posterior intercostal arteries to the first two intercostal spaces. The deep cervical artery passes to the back of the neck, where it ascends in the deep muscles and anastomoses with the descending branches of the occipital artery.

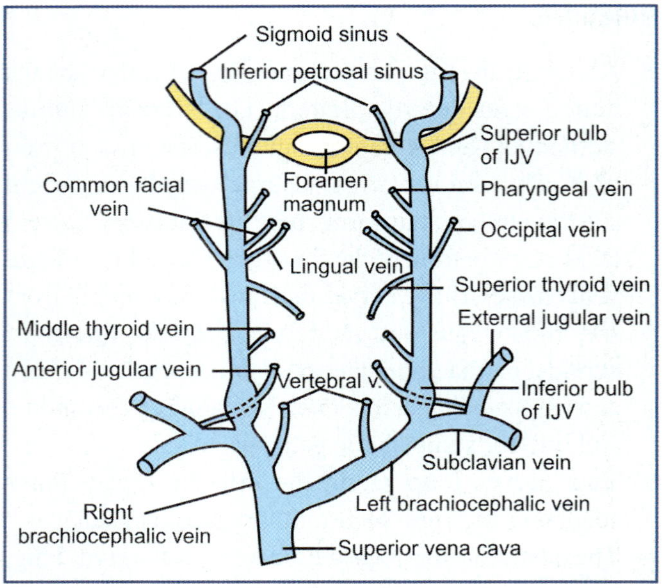

Fig. 74.3: Formation, tributaries and termination of internal jugular vein (IJV)

Branches of Third Part

Usually there are no branches but in a percentage of subjects the dorsal scapular artery takes origin from the third part and takes the place of the deep branch of the transverse cervical artery.

Veins of the Neck

The veins of the neck are the anterior jugular, external jugular, internal jugular and the subclavian veins. The anterior jugular veins are described with midline region of the front of the neck and the external jugular veins are described with the posterior triangle of neck. These two are the superficial veins of the neck.

Internal Jugular Vein (Fig. 74.3)

The internal jugular vein (IJV) is the major deep vein of the neck. It lies inside the carotid sheath. It begins as a continuation of the sigmoid sinus at the posterior part of the jugular foramen at the base of the cranium. At its origin it exhibits superior bulb, which is closely related to the floor of middle ear. The vein travels in the carotid sheath to the root of the neck, where it joins the subclavian vein to form the brachiocephalic vein medial to the medial border of the scalenus anterior and behind the medial end of the clavicle. At its termination it lies in the lesser supraclavicular triangle between the sternal and clavicular heads of the sternomastoid, where it can be easily approached. It presents the inferior bulb at its termination. The cervical lymph nodes belonging to the deep group lie in intimate relation of the internal jugular vein. The IJV may be injured during removal of the tuberculous or neoplastic (nodes involved in malignancy) lymph nodes.

Surface Marking

A broad band from the lobule of the ear to the medial end of the clavicle represents the IJV. Its inferior bulb is in the depression between the sternal and clavicular heads of the sternomastoid muscle.

Tributaries

Inferior petrosal sinus is the first tributary and opens in the superior bulb of the internal jugular vein. The other tributaries are, pharyngeal veins, common facial vein, lingual veins (deep lingual and dorsal lingual), superior thyroid and middle thyroid veins and occasionally the occipital vein.

Subclavian Vein

Each subclavian vein begins as the continuation of axillary vein at the outer border of first rib. It has two parts corresponding to the third and second parts of the subclavian artery. In the posterior triangle it lies anterior and inferior to the subclavian artery. This part of the vein lies in the anterior vascular groove on the superior surface of the first rib. The second part of the subclavian artery is separated from the vein by the scalenus anterior muscle. The subclavian vein ends by joining the internal jugular vein to form the brachiocephalic vein at the medial margin of the scalenus anterior muscle behind the medial end of the clavicle. External jugular vein is its main tributary in the posterior triangle.

Clinical Highlights

The internal jugular and the subclavian veins are usually used in clinical practice for central venous access. This is used for measuring the pulmonary artery and intracardiac pressures, for prolonged intravenous feeding and for introduction of cardiac pace makers.

a. The internal jugular vein is the most commonly used vein for central venous access. There are two approaches to the internal jugular vein. In the high approach the needle is introduced at the midpoint of an imaginary line joining the mastoid process and sternoclavicular joint. The point is immediately lateral to the carotid pulse or just lateral to the upper margin of thyroid cartilage. In low approach the needle is introduced through the apex of lesser supraclavicular triangle between the two heads of sternomastoid muscle.
b. The right internal jugular vein is an ideal venous manometer as it is in direct line with the right brachiocephalic vein, superior vena cava and the right atrium. There are no intervening valves in these veins. Therefore pressure in the IJV is the reliable indicator of the right atrial pressure. Normally when the subject is standing or sitting upright the internal jugular vein is collapsed. When the subject is lying flat the vein is completely filled. When the subject lies supine at 45 degrees the point at which jugular pulsation becomes visible is usually above the clavicle. A quick rule of thumb is, if jugular venous pulsation is visible above the clavicle with the subject bolt upright then the jugular venous pressure (JVP) must be raised. The common cause of raised jugular pressure is congestive cardiac failure.
c. The subclavian vein is the commonly used vein for central venous access for which infraclavicular approach is considered safer. The needle is inserted below the clavicle at the junction of its medial and middle thirds and then directed towards the posterior aspect of suprasternal notch to reach the vein.

75 Cervical Plexus

The cervical plexus lies in the upper part of the neck behind the prevertebral fascia and in front of the origin of the scalenus medius and levator scapulae muscles. It is formed by the ventral rami of upper four cervical spinal nerves. Each ventral ramus receives gray ramus from the superior cervical sympathetic ganglion.

Formation (Fig. 75.1)

There are three loops in the cervical plexus. Each ramus except the first divides in ascending and descending parts, which unite in communicating loops. The first loop is between C2 and C3, the second between C3 and C4, and the third between C4 and C5 rami, which connects the cervical and brachial plexuses. The C1 communicates with C2 but all C1 fibers leave this connection to join the hypoglossal nerve. The C1 ventral ramus has no cutaneous supply. The majority of the branches of the cervical plexus arise from the first and second loops.

Superficial or Cutaneous Branches (Fig. 65.2)	
Ascending	Lesser occipital (C2) Great auricular (C2,C3) Transverse cutaneous nerve of neck (C2,C3)
Descending	Medial, intermediate and lateral supraclavicular (C3,C4)

These six cutaneous branches pierce the prevertebral fascia and appear in the posterior triangle of neck at the nerve point of the posterior triangle along with the spinal accessory nerve. The nerve point is located just above the midpoint of the posterior margin of the sternomastoid.

a. The lesser occipital nerve hooks round the spinal accessory nerve at the nerve point and then ascends along the posterior margin of the sternomastoid muscle. It supplies the upper third of the medial aspect of the pinna of ear, the skin over the mastoid process and the skin in the posterior quadrant of scalp.
b. The great auricular nerve is the largest cutaneous branch of the cervical plexus. It emerges from the posterior margin of the sternomastoid and crosses the muscle to go towards the angle of mandible. It supplies the lower two-thirds of the medial surface of the pinna and the lateral surface of the lobule and also the skin over the mastoid process and the skin over the angle of mandible, masseter and parotid gland.
c. The transverse cutaneous nerve of neck or anterior cutaneous nerve of neck passes horizontally forwards on the sternomastoid muscle. At the anterior border of the muscle it pierces the deep fascia and splits in branches that supply the skin of the entire front of the neck.

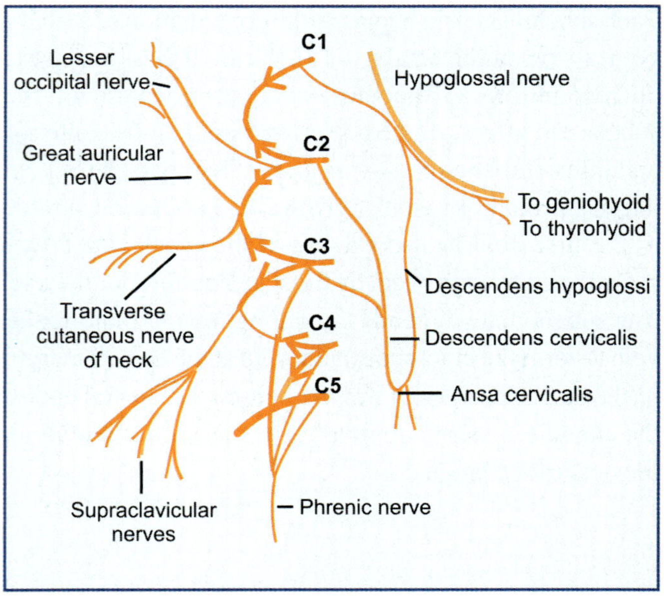

Fig. 75.1: Formation and branches of cervical plexus (Note that proprioceptive branches to sternomastoid, trapezius and levator scapulae are not shown)

d. The supraclavicular nerves emerge pierce the deep fascia above the clavicle and cross the clavicle or frequently pierce through it to enter the anterior wall of the chest and supply the skin as low as the level of sternal angle. In this region the cervical fourth dermatome comes to lie side by side with the thoracic second dermatome.

Deep or Muscular Branches	
Medial	Rectus capitis lateralis and anterior
	Longus capitis and longus colli
	Descendens cervicalis (C2,C3)
	Phrenic nerve (C3, C4, C5)
Lateral	Scalene muscles
	Levator scapulae
	Proprioceptive supply to trapezius and SCM

In addition to the cutaneous and muscular branches the cervical plexus receives communicating branches from the sympathetic chain and gives C1 fibers to the hypoglossal nerve as follows:

a. The superior cervical sympathetic ganglion gives postganglionic fibers to all four cervical rami via gray rami communicans.
b. The first loop of the plexus sends a communicating branch carrying C1 fibers to the hypoglossal nerve.

Ansa Cervicalis (Fig.75.1)

The C1 ventral ramus joins the hypoglossal nerve. A few of the C1 fibers leave the hypoglossal nerve as the superior root of ansa cervicalis. The fibers of C2 and C3 form the inferior root of the ansa. The superior and inferior roots unite with each other to form a nerve loop, which is embedded in the anterior wall of the carotid sheath. The remaining C1 fibers in the hypoglossal nerve, supply to the geniohyoid muscle by a branch of the hypoglossal nerve. The branches to the inferior belly of omohyoid, sternohyoid and sternothyroid arise from the loop. The superior limb supplies the superior belly of omohyoid muscle and thyrohyoid muscle (by a branch called thyrohyoid branch).

Phrenic Nerve (Fig. 41.1)

The phrenic nerve (C3, C4, C5) is described in the Section on Thorax in Chapter 41.

76 Sympathetic Chain in Neck

The cervical part of the sympathetic chain extends from the base of the cranium to the neck of the first rib, where it continues as its thoracic part. It has a straight course in the neck lying behind the carotid sheath and in front of the prevertebral fascia. It bears three ganglia, the superior, middle and the cervicothoracic or stellate, which is formed by the fusion of the inferior cervical and first thoracic ganglia. These ganglia send postganglionic sympathetic fibers to the cervical spinal nerves through gray rami communicans. They also give off cervical cardiac branches in addition to supplying the cervical viscera. The cranial continuation of the sympathetic chain is called internal carotid nerve, which forms a plexus along the internal carotid artery.

Superior Cervical Ganglion (Fig. 76.1)

The superior ganglion is the largest and is formed by fusion of upper four cervical ganglia. It lies in front of the transverse processes of vertebrae C2 and C3. It receives long preganglionic fibers from T1 to T4 segments of spinal cord, as these fibers pass uninterrupted through the corresponding thoracic and the inferior and middle cervical ganglia.

Branches

a. Gray rami to first to fourth cervical spinal nerves.
b. Laryngotracheal branches.
c. Superior cervical cardiac branch on the left side takes part in the superficial cardiac plexus and on the right side in the deep cardiac plexus.
d. Communicating branches to the cranial nerves at the base of skull.
e. Branches to the common and external carotid arteries form plexuses around these arteries. The plexus around the facial artery supplies the sweat glands and blood vessels of the face. Plexus around the middle meningeal artery sends branch to the otic ganglion and another branch called external petrosal nerve to the geniculate ganglion of the facial nerve.
f. Internal carotid nerve from the upper pole of the ganglion forms a plexus around the internal carotid artery. The plexus provides sympathetic supply to the dilator pupillae through the plexus around the ophthalmic artery or through the communicating branches to the nasociliary nerve. Thus, the long postganglionic fibers for the dilator pupillae pass through the internal carotid nerve to the sympathetic plexus around the internal carotid artery. This plexus may communicate with the nasociliary nerve from which the ciliary ganglion is suspended in the orbit. The sympathetic fibers pass through the ganglion and reach

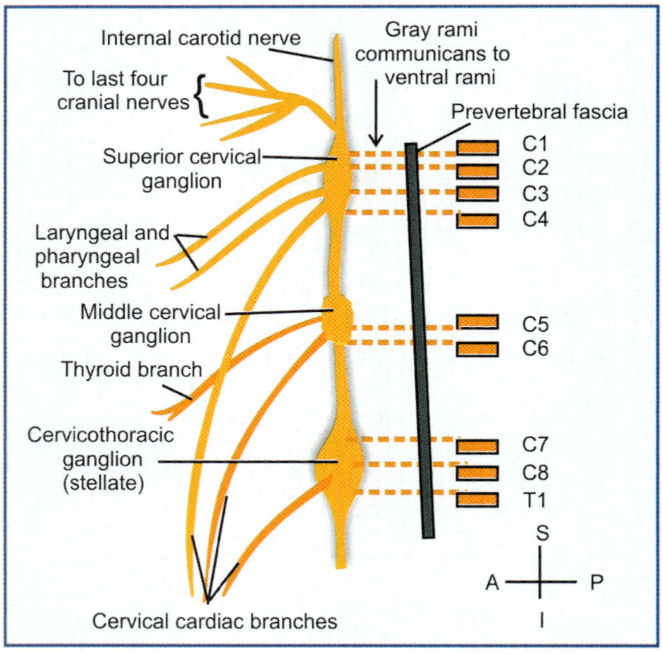

Fig. 76.1: Scheme to depict cervical sympathetic chain and its branches (Note that vascular branches of superior ganglion to extracranial arteries and those of other ganglia are not shown)

the dilator pupillae muscle via the short ciliary nerves. It must be understood that the course of the preganglionic as well as postganglionic sympathetic fibers of dilator pupillae muscle is very long (Fig. 4.2). Interruption of the fibers anywhere along this long route results in constriction of pupil, partial ptosis, loss of sweating and flushing on the same side of face (Horner's syndrome).

Middle Cervical Ganglion

This small ganglion lies in front of the transverse process of the sixth cervical vertebra. It is formed by fusion of fifth and sixth cervical ganglia. It lies on the inferior thyroid artery.

Branches

a. Gray rami to the fifth and sixth cervical spinal nerves.
b. Middle cervical cardiac branch of each side joins the deep cardiac plexus.
c. Branches to thyroid and parathyroid glands through the plexus around the inferior thyroid artery.
d. Ansa subclavia is a loop of fibers (Fig. 76.2) which winds round the subclavian artery and connects the middle and the cervicothoracic ganglia.

Cervicothoracic Ganglion

This is irregular in shape hence the name stellate ganglion. It is formed by the fusion of lower two cervical ganglia (inferior cervical) and first thoracic ganglion. It is located in the scalenovertebral triangle, where it lies behind the first part of the vertebral artery. Here the ganglion is related to the front of the neck of the first rib (Fig. 78.1).

Branches

a. Gray rami to cervical seventh and eighth nerves and first thoracic nerve for distribution to the upper limb.

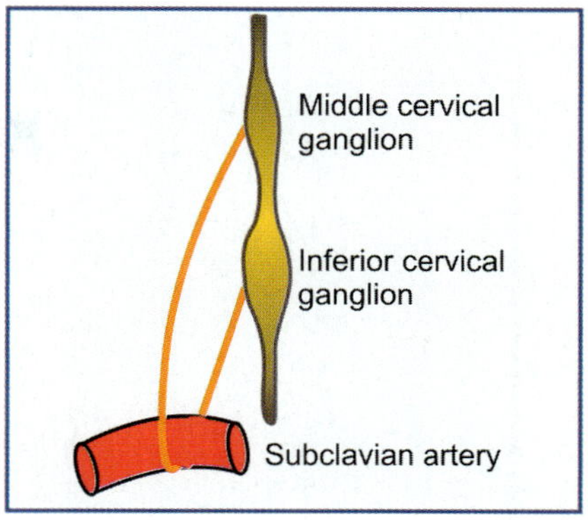

Fig. 76.2: Ansa subclavia connecting middle and inferior cervical sympathetic ganglia looping around subclavian artery

b. Inferior cervical cardiac branch to the deep cardiac plexus.
c. Branches that form plexus around the subclavian artery, which extends along the axillary artery.
d. Ansa subclavia connects it to the middle ganglion.
e. Branches, which form plexus around the vertebral artery.

Stellate Ganglion Block

For injecting anesthetic solution in the ganglion the needle is introduced at a point, which is 2 cm above the sternoclavicular joint and passed in a perpendicularly backward direction until it hits the transverse process of seventh cervical vertebra. This depth is usually 2.5 to 3 cm from the surface. The other method of stellate ganglion block is as follows. First the carotid tubercle (a large tubercle on the transverse process of the sixth cervical vertebra) is palpated. It lies about a fingerbreadth lateral to the cricoid cartilage. The carotid sheath and sternomastoid are pushed laterally. The needle is inserted at the skin over the carotid tubercle. The anesthetic is then injected in the lower direction.

77 Cervical Lymph Nodes

Of the total of nearly 800 lymph nodes in the body about 300 are located in the neck. Inflammation of the cervical lymph nodes is very common, especially due to tuberculosis. The secondary deposit in the lymph nodes from the primary cancer in the area of drainage of the nodes is another cause of lymph node enlargement. Cervical lymph nodes can be broadly divided in superficial and deep groups.

Superficial Group

This group consists of occipital, retroauricular or mastoid, preauricular or superficial parotid, deep parotid, submental, superficial nodes along the accessory nerve and along the external jugular and the anterior jugular veins.

Deep Group

This consists of the upper deep cervical group containing jugulodigastric nodes, the lower deep cervical group containing jugulo-omohyoid nodes, supraclavicular nodes, the anterior cervical nodes and the retropharyngeal nodes.

Superficial Lymph Nodes (Fig. 77.1)

a. The occipital nodes are located at the apex of the posterior triangle and drain the back of scalp. The efferent vessels drain in the deep cervical nodes. The occipital nodes are enlarged in German measles.
b. The posterior auricular or retroauricular nodes are located on the mastoid process and drain the back of scalp and posterior wall of external acoustic meatus. Its efferent vessels drain in the deep cervical nodes.
c. The superficial parotid nodes are located on the surface of parotid gland. Their area of drainage consists of upper part of face, anterior part of scalp, auricle and external acoustic meatus. These nodes drain in the superficial cervical nodes along the external jugular vein.
d. The deep parotid nodes are located in the substance of the parotid gland. The area of drainage is the temporal and infratemporal fossa, middle ear, auditory tube, upper molar teeth and gums. Their efferent vessels drain in the deep cervical nodes.
e. The submandibular nodes are embedded on the surface of the submandibular salivary gland. They drain the part of face below the line joining the medial angle of eye and the angle of mandible, submandibular and sublingual salivary glands, side of tongue and floor of mouth, teeth and gums, palate, part of nasal cavity. The buccal lymph nodes on the buccinator muscle also

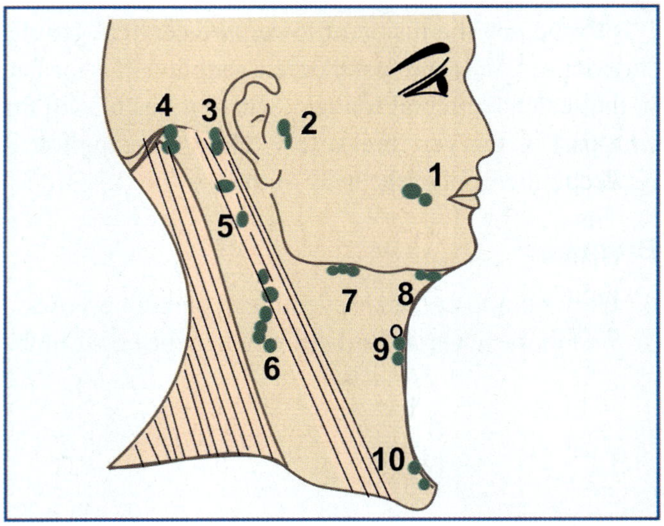

Fig. 77.1: Superficial lymph nodes of head and neck: 1—Buccal, 2—Preauricular, 3—Posterior auricular, 4—Occipital, 5—Superficial cervical, 6—Along accessory nerve, 7—Submandibular, 8—Submental, 9—Anterior cervical, 10—Inside suprasternal space

drain in these nodes. The efferent vessels drain in the deep cervical nodes.

f. The submental nodes are present in the submental triangle. Their area of drainage includes the tip of tongue, floor of mouth below the tip of tongue, incisor teeth and associated gums and central part of lower lip. The efferent vessels drain in the deep cervical nodes.

g. The superficial cervical nodes are located along the course of anterior jugular and external jugular veins. The nodes along the external jugular vein receive the lymph vessels from the parotid and the superficial tissues of the lower face and ear. The nodes along the anterior jugular vein receive lymph from the skin and muscles of the front of the neck to the deep cervical nodes.

Deep Lymph Nodes (Fig. 77.2)

a. The anterior cervical nodes include the prelaryngeal, pretracheal, paratracheal lymph nodes and the nodes in the suprasternal space of Burns. These nodes drain larynx, trachea and thyroid gland and their efferent vessels empty in the lower deep cervical nodes.

b. The retropharyngeal nodes lie in the space between the pharyngeal wall and prevertebral fascia. They receive lymph from the oropharynx, nasopharynx, palate, auditory tube, nasal cavity, paranasal sinuses and cervical vertebral column. These nodes are infected in tuberculosis of the cervical spine and form retropharyngeal abscess. Their efferents drain in the deep cervical nodes.

c. The upper and lower deep cervical nodes form a long chain on the carotid sheath almost embedded in the tunica adventitia of the internal jugular vein. Two nodes in this group are large compared to others. The upper is called the jugulo-digastric and is located in a triangle formed by posterior belly of digastric, common facial vein and internal jugular vein. It lies just below and behind the angle of the mandible. It receives lymph from the tonsil and the tongue. The jugulo-omohyoid node is located in relation to the intermediate tendon of the omohyoid and receives lymph mainly from the tongue.

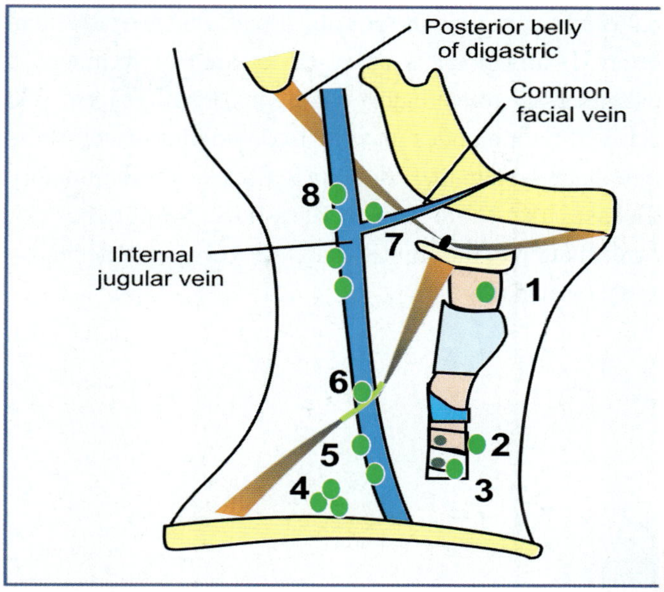

Fig. 77.2: Deep lymph nodes of neck: 1—Prelaryngeal, 2—Pretracheal, 3—Paratracheal, 4—Supraclavicular, 5—Lower deep cervical 6—Jugulo-omohyoid, 7—Jugulodigastric, 8—Upper deep cervical (Note that jugulodigastric node is located in a triangle bounded by IJV, common facial vein and posterior belly of digastric)

d. The supraclavicular nodes are located in the lower part of the posterior triangle in relation to the subclavian vessels and are palpated in the supraclavicular fossa (Fig. 65.5). Retrograde spread through the thoracic duct on the left side may be cause of their enlargement especially in cancer from the stomach, colon and both the testis, which spreads to the nodes of left side and not of the right side. The left supraclavicular lymph nodes are called Virchow's nodes.

The deep cervical lymph nodes receive lymph from the entire head and neck. The efferents from the deep group form the jugular lymph trunk on each side, which terminates on the right side in the right lymphatic duct or at the junction of right subclavian and right internal jugular veins. The left jugular trunk usually joins the thoracic duct or may join either the internal jugular or the subclavian vein.

Palpation of Cervical Lymph Nodes

The palpation of the cervical lymph nodes is part of the clinical examination of the patient. All the nodes are palpated starting at one point and proceeding in a sequential order. If any node is enlarged its area of drainage is examined for inflammatory conditions or malignancy. The cervical lymph nodes may be involved in diseases of the lymphatic system like Hodgkin's disease or inflammatory disease like tuberculosis or AIDS. Sometimes for confirmation of the clinical diagnosis cervical node biopsy is performed.

Block Dissection of Neck

The block dissection of the neck is a procedure in which all the lymph nodes of the neck along with the other structures like; sternomastoid muscle, internal and external jugular veins, submandibular salivary gland and accessory nerve are removed. The block dissection is usually required if cancer of tongue spreads to lymph nodes of the neck.

78 Paravertebral Muscles of Neck

The paravertebral muscles include the scalenus anterior, scalenus medius, scalenus posterior and scalenus minimus muscles.

Scalenus Anterior (Fig. 31.2)

This muscle is the key muscle of the root of the neck. It takes origin from the anterior tubercles of the transverse processes of the third to sixth cervical vertebrae and is inserted in to the scalene tubercle on the inner margin of the first rib and in to ridge on the superior surface of the first rib.

Important Relations

a. The phrenic nerve is plastered to the anterior surface of the muscle by the prevetebral fascia. The lateral part of the carotid sheath is related to the anterior surface. The transverse cervical and suprascapular arteries cross in front of the muscle. The subclavian vein crosses in front of the lower part of the muscle.
b. The lower part of the medial margin of the scalenus anterior muscle forms the lateral margin of the scalenovertebral triangle or triangle of vertebral artery. (Fig. 78.1). The triangle is bounded medially by the lateral margin of longus colli muscle. Its base is the first part of subclavian artery. This triangle contains the first part of vertebral artery, thyrocervical trunk and the sympathetic chain. The subclavian vein and the internal jugular vein unite to form the brachiocephalic vein medial to the medial margin of the scalenus anterior muscle behind the medial end if the clavicle. On the left side the thoracic duct is related to the medial margin as it arches down to open at the point of union of the left subclavian and left internal jugular veins.
c. The posterior aspect of scalenus anterior, superior surface of the first rib and anterior aspect of scalenus medius enclose scalene triangle at the insertion on the first rib (Fig. 31.1). This triangle contains second part of subclavian artery and lower trunk of brachial plexus.

Nerve Supply

The scalenus anterior receives direct branches from the anterior primary rami of the fourth, fifth and sixth cervical nerves.

Actions

a. Acting bilaterally the muscles fix the first rib during quiet inspiration.
b. Acting bilaterally the muscles lift the first ribs during forced inspiration.
c. Acting unilaterally the muscle bends the neck forwards and laterally thereby turning the face to the opposite side.

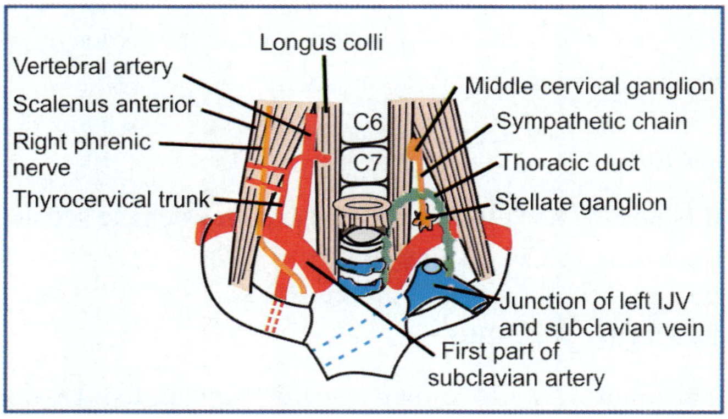

Fig. 78.1: Schematic depiction of the root of neck to show scalenovertebral triangle (Note that all contents of triangle are symmetrical, except thoracic duct. The figure also depicts crossing of right phrenic nerve anterior to internal thoracic artery)

Scalenus Anterior Syndrome

Hypertrophy or spasm of the muscle may compress the contents of the scalene triangle. The symptoms are similar to those produced by the cervical rib. Division of the muscle (scalenotomy) may relieve the symptoms.

Scalenus Medius

This muscle takes origin from the posterior tubercles of the second to seventh cervical vertebrae and is inserted into the upper surface of the first rib posterior to the groove for subclavian artery. The dorsal scapular nerve and the C5 and C6 roots of the long thoracic nerve pierce the muscle in the floor of the posterior triangle of neck.

Nerve Supply

Direct branches of the third to eighth cervical anterior primary rami supply the scalenus medius muscle.

Actions

The muscle bends the neck to its own side. It raises the first rib during forced inspiration.

Scalenus Posterior

It takes origin from the posterior tubercles of the transverse processes of the fourth, fifth and sixth cervical vertebrae and is inserted in the outer surface of the second rib.

Nerve Supply

The direct branches of primary rami of the lower three cervical nerves supply the muscle.

Actions

It bends the neck to its own side and elevates the second rib during forced inspiration.

Scalenus Minimus

This muscle is also known a scalenus pleuralis. It takes origin from the transverse process of the seventh cervical vertebra and is inserted into the inner margin of the first rib. Some of its fibers are continuous with the suprapleural membrane (Sibson's fascia) and the cervical pleura.

Prevertebral Muscles of Neck

These muscles are located in front of the cervical vertebral column and are covered with prevertebral layer of deep cervical fascia. These muscles consist of longus colli, longus capitis, rectus capitis anterior and rectus capitis lateralis muscles.

Longus Colli

This muscle consists of three parts, upper oblique part, middle vertical part and lower oblique part. The upper oblique part extends between the anterior arch of atlas to the transverse processes of the third, fourth and fifth cervical vertebrae. The vertical part arises from the bodies of the lower three cervical and the upper three thoracic vertebrae and is inserted in to the bodies of the second, third and fourth cervical vertebrae. The lower oblique part takes origin from the bodies of the upper three thoracic vertebrae and is inserted in to the anterior tubercles of the transverse processes of the fifth and sixth cervical vertebrae. This part forms the medial margin of the scalenovertebral triangle.

Nerve Supply

The muscle receives direct branches from the ventral rami of second to sixth cervical spinal nerves.

Actions

The longus colli flexes the cervical vertebral column.

Longus Capitis

This muscle takes origin from the anterior tubercles of the transverse processes of the third to sixth cervical vertebrae and is inserted in to the base of the cranium on either side and behind the pharyngeal tubercle.

Nerve Supply

The muscle receives branches from the ventral rami of the first, second and third cervical ventral rami.

Rectus Capitis Anterior

It arises from the lateral mass of atlas vertebra and is inserted in to the basilar part of the occipital bone.

Rectus Capitis Lateralis

It takes origin from the transverse process of atlas and is inserted in to the jugular process of the occipital bone.

Nerve Supply

Both the recti muscles are innervated by the loop of communication between the first and second cervical ventral rami.

79 Deep Muscles of the Back

The deep or intrinsic muscles of the back are a complex group of muscles extending from the sacrum to the skull. They are collectively called the postvertebral muscles and are very well developed in Man. In upright position the weight falls in front of the vertebral column because the line of gravity passes in front of it. Therefore, the postural tone of the postvertebral muscles is responsible for maintaining the normal curvatures of the vertebral column. All the deep muscles receive nerve supply from the dorsal rami of the spinal nerves.

Classification of the Deep Muscles of Back

From superficial to deeper level the muscles of the back are classified in four groups:

a. Splenius muscle is the one in which the fibers are directed upward and laterally.
b. Erector spinae group of muscles are those in which the fibers run vertically.
c. Transversospinalis group is the one in which muscle fibers run upward and medially.
d. Interspinales and intertransversarii are short segmental and the deepest muscles.

Splenius Muscles

The word splenius means a bandage. This muscle wraps round the other deep muscles of the neck like a bandage. The splenius consists of splenius capitis and splenius cervicis muscles.

a. Splenius capitis takes origin from the lower half of the ligamentum nuchae and spines of the seventh cervical and upper three to four thoracic vertebrae. It is inserted in the mastoid process and the lateral third of superior nuchal line. The splenius capitis appears in the upper part of the floor of the posterior triangle of the neck.
b. Splenius cervicis takes origin from the spines of third to sixth thoracic vertebrae and is inserted in the posterior tubercles of the transverse processes of the upper two to three cervical vertebrae.

Actions

Acting together the muscles of the two sides draw the head directly backward. Acting alone the muscle turns the head laterally (lateral flexion).

Erector Spinae or Sacrospinalis

This is a very long and complex muscle, composed of as many as nine muscles. It extends from the sacrum to the cranium. The posterior layer of thoracolumbar fascia covers its thoracolumbar part. The origin of erector spinae is U-shaped. The lateral limb of the U is attached to the posterior segment of iliac crest and lateral sacral crest. Its medial limb is attached to the median crest of sacrum, lumbar and lower thoracic spines and their supraspinous ligaments. In the lumbar region the muscle expands to form a thick fleshy mass, which can be felt in the living. This fleshy mass divides into three columns in the upper lumbar region. Each column is composed of three muscles. From lateral to medial side the columns are:

a. Iliocostocervicalis consists of iliocostalis lumborum, iliocostalis thoracis and iliocostalis cervicis.
b. Longissimus consists of longissimus thoracis, longissimus cervicis and longissimus capitis.
c. Spinalis consists of spinalis thoracis, spinalis cervicis and spinalis capitis.

These various muscles are inserted in the spines and transverse processes of thoracic and cervical vertebrae, lower ribs and in the cranium. The longissimus column alone is attached to the skull. The longissimus capitis is attached to the mastoid process.

Actions

a. When the right and left muscles act together they produce extension of vertebral column from the forward flexed position.
b. Acting singly the muscles cause lateral flexion of the trunk and rotation to the same side.

Importance of Erector Spinae

The erector spinae is very important postural muscle. If it becomes weak in old age or in persons, who do not take adequate exercise, the vertebral column tends to bend forward, which may predispose to disc prolapse. Exercise and brisk walking help in maintaining the tone of erector spinae.

Testing Muscle Function

The power of erector spinae is tested by asking the patient to lift shoulders and head against resistance while lying in prone position.

Transversospinalis

The muscles in this group lie deeper to the erector spinae. Their fibers run medially and upward from the transverse processes to the adjacent spinous processes. They help in stabilizing the vertebrae during movements. This group consists of three subgroups. The semispinalis subgroup consists of semispinalis thoracis, semispinalis cervicis and semispinalis capitis. Besides this, there are multifidus and rotators. They are supplied by dorsal rami of cervical and thoracic spinal nerves. Collectively they are the postural muscles. But they are extensors, lateral flexors and rotators of the head and spine.

Semispinalis Capitis

The semispinalis capitis is situated in the back of the neck under cover of the splenius capitis. It may appear in the floor of the posterior triangle of the neck nearer the apex and forms the roof of the suboccipital triangle in the back of the neck. The muscle takes origin from the tips of transverse processes of the upper six thoracic vertebrae and from the articular processes of the fourth, fifth and sixth cervical vertebrae. It travels upwards for insertion in to medial part of the area between the superior and inferior nuchal lines on the occipital bone. It receives branches from suboccipital nerve.

80 Suboccipital Triangle

The suboccipital triangle is situated in the back of the neck under cover of semispinalis capitis. The suboccipital muscles, which are the deep muscles joining the cranium, atlas and axis form the boundaries of the triangle.

Boundaries (Fig. 80.1)

The suboccipital triangle has superomedial, superolateral or lateral and inferior or inferomedial boundaries. The rectus capitis posterior major and minor muscles form the superomedial boundary and the obliquus capitis superior forms the superolateral or lateral boundary. The obliquus capitis inferior forms the inferomedial or inferior boundary. The semispinalis capitis muscle forms the roof. The greater occipital nerve winds around the obliquus capitis inferior and pierces the muscular roof to enter the scalp. The occipital artery crosses the roof of the triangle to reach the posterior quadrant of the scalp. The posterior atlanto-occipital membrane (upward continuation of ligamenta flava) and posterior arch of atlas lie in the floor.

Contents

The triangle contains the third part of the vertebral artery, suboccipital plexus of veins and dorsal ramus of first cervical nerve (suboccipital nerve).

Suboccipital Muscles

There are four small suboccipital muscles. The rectus capitis superior major and minor muscles are the extensors

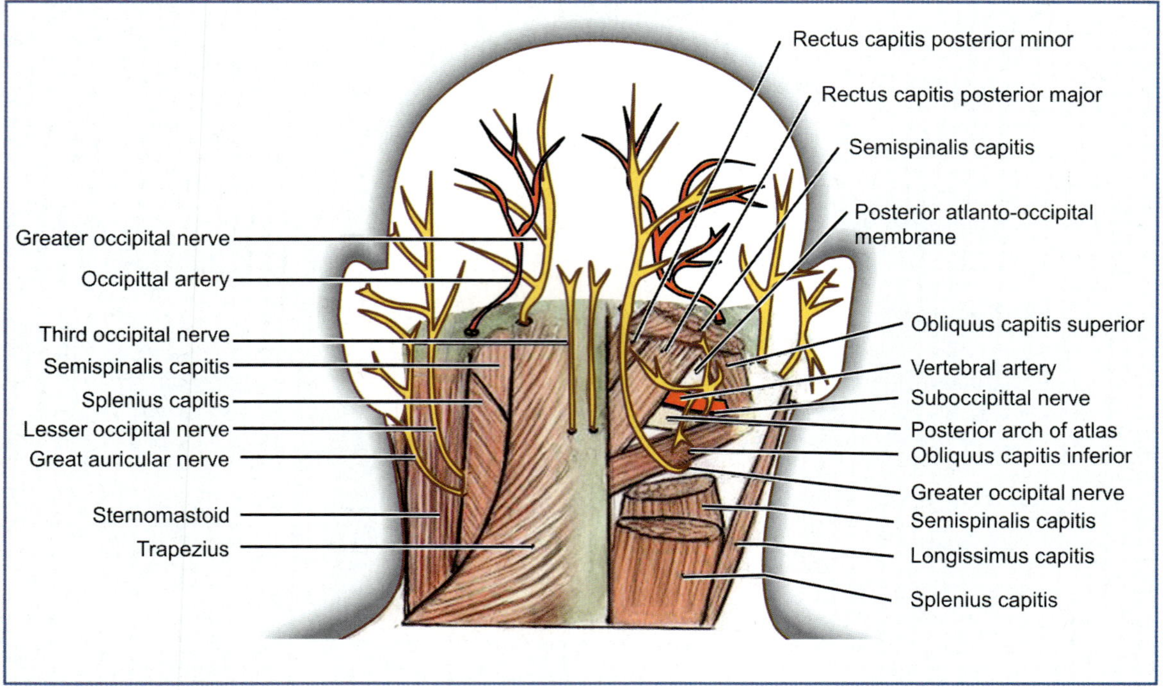

Fig. 80.1: Dissection of suboccipital region to show boundaries and contents of right suboccipital triangle (Note on the left side of figure, sensory nerves and artery of posterior quadrant of scalp and the upper part of posterior triangle of neck)

of the head at the atlanto-occipital joints. The oblique muscles rotate the head and the atlas on the axis at atlantoaxial joints.

a. The rectus capitis posterior major muscle originates from the spine of axis by a pointed tendon and is inserted in the lateral part of the inferior nuchal line.
b. The rectus capitis posterior minor muscle originates by a small pointed tendon from the tubercle on the posterior arch of atlas and is inserted in the lateral part of the inferior nuchal line.
c. The obliquus capitis superior muscle takes origin by tendinous fibers from the superior surface of the transverse process of atlas and is inserted in the occipital bone between the superior and inferior nuchal lines.
d. The obliquus capitis inferior muscle takes origin from the spine of the axis and is inserted in the posterior aspect of the transverse process of atlas.

Cisternal Puncture

This is a procedure to approach the cisterna magna in the posterior cranial fossa through the foramen magnum for obtaining a sample of CSF. The approach is via the suboccipital triangle by piercing the posterior atlanto-occipital membrane.

Suboccipital Nerve

The suboccipital nerve is the dorsal ramus of the first cervical spinal nerve. It is larger than the ventral ramus of the C1, which joins the hypoglossal nerve. The suboccipital nerve consists entirely of motor fibers (both the dorsal and ventral rami of first cervical nerve do not have sensory fibers). Hence there is no C1 dermatome. The nerve enters the suboccipital triangle by passing between the posterior arch of atlas and the vertebral artery and divides in muscular branches, which supply four suboccipital muscles and semispinalis capitis. It may communicate with the greater occipital nerve.

Suboccipital Venous Plexus

It is a dense plexus having plenty of connections. It unites with occipital vein, internal vertebral venous plexus, emissary vein traversing the posterior condylar canal, muscular veins, deep cervical vein and the plexus of veins around the vertebral artery.

81 Vertebral Artery

VERTEBRAL ARTERY

The vertebral artery (Fig. 81.1A) is a branch of the first part of the subclavian artery at the root of the neck. The area of supply of vertebral arteries includes parts posterior parts of cerebrum, brainstem, cerebellum and spinal cord. The vertebral artery has a very long course and hence is divisible in four parts.

a. The first part extends from its origin to the foramen transversarium of sixth cervical vertebra.
b. The second part lies within the foramina in the transverse processes of upper six cervical vertebrae.
c. The third part is located in the suboccipital triangle on the superior surface of the posterior arch of atlas. It extends from the foramen transversarium of atlas to the foramen magnum.
d. The fourth part is its intracranial part. The termination of the vertebral arteries is unique in that the arteries of the two sides unite at the ponto-medullary junction to form the midline basilar artery.

Course and Relations

a. The first part lies in the scalenovertebral triangle (Fig. 78.1). Here the artery is related anteriorly to the vertebral vein and the inferior thyroid artery and is crossed anteriorly by the thoracic duct on the left side below the loop of the inferior thyroid artery. Its posterior relations are ventral rami of seventh and eighth cervical nerves with the seventh transverse process between the two nerves. The stellate ganglion is partly behind the vertebral artery.
b. The second part is related posteriorly to cervical ventral rami in the intervals between the transverse processes of the adjoining vertebrae and is surrounded by the vertebral venous plexus and the sympathetic fibers (derived from the stelalte ganglion). At the foramen transversarium of the axis the vertebral artery takes a wide curve to turn laterally and upward to reach the foramen transversarium of atlas. This wide curve (loop) is necessary so that the artery is not compressed every time the head is laterally flexed and it also helps in reducing the intracranial arterial pressure.
c. The third part emerges from the foramen transversarium of atlas and turns medially to enter the suboccipital triangle (Fig. 80.1) where it grooves the superior surface of the posterior arch of the atlas and is closely related to the dorsal ramus of the first cervical nerve (suboccipital nerve). A rich venous plexus surrounds it here. It leaves the triangle by passing medially through the gap between the lateral margin of posterior atlanto-occipital membrane and the lateral mass of atlas.
d. The fourth part pierces the duramater and enters the foramen magnum. In the posterior cranial fossa the vertebral arteries lie on the anterior aspect of the medulla oblongata. The arteries of the two sides unite to form a single midline basilar artery at the pontomedullary junction.

Extracranial or Cervical Branches

a. The spinal branches arise from the second and third parts and enter the intervertebral foramina to take part in the supply the contents of the vertebral canal. The radicular branches of the spinal arteries supply the nerve roots.
b. The muscular branches supply the deep muscles in the upper part of the neck and form rich anastomoses with adjacent arteries.

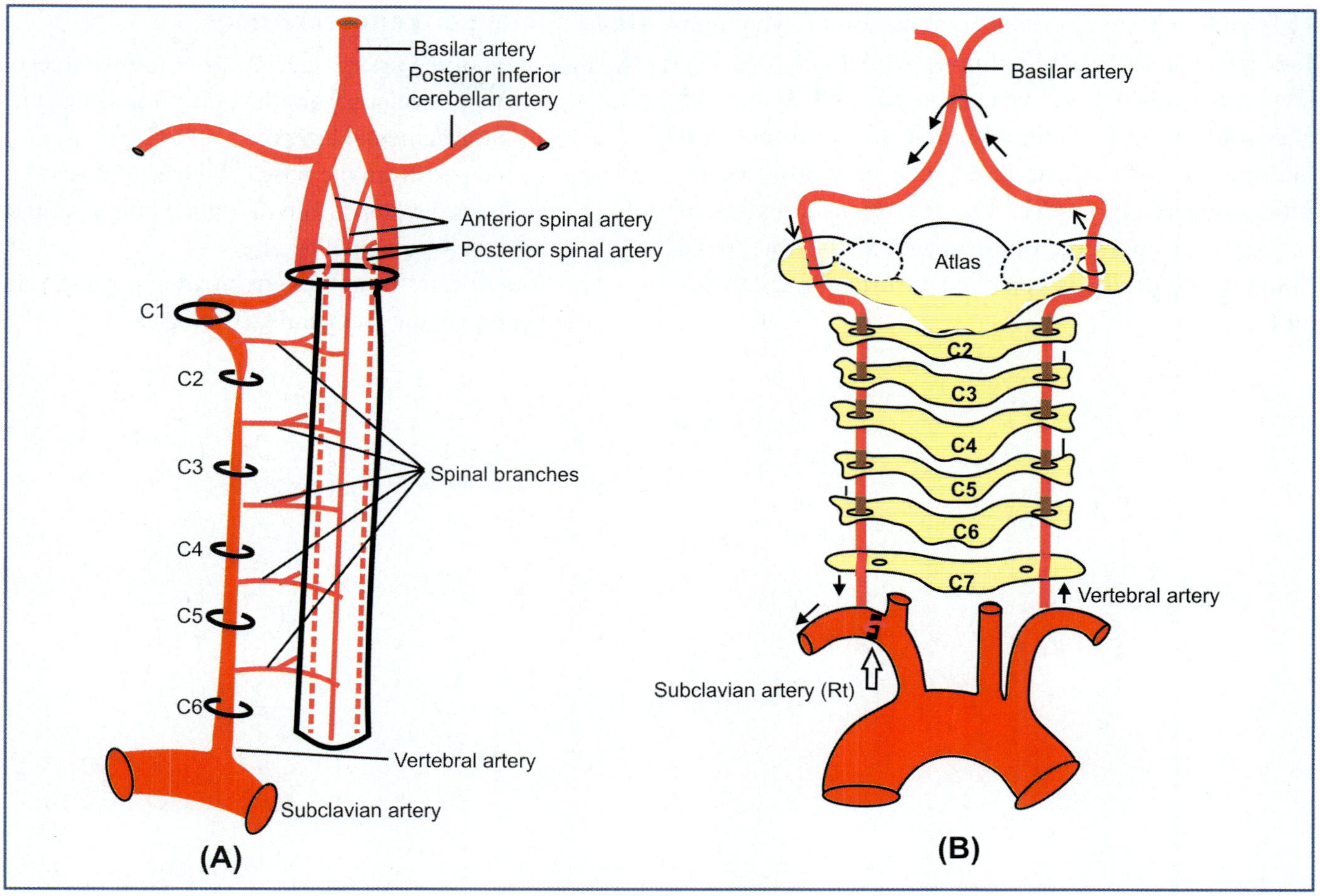

Fig. 81.1: (A) Showing origin, course and branches of vertebral artery. (B) Showing schematic representation of subclavian steal syndrome [Note that as result of stenosis of right subclavian artery (indicated by arrow) blood is syphoned from left to right vertebral artery across the midline at the union of two vertebral arteries]

Intracranial Branches

Each vertebral artery gives the meningeal, posterior spinal, anterior spinal and medullary branches apart from the large posterior inferior cerebellar artery (PICA).

Vertebral Vein

The venous plexus surrounding the vertebral artery in the suboccipital triangle accompanies the second part of the vertebral artery and enters the scalenovertebral triangle to become the vertebral vein, which opens into the brachiocephalic vein of its side.

Vertebral Angiography

It is a radiological procedure to visualize the vertebral artery and its branches.

Subclavian Steal Syndrome (Fig. 81.1B)

If the subclavian artery is narrowed at its origin from the arch of aorta or from the brachiocephalic trunk, the arterial supply of upper limb of that side is reduced. The narrowed subclavian artery is filled with blood in the most unusual way. The blood in the vertebral artery of the normal (opposite) side is shunted (at the point of the union of the two arteries inside the cranium) in to the vertebral artery of the affected side. There is reversal of blood flow in the vertebral artery of the affected side so that it is able to fill the subclavian artery beyond the stenosis. This is likely to result in shortage of blood to the brainstem especially during times of increased demand of blood in the upper limb (for example, exercise, etc.) of the affected side.

The syndrome presents as a combination of symptoms and signs due to ischemia of upper limb (pain, tingling, low blood pressure and weaker pulse) with symptoms of medullary insufficiency such as giddiness and fainting. Stenosis of the artery can be confirmed by subclavian angiography. The treatment consists of subclavian endarterectomy, in which the thickened lining of the artery is removed in order to dilate its lumen.

Development of Vertebral Artery

The four parts of the artery develop from four sources.

a. The first part develops from the dorsal branch of the seventh intersegmental artery.
b. The second part from the postcostal anastomosis.
c. The third part develops from the spinal branch of the first cervical intersegmental artery
d. The fourth part develops from the intracranial prolongation of the preneural anastomosis.

82 Clinicoanatomical Problems and Solutions

CASE 1

A one-year-old girl was brought to the hospital because her parents noticed that the child held her head to one side. On examination, it was found that the girl's head was tilted towards the right side and the face was turned towards the left side and upwards. The parents gave the history of birth trauma to the soft tissues of the neck.

Questions

a. Name the muscle and its side involved in birth injury in this case.
b. What is the clinical condition called?
c. Give the attachments and nerve supply of the above muscle.
d. Which blood vessel is present between the two heads of origin of this muscle?
e. Name the nerves related to the posterior margin of this muscle.
f. Describe the origin and course of the motor nerve related to the posterior margin.
g. Give the clinical importance of the anterior margin of this muscle.

Solutions

a. Right sternomastoid muscle
b. Torticollis
c. Sternal head arises from anterior surface of manubrium sterni and clavicular head from superior surface of the medial third of the clavicle. The muscle is inserted in to lateral surface of the mastoid process and lateral half of superior nuchal line. It is supplied by spinal accessory nerve.
d. Internal jugular vein is present in the interval between sternal and clavicular heads. This space is called lesser supraclavicular triangle.
e. About midpoint of the posterior margin of the sternomastoid seven nerves bunch together. Hence it is called nerve point of the neck. The nerves related are, spinal accessory, medial, intermediate and lateral supraclavicular nerves and great auricular, lesser occipital and transverse cutaneous nerve of neck.
f. Spinal accessory is the motor nerve related to the posterior margin. It supplies sternomastoid and trapezius muscles. Its root value is C1 to C5 as it takes origin from cervical 1 to 5 ventral rootlets (Fig. 125.10). The rootlets join in the cervical vertebral canal to form the trunk of the spinal accessory nerve, which enters the posterior cranial fossa via the foramen magnum. The spinal part joins the cranial part to form accessory or 11th cranial nerve, which leaves through the jugular foramen. Outside the cranium the accessory nerve splits. The cranial part joins the vagus and spinal part crosses the transverse process of atlas to enter the superolateral angle of the carotid triangle. Then it enters the substance of the sternomastoid muscle and descends to emerge around the midpoint of the posterior margin of the muscle. It crosses the posterior triangle lying close to the fascial roof and enters the trapezius muscle about 5 cm above the clavicle.
g. Along the anterior margin of sternomastoid branchial fistulae and cysts appear (Fig. 72.2).

CASE 2

A 12- year-old boy fell from a tree and suffered injury on the forehead near the hairline on the right side. Since there was severe bleeding the boy was rushed to the casualty, where the wound was sutured to control bleeding. After third day the boy was brought back to the hospital because his both eyes were black.

Questions

a. Black eyes develop due to presence of blood in which parts of the eyes?
b. Draw a diagram to show the communication between these parts of the eyes and the scalp.
c. Which layer of scalp contains nerves and blood vessels?
d. Why do scalp wound bleed profusely?
e. Name the sensory and motor nerves of the anterior quadrant of scalp.
f. Which vessels pass through the subaponeurotic layer of scalp and what is their clinical importance?
g. Differentiate between cephalhematoma and safety valve hematoma.

Solutions

a. Eyelids
b. Refer to Figure 57.2, which shows the continuity of subaponeurotic space with the upper eyelids. This space is closed posteriorly at the bony attachment of the occipitalis. Laterally it is closed by the attachment of galea aponeurotica at the superior temporal lines. Anteriorly the space extends in to the upper eyelids because of absence of bony attachments of the frontalis muscles. The blood from the upper eyelids may enter the lower ones also and after clotting it imparts black color to the eyes.
c. Superficial fascia or dense connective tissue layer.
d. There are two reasons for this. There are rich anastomoses between arteries of two sides hence they bleed from two ends when cut. The cut ends of the arteries do not contract because their walls are pulled by the dense connective tissue to which they are adherent.
e. There are four sensory nerves (supratrochlear, supraorbital, zygomaticotemporal and auriculotemporal). The only one motor nerve is temporal branch of facial nerve.
f. Emissary veins pass through this space. These veins are peculiar in that they connect the extracranial veins with intracranial venous sinuses and they are valveless. These veins may be torn in traction injuries of the scalp and give rise to bleeding in the subaponeurotic space. The emissary veins may act as conduits for spread of infection from the scalp to the meninges or brain.
g. Cephalhematoma is accumulation of blood under the pericranium due to rupture of periosteal blood vessels. This space is limited by the attachment of the pericranium to the sutural ligaments at the periphery of the concerned bone. Hence the shape cephalhematoma is like that of the subjacent bone. Safety valve hematoma occurs when there is minute fracture of the bone of the scalp and intracranial bleeding (usually due to birth trauma in the newborn). The symptoms of intracranial bleeding are delayed due to leakage of blood via the fracture site in to the subaponeurotic layer, which can expand to accommodate large quantity of blood. Since this hematoma delays the onset of symptoms of a serious condition it is called safety valve hematoma.

CASE 3

A 34-year-old woman came to the hospital with a nodular swelling in the midline in the neck. The swelling moved with swallowing. On examination, it was found that she had slight tremors on outstretched hands, her pulse rate was 100 per minute and there was slight bulging of the eyes.

Questions

a. Name the gland that is responsible for midline swelling in the neck and the clinical condition.
b. Give anatomical reason for the movement of swelling with swallowing.
c. Draw a diagram to show the parts of the gland.
d. What is the clinical importance of the capsules of the gland?
e. Give the surgical importance of the arterial supply of the gland.

f. Describe the lymphatic drainage of the gland.
g. Write briefly on the development of the gland.

Solutions

a. Thyroid gland. The clinical condition is toxic goiter or thyrotoxicosis.
b. The pretracheal fascia forms the false capsule. A thickening of the false capsule (ligament of Berry) connects the lobe of thyroid to the cricoid cartilage. Because of this firm anchorage to the laryngeal cartilage the thyroid moves with swallowing.
c. Refer to Figure 73.1.
d. The thyroid gland has two capsules, true and false. The veins pierce the capsules and form venous plexus underneath the true capsule. During thyroidectomy (surgical removal of gland) the veins are ligated and the gland is removed along the intercapsular plane to avoid injury to venous plexus.
e. The superior thyroid artery is in close relation to external laryngeal nerve except at the upper pole of the gland. Hence the surgeon ligates this artery as close to the upper pole of gland as possible. The inferior thyroid artery is closely related to the recurrent laryngeal nerve near the lower pole of the gland. Hence the surgeon ligates this artery as much away from the lower pole as possible.
f. Refer to Figure 73. 9.
g. The follicular cells of the thyroid gland develop from the endodermal thyroid diverticulum, which begins in the pharyngeal floor at the site of foramen cecum. The diverticulum becomes the thyroglossal duct, which passes downward through the developing tongue. The duct has peculiar relation to the hyoid bone. At first it passes in front of the bone then winds round it to come down to pass in front of the thyroid cartilage and cricoid arch. Having reached below thy cricoid cartilage by around 7 weeks the lower end of the duct divides to form lateral lobes and the connection is retained as isthmus. The lateral lobes receive cellular contributions from caudal pharyngeal complex (ultimobranchial complex). These give rise to parafollicular cells. The remaining thyroglossal duct normally disintegrates.

CASE 4

Two days following total thyroidectomy the patient experienced paraesthesia (altered sensation) around the mouth followed by tingling and numbness in fingers and toes and painful cramps in hands and feet. Blood calcium level was found to be very low.

Questions

a. Name the clinical condition giving its physiological basis.
b. Which structures were inadvertently removed by the surgeon during thyroidectomy?
c. How does the surgeon identify these structures during thyroid surgery?
d. Give the number and position of these structures.
e. Mention their development and comment on Di-George syndrome and Nazelof's syndrome.

Solutions

a. Tetany due to deficiency of parathormone.
b. Parathyroid glands
c. Branches of inferior thyroid artery supply the glands hence they are the surgeon's guide.
d. There are two pairs of parathyroid glands (superior and inferior). They are located posterior to the thyroid gland in side the false capsule. The superior pair is located at the level of junction of upper and middle one third of the thyroid lobe. The inferior pair is located near the lower end of the thyroid gland.
e. The superior parathyroid glands develop from the endoderm of fourth pouch and the inferior parathyroid from the endoderm of third pouch along with thymus. For the syndromes associated with development refer to Chapter 72.

CASE 5

A patient had swelling below the lower jaw on the right side. The swelling increased in size during eating. The surgeon inspected the sublingual papilla in floor of the mouth and did a bidigital examination by putting index finger inside the oral cavity and the thumb outside in front of the angle of the mandible.

Questions

a. Which salivary gland is palpated in this case?
b. Name the parts of this gland and the muscle that separates these parts.
c. What is the length of its duct and where does it open?
d. Where is the lumen of this duct narrowest?
e. Name the radiological investigation done to visualize the duct system of salivary glands.
f. Draw a diagram to show the relation of the lingual nerve to this duct.
g. Draw a diagram of secretomotor innervation of this gland.
h. Describe the relations of the medial surface of the gland.

Solutions

a. Submandibular salivary gland.
b. Its two parts are larger superficial and smaller deep. They are continuous with each other around the posterior free margin of mylohyoid muscle.
c. Wharton's duct is 5 cm. Long and it opens in the floor of the mouth at the summit of the sublingual papilla by the side of the frenulum of the tongue.
d. At the oral orifice.
e. Sialography
f. Refer to Figure 70.6
g. Refer to Figure 70.7
h. Refer to Figure 70.3 and related description in Chapter 70.

CASE 6

A middle-aged woman complained of pain, tingling and numbness along the medial side of the right forearm and hand. She had difficulty in gripping the objects firmly in the right hand. On examination the radial pulse seemed to be weak on the right side compared to the left. Adson's test was positive on right side. Plain X-ray showed presence of cervical rib on the same side.

To relieve the symptoms the cervical rib was removed along with its periosteum.

Questions

a. What is the morphology of cervical rib?
b. Which structures are likely to be compressed by the cervical rib?
c. Enumerate the steps in performing Adson's test.
d. What is the significance of positive Adson's test?
e. Compression of which structure results in inability to hold the objects tightly?
f. Give the extent of the compressed artery on the side of the lesion.
g. Name the nerves that loop around the right subclavian artery.
h. Explain why the cervical rib is surgically removed along with its periosteum?

Solutions

a. A cervical rib is the enlarged costal element of the 7th cervical vertebra (costotransverse bar, anterior tubercle and anterior root of the transverse process form the costal element).
b. The neurovascular structures, which are related to the superior surface of the first rib, namely, third part of subclavian artery and lower trunk of brachial plexus on the right side.
c. Adson's test is performed to assess the functional status of the arterial supply of upper limb. The patient sits on a stool. He or she is asked to take deep breath and then to turn the face towards the affected side. The force of the radial pulse is assessed.
d. In a positive Adson's test there is reduction in the force of radial pulse indicating compression of subclavian artery either by cervical rib or by hypertrophy of the scalenus anterior muscle.
e. Lower trunk of brachial plexus.
f. The right subclavian artery is one of the terminal branches of the brachiocephalic trunk. It extends from the sternoclavicular joint to the outer margin of the first rib.
g. Ansa subclavia and right recurrent laryngeal nerve.
h. If the periosteum is left behind during surgical removal of the rib its inner cellular layer will regenerate the rib.

CASE 7

A 58-year-old man presented with a complaint of rapidly growing painful swelling on the face below the ear lobule on the left side. On examination the left ear lobule was found to be lifted by the swelling. There was inability to close the left eye and to blow the cheek. The angle of mouth was deviated to the right side.

Questions

a. Name the gland that is swollen.
b. Name the major structures inside this gland.
c. Which of these structures is injured?
d. Draw a diagram to show the exit of the branches of this structure from the gland.
e. What is the reason for the inability to close the right eye and inability to blow the cheek?
f. Write briefly on the duct of this gland.
g. What is the clinical anatomy of fascial capsule of this gland?
h. Draw a diagram to show the surface marking of the gland and its duct.

Solutions

a. Parotid gland
b. The major structures are, facial nerve, retromandibular vein and external carotid artery.
c. Facial nerve
d. Refer Figure 62.4.
e. Inability to close the eye is due to paralysis or weakness of orbicularis oculi. Inability to blow the cheek is due to weakness or paralysis of buccinator muscle.
f. The parotid duct (Stensen's duct) collects serous secretions of the gland. It is about 5 cm long. It leaves the gland from its anterior margin and travels forward on the masseter muscle. Its superior relations are, upper buccal branch of facial nerve, transverse facial artery and accessory parotid gland. At the anterior margin of the masseter the duct turns inwards to pierce in succession the buccal pad of fat, buccopharyngeal fascia, buccinator and buccal mucosa. It opens in the vestibule of the oral cavity opposite the crown of upper second molar tooth.
g. The fascial capsule of the parotid gland is derived from the deep fascia of neck. It is called parotidomasseteric fascia. It is very tough and unyielding. Therefore if there is parotid swelling it is intensely painful (the tough fascia does not allow the swelling to expand). The parotid abscess unlike abscess in other locations does not show induration and fluctuation.
h. For surface marking of gland and the duct refer to Figure 62.2.

SINGLE BEST RESPONSE TYPE MCQs

1. **Which of the following lymph nodes are called Virchow nodes?**
   A. Right supraclavicular
   B. Left supraclavicular
   C. Right infraclavicular
   D. Left infraclavicular

2. **Which of the following veins pierces the fascial roof of posterior triangle?**
   A. External jugular **B.** Subclavian
   C. Transverse cervical **D.** Suprascapular

3. **Following are the derivatives of third arch mesoderm, *except:***
   A. Stylopharyngeus
   B. Palatopharyngeus
   C. Lower half of the body of hyoid bone
   D. Greater horn of hyoid bone

4. **Superior parathyroid glands develop from:**
   A. Mesoderm of third arch
   B. Mesoderm of fourth arch
   C. Endoderm of third arch
   D. Endoderm of fourth arch

5. **The ligament of Berry fixes the thyroid gland to:**
   A. Thyroid cartilage **B.** Cricoid cartilage
   C. First tracheal ring **D.** Hyoid bone

6. **Which statement is true about buccinator?**
   A. Origin from both bones of jaw
   B. Insertion in pterygomandibular raphe
   C. Supplied by buccal branch of mandibular nerve
   D. Tendon of tensor palati pierces it muscular part

7. **The hypoglossal nerve crosses in front of all the arteries in the carotid triangle, *except:***
   A. Occipital **B.** Lingual
   C. Internal carotid **D.** External carotid

8. **The absence of tears is due to lesion in:**
   A. Trigeminal ganglion
   B. Ciliary ganglion
   C. Sphenopalatine ganglion
   D. Superior cervical sympathetic ganglion

9. **Which is not a branch of superficial temporal artery?**
A. Zygomatico-orbital B. Zygomaticotemporal
C. Transverse facial D. Middle temporal

10. **Which structure is located behind the prevertebral layer of cervical fascia?**
A. Sympathetic chain B. Carotid sheath
C. Subclavian artery D. Subclavian vein

11. **The following is a content of suboccipital triangle:**
A. Vertebral artery
B. Membrana tectoria
C. Posterior atlanto-occipital membrane
D. Posterior arch of atlas

12. **Laryngeal prominence is formed by:**
A. Body of hyoid bone
B. Arch of cricoid cartilage
C. Oblique line of thyroid cartilage
D. Anterior margin of thyroid cartilage

13. **The following nerve hooks round the spinal accessory nerve:**
A. Great auricular B. Greater occipital
C. Lesser occipital D. Supraclavicular

14. **The philtrum of the upper lip develops from:**
A. Lateral nasal process
B. Globular process
C. Maxillary process
D. Fusion of maxillary and globular processes

15. **The suprasternal space contains all, *except:***
A. Interclavicular ligament
B. Jugular arch
C. Clavicular head of sternomastoid
D. Lymph node

16. **Which statement is untrue about sternomastoid muscle?**
A. Its anterior border forms the posterior boundary of carotid triangle
B. It is supplied by a nerve that passes through the foramen magnum
C. Bilateral contraction produces extension of head
D. Unilateral contraction brings the chin toward the contralateral shoulder

17. **Which one is not the tributary of internal jugular vein?**
A. Inferior petrosal sinus
B. Superior thyroid vein
C. Middle thyroid vein
D. Inferior thyroid vein

18. **A superficial incision on the posterior triangle of neck may cause difficulty in:**
A. Abduction of arm
B. Shrugging the shoulder
C. Rotation of head
D. Protraction of scapula

19. **Which of the following statements is false?**
A. The first cervical nerve is entirely motor
B. The dorsal ramus of the first cervical nerve is entirely motor
C. The ventral ramus of the first cervical nerve supplies strap muscles
D. C1 dermatome lies on the back of the head

20. **The external carotid artery divides at the level of:**
A. Superior margin of thyroid cartilage
B. Angle of mandible
C. Neck of mandible
D. Condyle of mandible

Key to MCQs—SBR

1 B	2 A	3 B	4 D	5 B	6 A	7 A
8 C	9 B	10 C	11 A	12 D	13 C	14 B
15 C	16 C	17 D	18 B	19 D	20 C	

MULTIPLE RESPONSE TYPE MCQs

Write true or false against each statement

1. **The mylohyoid muscle:**
A. is triangular in shape
B. originates from greater horn of hyoid bone
C. is related to geniohyoid superiorly
D. develops from mesoderm of second arch

2. **The pulse that is readily felt:**
A. facial at anteroinferior angle of masseter
B. subclavian at lateral third of clavicle
C. common carotid artery at lesser supraclavicular triangle
D. superficial temporal at preauricular point

3. **The frontalis muscle:**
   - **A.** on contraction produces expression of anger
   - **B.** is attached to frontal bone
   - **C.** merges with fibres of orbicularis oculi
   - **D.** is supplied by temporal branch of facial nerve

4. **The submandibular salivary gland:**
   - **A.** is a purely mucous gland
   - **B.** is related to facial vessels
   - **C.** is located in digastric triangle
   - **D.** its medial surface is related to mandible

5. **Structure leaving through the base of parotid gland:**
   - **A.** auriculotemporal nerve
   - **B.** superficial temporal artery
   - **C.** posterior auricular artery
   - **D.** posterior auricular nerve

6. **The posterior belly of digastric muscle:**
   - **A.** develops from mesoderm of first arch
   - **B.** originates from mastoid process
   - **C.** is related inferiorly to occipital artery
   - **D.** is supplied by posterior auricular nerve

7. **The superior cervical sympathetic ganglion:**
   - **A.** lies in front of prevertebral fascia
   - **B.** lies behind carotid sheath
   - **C.** continues as internal carotid nerve
   - **D.** receives first white ramus communicans

8. **The scalenus anterior muscle:**
   - **A.** is inserted into scalene turbercle
   - **B.** phrenic nerve is plastered to its anterior surface
   - **C.** its lateral margin is related to thoracic duct
   - **D.** is supplied by phrenic nerve

9. **The components of secretomotor path of lacrimal gland:**
   - **A.** nervus intermedius
   - **B.** sphenopalatine ganglion
   - **C.** lesser petrosal nerve
   - **D.** nerve of pterygoid canal

10. **The carotid triangle:**
    - **A.** is bounded anterosuperiorly by superior belly of omohyoid
    - **B.** superior constrictor is its floor muscle
    - **C.** is a site of pulsations of all carotid arteries
    - **D.** contains spinal accessory nerve

83 Vertebral Column

The vertebral column is also described by the terms such as the spine or spinal column or backbone. It forms the central axis of the body. It consists of a number of vertebrae joined to each other by a series of articulations. The vertebral column is a flexible but strong pillar that supports the skull, trunk, and limbs. It transmits body weight to the lower extremity through the sacroiliac joints. It provides a large site for attachment of the muscles of posture and locomotion. The bodies of the vertebrae are active sites of haemopoesis throughout life. The vertebral column encloses a canal, in which the spinal meninges, spinal cord and the cauda equina are protected.

Length of Vertebral Column

The average length of the vertebral column in adult male is 70 cm and in adult female is 60 cm. The vertebral bodies contribute the four-fifths and the intervertebral discs contribute one fifth of the total length of the column.

Vertebrae

There are seven cervical, twelve thoracic and five lumbar vertebrae. The sacrum consists of a single piece made of five fused sacral vertebrae. The coccyx consists of four fused coccygeal vertebrae. Thus, there are twenty-four movable vertebrae and nine non-movable vertebrae. The vertebra consists of a centrum or body anteriorly and the vertebral arch posteriorly. The body and the arch enclose the vertebral foramen. In the articulated column the vertebral foramina of all the vertebrae make up the vertebral canal. The vertebral arch consists of two pedicles and two laminae, which bear seven processes, namely, two pairs of articular processes (zygapophyses), one pair of transverse processes and a spinous process. The pedicles connect the body to the laminae and bear the superior and inferior vertebral notches. The bodies of adjacent movable vertebrae articulate with each other by fibrocartilaginous discs. There is a thin disc between the sacrum and coccyx. The first cervical vertebra (atlas) has no body hence there is no disc between the atlas and the second cervical (axis) vertebra.

Variations

a. Sacralization of the fifth lumbar vertebra is the condition in which the fifth lumbar vertebra fuses with the sacrum reducing the number of movable vertebrae to twenty-three.
b. Lumbarization of first sacral vertebra is a condition in which the first sacral vertebra separates from the sacrum and assumes the features of the lumbar vertebra. In such cases the number of movable vertebrae is increased to twenty-five.
c. Occipitalization of atlas is a condition in which atlas is fused with occipital bone.

Development of Vertebra (Fig. 83.1)

The sclerotome part of the somite is the developmental basis of the vertebra. The mesenchyme of the bilateral sclerotomes condenses around the notochord. Each vertebra passes through three stages of development called, blastemal, cartilaginous and ossific. In the blastemal stage the vertebral body is formed from the fusion of caudal half of cranial sclerotome and an equal contribution of the cranial half of the succeeding sclerotome. This is followed by appearance of chondrification centers in the blastemal vertebra in the sixth week. In the ossific stage the primary centers of ossification appear in the centrum of vertebra during seventh to eighth weeks. The secondary centres appear at the age of puberty.

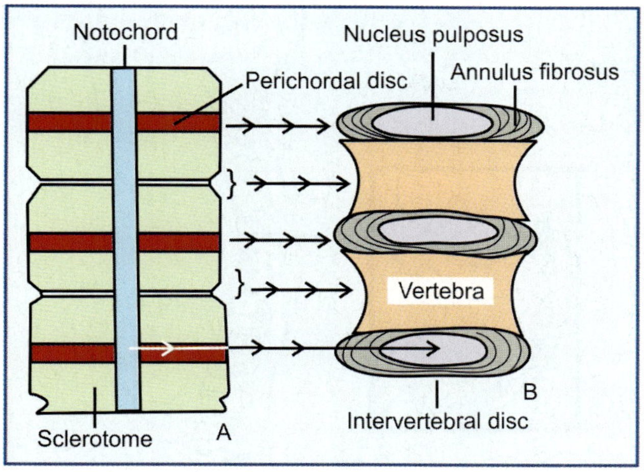

Fig. 83.1: Development of vertebra and disc. Figure A shows sclerotome and notochord which are the embryonic basis of vertebral column shown in Figure B

Costal Elements of Vertebrae

The costal element is the anterior part of the vertebral arch of the developing vertebra. It may form a rib or it may remain incorporated in the transverse process of the definitive vertebra. The true transverse process is the posterior part of the vertebral arch.

Thoracic Vertebra

The costal element forms the rib. The true transverse process forms the entire transverse process.

Cervical Vertebra

The costal element forms major part of the transverse process (anterior root, anterior tubercle, costotransverse bar and posterior tubercle). The true transverse process is limited to the medial part of the posterior root of the transverse process. Sometimes, the costal element of the seventh cervical vertebra enlarges to form a cervical rib, which may be complete or incomplete or merely represented by a fibrous cord and give rise to symptoms.

Lumbar Vertebra

The costal element becomes the transverse process and the true transverse process becomes the accessory process of the vertebra. Very rarely the first lumbar vertebra may show a lumbar rib.

Sacrum and Coccyx

The costal elements of the upper two to three pieces form the anterior part of the lateral mass of the sacrum while the true transverse processes form the posterior part of the lateral mass. In the coccygeal vertebrae the costal elements are absent.

Congenital Anomalies of Vertebrae

a. Spina bifida results from the failure of fusion of the right and left centers of ossification of the vertebral arches. If it is not associated with spinal cord defects it is called spina bifida occulta.
b. Occasionally, the defect in the vertebral arches is so large that the spinal meninges or spinal cord may protrude through it, which may give rise to a swelling in the back (Fig. 88.3). If the meninges of the spinal cord protrude it is called meningocele or if the meninges and part of spinal cord protrude then it is known as meningomyelocele.
c. Spondylolisthesis is the anterior displacement of the vertebral column, usually at the lumbosacral articulation. The fifth lumbar vertebra is in two pieces due to the developmental defect in its pedicle. The body of the vertebra and the superior articular processes form one piece. This piece migrates forwards and carries the entire vertebral column with it. The spine, inferior articular processes and laminae form the second piece, which is retained in contact with the sacrum. This may result in stretching of S1 nerve roots causing symptoms like backache and root pain.

Intervertebral Joints

a. The joints between the bodies of adjacent vertebrae (intervertebral joints) are the secondary cartilaginous joints or symphyses.
b. The zygapophyseal or facet joints between the articular processes of adjacent vertebrae are synovial joints.
c. The joints between the laminae of adjacent vertebrae (the laminae being connected by ligamenta flava) are called vertebral syndesmoses.

Boundaries of Intervertebral Foramina

In an articulated vertebral column the boundaries of the intervertebral foramen are, superiorly the inferior vertebral notch of the vertebra above, inferiorly the superior vertebral notch of the vertebra below, anteriorly the intervertebral disc and adjacent vertebral bodies and posteriorly the capsule of the zygapophyseal or facet joint.

Contents of Intervertebral Foramen

The intervertebral foramen gives passage to the corresponding spinal nerve, its recurrent meningeal branch, spinal branches of regional arteries and the intervertebral veins. The spinal nerve or nerves may be compressed or irritated in the foramen due to the stenosis or narrowing of the foramen (prolapse of the intervertebral disc, osteoarthritis of the facet joints, the presence of osteophytes (bony spurs) in cervical spondylosis and fractures or diseases of the vertebral bodies. This will give rise to shooting pain.

Vertebral Canal

The vertebral canal is continuous superiorly with the posterior cranial fossa through the foramen magnum. In the cervical and lumbar regions, which exhibit free mobility the vertebral canal is large and triangular. In the thoracic region, where movement is restricted it is small and circular. The lumbar vertebral canal becomes continuous with sacral canal. The caudal opening of the sacral canal is the sacral hiatus. The spinal cord and its three meninges lie in the vertebral canal up to the level of the lower border of L1 vertebra. Below this level the lumbar canal and the sacral canal contain the cauda equina with outer two layers of meninges. The arachnoid mater and the dura mater cover the cauda equina upto the lower border of sacral second vertebra, beyond which the sacral canal contains the filum terminale, fifth sacral and coccygeal nerve roots, which exit via the sacral hiatus.

Curvatures of Vertebral Column (Fig. 83.2)

In the intrauterine life the vertebral column has forward concavity because the fetus lies in the position of universal flexion. After birth the vertebral column shows two types of curvatures. The primary curvature with forward concavity is retained in the thoracic and sacral parts. The secondary curvatures with forward convexity in cervical and lumbar regions are called postural curvatures. The cervical curvature develops when the child begins to hold the head upright by about third months after birth. The lumbar curvature develops when the child begins to sit by about six or seven months of age and is more marked when the child begins to walk.

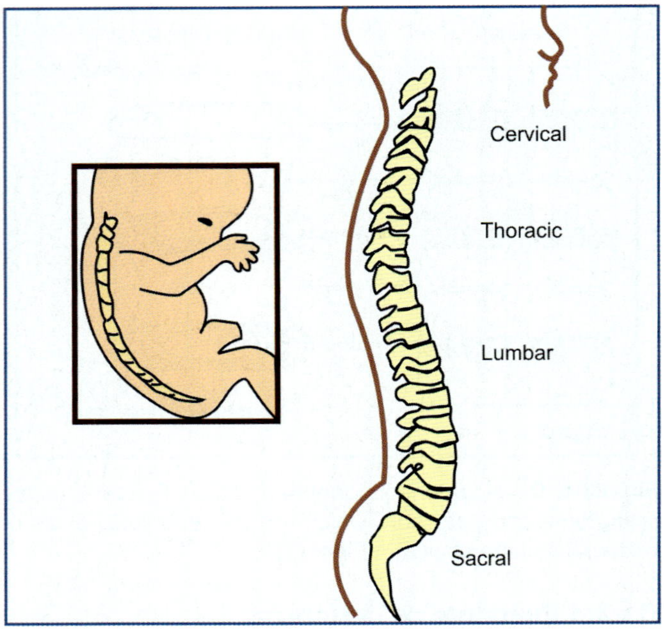

Fig. 83.2: Curvatures of vertebral column (Note: The concavity of primary curvature in fetal life (inset). Anterior convexity of cervical and lumbar regions develops secondarily after birth)

Abnormal Curvatures

a. Kyphosis (hunchback) means anterior concavity of the vertebral column. In the thoracic region the concavity is exaggerated while in cervical and lumbar regions the convexity is reduced. In old age, due to osteoporosis of the vertebrae and degeneration of the discs the vertebral column loses its forward convexity in lumbar and cervical regions.
b. Lordosis (swayback) means the posterior concavity of the vertebral column. The normal lumbar lordosis is exaggerated in pregnancy.
c. Scoliosis means the lateral curvature of the vertebral column as a result of maldevelopment of a vertebra for example, hemivertebra.

Ligaments of Vertebral Column (Fig. 83.3)

a. The anterior longitudinal ligament is a strong and broad band, which is attached to the anterior surfaces of the vertebral bodies and the discs. It extends from the sacrum to the anterior tubercle of atlas, from where it

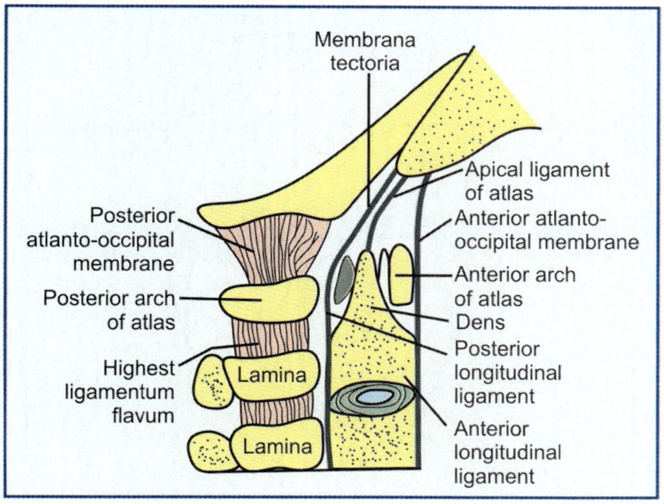

Fig. 83.3: Median section through upper cervical column showing upward continuity of vertebral ligaments

continues upwards as anterior atlanto-occipital membrane.

b. The posterior longitudinal ligament is located inside the vertebral canal. It is attached to the posterior surfaces of the discs and adjacent margins of the vertebral bodies. It is not attached to the posterior surfaces of the bodies because the basivertebral veins emerge from the vertebral bodies on this aspect and empty in to the internal vertebral venous plexus. This ligament extends from the sacrum to the lower margin of the posterior surface of the body of axis, from where it continues as the membrana tectoria, which passes through the foramen magnum to attach to the basilar part of occipital bone near the margin of the foramen magnum.
c. The ligamentum flavum derives the name from its yellow color (flavum means yellow). The ligamenta flava consisting of thick bands of yellow elastic tissue connects the adjacent laminae to each other. The elasticity of the ligamenta flava restores the vertebral column to erect posture after flexion. These ligaments are described as muscle sparers. The uppermost ligamentum flavum is attached to the posterior arch of atlas from where it is continued upwards as the posterior atlanto-occipital membrane to be attached to the posterior margin of foramen magnum.
d. The interspinous ligaments connect the adjacent spines to each other.
e. The supraspinous ligaments connect the tips of the adjacent spines to each other.
f. The ligamentum nuchae is the greatly thickened interspinous and supraspinous ligaments in the cervical column. The upper attachment of the ligamentum nuchae is to the external occipital crest.

Intervertebral Discs

The intervertebral discs are the main connecting bonds between the bodies of adjacent vertebrae. The discs are thickest and wedge shaped in the cervical and lumbar regions, where the vertebral column is highly mobile. They are absent between atlas and axis, in the sacrum and coccyx.

Parts of Disc

The disc has two parts. The inner nucleus pulposus is the remnant of notochord and outer annulus fibrosus is a fibrocartilage. The nucleus pulposus is a mass of gelatinous material containing mucopolysachharides with large amount of water. It is normally under pressure. It is situated slightly towards the posterior margin of the disc. The semifluid nature of the nucleus pulposus allows the disc to change shape and permit movement of one vertebra over the other. It also enables the discs to act as shock absorbers. The outer annulus fibrosus forms a tough casing for the nucleus pulposus.

Diurnal Variation

Diurnal variation means changes in the disc during the course of a day due to changes in its water content. During daytime, when the individual is up and about the water content gradually reduces, thus reducing the height of the individual by half to one cm. The loss is made up by reabsorption of water during the night, when the individual is resting. Therefore, the height is highest in early morning and lowest at the end of the day (before retiring to bed).

Age Changes

In old age the nucleus pulposus is gradually invaded by fibrocartilage. This reduces the elasticity of the vertebral column. There is degeneration of the collagen fibers of annulus fibrosus. Therefore, in old age the discs become thin and less elastic. The shrinking height and kyphotic deformity in old age are due to atrophy of discs and osteoporosis of vertebrae.

Development

The nucleus pulposus develops from the notochord and the annulus fibrosus develops from the sclerotome of the somite.

Disc Prolapse (Fig. 83.4)

The disc prolapse is also known by herniation of disc or slipped disc. This is very common in the lumbar vertebral column (between L4 and L5). The nucleus pulposus protrudes through the crack in the annulus fibrosus in disc prolapse. The weakest part of the annulus lies just lateral to the posterior longitudinal ligament on either side. This part of the annulus is thin due to lack of support by strong ligaments. Hence, the annulus ruptures at this point as a result of exertion like lifting heavy weight. The nucleus pulposus herniates in posterolateral direction and narrows the intervertebral foramen compressing the spinal nerve. The patient experiences severe back pain and sciatica. The pain increases on coughing or sneezing. The movements of vertebral column are restricted due to muscle spasm. The prolapse of the disc between vertebrae L4 and L5 results in compression of L5 spinal nerve. This may cause diminished sensation in L5 dermatome and weakness of extensor muscles of the leg. MRI scanning demonstrates the disc and its prolapse very clearly.

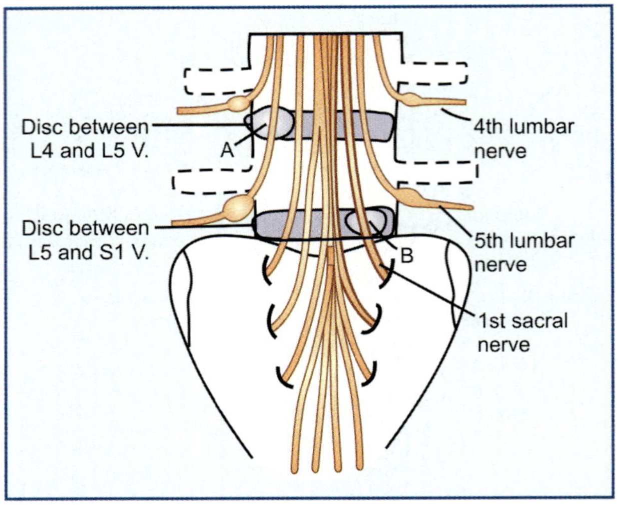

Fig. 83.4: Posterolateral disc prolapse in lumbar region (Note that disc prolapse at A compresses 5th lumbar nerve and at B 1st sacral nerve)

Craniovertebral Joints

These are the joints between the atlas, axis and occipital bone. The two atlanto-occipital joints are the uppermost joints of the vertebral column. There are three joints between the atlas and axis, a median and lateral atlanto-axial joints. The atlanto-occipital joints permit movements of flexion and extension of head around a transverse axis while the atlantoaxial joints permit rotation of the head around a vertical axis. Thus we nod "yes" at the atlanto-occipital joints and "no" at atlantoaxial joints. These movements of the head are adapted for eye-head coordination.

a. In the atlanto-occipital joint the kidney shaped large superior articular facets on the atlas articulate with the similar facets on the occipital condyles. The anterior and posterior atlanto-occipital membranes strengthen the fibrous capsule of the joint. The right and left joints act as one unit in producing the flexion and extension of head.
b. The atlanto-axial joints consist of three synovial articulations. The lateral joints are between the inferior articular processes of the atlas and the superior articular processes of the axis. The median joint is between the facet on the anterior arch of atlas and the dens of axis. It is a pivot type of joint, in which the dens rotates in the ring formed by the articular facet and the transverse ligament of the atlas. The movements of rotation of head take place in the three joints simultaneously.

Ligaments Connecting Axis and Occipital Bone

a. Apical ligament passes through the foramen magnum. It connects the tip of the dens to the basilar part of occipital bone closer to foramen magnum. It is a remnant of notochord.
b. Alar ligaments are attached to the sides of the dens. Superiorly they are attached to the medial sides of the occipital condyles.
c. Membrana tectoria extends from the posterior surface of the body of axis to the upper surface of basilar part of occipital bone. Like the apical ligament it too passes

through the foramen magnum. It is the upward continuation of posterior longitudinal ligament.

d. Cruciate ligament has a strong transverse part, which is the transverse ligament of atlas. It has a vertical part consisting of a strong upper part and a lower weak part. The upper part of the vertical limb is attached to the anterior margin of foramen magnum while the lower part is attached to the dens.

Lumbosacral Joint

This is the joint between the fifth lumbar vertebra and the base of the sacrum. It is the intervertebral joint of secondary cartilaginous variety. The intervertebral disc is thicker in front compared to its posterior part, because of which the lumbosacral angle is prominent. This is the reason for the normal lumbar lordosis, which is exaggerated in pregnancy. The lumbosacral joint is supported by the iliolumbar ligament, which extends from the tip of the fifth lumbar transverse process to the iliac crest and by the lumbosacral ligament, which is the lower part of iliolumbar ligament and is attached to the posterior part of ala of sacrum.

Sacrococcygeal Joint

This is an intervertebral joint between the last piece of sacrum and the coccyx. Its disc is thin. The ventral sacrococcygeal ligament is present in place of the anterior longitudinal ligament. The dorsal sacrococcygeal ligament is divided in superficial and deep parts, which close the sacral hiatus. The intercornual ligaments connect the sacral and coccygeal cornua.

Movements of Vertebral Column

The movements of the vertebral column are, the flexion, extension, lateral flexion and rotation. Flexion, extension and lateral flexion are extensive in cervical and lumbar regions. The movements of thoracic region are limited because of the ribs and their attachments to the sternum. The rotation is severely restricted in lumbar region because the articular facets have characteristic orientation. There is no common centre of curvature for right and left articular facets and the superior articular facets face medially while the inferior ones laterally in the case of lumbar vertebrae.

Cervical Region

a. The flexion of vertebral column is by the longus cervicis, scalenus anterior and sternomastoid muscles of both sides.
b. The extension is by the splenius capitis and erector spine muscles of both sides.
c. The lateral flexion is due to contraction of the scalenus anterior and medius, sternomastoid and trapezius muscles of one side.
d. The rotation is the combined action of the sternomastoid of one side and splenius cervices of opposite side.

Thoracic Region

The rotation is by the actions of the semispinalis thoracis, multifidus and rotators. The anterolateral muscles of the anterior abdominal wall assist them.

Lumbar Region

a. The flexion is by rectus abdominis and psoas major muscles. In flexion against resistance (e.g., when raising head and shoulder from supine position, the anterolateral muscles of the abdomen contract.
b. The extension is by the erector spinae and transversospinalis group of muscles.
c. The lateral flexion is by the erector spinae, transversospinalis group, quadratus lumborum, and oblique muscles of anterior abdominal wall.

Blood Supply of Vertebrae

The vertebrae receive rich blood supply because their marrow is a site of erythropoesis. They receive blood from the paired spinal branches (of regional arteries), which enter the intervertebral foramina. The discs are avascular structures. They are nourished by diffusion from the adjoining vertebrae.

The venous drainage of the vertebral column has considerable clinical importance. The extradural space (epidural apace) in the vertebral canal contains the internal vertebral venous plexus, which is devoid of valves (Batson's vertebral venous plexus). This plexus receives blood from the vertebral bodies via the basivertebral veins. The external vertebral venous plexus communicates with the internal plexus through plexuses by intervertebral veins by passing through the intervertebral foramina. The external vertebral plexus drains into the segmental veins at different regions of the vertebral column.

Basivertebral Veins (Fig. 83.5)

These veins have physiological, clinical and embryological importance. The large size of the veins reflects the importance of their function as they carry the products of haemopoesis from the vertebral body to the internal vertebral venous plexus. They are responsible for venous metastasis in the vertebral bodies from the primary at some distant site. The retrograde flow of venous blood in pelvic veins or posterior intercostal veins may bring malignant cells from the primary in the prostate or the breast to the vertebral venous plexus and to the basivertebral veins may deposit the malignant cells to the vertebral bodies. The embryologically the basivertebral veins are segmental in location as is evident by the centrally placed location of the foramen in the vertebral body. This indicates that the vertebral body is intersegmental and hence derived from two adjacent sclerotomes.

Internal Vertebral Venous Plexus of Batson

These veins show temporary retrograde flow in situations of raised intrathoracic or intra-abdominal pressure because of absence of valves in them. When the flow is reversed the segmental veins bring blood from the vena caval system to the vertebral venous plexus. This can become a route for the malignant cells from the cervical, thoracic or pelvic regions to reach the vertebral column. The malignant cells can also deposit in skull bones because of the communication of the internal vertebral venous plexus with the venous sinuses in the cranium.

Radiology of Vertebral Column

The vertebral column can be examined in AP and lateral radiographs but MRI scan of the vertebral column is the best method of imaging the anatomical parts of the vertebrae and the intervertebral discs.

Lumbar Puncture (Fig. 83.6)

It is a procedure by which CSF sample is withdrawn from the subarachnoid space or anaesthetic solution is introduced in it. The patient lies on his or her side curled up tightly to flex the lumbar spine so as to open up the interval between the laminae of the lumbar vertebrae. The line passing through the highest points of the iliac crests cuts the midline between the spines of L3 and L4. The needle inserted at this point in the midline passes through, skin, fasciae, supraspinous ligament, interspinous ligament, ligamentum flavum, duramater and arachnoid mater before reaching subarachnoid space.

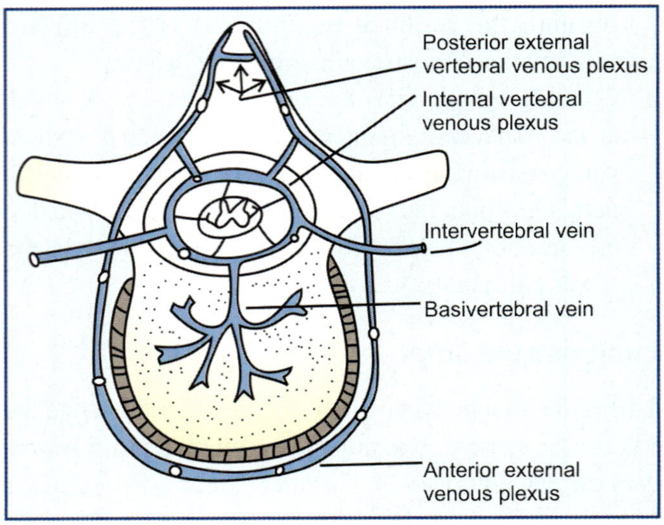

Fig. 83.5: Vertebral system of veins (Note that the basivertebral vein drains products of hemopoesis from vertebral body into internal vertebral venous plexus)

Caudal (Sacral) Analgesia (Fig. 83.7)

The caudal analgesia or anesthesia is given in obstetric practice for painless labor. To carry out the procedure at first the sacral hiatus is identified by palpating the sacral cornua about 5 cm above the tip of coccyx. The other method is to join the two posterior superior iliac spines by a line, which forms the base of the equilateral triangle. The apex of the triangle lies over the sacral hiatus. The needle passes through the posterior sacrococcygeal ligament to enter the sacral hiatus. The volume of sacral canal is 20 to 25 ml and this much quantity of anesthetic solution is sufficient to block the sacral spinal nerves supplying the perineum and the uterus.

Clinical Highlights

a. Pott's spine or tuberculosis of the vertebral column is very common in thoracic spine. It causes pain, restriction of movements and deformity. Retro-

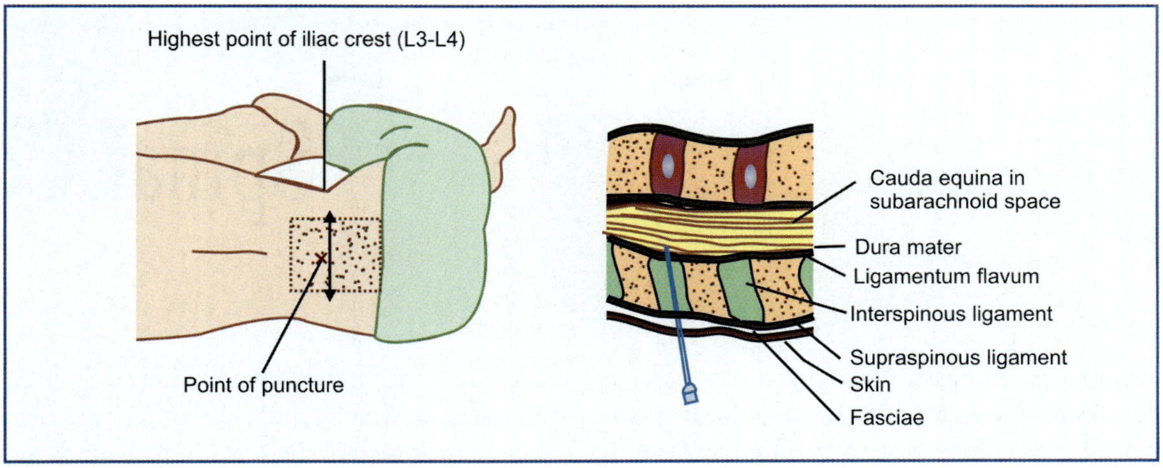

Fig. 83.6: Anatomy of lumbar puncture (Note that the patient lies in left lateral position. The vertebral column is flexed to increase the space between the spines of L3 and L4 V. The needle inserted at this site traverses the anatomical layers shown in the right side figure. Note that arachnoid mater is not labeled)

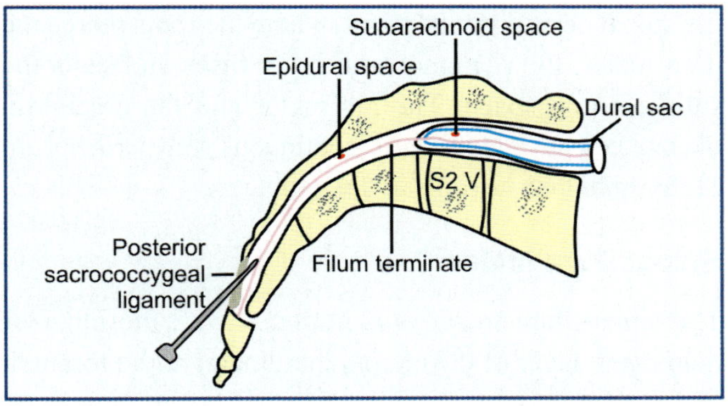

Fig. 83.7: Median section of the sacral canal to depict anatomical basis of caudal analgesia (Note that the needle pierces posterior sacrococcygeal ligament to enter sacral hiatus. The anesthetic solution is injected in epidural space)

pharyngeal abscess, psoas abscess and paraplegia are common complications. Flexion test (picking a coin from the floor) is a valuable test for Pott's disease. A patient suffering from this disease is unable to bend the spine.

b. Cervical spondylosis is a condition characterized by the degeneration of the facet joints in the lower cervical vertebrae and formation of osteophytes. It is common in those whose occupation involves prolonged flexion of neck. The patient presents with pain in the neck with or without radiation to the arm. The cervical collar is often advised for relief of symptoms.

c. The fracture of the vertebrae is met with in accidents. It is common in coconut tree climbers, miners and construction workers. The most feared complication of the fracture is the injury to the spinal cord or cauda equina. First aid to a patient with injury to the vertebral column is very important. The patient must be carefully shifted in the face down position so as to prevent injury to the spinal cord by flexion of the vertebral column.

84 Spinal Cord

The spinal cord is the elongated part of the central nervous system. It is located inside the upper two-thirds of the vertebral canal. The spinal cord gives origin to 31 pairs of spinal nerves, which provide sensory and motor innervation to the entire body excluding the head region. The cord also contains the preganglionic sympathetic neurons (thoracolumbar outflow) for the sympathetic nerve supply of the entire body including the head region.

Development of Spinal Cord

It is described in Chapter 88 along with Development of Nervous System.

Extent

The spinal cord begins as the continuation of the medulla oblongata. It extends from the level of upper border of the posterior arch of atlas to the lower margin of first lumbar vertebra in the adult. The lower tapering end of the spinal cord is called the conus medullaris. Till third month of intrauterine life the spinal cord and vertebral column coincide in length. At birth, the tip of the conus medullaris is at the level of lower margin of third lumbar vertebra. The spinal cord shows enlargements, where it gives origin to nerves that take part in nerve plexuses in cervical and lumbosacral regions.

Length

The length of spinal cord is about 45 cm long in the adult male and 42 cm in adult female.

Spinal Meninges (Fig. 84.1)

The spinal cord is surrounded by three meninges and three spaces related to the meninges. From without inwards the meninges are, dura mater, arachnoid mater and pia mater and the spaces are, epidural, subdural and subarachnoid (which contains CSF). The dura mater sends tubular coverings for the roots of the spinal nerves. It is attached to the margins of the intervertebral foramina, where it is continuous with the epineurium of the spinal nerves. The arachnoid mater and the pia mater (spinal pia-arachnoid) extend as thin sheaths around the roots of the spinal nerves. At the point, where the roots pierce the dura mater, the pia-arachnoid layer fuses and seals the subarachnoid space. The pia mater and the arachnoid mater are believed to become continuous with perineurium of the spinal nerve roots at this point.

Spinal Dura Mater

The spinal dura mater is continuous with the inner or meningeal layer of the cranial dura mater at the foramen magnum. The dura mater lies free in the vertebral canal as the epidural space separates it from the periosteum of the vertebrae. It ends as a blind tube at the level of lower

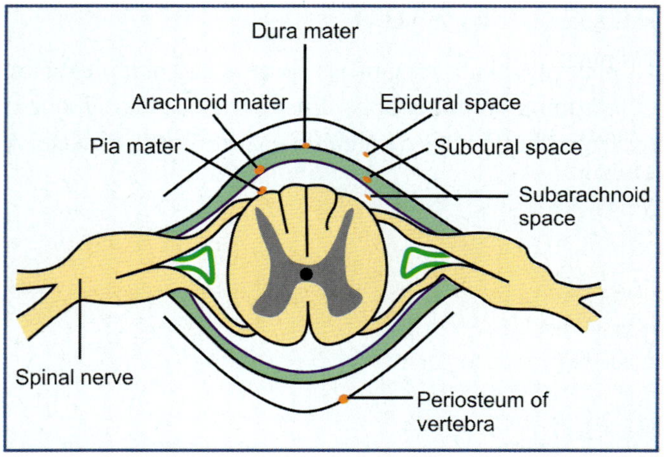

Fig. 84.1: Scheme to depict meninges and spaces surrounding spinal cord (Note that the meninges extend along the dorsal and ventral roots of the spinal nerve)

margin of S2 vertebra. This blind dural tube is pierced by filum terminale, fifth sacral and first coccygeal nerves. The nerve supply of spinal dura mater is derived from the recurrent meningeal branches of the spinal nerves.

Epidural Space

The epidural space contains loose areolar tissue, internal vertebral venous plexus, roots of spinal nerves, spinal branches of regional arteries, recurrent meningeal branches of spinal nerves and semi fluid fat. The epidural anesthesia can be given in this space to numb the spinal nerves that traverse the space. This approach is used in relief of pain in cancer patients, in whom analgesics or pain relieving medicines have no effect. Beyond the lower limit of dura mater the wide epidural space in the sacral canal extends up to the sacral hiatus. The anesthetic is introduced in this space through the sacral hiatus (caudal analgesia) for painless labor.

Subdural Space

This space is the potential space between the dura mater and arachnoid mater.

Arachnoid mater

This is a transparent and avascular membrane continuous with the cranial arachnoid mater above. It extends upto the second sacral vertebra.

Subarachnoid Space

This space containing CSF lies between arachnoid mater and pia mater. It is of uniform size up to the lower end of spinal cord beyond which it expands. This happens because the vertebral canal below the first lumbar vertebra is occupied by the cauda equina, which is a bunch of nerves surrounding the filum terminale. The enlarged subarachnoid space is called lumbar cistern, which extends up to S2 vertebra. The lumbar cistern is approached to collect CSF or to inject spinal anesthetic through the disc between the L3 and L4 vertebrae.

Pia mater

It is a vascular membrane that closely invests the surface of the spinal cord. The pia mater is modified in some places as follows:

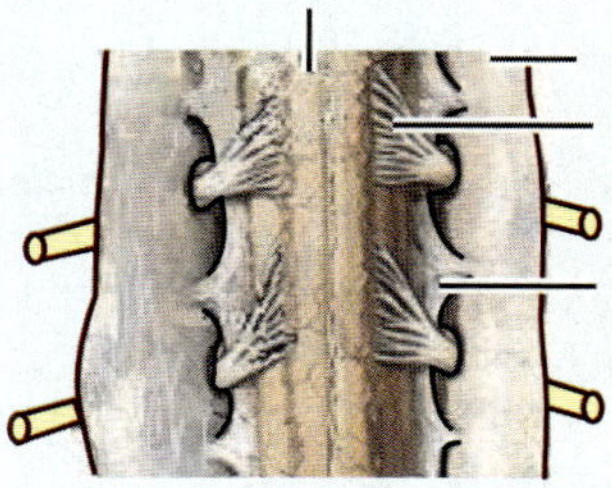

Fig. 84.2: Spinal pia mater seen from the posterior aspect (Dura mater and arachnoid mater have been reflected. Note the extension of pia mater and ligamenta denticulata attaching it to dura mater)

a. Filum terminale is a slender filament of pia mater beyond the conus medullaris. It is about 20 cm long. It pierces the blind end of the dural tube and is subdivided in filum terminale internum inside the dural sac (15 cm) and filum terminale externum outside the dural sac (5 cm). It leaves the sacral canal through the sacral hiatus and is fused with the dorsal surface of the first piece of coccyx.
b. Linea splendens is a thickened band of pia mater along the anterior median fissure of the spinal cord.
c. The ligamenta denticulata (Fig. 84.2) are two ribbon like lateral extensions of the pia mater between the attachments of the ventral and dorsal nerve roots. Each band sends 21 tooth like projections, which pass through the subarachnoid space to gain attachment to the inner surface of the dura mater. The last or the twenty-first ligamentum denticulatum extends obliquely downwards between T12 and L1 spinal nerves. Its identification helps the surgeon in locating the first lumbar nerve during operation.

Surface Features of Spinal Cord

The surface of the spinal cord shows the anterior median fissure and a posterior median sulcus. The rootlets of the dorsal roots enter the cord at the posterolateral sulcus while the rootlets of the ventral roots leave through the anterolateral sulcus.

Spinal Nerves

There are 31 pairs of spinal nerves, 8 cervical, 12 thoracic, 5 lumbar, 5 sacral and 1 pair of coccygeal nerve. The spinal nerve is formed by the union of ventral and dorsal roots in the intervertebral foramen. The dorsal root bears

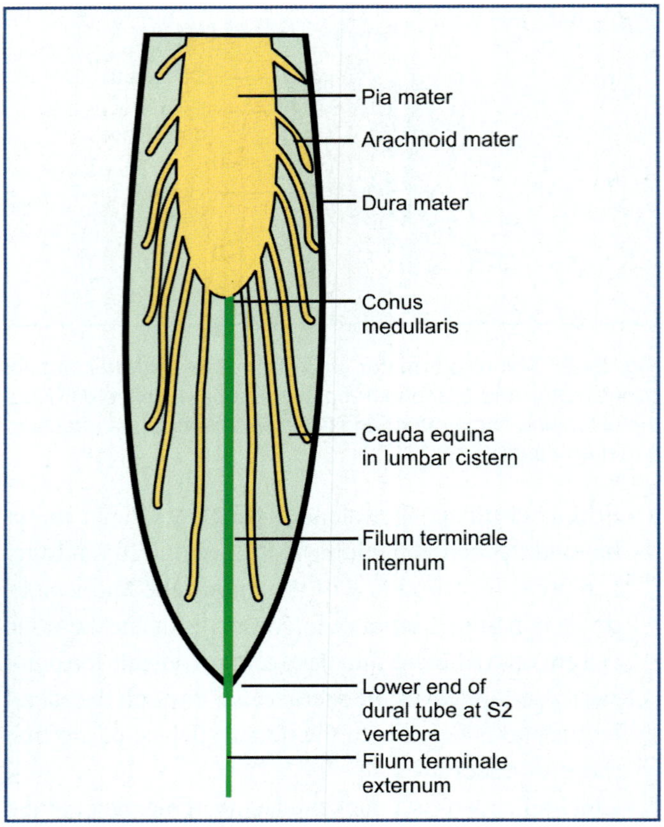

Fig. 84.3: Lumbar cistern with cauda equina

a dorsal or spinal ganglion just before its union with the ventral root. The ventral root carries somatic efferent fibers from the anterior horn cells and the general visceral efferent fibers in the case of thoracic and first two lumbar ventral roots. The dorsal root carries the sensations from the skin, joints, and muscles and from visceral structures brought first to the dorsal root ganglia, and then from here to the spinal cord by the central processes of the ganglion cells. The fibers in the dorsal root belong to general somatic afferent and general visceral afferent functional group. Each spinal nerve divides into a dorsal and a ventral ramus and each ramus contains all the four functional types of fibers.

All the thoracic and first two lumbar spinal nerves give white rami communicantes (14 pairs), through which preganglionic sympathetic fibers are carried to the entire the sympathetic chain. The sympathetic ganglia of all the regions give gray rami communicantes (31 pairs) to respective spinal nerves. In this way, the postganglionic sympathetic fibers are given to the 31 pairs of spinal nerves.

Spinal Segments

A part of spinal cord giving origin to a pair of spinal nerves is called the spinal segment. There are 31 segments of spinal cord. The area of skin supplied by one spinal segment or its dorsal root is called a dermatome. The C1 dermatome does not exist since the C1 spinal nerve has no sensory fibers in it. Only in the trunk, each dermatome is supplied directly by a single spinal nerve. In the case of limbs, the sensory fibers of the ventral ramus of the spinal nerve supply each dermatome. The places, where discontinuous dermatomes meet are called axial lines.

On the trunk, the C4 and T2 dermatomes meet at the sternal angle, which coincides with the ventral axial line of upper limb dermatomes. At the junction of the anterior one-third and posterior two-thirds of the scrotum or labium majus, the L1 and S3 dermatomes meet. This junctional zone coincides with the ventral axial line of lower limb dermatomes. The working knowledge of dermatomes is essential for neurological examination of a patient. In viral infection of dorsal root ganglion (herpes zoster) of a spinal nerve, the cutaneous eruptions appear on the dermatomal area of corresponding spinal segment.

Vertebral Levels of Spinal Segments

Since the spinal cord is shorter than the vertebral column the segments of the spinal cord do not coincide with the overlying vertebrae. This has clinical significance while determining the level of vertebral injury from signs of injury to the spinal segment or vice versa. A simple working rule to identify the vertebral levels of spinal segments is as follows. Add two to the number of vertebra with respect to vertebrae C2 to T10 to find the corresponding spinal segments (for example C2 vertebral spine corresponds to C4 spinal segment). The spines of T11 and T12 correspond to all five lumbar segments and L1 spine corresponds to all five sacral and coccygeal segments.

The shortening of the spinal cord relative to the vertebral column has the effect on the length and direction of the spinal nerve roots. The lower roots are pulled up along with the spinal cord. However, to reach the corresponding intervertebral foramina these nerves have to travel longer in the lateral and downward direction. This also results in formation of cauda equina at the lower

Section three

end of the conus medullaris. The cervical roots are short and horizontal. The rest of the roots become progressively longer and oblique.

Exit of Spinal Nerves

Each spinal nerve emerges through the intervertebral foramen except the following four nerves. The first cervical nerve lies above the posterior arch of the atlas. The second cervical nerve emerges between the posterior arch of atlas and the vertebral arch of axis. The fifth sacral and coccygeal nerves leave through the sacral hiatus. The first to seventh cervical nerves leave in relation to the superior aspect of the numerically corresponding vertebra. The eighth cervical nerve leaves through the foramen above the first thoracic vertebra. The exit of the remaining spinal nerves takes place through the foramina below the numerically corresponding vertebra.

Cauda Equina

The meaning of the term cauda equina is tail of a horse. A leash of nerves suspended from the conus medullaris in the lumbar cistern, is called the cauda equina (Fig. 84.3). It is composed of lumbar, sacral and coccygeal nerve roots (both dorsal and ventral) surrounding the filum terminale. The second to fourth sacral ventral roots carry with them preganglionic parasympathetic fibers. The dura mater and arachnoid mater surround the cauda equina up to the level of second sacral vertebra. The lumbar cistern is approached in the interval between L3 and L4 spines by lumbar puncture. This avoids the injury to the spinal cord by the needle because the roots of cauda equina slip away from the needle or even if injured they have the capacity for regeneration.

Internal Structure of Spinal Cord (Fig. 84.4)

The spinal cord has an H-shaped core of gray matter consisting of the cell bodies of neurons and the neuroglia. The white matter surrounds the gray matter and consists of myelinated and unmyelinated nerve fibers and neuroglia. The gray matter is divisible in a larger anterior column or horn and a narrow elongated posterior column or horn, on each side. A horizontal bar of gray matter known as gray commissure connects the right and left halves of the gray matter. The white matter is divided in two-halves by the anterior median fissure and the posterior median septum.

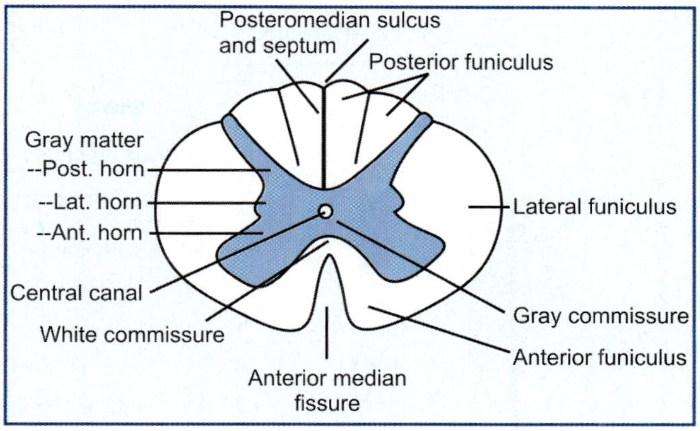

Fig. 84.4: External and internal features of spinal cord as seen in cross-section

Each half of the white matter is subdivided in the anterior, lateral and posterior funiculi. A small strip of white matter in front of the gray commissure is called white or anterior commissure, which is the connecting link between the white matter of the two sides. The central canal of the spinal cord containing CSF traverses the gray commissure. The lining of the canal belongs to ciliated simple columnar epithelium. Superiorly the canal is continuous with the central canal of the closed part of medulla oblongata and through it with the cavity of the fourth ventricle. In the conus medullaris the canal expands slightly to form terminal ventricle.

Gray Matter (Fig. 84.5)

Groups of cell bodies of the multipolar neurons predominantly and plenty of interneurons including Renshaw cells make up the gray matter of the spinal cord. The gray matter is divided into three horns, anterior (or motor), intermediolateral (or visceral) and posterior (or sensory).

The anterior horn is short and bulbous. The neurons in the anterior horn are the lower motor neurons, which are subdivided into alpha neurons and gamma neurons. The alpha neurons supply the extrafusal fibers of skeletal muscles. The gamma neurons supply the intrafusal fibers of neuromuscular spindles in the skeletal muscles.

The anterior horn shows central, medial and lateral groups of neurons. The neurons of the central group in the upper five cervical segments form the spinal nucleus of accessory nerve and those mainly of the fourth cervical segment form the phrenic nucleus. The neurons in the medial group extend throughout the cord and supply the

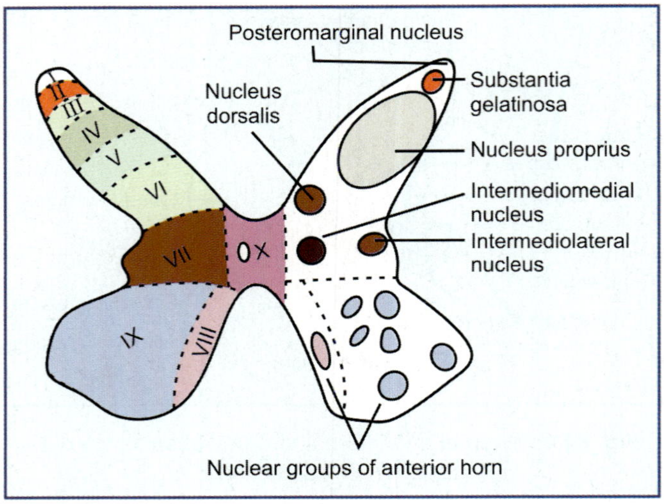

Fig. 84.5: Laminae of Rexed and corresponding nuclear groups in spinal gray matter (I through X-Rexed's laminae) (Note that the lamina X surrounding the central canal consists of gray commissure and substantia gelatinosa centralis)

striated muscles of the neck and trunk. The lateral group neurons are confined to the cervical and lumbar enlargements of the spinal cord and are involved in the supply of limb muscles. A ventrolateral group in first and second sacral segments only is named after Onuf. The neurons in this group supply perineal muscles (anal and urethral muscles). Hence, damage to this nucleus results in rectal and urinary incontinence.

The posterior horn is narrow and reaches the surface of the cord. It is divisible in apex, head, neck and base and contains sensory neurons. The neuronal groups in this horn are, substantia gelatinosa, nucleus proprius, nucleus dorsalis or Clarke's column and visceral afferent.

The intermediate or lateral horn is composed of intermediolateral and intermediomedial nuclei. The intermediolateral nucleus is equal to the preganglionic sympathetic nucleus, in the T1 to L2 segments of the cord (thoracolumbar outflow). The intermediomedial nucleus is present in S2 to S4 segments of spinal cord. It is equal to the preganglionic parasympathetic nucleus (sacral parasympathetic outflow).

Laminae of Rexed

The gray matter is divisible in ten laminae, which are indicated by Roman numerals.

a. Lamina I is at the tip of the posterior horn (pericornual cells).
b. Lamina II corresponds to the substantia gelatinosa.
c. Laminae III, IV, V and IV correspond to the nucleus proprius.
d. Lamina VII corresponds to intermediate or lateral horn in the T1 to L2 segments, where it extends in the base of the anterior horn. This lamina also contains the Clarke's nucleus or dorsal nucleus in the C8 to L3 segments and spinal border cells of Cooper-Sherrington in the L2 to S3 segments.
e. Lamina VIII occupies most of the anterior horn in the thoracic segments but in cervical and lumbar segments it occupies the medial part of the anterior horn.
f. Lamina IX consists of the groups of motor neurons in the ventral horn.
g. Lamina X corresponds to the substantia gelatinosa centralis (gray matter surrounding the central canal).

White Matter (Fig. 84.6)

The spinal white matter consists of ascending and descending spinal tracts. It is divided by sulci into three funiculi. The dorsal funiculus is located between the posterior median septum and posterior gray horn. Above the level of sixth thoracic segment it presents two fasciculi, medially placed fasciculus gracilis and laterally placed

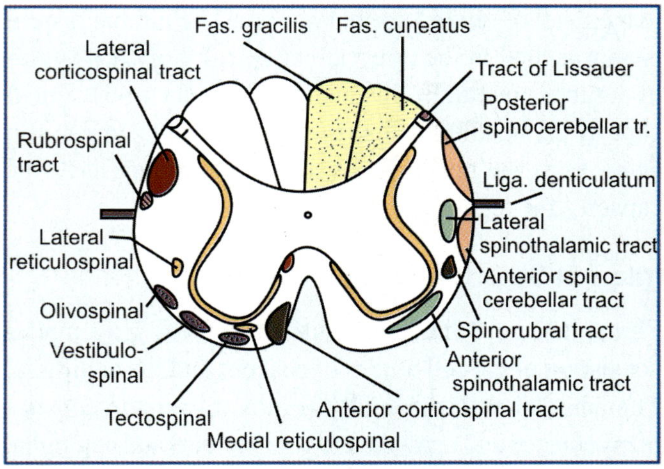

Fig. 84.6: Cross-section of spinal cord showing the location of ascending tracts in left half and of descending tracts in right half. (Note that the intersegmental tract (fasciculus proprius) surrounds the gray matter of spinal cord. Lateral spinothalamic tract is anterior to and lateral corticospinal tract is posterior to the plane of ligament denticulatum

fasciculus cuneus. The lateral funiculus is located between the posterior gray horn and the anterior gray horn. It contains a number of tracts. The ventral funiculus is located between the ventral median fissure and anterior gray horn. The white (anterior) commissure gives passage to the crossing fibers of the anterior (ventral) and lateral spinothalamic, anterior (ventral) spinocerebellar and anterior (ventral) corticospinal tracts.

Major Ascending Tracts

The ascending or sensory tracts usually consist of a chain of the first, second, and third order neurons. The first order neuron is always the pseudounipolar neuron in the dorsal root ganglion.

Spinothalamic Tracts (Fig. 84.7)

a. The anterior (ventral) spinothalamic tract carries light (simple non-discriminative) touch. The first order neurons are located in the dorsal root ganglia of the spinal nerves. The central processes of these neurons enter the spinal cord close to the posterior horn in dorsal funiculus and ascend ipsilaterally for about 7 segments to terminate on the second order neurons, located in laminae IV to VI in the posterior horn. The axons of the second order neurons decussate in the narrow white commissure and ascend in contralateral anterior funiculus as anterior spinothalamic tract. After passing through the brainstem, they terminate in the third order neurons, which are present in the VPL nucleus of thalamus. The axons of the third order neurons (forming superior thalamic radiation) project via the posterior limb of internal capsule and corona radiata to the postcentral gyrus (areas 3,1,2) of cerebral cortex.
b. The lateral spinothalamic tract carries pain and temperature sensations from the free nerve endings and thermal receptors in the skin. The first order neurons are found in the dorsal root ganglia of the spinal nerves. The central processes of these neurons enter the spinal cord via the dorsolateral tract of Lissauer and ascend ipsilaterally for two segments before terminating on the second order neurons in laminae IV to VI. The axons of the second order neurons decussate in the white commissure and ascend in the anterior part of the lateral funiculus as the lateral spinothalamic tract (It is important to understand that a lesion in white commissure at C8 segment will lead to loss of pain and temperature sensation in T2 dermatome since T2 fibers cross at C8 segment). In its further course in the brainstem the lateral spinothalamic tract ascends as part of spinal lemniscus, (which is formed by merging of lateral spinothlamic, anterior spinothalamic and spinotectal tracts) to terminate in nucleus VPL of thalamus, the third order neurons. Its further projection to the cerebral cortex is like that of the anterior spinothalamic path.

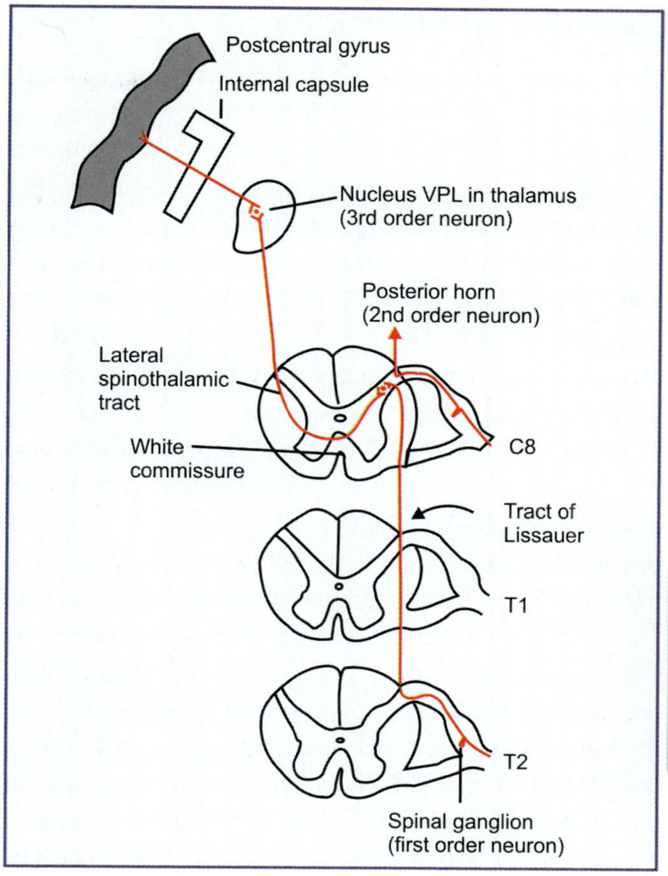

Fig. 84.7: Scheme to show course of lateral spinothalamic tract

The lesion of the lateral spinothalamic tract results in contralateral loss of pain and temperature sensations in two segments below the level of lesion. Surgical sectioning of the lateral spinothalamic tract is called anterolateral cordotomy, which may at times be necessary to relieve intractable pain. In this procedure, the incision is placed in front of the ligamentum denticulatum to access the lateral spinothalamic tract.

Posterior Column Tracts (Fig. 84.8)

There are two tracts in the posterior column, medial, fasciculus gracilis (tract of Gall) and lateral, fasciculus cuneatus (tract of Burdach). They carry the sensations of discriminative or fine touch, pressure, vibration, and conscious sense of position and movements (conscious proprioception) and stereognosis. The tract of Burdach carries all the above sensations from the upper limb and upper part of the trunk. However, the tract of Gall carries all the sensations except that of conscious proprioception, from the lower limb and lower part of trunk. The first order neurons in the spinal ganglia, receive the sensations. The central processes of these neurons enter the spinal cord via the medial bundle of dorsal roots to travel upwards in fasciculus gracilis and fasciculus cuneatus in the dorsal funiculus to terminate in the gracile and cuneate nuclei respectively in the lower part of medulla oblongata. The axons of second order neurons present in these nuclei are called internal arcuate fibers, which cross over in the medulla in the sensory decussation to give rise to medial lemniscus on each side. The medial lemniscus ascends to terminate in the third order neurons, which are present in the nucleus VPL of thalamus. The axons of these neurons pass through the posterior limb of internal capsule and corona radiata to the postcentral gyrus of cerebral cortex.

The lesion of fasciculus gracilis and cuneatus results in loss of conscious proprioception in upper limb and upper trunk, loss of fine touch and vibration ipsilaterally below the level of lesion.

(Landgren and Silfvexius in 1971 propounded the theory of an alternate path for conscious proprioception from the lower limb. This theory is gaining support among neuroscientists. This path is unique as it is a 4-neuron path. The sensation is carried via the central processes of first order neurons (dorsal ganglion) to the neurons of Clarke's column (second order neurons). Further, the sensation is carried upwards through the fibers in the dorsal spinocerebellar tract to the medulla oblongata, where they terminate in nucleus Z of Brodal and Pompieano (third order neurons). Nucleus Z is located at the cranial end of nucleus gracilis. The axons of the neurons in nucleus Z join the medial lemniscus to reach the nucleus VPL of thalamus (fourth order neurons). The observation that lesion of fasciculus gracilis spares conscious proprioception from lower limb lends support to the existence of an alternate path).

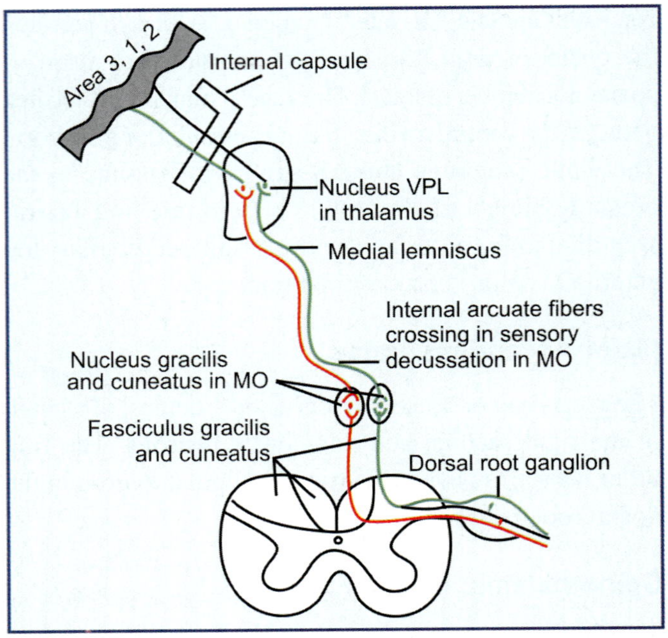

Fig. 84.8: Posterior column pathway (Note that this is three neuron pathway first order neuron—dorsal root ganglion, second order neuron-nucleus gracilis and cuneatus, third order neuron—VPL of thalamus)

Spinocerebellar Tracts

The spinocerebellar tracts (Fig. 84.9) are two neuron paths that carry proprioceptive impulses from muscle spindles and Golgi tendon organs to the cerebellum. This is described as unconscious proprioception. There are four tracts, which carry these sensations, posterior spino-cerebellar, anterior spinocerebellar, cuneocerebellar and rostral spinocerebellar.

a. The posterior (dorsal) spinocerebellar tract carries unconscious proprioceptive sensation from the lower extremity and trunk. The first order neurons are located in dorsal root ganglia of C8 to L3 spinal nerves. The central processes of the ganglion cells terminate on the nucleus dorsalis of Clarke (lamina VII), which are the second order neurons in C8 to L3 levels. The axons of these neurons ascend in the posterior spinocerebellar tract, which is situated in the lateral funiculus. The tract passes through the medulla oblongata and reaches the cerebellum via inferior

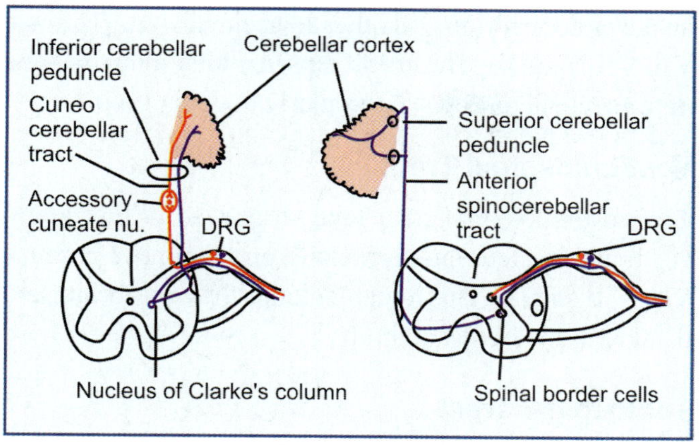

Fig. 84.9: Two-neuron spinocerebellar and cuneocerebellar tracts

cerebellar peduncle. It terminates ipsilaterally in the cerebellar cortex as mossy fibers. The function of this tract is fine coordination of posture and movements of individual muscles of lower extremity and lower half of the trunk.

b. The anterior (ventral) spinocerebellar tract is concerned with coordinated movement and posture of the entire lower extremity. The first order neurons on this tract are the cells of dorsal root ganglia in L2 to S3 spinal nerves. The central processes of these neurons terminate on the cells of Clarke's column or on spinal border cells of Cooper-Sherrigton in lamina VII at the base of the anterior horn in L2 to S3 segments. These are the second order neurons and their axons decussate in white commissure to ascend as anterior spinocerebellar tract in the lateral funiculus. This crossed tract passes through the medulla oblongata and the pons to reach the midbrain, where it enters the superior cerebellar peduncle and terminates in the contralateral cerebellar hemisphere as mossy fibers. A few fibers cross back to the ipsilateral cerebellum.

c. The cuneocerebellar tract is part of fasciculus cuneatus. It carries unconscious proprioceptive sensation from the upper half of the trunk and upper limb. The first order neurons are located in C2 to T8 dorsal root ganglia. The central processes of these neurons are very long. They enter the spinal cord and ascend along with fasciculus cuneatus to terminate on the neurons of accessory cuneate nucleus (on the surface of cuneate tubercle in the lower part of medulla oblongata). The axons of the neurons in this nucleus are called the posterior external arcuate fibers (cuneocerebellar tract). They reach the cerebellum through the inferior cerebellar peduncle. The accessory cuneate nucleus is equivalent to the nucleus dorsalis of Clarke and cuneocerebellar tract is equivalent to the posterior spinocerebellar tract.

d. The rostral spinocerebellar tract serves the upper limb and upper half of the trunk and is equivalent to the anterior spinocerebellar tract of the lower limb. The location of the neurons of its origin in the cervical spinal cord is not confirmed. The tract reaches the cerebellum via the inferior and superior cerebellar peduncles.

Lissauer's Tract

The dorsolateral bundle or Lissauer's tract is situated between the apex of posterior horn and the surface of the spinal cord. It is present throughout the spinal cord. The tract is formed by lateral bundles of dorsal roots carrying pain and temperature sensations, which divide in ascending and descending fibers. The ascending fibers travel two segments of the spinal cord before terminating in the posterior horn cells. The tract is continuous above with the spinal tract of trigeminal nerve.

Major Descending Tracts

The descending spinal tracts influence the motor neurons in the spinal cord. Their cells of origin are located either in the cerebrum or in the brainstem.

Corticospinal (Pyramidal) Tract (Fig. 84.10)

The two corticospinal tracts are, the anterior and lateral corticospinal tracts. They begin in the medulla oblongata after the pyramidal decussation. The corticospinal fibers from the cerebral cortex pass through various parts of the cerebrum and the brainstem to reach the medulla oblongata, where 80-85 percent fibers decussate to form lateral corticospinal tract. The uncrossed fibers descend as anterior corticospinal tract. These uncrossed fibers finally cross by passing through the white commissure.

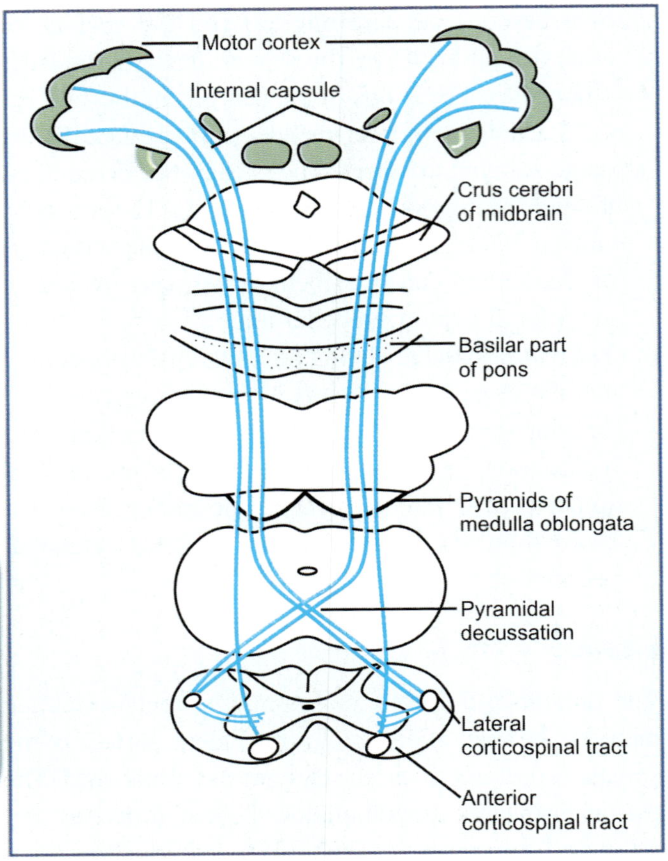

Fig. 84.10: Pyramidal tracts—origin, course and termination of corticospinal fibers

The majority of corticospinal fibers influence the anterior horn cells via the internuncial neurons. Only about 10 percent of fibers directly terminate on the anterior horn cells. Thus the corticospinal fibers control the voluntary skilled movements of the opposite side of body through the anterior horn cells. The detailed description of the tract is given in Chapter 98 on white matter of brain.

Descending Autonomic Pathways

These tracts begin in the higher centers of autonomic functions (hypothalamus and reticular formation) and terminate on the intermediolateral column in T1 to L2 segments of spinal cord for sympathetic control and in S2-S4 segments for parasympathetic control.

Rubrospinal Tract

The rubrospinal tract is a crossed tract from red nucleus of midbrain and is located in lateral funiculus. It extends along the entire length of the spinal cord and terminates on the motor neurons and other adjacent neurons (laminae VII, VIII and IX). This tract helps in maintaining the tone of the skeletal muscles, particularly in upper limb.

Vestibulospinal Tract

The vestibulospinal tract takes origin from the lateral vestibular nucleus and terminates on neurons in laminae VII, VIII and IX. This tract maintains the equilibrium and posture of the body and limbs

Tectospinal Tract

The tectospinal tract begins in the midbrain from the dorsal tegmental decussation of the fibers from the superior colliculi. It travels down in the brainstem and occupies the anterior funiculus. The fibers terminate like the rubrospinal and vestibulospinal tracts.

Olivospinal Tract

The olivospinal tract originates in the inferior olivary nucleus in the medulla oblongata and terminates in relation to the anterior horn cells.

Reticulospinal Tract

The reticulospinal tracts (lateral and medial) originate in the reticular formation of the pons and medulla oblongata and descend in to the spinal cord to terminate in relation of the anterior horn cells. These tracts play a role in maintenance of muscle tone.

Fasciculus Proprius (Intersegmental Tract)

These are short ascending and descending tract that interconnect the neurons of the adjacent segments of spinal cord. They are centrally located in all the three funiculi since they surround the gray matter of the spinal cord. The ventral fasciculus proprius is in continuation with the lower end of the medial longitudinal fasciculus (MLF) of brainstem.

Regional Variation in Internal Appearance of Spinal Cord

a. In the cervical cord, the anterior horns are broad and blunt but the posterior horns are relatively tapering. There is no lateral horn. All the funiculi are well-developed. The central canal is pushed toward the anterior surface due to the large size of the posterior columns.

b. In the thoracic cord, the anterior and the posterior horns are typical H-shaped. The lateral horn is present. The white matter is more compared to the gray matter. The central canal is nearer the anterior surface.

c. In the lumbar cord, both the horns are broad but anterior is broader than the posterior. The lateral horn is present in upper two segments only. White matter is less in proportion to gray matter and the central canal is in the center.

d. In the sacral cord, the white matter is very scanty and proportionately the gray matter is large. The central canal is present in the center. Separate lateral horn is not discernable. The overall size of the spinal cord is greatly reduced.

Arterial Supply

Being an elongated structure, the spinal cord receives arteries from several sources (Fig. 84.11). A few of these arteries may be supplying a large part of the spinal cord and if this major source is diseased or damaged the spinal cord undergoes necrosis. This will lead to serious complications like paraplegia (paralysis of both upper or lower limbs) or monoplegia (paralysis of a single limb). The arterial supply of the cord is derived from the anterior spinal artery and two pairs of posterior spinal arteries. These arteries are replenished at regular intervals by the radicular arteries.

a. A single midline anterior spinal artery is formed in the posterior cranial fossa by the union of the right and left anterior spinal arteries, which are the branches of the fourth part of the vertebral artery. This artery descends through the foramen magnum and runs down in the anterior median fissure of the spinal cord.

b. The right and left posterior spinal arteries are the branches of the fourth part of the vertebral arteries. Each posterior spinal artery descends through the foramen magnum as two branches, which pass one in front, and one behind, the dorsal roots of the spinal nerves.

c. The paired anterior and posterior radicular arteries originate from spinal branches of second and third parts of vertebral arteries, ascending cervical arteries

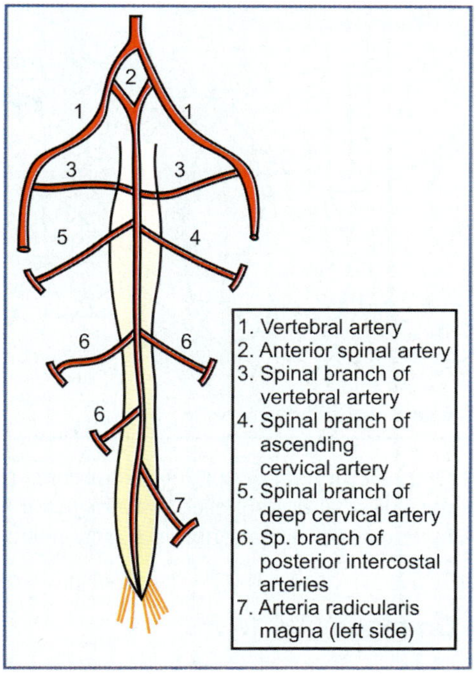

Fig. 84.11: Anterior view showing sources of arterial supply of spinal cord

(from inferior thyroid), deep cervical arteries (from costocervical trunk), posterior intercostal arteries (from thoracic aorta), lumbar arteries (from abdominal aorta) and lateral sacral arteries (from posterior division of the internal iliac artery). The majority of the radicular arteries do not reach the longitudinally oriented spinal arteries because they are exhausted in the supply of the roots of the spinal nerves. However, a few of them are larger and take part in the supply of spinal cord. One of the anterior radicular branches (usually on the left side) is very large and hence is called the arteria radicularis magna of Adamkiewicz. The position of this vessel is variable. It may take origin from the tenth or eleventh posterior intercostal or subcostal arteries. It is sometimes the main supply to the lower two-thirds of the spinal cord. The central branches of the radicular arteries supply the gray and white matter of the spinal cord. The central branches of the anterior spinal artery (replenished by arteria radicularis magna) supply about anterior two-thirds of the cross-sectional area of the spinal cord. It includes the anterior gray matter, part of dorsal gray matter, anterior and lateral funiculi. The central branches of the posterior spinal arteries supply the posterior horn and the posterior funiculus (Fig. 84.12).

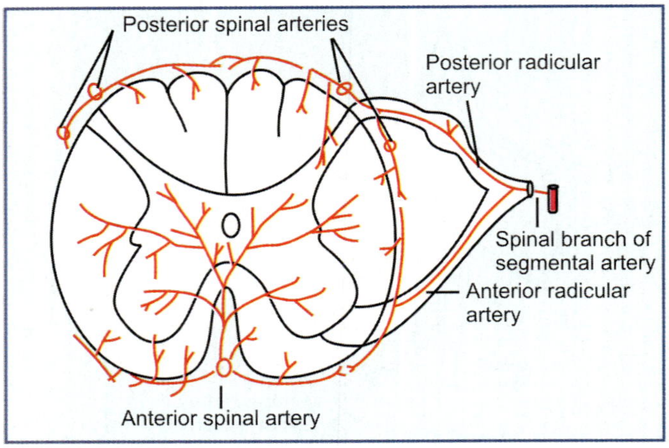

Fig. 84.12: Intrinsic arterial supply of spinal cord (Note that single anterior spinal artery supplies anterior two-third of the cord while two posterior spinal arteries supply posterior one-third)

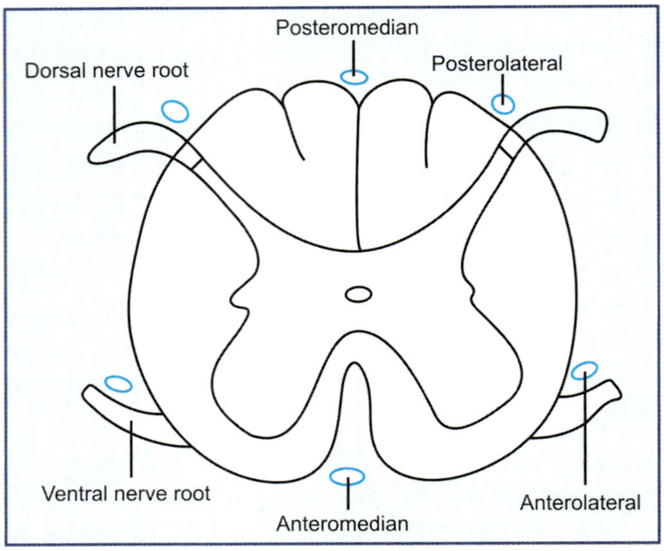

Fig. 84.13: Site of six longitudinal venous channels draining spinal cord

Venous Drainage (Fig. 84.13)

The spinal veins drain in six plexiform longitudinal channels, which surround the cord. The anteromedian and posteromedian channels run in the respective fissure or sulcus. The paired anterolateral and posterolateral channels run anterior and posterior to the ventral and dorsal roots of the spinal nerves. Superiorly, the venous channels are continuous with the cranial venous sinuses and they communicate with the internal vertebral venous plexuses, which drain via the intervertebral veins into the regional veins.

Radiology of Spinal Cord

The subarachnoid space is outlined by the injection of contrast media (iodized oil) in the subarachnoid space by lumbar puncture. The normal myelogram shows the pointed lateral projections at regular intervals at the intervertebral space, where the lateral extensions of the subarachnoid space around the spinal nerves are present. The presence of a tumor or the prolapsed disc will obstruct the movement of the contrast medium. The MRI and CT scans are the modern methods to visualize spinal cord.

Clinical Highlights

a. The arteria radicularis magna may be injured during surgery. The occlusion of the feeder artery (the artery that gives origin to the radicular artery) may result in poor blood flow in the radicular artery. The examples of feeder artery diseases are, atherosclerosis of vertebral arteries, dissecting aneurysm of thoracic aorta, emboli from the heart and sickle cell disease. In the event of the disease of the feeder artery or injury to the arteria radicularis magna, the midthoracic region of the cord will be deprived of the blood supply resulting in the infarction of the entire anterior half or more of the spinal cord (anterior spinal artery syndrome). It presents clinically as acute flaccid paraplegia below the level of lesion, bilateral loss of pain and temperature below the level of lesion but complete preservation of joint position sense, touch and stereognosis.
b. The spinal cord may show upper motor neuron and/or lower motor neuron lesions. The upper motor neuron (UMN) means the neuron, which is located in the motor area of cerebral cortex and its axon (Fig. 84.14). The term lower motor neuron (LMN) means the anterior horn cell of spinal cord and its axon, which supplies the skeletal muscle. The upper and lower motor neuron injuries result in different clinical signs, although both result in paralysis. The fundamental difference in UMN and LMN lesions is that UMN lesions result in paralysis of voluntary movements but LMN lesions cause paralysis of individual muscles or muscle groups. The UMN lesion causes spastic paralysis. The spasticity is due to increased tone of the muscles as

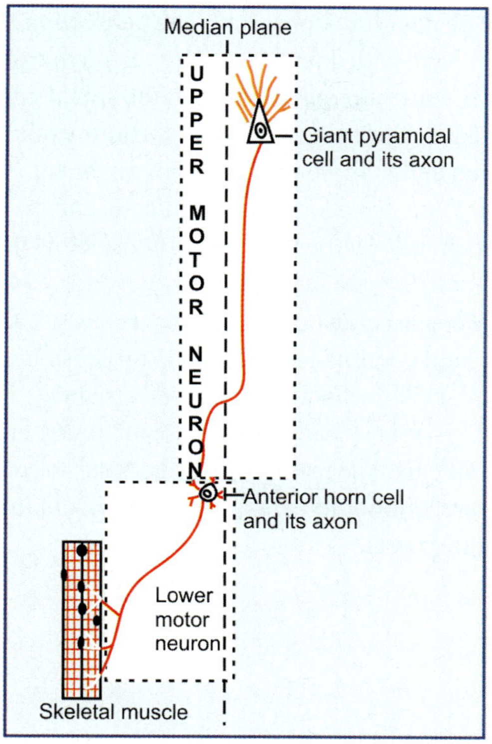

Fig. 84.14: Scheme to show upper motor neuron (UMN) and lower motor neuron (LMN)

result of continuous activity of the monosynaptic stretch reflex. The alpha and gamma motor neurons involved in stretch reflex are not under the inhibiting influence of corticospinal tracts and extrapyramidal tracts in UMN lesion. In addition, there is hyper-reflexia (exaggerated deep tendon reflexes) and positive Babinski sign (refer to pyramidal tract in Chapter 98). On the other hand, the LMN lesion causes flaccid paralysis, (flaccidity is due to loss of tone in the muscles), wasting or atrophy of muscles and loss of tendon reflexes. In the spinal cord lesion, of both UMN and LMN can coexist if there is involvement of corticospinal tracts and anterior horn cells.

Lesions of Spinal Cord (Fig. 84.15)

a. Syringomyelia is a degenerative disease of the gray and white commissures usually in the cervical region. There is cavitation in the gray commissure causing enlargement of the central canal, which extends in ventral direction destroying the crossing spinothalamic fibers in the white commissure. So, syringomyelia in cervical cord presents as bilateral loss of pain and temperature (without loss of touch sensation) in the shoulder area. The dissociated sensory loss is the hallmark of this disease. With progression of the disease the anterior horn cells and the lateral corticospinal tracts may be involved. At this stage, the characteristic clinical picture is the combination of upper and lower motor neuron paralysis and the dissociated sensory loss.

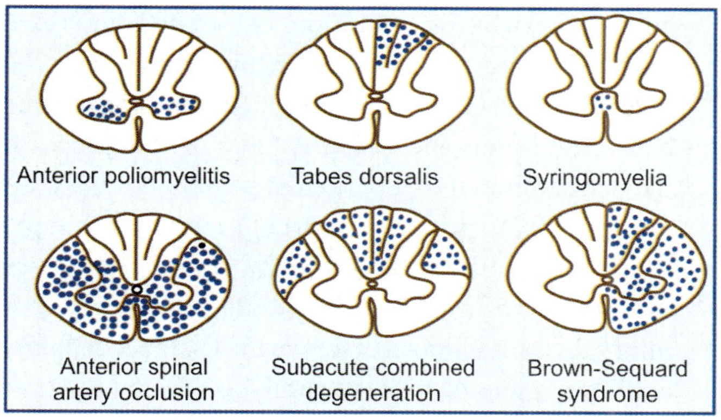

Fig. 84.15: Sites of lesions of spinal cord

b. The tabes dorsalis or tertiary syphilis affects the intraspinal part of posterior root and posterior column tracts, which results in loss of position sense, vibratory sense, sense of stereognosis, two-point discrimination on the same side, below the level of lesion. Romberg's sign is positive, in which on closing the eyes the patient becomes ataxic.
c. The subacute combined degeneration of spinal cord occurs in vitamin B_{12} deficiency. One of the causes of this deficiency is pernicious anaemia. The posterior columns and the lateral corticospinal tracts undergo degeneration on both sides. It usually affects the lumbosacral region of the cord. The clinical manifestation is bilateral loss of position and vibratory sense and spastic paraplegia with exaggerated tendon reflexes and positive Babinski sign.
d. Brown-Sequard syndrome or hemisection of spinal cord is characterized by ipsilateral spastic paralysis (UMN) due to lesion of corticospinal tract. The sensory deficits due to involvement of spinothalamic and dorsal column tracts below the level of lesion are as follows, contralateral loss of pain and temperature sensation and ipsilateral loss of conscious proprio-

ception, joint sense, vibration, etc. In addition there may be ipsilateral lower motor neuron paralysis at the level of the lesion due to injury to anterior horn cells and ventral roots and ipsilateral loss of sensations on the dermatome of that particular segment of the cord due to injury to posterior horn cells and dorsal roots.

e. The complete transection of the spinal cord gives different clinical pictures depending on the level of injury. In transection at or above the C4 level of spinal cord the patient dies due to paralysis of diaphragm. If the cervical cord below the level of C5 is transected the effect is quadriplegia in which all the four limbs are paralysed. Transection in the thoracic segments of the spinal cord leads to paraplegia. In both quadriplegia and paraplegia the voluntary control over the bladder function is lost. The transection at T1 level will have added feature of Horner's syndrome due to involvement of lateral horn of the spinal gray matter.

f. The anterior spinal artery occlusion results in motor signs and symptoms due to involvement of cortico-spinal tracts and anterior horn cells and bilateral loss of pain and temperature sensations below the level of lesion.

g. The cauda equina syndrome occurs due to compression of cauda equina (in acute disc prolapse between the L2/3 levels or fracture of lumbar vertebrae). This gives rise to severe pain in both lower limbs and flaccid paraplegia. The retention of urine is due to compression of preganglionic parasympathetic fibers in S2 to S4 ventral roots.

85 Cranial Meninges

There are three meningeal layers inside the cranium. The dura mater or pachymeninx is the outermost layer followed internally by the arachnoid mater and then the pia mater. The arachnoid and pia mater together are called the leptomeninges. The meninges are related to three spaces. The extradural (epidural) space is a potential space between the outer layer of the dura mater and the adjacent bone. This space becomes apparent when bleeding takes place due to rupture of the meningeal vessels (extradural/ epidural hemorrhage or hematoma). The subdural space lies between the dura mater and the arachnoid mater. The superior cerebral veins pass through it and rupture of these veins is the cause of subdural hemorrhage. The subarachnoid space between the arachnoid mater and the pia mater contains CSF. The rupture of cerebral arteries or their branches at the base of brain is the cause of the subarachnoid hemorrhage.

Cranial Dura Mater

The peculiarity of the cranial dura mater is that it is divisible in outer and inner layers. The outer layer is the endosteal layer hence it is very close to the cranial bones. The endosteal layer is actually the endocranium of the cranial bones. The inner layer is called the meningeal layer. The two layers of the dura mater are adherent to each other except in places, where the dural venous sinuses are present and where the inner layer is reduplicated to form dural folds. At the foramen magnum, the meningeal layer of dura mater is continuous with the spinal dura mater. The endosteal layer of dura mater is continuous with the pericranium at the foramina in the cranial cavity and at the foramen magnum it is continuous with the pericranium covering the occipital bone. The branches of middle meningeal artery and accompanying veins ascend on the external surface of the endosteal layer in the extradural space.

Dural Folds

The cranial dura mater forms four folds by reduplication of its inner layer, falx cerebri, tentorium cerebelli, diaphragma sellae, and falx cerebelli. The folds help in stabilizing the brain during movements of the head. If the brain moves within the cranial cavity it may exert strain on the thin walled, veins that pass through the subdural space. Therefore, to prevent the rupture of these veins it is necessary to have strong dural folds inside the cranial cavity.

a. The falx cerebri is so named because of its sickle shape. It forms a vertical partition in the longitudinal fissure between the cerebral hemispheres. The falx cerebri is attached anterioly to the frontal crest of frontal bone and crista galli of ethmoid bone. Superiorly, it is attached to the midline of the vault as far back as the internal occipital protuberance. Inferiorly, it presents a free margin anteriorly and is attached to the tentorium cerebelli posteriorly. There are three venous sinuses inside the falx cerebri. Its attached superior margin encloses the superior sagittal sinus. Its free inferior margin encloses the inferior sagittal sinus and the straight sinus is enclosed along the line of attachment of the falx cerebri and the tentorium cerebelli.
b. The tentorium cerebelli is a tent-shaped fold of dura mater, which roofs the posterior cranial fossa. It forms a partition between the cerebellar lobes and the occipital lobes of the cerebrum. It helps to take the weight of the cerebrum off cerebellum. This fold is attached to the posterior clinoid process, superior margin of the petrous temporal bone and the internal

surface of the occipital bone and to the inferior margin of the falx cerebri in the midline. The attached margin contains three venous sinuses. The superior petrosal sinus lies along the line of attachment to the superior margin of the petrous temporal bone. The transverse sinus lies along the attachments to the lips of the sulcus, from the internal occipital protuberance to the base of the petrous temporal bone. The straight sinus lies along its line of attachment to the falx cerebri. The free and attached margins of the tentorium cerebelli cross each other at the apex of the petrous temporal bone.

The free margin of the tentorium cerebelli encloses a U-shaped tentorial notch (Fig. 85.1), which gives passage to the midbrain, oculomotor nerves and the posterior cerebral arteries. The narrow subarachnoid space between the boundary of the notch and the midbrain is the only communication between the subarachnoid space of supratentorial and infratentorial compartments of the cranial cavity. Obstruction of the subarachnoid space in the tentorial notch will give rise to communicating hydrocephalus. For clinical anatomy of the tentorial notch refer to Chapter 86. A large extradural hemorrhage (Fig. 86.2) in the supratentorial compartment may cause herniation of the uncus of the temporal lobe through the notch.

c. The diaphragma sellae is a circular dural fold. It forms the roof the hypophyseal fossa and is pierced by the infundibulum of the pituitary gland. The fold is attached to the tuberculum sellae in front and dorsum sellae behind. It encloses the anterior and posterior intercavernous sinuses in its attached margins.

d. The falx cerebelli lies in the posterior cranial fossa. It is attached to the inferior surface of the tentorium cerebelli and to the internal occipital crest. It contains the occipital sinus.

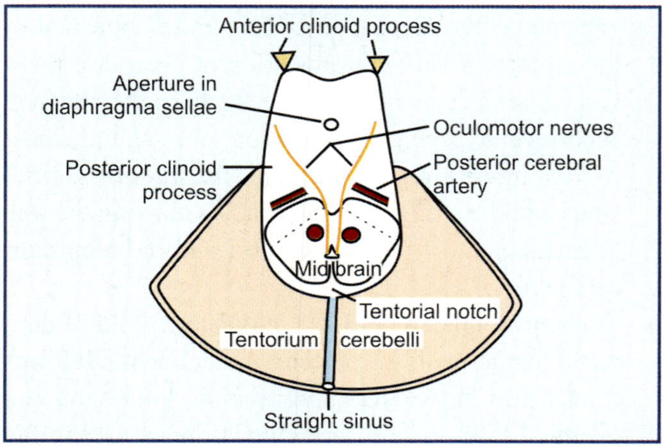

Fig. 85.1: Scheme depicting the attachments of tentorium cerebelli (Note: U-shaped tentorial notch through which midbrain, oculomotor nerves and posterior cerebral arteries pass)

Nerve Supply

a. The dura mater in the anterior cranial fossa receives sensory supply from the anterior and posterior ethmoidal nerves and the anterior filaments of the meningeal branches of maxillary and mandibular nerves.
b. The dura mater of the middle cranial fossa receives sensory supply from the nervus spinosus, which is the meningeal branch of the mandibular nerve. The meningeal branches of the maxillary nerve and the direct branches from the trigeminal ganglion also provide additional branches.
c. The dura mater of posterior cranial fossa receives twigs from the ascending meningeal branches of upper cervical nerves. The tentorium cerebelli receives branches from the tentorial nerve, which is the recurrent meningeal branch of ophthalmic division of trigeminal nerve. The meningeal branches of vagus and hypoglossal nerves also contribute.

Blood Supply

The meningeal branches of the anterior and posterior ethmoidal arteries and of the middle meningeal artery, supply the dura mater in the anterior cranial fossa. The dura mater of the middle cranial fossa receives arterial blood from the middle and accessory meningeal arteries, ascending pharyngeal artery, internal carotid artery and the recurrent branch of lacrimal artery. The dura mater of the posterior cranial fossa receives twigs from the occipital artery, vertebral artery and meningeal branch of ascending pharyngeal artery.

Dural Venous Sinuses

The dural venous sinuses are enclosed between the two layers of the dura mater. They drain blood from the brain, meninges and the cranial bones. They are lined by endothelium, are devoid of muscular tissue in their walls and do not possess valves.

Classification

The dural venous sinuses are broadly classified into the posterosuperior group and the anteroinferior group (Fig. 85.2).

Posterosuperior group	*Anteroinferior group*
Superior sagittal sinus	Cavernous sinus
Inferior sagittal sinus	Inferior petrosal sinus
Straight sinus	Sphenoparietal sinus
Transverse sinus	Superior petrosal sinus
Sigmoid sinus	Intercavernous sinuses
Occipital sinus	Basilar venous plexuses

Superior Sagittal Sinus

This sinus is present along the attached margin of the falx cerebri. It lies deep to the bregma and the sagittal suture. In children up to the age of one and half years, in place of bregma there is a soft anterior fontanelle. So the sinus lies subjacent to the anterior fontanelle, through which it may be approached if other veins are collapsed.

Origin and Termination

The superior sagittal sinus begins at the crista galli in front and ends at the internal occipital protuberance behind. Usually it ends by continuing as the right transverse sinus but in some cases it may become the left transverse sinus or joins both sinuses. At the termination of the superior sagittal sinus there is a dilatation known as confluence of sinuses, where as many as five sinuses may communicate (superior sagittal, straight, right and left transverse and the occipital).

Surface Marking

The sinus can be marked on the surface by a line joining the glabella to the inion.

Tributaries

About ten to twelve superior cerebral veins open against the flow of blood in the superior sagittal sinus. These veins are extremely thin-walled. They cross the subdural space to enter the superior sagittal sinus through the duramater. The veins enter the sinus obliquely so that

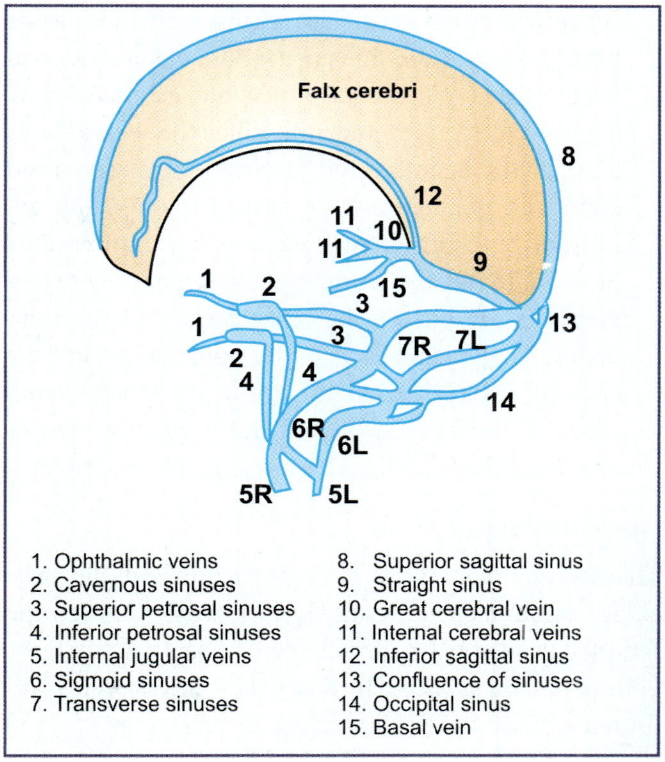

Fig. 85.2: Dural venous sinuses

their openings are directed anteriorly. This unusual feature has functional importance. It helps the superior cerebral veins to remain patent.

Special Features of Superior Sagittal Sinus

a. The lateral venous lacunae are cleft like lateral extensions of the sinus between the two layers of the dura mater. The lacunae are seen in three locations. A small frontal lacuna lateralis is the most anteriorly placed. The parietal lacuna lateralis is the largest and overlies the upper part of the motor area of brain. The occipital lacuna lateralis is intermediate in size. The lacunae absorb the CSF through the arachnoid granulations that project inside them. Besides, they receive the diploic and meningeal veins. The lacunae and the arachnoid granulations increase in size with age. These three lacunae unite to form a single large lacuna, which may produce shallow depressions on the inner aspect of the skull on either side of the superior sagittal sinus.
b. The arachnoid granulations, which are the projections of the arachnoid mater, are most numerous in the

superior sagittal sinus. The arachnoid matter passes through minute apertures in the dura mater to project in the sinuses. Where such projections are microscopic they are called arachnoid villi. When the aggregations of the villi become macroscopic they are called arachnoid granulations. In early life only villi are present but with advancing age the granulations develop. In old age, the granulations are so large that they produce pits on the inner surface of the skull bones. The arachnoid villi and granulations are the sites of absorption of CSF from the subarachnoid space in the venous blood. These valvular bodies prevent reflux of blood in the subarachnoid space.

Communications

The superior sagittal sinus communicates with the nasal cavity through the emissary vein passing through the foramen cecum and with the veins of scalp through the emissary vein passing through the parietal emissary foramen. The superior anastomotic vein connects it to the superficial middle cerebral vein. Infection can reach the sinus through the nasal cavity or scalp or through the infected sigmoid or transverse sinuses.

Clinical Highlights

In thrombosis of the superior sagittal sinus the absorption of the CSF is interfered with leading to higher pressure of CSF and consequent rise in intracranial pressure.

Inferior Sagittal Sinus

This sinus is located in the inferior margin of the falx cerebri. It joins the great cerebral vein of Galen to form the straight sinus. Another way of describing its termination is that it continues as the straight sinus. According to this description the great cerebral vein becomes the tributary of the straight sinus.

Straight Sinus

This sinus lies in the junction of falx cerebri and the tentorium cerebelli. It runs in the posteroinferior direction in the line of union of the two dural folds. It becomes continuous usually with the left transverse sinus at the internal occipital protuberance. The area of drainage of the straight sinus includes veins from the posterior and central parts of the cerebrum, falx cerebri and tentorium cerebelli. The great cerebral vein is the important vein draining the interior of the brain. The termination of this vein in the straight sinus is guarded by a small mass of sinusoidal plexus of vessels. This acts like a valve when engorged, thus, preventing outflow of venous blood from the vein in the sinus. This is probably to reduce the formation of CSF in the ventricles.

Occipital Sinus

It is a small venous sinus situated in the attached margin of the falx cerebelli. It extends from the foramen magnum to the internal occipital protuberance. Its anterior end bifurcates to communicate with the sigmoid sinus of each side. Its posterior end opens in the confluence of sinuses. The occipital sinus communicates with the internal vertebral venous plexus.

Transverse Sinuses

The right and left transverse sinuses begin at the internal occipital protuberance. The right sinus is the continuation of superior sagittal sinus in the majority of cases and the left is the continuation of the inferior sagittal sinus. Accordingly, the size of the right transverse sinus is larger than the left. The transverse sinus lies in the attached margin of the tentorium cerebelli grooving the inner surface of the occipital bone. It terminates by becoming the sigmoid sinus at the posteroinferior angle of parietal bone, which is also grooved. The sinus is related to the occipital lobe of the cerebrum above and to the cerebellum below.

Tributaries

The tributaries of the transverse sinus are, inferior cerebral veins, diploic veins, inferior anastomotic vein connecting to the superficial middle cerebral vein, inferior cerebellar veins and superior petrosal sinus.

Surface Marking

A line that begins at the inion and ends at the base of the mastoid process represents the sinus on the surface.

Sigmoid Sinuses

The sigmoid sinuses are S-shaped. They are the continuations of the transverse sinuses. Each sinus deeply grooves the mastoid part of temporal bone. In this location, it is very close to the mastoid air cells laterally. The mastoid antrum and the vertical part of the facial nerve lie anterior to it while the cerebellum lies posteriorly. These close relations have clinical importance. The sigmoid sinus thrombosis, internal jugular vein thrombosis or cerebellar abscess are the complications of mastoiditis. The sigmoid sinus curves forwards to enter the posterior compartment of the jugular foramen, where it becomes the superior bulb of the internal jugular vein. It receives veins from the cerebellum.

Communications

It communicates with the scalp veins by emissary veins passing through mastoid emissary foramen and with suboccipital venous plexus by condylar emissary veins.

Surface Marking

It starts at the base of the mastoid process and passes down just anterior to the posterior border of the mastoid to reach a point 1 cm above its tip.

Cavernous Sinuses

These venous sinuses are located in the middle cranial fossa on the side of the body of sphenoid bone. The name cavernous is derived from the trabeculated or spongy appearance of the interior of sinus. Each sinus extends from the medial end of the superior orbital fissure to the apex of the petrous temporal bone. It is two cm long and one cm wide.

According to some descriptions, the sinus has a roof, floor, lateral and medial walls. The meningeal layer of dura mater forms the roof and lateral wall and endosteal layer forms the floor and medial wall of the sinus.

Close Relations of Sinus (Fig. 85.3)

a. Four nerves travel in the lateral wall of the sinus. From above downward, they are, oculomotor, trochlear, ophthalmic and maxillary nerves.
b. The internal carotid artery surrounded by sympathetic plexus passes forwards through the sinus in close contact with the floor (the artery produces a groove on the body of the sphenoid bone). The abducent nerve passes forwards in inferolateral relation to the artery.

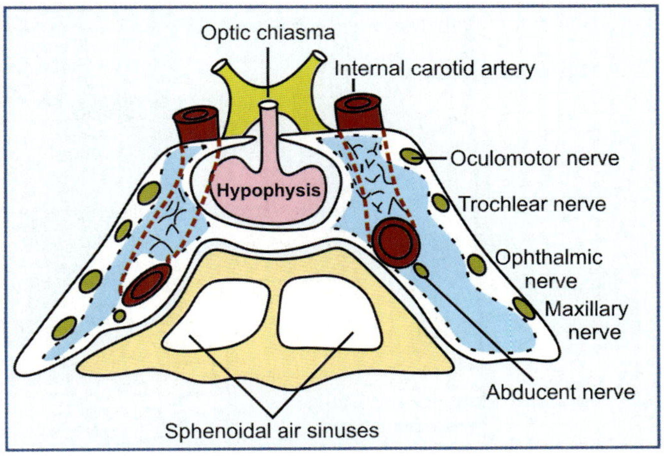

Fig. 85.3: Relations of cavernous sinus

Both the artery and the nerve are separated from the interior of the sinus by endothelium. The internal carotid artery comes out of the sinus by piercing its roof.
c. Medially, the cavernous sinus is in relation to the sphenoid air sinus and hypophysis cerebri.

Relations of the Sinus with Surrounding Structures

a. The hypophysis cerebri is related medially and the body of the sphenoid with contained air sinus is related inferomedially.
b. The trigeminal ganglion and mandibular nerve are related posterolaterally.
e. The optic chiasma and internal carotid artery (after it emerges from the roof of the sinus) are present above it.

Tributaries (Fig. 85.4)

The tributaries are, superior ophthalmic vein, inferior ophthalmic vein, middle meningeal sinus (vein), central vein of retina and sphenoparietal sinus, (which lies along the lesser wing of sphenoid).

Draining Channels

The superior petrosal sinus drains the cavernous sinus into the junction of transverse and sigmoid sinuses. The inferior petrosal sinus empties into the internal jugular vein after coming out of cranium through the jugular foramen.

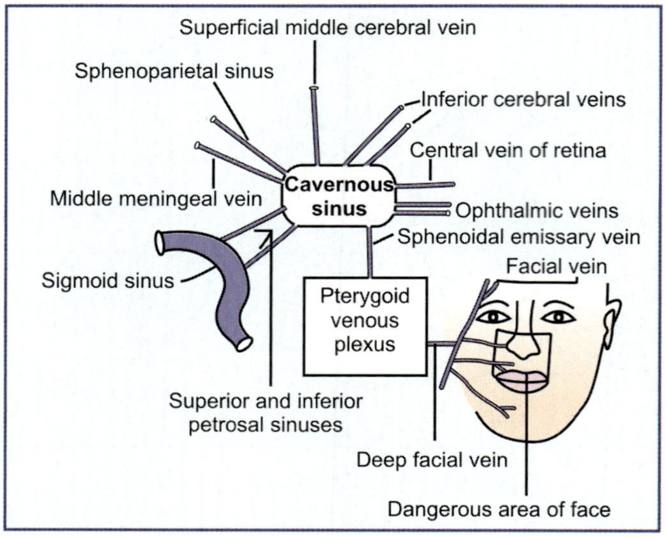

Fig. 85.4: Scheme to depict tributaries and communications of cavernous sinus (Note: The venous route of spread of infection from the dangerous area of face to the cavernous sinus)

Communications

a. The cavernous sinus communicates with the pterygoid venous plexus (in the infratemporal fossa) by an emissary vein passing through either the foramen ovale or the emissary sphenoidal foramen or Vesalius foramen. This route communicates cavernous sinus with dangerous area of face.
b. The superior ophthalmic veins connect it with the facial vein.
c. The two cavernous sinuses interconnect by intercavernous sinuses.
Note the difference between the tributaries, draining channels and communications.

Clinical Highlights

a. Cavernous sinus thrombosis occurs usually from the infection on the dangerous area of the face. The symptoms and signs of the cavernous sinus thrombosis are due to involvement of the structures in its close relation. Exophthalmos or proptosis occurs due to engorgement of ophthalmic veins. The papilledema is due to engorgement of central vein of retina. The paralysis of extraocular muscles (ophthalmoplegia) is due to involvement of third, fourth and sixth cranial nerves. The dilated and fixed pupil and ptosis are due to injury to oculomotor nerve. There are sensory disturbances in the areas of ophthalmic and maxillary divisions of the trigeminal nerve.
b. Pulsating exophthalmos occurs due to an abnormal communication between the cavernous sinus and the internal carotid artery (arteriovenous fistula or the arteriovenous aneurysm). The cause may be a severe blow or the fall on the head. The eyeball is protruded and the conjunctival blood vessels are dilated. The exophthalmos pulsates synchronously with the arterial pulse. The patient complains of rumbling sound in the orbit, which can be heard on auscultation over the eye or the orbit. The venous congestion gives rise to papilledema leading to impaired vision.

Superior Petrosal Sinuses

Each sinus begins from the posterior end of the cavernous sinus. It runs backward and laterally in the attached margin of tentorium cerebelli along the superior margin of petrous temporal bone and ends by joining the transverse sinus at its junction with the sigmoid sinus. It receives veins from cerebrum, cerebellum and middle ear.

Inferior Petrosal Sinuses

Each sinus begins at the posterior end of the cavernous sinus and ends in the internal jugular vein. It lies in the groove between the petrous part of temporal bone and basilar part of occipital bone. The inferior petrosal sinus is the only dural venous sinus that leaves the cranium. It passes through the anterior compartment of the jugular foramen to join the internal jugular vein and to become the first tributary of the internal jugular vein. The sinus receives veins from the internal ear, medulla, pons and inferior surface of cerebrum. The right and left inferior petrosal sinuses are interconnected by basilar venous plexuses, which lie on the anterior surface of clivus between the layers of dura mater. The basilar venous plexuses are in communication with the internal vertebral venous plexus.

Emissary Veins

These tiny veins pass through the foramina of the cranium and connect the intracranial venous sinuses with the extracranial veins. The function of the emissary veins is to equalize the venous pressure within and outside the cranium. Being valveless blood can flow in both directions in them. The importance of these veins lies in the fact that they are the vehicles of infection from outside in to the intracranial sinuses leading to venous thrombosis.

Examples of Emissary Veins

a. Mastoid emissary vein passes through the mastoid foramen and connects the sigmoid sinus to the scalp veins (posterior auricular and occipital veins).
b. The superior sagittal sinus is connected to the veins of scalp through the parietal emissary vein and to the veins of nasal cavity by emissary veins passing through the foramen cecum.
c. The cavernous sinus is connected to the pterygoid venous plexus by emissary vein passing through the emissary sphenoidal foramen of Vesalius, emissary vein passing through foramen lacerum and through foramen ovale.
d. Anterior condylar emissary vein connects the sigmoid sinus to the internal jugular vein.
e. Posterior condylar emissary vein connects the veins of suboccipital triangle to the sigmoid sinus.

Diploic Veins

These veins drain the diploë of the skull bones. The diploë are the venous spaces between the outer and inner tables of the flat bones of the skull. They are valveless.

Cranial Pia-arachnoid

The arachnoid mater is separated from the dura mater by a thin film of fluid in the potential subdural space. The arachnoid mater is very thin, avascular and transparent membrane. It lines the internal surface of the dura mater. It projects as villi and granulations in the venous sinuses. The arachnoid granulations or Pacchionian bodies are the hypertrophied arachnoid villi.

Subarachnoid Space

This space is filled with CSF and lies between the arachnoid mater and pia mater. This fluid-filled space around the semifluid soft brain acts as a buffer in protecting it from injury. The two meningeal layers are held tightly to each other by dense trabeculae. The subarachnoid space contains the larger arteries and veins of the brain.

Subarachnoid Cisterns

There are certain locations where the arachnoid mater is separated from the pia mater by wide subarachnoid space. In such locations, the subarachnoid space is wider and hence called cistern, which contains pool of CSF.

a. The cerebello-medullary cistern is the biggest subarachnoid cistern and hence called the cisterna magna. It occupies the interval between the inferior surface of cerebellum and the posterior aspect of medulla oblongata. It receives the median aperture of the fourth ventricle called foramen of Magendie. This cistern is approached to collect CSF samples (cisternal puncture) via the suboccipital triangle.
b. The cisterna pontis lies in front of the pons and medulla oblongata and contains the vertebral and basilar arteries.
c. The interpeduncular cistern is seen at the base of the brain in the interpeduncular fossa. It contains the circle of Willis. The pulsations of the cerebral arteries taking part in the arterial circle help the propulsion of the CSF to the surface of the cerebral hemisphere.
d. The cistern of the lateral sulcus is formed by the arachnoid bridging the lips of the lateral sulcus. It contains the middle cerebral vessels.
e. The cistern of the great cerebral vein (cisterna ambiens) lies inferior to the splenium of the corpus callosum. The great cerebral vein is its content and the pineal gland protrudes in it.

Subarachnoid Hemorrhage

The subarachnoid hemorrhage results from rupture of a congenital berry aneurysm at the base of the brain. The symptoms are of sudden onset. They include severe headache, stiffness of neck and loss of consciousness. The diagnosis is established by the presence of blood in the CSF.

Pia Mater

The cranial pia mater is a delicate highly vascular membrane that closely invests the surface of the brain. It dips in the cerebral sulci. Between the pia mater and the surface of the brain there is a subpial space. The pial plexus of blood vessels supplies branches to the brain. The older concept that the blood vessels entering the brain are encircled by perivascular space filled with CSF is no longer valid. The special modifications of the cranial pia mater are the tela choroidea and choroid plexuses. Tela choroidea is a vascularized double fold of pia mater. The choroid plexus is formed, when the tela choroidea is covered with ependyma and extends in to the ventricle to secrete CSF.

86 Middle Meningeal Artery

The middle meningeal artery takes origin from the first part of the maxillary artery in the infratemporal fossa (Fig. 105.3). At its origin, two roots of the auriculotemporal nerve encircle the artery. The middle meningeal artery ascends towards the roof of the infratemporal fossa, where it enters the middle cranial fossa via the foramen spinosum accompanied by the nervus spinosus (meningeal branch of the mandibular nerve). In the middle cranial fossa, the trunk of middle meningeal artery and its branches are located in the extradural space. The artery passes anterolaterally on the floor of the middle cranial fossa and then divides into anterior and posterior branches on the greater wing of the sphenoid. The anterior or frontal branch lies in a groove on the greater wing of sphenoid at the pterion. Thereafter, it breaks up in branches that supply the dura mater and the cranial bones as far back as the vertex. One branch grooves the anteroinferior angle of the parietal bone and overlies the precentral gyrus. The parietal or posterior branch arches backward on the squamous part of temporal bone to supply the dura mater and the cranial bones as far as the lambda.

Branches

The middle meningeal artery primarily supplies the cranial bones, diploë and the dura mater. Apart from this, it has the following named branches:

a. Ganglionic branches supply the trigeminal ganglion.
b. Petrosal branch passes through the greater petrosal hiatus to enter the petrous temporal bone and supply the facial nerve, geniculate ganglion and the middle ear.
c. Superior tympanic branch enters the middle ear along the canal for tensor tympani muscle.
d. Anastomotic branch enters the orbit through the lateral part of superior orbital fissure to anastomose with the recurrent meningeal branch of lacrimal artery.
e. Temporal branches enter the temporal fossa to anastomose with deep temporal branches of maxillary artery.

Surface Marking (Fig. 86.1)

A line joining the preauricular point to a point two cm above the middle of the zygomatic arch represents the trunk of the middle meningeal artery. The anterior branch is represented by a line, which begins at the upper end of the trunk of the middle meningeal artery and passes forward and upward to the pterion and then passes upward and backward to a point that lies midway between the nasion and inion. The pterion lies at a point about four cm above the zygomatic arch and 3.5 cm behind the frontozygomatic suture. The posterior branch corresponds to a line starting at the upper end of the trunk to the lambda, which lies about seven cm above the inion.

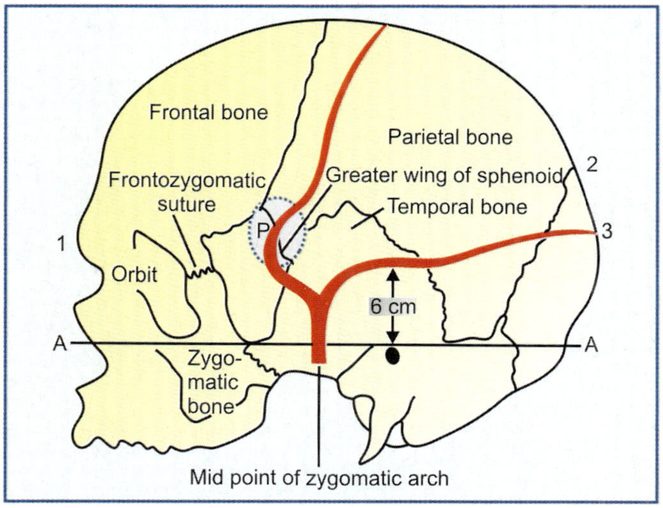

Fig. 86.1: Surface marking of middle meningeal artery (Note that pterion (P) is the meeting point of 4 bones and lies 3.5 cm behind frontozygomatic suture and 4 cm above zygomatic arch. 1–Nasion, 2–Lambda, 3–Inion AA–Reid's base line

Extradural Hemorrhage

The fracture of the side of the skull involving the pterion is likely to tear the anterior branch of middle meningeal artery. The arterial injury causes gradual accumulation of blood in the extradural space. Initially, the symptoms of confusion and irritability are seen. Later on, a hematoma may form and it may exert pressure on the underlying precentral gyrus. A large and long-standing extradural hemorrhage (Fig. 86.2) in the supratentorial compartment may cause herniation of the uncus of the temporal lobe through the notch. In such cases, midbrain is shifted to the opposite side and its crus cerebri is compressed by the sharp edge of the tentorium (Kernohan's notch). If this happens, clinical signs of compression of corticospinal fibers in the crus cerebri will become apparent in addition to signs of compression of the third cranial nerve and the posterior cerebral artery. To prevent these serious complications, immediate treatment consists of ligating the bleeding vessel through a burr hole at about 2.5 to 4 cm above the midpoint of the zygomatic arch.

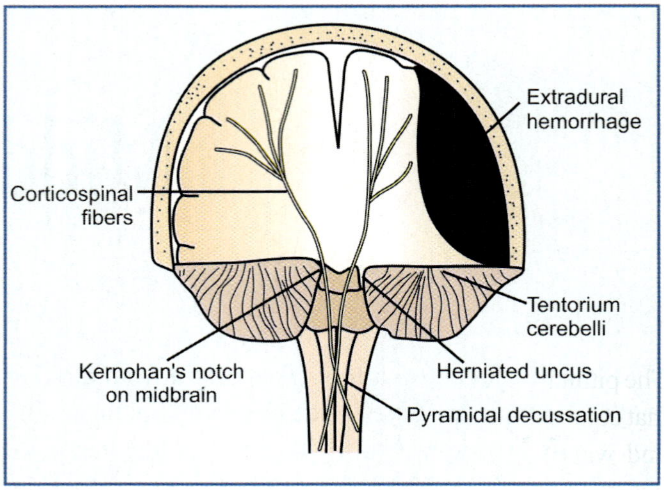

Fig. 86.2: Schematic diagram depicting effects of large extradural hematoma—left side (Note: The herniation of left uncus through tentorial notch and the shift of midbrain to right. Also the compression of corticospinal fibers at Kernohan's notch causing limb weakness on the side of the lesion)

Middle Meningeal Vein or Sinus

The vein accompanying the middle meningeal artery is called the middle meningeal sinus. It behaves more like an emissary vein. It opens in the lateral lacuna of the superior sagittal sinus. Its frontal and pareital tributaries groove the inner aspects of the parietal bone (the veins being actually in contact with the bone). The termination of the two tributaries is variable. The parietal tributary passes through the foramen spinosum to open in pterygoid venous plexus. The frontal tributary may reach the pterygoid plexus through the foramen ovale or it may open in the sphenoparietal or cavernous sinus. The middle meningeal sinuses receive diploic and cerebral veins.

87 Pituitary Gland

The pituitary gland or the hypophysis is the endocrine gland that controls the growth, metabolism, reproductive function and water conservation in the body. The pituitary is a pea-shaped gland weighing about 500 mg. It consists of two lobes (adenohypophysis and neurohypophysis), which are anatomically, structurally and developmentally different from each other. The adenohypophysis is larger than the neurohypophysis and accounts for 75 percent of the total weight of the gland.

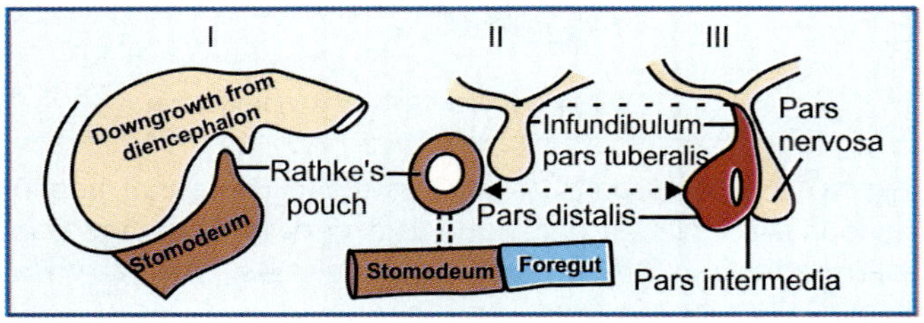

Fig. 87.1: Stages in the development of pituitary glang (Note: The intraglandular cleft in the adenohypophysis. It is a remnant of the cavity of Rathke's pouch)

Location

The pituitary is placed inside the hypophyseal fossa of the sphenoid bone. It is suspended from the floor of the third ventricle (hypothalamus) by the stalk.

Development (Fig. 87.1)

The pituitary develops from two sources, adenohypophysis from ectoderm of stomodeum and neurohypophysis from neuroectoderm of diencephalon.

a. The adenohypophysis develops from Rathke's pouch, which extends from the roof of the stomodeum towards the base of the diencephalon. The anterior wall of the Rathke's pouch proliferates to form pars distalis and the thin posterior wall forms the pars intermedia. The original cleft largely obliterates but its remnant (colloid follicles) are present between pars distalis and pars intermedia (some regard the intraglandular cleft as persistent part of Rathke's pouch). The original site of attachment of the Rathke's pouch in the stomodeum, shifts posteriorly in the roof of the nasopharynx and is indicated by a dimple in the mucosa above the nasopharyngeal tonsil in the adult.
b. The neurohypophysis develops from the downgrowth from the base of diencephalon towards Rathke's pouch.

Congenital Anomalies

If a remnant of the Rathke's pouch is left in the roof of nasopharynx it is called accessory anterior lobe in pharyngeal wall or pharyngeal hypophysis. Remnants of Rathke's pouch may give origin to tumors called craniopharyngiomas, which are found inside the sphenoid bone.

Subdivisions (Fig. 87.2)

a. The adenohypophysis consists of three parts, namely, the pars distalis or pars anterior or anterior lobe, pars intermedia and pars tuberalis.
b. The neurohypophysis consists of three parts, namely, pars nervosa or posterior lobe, infundibular stem and median eminence, which is the part of tuber cinereum from which infundibular stem begins.

Infundibulum

The infundibulum belongs to both subdivisions of the pituitary. The stem of the infundibulum carries neural

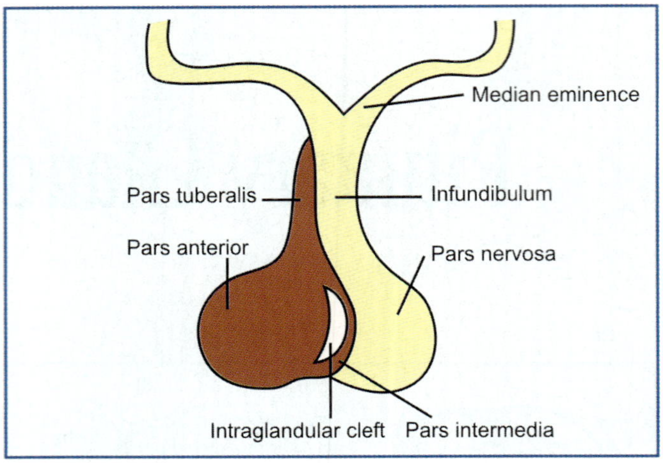

Fig. 87.2: Subdivisions of pituitary gland (Note that adenohypophysis includes pars tuberalis, pars anterior and pars intermedia and neurohypophysis includes pars nervosa, infundibulum and median eminence)

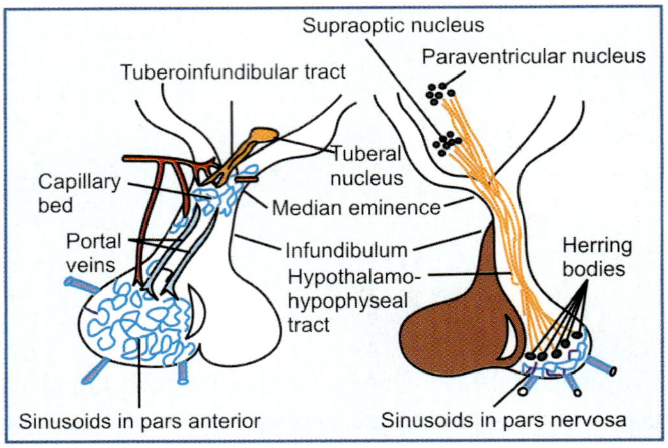

Fig. 87.3: Scheme showing connections of anterior and posterior lobes of pituitary with hypothalamus (Note that there is vascular connection with pars anterior and neural connection with pars nervosa)

fibers from the hypothalamus to the pars nervosa. The part of adenohypophysis that surrounds the infundibular stem is known as pars tuberalis. The infundibulum is composed of the infundibular stem (hypothalamo-hypophyseal tract), hypophyseal portal vessels and pars tuberalis.

Relations (Fig. 85.3)

a. The dural relations of the gland are noteworthy. The diaphragma sellae separates the pituitary from the hypothalamus. The infundibulum, which is a functional link between the hypothalamus and the pituitary, passes through the central aperture in the diaphragma sellae. The gland is surrounded by dura mater all around. The capsule of the gland is adherent to the dura mater. Hence, subdural and subarachnoid spaces are absent around the gland. This is to ensure that the gland is protected from the effects of high CSF pressure. The empty sella syndrome occurs, when the central aperture in the diaphragma sellae is large and the pia-arachnoid herniates through it in the pituitary fossa. This leads to accumulation of CSF in the herniated subarachnoid space with consequent compression and atrophy of the gland.
b. Inferiorly, the gland is related to the sphenoidal air sinuses.
c. The optic chiasma is located very close anteriorly and superiorly and hence pituitary growths present with visual symptoms.
d. On either side, it is related to the cavernous sinus and its contents.

Connections with Hypothalamus (Fig. 87.3)

a. The neurophypophysis is directly connected to the supraoptic and paraventricular nuclei of the hypothalamus via the hypothalamohypophyseal or supraopticohypophyseal tract. Vasopressin and ADH produced by the neurons in these nuclei are transported by the nerve fibers in the tract and are stored in the nerve terminals (Herring bodies) of these fibers in the neurohypophysis. The hormones are released in the venous sinusoids as and when necessary.
b. The adenohypophysis communicates with the hypothalamus via the portal blood vessels, which transport releasing hormones and release inhibiting hormones to the adenohypophysis. These hormones are secreted by the tuberal infundibular or arcuate) nuclei and are carried by the tuberoinfundibular tract to the capillary bed in the median eminence. The hypothalamohypophyseal portal veins begin in this capillary bed and carry these hormones to the cells in the anterior pituitary. Figure 87.4 illustrates the role of

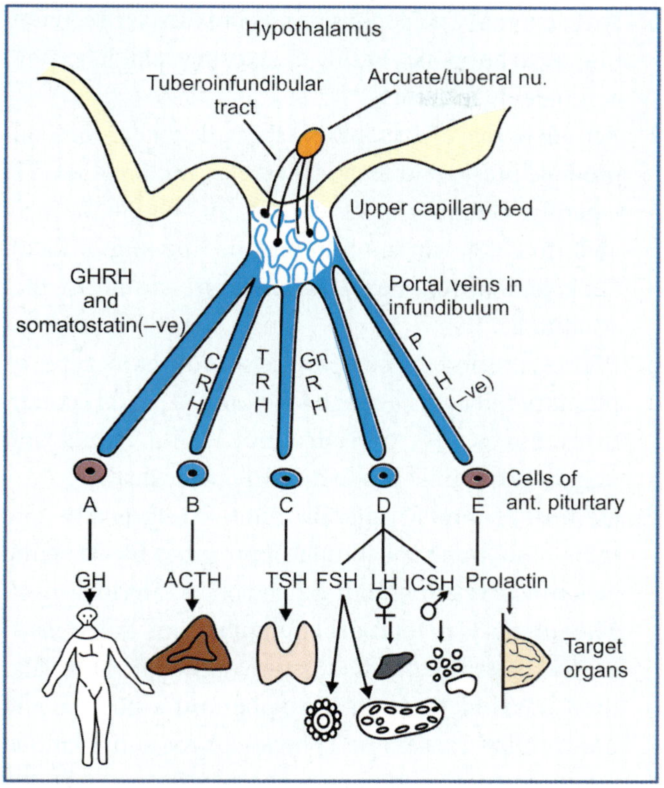

Fig. 87.4: Graphic representation of structural and functional inter-relationship between hypothalamus, anterior pituitary and target organs (Note: The cellular source of pituitary hormones, A-Somatotroph, B-Corticotroph, C-Thyrotroph, D-Gonadotroph, E-Mammotroph)

hypothalamus as master orchestrator of endocrine system.

Blood Supply (Fig. 87.5)

a. The adenohypophysis receives blood from two sources (arterial and portal venous). The superior hypophyseal arteries are the branches of the internal carotid artery. The long and short portal veins originate in the primary plexus formed by the superior hypophyseal arteries in the vicinity of the median eminence and reach the pars distalis through the infundibulum. The portal veins break up in the secondary plexus in the substance of the pars distalis. Thus, the hypophyseal portal veins begin in the capillary bed at the median eminence and terminate in the capillary bed in the adenohypophysis and carry the releasing and release inhibiting hormones (factors) from the hypothalamus to the adenohypophysis.

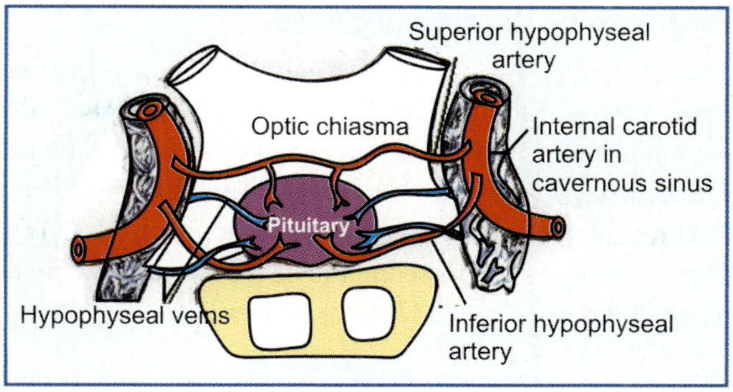

Fig. 87.5: Arterial supply and venous drainage of pituitary gland

b. The neurohypophysis receives arterial blood from the inferior hypophyseal arteries, which are the branches of internal carotid artery.
c. The veins of the pituitary drain into the cavernous or intercavernous sinuses.

Structure of Adenohypophysis

Three types of cells are observed on routine hematoxylin and eosin staining in the highly cellular adenohypophysis. The cells are, the chromophobes, acidophils and basophils. Two cells come under acidophils, somatotrophs (which secrete growth hormone or somatotropin) and mammotrophs (which secrete lactogenic hormone or prolactin or PRL). The somatotrophs are under the dual control of growth hormone releasing hormone and somatostatin (an inhibitory hormone). The mammotrophs are under dual control. They are under the dominant inhibitory control of prolactin inhibitory hormone (PIH), which is a dopamine. The stimulation of mammotrophs is by TRH. Three cells fall under the basophils. The gonadotrophs secrete FSH (follicle stimulating hormone), LH (leutinising hormone) or ICSH (interstitial cell stimulating hormone). They are regulated by gonadotropin releasing hormone. The thyrotrophs secrete TSH (thyroid stimulating hormone), which is controlled by thyrotropin releasing hormone. The corticotrophs secrete ACTH, which is regulated by corticotropin release hormone. The cells of pars intermedia secrete MSH (melanocyte stimulating hormone). These cells are believed to be under the control of both MSH release and MSH-inhibitory factors.

Structure of Neurohypophysis

The neurohypophysis consists mainly of unmyelinated nerve fibers of the hypothalamohypophyseal tract. The neuroglial cells called pituicytes support these nerve fibers. The neurohypophysis does not secrete any hormones but it stores and releases oxytocin and aldosterone (ADH). These hormones are stored in the nerve terminals, which when dilated, are called Herring bodies.

Clinical Highlights

a. The commonest tumor of the pituitary is adenoma arising from chromophobe cells. It compresses the structures in relation to the gland leading to diverse signs and symptoms. The pressure on the central part of the optic chiasma results in loss of right and left temporal fields of vision (bitemporal hemianopia). Pressure on the cavernous sinus gives rise to exophthalmos and paralysis of the muscles of the eyeball supplied by third, fourth and sixth cranial nerves. Downward growth of the tumor may break the sella turcica and cause the enlargement of the hypophyseal fossa, which is seen on a plain radiograph of the cranium as ballooning of the sella turcica.

b. An adenoma of acidophils results in excessive secretion of growth hormone causing gigantism in childhood and acromegaly in adults.

c. An adenoma of basophils is small hence does not produce pressure effects. It secretes excess of ACTH causing Cushing's syndrome, in which there is abnormal deposition of fat on face (moonig of face), neck and trunk. Females are more prone to this condition.

d. PRL secreting tumors are also common type of pituitary tumors. The high level of PRL in this condition causes loss of reproductive functions and inappropriate milk production (galactorrhea).

e. Quite often pituitary gland is removed surgically. The trans-nasal trans-sphenoidal approach is based on the anatomical relations of the gland on its inferior aspect. The pituitary is approached via the roof of the nasal cavity (by removing the rostrum of the sphenoid) and then passing through the sphenoid sinus. In the transorbital-transethmo-sphenoidal route the lamina papyracea of the ethmoid is entered first to reach the ethmoidal sinuses. Then the partitions of the ethmoidal air cells are broken.

88 Development of Nervous System

The central nervous system develops from the neural plate, which is the thickened area of ectoderm overlying the notochord in the embryonic trilaminar germ disc during third week.

Development of Neural Tube

The neural plate shows a depression in the midline called a neural groove, which is flanked on either side by the neural folds. The closure of the neural folds in the midline leads to formation of the neural tube, which soon separates from the surface ectoderm. The neural tube is the forerunner of the brain and spinal cord. The neural crest cells are spilled off from the neural tube in the angle between the surface ectoderm and the neural tube (before its separation).

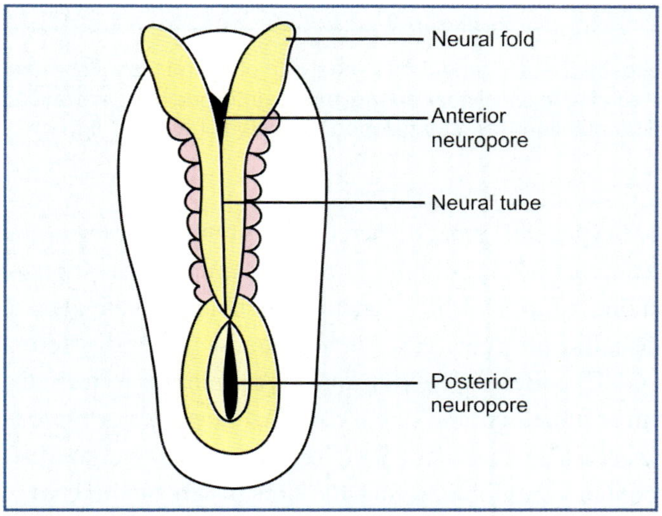

Fig. 88.1: Dorsal view of 23-day-old human embryo showing formation of neural tube (Note that the cranial and caudal ends are open at this stage. Note the somites on either side of the neural tube)

Derivatives of Neural Crest

The neural crest cells give rise to the following: sensory ganglia belonging to spinal and cranial nerves, autonomic ganglia (sympathetic and parasympathetic ganglia), medulla of suprarenal gland, Schwann cells, leptomeninges (pia-arachnoid) and melanocytes and odontoblasts.

Neural Tube

The neural tube is open at its cranial and caudal ends (anterior and posterior neuropores), through which it communicates with the amniotic cavity. Figure 88.1 shows a 23-day-old human embryo, in which the neuropores of the neural tube are fairly wide. The anterior neuropore closes on the twenty-fifth or twenty-sixth day. The lamina terminalis represents the cranial end of the neural tube. The posterior neuropore closes on the twenty-seventh day.

There are three layers in the wall of the neural tube. The inner neuroepithelial layer gives origin to the neuroblast and spongioblast cells, which enter the mantle layer. The neuroblasts give rise to the neurons and the spongioblasts give rise to the oligodendrocytes and astrocytes. Thus, the middle mantle layer is the forerunner of the gray matter. The outer marginal layer is the forerunner of the white matter (Fig. 88.2).

The neural tube has a central canal, roof plate, a floor plate and the lateral walls (Fig. 88.2). The central canal is diamond shaped to begin with. The roof and floor plates are thin and non-neural.

Development of Spinal Cord (Fig. 88.2)

The caudal part of the neural tube develops into the spinal cord. Appearance of sulcus limitans divides the mantle layer into two parts, the alar (dorsal or sensory) lamina and the basal (ventral or motor) lamina. The alar lamina gives origin to sensory neurons, which functionally belong

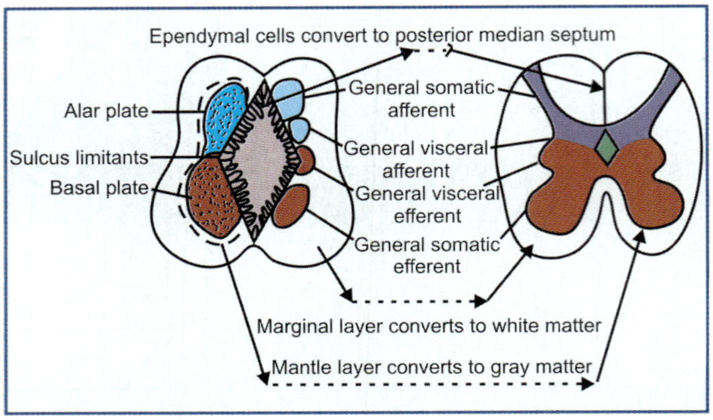

Fig. 88.2: Histogenesis of caudal part of neural tube (Note that neural tube consists of ependymal, mantle and marginal layers. The mantle layer is enveloped by dotted line in the figure)

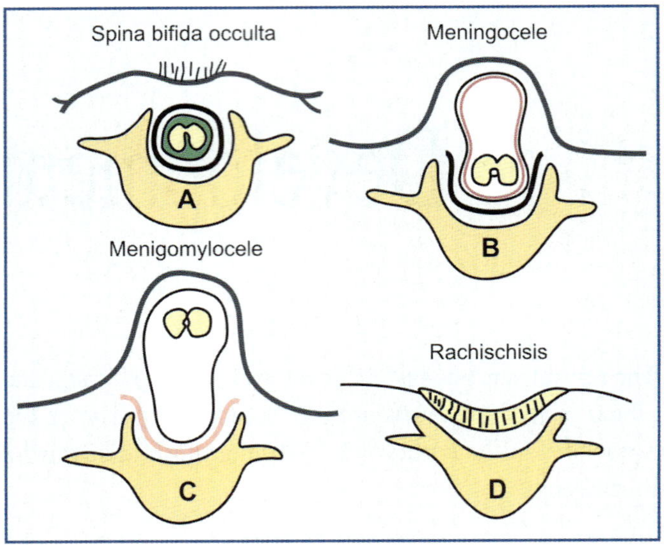

Fig. 88.3: Scheme to show types of spina bifida defects. In A the meninges are intact so the defect is without symptoms. In B pia-arachnoid protrude forming a sac filled with CSF. In C pia-arachnoid and spinal cord protrude forming a sac. In D the neural tissue is exposed to the surface of the back

to the general somatic afferent (GSA) and general visceral afferent (GVA) column. The basal lamina gives origin to motor neurons, which functionally belong to the general somatic efferent (GSE) and general visceral efferent (GVE) column. The marginal layer enlarges to form the three funiculi of the spinal cord. As the posterior funiculi increase in thickness their medial surfaces come into contact, thus obliterating the dorsal part of the central canal of the neural tube. The ependymal lining of the obliterated central canal forms the posterior median septum, which is composed of neuroglial tissue only.

Positional Changes in Spinal Cord

Till the third month of intrauterine life the spinal cord extends the entire length of the vertebral column. After this stage the vertebral column grows faster than the spinal cord, as a result of which at birth the lower end of the spinal cord is at level of the lower border of the third lumbar vertebra. In the adult the spinal cord ends at the lower border of first lumbar vertebra. Below this point the vertebral canal contains cauda equina, which is composed of filum terminale and the roots of the lumbar, sacral and coccygeal nerves.

Congenital Anomalies (Fig. 88.3)

The neural tube defects (NTD) called the spina bifida usually occur in the sacrolumbar region. There are various degrees of this defect. Spina bifida occulta is a defect in the vertebral arch without a defect in the spinal cord. Spina bifida with meningocele occurs when the meninges protrude through the vertebral defect forming a sac filled with CSF. Spina bifida with meningomyelocele occurs when the meninges and spinal cord project through the defect, forming a sac. Spina bifida with myeloschisis or rachischisis is the most severe anomaly, in which the neural tube is exposed on the surface of the back. This is due to failure of the closure of the posterior neuropore. The cause of the defect is deficiency of folic acid in the mother. Periconceptional (around the time of the fertilization) folic acid therapy to mothers is widely practised to prevent the occurrence of neural tube defects.

Development of Brain

The cranial part of the neural tube dilates to form three primary brain vesicles, the prosencephalon or forebrain, mesencephalon or midbrain, and rhombencephalon or hindbrain (Fig. 88.4). There are two bends or flexures in the neural tube at this stage, which are concave ventrally. The cervical flexure is present at the junction of spinal cord and rhombencephalon. The cephalic flexure is located in the region of mesencephalon. When the embryo is five weeks old, five secondary brain vesicles appear. The prosencephalon divides in to the telencephalon and diencephalon (which gives rise to optic vesicles). The rhombencephalon divides by an acute pontine flexure

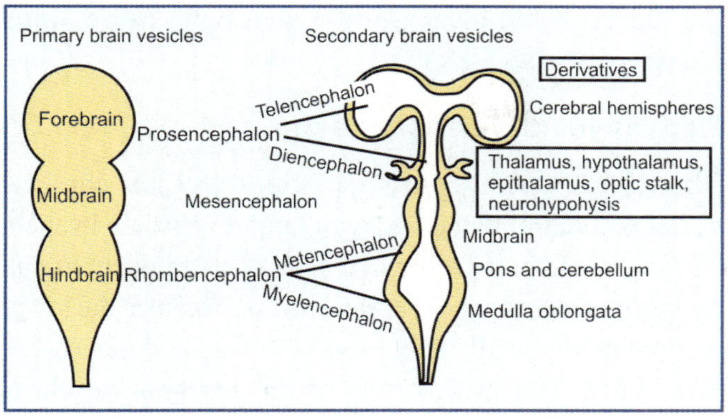

Fig. 88.4: Subdivisions of cranial part of neural tube and their derivatives

(concave dorsally), in to the cranial metencephalon and the caudal myelencephalon. The cavity of the rhombencephalon or hindbrain becomes the fourth ventricle. The cavity of the mesencephalon becomes the cerebral aqueduct. The cavity of diencephalon becomes the third ventricle. The cavity of each telencephalic vesicle becomes the lateral ventricle.

Effect of Pontine Flexure

The roof plate of the hindbrain (rhombencephalon) is stretched in lateral directions due to the acute pontine flexure in such a way that the position of alar and basal laminae in the wall is altered. The alar laminae come to lie dorsolateral to the basal laminae. Therefore both the laminae lie in the floor or anterior wall of the fourth ventricle.

Functional Classification of Neurons in the Brainstem (Fig. 88.5)

a. The basal or motor lamina gives rise to three types of motor neurons. The general somatic efferent (GSE) neurons lie closer to the midline and supply the skeletal muscles developed from somites. The nuclei belonging to this group are hypoglossal, abducent, trochlear and oculomotor nuclei. The special visceral efferent (SVE) or branchial efferent (BE) neurons, which are lateral to GSE column, supply the skeletal muscles developed from the mesoderm of the branchial arches. The nuclei belonging to this group are nucleus ambiguus, motor nucleus of facial nerve and motor nucleus of trigeminal nerve. The general visceral efferent (GVE) neurons

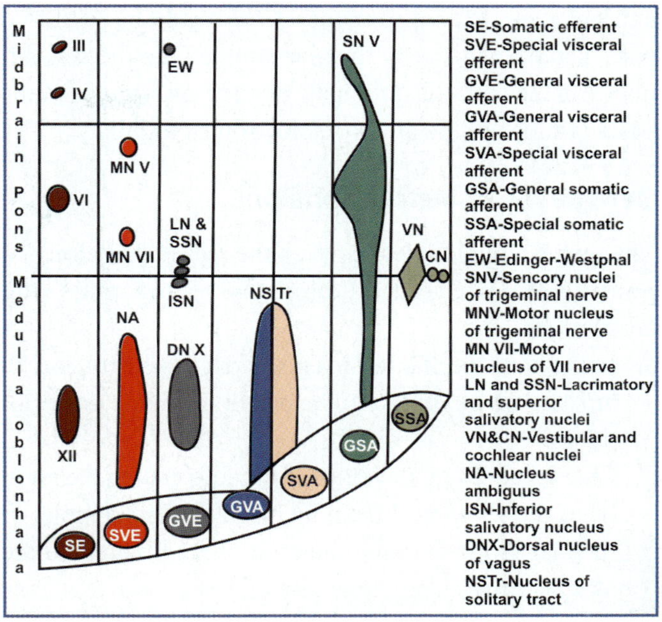

Fig. 88.5: Functional classification of cranial nerve nuclei in brainstem

consist of parasympathetic cranial outflow for the glands and smooth muscles. The nuclei belonging to this group are, dorsal nucleus of vagus, inferior salivatory nucleus, superior salivatory nucleus and Edinger-Westphal nucleus.

b. The alar or sensory lamina gives origin to four types of sensory neurons. The general visceral afferent (GVA) neurons receive sensations from the viscera. The nucleus of tractus solitarius and dorsal nucleus of vagus represent this group. Special visceral afferent (SVA) neurons receive sensation of taste. The nucleus of tractus solitarius receives taste fibers from the facial, glossopharyngeal and vagus nerves. General somatic afferent (GSA) neurons receive sensations from skin of head and face via the trigeminal nerve. The nuclei belonging to this group are nucleus of spinal tract, principal sensory nucleus and mesencephalic nucleus of trigeminal nerve. Special somatic afferent (SSA) neurons receive sensations of hearing and balance and are present in the cochlear and vestibular nuclei.

Derivatives of Myelencephalon

The myelencephalon lies between the pontine and cervical flexures. It becomes the medulla oblongata and contains the caudal or medullary half of the floor of fourth ventricle and the central canal of medulla oblongata in its closed part. The derivatives of the alar laminae are the sensory nuclei in the medulla oblongata and the derivatives of the basal lamina are the motor nuclei of the medulla.

Derivatives of Metencephalon

The metencephalon lies between the mesencephalon and pontine flexure and develops in to the pons and cerebellum.

a. In the pons the alar lamina gives rise to sensory nuclei and the basal lamina gives origin to motor nuclei of pons.
b. The cerebellum develops from the metencephalon from the rhombic lips, which are the thickenings of the alar laminae at the junction of roof plate and the alar laminae. The right and left rhombic lips fuse across the roof to form a dumb-bell shaped cerebellar rudiment. The midline part of the cerebellar rudiment forms the vermis and the lateral portions form the cerebellar hemispheres. The fissura posterolateralis is the first fissure to develop as it separates the flocculonodular lobe (archicerebellum) from the rest of the cerebellum. The second fissure to develop is the fissura prima and it separates the anterior lobe (spinocerebellum) from the middle lobe (neo-cerebellum). Subsequently a number of fissures develop.

Derivatives of Mesencephalon

The narrow central cavity of the mesencephalon becomes the cerebral aqueduct. The derivatives of the alar lamina are the colliculi and substantia nigra. The basal lamina gives origin to motor nuclei. The mesencephalic nucleus of trigeminal nerve is unique in being the only nucleus in the brainstem, which is composed of pseudounipolar neurons, derived from the neural crest. These neurons are functionally equivalent to the dorsal root ganglia.

Derivatives of Diencephalon

In the region of the diencephalon the neural tube does not possess basal lamina. So the derivatives of the diencephalon (epithlamus, thalamus, hypothalamus, metathalamus and subthalamus) originate from the alar lamina. The optic vesicles (optic cup and optic stalk) from the diencephalon give rise to retina, optic nerve, optic chiasma and optic tract.

Derivatives of Telencephalon

The telencephalon consists of right and left cerebral vesicles containing the cavity of lateral ventricle in each. The wall of the cerebral vesicle is composed of the ependymal, mantle and marginal layers, except at the lower edge of medial wall, where it is composed of ependymal layer only. The wall of rest of the cerebral vesicle is considerably thickened to form pallium. The cerebral vesicle expands in all directions to form the temporal, occipital, parietal and frontal lobes. The choroid fissure develops along the medial ependymal wall of the hemisphere. In this location the vascularized piamater comes in direct contact with the ependyma so as to facilitate the entry of choroid plexus in to the interior of the ventricle.

Corpus Striatum

The corpus striatum appears in the floor of the cerebral vesicle from the mantle layer. The projection fibers of neocortex pass through the corpus striatum and divide it in to the caudate and lentiform nuclei.

Cerebral Cortex

The thickened wall of the cerebral vesicle is called pallium, which differentiates in the cerebral cortex. The definitive cortex is first formed in hippocampus during the seventh week. Hence the hippocampus is called the archipallium. The piriform cortex with predominantly olfactory connections develops next and is called paleopallium. The archipallium and paleopallium are three layered unlike the neopallium or neocortex, which is six layered and last to develop. In the fully-developed brain the archipallium is represented by hippocampus and dentate gyrus and the paleopallium is represented by piriform lobe, which includes uncus, anterior part of parahippocampal gyrus and anterior perforated substance. The neopallium is represented by the entire cerebral cortex except the piriform lobe. The first sulcus to appear in the fourth month is the lateral sulcus. The cortex surrounding the lateral sulcus grows faster so that the cortex of the lateral sulcus gets submerged to form the insula. By sixth month the parieto-occipital, central, cingulate and calcarine sulci appear and the rest of the sulci appear by seventh month.

Commissures of Brain

The fibers connecting the neurons of the two cerebral vesicles pass through the lamina terminalis, which forms the commissural plate. The anterior commissure develops first followed by the hippocampal commissure. The corpus callosum is the third commissure to appear during the tenth week. As the fibers increase in number the corpus callosum at first grows forwards and then arches backwards above the fornix. The part of the lamina terminalis that is pulled backwards between the corpus callosum and fornix develops in to the septum pellucidum.

Congenital Anomalies

a. Anencephaly is one of the common types of open neural tube defect (NTD), where the cranial vault is fully or partially absent (Fig. 88.6). It results from failure of anterior neuropore to close. Anencephalic fetuses usually are born dead or die within a few days or hours after birth. There is no normal development of brain. The exposed brain is represented by a discoid mass of highly vascularised tissue consisting of rudimentary cerebral hemispheres. Due to brain malfunction the fetus lacks the mechanism of swallowing. This results in hydramnios. Assessing the level of AFP (alpha fetoprotein) in amniotic fluid helps in prenatal diagnosis of NTD (AFP level is high in NTD). Periconceptional folic acid therapy to the mother (giving folic acid tablets to the mother around the time of conception) is an effective method of prevention of NTD.

b. Arnold-Chiari syndrome occurs due to cerebello-medullary malformation in which cerebellar tonsils and medulla oblongata herniate through either a congenitally large foramen magnum or due to spina bifida resulting in a wide spectrum of deficits. Blockage of foramina in the roof of fourth ventricle results in internal hydrocephalus. Other signs and symptoms are due to pressure on cerebellum and medulla and traction on the last four cranial nerves.

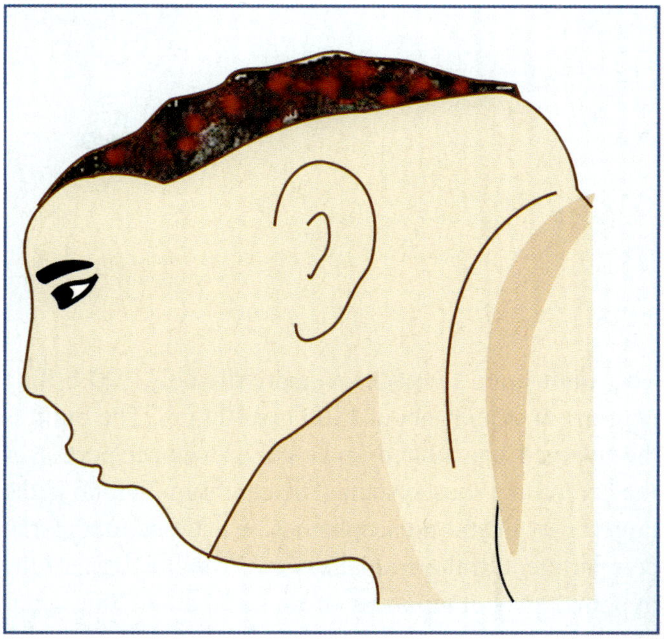

Fig. 88.6: Side view of the head of a newborn with anencephaly. The absence of bones of the vault of the skull is responsible for exposure of discoid vascularized mass of degenerated brain tissue

c. Dandy-Walker syndrome is the congenital dilatation of the fourth ventricle due to atresia of foramina of Luschka and Magendie. It is associated with cranial meningocele, agenesis of cerebellar vermis and agenesis of the splenium of corpus callosum.

d. Lissencephaly or agyria is the absence of sulci and gyri in the cerebral cortex.

89 Brain

The adult brain is made of approximately 100 billion neurons. It weighs about 1300 to 1400 gm. The brain is the enlarged, convoluted, and highly developed portion of the central nervous system. The cerebrum, which is the largest part and the diencephalons lie in the supratentorial compartment of the cranial cavity. From the base of the hypothalamus component of diencephalons, the hypophysis cerebri is suspended by the infundibulum. The hindbrain is located in the posterior cranial fossa below the tentorium cerebelli and consists of the pons, medulla oblongata and the cerebellum. Between the pons and the diencephalon and the cerebrum lies the midbrain. The brainstem consists of midbrain, pons and medulla oblongata. In the living state, the brain is very soft and gelatinous. It is protected by the rigid cranial cavity inner to which, it is covered by a succession of three meninges. The CSF filled subarachnoid space, which acts as a shock absorber, gives added protection, when the head receives jolts. The fluid also buoys the brain so that it floats in the cranial cavity.

Main Parts of Brain

Embryonic subdivision of brain	*Derivatives*	*Cavity*
1. Telencephalon	Right and left cerebral hemispheres	Right and left lateral ventricles
2. Diencephalon	Thalamus, hypothalamus metathalamus and epithalamus, subthalamus	Third ventricle
3. Mesencephalon	Midbrain	Cerebral aqueduct
4. Rhomb-encephalon	Hindbrain (cerebellum, pons and medulla oblongata)	Fourth ventricle

Gray and White Matter

In the cerebrum and cerebellum the gray matter is on the surface and is called cortex while the white matter forms the core. The brainstem shows arrangement like that of the spinal cord in having the white matter outside and the gray matter inside.

Base of Brain

The base of the brain is its inferior aspect, which lies between the two cerebral hemispheres. A pair of olfactory bulbs and tracts is present most anteriorly. Behind this, a prominent landmark is the optic chiasma, where the optic nerves partially decussate and the optic tracts begin. The lamina terminalis is a thin structure, which stretches between the dorsum of optic chiasma and the rostrum of corpus callosum. The vallecula of the cerebrum lies lateral to the optic chiasma. The relations of the vallecula are as follows. Anterior perforated substance forms the roof of the vallecula and is pierced by the anterolateral group of central branches of the circle of Willis. Laterally, the vallecula is continuous with the limen insulae of the insula. Above, it is continuous directly with the head of caudate nucleus providing the only link between the surface gray matter and the intracerebral gray matter. The stem of the lateral sulcus begins in the vallecula lateral to the anterior perforated substance. The internal carotid artery terminates into the anterior and middle cerebral arteries at the vallecula. The middle cerebral artery enters the stem of the lateral sulcus and the anterior cerebral artery turns medially to enter the longitudinal fissure. The basilar vein is formed at this site by the union of deep middle cerebral vein, anterior cerebral vein and striate veins (coming out of the anterior perforated substance).

Interpeduncular Fossa

This is a depressed area at the base of the brain. The interpeduncular cistern of subarachnoid space lies in the fossa. The circle of Willis lies in this cistern.

Boundaries (Fig. 89.1)

The optic chiasma forms the anterior boundary and the optic tract forms the anterolateral boundary on each side. The crus cerebri of the midbrain bound the fossa posterolaterally on each side. The small midline part of the upper border of pons forms the posterior boundary.

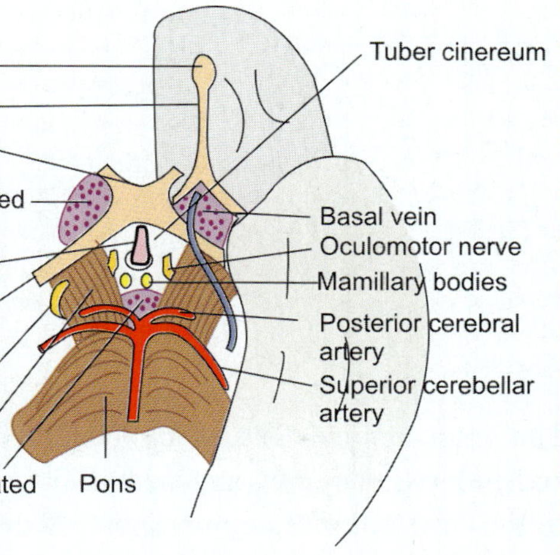

Fig. 89.1: Base of brain and interpeduncular fossa

Structures in the Fossa

a. The oculomotor nerves emerge from the medial side of the crura and pierce the dura mater here.
b. The posterior perforated substance lies in the midline between the right and left crura cerebri and the upper margin of pons. Posteromedian group of central arteries from the circle of Willis pierces it.
c. The mamillary bodies are two rounded swellings, which are part of hypothalamus and lie anterior to the posterior perforated substance.
d. The tuber cinereum is the raised area of gray matter bounded anteriorly by optic chiasma, laterally by optic tracts and posteriorly by mamillary bodies. It forms the floor of third ventricle. The infundibulum and median eminence are its named parts. The infundibulum extends downwards from the tuber cinereum to the neurohypophysis. The median eminence is between the infundibulum and the mamillary bodies. It contains capillary plexus of hypophyseal portal vessels and it contains specialized cells called tanicytes, which presumably monitor the hormone concentration of blood.

It should be noted that in the interpeduncular fossa, a portion of hypothalamus is visible as a surface cortex (the only area where the hypothalamus is visible on the surface). The parts of hypothalamus seen here are mamillary bodies and tuber cinereum.

90 Brainstem

The brainstem consists of the medulla oblongata, pons and midbrain. The pons and medulla oblongata are located in the infratentorial compartment of the cranial cavity and the midbrain passes through the tentorial notch. The brainstem gives passage to the various ascending and descending tracts besides housing nuclei of third to twelfth cranial nerves. Figure 90.1 shows the sites of emergence of these cranial nerves from the surface of the brainstem. The three components of the brainstem are connected to the cerebellum by means of three separate peduncles. The functional and clinical significance of the brainstem is that it houses the vital centres for the control of respiration, cardiovascular activity and alertness.

Medulla Oblongata

The cone-shaped medulla oblongata extends from the lower margin of pons to the upper end of spinal cord at the level of superior border of posterior arch of atlas. The inferior cerebellar peduncle connects the medulla to the cerebellum. The term "bulb" was earlier used for medulla oblongata. Hence one comes across terms like corticobulbar fibers and clinical conditions referred to as bulbar palsy and bulbar poliomyelitis.

Location

The medulla oblongata is located in the posterior cranial fossa. Its anterior surface is in contact with the clivus (basisphenoid). The upper part of its posterior surface forms the floor of fourth ventricle while the lower part of the posterior surface in contact with the cerebellum. In a patient with tumor in posterior cranial fossa there will be rise in intracranial tension, which will favor the herniation of medulla oblongata and cerebellar tonsils into the foramen magnum and below. This will cause traction on the last four cranial nerves initially. Further herniation into the vertebral canal may endanger the life due to sudden compression of cardiovascular and respiratory vital centres in the medulla oblongata.

Subdivisions

The medulla oblongata is divisible in upper open part and the lower closed part. The posterior wall of the open part of medulla oblongata is covered with the gray matter of the floor of fourth ventricle. The closed part of medulla encloses the central canal, which is continuous above with the fourth ventricle and below with the central canal of the spinal cord.

Surface Features

The anterior surface (Fig. 90.1) presents a prominent median sulcus and an anterolateral sulcus on each side. The pyramid lies between these two sulci. Lateral to the anterolateral sulcus lies the prominence of the olive. The posterior aspect has a posterior median sulcus and posterolateral sulcus on each side. The posterolateral sulcus separates the olive and the inferior cerebellar peduncle. The rootlets of the hypoglossal nerve are attached to the anterolateral sulcus between the olive and the pyramid. The rootlets of the ninth, tenth and cranial part of eleventh cranial nerves are attached to the posterolateral sulcus. The abducent nerve is attached at the upper end of pyramid. The seventh and eighth cranial nerves with a small nervus intermedius are attached at the upper end of the olive at the pontomedullary junction.

a. The pyramids are formed by bundles of corticospinal fibers, which connect the upper motor neurons of motor cortex to the lower motor neurons in the anterior horn cells of spinal cord. At the lower part of medulla oblongata, about 75 to 90% corticospinal fibers cross in the pyramidal decussation. The crossed and

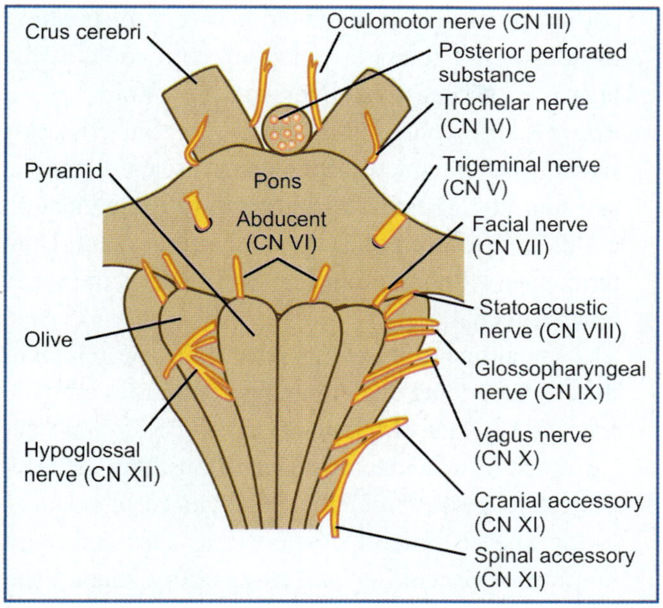

Fig. 90.1: Sites of attachment of cranial nerves to ventral surface of brainstem (Note that trochiear nerve alone is attached the dorsal surface of midbrain. The spinal part of accessory nerve ascends to join its cranial part)

uncrossed fibers form the lateral and anterior corticospinal tracts respectively. The arcuate nucleus lies on the surface of the pyramid. It gives rise to anterior external arcuate fibers, which pass in front of the olive laterally to enter the inferior cerebellar peduncle. The arcuate nucleus is a collection of displaced pontine nuclei. Hence the anterior external arcuate fibers are displaced pontocerebellar fibers.

b. The olive overlies a large inferior olivary nucleus, which lies deep in the medulla. The olive is flanked by the rootlets of hypoglossal nerve on the medial and rootlets of the ninth, tenth and eleventh cranial nerves on the lateral side.

c. The inferior cerebellar peduncle (also referred to as restiform body) is the connecting link between medulla oblongata and cerebellum. Its fiber contents are described with cerebellum.

d. The gracile and cuneate fasciculi are present on the posterior surface of the closed part of the medulla. The fasciculus gracilis (tract of Gall) is the medial tract and ends superiorly in the gracile tubercle, which overlies the gracile nucleus. The fasciculus cuneatus (tract of Burdach) is lateral in position and ends in cuneate tubercle, which overlies the cuneate nucleus. The fasciculus gracilis carries the sensation of discriminatory touch, vibration and pressure from the lower half of body and the fasciculus cuneatus caries conscious proprioception in addition to above sensations from the upper half of the body. The accessory cuneate nucleus (which lies on the lateral aspect of cuneate tubercle) receives fibers carrying unconscious proprioception from the upper limb through the fasciculus cuneatus. The efferent fibers from this nucleus are called the posterior external arcuate fibers or cuneocerebellar tract. Thus, the accessory arcuate nucleus is the equivalent of Clarke's column of the posterior horn of spinal cord and the posterior external arcuate fibers are the equivalent of dorsal spinocerebellar tract.

d. The tuberculum cinereum (when present) is a raised area antero-lateral to the fasciculus cuneatus. It is produced by the spinal tract of the trigeminal nerve. The importance of this surface feature is that it could easily be approached surgically.

Internal Structure

The internal structure of the medulla oblongata is not uniform through out. The arrangement and number of nuclei and fiber tracts vary at various levels. These structural differences in the medulla are due to presence of pyramidal and sensory decussations in the closed part and the presence of seven groups of functionally different nuclei of cranial nerves in addition to a large inferior olivary nucleus in its open part. Therefore, it is customary to study the internal structure from below upwards as follows, at pyramidal decussation, at sensory decussation and at mid-olivary level (open part).

Transverse Section at the Level of Pyramidal Decussation (Fig. 90.2)

The medulla oblongata more or less resembles the spinal cord in cross-section at this level. The gray matter surrounds the central canal. However, a small part of the anterior gray matter is cut off from the central gray matter by the decussating pyramidal fibers. The white matter is relatively more and consists of the reticular formation and the ascending and descending tracts seen in the spinal cord.

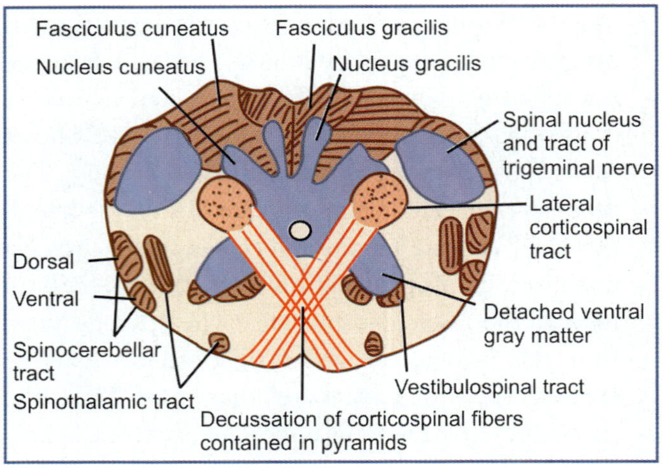

Fig. 90.2: Transverse section of medulla oblongata at the level of pyramidal decussation (Note: The position of the central canal in the central gray matter. The medial longitudinal fasciculus and tectospinal tract are medial to the detached gray matter)

Gray Matter

a. Nuclei gracilis and cuneatus appear as the posterior projections of the central gray matter
b. Lateral ends of the gray matter contain the nucleus of the spinal tract of trigeminal nerve. This nucleus extends in the upper two cervical segments of the spinal cord, where it is continuous with the substantia gelatinosa located at the posterior gray horn of spinal cord.
c. The detached anterior gray matter is the junctional gray matter. It is divisible in supraspinal nucleus and the accessory nucleus. The supraspinal nucleus is continuous above with hypoglossal nucleus and below with the anterior horn cells of the first spinal segment. The accessory nucleus is continuous above with the nucleus ambiguus and below with the spinal nucleus of the accessory nerve (spinal accessory nerve takes origin from anterior horn cells of first five segments of spinal cord).

White Matter

a. The most prominent feature is the decussation of the pyramidal or corticospinal fibers in front of the central gray matter. Majority of fibers (between 75 to 90%) cross to the opposite side to form lateral corticospinal tracts. The uncrossed fibers are named anterior corticospinal tracts. The anterior part corresponding to the anterior funiculus of spinal cord contains the uncrossed corticospinal fibers in the pyramid.
b. The posterior part corresponding to the posterior funiculus of the spinal cord contains fasciculus gracilis and cuneatus. These tracts are the upward continuation of the posterior column tracts of spinal cord. They terminate in the gracile and cuneate nuclei at the upper level of medulla.
c. The spinal tract of trigeminal nerve lies peripheral to the corresponding nucleus and is continuous with the tract of Lissauer of the spinal cord. The spinal tract carries pain and temperature sensations from the face.
d. The lateral parts of medulla oblongata corresponding to the lateral funiculi of the spinal cord contain a number of ascending and descending tracts. The descending tracts include the lateral corticospinal tract, rubrospinal tract, tectospinal tract, olivospinal tract, vestibulospinal tract and the reticulospinal tract on each side. The medial longitudinal fasciliculus (MLF) is continuous with the anterior intersegmental tract of the spinal cord. The ascending tracts include, the lateral and anterior spinothalamic tracts, posterior and anterior spinocerebellar tracts, spinotectal tract, spino-olivary tract and spinoreticular tract.

Transverse Section at the Level of Sensory Decussation (Fig. 90.3)

The level of sensory decussation is higher than that of pyramidal decussation. The most prominent feature of the medulla at this level is the decussation of the internal arcuate fibers (which are the axons of the cells of the gracile and cuneate nuclei) anterior to the central gray matter. The reticular formation occupies the space between the fiber tracts and nuclear groups.

Gray Matter

a. The medially placed nucleus gracilis is large and occupies posterior position in relation to the central gray matter. Nucleus Z at the upper pole of nucleus gracilis receives input from dorsal spinocerebellar tract carrying sensations of conscious proprioception from lower limb. The nucleus cuneatus lies lateral to the gracile nucleus. The accessory cuneate nucleus

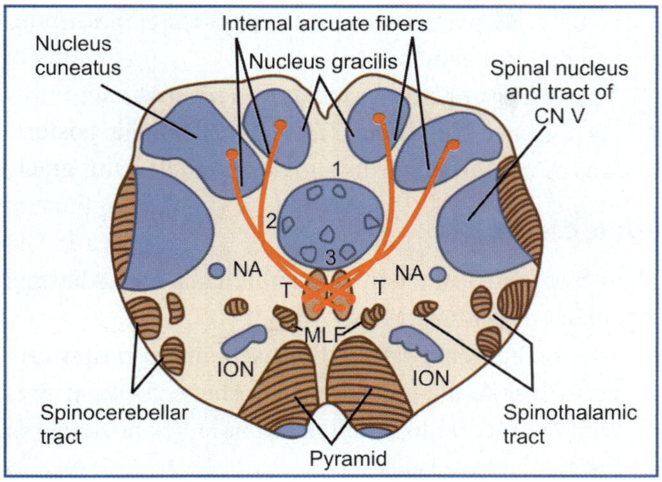

Fig. 90.3: Transverse section of medulla oblongata at the level of sensary decussation (Note: The crossing of internal arcuate fibers to form medial lemniscus. Nuclei in the central gray matter are: 1–Nucleus of tractus solitarius, 2–Dorsal nucleus of vagus, 3–Hypoglossal nucleus, NA–Nucleus ambiguus, T–Tecto-spinal, tract, ION—Inferior olivary nucleus)

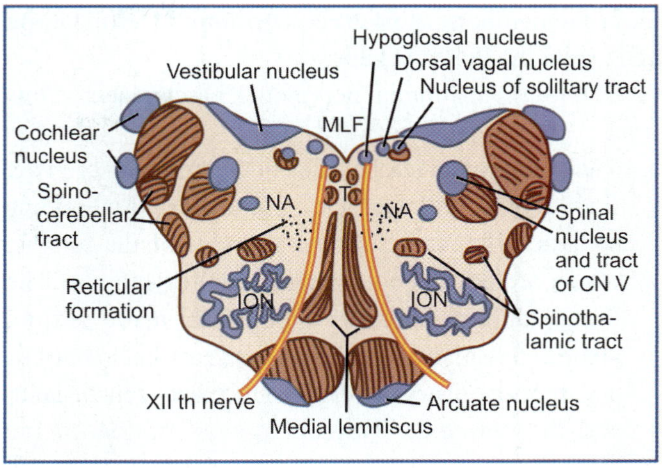

Fig. 90.4: Transverse section of medulla oblongata at the level of Inferior olivary nucleus (MLF–Medial longitudinal fasciculus, T–Tectospinal tract, NA–Nucleus ambiguus, ION–Inferior olivary nucleus)

projects from the lateral aspect of cuneate nucleus on each side.

b. The nucleus of the spinal tract of trigeminal nerve is located anterolateral to the cuneate nucleus.
c. The central gray matter contains the hypoglossal nuclei, dorsal nuclei of vagus and nuclei of solitary tract of both sides.
d. Nucleus ambiguus is present between the central gray and the spinal nucleus of trigeminal nerve.
e. The inferior olivary nucleus makes its appearance at this level posterolateral to the pyramid.
f. The arcuate nuclei, which are the displaced pontine nuclei, lie in front of the pyramids.

White Matter

a. The internal arcuate fibers originating in the gracile and cuneate nuclei cross in the sensory decussation in front of the central gray. The decussating internal arcuate fibers form the medial lemniscus on the opposite side. The medial lemniscus is located anterior to the central gray closer to the midline. It carries sensation of conscious proprioception, two-point discrimination, vibration and pressure to nucleus VPL of thalamus.
b. The pyramids occupy the anterior region close to the midline. They are very prominent at this level and contain ipsilateral corticospinal and corticonuclear fibers.
c. The spinal tract of the trigeminal nerve produces a surface elevation called the tuberculum cinereum.
d. All the descending tracts are present except the corticospinal tracts.
e. All other ascending tracts from spinal cord are present at this level.

Transverse Section at Mid-olive Level (Fig. 90.4)

Since this is the open part of the medulla oblongata its posterior surface is lined with the gray matter of the fourth ventricle.

Gray Matter

The inferior olivary nucleus is a large crumpled mass of gray matter on each side. The olivary nuclei receive fibers from the red nucleus and peri-aqueductal gray in the midbrain through the central tegmental tract. The other afferents to the nucleus come from cerebral cortex, cerebellum and spinal cord (spino-olivary tract). The olivo-cerebellar fibers originate in the inferior olivary nucleus and leave through the medially directed hilum. They cross to enter the opposite inferior cerebellar peduncle to reach the cerebellum. These fibers become

Section three

the climbing fibers inside the cerebellum and terminate on and excite the Purkinje cells.

The following cranial nerve nuclei are present at this level:

a. The hypoglossal nucleus lies in the gray matter in the floor of the fourth ventricle close to the midline. Being somatic efferent it supplies muscles of the tongue, which are developed from occipital myotomes. The intramedullary fibers of hypoglossal nerve pass in anterior direction at first between the medial lemniscus and inferior olivary nucleus and then between the latter and the pyramid. They emerge as rootlets of the hypoglossal nerve through the anterolateral sulcus on the surface of medulla.
b. The nucleus ambiguus lies in the reticular formation posterior to the inferior olivary nucleus. This nucleus sends branchial efferent fibers to the ninth, tenth and cranial part of the eleventh cranial nerves for the supply of striated muscles that develop from mesoderm of 3rd, 4th and 6th branchial arches. From its embryonic position lateral to hypoglossal nucleus at the floor of fourth ventricle the nucleus ambiguus moves towards spinal nucleus of trigeminal nerve due to forces of neurobiotaxis.
c. The dorsal motor nucleus of vagus lies lateral to the hypoglossal nucleus in the gray matter of the floor of the fourth ventricle. It is the largest of the general visceral efferent nuclei of the brainstem. Its axons form the preganglionic component of the parasympathetic innervation to the glands and smooth muscles and glands in the thoracic and abdominal viscera (derivatives of foregut and midgut only).
d. The nucleus of the tractus solitarius or solitary nucleus receives general visceral afferent fibers from the vagus and glossopharyngeal nerves. Its upper pole (called the gustatory nucleus belonging to special visceral afferent functional group) receives taste fibers via the seventh, ninth and tenth cranial nerves.
e. The spinal nucleus of the trigeminal nerve belonging to general somatic afferent functional group receives general sensations of pain and temperature from the face. It lies a little deeper in the medulla, medial to the inferior cerebellar peduncle.
f. The lower ends of the vestibular and cochlear nuclei, belonging to special somatic afferent functional column, are placed in the lateral part nearer the inferior cerebellar peduncle.
g. The nuclei of cardiovascular and respiratory centres are present in the reticular formation adjoining the nucleus of tractus solitarius and dorsal nucleus of vagus.

White Matter

The white matter of the medulla oblongata at this level is organized in distinct tracts.

a. The medial lemniscus is disposed antero-posteriorly very close to the median plane. The tectospinal tract with the medial longitudinal bundle lies posterior to the medial lemniscus.
b. The corticospinal fibers occupy the pyramids anteriorly.
c. In the lateral region the major tracts are placed as follows. The spinothalamic tracts lie postero-lateral to the inferior olivary nucleus. The anterior spinocerebellar tract is closer to the surface between the inferior cerebellar peduncle and the inferior olivary nucleus. The spinal tract of trigeminal nerve along with its nucleus lies posterior to the olivary nucleus. The spinal tract contains fibers belonging to all the three subdivisions of the trigeminal nerve. These fibers are arranged as follows, mandibular fibers are most posterior, the maxillary fibers are in the middle and the ophthalmic fibers are most anterior. The mandibular fibers are present only in the open part of the medulla hence they end at the level of obex. The other ascending and descending tracts are similar to those present at the lower level.

Arterial Supply

a. Medullary branches of anterior spinal artery supply the medial region of the medulla oblongata, which includes the hypoglossal nucleus, medial lemniscus and the pyramid.
b. The branches of posterior inferior cerebellar artery (PICA) supply the posterolateral region of the medulla, which includes nucleus ambiguus, nucleus of tractus solitarius, vestibular nucleus, spinal nucleus and tract of fifth nerve, spinothalamic tracts, inferior cerebellar peduncle and descending sympathetic fibers.
c. The posterior region, which includes the gracile and cuneate tubercles, receives supply from the branches of the posterior spinal artery.

Clinical Highlights

a. The medial medullary syndrome is due to deficient arterial supply to the medial region of medulla oblongata as a result of the thrombosis of anterior spinal artery (branch of vertebral artery).

Neurological Effects

Structure involved	*Resultant signs and symptoms*
Pyramid	Contralateral hemiplegia- UMN
Intramedullary hypoglossal nerve	Ipsilateral paralysis of tongue-LMN
Medial lemniscus	Contralateral loss of conscious proprioception, discriminative touch and vibration from the body

b. The lateral medullary of Wallenberg or PICA syndrome is due to deficient arterial supply to the postero-lateral region of medulla oblongata due to occlusion of posterior inferior cerebellar artery (branch of vertebral artery).

Neurological Effects

Structure involved	*Resultant signs and symptoms*
Spinothalamic tract	Contralateral loss of pain and temperature sensation from the body
Spinal tract and nucleus	Ipsilateral loss of pain and temperature sensation on face
Nucleus ambiguus	Ipsilateral paralysis of laryngeal, pharyngeal and palatal muscles resulting in hoarseness of voice, dysphagia, dysarthria and deviation of uvula opposite to the side of lesion.
Vestibular nucleus	Vertigo, nausea, nystagmus
Inferior cerebellar peduncle	Ipsilateral ataxia
Descending sympathetic fibers in reticular formation	Ipsilateral Horner's syndrome

PONS

The pons forms a bridge between the hindbrain and midbrain. It appears as a protuberance above the medulla and anterior to the cerebellum. The anterior surface of the pons presents a transversely ridged appearance due to the underlying transversely disposed ponto-cerebellar fibers. Its posterior surface is lined with gray matter and forms the upper half of the floor of the fourth ventricle. The pons is connected to the cerebellum by middle cerebellar peduncle.

External Features

Anterior surface of pons lies in contact with the upper part of the clivus. It bears a midline sulcus, which contains the basilar artery. The superior cerebellar, anterior inferior cerebellar and labyrinthine arteries, (the branches of basilar artery) run on its anterior surface. The basilar artery divides into its terminal branches at the upper margin of pons. The right and left crus cerebri, which are the anterior parts of the midbrain, appear to emerge and diverge from the upper margin of pons. The following cranial nerves emerge from the surface of the pons. The trigeminal nerve is attached to the junction of basilar part of pons and the middle cerebellar peduncle by a large sensory root and small motor root. The abducent nerve emerges near the midline at the ponto-medullary junction and it ascends on the anterior surface pons before piercing the duramater. The facial and vestibulocochlear nerves emerge laterally in the cerebellopontine angle.

Cerebellopontine Angle (CP Angle)

The cerebello-pontine angle lies in a shallow triangular area, which is bounded by the lateral aspect of pons, superior part of cerebellum and the medial third of the superior margin of petrous temporal bone. There are two openings at this site, internal acoustic meatus and lateral aperture of the fourth ventricle (foramen of Luschka). The CP angle contains the facial nerve, vestibulocochlear nerve, labyrinthine artery and the protruding choroid plexus of the fourth ventricle. The tumor arising from the Schwann cells in the neurilemmal sheath of the eighth nerve (acoustic neurinoma) is the common cause of cerebellopontine angle lesion. It compresses the eighth nerve initially and the seventh nerve gradually. At a later stage the tumor may compress the pons and the cerebellum. The symptoms include persistent tinnitus, deafness and vertigo due to eighth nerve dysfunction; facial palsy, ataxia due to cerebellar involvement and the advanced cases may show symptoms of involvement of the fifth and ninth cranial nerves.

Internal Structure

The pons is subdivided in anterior or basilar part and posterior or tegmental part. The contents of the two parts are different. The basilar part shows uniform structure throughout the pons but the tegmental region differs at the upper and lower levels of pons.

Basilar Part of the Pons

The basilar part of the pons contains scattered pontine nuclei, which receive ipsilateral corticopontine fibers from all parts of the cerebrum. The pontine nuclei give rise to pontocerebellar fibers, which cross to the opposite side and reach the cerebellum through the middle cerebellar peduncle. In this way the cerebro-ponto-cerebellar path controls the contralateral cerebellum. The basilar part of the pons also contains corticospinal fibers and the cortico-nuclear (corticobulbar) fibers, which terminate on the cranial nerve nuclei. The longitudinal fibers in the pons are the corticospinal, cortico-nuclear and cortico-pontine. The transverse fibers in the pons are the ponto-cerebellar fibers.

Tegmentum at Lower Pons (Fig. 90.5)

The tegmentum at the lower level consists of gray matter and white matter.

Gray Matter

The following nuclei cranial nerve nuclei are present:

a. The vestibular nuclei are located partly in pons and partly in medulla. They are divided in four groups called superior, lateral (Deiter's), medial and inferior vestibular nuclei. The main afferent connection of the vestibular nuclei is the vestibular nerve. Their efferent connections are divisible in three sets.
   i. The vestibulo-cerebellar fibers reach the flocculonodular lobe of cerebellum through the inferior cerebellar peduncle.
   ii. The medial longitudinal fasciculus (MLF) connects the vestibular nuclei to the cranial nerve nuclei supplying the muscles of eyeball. The lower continuation of MLF, known as anterior intersegmental tract connects the motor neurons in the cervical spinal cord to the vestibular nuclei. These connections are responsible for the coordination between the eyes and neck and head in response to position of the body.

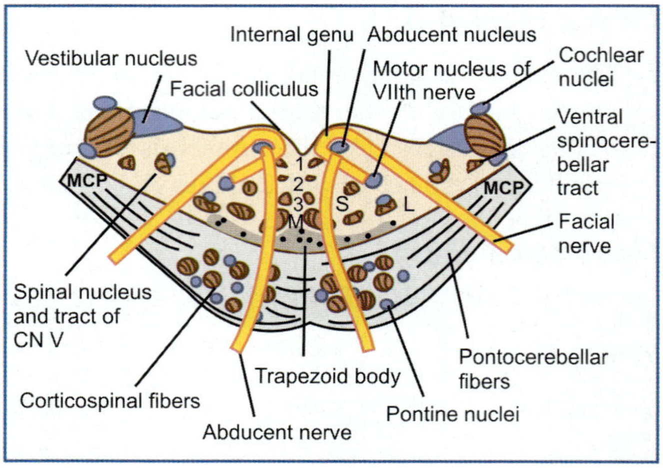

Fig. 90.5: Transverse section through the lower part of pons 1–Medial longitudinal fasciculus, 2–Tectospinal tracts, 3–Rubrospinal tracts, M–Medial lemniscus, S–Spinal lemniscus, L–Lateral lemniscus

   iii. The vestibulospinal tract arises from the lateral vestibular nucleus and terminates on the motor neurons in the spinal cord.

b. The cochlear nuclei are located partly in pons and partly in medulla. They consist of dorsal and ventral cochlear nuclei. The fibers of the cochlear nerve terminate in these nuclei. The majority of the axons of the cochlear nuclei cross to the opposite side. The crossing fibers form a large mass of fibers called trapezoid body. The majority of crossed fibers end in contralateral superior olivary nucleus. Others end either in trapezoid nuclei or in nucleus of lateral lemniscus. The lateral lemniscus is an ascending tract consisting of axons arising in the superior olivary nucleus and the nuclei of trapezoid body and lateral lemniscus. It carries fibers from both sides. The uncrossed fibers end in the ipsilateral superior olivary nucleus or the nucleus of the lateral lemniscus.

c. The abducent nucleus is located in the gray matter of the floor of fourth ventricle near the midline underneath the facial colliculus. The axons of the abducent nuclei pass in anterior direction through the reticular formation, trapezoid body and medial lemniscus to emerge on the anterior aspect of the lower margin of pons. The para-abducent neurons (internuclear neurons or interneurons) are part of the abducent nucleus. Their axons cross the midline and ascend in the medial longitudinal fasciculus to the part of the oculomotor nucleus supplying the medial rectus muscle. This connection coordinates the simultaneous contraction of the lateral rectus of one eye and the medial rectus of the opposite eye. This is called horizontal conjugate or lateral gaze movement (Fig. 90.10A). The cells of PPRF (paramedian pontine reticular formation lying close to the abducent nucleus) control the horizontal gaze.

d. The motor nucleus of the facial nerve lies in the deeper part in the reticular formation. The axons begin in the facial nucleus and incline posteromedially towards the abducent nucleus to ascend in medial relation to it. Then, they curve antero-laterally round the upper pole of the abducent nucleus forming the internal genu of the facial nerve. Finally they descend anterolaterally through the reticular formation passing between seventh nerve nucleus and the spinal nucleus of the trigeminal nerve on way out of the pons. This unusual course of the facial nerve fibers in the pons is an example of neurobiotaxis, which is a term used for the tendency of neurons to migrate towards major sources of stimuli in embryonic life.

e. The superior salivatory nucleus lies just above the ponto-medullary junction. It sends preganglionic parasympathetic fibers to the nervus intermedius of facial nerve for secretomotor supply of lacrimal gland, submandibular and sublingual salivary glands.

f. The spinal nucleus of trigeminal nerve continues upwards to terminate in the principal sensory nucleus. Its ventral trigeminothalamic tract crosses to the opposite side to form the trigeminal lemniscus.

g. Pneumotaxic center is located in the reticular formation of pons.

White Matter

a. Lemniscal system consists of the major ascending tracts, which are disposed as a transverse band in the pons on either side of the midline. From the midline to lateral, the lemnisci are arranged as follows, medial lemniscus, trigeminal lemniscus, spinal lemniscus and lateral lemniscus.

b. Trapezoid body is composed of crossing fibers of the cochlear nuclei.

c. Medial longitudinal fasciculus lies in paramedian position medial to the abducent nucleus.

d. Other ascending (except the olivospinal tract) and descending tracts except the corticospinal fibers, as seen in upper medulla, are present in the tegmentum of pons.

e. Olivocochlear fibers originate in the olivocochlear cells in the superior olivary complex. They leave the pons along with the vestibular nerve. The fibers are passed on to the cochlear nerve in the internal acoustic meatus through vestibulocochlear anastomosis of Oort.

Tegmentum at Upper Pons (Fig. 90.6)

The tegmentum at this level contains all the four nuclei of the trigeminal nerve. The other contents are similar to those of the lower level of pons. The motor nucleus of the

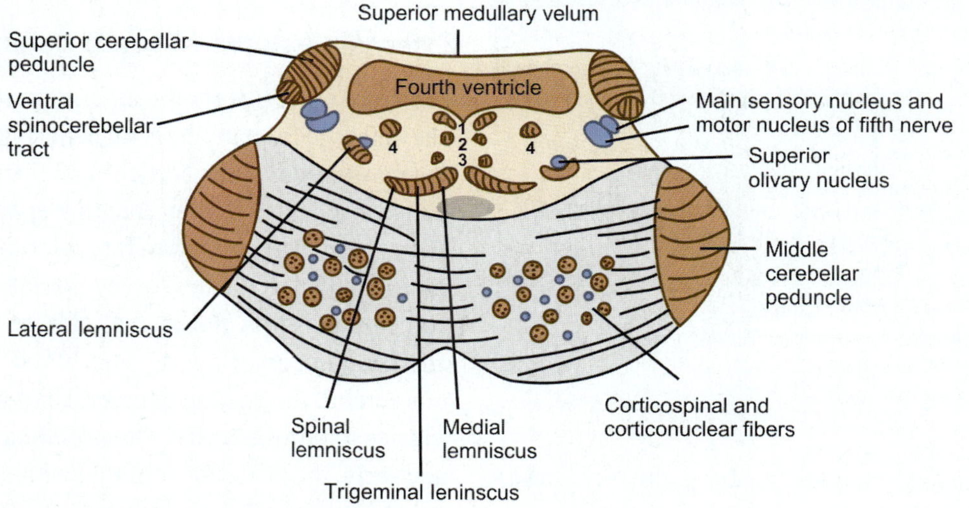

Fig. 90.6: Transverse section through upper part of pons: 1-Medial longitudinal fasciculus, 2-Tectospinal tract, 3-Rubrospinal tract, 4-Central tegmental tract

trigeminal nerve lies deep in the lateral part of the tegmentum. The principal sensory nucleus of trigeminal nerve is located lateral to the motor nucleus. It is continuous superiorly with the mesencephalic nucleus and inferiorly with the spinal nucleus. The terminal part of the spinal nucleus joins the principal nucleus at this level. The initial part of the mesencephalic nucleus is apparent at this level. All the four lemnisci and other tracts are present except the anterior spinocerebellar, which enters the superior cerebellar peduncle.

Arterial Supply

The pontine branches of the basilar artery and the pontine branches of anterior inferior cerebellar and superior cerebellar arteries, supply the pons. The paramedian penetrating arteries supply the anterior part and the peripheral circumferential arteries supply the posterolateral region of the pons.

Clinical Highlights

a. Anterior inferior cerebellar artery syndrome (AICA syndrome) is also known as lateral inferior pontine syndrome as it involves the structures of the lateral portion of the pons at the inferior level.

Neurological Effects

Structure involved	*Resultant signs and symptoms*
Facial nucleus	Ipsilateral facial paralysis-LMN
Solitary nucleus	Ipsilateral loss of taste sense from anterior 2/ 3rd of tongue
Cochlear nucleus	Clinically asymptomatic (ipsilateral weak hearing identified only by sophisticated audiometric tests
Vestibular nucleus	Vertigo, nausea, nystagmus
Spinal tract and nucleus of CN V	Ipsilateral loss of pain and temperature on face
Spinothalamic tract	Contralateral loss of pain and temperature from the body
Descending sympathetic fibers in reticular formation	Ipsilateral Horner's syndrome

b. In Millard Gubler syndrome (medial pontine syndrome) the lesion is in the basilar part of lower pons.

Neurological Effects

Structure involved	*Resultant signs and symptoms*
Corticospinal fibers	Contralateral hemiplegia-UMN
Intrapontine abducent nerve	Ipsilateral internal squint and diplopia on looking laterally
Intrapontine facial nerve	Ipsilateral facial paralysis-LMN

MIDBRAIN

The midbrain is the shortest and uppermost part of the brainstem. It connects the hindbrain in the infratentorial compartment with the cerebrum in the supratentorial compartment of the cranial cavity. It passes through the tentorial notch along with the oculomotor nerves and posterior cerebral arteries. The tubular cavity passing through the midbrain is called cerebral aqueduct. The midbrain consists of tectum and cerebral peduncles. The tectum is the part that lies posterior to the cerebral aqueduct. It consists of one pair of superior colliculi and one pair of inferior colliculi. The right and left cerebral peduncles lie in front of the cerebral aqueduct. Each cerebral peduncle is divided in to three parts, the crus cerebri anteriorly, followed by substantia nigra and tegmentum posteriorly. The crura and substantia nigra are separate but the tegmentum is single and is traversed by cerebral aqueduct. The crus cerebri is continuously superiorly with the internal capsule inside the cerebral hemisphere and the tegmentum is continuous with the subthalamus.

External Features of Crura Cerebri

The crura cerebri form the anterior part of the midbrain. They emerge from the cerebral hemispheres as thick rope-like masses containing corticofugal fibers. They converge to meet each other as they enter the upper margin of pons. They form the postero-lateral boundaries of the interpeduncular fossa. The oculomotor nerve emerges from the fossa on the medial side of the crus on each side. A number of nerves and blood vessels cross the crus cerebri, the posterior cerebral and superior cerebellar arteries mediolaterally, the trochlear nerve postero-anteriorly, the posterior communicating artery, basal vein and the optic tract antero-posteriorly (Fig. 89.1).

External Features of Tectum

The superior and inferior pairs of colliculi are separated from each other by a cruciform sulcus, which has a vertical limb and a transverse limb. The pulvinar of thalamus and the pineal gland are related superiorly to the tectum. The superior cerebellar peduncles enter the midbrain distal to the inferior colliculi. The frenulum veli is a median ridge starting from the lower end of the vertical limb of the cruciform sulcus. It continues on the posterior surface of superior medullary velum, which spans the two superior cerebellar peduncles. The trochlear nerves decussate in the superior medullary velum and then emerge on the side of the frenulum veli. The trochlear nerve is the only cranial nerve with posterior attachment to the brainstem and which crosses to the opposite side before emerging. The superior brachium, which is a raised band of fibers, connects the superior colliculus to the lateral geniculate body and the inferior brachium connects the side of the inferior colliculus to the medial geniculate body.

Internal Structure of Midbrain

The crus cerebri and substantia nigra have same structure at all levels but the tegmentum differs at the superior and inferior collicular levels.

a. The crus cerebri or basis pedunculi give passage to the fibers originating in cerebral cortex. These cortical fibers are arranged in specific order. The corticospinal and corticonuclear (corticobulbar) fibers run in the middle part of the crus. The medial part contains the frontopontine fibers and the lateral part contains the temporopontine, parietopontine and occipitopontine fibers.
b. The substantia nigra is a band of medium-sized pigmented neurons situated between the crus cerebri and tegmentum on both sides. Because of the presence of melanin pigment in the neurons the substantia nigra appears dark in macroscopic sections. The neurons are arranged in two zones. The pars compacta is adjacent to tegmentum and pars reticularis is adjacent to crus cerebri. The pars reticularis receives the striatonigral fibers mainly from the caudate nucleus and putamen. It also receives a few pallidonigral fibers arising from globus pallidus. The corticonigral fibers terminate on the pars reticularis but a large number of them pass through the substantia nigra to reach the red nucleus. The nigrostriatal fibers originate in pars compacta and terminate in caudate nucleus and putamen. These fibers are dopaminergic. So dopamine is present in both substantia nigra and corpus striatum. The nigrostriatal fibers exert an inhibitory influence on the neurons of the striatum so as to bring about smooth voluntary movements. It is one of the components of the extrapyramidal system. In Parkinson's disease there is degeneration of the pigmented neurons in the substantia nigra, causing deficiency of dopamine in the corpus striatum. This disease is the disorder of movements of the body. The patient experiences involuntary tremors while doing work. Levodopa, which is the precursor of dopamine, is helpful in some patients. Levodopa crosses the blood brain barrier and is concentrated in nigrostriatal system. In this way the reduced dopamine is replenished. Transplantation of embryonic suprarenal medulla and stem cells, into substantia nigra have been tried with varying results.

Tegmentum at the Level of Inferior Colliculi (Fig. 90.7)

Besides the gray matter and tracts the tegmentum contains reticular formation.

a. The gray matter of the midbrain surrounds the cerebral aqueduct. The nucleus of trochlear nerve is located in ventral part of periaqueductal gray close to the midline. Its axons wind round the peri-aqueductal gray in posterior direction and decussate in the upper end of superior medullary velum with similar fibers of opposite side before emerging out. The mesencephalic nucleus of trigeminal nerve lies in lateral position in the central gray matter throughout the midbrain. The unusual feature of this nucleus is that it is the only nucleus in entire CNS that contains pseudounipolar neurons similar to those of sensory ganglia. The peripheral processes of these neurons are believed to bring proprioceptive sensations from the muscles of mastication, eyeball, face and tongue. Their central processes descend to end in motor nucleus of trigeminal nerve on both sides. Thus, the mesencephalic nucleus plays a role in mediating jaw reflex.
b. The white matter of the midbrain at the level of inferior colliculus contains all the fiber tracts present at the

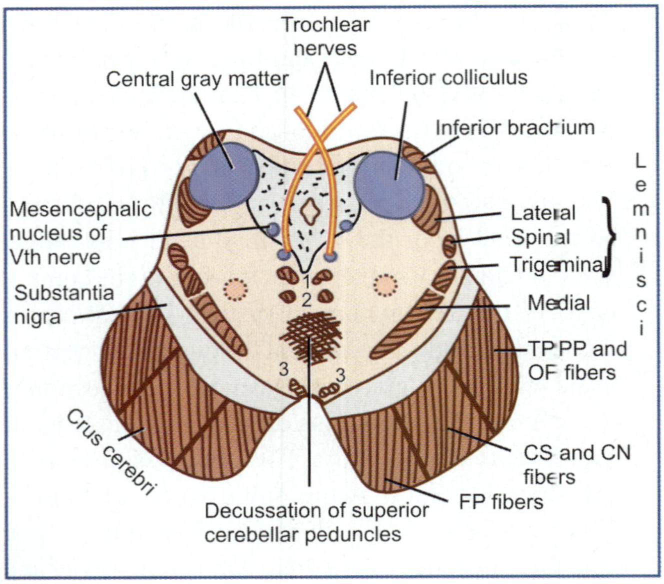

Fig. 90.7: Transverse section through midbrain at the level of inferior colliculus (1–MLF, 2–Tectospinal tract, 3–Rubrospinal tract, TP–Temporopontine, PP–Parietopontine, OP–Occipito-pontine, FP–Frontopontine, CS and CN–Corticospinal and corticonuclear fibers)

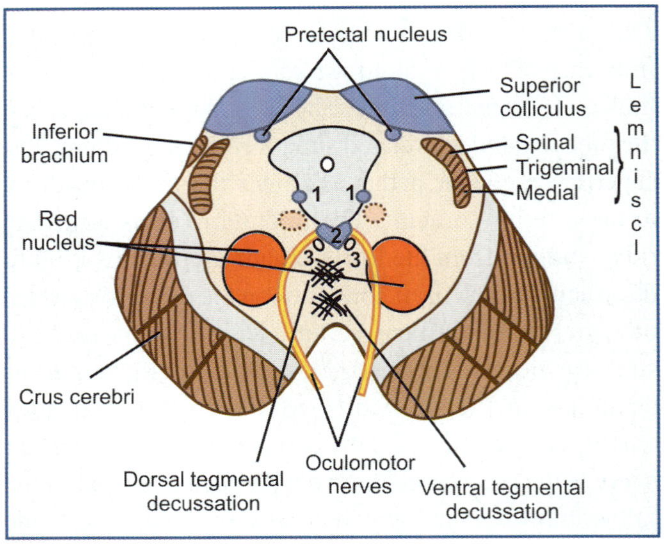

Fig. 90.8: Transverse section through midbrain at the level of superior colliculus (1–Mesencephalic nu of vth nerve, 2–Oculomotor nuclei, 3–MLF, SN–Substantia nigra)

upper pons. The most significant feature of the white matter is the presence of a large decussation of the fibers of the superior cerebellar peduncle in the midline. This is located at the level of the medial ends of the substantia nigra. The crossed fibers ascend to end in the red nucleus and a few ascending fibers go to the nucleus ventralis lateralis of thalamus. Through these connections the cerebellar nuclei are brought in contact with the red nucleus and the thalamus of the opposite side. The rubrospinal tracts lie in the midline in front of the cerebellar decussation, while the tectospinal tracts lie behind the decussation. The rubrospinal and tectospinal tracts begin at this level from the fibers originating in the red nucleus and the superior colliculus respectively, of the opposite side. The medial longitudinal fasciculus lies in front of the trochlear nucleus. The medial, trigeminal, spinal and lateral lemnisci form a curved band of fibers lying posterolateral to the substantia nigra. Some fibers of the lateral lemniscus end in the inferior colliculus. The remaining fibers of the lateral lemniscus and the fibers originating in inferior colliculus enter the inferior brachium to be carried to the medial geniculate body.

Tegmentum at the Level of Superior Colliculi (Fig. 90.8)

The central gray matter around the aqueduct contains a single oculomotor complex, which lies in the midline in front of the aqueduct. The oculomotor nucleus is divided in neuronal groups for the innervation of specific extra-ocular muscles. The Edinger-Westphal nucleus (which supplies parasympathetic innervation to the sphincter pupillae and ciliaris muscles) lies in association with the oculomotor complex. The fibers of the oculomotor nerve pass anteriorly through the red nucleus and the medial ends of substantia nigra and the crus cerebri to emerge at the medial surface of the latter in the interpeduncular fossa. The mesencephalic nucleus of the trigeminal nerve is present laterally in the central gray matter. The pretectal nucleus is present in relation to the upper part of the superior colliculus. It is part of the path of pupillary light reflex.

Red Nucleus

a. The red nucleus forms a prominent feature in the anterior part of the tegmentum closer to the midline at the level of superior colliculi. The red color is due to presence of ferric iron in the neurons. Its main afferent connections are, the cerebello-rubral fibers, which originate in the emboliform, globose and dendate nuclei of the cerebellum and the cerebro-rubral fibers. The efferent fibers from the red nucleus form the rubrospinal tract. The red nucleus also communicates with ventralis lateral (VL) nucleus of thalamus by rubrothalamic projection. Besides, it sends fibers to reticular formation, cranial nerve nuclei and inferior olivary nucleus. The red nucleus is an integrating and relay centre on the cerebello-rubro-spinal, cortico-rubro-spinal and cortico-rubro-nuclear pathways. Since it is part of the extrapyramidal system the red nucleus has a role in maintaining the tone of the voluntary muscles.

b. The white matter in the midline region consists of the ventral and dorsal tegmental decussations. The dorsal tegmental decussation of Meynert consists of decussating tectospinal fibers from the superior colliculi. After crossing the fibers form tectospinal tract. The ventral tegmental decussation of Forel consists of decussating fibers (from the red nucleus), which after crossing form the rubrospinal tracts. The cerebellum influences the spinal cord of the same side by way of the two decussations on the cerebello-rubro-spinal pathway. The first decussation is the decussation of the fibers of superior cerebellar peduncle and the second one is the ventral tegmental decussation. The medial longitudinal fasciculus lies in close relation to the oculomotor complex. The bundle of ascending tracts consists of medial lemniscus, trigeminal lemniscus and spinal lemniscus from anterior to posterior order. The position of the ascending tracts is shifted laterally posterior to the substantia nigra and nearer the surface of the midbrain.

Medial Longitudinal Fasciculus (MLF)

MLF is a compact bundle of fibers, which retains its medial position throughout the brainstem (Fig. 90.9). Superiorly it ascends to the rostral interstitial nucleus of MLF, which lies just above the upper extremity of cerebral aqueduct. This nucleus is in association with interstitial nucleus of Cajal and Darkshewitsch. It forms the premotor centre of vertical gaze movements of the eyes through connections with nuclei of third and fourth cranial nerves. Inferiorly the MLF becomes continuous with anterior intersegmental tract of spinal cord (fasciculus proprius).

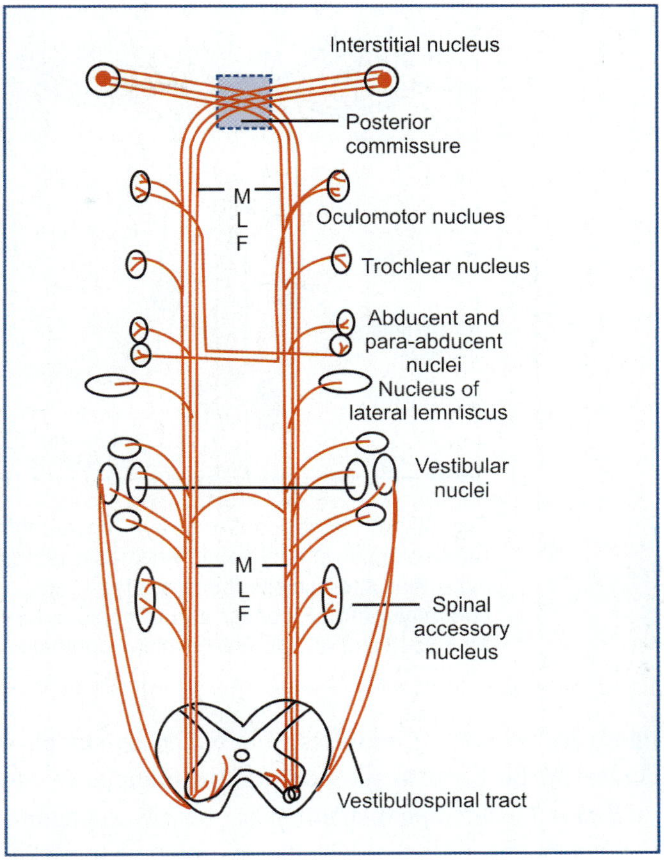

Fig. 90.9: Scheme to depict formation and connections of medial longitudinal fasciculus (Note: The course of fibers from para-abducent nucleus to contralateral oculomotor nucleus)

The MLF receives a large contribution from the vestibular nuclei through which it interconnects the oculomotor, trochlear, abducent, spinal accessory and nuclei of lateral lemniscus. It makes connections with anterior horn cells of cervical spinal cord through fasciculus proprius. It also carries the axons of paraabducent nucleus to the contra-lateral oculomotor nucleus (for controlling the action of medial rectus muscle) and has connections with pontine paramedian reticular formation (PPRF), which is the horizontal gaze centre. The rostral interstitial nuclei of MLF and the MLF of the two sides are connected by the posterior commissure. The MLF plays a role in co-ordination of vertical and horizontal conjugate eye movements. It is also important in coordinating the movements of eyes and head in response to vestibulocochlear stimulation.

Lesions of MLF

Internuclear ophthalmoplegia (Fig. 90.10) results due to unilateral damage to MLF in midbrain or pons. This

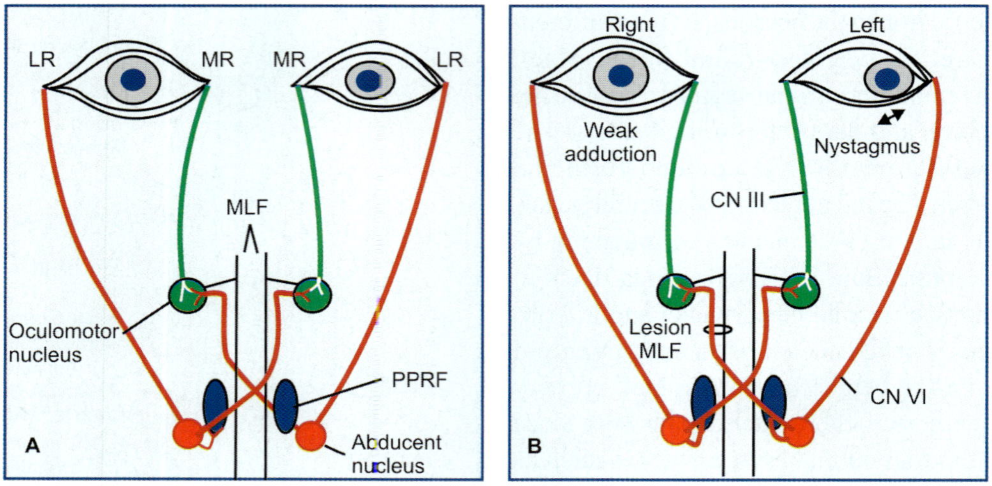

Fig. 90.10: Neural control of eye movement in conjugate lateral gaze. 'A' is diagrammatic representation of nerve supply of medial rectus (MR) and lateral rectus (LR) muscles of eyeball. Note that internuclear fibers arising in para-abducent neurons and PPRF and passing via contralateral MLF control part of oculomotor nucleus supplying MR. 'B' shows lesion in right MLF resulting in right internuclear ophthalmoplegia

interrupts the path of impulses from the horizontal gaze centre in the pons to the oculomotor nucleus in the midbrain. On attempted lateral gaze, there is nystagmus (jerky movements) in the abducting eye (contralateral eye) and slow or absent adduction in the affected side. That means the lesion of right MLF will cause slow or absent adduction in right eye and nystagmus in the left eye during attempted lateral gaze to the left. Lesion in the PPRF and MLF on the same side will result in one and half syndrome, in which there is failure of lateral conjugate gaze on the side of lesion together with impairment of adduction and nystagmus on abduction in the opposite eye. So in this lesion the eye on the side of the lesion has totally lost the capacity of horizontal movement and the eye on the opposite eye can move horizontally only on abduction (loss of one and half lateral movements).

Lesion of the Vertical Gaze Center

This gives rise to defects in the up-gaze or down- gaze or both. Lesion of posterior commissure and its nuclei causes disturbances of up-gaze. The lesion of interstitial nucleus of Cajal may cause paralysis of downward gaze.

Tectum

a. The inferior colliculi are a pair of ovoid masses of gray matter forming the lower part of tectum. Each inferior colliculus is a relay centre in the auditory pathway. The inferior colliculi of two sides are reciprocally connected to each other. The inferior colliculus receives the auditory impulses from both ears through the lateral lemniscus and the fibers from the ipsilateral medial geniculate body via the inferior brachium. It projects on the medial geniculate body through the inferior brachium. Some connections are believed to exist with the superior olivary nucleus and cochlear nuclei. The inferior colliculi are the reflex centres for responses to auditory stimuli. They are important in locating the source of sound.
b. The superior colliculi are a pair of ovoid masses of gray matter located above the inferior colliculi. Each superior colliculus is connected to the lateral geniculate body of its side by superior brachium. It receives retinotectal fibers, which travel in the optic tract, reach the lateral geniculate body but leave it to travel in the superior brachium to finally terminate in the superior colliculus. It also receives the spinotectal fibers from the spinal cord and the corticotectal fibers from occipital and temporal lobes. Its efferent connections are as follows. The tectospinal fibers cross-over in the dorsal tegmental decussation in the midbrain and reach the gray matter of the opposite side in the spinal cord. The tectothalamic fibers end in the pulvinar of thalamus

and the tectocortical fibers reach the occipital cortex. The superior colliculi are the reflex centers for the movements of the eyes and the head in response to the visual stimuli. With multiple connections it is possible that the superior colliculi play an integrating role between the visual inputs and various activities of the body.

Arterial Supply

The midbrain is supplied by posterior cerebral and superior cerebellar arteries, which are the branches of basilar artery. In addition direct branches from the basilar artery and from posterior communicating arteries are also received. These arteries give off paramedian and circumferential branches, which penetrate the midbrain. One of the circumferential arteries supplying the tectum is called quadrigeminal artery (the older name of colliculi was corpora quadrigeminia).

Clinical Highlights

a. Weber's syndrome results due to infarction in basal region of cerebral peduncle following occlusion of a branch of posterior cerebral artery. This causes contralateral hemiplegia and ipsilateral paralysis of muscles supplied by third nerve.
b. Benedikt's syndrome results due to lesion of the tegmentum involving red nucleus, fibers of third nerve and medial lemniscus. This syndrome consists of ipsilateral paralysis of muscles supplied by third nerve, contralateral hemianesthesia (loss of proprioception, discriminative touch and vibration sense) and involuntary movements like chorea and athetosis on the side of lesion.
c. Perinaud's syndrome is caused due to compression of the uppermost dorsal region of the midbrain including the superior colliculi either by vascular lesion or by the pineal tumor. It presents as a combination of impaired upward or downward gaze (due to compression of vertical gaze center), pupillary abnormality or loss of accomodation reflex. If the cerebral aqueduct is compressed, it causes dilatation of third and lateral ventricles.
d. Herniation of the uncus of temporal lobe through the tentorial notch (Fig. 86.2) results in compression of midbrain and its displacement to the opposite side. The commonest cause of tentorial herniation is the supratentorial extradural hematoma (due to middle meningeal artery rupture). This results in following neurological deficits. Compression of oculomotor nerve leads to ipsilateral dilated and fixed pupil. Shifting of the midbrain to the opposite side causes the notching of opposite crus cerebri (Kernohan's notch) by the free edge of tentorium cerebelli. This leads to ipsilteral hemiplegia due to compression of uncrossed corticospinal fibers in opposite crus cerebri. The compression of posterior cerebral artery leads to infarction of occipital lobe (homonymous hemianopia). The obstruction to the flow of CSF surrounding the midbrain causes communicating hydrocephalus, where there is internal hydrocephalus in supratentorial compartment but external hydrocephalus in the infratentorial compartment.

91 Cerebellum

The cerebellum lies posterior to the medulla oblongata and pons and inferior to the occipital lobes of cerebrum in the posterior cranial fossa. The tentorium cerebelli intervenes between the cerebellum and cerebrum. The cerebellum is the largest part of hindbrain (weight about 150 gm). Each hemisphere is connected to the three components of the brainstem by three cerebellar peduncles. The gray matter on the surface of the cerebellum is known as the cerebellar cortex, which is of uniform thickness. The gray matter inside the cerebellum is disposed as four intracerebellar nuclei. The cortex is folded in such a way that surface of cerebellum presents characteristic transverse fissures, which enclose between them leaf like areas (folia) of gray and white matter. The central core of white matter of the folium presents the pattern of a branching tree hence the name, arbor vitae cerebelli.

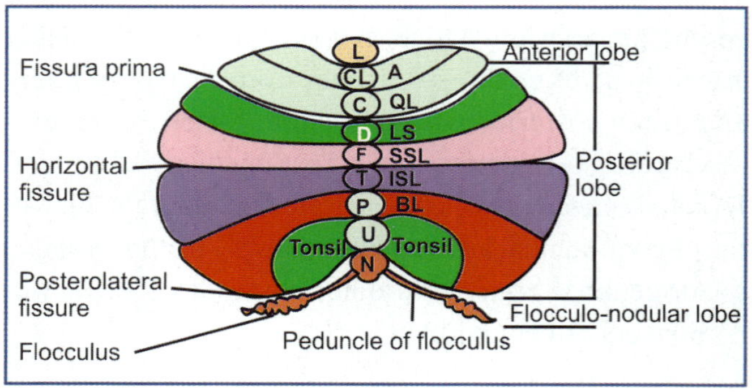

Fig. 91.1: Schematic representation of anatomical and functional subdivisions of cerebellar hemispheres and vermis (L—lingula, U—uvula, N—nodule, A—ala of CL, QL—quadrate lobule, LS—lobulus simplex, SSL—superior semilunar lobule, ISL—inferior semilunar lobule, BL—biventral lobule

Parts of Cerebellum

The cerebellum consists of right and left hemispheres, joined by the midline vermis, which has worm like appearance. Each hemisphere is divided in superior and inferior surfaces by the horizontal fissure. The vermis is also divided into superior and inferior vermis. The superior vermis is almost on the same plane as that of the superior surface of the cerebellum. The inferior vermis is situated in a depression between the inferior surfaces of the two hemispheres called vallecula.

Anatomical Lobes (Fig. 91.1)

The cerebellum is divided in three lobes with the help of the deep fissures like the fissura posterolateralis and the fissura prima. The fissura postero-lateralis on the inferior aspect, demarcates the flocculonodular lobe from the middle (posterior) lobe. The fissura prima on the superior surface demarcates the anterior lobe from the middle (posterior) lobe. These lobes and their components are shown in the following table.

Lobes	*Part of vermis*	*Part of cerebellar hemisphere*
Anterior	Lingula, central lobule, culmen	Ala of central lobule quadrangular lobule
Posterior	Declive to uvula	Lobulus simplex, superior and inferior semilunar lobules, biventral lobule and tonsil
Flocculonodular	Nodule	Flocculus

Functional Lobes

Based on connections and functions the cerebellum is divisible in three lobes, which do not exactly coincide with the anatomical lobes.

a. Archicerebellum or vestibulocerebellum is phylogenetically the oldest part. It consists of flocculonodular lobe and the lingula. It receives predominantly vestibulocerebellar fibers from the vestibular nuclei and a few fibers directly from the vestibular nerve. The archicerebellum projects on the nucleus fastigii. The efferent fibers from this nucleus mainly terminate on the vestibular nuclei and the reticular formation of the brainstem. These connections influence the cranial nerve nuclei supplying the muscles that move the eyeball via the medial longitudinal fasciculus. The anterior horn cells of spinal cord are influenced via the vestibulospinal and reticulospinal tracts. Through these connections, the archicerebellum maintains the posture and coordinates the eye movements during changes in the posture of the body.

b. Paleocerebellum or spinocerebellum consists of anterior lobe without lingula but with pyramid and uvula. It receives impulses mainly from the spinal cord via the spinocerebellar and cuneocerebellar (posterior external arcuate fibers) tracts. The paleocerebellum projects on the globose and emboliform nuclei. The efferent fibers from these nuclei pass to the brainstem centres from which the rubrospinal, reticulospinal and olivospinal tracts arise. These tracts in turn influence the anterior horn cells of the spinal cord. The paleocerebellum is responsible for maintenance of posture and muscle tone.

c. Neocerebellum or cerebro-cerebellum consists of the middle (posterior) lobe without the pyramid and uvula. It receives cortico-ponto-cerebellar connections from the opposite cerebrum and olivocerebellar and tectocerebellar fibers from the brainstem. The neocerebellum projects on the dentate nucleus. The efferent fibers from this nucleus end in the red nucleus of the midbrain and the ventralis lateral (VL) nucleus of the thalamus. The dentato-thalamo-cortical projection controls the lower motor neurons through the corticospinal, corticonuclear and cortico-olivary tracts. The neocerebellum is responsible for the smooth and coordinated movements.

Cerebellar Peduncles

a. The inferior cerebellar peduncle or restiform body connects the cerebellum to the medulla oblongata. It is composed of a large number of afferent fibers and a few efferent fibers.

The afferent fibers are:

i. Dorsal or posterior spinocerebellar tract
ii. Cuneocerebellar tract or posterior external arcuate fibers
iii. Olivocerebellar fibers
iv. Vestibulocerebellar fibers
v. Trigeminocerebellar fibers
vi. Anterior external arcuate fibers and striae medullaris
vii. Reticulocerebellar fibers.

The efferent fibers are cerebello-vestibular fibers and cerebelloreticular fibers.

b. The middle cerebellar peduncle or brachium pontis connects the cerebellum to the pons and consists of pontocerebellar fibers only. These fibers arise in the pontine nuclei and reach the cerebellum of the opposite side.

c. The superior cerebellar peduncle or brachium conjunctivum connects the cerebellum to the midbrain and is composed of both afferent and efferent fibers. The afferent fibers consist of (i) Anterior (ventral) spinocerebellar tract, (ii) Tectocerebellar fibers iii. Trigeminocerebellar fibers.
The efferent fibers are dentato-thalamic fibers and dentato-rubral fibers.

Histology of Cerebellar Cortex

There are three layers in the cerebellar cortex, which consists of five types of neurons. The molecular layer contains stellate and basket cells. The Purkinje cells, which are large flask-shaped cells, are arranged as a single row in the middle layer. The granule cell layer is composed of granule cells and Golgi cells. The dendrites of the Purkinje cells enter the molecular layer, where they synapse with parallel fibers of granule cells (axons of granule cells), stellate cells, basket cells and with the climbing fibers (olivocerebellar fibers). The axons of the Purkinje cells project on the intracerebellar nuclei. The axons of the granule cells form parallel fibers, which synapse with dendrites of Purkinje cells, Golgi cells, basket and stellate cells in the molecular layer. The dendrites of the granule cells end in claw- like endings in the cerebellar glomeruli, where they synapse with the rosette of the mossy fibers directly and with the axons and dentrites of Golgi cells indirectly.

Neuronal Circuitry in Cerebellar Cortex

The neuronal connections of the cerebellum are shown in Figure 91.2. The excitatory climbing fiber (olivocerebellar fiber) makes synaptic contacts with the dendrites of one Purkinje cell in the molecular layer. The mossy fibers consisting of rest of the afferent fibers branch profusely within the granular layer of the cortex. Each branch of the mossy fiber terminates in an expanded end called rosette, which forms a complex synapse (cerebellar glomerulus) with the dendrites of the granule cells. The axons of the Golgi cells indirectly synapse with the rosette via connections with the dendrites of the granule cells. The dendrites of the Golgi cells also take part in the synapse. The neuroglial capsule covers the entire glomerulus. The mossy fibers influence the Purkinje cells through the granule cells and like the climbing fibers are excitatory to the Purkinje cells. To sum up, in the cerebellar cortex the granule cells are the only excitatory neurons, which excite the other four cell types. The stellate, basket and Golgi cells are inhibitory interneurons. The Purkinje cells are inhibitory to the intracerebellar nuclei. The cerebellum is unique in having largest population of inhibitory neurons in the CNS.

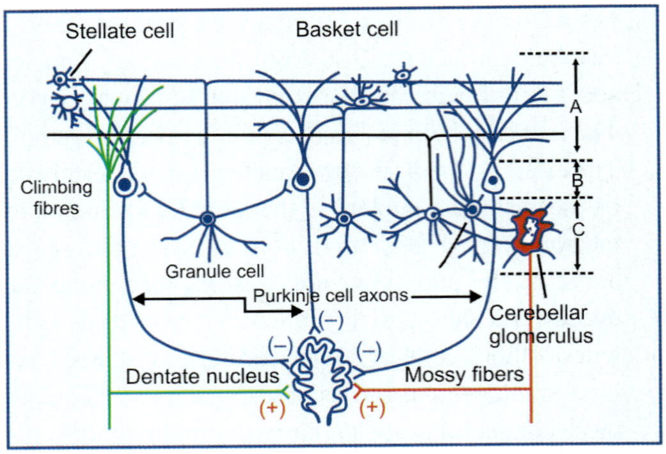

Fig. 91.2: Schematic diagram of the connections of the nerve cell in cerebellar cortex (Note that granule cells are the only excitatory neurons, while the other four are inhibitory-Purkinje cells are the only output neurons inhibitory)

Cerebellar Nuclei

The cerebellar nuclei or deep cerebellar nuclei (Fig. 91.3) are described as the output neurons of the cerebellum. They consist of four nuclei per hemisphere. From lateral to medial side they are, the dentate nucleus, emboliformis, globosus and the fastigial or roof nucleus. The deep nuclei receive axons of the Purkinje cells (inhibitory). In addition they receive collaterals from the climbing and mossy fibers (excitatory).

a. The fastigial nuclei are the smallest and belong to the archicerebellum. They receive axons of the Purkinje cells of the vermal cortex and flocculonodular lobe. The efferents from these nuclei form the cerebellovestibular and cerebelloreticular fibers, which leave through the inferior cerebellar peduncle.
b. The emboliform and globosus (nucleus interpositus) nuclei belong to the paleocerebellum. They receive axons of the Purkinje cells of the paravermal cortex. The efferent fibers from these nuclei form the cerebellorubral fibers, which leave the cerebellum through the superior cerebellar peduncle. These fibers influence the spinal cord through the rubrospinal tracts.
c. The dentate nucleus belongs to the neocerebellum and receives axons of the Purkinje cells of the lateral parts

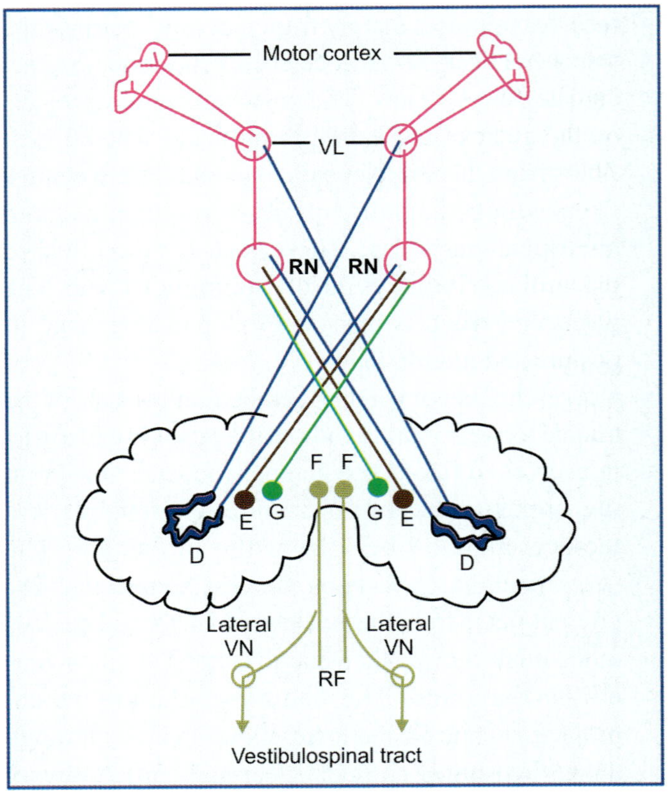

Fig. 91.3: Connections of intracerebellar nuclei
D–dentate nucleus, E–emboliform nucleus, G–globosus nucleus, F–fastigeal nucleus, VN–vestibular nucleus, RF–reticular formation, RN–red nucleus, VL–ventralis lateral nucleus of thalamus

of the hemisphere. The axons of the dentate nucleus form the dentato-rubro-thalamic tract. These fibers and the axons of the nucleus interpositus decussate in the midbrain at the level of inferior colliculus to cross to the opposite side. Some of the crossed fibers ascend to terminate in the red nucleus and in the intermediate nucleus of thalamus. Some fibers descend in the brainstem to end on inferior olivary nuclei and reticular formation.

Arterial Supply

The cerebellum receives blood from three pairs of cerebellar arteries. The superior cerebellar artery (a branch of basilar artery) supplies the superior surface of the cerebellum. The anterior inferior cerebellar artery (AICA) is also a branch of basilar artery and supplies the anterior part of inferior surface. The posterior inferior cerebellar artery (PICA) is a branch of vertebral artery and supplies the posterior part of inferior surface of cerebellum.

Functions

a. The cerebellum plays a crucial role in precise coordination of the voluntary movements of the body by controlling the strength, duration and force of contraction.
b. It is responsible for the maintenance of tone of the skeletal muscles and of equilibrium of the body. The cerebellum thus acts as a regulatory system that modifies motor acts initiated by other regions of CNS.

Clinical Highlights

a. The dysfunction of cerebellar hemispheres produces typical signs and symptoms (described as cerebellar syndrome), which manifest on the side of the lesion.
   i. Generalized muscular hypotonia.
   ii. Intention tremor at the end of a voluntary act.
   iii. Dysmetria or loss of control over the voluntary act as for example, when reaching the finger to the nose, the finger overshoots the nose.
   iv. Adiadochokinesis or inability to perform rapidly alternating opposite movements like pronation-supination
   v. Speech defect like dysarthria and thick monotonous speech
   vi. Jerky nystagmus in horizontal plane due to defective postural fixation of conjugate gaze.
   vii. Swaying towards the side of lesion on walking.
   viii. Falling on the side of lesion on closing the eyes (Romberg's sign).
b. Medulloblastoma is a highly malignant tumor of childhood. It arises from the granule cells of the cerebellar vermis. It usually damages the vermis and flocculonodular lobe, resulting in signs and symptoms, which collectively are called vermis syndrome. There is disturbance in equilibrium causing truncal ataxia. The child walks in a peculiar broad based gait. There is difficulty in holding the head steady. Romberg's sign is positive. When the tumor enlarges it may project in the cavity of the fourth ventricle. If it encroaches on the cerebello-pontine angle it may compress the facial and statoacoustic nerves.
c. The rise in intracranial pressure due to, for example, the posterior fossa tumor may displace the cerebellar tonsils downward into the foramen magnum, where the tonsils get impacted causing compression of the medulla oblongata. This may lead to loss of consciousness and injury to the lower four cranial nerves.
d. Arnold-Chiari malformation is characterised by the herniation of cerebellar tonsil with or without the medulla in the upper part of vertebral canal. This is one of the causes of hydrocephalus in infancy. Contrast myelography demonstrates the obstruction to the flow of CSF.

92 Fourth Ventricle

The fourth ventricle is the cavity of the hindbrain hence it is bounded by the medulla oblongata, pons and the cerebellum. It is located posterior to the posterior surfaces of the pons and upper half of medulla oblongata and anterior to the cerebellum (Fig. 92.1). The cavity is lined by the ependyma and contains CSF. At its upper end, the ventricle is continuous with the cerebral aqueduct and at its lower end it is continuous with the central canal of the closed part of medulla oblongata. The CSF in the fourth ventricle enters the subarachnoid space through the median aperture (foramen of Magendie) and the lateral apertures (foramina of Luschka).

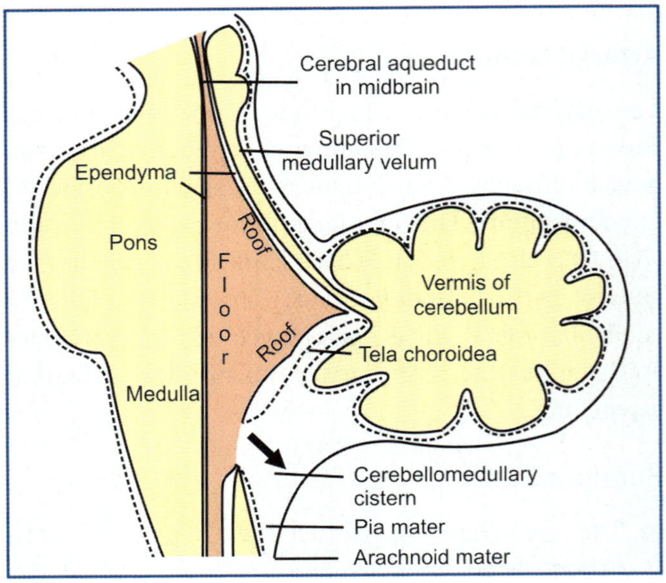

Fig. 92.1: Median section through brainstem and cerebellum to show location of IVth ventricle (Note the continuity of the ventricle with cerebral aqueduct above and with central canal of closed part of medulla below. The arrow indicates the median aperture in the roof)

Parts

The main parts of the fourth ventricle are, a cavity, lateral walls, roof or posterior wall and floor or anterior wall. The cavity has three apertures, two lateral recesses and three dorsal recesses in the roof. The cavity extends laterally on each side as the lateral recess, which passes between the inferior cerebellar peduncle and the peduncle of the flocculus. Each recess reaches upto the flocculus, where it opens in the subarachnoid space by the lateral aperture.

Lateral Walls

The upper part of each lateral wall is formed by superior cerebellar peduncles and the lower part is formed on each side by the inferior cerebellar peduncle and also by the gracile and cuneate tubercles.

Roof (Fig. 92.2)

The roof of the fourth ventricle is tent-shaped. The upper and the lower parts of the roof meet at the apex, which projects in the white core of the cerebellum as the median dorsal recess (Fig. 92.1).

a. The upper half of the roof is formed by the converging superior cerebellar peduncles and by the superior medullary velum.
b. The lower part of the roof is mainly formed by the tela choroidea of the fourth ventricle. The tela choroidea consists of the ependyma and a double fold of pia mater. The inferior medullary velum is present on each side in the roof lying in anterior relation to the cerebellar tonsil, where it becomes continuous with the white matter of the cerebellum. The peduncle of the flocculus is the upper thickened margin of the inferior medullary velum. Below the tela choroidea the roof presents a big midline aperture called foramen of Magendie, through which ventricular cavity communicates with cisterna magna.

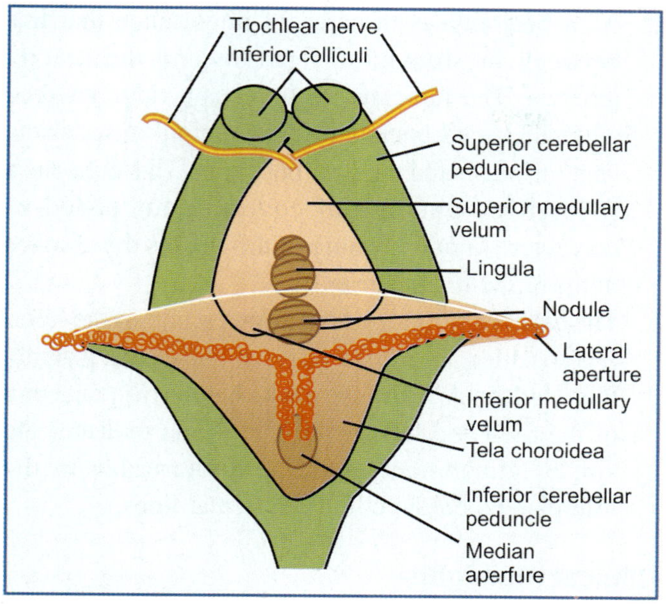

Fig. 92.2: Simplified diagram of the roof of IV th ventricle. The transverse white line represents white matter of cerebellum (Note the 'T' shaped choroid plexus entering through lower part of the roof and protruding through the lateral apertures. Note also the decussation of trochlear nerves in the uppermost end of superior medullary velum)

Recesses

a. There are three recesses in the roof. The median dorsal recess extends in the white core of the cerebellum and lies just superior to the nodule. The right and left lateral dorsal recesses project in the white matter lateral to the nodule but above the inferior medullary velum.
b. The right and left lateral recesses extend laterally between the inferior cerebellar peduncle and peduncle of flocculus to reach the flocculus and open in the subarachnoid space at the cerebellopontine angle by a lateral aperture called foramen of Luschka.

Choroid Plexuses (Fig. 92.2)

The tela choroidea of the roof is vascularized to form choroid plexuses. A branch of posterior inferior cerebellar artery supplies the choroid plexus on each side. The right and left plexuses protrude in to the cavity as vertical limbs (separated by foramen Magendie) and then extend on either side as horizontal limb in to the lateral recesses. Thus the plexus presents a T-shaped appearance. The horizontal limb of the plexus projects through the lateral aperture. The lower ends of the vertical limbs project through the median aperture into the subarachnoid space.

Floor (Rhomboid Fossa)

The floor of the fourth ventricle is diamond-shaped. It is covered by a thick layer of gray matter, which contains the nuclei of some of the cranial nerves. The ependyma covers the gray matter of the floor.

Subdivisions (Fig. 92.3)

The floor is divisible into two triangular parts, the upper pontine and lower medullary, by the striae medullaris. These fibers originate in arcuate nuclei and reach the inferior cerebellar peduncle via the floor of the fourth ventricle. They are aberrant pontocerebellar fibers. The floor is divided into right and left halves by a median sulcus. Just lateral to the median sulcus, there is a longitudinal elevation of gray matter called the medial eminence, which is limited laterally by the sulcus limitans. The region lateral to the sulcus limitans is called vestibular area since it overlies vestibular nuclei. The vestibular area is seen on both pontine and medullary parts and extends in the lateral recess, where it is continuous with the auditory (acoustic) tubercle (located on the inferior cerebellar peduncle). This tubercle overlies the dorsal cochlear nucleus and forms anterior boundary of foramen of Luschka.

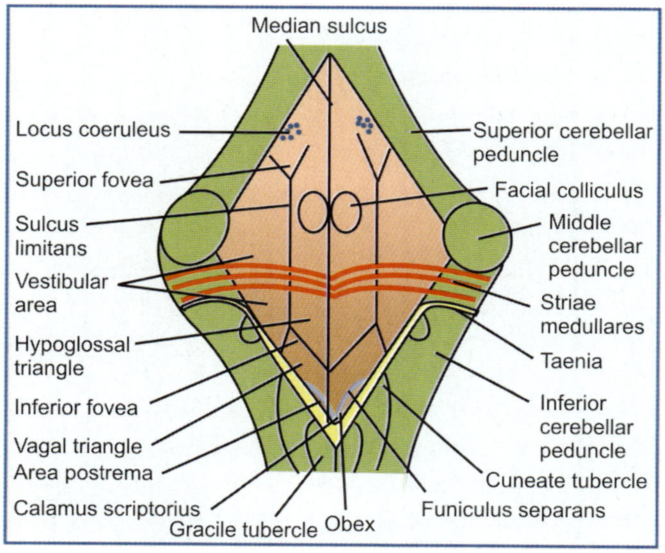

Fig. 92.3: Features of the floor of fourth ventricle

Section three

Features of Pontine Part

a. The facial colliculus is a small swelling in the lower part of the medial eminence. It indicates the position of the subjacent abducent nucleus but is produced by the recurving fibers (internal genu) of the facial nerve around the abducent nucleus.
b. The superior fovea is the depression of the sulcus limitans lateral to the facial colliculus.
c. Locus coeruleus is a small bluish area above the superior fovea. It overlies the pigmented neurons of pontine reticular formation. These pigmented neurons constitute substantia ferruginea.

Features of Medullary Part

a. The inferior fovea is an inverted V-shaped area at the lower end of sulcus terminalis.
b. The vagal triangle is the area below the inferior fovea. It overlies the dorsal nucleus of vagus.
c. The hypoglossal triangle lies medial to the inferior fovea and overlies the hypoglossal nucleus.
d. Area postrema is the area of importance that lies between the funiculus separans and the gracile tubercle. The funiculus separans is a ridge covered with thickened ependyma intervening between the vagal triangle and the area postrema. This area has a specialized ependymal covering composed of tanycytes. Another feature of this area is the absence of the blood-brain barrier.
e. The calamus scriptorius is the lowest part of the floor. It is so called because of its resemblance to a pen nib. It is overlapped by the obex, which is the meeting point of the right and left taenia. The taenia indicates the site of attachment of the tela choroidea to the inferolateral border of the ventricular floor.

Clinical Highlights

The most common tumor of the fourth ventricle is ependymoma, which arises from the ependymal cells. This tumor causes obstruction to the flow of CSF leading to internal hydrocephalus.

93 Diencephalon

The diencephalon is the part of the forebrain, which is more or less surrounded by the cerebrum. The only part of the diencephalon that is exposed to the surface is at the base of the brain in the interpeduncular fossa. The diencephalon is divided into two symmetrical halves by the cavity of the third ventricle. The line of demarcation between the midbrain and the diencephalon passes through the posterior commissure.

Subdivisions

The diencephalon is subdivided into five parts, thalamus (dorsal thalamus), epithalamus, hypothalamus, subthalamus (ventral thalamus) and metathalamus (lateral and medial geniculate bodies).

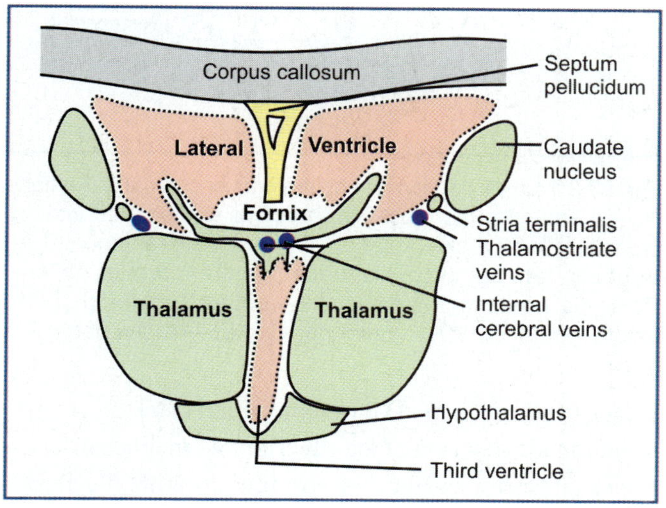

Fig. 93.1: To show the position of thalamus in relation to third and lateral ventricles (Note: The superior relations of thalamus and the location of choroid fissure between fornix and thalamus)

Thalamus (Figs 93.1 and 93.2)

The thalamus is a large mass of gray matter. The right and left halves of the thalamus are completely separate except for the interthalamic adhesion (found only in approximately 70% of brains). The thalamus receives all the sensory information from the body through the lemnisci or ascending tracts. It processes the sensory input for onward transmission to the sensory areas of the cerebral cortex via the thalamic radiations.

Each thalamus has an anterior narrow end called the anterior tubercle, which forms the posterior boundary of the interventricular foramen. The posterior expanded end is called the pulvinar, which lies just above and lateral to the superior colliculus of midbrain. The pulvinars of the two sides are separate from each other and overhang the tectum of the midbrain. Below the pulvinar and lateral to the superior colliculus, the lateral and medial geniculate bodies come in close relation to the thalamus.

a. The medial surface of the thalamus is covered with ependyma as it forms the greater part of lateral wall of the third ventricle. The interthalamic adhesion made of gray matter, connects a small area on the medial surfaces of the two sides though there is no structural continuity between the two sides. The medial surface of the thalamus is demarcated from that of hypothalamus by the hypothalamic sulcus.
b. The lateral surface is related to the posterior limb of the internal capsule (Fig. 98.2).
c. The superior or dorsal surface is divisible into lateral and medial parts by the fornix, which lies in close contact with this surface. The superior surface of the thalamus and the inferior surface of the fornix bound a narrow space called the choroid fissure (Fig. 93.2). The lateral part of the superior surface forms the floor of the central part of lateral ventricle hence it is covered with ependyma. The medial part of the superior surface is covered with the tela choroidea of

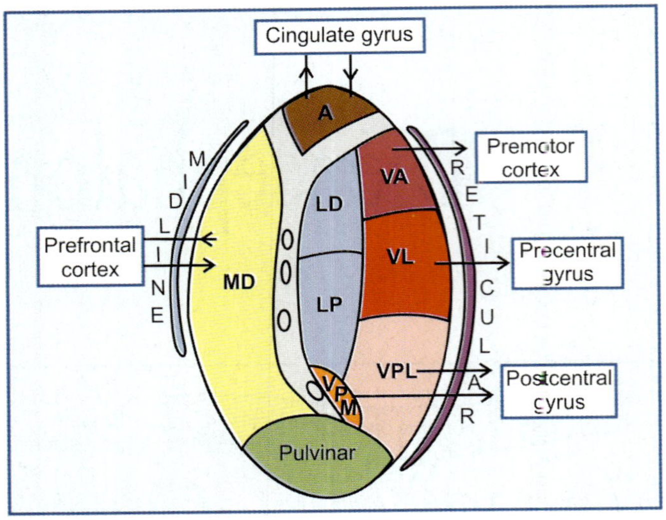

Fig. 93.2: Nuclei of thalamus and their major cortical projections Note the intralaminar nuclei in the stem of Y-shaped internal medullary lamina. A—Anterior, VA—Ventralis anterior, VL—Ventralis lateral, VPL—Ventralis postero-lateralis, VPM—Ventralis posterior medialis, LP—Lateral posterior, LP—Lateral posterior, LD—Lateral dorsal, MD—Medial dorsal

the third ventricle. The stria medullaris thalami courses along the junction of the superior and medial surfaces.

d. The inferior surface is continuous with the hypothalamus, subthalamus, and tegmentum of midbrain from before backwards.

Nuclear Groups

The thalamic gray matter is divisible into three main groups of nuclei by a Y-shaped internal medullary lamina. In addition, three nonspecific groups of nuclei are present in the thalamus. Thus, thalamus consists of a total of six groups of nuclear masses. The white matter of the thalamus is minimal and consists of two medullary laminae. The external medullary lamina covers the lateral surface of the thalamus.

Main Nuclear Groups (Fig. 93.2)

The three main groups are, the anterior, medial or dorsomedial (DM) and the lateral groups. The lateral group is further subdivided in ventral and dorsal parts. The ventral part consists of three nuclei from before backwards:

a. Ventralis anterior (VA)
b. Ventral lateral (VL)
c. Ventralis posterior (VP).

Which is further, divided in ventralis posterolateralis (VPL) and ventralis posteromedialis (VPM). The dorsal (lateral) part consists of three nuclei from before backward:

a. Lateral dorsal (LD)
b. Lateral posterior (LP)
c. Pulvinar (P).

Minor Groups (Nonspecific Thalamic Nuclei)

The minor groups of thalamic nuclei are the intralaminar nuclei, the midline nuclei and the reticular thalamic nuclei. The intralaminar nuclei are present in the substance of internal medullary lamina and consist of, centromedian nucleus (CM) and parafascicular nucleus (PF). The midline nuclei (MLN) lie between the medial dorsal group and the ependymal wall of the third ventricle. The reticular thalamic nuclei (RTN) are located between the external medullary lamina and the posterior limb of internal capsule.

Connections of Nuclei

a. Anterior nucleus receives the mamillothalamic tract from the mamillary body and the projection fibers (fornix) from the hippocampus. It projects to the cingulate gyrus via the anterior thalamic radiation. The anterior nucleus and its connections are part of the Papez circuit (Fig. 101.2) of the limbic system. They play role in the emotional behavior and recent memory.

b. The dorsomedial (DM) group receives fibers mainly from the prefrontal cortex. In addition, it receives afferents from the amygdaloid body, hypothalamus, corpus striatum and the piriform cortex.

   The major projection from the DM is to the prefrontal cortex. A few efferent fibers terminate on the intralaminar nuclei and the corpus striatum. The DM group plays an important role in emotion and behavior. Damage may lead to decrease in anxiety, tension, aggression and temporary amnesia (personality changes similar to those seen in prefrontal lobotomy). It is regarded as an integrating centre of somatic and visceral impulses.

c. The ventralis anterior (VA) nucleus receives afferent fibers from globus pallidus, deep cerebellar nuclei and substantia nigra. It sends diffuse projections to the striatum and sensory and motor cortices. The VA nucleus plays a central role in transmission of the cortical recruiting response.

d. The ventralis lateral (VL) nucleus receives fibers from the cerebellar nuclei, red nucleus, globus pallidus and substantia nigra. It projects to the motor and premotor cortex. The VL nucleus has an important role in regulation of voluntary movements and maintenance of muscle tone. It is an integrating centre for inputs from cerebellum, striatum and cerebral cortex. Surgical ablation of this nucleus is sometimes used in the treatment of Parkinson's tremor.
e. The ventralis posterolateralis (VPL) nucleus receives afferent connections from medial lemniscus, spinal lemniscus and parietal lobe. It projects to the postcentral gyrus through the superior thalamic radiation. It is a relay station for sensations of touch, pain, temperature and proprioceptive sensations from the contralateral body except the face.
f. The ventralis posteromedialis (VPM) receives sensations from the trigeminal lemniscus, solitary nucleus and the parietal lobe. It projects to the postcentral gyrus through the superior thalamic radiation. The VPM is a relay station for the touch, pain, temperature and proprioceptive sensations from the contralateral face and for taste.
g. The lateral dorsal (LD) nucleus receives fibers from the pretectum, superior colliculus, other thalamic nuclei, cingulate gyrus, posterior parahippocampal cortex and hippocampus. It projects to the cingulate gyrus, precuneus and parahippocampal gyrus.
h. The lateral posterior (LP) nucleus receives afferent connections from the superior colliculi and parietal lobe. Its efferent connections are to the superior and inferior parietal lobules, cingulate gyrus and parahippocampal gyrus.
i. The pulvinar receives afferents from the superior colliculi, lateral and medial geniculate bodies and amygdaloid bodies. It has reciprocal connections with the occipital cortex, parietal cortex, temporal cortex, prefrontal and orbitofrontal cortex. The function of the pulvinar is to integrate the visual, somatic sensory and auditory inputs.
j. The centromedian and parafascicular nuclei are part of ascending reticular activating system since they receive large input from the reticular formation. Besides this, they receive fibers from the corpus striatum, cerebellum, other thalamic nuclei, amygdaloid nucleus and hypothalamus. They project on the striatum, and through it, establish diffuse connections with the entire cortex.
k. The reticular thalamic nuclei do not project to the cortex but receive input from the cortex and other thalamic nuclei. It is probably concerned with regulation of intrathalamic activity.

Thalamic Radiations

There are four thalamic radiations, anterior, superior, inferior and posterior. The thalamus establishes to and fro connections with the cerebral cortex via the thalamic radiations, which pass through the internal capsule.

a. The anterior thalamic radiation connects the frontal lobe to the dorsomedial (DM), VA, VL group of nuclei and the anterior nuclei. It also contains reciprocal frontothalamic fibers. It passes through the anterior limb of internal capsule.
b. The superior thalamic radiation connects the VPM and VPL nuclei to the postcentral gyrus (parietal lobe). It contains reciprocal parietothalamic fibers and corticothalamic fibers for other thalamic nuclei. It passes through the posterior limb of internal capsule.
c. The inferior thalamic radiation passes through the sublentiform part of internal capsule and connects the medial geniculate body to the temporal lobe. It also contains temporothalamic fibers and corticothalamic fibers for other thalamic nuclei.
d. The posterior thalamic radiation passes through the retrolentiform part of internal capsule and connects the lateral geniculate body to the occipital lobe. It contains reciprocal fibers and corticothalamic fibers for other thalamic nuclei.

Arterial Supply

The branches of posterior communicating, posterior cerebral and basilar arteries supply the thalamus.

Functions

The thalamus is a relay station of fine sensations but crude sensations (pain and temperature) are perceived in the thalamus. It maintains state of wakefulness and alertness through the connections of the intralaminar nuclei to the ascending activating reticular system on one hand and cerebral cortex on the other hand via the striatum. It regulates the motor activities by linking cerebellum and globus pallidus to the motor and premotor cortex.

Thalamic Syndrome

The thalamic syndrome is the disturbance of the sensory functions of the thalamus, usually due to vascular lesion. The threshold for touch, pain and temperature sensations is raised on the opposite side of the lesion. When the sensations are felt they are perverted, exaggerated and exceptionally disagreeable. There is emotional instability with spontaneous crying and laughing. It has been hypothesized that thalamic syndrome is due to abnormal activity in thalamic and cortical neurons that have been deprived of their normal afferents.

Epithalamus (Fig. 93.1)

The epithalamus lies in relation to the posterior part of the roof and lateral wall of the third ventricle. It consists of pineal gland, habenular nuclei with their connections and the posterior commissure.

Pineal Gland

The pineal gland (epiphysis cerebri) is a small gland, which is located just below the splenium of corpus callosum in a depression between the superior colliculi. It is attached to the roof the third ventricle by pineal stalk, which contains superior and inferior laminae separated by the pineal recess of the third ventricle. The superior lamina gives passage to the habenular commissure and the inferior lamina to the posterior commissure.

Nerve Supply

a. The nervus conarii consists of postganglionic sympathetic fibers, which run subendothelially in the wall of the straight sinus in the tentorium cerebelli and enter the pineal gland to supply the pinealocytes.
b. Nervus pinealis is vestigial as it makes a brief appearance in the fetal stage only. It is homologous with sensory pineal nerve of fish and amphibians, whose pineal gland contains photoreceptors.

Structure and Function

The pineal gland is composed of the pinealocytes, neuroglial cells and a rich network of fenestrated capillaries. There is no blood-brain barrier in pineal gland. The gland exerts an inhibitory effect on the gonads. It secretes melatonin and serotonin. The aggregations of calcium and magnesium phosphates and carbonates form the corpora arenacea or brain sand from early age. The presence of the brain sand in the midline is detectable on radiographs. Displacement of the gland to one side of the midline is indicative of space occupying lesion in the cranium. The tumor of pineal gland causes lowered activity in gonads. Destruction of pineal gland in childhood results in precocious puberty.

Habenular Nucleus and Commissure

The habenular nucleus is located in the habenular triangle, which is bounded superomedially by stria medullaris thalami, inferiorly by superior colliculus and laterally by pulvinar. The habenular nucleus receives afferent connections through the stria medullaris thalami from neurons in the septal area, basal nucleus of Meynert in the basal forebrain and preoptic hypothalamus. The efferent connections of the habenular nucleus form the fasciculus retroflexus, which ends in interpeduncular nucleus, which projects on the midbrain reticular formation. The habenula is responsible for integration of olfactory and visceral functions hence it is part of the limbic system. Also, habenula is olfacto-somatic correlation centre as is apparent from the fact that there is reflex movement of the neck and body towards or away from source of olfactory stimuli. After reaching the habenular nucleus some fibers of the stria medullaris thalami pass through the superior lamina of the pineal stalk to reach the habenular nucleus and through it the septal area of the opposite side. These fibers constitute the true habenular commissure since they communicate the septal areas of the two hemispheres.

Posterior Commissure

This commissure connects the pretectal nuclei, interstitial nuclei of posterior commissure, interstitial nucleus of Cajal, nucleus of Darkshewitsch and rostral interstitial nuclei of medial longitudinal fasciculus of the two sides.

The pinealomas may compress the vertical gaze center located here and present as Perinaud's syndrome.

Hypothalamus

The hypothalamus is a small mass of gray matter below the thalamus. It forms the floor and anterior parts of the walls of the third ventricle. Superiorly it is continuous with the thalamus at the hypothalamic sulcus and inferiorly it is continuous with the tegmentum of midbrain. The hypothalamus controls the endocrine glands, autonomic nervous system and the limbic system. It is regarded as the biological clock of the body.

Location of Hypothalamus on the Surface of Brain

It is visible only at the base of the brain in the interpeduncular fossa behind the optic chiasma. It includes tuber cinereum and mamillary bodies.

Arterial Supply

The circle of Willis provides ample blood supply as it is in close relation to the hypothalamus.

Hypothalamic Nuclei (Table 93.1)

a. The lateral hypothalamic area contains a nucleus, which on stimulation induces eating. The lesions of this nucleus cause anorexia and starvation.
b. The preoptic nucleus regulates the release of gonadotrophic hormones from the adenohypophysis. So, it is the only nucleus of the hypothalamus that is sexually dimorphic.
c. Paraventricular and supraoptic nuclei contain neurosecretory neurons, which secrete ADH and oxytocin. The axons of these neurons form hypothalamo-hypophyseal tract, which projects to the neurohypophysis. The neurosecretory granules are stored in the nerve terminals of the axons (Herring bodies) in the neurohypophysis. Lesion of these nuclei for example a tumor or trauma, causes diabetes insipidus which is characterized by polyuria (excess of urination) and polydipsia (excessive thirst).
d. Arcuate or infundibular nucleus is located in tuber cinereum. It contains neurons that produce hypothalamic-releasing and release inhibiting hormones and give rise to tubero-hypophyseal tract, which terminates on hypophyseal portal vessels in the median eminence. Thus, it influences the release or release inhibition of the hormones of the adenohypophysis.
e. Mamillary nuclei receive input from the hippocampus through the anterior column of fornix and project to the anterior nucleus of thalamus.

Afferent Connections

a. Septal area and nuclei belonging to the limbic system by medial forebrain bundle.
b. Hippocampal formation of the limbic system by fornix.
c. Amygdaloid complex by stria terminalis and ventral amygdalofugal pathway.
d. Primary olfactory cortex by medial forebrain bundle.
e. Dorsomedial nucleus (DM) of thalamus by thalamic radiations.
f. Brainstem nuclei like tegmental nuclei, raphe nuclei and locus cereruleus of reticular formation by medial forebrain bundle.

Efferent Connections

a. Septal area and nuclei via medial forebrain bundle.
a. Anterior nucleus of thalamus.
b. Dorsomedial nucleus of thalamus.
c. Amygdaloid complex.
d. Brainstem reticular formation.
e. Brainstem nuclei and spinal cord by dorsal longitudinal fasciculus for connecting to the parasmpathetic and sympathetic neurons.
f. Adenohypophysis by hypothalamo-hypophyseal portal vessels.
g. Neurohypophysis by hypothalamo-hypophyseal neural pathways.

Functions

a. The anterior hypothalamus has an excitatory effect on the parasympathetic neurons while posterior hypothalamus has similar effect on sympathetic neurons.
b. The anterior hypothalamus helps in temperature regulation.
c. The water balance of the body is maintained by action of ADH secreted in the hypothalamic cells.

Table 93.1: Nuclear source of hypothalamic hormones (factors) and their effects on anterior pituitary

Hypothalamic hormone	*Nuclear origin*	*Anterior pituitary hormone*	*Final effect*
GHRH	Arcuate	Growth hormone	Stimulation of growth cartilage
GHIH- somatostatin	Suprachiasmatic	Growth hormone	Reduction in activity of growth cartilage
CRH	Paraventricular	ACTH	Production of adrenal cortical hormones
TRH	Paraventricular	TSH	Production of thyroxine
PIH (dopamine)	?	Prolactin- LTH	Reduction of lactogenesis
GnRH and LHRH	Preoptic	FSH and LH/ ICSH	Production of sex hormones in respective sex

d. The food intake is regulated by hypothalamic nucleus in the tuberal region, which lies dorsal to the tuber cinereum. It is called ventromedial nucleus. It inhibits the urge to eat and hence called satiety center. Bilateral destruction results in hyperphagia and obesity. The lateral hypothalamic nucleus is called hunger or feeding center. Its destruction causes starvation and emaciation.
e. The hypothalamus is aptly described as master orchestrator of endocrine system of the body through its control of anterior pituitary (Fig. 87.4).
f. Oxytocin secreted by hypothalamus causes contraction of smooth muscle of uterus and myoepithelial cells of the lactiferous ducts of mammary glands.

Subthalamus

The subthalamus is a very complex region. It is situated ventral to the thalamus and lateral to the hypothalamus overlying the inferior part of the internal capsule. It lies superior to the substantia nigra and red nucleus. The subthalamus contains gray matter and fiber tracts.

Gray Matter and Fiber Tracts in Subthalamus

a. Subthalamic nucleus of Luys has reciprocal connections with the globus pallidus through the fasciculus subthalamicus.
b. Zona incerta is a thin sheet of gray matter between the thalamus and subthalamic nucleus.
c. Field H1 of Forel is the area between the zona incerta and thalamus. Fasciculus lenticularis, ansa lenticularis and dentato-rubro-thalamic tracts meet here to form thalamic fasciculus.
d. Field H2 of Forel is the area between the zona incerta and subthalamic nucleus and is traversed by fasciculus lenticularis.
e. Field H of Forel or prerubral field lies below and medial to the zona incerta. The fasciculus lenticularis and ansa lenticularis are assembled here.

Lesion of the subthalamic nucleus produces hemiballismus in the opposite side. The involuntary and violent movements (of throwing or flailing type) affecting usually the proximal part of the upper limbs are the characteristic features of this condition.

Metathalamus

The lateral geniculate body is described with optic pathway and the medial geniculate body with auditory pathway in Chapter 125.

94 Third Ventricle

The third ventricle is the cavity bounded by the thalamus and hypothalamus (Fig. 93.1). It is a narrow slit-like cavity lined with ependyma. The third ventricle communicates with the lateral ventricles through the interventricular foramina and with the fourth ventricle through the cerebral aqueduct. It is visible radiologically in CT scan and MRI as a narrow midline space.

Boundaries (Fig. 94.1)

a. A layer of ependyma stretching across the two thalami forms the roof. The ependyma of the roof comes in contact with the vascular pia mater (tela choroidea) in two places and they invaginate as linear choroid plexuses in the cavity of the ventricle (Fig. 93.2). Anterior and posterior choroidal arteries supply the choroid plexuses of the third ventricle and the internal cerebral veins pass posteriorly lying within the tela choroidea.
b. The anterior wall of the third ventricle is formed by the lamina terminalis, which stretches between the optic chiasma and the rostrum of the corpus callosum. The anterior commissure lies in the superior part of the lamina terminalis. The anterior column of fornix lies behind the lamina terminalis on each side. The interventricular foramen of Monro is located between the column of fornix and the anterior tubercle of thalamus. This foramen is a communication between the third ventricle and the lateral ventricle of each side. The choroid plexuses of the third ventricle are continuous with those of lateral ventricles through the interventricular foramen. Hypertrophy of the choroid plexus may block the interventricular foramen with resultant accumulation of CSF in the lateral ventricles. The unilateral hydrocephalus of the lateral ventricle may compress the opposite hemisphere thus shifting the midline structures towards the opposite side.
c. The lateral wall of the third ventricle is traversed by hypothalamic sulcus, which extends from the interventricular foramen to the cerebral aqueduct. The hypothalamic sulcus demarcates the thalamus above and the hypothalamus below. The medial surfaces of the two thalami often fuse with each other at a localized interthalamic adhesion, which lies above the hypothalamic sulcus.
d. The floor of the third ventricle is formed by the optic chiasma, infundibulum, tuber cinereum, mamillary bodies, posterior perforated substance and the upper end of the tegmentum of midbrain.
e. The posterior wall consists of the pineal body, posterior commissure, habenular commissure and cerebral aqueduct.

Recesses (Fig. 94.1)

The recesses of the third ventricle are the prolongations of its cavity. There are four recesses.

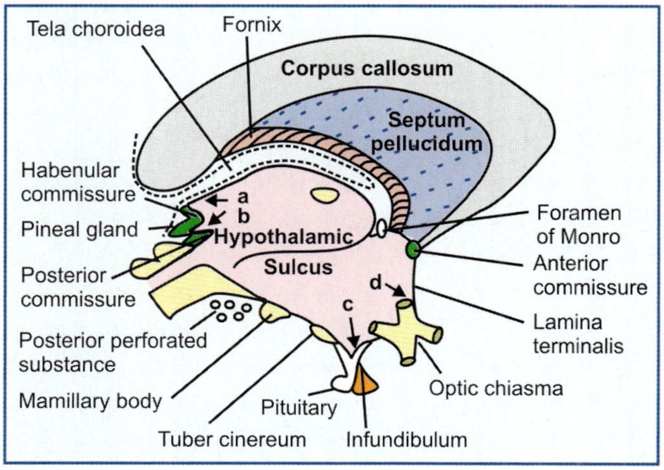

Fig. 94.1: Boundaries and recesses of third ventricle. Recesses: a–Suprapineal, b–Pineal, c–Infundibular, d–Optic

a. Infundibular recess is a funnel-shaped extension in the infundibulum.
b. Optic recess is an angular diverticulum just above the optic chiasma.
c. Pineal recess projects into the stalk of the pineal gland
d. Suprapineal recess is a diverticulum of the roof of the ventricle above the habenular commissure.

Circumventricular Organs

These are a group of specialized structures composed of tufts of fenestrated (highly permeable) capillaries, a few neuroglial cells and neurons. They are covered with ependymal cells and are devoid of blood-brain barrier. They are located in the vicinity of the ventricles. These include median eminence (described with interpeduncular fossa), organum vasculosum laminae terminalis (OVLT), subfornical organ and area postrema (described with fourth ventricle).

OVLT is embedded in the lamina terminalis. It plays a role in regulation of sodium metabolism by way of appetite for salt. It is believed to be implicated in mechanisms of fever.

The subfornical organ is located close to the interventricular foramen. It probably helps in osmo-regulation by acting as drinking center.

95 Reticular Formation

The reticular formation is a diffuse network of neurons and nerve fibers extending through out the brainstem. It lies in the tegmentum of midbrain, dorsal part of pons and retro-olivary region in medulla oblongata. Inferiorly, it makes connections with the neurons in lamina VII of spinal cord via the reticulospinal tracts. Superiorly, it extends in the diencephalon (intralaminar and ventral anterior nuclei of thalamus, hypothalamus and zona incerta of subthalamus) via the central tegmental tracts. The reticular formation is connected to all parts of the cerebral cortex, basal ganglia, limbic system and cerebellum. All the ascending and descending pathways of the reticular formation are polysynaptic.

Functions

The reticular formation is necessary for maintenance of alertness and wakeful state. It is required for arousal from sleep to consciousness and is responsible for slow sleep and REM sleep. It controls the cardiac and respiratory functions and maintains the tonic and phasic motor activities. Apart from these functions, it controls the vertical and horizontal gaze centers in the brainstem and modulates pain sensation.

Arrangement of Neurons

The neurons of the reticular formation are arranged in three longitudinal columns (median, medial or paramedian and lateral) in the brainstem on each side.

a. The median columns consist of serotoninergic raphe nuclei. The projection of dorsal raphe nucleus located in the periaqueductal gray, to the spinal cord forms a pain controlling system. It is observed that electrical stimulation of periaqueductal gray results in profound analgesia lasting for several hours through effect of enkephalin produced by substantia gelatinosa of posterior horn of spinal cord.
b. The medial or paramedian column is composed of neurons of large size. These neurons give origin to polysynaptic reticulospinal tracts, which control muscle tone. In the pons, this column contains horizontal gaze center in the vicinity of abducent nucleus.
c. The lateral column is composed of neurons of small size as well as large size. It includes locus coeruleus, pedunculopontine nucleus, parabrachial nuclei and Kolliker-Fuse nucleus. Some areas of this column control the cardiovascular, respiratory and gastro-intestinal functions.

Attention Center

The locus coeruleus contains the largest concentration of noradrenergic melanin containing neurons in CNS. Since it has diverse to and fro cranial and caudal connections its functions can be postulated as follows. It possibly functions as an attention center that helps to increase the speed of reflex responses and general level of alertness. It is observed that firing rates of its neurons rise to peak in wakeful state and are further enhanced in the presence of novel stimuli. Thus, locus coeruleus plays a role in enhancing the signal processing capacity of target neurons by increasing their signal-to-noise ratio. Yet another function attributed to locus coeruleus is that it triggers the onset of REM sleep (paradoxical sleep) by releasing noradrenaline.

Respiratory Centers

The inspiratory and expiratory centers are present in the medulla oblongata while the pneumotaxic center is in the pons. The inspiratory center is located at obex of the fourth ventricle ventrolateral to nucleus solitarius. The neurons in the inspiratory center are excitatory to lower motor neurons of the phrenic and intercostal nerves via the reticulospinal tracts. The expiratory center is found in association with nucleus ambiguus in medulla oblongata. This center functions only in forced expiration. The pneumotaxic center (parabrachial nuclei and Kolliker-Fuse nucleus in pons) influences the rate of breathing. It inhibits the inspiratory center and shortens the respiratory cycle. The respiratory centers in brainstem maintain automatic breathing in sleeping state. In destruction of medullary centers, the patient is able to maintain breathing through pyramidal tract in the waking state but if the patient falls asleep, for want of automatic breathing the patient will die. This clinical condition, where there is loss of automatic control of breathing without loss of voluntary control is called Ondine's curse.

Gaze Centers in the Brainstem

The gaze centers for horizontal movements of the eyes are located in pons near the abducent nucleus in paramedian pontine reticular formation (PPRF). Each center controls conjugate movements towards its own side. The stimulation of left abducent nucleus brings about contraction of left lateral rectus muscle and simultaneous stimulation of the right oculomotor nucleus through the medial longitudinal fasciculus (MLF), brings about the contraction of right medial rectus muscle. In this way, both eyes turn to the left. Lesion in the horizontal gaze center leads to total ipsilateral loss of horizontal conjugate gaze. The gaze centers for vertical movements of the eye lie in the midbrain in the rostral interstitial nucleus of MLF and nucleus of Cajal and neurons in tegmentum of midbrain. Lesions in this part produce paralysis of vertical gaze either up-gaze or down-gaze.

Sleep Inducing or Hypnogenic Center

The serotoninergic raphe nuclei at pontomedullary region act as hypnogenic centers because on stimulation they induce slow sleep.

Ascending Reticular Activating System (ARAS)

The ARAS consists of reticular formation, ascending sensory tracts in the brainstem (spinothalamic, trigemino-thalamic, gustatory path, auditory path, etc.), nonspecific thalamic nuclei and diffuse thalamo-cortical projections. The ascending tracts give off collaterals, which terminate on the lateral column of the reticular formation. The ascending fibers from the reticular formation terminate mainly in intralaminar nuclei of thalamus, which project on wide areas of cerebral cortex and limbic system. These ascending reticular fibers forming ARAS are believed to be responsible for arousal from sleep. When the ARAS is stimulated the cerebral cortex is alerted. Supression of impulse transmission through ARAS produces drowsiness and sleep. Epinephrine and smelling salts stimulate ARAS activity while barbiturates, general anesthetics and largactil supress it.

96 Cerebrum

The cerebrum is the largest part of the brain. It has an ovoid shape, as it is broad behind and narrower in front. It consists of two incompletely separated cerebral hemispheres.

Cerebral Hemisphere

The outer surface of the cerebral hemisphere is covered with cortex, which is highly folded due to the presence of sulci and gyri. It is estimated that the surface area of human cortex is 2200 sq. cm and it is composed of about ten thousand million neurons. The core of the hemisphere consists of white matter, which contains a group of nuclei called basal ganglia. The cavity inside each hemisphere is called the lateral ventricle. The longitudinal fissure of cerebrum intervenes between the medial surfaces of the right and left hemispheres. At the bottom of the fissure lies the corpus callosum, which is a connecting bond between the hemispheres. The contents of the longitudinal fissure are, falx cerebri and the accompanying arachnoid mater, pia mater covering the medial surfaces of the hemispheres, anterior cerebral vessels and the indusium griseum on the superior surface of corpus callosum.

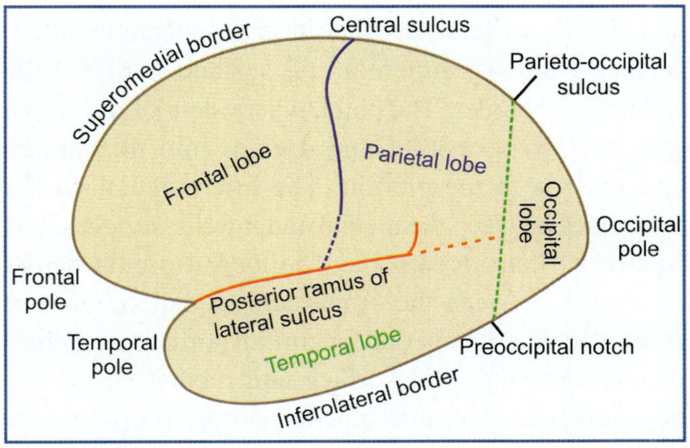

Fig. 96.1: Superolateral surface of cerebral hemisphere showing poles, borders and demarcation of lobes

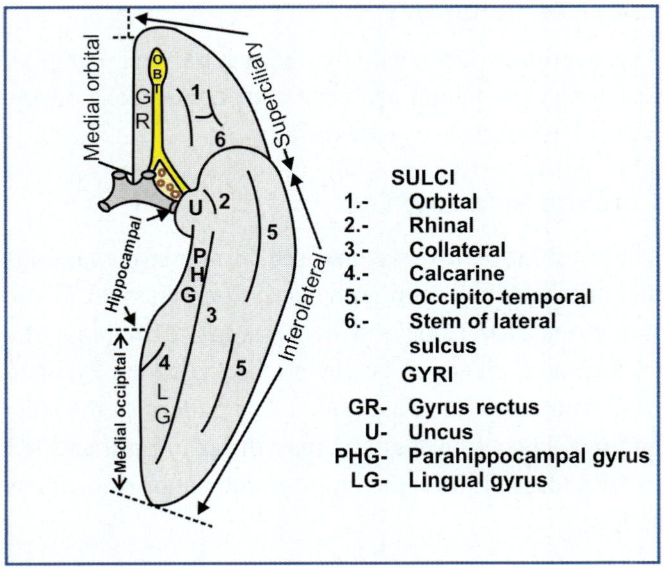

Fig. 96.2: Sulci and gyri on inferior (tentorial and orbital) surface of left cerebral hemisphere (Note that olfactory bulb and tract (OBT) lie in olfactory sulcus, which is not labeled. The figure also shows borders as seen on the inferior surface)

External Features (Figs 96.1 and 96.2)

Each cerebral hemisphere has three poles, three surfaces and three borders.

a. The frontal pole is the pointed anterior extremity of the cerebral hemisphere. Its surface marking is the junction of the root of the nose and the medial end of superciliary arch. The occipital pole is the pointed posterior extremity of the cerebral hemisphere. A point superolateral to the external occipital protuberance indicates its position on the surface. The temporal pole is the anterior end of the temporal lobe. It lies in the middle cranial fossa under cover the lesser wing of sphenoid.

b. The surfaces of the cerebral hemisphere are, superolateral, medial (or vertical) and inferior. The right and left medial surfaces enclose the longitudinal fissure. The inferior surface is subdivided into orbital and tentorial surfaces by the stem of the lateral sulcus.
b. The superomedial border lies between the medial and superolateral surfaces. It is indicated on the surface by a paramedian line from a point just superolateral to inion to a point just superolateral to nasion.

The inferolateral border lies between the superolateral and inferior surfaces. Its anterior part separating orbital surface from the superolateral surface is called the superciliary border. The point, where stem of the lateral sulcus cuts this border and divides into three rami, corresponds to the pterion. The inferomedial border intervenes between the medial and inferior surfaces. It is subdivided into three parts. The medial orbital border intervenes between the orbital and medial surfaces of frontal lobe. The medial occipital border intervenes between the tentorial surface and medial surface of occipital lobe. The inferomedial border proper or the hippocampal border (formed by uncus and parahippocampal gyrus) is present between the previous two.

Lobes of Cerebrum

There are four lobes namely, frontal, parietal, occipital and temporal, which are very well demarcated on the superolateral surface (vide infra).

Cerebral Sulci and Gyri

The cerebral cortex is composed of numerous neurons and neuroglia and minimum nerve fibers. It is thrown in numerous elevations and depressions to increase the surface area greatly. The elevations are called gyri and depressions are known as sulci. The pattern of the sulci and gyri is not constant and may differ in right and left hemispheres of the same brain. Some major sulci are as follows.

Lateral Sulcus or Sylvian Fissure

The lateral sulcus is located on the inferior and superolateral surfaces. It consists of a stem and three rami. The stem begins at the base of the brain in the vallecula and extends laterally to cut the inferolateral border. On reaching the superolateral surface, it divides into three rami (Fig. 96.3). The posterior ramus of the lateral sulcus is long and continues backwards in the parietal lobe. It can be marked on the surface by drawing a seven cm long line from the pterion to the parietal eminence. The anterior and ascending rami are short. They project in the inferior frontal gyrus. The insula or island of Reil and the limen insulae are in the floor of the lateral sulcus. The parts of cerebral hemisphere surrounding the lateral sulcus on the superolateral surface are called opercula since they cover the insula.

Contents of Lateral Sulcus

The lateral sulcus contains free margin of lesser wing of sphenoid, sphenoparietal sinus, middle cerebral artery and its cortical branches in addition to deep and superficial middle cerebral veins

Central Sulcus or Fissure of Rolando

This sulcus is an important landmark for demarcating the sensory and motor cortex on the superolateral surface. It begins at the superomedial border slightly (one cm) behind the midpoint and passes downward, forward and laterally at an angle of 70° to the median plane. Its lower end lies slightly above the posterior ramus of lateral sulcus.

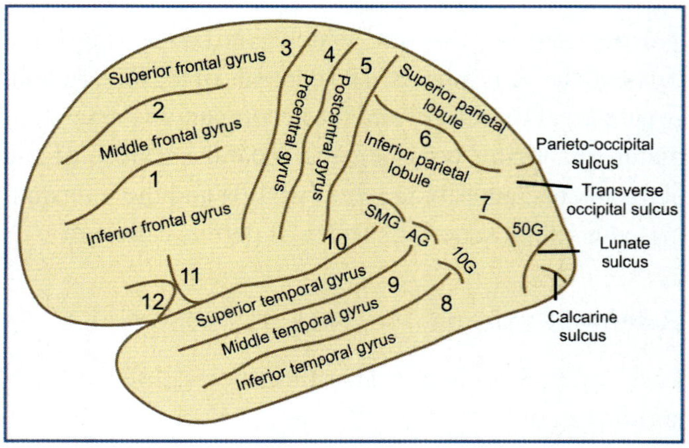

Fig. 96.3: Sulci and gryi on superolateral surface of cerebral hemispheres. (1) Inferior frontal sulcus, (2) Superior frontal sulcus, (3) Precentral sulcus, (4) Central sulcus, (5) Post-central sulcus, (6) Intraparietal sulcus, (7) Lateral occipital sulcus, (8) Inferior temporal sulcus, (9) Superior temporal sulcus, (10) Posterior ramus of lateral sulcus, (11) Ascending ramus of lateral sulcus, (12) Anterior ramus of lateral sulcus (SMG-Supramarginal gyrus, AG-Angular gyrus, SOG-Superior occipital gyrus, IOG-Inferior occipital gyrus)

Surface Marking

Take a point about one cm behind the midpoint of the line joining the nasion and inion. Draw another line from this point at an angle of 70° directed downward, forward and laterally for a distance of eight to ten cm.

Parieto-occipital Sulcus

This sulcus lies on the medial surface mainly but cuts the superomedial margin about four cm in front of the occipital pole and appears for a short distance on the superolateral surface.

Demarcation of Lobes on Superolateral Surface (Fig. 96.1)

With the help of the lateral, central and parieto-occipital sulci, the preoccipital notch and two imaginary lines, it is possible to divide the superolateral surface of the cerebrum in four lobes. The central sulcus is prolonged till it touches the posterior ramus of lateral sulcus. An imaginary vertical line is drawn from the point of parieto-occipital sulcus on the superomedial border to the preoccipital notch on the inferolateral margin (preoccipital notch lies about five cm in front of the occipital pole). The posterior ramus of the lateral sulcus is extended to touch the vertical line.

a. The frontal lobe lies in front of the central sulcus and above the posterior ramus of lateral sulcus.
b. The parietal lobe is bounded in front by central sulcus, behind by the vertical imaginary line, above by superomedial border and below by posterior ramus of lateral sulcus and its backward extension.
c. The occipital lobe lies behind the vertical imaginary line
d. The temporal lobe lies below the posterior ramus of the lateral sulcus and its extension. It is limited behind by the lower part of the vertical line.

Sulci and Gyri on Superolateral Surface (Fig. 96.3)

Frontal Lobe

a. The precentral sulcus runs parallel to and one fingerbreadth in front of the central sulcus. The cortex between the precentral and central culcu is known as precentral gyrus.
b. In front of precentral sulcus the frontal lobe presents superior and inferior frontal sulci, which run horizontally forwards. These two sulci, subdivide the frontal lobe into superior, middle and inferior frontal gyri, which are disposed in anteroposterior plane.
c. The inferior frontal gyrus is subdivided into following three parts by the ascending and anterior rami of the lateral sulcus: pars orbitalis below the anterior ramus, pars triangularis (frontal operculum) between the anterior and ascending rami and pars operculris posterior to ascending ramus.

Parietal Lobe

a. The postcentral sulcus runs parallel to and one fingerbreadth behind the central sulcus. The cortical area between these two sulci is known as postcentral gyrus.
b. Behind the postcentral sulcus the parietal lobe presents an intraparietal sulcus, which divides the lobe into superior and inferior parietal lobules.
c. The inferior parietal lobule shows three gyri: supramarginal, angular and arcus parietotemporalis. The supramarginal gyrus surrounds the upturned posterior end of posterior ramus of lateral sulcus. The angular gyrus and arcus parietotemporalis surround the posterior ends of the superior and inferior temporal sulci.

Temporal Lobe

Below the posterior ramus of lateral sulcus, the temporal lobe shows superior and inferior temporal sulci, which subdivide the lobe into superior, middle and inferior temporal gyri.

Occipital Lobe

a. The lunate sulcus in front of the occipital pole. It is very much curved with forward convexity.
b. The lateral occipital sulcus runs forwards from the lunate sulcus towards the line of demarcation between parietal and occipital lobes.
c. A small transverse occipital sulcus enters the occipital lobe from the superomedial border just behind the parieto-occipital sulcus.
d. Calcarine sulcus may cut the occipital lobe and reach the superolateral surface. In such cases the end of the calcarine sulcus is surrounded by the lunate sulcus.

e. The upper end of the parieto-occipital sulcus cuts the superomedial border and the area surrounding it is called the arcus parieto-occipitalis (so named since it belongs to both occipital and parietal lobes).

Insula (Island of Reil)

The word insula means hidden. The insula is the submerged part of the cerebral cortex in the depths of the stem and posterior ramus of the lateral sulcus. It forms the floor of the lateral sulcus. It is surrounded by the circular sulcus except at its apex. The surface of the insula is marked by a number of sulci and gyri. The middle cerebral blood vessels lie on its surface. The insular cortex is continuous with the anterior perforated substance at the limen insulae or gyrus ambiens, which forms the apex of the insula. On its internal aspect the insular cortex is very close to the lateral surface of the lentiform nucleus, the structures intervening between the two, being, extreme capsule, claustrum and the external capsule. There is considerable uncertainty about the function of insula. It is assumed that parainsular cortex bears the gustatory area.

Opercula of Insula

The parts of the superolateral surface covering the insula are called opercula or lids. The frontal operculum lies between the anterior and ascending rami of the lateral sulcus. The frontoparietal operculum is between ascending and posterior rami. The temporal operculum lies below the posterior ramus of lateral sulcus. The cortex of the insula is continuous with that of its opercula at the circular sulcus.

Medial Surface of Cerebral Hemisphere

The features of the medial surface include the sulci and gyri as well as the corpus callosum and the midline structures below it (Fig. 96.4). The most prominent landmark on the medial surface is the corpus callosum, which connects the right and left hemispheres. It consists of the genu, trunk and the splenium. The genu is the anterior curved part of the corpus callosum. It continues backward and inferiorly as the rostrum, which reaches the upper end of lamina terminalis. The septum pellucidum stretches between the concave surfaces of the trunk, genu and rostrum of corpus callosum and the fornix, which is a curved band of white matter lying on the superior surface of thalamus. The thalamus and hypothalamus lie below the fornix and form the lateral wall of the third ventricle. At the anterior extremity of the thalamus, the interventricular foramen is located between the anterior column of fornix in front and the anterior tubercle of thalamus behind. In the anterior wall of the third ventricle, (formed by the lamina terminalis) there is anterior commissure at the point of continuity between the lamina terminalis and rostrum of corpus callosum. The lower end of the lamina terminalis is attached to the optic chiasma. The hypophysis is suspended from the floor of the third ventricle and the pineal gland is related to its posterior wall.

Sulci and Gyri on Medial Surface (Fig. 96.4)

a. The long cingulate sulcus is located 1 cm above and parallel to the corpus collosum. Its curved anterior end starts below the genu and it posterior end turns towards the superomedial border just behind the paracentral lobule. The cingulate gyrus lies between the cingulate sulcus and the callosal sulcus (seen just above the corpus collosum).
b. The paracentral lobule is located around the central sulcus. It is continuous with both the precentral and postcentral gyri across the superomedial border. Hence, paracentral lobule belongs to both frontal and perietal lobes.
c. The medial frontal gyrus is the large anterior part of the medial surface of the frontal lobe.
d. The paraterminal gyrus lies in front of the lamina terminalis and parolfactory gyrus lies in front of the paraterminal gyrus. The anterior and posterior parolfactory sulci bound the parolfactory gyrus.

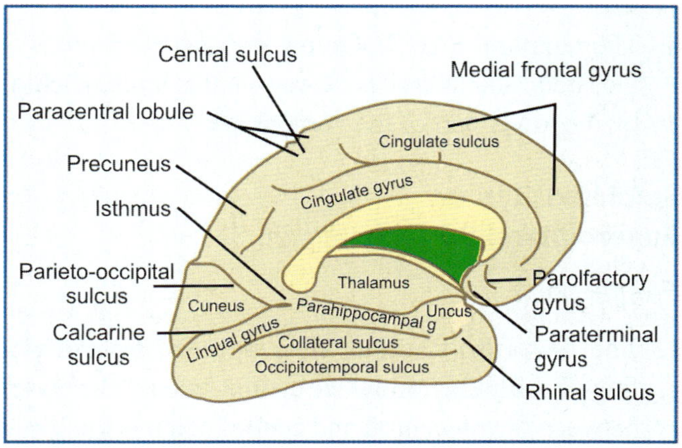

Fig. 96.4: Sulci and gryi on medial and tentorial surfaces of left cerebral hemisphere

e. The parieto-occipital sulcus lies on the posterior part of the medial surface. It begins on the superomedial border about five cm anterior to the occipital pole and descends anteriorly to meet the calcarine fissure below and behind the splenium. This sulcus demarcates the perietal and occipital lobes on the medial surface.
f. The calcarine sulcus starts near the occipital pole and extends forward lying a little above the medial occipital border. It ends by joining the parieto-occipital sulcus. It is very deep and projects in the posterior horn of lateral ventricle as calcar avis.
g. The precuneus is the quadrilateral area in front of the parieto-occipital sulcus and the upturned end of the cingulate sulcus. It forms the medial surface of the parietal lobe.
h. The cuneus is a triangular area of cortex bounded by the superomedial border, parieto-occipital sulcus and the calcarine sulcus. It forms the medial surface of the occipital lobe.

Sulci and Gyri on Inferior Surface (Fig. 96.2)

Orbital Surface

a. The olfactory sulcus is present close to the medial margin. The olfactory bulb and tract lie in this sulcus.
b. Gyrus rectus is the area medial to the olfactory sulcus.
c. The remaining orbital surface is divided into anterior, posterior, medial and lateral orbital gyri by an H-shaped orbital sulcus.

Tentorial Surface

a. The collateral sulcus is a long sulcus that begins near the occipital pole and runs forward almost parallel to the calcarine sulcus. It reaches as forward as the rhinal sulcus, which demarcates the uncus on the medial surface of the temporal lobe from the temporal pole. The collateral sulcus projects in the inferior horn of the lateral ventricle as the collateral eminence.
b. The lingual gyrus lies between the collateral and calcarine sulci.
c. The parahippocampal gyrus lies medial to the collateral sulcus. It is continuous anteriorly with the uncus and posteriorly with the cingulate gyrus through the isthmus, which winds round the splenium and forms a connecting link between the medial and inferior surfaces.

Types of Sulci

There are four main types of sulci on the cerebral hemisphere.

a. Limiting sulcus separates the areas of cortex differing in structure and functions, for example, the central sulcus.
b. Axial sulcus develops in the long axis of a rapidly growing cortical area. The posterior part of the calcarine sulcus, which is a mere fold in the center of the visual cortex, is the example of the axial sulcus.
c. Complete sulcus is the one that reaches the wall of the ventricle to produce an elevation there. There are two examples of this type. The posterior part of the calcarine sulcus produces calcar avis in the posterior horn and the collateral sulcus produces collateral eminence in the inferior horn of the lateral ventricle.
d. Secondary sulcus is the one that depends on other factors for its formation. Examples of the secondary sulci are the lateral sulcus and the parieto-occipital sulcus. The submerging of insula is responsible for the formation of lateral sulcus and the backward growth of corpus callosum is responsible for the formation of parieto-occipital sulcus.

Functional Areas of Cerebral Cortex

Different areas of cerebral cortex perform different functions. The functional areas are classified according to Brodmann in terms of numbers.

Motor Areas (Figs 96.5 and 96.6)

a. The primary motor area (area 4) occupies the entire precentral gyrus and the anterior part of the paracentral lobule on the medial surface of the hemisphere.

   Histologically, it is characterized by presence of giant pyramidal cells of Betz in the inner pyramidal layer (fifth layer) of the cerebrum. The pyramidal cells that give origin to the corticospinal and corticonuclear (corticobulbar) fibers are known as upper motor neurons. Majority of corticospinal fibers ends on the anterior horn cells of spinal cord indirectly via internuncial neurons. The corticonuclear fibers end on the motor nuclei of the cranial nerves in the brainstem. The motor area controls the voluntary movements of the opposite half of the body. The body is represented upside down. The sequence from below upwards, is

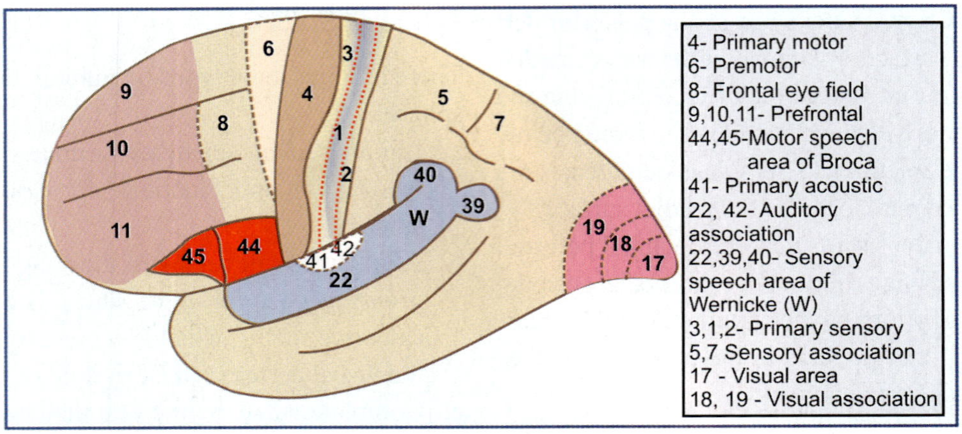

Fig. 96.5: Functional areas of Brodmann on superolateral surface of left cerebral hemisphere

pharynx, larynx, tongue, lips, face, neck, fingers with hand, wrist, elbow, shoulder, trunk, and hip in the precentral gyrus. The leg and perineum are represented in the paracentral lobule. The extent of the cortical area for the movements depends on the skill of movements. Thus, in the upper limb the hand has larger representation and among fingers the thumb has the largest representation. The representation of the human body in proportion to the area of the motor cortex is known as motor homunculus, which in Latin means "the little man inside."

The motor area is supplied by cortical branches of middle cerebral and of anterior cerebral arteries. Injury to the motor cortex due to vascular lesions results in upper motor neuron (UMN) paralysis of either the face or the hand or one limb (monoplegia) on the opposite side of the body.

b. Premotor cortex (area 6) is located in front of the precentral gyrus. It occupies the posterior parts of the superior, middle and inferior frontal gyri. The neurons in this area give origin to corticospinal and cortico-nuclear fibers, which descend along with the similar fibers of the motor cortex. This area is responsible for the performance of skillful acts, which are learnt through repetitive efforts. Lesion in this area leads to apraxia, which is characterized by impairment of performance of skillful movements in the absence of voluntary motor paralysis.
c. Supplementary motor area is present on the medial surface in the medial frontal gyrus. The body is represented in anteroposterior direction (in head to foot order).

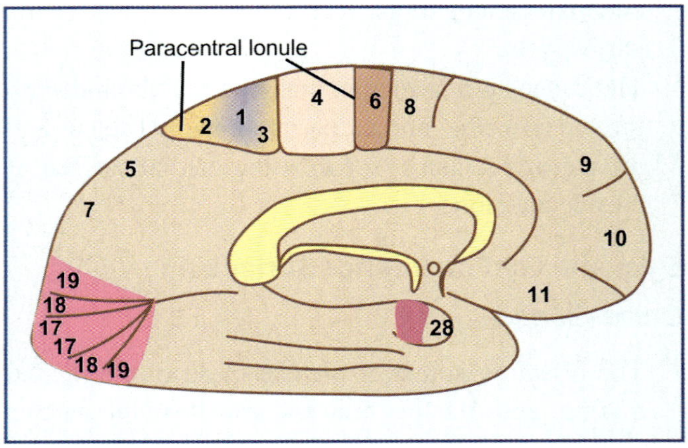

Fig. 96.6: Functional areas of Brodmann on medial surface of left cerebral hemisphere (Note that paracentral lobule is highly exagerrated in the figure. Area 28 is entorhinal area. For other areas refer to Figure 96.5)

d. Frontal eye field (area 8) lies in front of the premotor area in the middle frontal gyrus. It is connected to the visual cortex of the same side and of the opposite side. It is projected to the superior colliculi and pontine gaze center in the reticular formation and other oculomotor related nuclei in the brainstem. It is necessary for the conjugate movements of the eyes (stimulation causes movements of both eyes to the opposite side). Lesion in this area results in difficulty in voluntarily moving the eyes to the opposite side. So, the eyes move towards the side of lesion.
e. Prefrontal cortex (areas 9, 10, 11 and 12) occupies the anterior part of frontal lobe (area 12 is largely present on orbital surface of frontal lobe). It is regarded as the association cortex. It has numerous connections with cortex of the other three lobes. There are to and

fro connections with dorsomedial thalamic nucleus. Lesion in prefrontal cortex results in personality change due to impaired capacity in abstract thinking, judgement, foresight and tactfulness.

f. Motor speech area of Broca (area 44, 45) occupies the opercular and triangular portions of the inferior frontal gyrus of the dominant hemisphere. Detail description of motor speech area is given with cortical speech areas (vide infra).

Sensory Areas (Figs 96.5 and 96.6)

a. Primary sensory area occupies the postcentral gyrus and extends in the posterior part of the paracentral lobule. The Brodmann's areas 3,1,2 are arranged in anteroposterior order in these gyri. The sensory cortex is granular in type since it contains more granule cells and less pyramidal cells. It receives profuse thalamocortical connections from the nuclei VPM and VPL of thalamus. The contralateral body is represented upside down in the sensory cortex (sensory homunculus). Injury to sensory cortex results in altered or impaired sensations and not loss of sensations in the opposite half of body.
b. Sensory association area (5 and 7) is located in superior parietal lobule on the superolateral surface.
c. Visual or striate area (area 17) includes the calcarine sulcus, cuneus and lingual gyrus in the occipital lobe. The visual cortex is very thin hence it is possible to see the stria of Genneri on macroscopic sectioning of the cortex in the calcarine sulcus. The stria consists of the thick outer band of Baillarger in the fourth or inner granular layer of the cortex. The visual cortex receives the optic radiation, which brings impulses from the temporal half of ipsilateral retina and nasal half of contralateral retina. Thus, the left half of field of vision is represented in right visual area and right half is represented in left visual area. Macula lutea of retina (area of highest visual acuity) is represented in the occipital pole.
d. The visual association cortex or parastriate and peristriate cortex (area 18 and 19) surround the striate cortex. The association areas help in interpretation of visual impulses in the light of past experiences. Areas 18 and 19 form the occipital eye field. The corticotectal fibers originate in both the visual and visual association areas and terminate on the superior colliculi. Entire visual area is supplied by cortical branches of posterior cerebral artery.
e. Primary acoustic or auditory cortex (area 41 and 42) is concealed from superolateral surface because it occupies the anterior transverse temporal gyri (Heschl's gyri) on the superior aspect of the superior temporal gyrus. The acoustic cortex receives auditory radiations from both sides. The acoustic association area lies in the posterior transverse temporal gyri and area 22 lies on the lateral aspect of the superior temporal gyrus. The association areas are essential for the interpretation of the sound impulses in the light of past experiences.
f. The entorhinal or olfactory area (Brodmann's area 28) is located in the uncus, which is the anteromedial part of parahippocampal gyrus. It is bounded by rhinal sulcus laterally and anterior perforated substance medially.

Cortical Speech Areas

The cortical areas of speech are present on the dominant hemisphere. So, in a right-handed person the left cerebral hemisphere is responsible for language function. The dominant hemisphere is referred to as the verbal or talking hemisphere. There are two types of speech areas, motor and sensory. The motor speech centre is located in front of the central sulcus while the sensory speech centers are located behind the central sulcus. All the cortical speech centers receive arterial blood from the middle cerebral artery.

Motor Speech Area

The motor speech area or Broca's area is located in the inferior frontal gyrus. It corresponds to Brodmann's areas 44 and 45 in the dominant hemisphere. It is connected to the motor area controlling the movements of the vocal cords in the precentral gyrus. It is also connected to the sensory speech areas by arcuate fasciculus (a bundle of association fibers). The Broca's area is responsible for spoken speech (fluency of speech).

Sensory Speech Areas

There are three areas for sensory speech. Area 22 is located on the posterior part of superior temporal gyrus.

The angular gyrus (area 39) and supramarginal gyrus (area 40) are located on the inferior parietal lobule. There are different views as to the location and definition of Wernicke's speech area. Some believe that it coincides with posterior part of superior temporal gyrus. According to 38th edition of Grey's Anatomy and Davidson's Principles and Practice of Medicine, Wernicke's area occupies a large parieto-temporal area, which includes area 22 (posterior part of superior temporal gyrus), area 39 (angular gyrus) and area 40 (supramarginal gyrus). This area is important in comprehension of received speech and selection of words to express ideas. It can be equated to a dictionary. Area 22 comprehends spoken language and recognizes familiar sounds. Area 39 is responsible for visual speech or reading and area 40 is responsible for recognition of and naming of the objects by touch and proprioception. All these areas are interconnected and connected to the motor speech area by the arcuate fasciculus.

Clinical Highlights

Aphasia means disturbance in the ability to speak or comprehend or write or read the words.

a. The lesion of Broca's area causes motor aphasia (expressive or nonfluent aphasia). It is characterized by distorted and hesitant speech even though the peripheral speech apparatus is normal. However, the comprehension is preserved.
b. The lesion of area 22 produces word deafness (fluent aphasia), in which the patient speaks without understanding what is spoken.
c. The lesion of area 39 gives rise to word blindness in which there is reading difficulty (alexia) and writing difficulty (agraphia). In addition, the patient experiences right-left confusion, finger agnosis (inability to select or name own or another's finger) and dyscalculia (difficulty with simple mathematics).
d. The lesion of area 40 causes tactile agnosia (inability to name objects by touch).
e. The lesion in the arcuate fasciculus results in conduction aphasia, where repetition of spoken language is extremely difficult though comprehension is intact and speech is fluent.
f. Lesion of both sensory and motor speech areas results in global aphasia in which the patient neither can speak nor can understand spoken speech.

97 Blood Supply of Brain

The brain is richly supplied with blood through the vertebrobasilar and internal carotid arteries. The oxygen consumption of the neural tissue is very high (25% of the oxygen that is breathed in is cerebrally used!). Acute arrest of circulation produces loss of consciousness in about seven seconds. The cerebrovascular accidents (CVA) due to infarction, hemorrhage and embolism result in stroke, in which the entire half of the body or a limb or one-half of the face is suddenly paralyzed. The persons in whom there is narrowing of cerebral arteries (due to hypertension, atherosclerosis and diabetes) are more prone to stroke. The common causes of cerebral hemorrhage are aneurysm of major arteries or small aretriolar aneurysms due to hypertension or arteriovenous malformations. Stroke, either causes death or results in paralysis. In this condition, neural tissue is rapidly lost for want of oxygen. According to Jeffrey L Saver, when someone suffers from stroke, 1.9 million nerve cells die each minute, resulting in the loss of around 15 billion synapses and 7.5 miles of nerve fibers. This tells us the importance of the blood supply of the brain.

Intracranial Course of Internal Carotid Artery (ICA)

The internal carotid artery ascends in the carotid canal and enters the middle cranial fossa through the opening of the foramen lacerum. It runs forwards lying close to the floor of cavernous sinus. Here, it is accompanied by the abducent nerve. It pierces the dural roof of the cavernous sinus and bends sharply backwards and upwards to terminate at the vallecula of cerebrum into the middle and anterior cerebral arteries. Thus, the intracranial course of the artery can be divided into intrapetrous, intracavernous and supraclinoid parts. The artery shows multiple bends, which produce S-shaped shadow called the carotid siphon on an angiography. These bends in the artery help in damping down its pulsations in the cranial cavity. The aneurysm of the intracavernous and supraclinoid parts of ICA may compress the optic chiasma. Trauma to the ICA in cavernous sinus leads to the formation of arterio-venous fistula that results in pulsating exophthalmos.

Branches

a. The intrapetrous part gives origin to superior and inferior carotico-tympanic branches which enter the middle ear. The pterygoid artery is inconstant. When present it anastomoses with the artery of the pterygoid canal (from the maxillary or its greater palatine branch) in the perygoid canal.
b. The intracavernous part gives branches to the trigeminal ganglion, hypophyseal branches to the pituitary gland and meningeal branches.
c. The branches of supraclinoid part (Fig. 97.1) are, ophthalmic artery, posterior communicating artery, anterior choroidal artery, direct branches to the genu of internal capsule and the terminal branches (anterior and middle cerebral arteries).

Vertebrobasilar Arteries (Fig. 97.1)

The right and left vertebral arteries unite with each other at the lower margin of pons to form the basilar artery. The branches of fourth or intracranial part of vertebral artery supply not only the hindbrain but also the spinal cord (for description of Vertebral Artery refer Chapter 81).

Basilar Artery

The basilar artery runs on the median sulcus on the ventral surface of pons and divides into right and left posterior

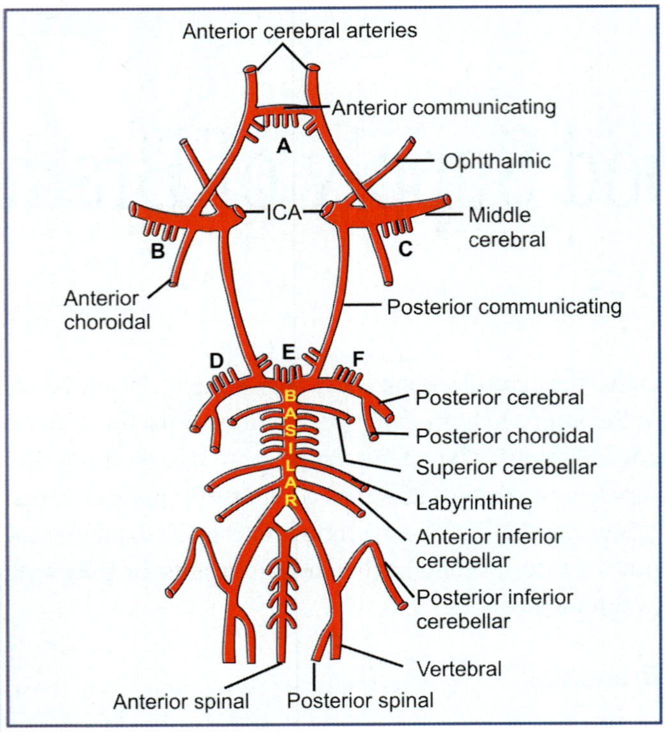

Fig. 97.1: Circle of Willis and intracranial branches of internal carotid and vertebrobasilar arteries. Groups of central branches of circle of Willis: A-Anteromedian, B and C-Anterolateral, D and F-Posterolateral, E-Posteromedian

cerebral arteries at upper margin of pons. Its bilateral branches include superior cerebellar, pontine, anterior inferior cerebellar (AICA) and labyrinthine. In 83 percent of cases, labyrinthine artery originates from the anterior inferior cerebellar artery for which reason AICA is termed as cerebellolabyrinthine artery.

Circle of Willis (Circulus Arteriosus)

The arterial circle at the base of the brain is an anastomosis between the internal carotid and the vertebrobasilar system of arteries. It is polygonal in shape and is located in the interpeduncular cistern.

Formation (Fig. 97.1)

The anterior communicating artery, which connects the right and left anterior cerebral arteries, forms anterior boundary of the circle of Willis. The anterior cerebral artery forms the anterolateral part on each side. The lateral part is formed by the termination of internal carotid artery on each side. The circle is completed posteriorly by the bifurcation of basilar artery into the right and left posterior cerebral arteries. Posterolaterally, the posterior communicating artery is the connecting link between the internal carotid and posterior cerebral arteries (note that middle cerebral artery does not enter into the formation of the circle).

Functional Importance

This arterial circle equalises the pressure of the blood flow to the two sides of the brain, as it is the main collateral channel.

Variations

Variations are very common in the circle of Willis. One of the arteries may be underdeveloped or absent. The hemodynamic balance of the circle is disturbed by such variations. The posterior communicating artery enlarges to compensate for the absent or the unusually small proximal segment of posterior cerebral artery. Similarly, the anterior communicating artery enlarges to compensate for the absent or unusually small anterior cerebral artery. Sometimes, the anterior communicating channel may be double.

Berry Aneurysm (Fig. 97.2)

The berry aneurysm is a localized dilatation on one of the arteries of the circle of Willis due to congenital muscular

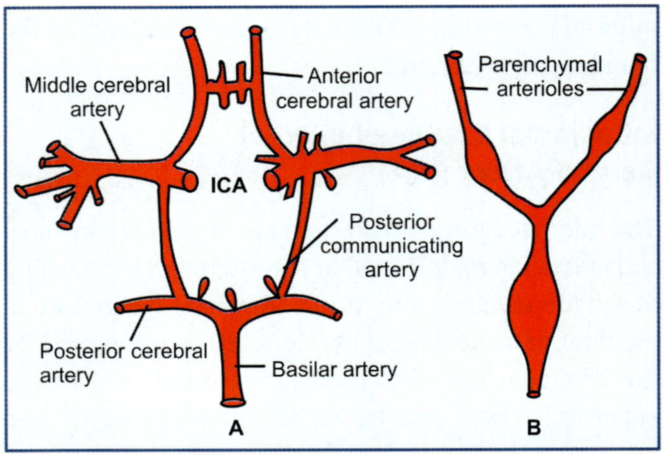

Fig. 97.2: Types and locations of aneurysms in arteries supplying brain. 'A' depicts berry (saccular) aneurysms occuring at branch points on circle of Willis. 'B' depicts Charcot-Bouchard aneurysms due to chronic hypertension occuring in parenchymal arterioles of lenticulostriate arteries

weakness. This is of common occurrence at the junction of anterior cerebral and anterior communicating arteries and at the bifurcation of internal carotid arteries. Rupture of berry aneurysm may cause life-threatening subarachnoid hemorrhage.

Branches of Circle of Willis

The central branches of the circle of Willis supply the interior of the hemisphere and hence penetrate the base of the brain at specific points. There are six groups of central branches.

a. Anteromedian branches arise from the anterior communicating and anterior cerebral arteries and perforate the lamina terminalis to supply the anterior hypothalamus.
b. The right and left anterolateral or striate branches originate mainly from the middle cerebral artery of the corresponding side (with few medial striate arteries from the anterior cerebral artery) and pierce the anterior perforated substance. The striate arteries are divided in lateral and medial groups. The medial striate branches arise from both middle cerebral and anterior cerebral arteries. The lateral striate branches arise from the middle cerebral artery.

i. The medial striate arteries of the middle cerebral artery, ascend to enter the lentiform nucleus to supply it and also the caudate nucleus and internal capsule. A large medial striate artery called recurrent artery of Heubner takes origin from the anterior cerebral artery, enters the medial part of the anterior perforated substance to supply the head of caudate nucleus, part of putamen, anterior limb of the internal capsule including the genu.
ii. The lateral striate arteries (lenticulo-striate) ascend in the external capsule to pierce the lateral surface of the lentiform nucleus. They pass through this nucleus and the internal capsule in latero-medial direction to end in the caudate nucleus (one of the lateral striate arteries, which is usually the longest, was termed by Charcot as artery of cerebral hemorrhage). The structures supplied by the lateral striate arteries are, part of anterior limb of internal capsule, part of posterior limb of internal capsule, caudate nucleus, putamen and part of globus pallidus. One of the lateral striate arteries is very long and is called deep optic artery. It supplies the optic radiation. Microaneurysms develop in the lenticulo-striate arteries in the presence of long-standing hypertension. Such aneurysms are called Charcot-Bouchard aneurysms (Fig. 97.2) and their rupture results in cerebral hemorrhage.

c. Posteromedian central arteries originate from posterior communicating and posterior cerebral arteries. They are divided in two groups. The rostral group of arteries pierces the hypophysis, infundibulum and tuberal region of hypothalamus. A few of these, called thalamoperforating arteries supply the thalamus. The caudal group of arteries pierces the posterior perforated substance to supply the mamillary bodies, subthalamus and thalamus.
d. The right and left posterolateral central branches are called thalamogeniculate arteries. They take origin from the posterior cerebral arteries and pierce the cerebral peduncle and lateral geniculate body to supply the caudal half of thalamus, geniculate bodies and most of the lateral nuclear mass of thalamus.

Choroidal Arteries

The anterior and posterior choroidal arteries are regarded as central arteries since they supply the structures inside the cerebral hemispheres.

a. The anterior choroidal artery is a branch of the internal carotid artery. From its origin, the artery passes backwards along the edge of the optic tract and crosses it twice, hence it is called the satellite artery of the optic tract. Then, it enters the inferior horn of lateral ventricle through the choroid fissure to supply the choroid plexus. In addition, it supplies the optic tract, amygdaloid complex, tail of caudate nucleus, globus pallidus, hippocampus and posterior limb of internal capsule including its retrolentiform and sublentiform parts. The anterior choroidal artery is prone to thrombosis due to its small caliber and long subarachnoid course. Its thrombosis may result in contralateral hemianesthesia, hemiparesis and hemianopia accompanied by loss of recent memory.
b. The posterior choroidal artery is a branch of the posterior cerebral artery in the region of the splenium. There are three posterior choroidal branches, one medial and two lateral. The medial posterior choroidal

artery supplies the tectum, choroid plexus of third ventricle, and thalamus. The lateral posterior choroidal arteries enter the choroid fissure and supply the choroid plexus of the central part and inferior horn of the lateral ventricle. These arteries supply the pulvinar, lateral geniculate bodies and fornix. Clinical evidence suggests that posterior choroidal arteries supply the hippocampus.

Blood Supply of Cerebral Cortex

The cortical branches of the anterior, middle and posterior cerebral arteries supply blood to the cerebral cortex (Figs 97.3 to 97.5).

Anterior Cerebral Artery

This artery arises from the internal carotid artery below the anterior perforated substance and lateral to the optic chiasma. It crosses the optic chiasma to reach the longitudinal fissure. At the anterior end of the longitudinal fissure the anterior communicating artery connects the right and left anterior cerebral arteries. Further, it winds round the front of the genu of the corpus callosum and then runs posteriorly on the superior aspect of the body of corpus callosum.

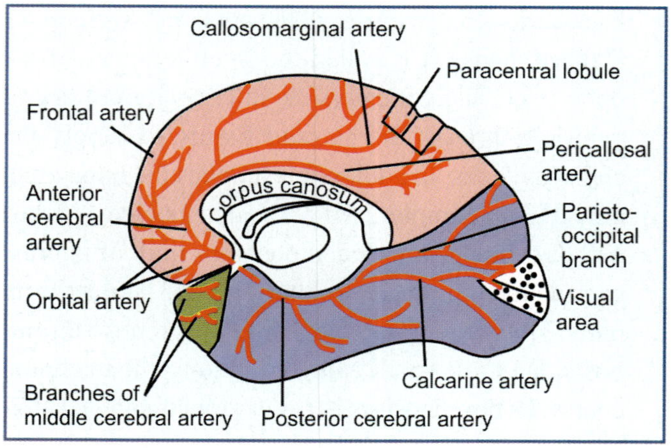

Fig. 97.3: Arterial supply of medial (inferomedial) surface of right cerebral hemisphere (Note: The course and branches of anterior cerebral artery, which supplies paracentral lobule containing motor and sensory areas for leg and perineum. The visual area receives blood from posterior cerebral artery

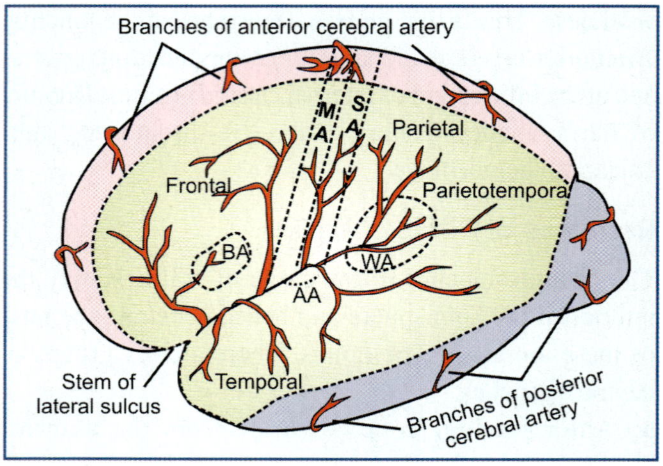

Fig. 97.4: Arterial supply of superolateral surface of left cerebral hemisphere (Note that the named branches of middle cerebral artery supply the largest territory. Note also arterial supply of functional areas. BA–Broca's area, WA–Wernicke's area, AA–Auditory area, MA–Motor area, SA–Sensory area)

Distribution

The orbital branches supply the medial half of orbital surface of the frontal lobe (olfactory bulb, olfactory gyrus and medial olfactory gyri).

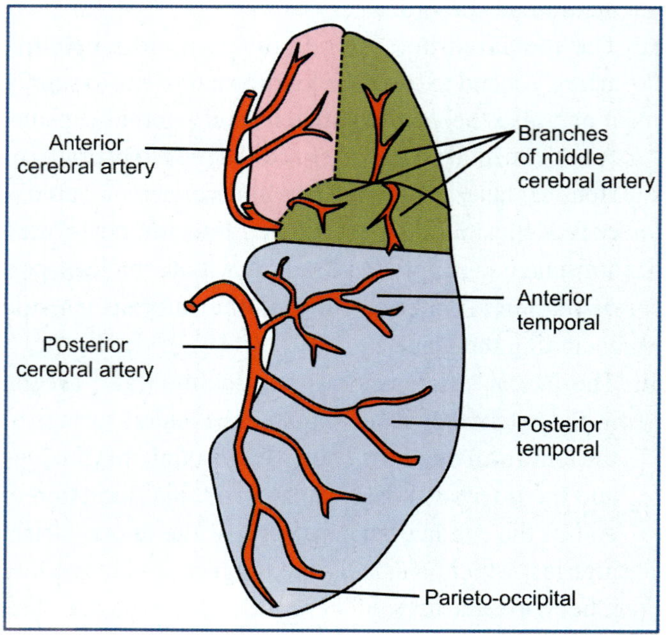

Fig. 97.5: Arterial supply of inferior surface of left cerebral hemisphere (Note that posterior cerebral artery supplies largest territory including the uncus and the temporal pole is supplied by middle cerebral artery)

The frontal branches supply the medial surface of the frontal and the parietal lobes including the paracentral lobule, cingulate gyrus, and corpus callosum.

The parietal branches supply the precuneus. The area of supply of the anterior cerebral artery flows over the superomedial margin to include one to two cm of the superolateral surface of the frontal and parietal lobes. The functional areas that receive blood from anterior cerebral artery are the motor and sensory areas for lower limb and perineum.

Middle Cerebral Artery

This artery is a continuation of internal carotid artery beyond the origin of anterior cerebral artery. It turns laterally on the anterior perforated substance to enter the stem of the lateral sulcus, where it divides into a handful of cortical branches on the surface of insula.

Distribution

The orbital branches supply the lateral half of orbital surface of frontal lobe. The frontal branches supply the superolateral surface of frontal lobe (precentral, middle and inferior frontal gyri) excluding the area supplied by anterior cerebral artery. The parietal branches supply the postcentral gyrus, inferior parietal lobule and superior parietal lobule excluding the area supplied by the anterior cerebral artery. The temporal branches supply the lateral surface of the temporal lobe excluding the inferior temporal gyrus but including the temporal pole. The functional areas that receive blood from the middle cerebral artery are, the motor and sensory areas (upper limb, trunk and face), premotor area, frontal eyefield, auditory area and the speech centers in the dominant hemisphere.

Posterior Cerebral Artery

The right and left posterior cerebral arteries are the terminal branches of basilar artery. Each passes laterally around the crus cerebri of the midbrain, where it receives the posterior communicating artery. It continues along the lateral aspect of the midbrain and enters the supratentorial compartment through the tentorial notch. Then, it courses on the tentorial surface of temporal lobe lying on the parahippocampal gyrus giving cortical branches, which supply the tentorial surface including the uncus and the medial surface of occipital lobe.

Distribution

The posterior temporal branches supply to the inferior surface of temporal lobe, uncus, and occipito-temporal and lingual gyri. They also send twigs to inferior temporal gyrus excluding the temporal pole. The calcarine and parieto-occipital branches supply the medial surface of the occipital lobe, which includes the cuneus. These cortical branches send twigs to superolateral surface of the occipital lobe. The visual cortex is the important functional area supplied by the posterior cerebral artery. The occipital pole receives blood from the anastomosis between the branches of posterior cerebral and middle cerebral arteries. Therefore, in the occlusion of the posterior cerebral artery there is macular sparing.

Clinical Highlights

It is essential to understand the effects of loss of blood supply due to occlusion of central branches and due to occlusion of cortical branches of the three main cerebral arteries.

Occlusion of Anterior Cerebral Artery

a. The loss of cortical supply to paracentral lobule results in contralateral spastic monoplegia (lower limb), altered sensorium in lower limb and urinary incontinence. There may be gradual change in personality and impaired cognition due to damage to orbital cortex of prefrontal lobe.
b. Occlusion of medial striate branches (Heubner's artery) may lead to contralateral paresis of upper limb, tongue and lower facial weakness due to deficient blood supply to genu of internal capsule.

Occlusion of Middle Cerebral Artery

a. The loss of cortical supply results in contralateral spastic paralysis of trunk, upper limb and lower part of face with altered sensorium, conjugate deviation of the eyes to the side of the lesion (due to involvement of posterior part of middle frontal gyrus), global aphasia (if dominant hemisphere is affected) and hemi-attention or neglect (if non-dominant hemisphere is affected).

b. There may be gradual changes in personality due to loss of arterial supply to prefrontal lobe.
c. Occlusion of deep optic artery (longest lenticulostriate artery) manifests as homonymous hemianopia.
d. Occlusion of lenticulostriate arteries results in loss of supply to internal capsule leading to contralateral spastic hemiplegia, paralysis of lower half of face and altered sensorium.

Occlusion of Posterior Cerebral Artery

The loss of cortical supply results in contralateral homonymous hemianopia with macular sparing. Damage to association cortex of visual area results in visual hallucinations (distortion of color vision).

Cerebral Angiography

Both internal carotid and vertebral arteries are used for cerebral angiography. The carotid angiography is performed by direct needle puncture of the internal carotid arteries. The right vertebral artery is approached by passing a catheter in succession through the femoral, external iliac, common iliac, abdominal aorta, thoracic aorta, arch of aorta, brachiocephalic and right subclavian arteries. For the left vertebral artery after the arch of aorta the catheter passes into the left subclavian artery. The contrast material is injected under general anesthesia and serial films are taken.

Venous Drainage of Cerebrum

The veins of the cerebrum are divided into external (superficial) and internal (deep) sets. The veins of the superficial set drain the surface of the cerebrum while those of deep set drain the interior of the cerebrum.

External or Superficial Veins of Cerebrum

a. The superior cerebral veins, about eight to ten in number, drain the superolateral and medial surfaces of the cerebrum. They run in forward direction to empty in the superior sagittal sinus against the flow of blood in the sinus. Tear of the superior cerebral vein results in subdural hemorrhage.
b. The superficial middle cerebral vein begins on the superolateral surface and enters the posterior ramus and the stem of the lateral sulcus. On reaching the inferior surface, it terminates in the cavernous sinus. This vein is connected to the superior sagittal sinus by a superior anastomotic vein of Trolard and to the transverse sinus by inferior anastomotic vein of Labbe.
c. The deep middle cerebral vein receives veins from the insula in the depths of the lateral sulcus and runs medially to reach the base of the brain at the vallecula.
d. The anterior cerebral vein accompanies the anterior cerebral artery on the superior aspect of corpus callosum. It reaches the anterior perforated substance at the base of the brain.
e. The basal vein is formed at the valleculla of cerebrum on the anterior perforated substance by the union of anterior cerebral vein, deep middle cerebral vein and the striate veins, which come out through the anterior perforated substance. It runs posteriorly along with the optic tract and crosses the crus cerebri to open in the great cerebral vein under the splenium. It receives tributaries from the interpeduncular fossa, inferior horn of lateral ventricle, parahippocampal gyrus and midbrain.
f. The inferior cererbral veins drain the orbital and tentorial surfaces. Those of the orbital surface join the superior cerebral veins to open in superior sagittal sinus. Those on the tentorial surface open in basal vein and mainly empty in transverse sinus.

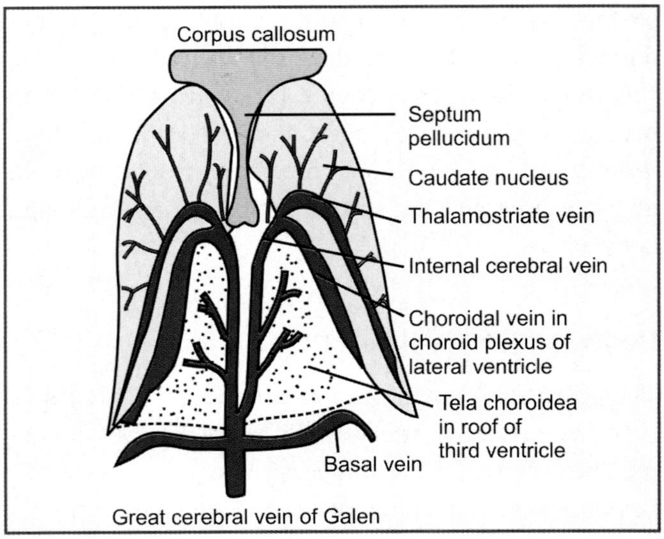

Fig. 97.6: Formation, course and termination of internal cerebral veins

Deep Veins of Cerebrum (Fig. 97.6)

a. The thalamostriate vein travels in the floor of the lateral ventricle between the thalamus and the caudate nucleus up to the level of the interventricular foramen. It drains the corpus striatum, internal capsule, thalamus, fornix and septum pellucidum.
b. The choroidal vein spirals along the entire choroid plexus of the lateral ventricle. It receives veins from the hippocampus, fornix, and corpus callosum on its way to the interventricular foramen.
c. The internal cerebral vein is formed on each side at the level of the interventricular foramen by the union of thalamostriate and choroidal veins. The right and left internal cerebral veins run backwards in the tela choroidea of the third ventricle and unite with each other below the splenium to form the great cerebral vein.
d. The great cerebral vein of Galen is a very short vein, which is located in the cisterna ambiens under the splenium. Its main tributaries are the right and left basal veins. It also receives veins from cerebellum, pineal gland and tectum. It emerges from beneath the splenium to open in the anterior end of the straight sinus. The site of its junction with the straight sinus is marked by a sinusoidal plexus, which regulates the blood flow from the great cerebral vein into the straight sinus.

98 White Matter of Cerebrum

The interior of each cerebral hemisphere consists of a core of white matter, which is made of myelinated nerve fibers. These fibers are of three types.

Classification of White Matter

a. The association fibers connect the different parts of the cerebral cortex of the same hemisphere, to each other. The short association fibers connect the adjacent gyri to each other. The long association fibers connect the gyri located at a distance from each other.
b. The commissural fibers cross the midline and connect the identical parts of the two hemispheres.
c. The projection fibers connect the cerebral cortex to other regions of central nervous system by corticopetal or ascending and corticofugal or descending fibers.

Examples of Long Association Fibers (Fig. 98.1)

a. The cingulum (girdle shaped) lies within the cingulate gyrus. It extends from the paraterminal gyrus to the uncus. The cingulum is part of the Papez circuit, which is part of the limbic system.
b. The uncinate fasciculus (arcuate fasciculus) is a curved fiber bundle, which connects the inferior frontal gyrus and the orbital gyri of the frontal lobe to the cortex of the temporal lobe. Thus, it connects the sensory and motor speech areas to each other in the dominant hemisphere.
c. The superior longitudinal fasciculus is a long bundle that begins in the frontal lobe and arches back via the parietal lobe to the occipital lobe from where it turns in the temporal lobe. Thus, it connects the occipital lobe to the frontal eye field.
d. The inferior longitudinal fasciculus connects the occipital lobe to the temporal lobe.

Examples of Commissural Fibers

a. The anterior commissure connects the right and left temporal lobes. It is of the shape of a cupid's bow. It crosses the midline in the upper part of the lamina terminalis anterior to the columns of fornix. Its fibers divide in anterior and posterior bundles. The anterior bundle connects the anterior perforated substance and the olfactory tracts of the two sides. The posterior bundle at first passes through the head of the caudate nucleus and then inclines posteriorly in the lentiform nucleus to enter the middle and inferior gyri of the temporal lobe.
b. The posterior and habenular commissures are part of epithalamus and lie in the posterior part of the roof of third ventricle.
c. The hippocampal commissure connects the hippocampus of the two sides to each other.
d. The corpus callosum is the largest commissure of the brain.

Corpus Callosum

This is located in the floor of the longitudinal fissure. It is of the shape of an arch. The corpus callosum consists

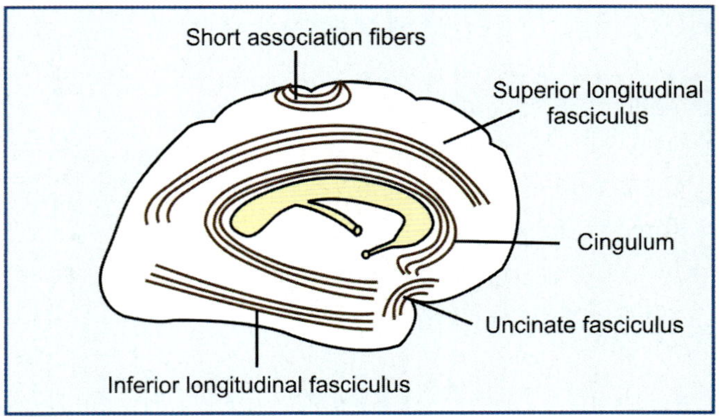

Fig. 98.1: Association fibers in the white matter of cerebrum

of four parts. Its anterior end is called the genu, the central part is the trunk and the posterior bulbous part forms the splenium. The fourth part is the rostrum, which is the prolongation from the genu to the upper end of lamina terminalis.

Relations

a. The superior aspect of the corpus callosum is covered with indusium griseum, in which medial and lateral longitudinal striae are embedded. The induseum griseum is the rudimentary gray matter.
b. Below the splenium, between it and the superior colliculi and pineal gland lies the transverse fissure through which the tela choroidea of the third and lateral ventricles, enters. The posterior choroidal arteries enter the fissure and the internal cerebral veins leave it to unite in the cisterna ambiens to form the great cerebral vein beneath the splenium.
c. The anterior and superior aspects of the corpus callosum are in close relation to the anterior cerebral vessels.
d. The inferior aspect of the corpus callosum gives attachment to the septum pellucidum anteriorly and the fornix posteriorly.
e. The rostrum and genu form the boundaries of the anterior horn and the trunk forms the roof of the central part of the lateral ventricle.

Connections (Fig. 98.2)

The fibers of the corpus callosum interconnect the corresponding parts of all lobes of the two hemispheres.

a. The fibers passing through the rostrum connect the orbital surfaces of the frontal lobes.
b. The fibers passing through the genu interconnect the two frontal lobes and they form a fork-like bundle called forceps minor.
c. The fibers passing through the splenium interconnect the occipital lobes and form the forceps major. The forceps major bulges in the medial wall of the posterior horn of lateral ventricle to give rise to an elevation called the bulb.
d. Majority of fibers from the trunk run transversely and intersect with the fibers of the corona radiata. Some fibers of the trunk and adjacent splenium, which do not intersect with corona radiata, are known as the tapetum. The tapetum turns inferiorly and forms the roof and lateral wall of the posterior horn and lateral wall of inferior horn of the lateral ventricle.

Arterial Supply

The rostrum, genu and body of corpus callosum receive bilateral branches from anterior cerebral artery. The splenium receives branches from the posterior cerebral arteries.

Split-brain Syndrome (Disconnection Syndrome)

Commissurotomy or transection of corpus callosum causes split-brain syndrome. The non-dominant hemisphere (right) is dissociated from the dominant hemisphere (left). The patient is unable to match an object held in one hand with that in the other, when blindfolded and is unable to correctly name objects placed in the left hand (anomia). There is alexia in the left visual field in which the verbal symbols received in the right visual cortex have no access to the language centres in the left hemisphere. Therefore, the patient can write but cannot read what is written. This symptom of alexia without agraphia also occurs in infarction of the splenium in occlusion of pericallosal branch of posterior cerebral artery in dominant hemisphere.

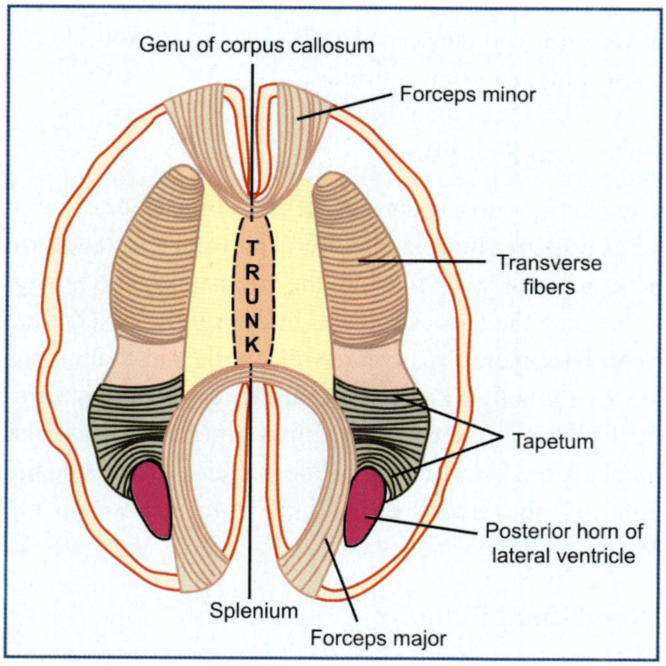

Fig. 98.2: To show course of commissural fibers passing through genu, trunk and splenium of corpus callosum

Examples of Projection Fibers

a. Corona radiata (Fig. 98.3) is a mass of white matter composed of the projection fibers, which converge from the cerebral cortex to the internal capsule and fan out from the internal capsule towards the cortex.
b. The internal capsule gives passage to the descending fibers, which arise in the cortex and terminate in the lower motor neurons. The corticospinal, corticonuclear and corticopontine fibers are the examples of descending fibers. The internal capsule gives passage to ascending fibers, which arise in the neurons of the thalamus as part of the thalamic radiations, which also contain the corticothalamic descending fibers. The knowledge of the reciprocal connections between the thalamus and cerebral cortex is necessary to understand the ascending fibers in the internal capsule.
c. The fornix is composed of projection fibers, which take origin from the hippocampus. The fibers in the fornix are connected to the neurons of the mammillary body.

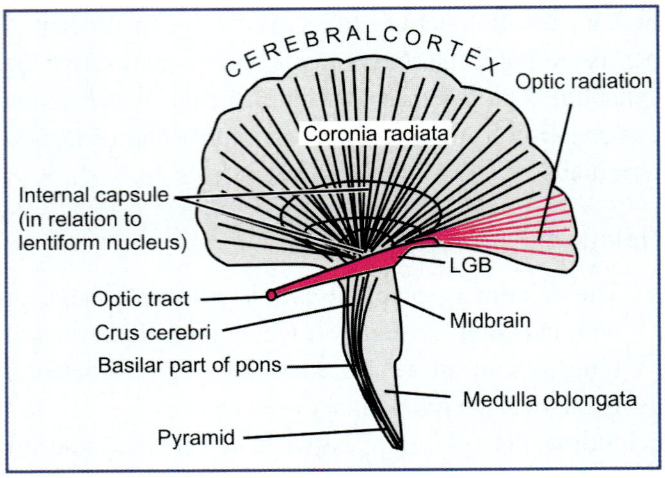

Fig. 98.3: Diagram showing projection fibers (corona radiata and internal capsule) in white matter of cerebrum (Note the continuity of corticospinal fibers from corona radiata to pyramid. These fibers are widely separated in corona radiata below which they congregate)

Internal Capsule

The internal capsule (Fig. 98.4) is a curved and compact mass of projection fibers situated deep inside the hemisphere. All projection fibers of the cerebrum are concentrated in the internal capsule. Therefore, a small lesion in it can cause widespread paralysis and altered sensorium in the opposite side.

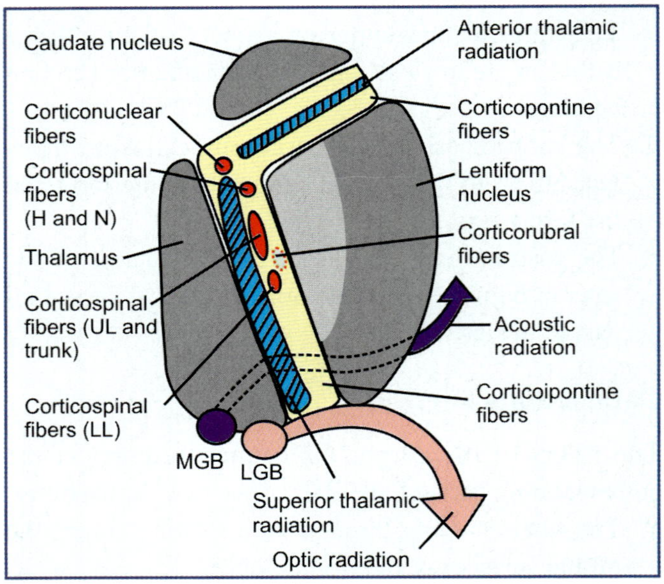

Fig. 98.4: Location and constituent fibers of internal capsule

Parts and Relations

The internal capsule consists of five parts, anterior limb, genu, posterior limb, sublentiform part and retrolentiform part. Superiorly the fibers in the internal capsule fan out to become the corona radiata. Inferiorly the descending fibers pass in the crus cerebri while the thalamic radiations are in continuity with the thalamus. Laterally the lentiform nucleus fits in the concavity of the internal capsule and medially the head of the caudate nucleus is related to the anterior limb and the thalamus is in relation to the posterior limb.

Constituent Fibers

The corticospinal, corticonuclear, corticoreticular, corticorubral and corticopontine fibers are the descending fibers and the thalamic radiations are the reciprocal fibers containing both ascending and descending fibers between thalamus and cortex.

Anterior Limb

a. The descending fibers consist of the frontopontine fibers that originate in the frontal cortex and terminate on the nuclei pontis.

b. The anterior thalamic radiation consists of ascending fibers from the following nuclei of thalamus, from the dorsal medial (DM) nucleus to the prefrontal cortex, from the ventralis anterior (VA) nucleus to the premotor area, from VL to the motor area and from the anterior nuclei to the cingulate gyrus. The frontothalamic fibers are the descending fibers in this radiation from the frontal lobe to the same nuclei of the thalamus.

Genu

a. The descending fibers in the genu are the corticonuclear fibers, which arise in area 4 (precentral cortex) and terminate on the motor nuclei of the cranial nerves in the brainstem. The frontopontine and corticoreticular are the other descending fibers in the genu.
b. A few fibers of the superior thalamic radiation containing ascending fibers from the nuclei VPM and VPL of the thalamus and parietothalamic fibers to same nuclei pass through the genu.

Posterior Limb

a. The descending fibers consist of the corticospinal fibers arising mainly from the precentral gyrus. They are located in discrete bundles more towards the anterior part of the posterior limb. From antero-posterior direction the arrangement of fibers is, upper limb, trunk and lower limb. These fibers are part of the pyramidal tract, which is described separately below. The other descending fibers are the corticorubral, corticoreticular and frontopontine.
b. The superior thalamic radiation consists of projections from the VPL and VPM nuclei to the postcentral gyrus. This radiation also contains ascending fibers from other thalamic nuclei (pulvinar) and the descending fibers from the parietal cortex to the same thalamic nuclei and other nuclei of thalamus including pulvinar.

Sublentiform Part

a. The descending fibers include the parietopontine and temporopontine fibers to the pons.
b. The inferior thalamic radiations mainly consist of auditory radiation from the medial geniculate body to the anterior transverse gyri and superior temporal gyrus. The temporothalamic fibers are the descending fibers in this radiation.

Retrolentiform Part

a. The descending fibers are the parietopontine, occipitopontine and occipitotectal fibers.
b. The posterior thalamic radiations mainly consist of the optic radiation from the lateral geniculate body to the visual cortex in the occipital lobe. The other ascending fibers are thalamocortical projection from other thalamic nuclei including the pulvinar. The reciprocal corticothalamic fibers are also present in the posterior thalamic radiation.

Arterial Supply (Fig. 98.5)

a. The upper part of the anterior limb receives blood from the striate branches of middle cerebral artery and its lower part from the recurrent branch of anterior cerebral artery (Heubner's).
b. The upper part of the genu receives blood from the striate branches of middle cerebral artery and the lower part from the direct branches of internal carotid and recurrent branch of anterior cerebral arteries.
c. The upper part of the posterior limb receives arterial supply from the striate branches (lenticulostriate) of middle cerebral artery and its lower part by anterior choroidal artery.

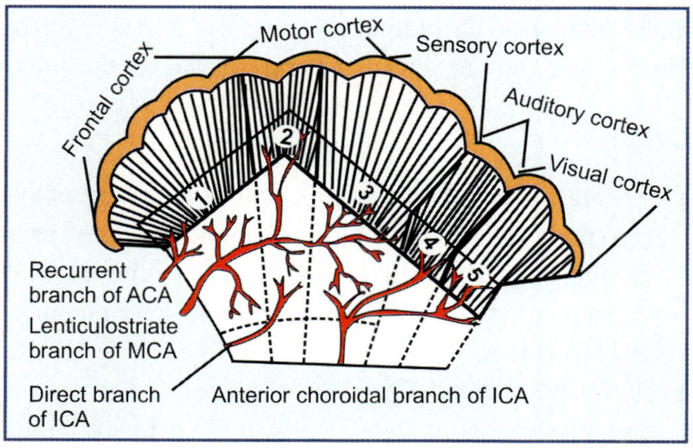

Fig. 98.5: Scheme showing arterial supply of parts of internal capsule. 1–Anterior limb, 2–Genu, 3–Posterior limb, 4–Sublentiform, 5–Retrolentiform

d. The retrolentiform and sublentiform parts receive branches from the anterior choroidal artery.

Clinical Highlights

a. Microaneurysms (Charcot-Bouchard) usually develop in the intracerebral arterioles of lenticulostriate branches of middle cerebral arteries especially in the presence of long-standing hypertension (Fig. 97.2). The rupture of such aneurysms is a common cause of hemorrhage (stroke) with consequent contralateral hemiplegia and contralateral impaired sensations in the body. The hemiplegia is usually associated with contralateral paralysis of lower half of face. This is an upper motor neuron type of paralysis in which there is increased muscle tone (spastic paralysis), increased tendon reflexes and positive Babinski response.
b. The thrombosis of recurrent branch of anterior cerebral artery (Heubner's) may result in paresis of contralateral lower face and upper limb.
c. The thrombosis of anterior choroidal artery may by symptomless in the presence of adequate collateral circulation or it may present as contralateral hemiparesis and impaired loss of sensations and homonymous hemianopia.

Pyramidal Tract (Fig. 84.10)

The pyramidal tract constitutes the motor pathway, which controls the voluntary movements of the body. It consists of corticonuclear fibers and corticospinal fibers. The function of the pyramidal tract is to control the lower motor neurons in the brainstem and spinal cord to regulate the voluntary movements in the opposite side of the body.

Origin

a. The corticonuclear fibers originate as the axons of the pyramidal cells of the motor and premotor cortex, pass through the corona radiata and genu of the internal capsule to terminate at various cranial nerve nuclei in the brainstem.
b. The corticospinal fibers are the axons of the giant pyramidal cells or Betz's cells in the primary motor area 4 (precentral gyrus and the anterior part of paracentral lobule) and pyramidal cells of premotor area 6 (posterior parts of superior, middle and inferior frontal gyri and corresponding area extending on medial surface of frontal lobe). It is believed that a few pyramidal cells of sensory cortex (area 3, 1, 2) also contribute to the corticospinal fibers.

Motor Homunculus

In the motor cortex, the body is represented upside down. The corticospinal tract controlling movements of perineal muscles and leg originate in anterior part of paracentral lobule. Those controlling the hip originate in the upper most part of precentral gyrus. This is followed downwards by trunk, neck, head, shoulder, elbow, wrist, hand and fingers, face, lips, tongue, larynx and pharynx. The area of vocalization muscles is close to Broca's area.

Course of Corticospinal Fibers

The corticospinal fibers pass through the corona radiata and aggregate towards the anterior two-thirds of the posterior limb of the internal capsule, where fibers form discrete bundles. The bundle for head and neck is placed most anteriorly followed by upper limb, trunk and the lower limb. From the internal capsule, the corticospinal fibers descend through the middle two-thirds of the crus cerebri of midbrain, where they are in close approximation with the oculomotor nerve. In their further descent, the corticospinal fibers enter the ventral or basilar part of the pons, where they break up into smaller fascicles and interlace with crossing pontocerebellar fibers and pontine nuclei. In the pons, the fibers are in close relation to the abducent and a little laterally to the facial nerve. As they enter the medulla oblongata, the scattered fascicles aggregate to form pyramids on the ventral surface of medulla oblongata. At the level of pyramidal decussation, about seventy to ninety percent of fibers cross over the opposite side to form lateral corticospinal tract on each side. This tract extends through the entire length of the spinal cord and terminates directly or indirectly on the anterior horn cells. The uncrossed fibers continue downwards as anterior corticospinal tracts and at different levels of spinal cord cross to the opposite side via the anterior commissure to terminate like the lateral corticospinal tract. The anterior corticospinal tract extends upto the mid-thoracic level of the cord. Thus, it should be understood that upper motor neurons control the lower motor neurons through the pyramidal tracts.

Upper and Lower Motor Neurons

a. The cell bodies of the giant pyramidal neurons and their axons together comprise the upper motor neurons (UMN), which are very long cells extending from the cerebrum to the anterior horn cells (lower motor neurons) at various levels of spinal cord.
b. The motor nuclei of the cranial nerves in the brainstem and the anterior horn cells of spinal cord are the lower motor neurons. The axons of these neurons constitute the motor component of the cranial and spinal nerves, through which they are innervate the striated muscles.

Comparative Features of UMN and LMN Lesions

Sign	Upper motor neuron (for example-lesion of internal capsule due to cerebral hemorrhage)	Lower motor neuron (for example-lesion of anterior horn cells due to poliomyelitis)
Type of paralysis	Spastic	Flaccid
Tone of muscles	Hypertonia	Hypotonia
Superficial reflexes	Absent or decreased	Absent or decreased
Deep tendon reflexes	Exaggerated	Absent or decreased
Fasciculations	Absent	Present
Muscle wasting	Less atrophy	Marked atrophy
Plantar response	Extensor (Babinski sign +)	Flexor

Plantar Response

It is elicited as follows. The outer aspect of the sole (S1 dermatome) is firmly stroked with a blunt point (for example, a key). The normal plantar response is the flexion of the metatarsophalangeal joint of great toe and flexion and closing together of other toes. The Babinski sign consists of extension of great toe and the fanning out of other toes. This occurs in upper motor neuron lesion (UMN). The Babinski sign is positive in newborn and infants due to incomplete myelination of corticospinal fibers.

Clinical Highlights

a. Cortical lesions are produced due to thrombosis in middle cerebral artery or anterior cerebral artery. This may cause contralateral localized paralysis, for example of face or one limb. This may be accompanied by altered sensorium, convulsions, aphasia and abnormality of higher functions.
b. Vascular lesions at internal capsule are very common, especially in hypertensive patients. Small lesion of posterior limb of internal capsule results in contralateral hemiplegia and contralateral upper motor neuron type of facial palsy affecting lower part of face, due to crowding of fibers here.
c. In the midbrain, the lesion of corticospinal fibers is accompanied by lesion of oculomotor nerve resulting in a combined LMN and UMN lesions. There is ipsilateral LMN paralysis due to third nerve lesion and contralateral hemiplegia due to lesion of corticospinal fibers (Weber's syndrome).
d. In pons, there is combination of UMN and LMN lesions. Contralateral hemiplegia is accompanied by either the abducent nerve palsy or facial nerve palsy.
e. In medulla oblongata, the thrombosis of anterior spinal artery leads to medial medullary syndrome in which there is contralateral hemiplegia accompanied by ipsilateral hypoglossal nerve palsy and contralateral loss of conscious proprioception in the body.
f. In lesions of spinal cord, the corticospinal tracts are involved. These tracts are crossed hence their lesion produces ipsilateral UMN paralysis on the same side of the lesion. If the anterior horn cells and lateral corticospinal tracts show degeneration it will result in combined UMN and LMN paralysis.

Localization of Lesions in CNS

Localization of lesion in CNS involves two steps. In the first step, the lesion is placed in the longitudinal plane, which means whether it is located in the spinal cord, brainstem, cerebellum, thalamus, internal capsule or cerebral cortex. In the second step, the lesion is placed in the transverse plane, which means whether it is central or peripheral, anterior (ventral) or posterior (dorsal) and right or left. All the signs and symptoms can be explained on the basis of a single lesion.

The following principles help in precise localization:

a. Cerebral hemispheres control the contralateral half of the body while the cerebellar hemispheres control the ipsilateral half.
b. By and large, the ascending or sensory tracts and descending or motor tracts are ipsilateral and decussate to become contralateral at some level in the CNS. Therefore, precise knowledge of the site of decussation is important. Lesion of both descending and ascending tracts below the level of decussation gives rise to ipsilateral signs and symptoms and lesion above the level of decussation, contralateral signs and symptoms.
c. Complete loss of sensations indicates infra-thalamic lesion (brainstem and spinal cord).
d. Increased threshold of some sensations and exaggerated and often disagreeable perception is found in lesion of thalamus.
e. Suprathalamic lesion (cortex and internal capsule) is characterized by impaired or altered sensations (inability to localize the source of sensory stimuli and to appreciate the quality of sensations) in the contralateral half.
f. The cortical lesion may present as contralateral paralysis of upper limb and lower face accompanied by seizures, impaired sensations, aphasia or deviation of the eyes to the side of lesion (due to lesion in precentral gyrus, postcentral gyrus, frontal eye field and speech area in dominant hemisphere respectively). It may also present as spastic monoplegia of lower limb along with impaired sensation in the same limb and impaired bladder function (lesion in paracentral lobule). Therefore, knowledge of sensory and motor homunculus is essential.
g. Localized lesions of internal capsule are very common. There is contralateral spastic hemiplegia accompanied by UMN facial palsy (due to involvement of cortico-nuclear fibers) and altered sensorium in contralateral body. The lesion of internal capsule does not cause aphasia because the connections of speech centres to the opposite hemisphere are intact.
h. Brainstem lesions present as combination of involvement of pyramidal tract and cranial nerves or their nuclei. Hence, it is essential to be familiar with the position of these nuclei.
i. Dissociated sensory loss localizes the lesion to pons, medulla oblongata or spinal cord. It means loss of one type of sensation in one half of the body and another type in other half, like what happens in Wallenberg syndrome (contralateral loss of sensation of vibration and discriminative touch in the body and ipsilateral loss of pain and temperature in the face). Dissociated sensory loss also manifests as loss of same sensation on the contralateral body and ipsilateral face as found in Wallenberg syndrome regarding pain and temperature sensations.

99 Basal Ganglia

The basal ganglia or the basal nuclei are the collections of gray matter situated inside the cerebral hemisphere. The basal ganglia belong to the extrapyramidal system and their lesion results in movement disorders in the body.

Component Nuclei (Fig. 99.1)

Broadly, the basal ganglia consist of four nuclei, the caudate nucleus, lentiform nucleus, claustrum (which is a small strip of gray matter between lentiform nucleus and insular cortex) and the amygdaloid nucleus, which is located in the temporal lobe deep to the uncus. The amygdaloid nucleus has complex chemical connections with the limbic system and hence functionally belongs to the limbic system.

Lentiform Nucleus

The lentiform nucleus consists of the lateral part called, putamen and the medial part called, globus pallidus. The structure and functions of the putamen and globus pallidus are different.

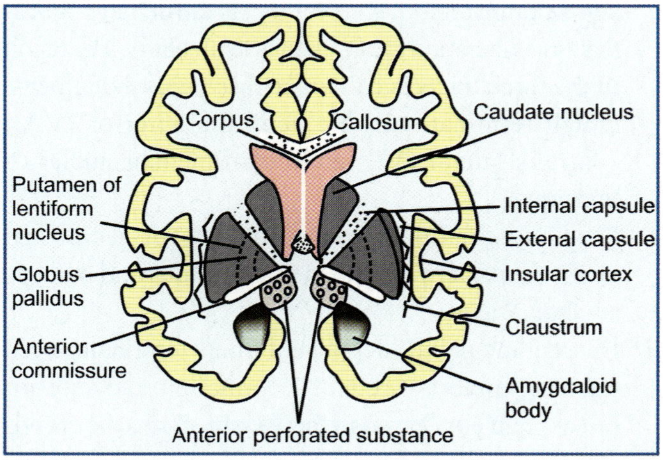

Fig. 99.1: Basal ganglia as seen in coronal section passing through anterior perforated substance (Note: The continuity of surface gray matter with basal ganglia at anterior perforated substance)

Corpus Striatum

The corpus striatum includes the caudate nucleus and the lentiform nucleus.

Striatum

The caudate nucleus and the putamen of the lentiform nucleus are similar in structure and connections. Therefore, together they are called the striatum.

Pallidum

The globus pallidus is known as the pallidum.
The main receiving station of the corpus striatum is the striatum but its main output is through the pallidum.

Caudate Nucleus (Fig. 99.2)

This is a comma-shaped nucleus having three parts, the head, body and tail. The head bulges in the lateral part of the floor and the lateral wall of the anterior horn. It is related laterally to the anterior limb of the internal capsule, which separates it from the lentiform nucleus. Below the head, a band of gray matter connects the caudate nucleus with the putamen. This band of gray matter is continuous with the anterior perforated substance through aggregations of gray and white matter called substantia innominata. This is the only place, where the surface gray matter is continuous with the intracerebral gray matter. The body of the caudate nucleus extends backward from the head at the level of interventricular foramen and lies in the floor of the central part of the lateral ventricle. The thalamostriate vein and stria terminalis lie in the groove between the body and the thalamus. The tail continues

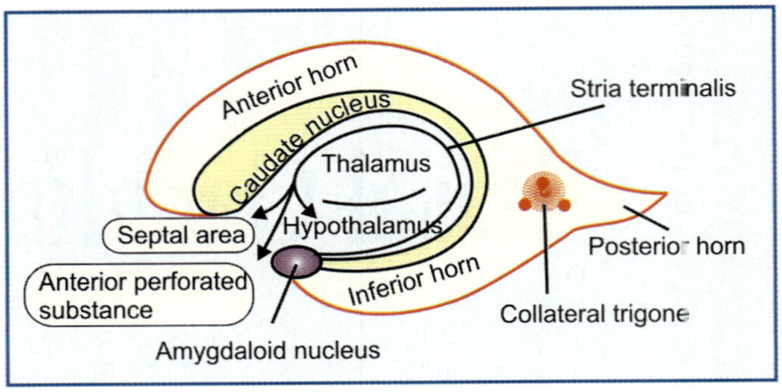

Fig. 99.2: Relation of caudate nucleus to the cavity of lateral ventricle (Note: The origin and termination of stria terminalis)

forwards and downwards in the roof of the inferior horn of the lateral ventricle along with stria terminalis and ends in the amygdaloid nucleus at the tip of the inferior horn.

Lentiform Nucleus

The lentiform nucleus has the shape of a biconvex lens.

Relations

It has a highly convex medial surface and a lateral surface. The structures intervening between the lateral surface and the insular cortex are, external capsule, claustrum and the extreme capsule (from medial to lateral side). A few of the lateral striate arteries pierce the lateral surface and pass through the substance of lentiform nucleus. The medial surface is intimately related to the anterior limb of internal capsule anteriorly and the posterior limb of internal capsule posteriorly (the genu being in contact with the apex). Inferiorly, the lentiform nucleus is connected by a band of gray matter to the head of the caudate nucleus and is continuous with the anterior perforated substance. Its inferior aspect is deeply grooved by fibers of anterior commissure.

Subdivisions

A vertical line of white matter called external medullary lamina divides the lentiform nucleus into larger lateral putamen and smaller medial globus pallidus. The putamen is darker in color compared to globus pallidus, which is pale. The globus pallidus is called pallidum because of its color (pallidum means pale). It is divided into outer and inner segments by internal medullary lamina of white matter. The globus pallidus is the only output nucleus of corpus striatum.

Afferent Connections of Striatum

a. Corticostriate fibers from the sensory and motor cortices are excitatory and cholinergic.
b. Thalamo-striate fibers from the centro-median nucleus, midline and intralaminar nuclei and the nucleus dorsalis medialis of the thalamus are considered to be excitatory.
c. Nigrostriate fibers from the substantia nigra are dopaminergic and inhibitory to the striatum.

Efferent Connections of Striatum

Major output is striatopallidal fibers, which terminate in globus pallidus.

Afferent Connections of Pallidum

The pallidum receives fibers from the striatum, substantia nigra and the subthalamic nucleus.

Efferent Connections of Pallidum

The pallidofugal fibers form four separate bundles:

a. Fasciculus lenticularis arises from the inner segment of the globus pallidus and enters the subthalamic region.
b. Ansa lenticularis arises from both the inner and outer segments of the globus pallidus and enters the subthalamic region, where it meets the dentato-rubro-thalamic fibers and the fasciculus lenticularis. The union of the three tracts is called the fasciculus thalamicus, which terminates in the ventralis anterior (VA), ventralis lateral (VL) and centromedian nuclei of thalamus.
c. Fasciculus subthalamicus consists of reciprocal connections between the globus pallidus and nucleus subthalamicus.
d. Descending pallido-tegmental fibers terminate in red nucleus, midbrain reticular formation and inferior olivary nucleus. Through these connections the corpus striatum exerts influence on the lower motor neurons (rubrospinal, reticulospinal and olivospinal tracts, rubrobulbar, reticulobulbar and olivobulbar connections).

Functions of Corpus Striatum

The basal ganglia mediate the enormous number of automatic activities involved in normal motor functions. For example, the maintenance of erect posture when sitting or standing requires coordinated contraction of many muscles. This coordination is under subconscious control and is mediated by the extrapyramidal system.

The basal ganglia provide the crucial physiological link between the "idea of movement" and the "motor execution of that idea." Their influence on the motor action is indirect as they affect the motor regions of the cerebral cortex before motor commands are sent to the brainstem and spinal cord.

Clinical Highlights

Lesions in the basal ganglia cause disturbances in the initiation and cessation of a motor event. This results in to various kinds of abnormal movement (movement disorders).

a. Parkinson's disease is associated with degeneration of neurons of substantia nigra with resultant depletion of dopamine in corpus striatum. This gives rise to increased muscle tone with slow and abnormal movements. The characteristic features of this disease are, cogwheel rigidity and resting tremor (pill-rolling tremor). Mask-like facies with no emotional response and shuffling gait are the other characteristic features.
b. Huntington's chorea is an autosomal dominant disorder associated with severe degeneration of neurons in caudate nucleus and putamen. It is accompanied by gyral atrophy in frontal and temporal lobes. It leads to movements, which are brisk, jerky and purposeless resembling fragments of voluntary movements and progressive mental deterioration.
c. Sydenham's chorea or St. Vitus' dance occurs as a result of minute hemorrhages and capillary emboli in the corpus striatum. The abnormal movements similar to Huntington chorea are the cardinal sign of this disease.
d. Hepatolenticular degeneration or Wilson's disease is an autosomal recessive disease due to defect in copper metabolism. Lesions are found in liver and lentiform nucleus. Deposition of copper in cornea gives rise to characteristic Kayser-Fleischer ring. The clinical manifestations are tremor, rigidity and impairment of voluntary movements.

100 Lateral Ventricle

The lateral ventricle is the ependyma-lined cavity inside each cerebral hemisphere. It contains choroid plexus and CSF. Each lateral ventricle communicates with the third ventricle through the interventricular foramen of Monro. The lateral ventricle is roughly a C-shaped cavity with an extension from the back of the C.

Subdivisions (Fig. 99.2)

The ventricle consists of a central part, which lies in the parietal lobe. From the central part, anterior horn extends in the frontal lobe from the level of interventricular foramen. The inferior horn extends in the temporal lobe and the posterior horn extends in the occipital lobe.

Central Part

The central part extends from the interventricular foramen to the splenium of corpus callosum. It presents a medial wall, roof and floor.

a. The medial wall (Fig. 93.1) decreases in height from anterior to posterior direction. The septum pellucidum and the fornix below it, form the anterior part of the medial wall but the fornix alone is present in the posterior part. The septum pellucidum (septum lucidum) consists of right and left laminae, which connect the fornix and the corpus callosum. Its two laminae may be separated by a cavity of the septum pellucidum, which is also known as the fifth ventricle. This septum contains a few septal nuclei.
b. The trunk of the corpus callosum forms the roof.
c. The floor consists of six structures (Fig. 93.2). From lateral to medial they are, the body of caudate nucleus, thalamostriate vein, stria terminalis, a narrow strip of superior surface of thalamus, the choroid plexus and the fornix. At the posterior end, the floor has a triangular area, called the collateral trigone, where the inferior and posterior horns diverge from the central part of the ventricle.

Anterior Horn

The anterior horn has the roof, floor, anterior medial and lateral walls.

a. The roof is formed by the trunk of the corpus callosum.
b. The anterior wall is formed by the genu of the corpus callosum.
c. The medial wall is formed by the septum pellucidum.
d. The floor consists mainly of the head of caudate nucleus laterally and the rostrum of the corpus callosum medially.
e. The lateral wall contains the head of the caudate nucleus.
   (Note that the head of the caudate nucleus is related to the lateral wall and the floor).

Inferior Horn (Fig. 100.1)

The anterior end of the inferior horn reaches very close to the uncus in the temporal lobe. The inferior horn has the roof, lateral wall and the floor.

a. The roof contains the tail of caudate nucleus and stria terminalis, which enter the roof of inferior horn from the central part of the lateral ventricle. The tail of the caudate nucleus joins the amygdaloid nucleus and the stria terminalis begins in the same nucleus, which overlies the tip of the inferior horn in the uncus.
b. The tapetum forms the lateral wall, which is closely related to the looping fibers (Meyer's loop) of the optic radiations. Enlarged inferior horn may compress these fibres giving rise to visual defect known as contralateral upper homonymous quadrantinopia.
c. The floor shows the bulge of the hippocampus covered by a white sheet called alveus and the fimbria medially

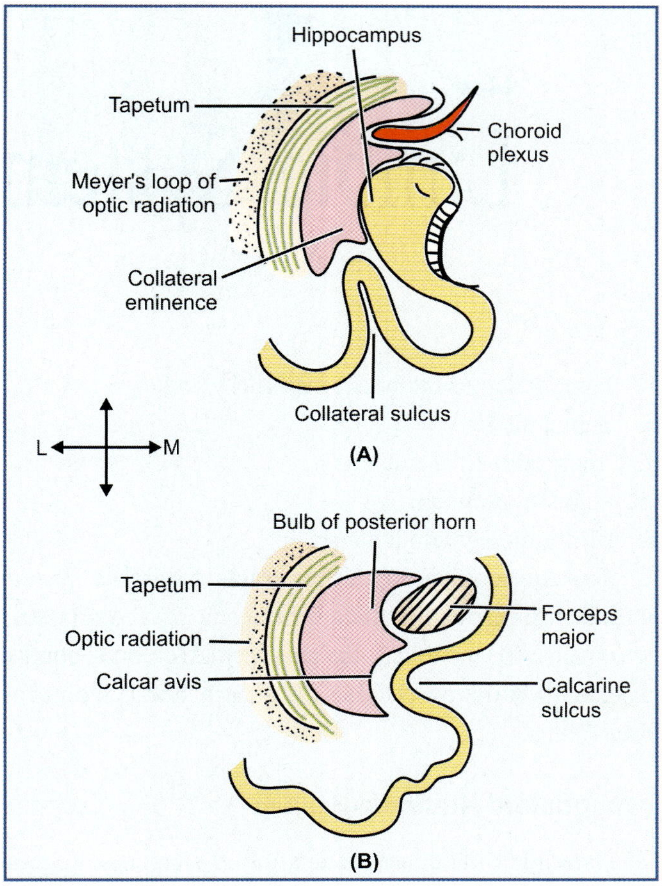

Fig. 100.1: Coronal section of lateral ventricle to show features of inferior horn (A) and of posterior horn (B)

and the collateral eminence produced by the collateral sulcus laterally.

Posterior Horn

The posterior horn may be asymmetrical in adults or sometimes absent. It has a roof, medial wall and a lateral wall.

a. The roof and the lateral walls are formed by the tapetum.
b. The medial wall is invaginated by the forceps major, which produces the bulb of posterior horn above and by the calcarine sulcus, which gives rise to the calcar avis below (Fig. 100.1).

Choroid Fissure

The choroid fissure is the space through which a vascular sheet of piamater enters the lateral ventricle. The ependyma and tela choroidea come in direct contact with each other in this space. The ependyma-covered tela choroidea forms the choroid plexus of the lateral ventricle. The choroid fissure is a C-shaped gap having upper and lower parts. The upper part of the choroid fissure is related to the central part of the lateral ventricle and is bounded by fornix above and superior surface of thalamus below. The lower part of the choroid fissure is related to the inferior horn of the lateral ventricle and is bounded by the fimbria below and the structures in the roof of the inferior horn above.

Choroid Plexus (Fig. 97.6)

The tela choroidea enters the transverse fissure to reach the superior surface of the thalamus. Here it comes in direct contact with the ependyma of the roof of the third ventricle and at the choroid fissure with the ependyma of the lateral ventricle. The choroid plexuses thus formed, project through the roof of third ventricle and through the choroid fissure of lateral ventricle. Anterior and posterior choroidal arteries supply choroid plexuses of both the ventricles. The choroid plexuses are present in central part and inferior horn only since the choroid fissure is confined to these parts of the lateral ventricle. The anterior and posterior horns are devoid of choroid plexuses.

Radiological Visualization

Pneumoencephalography and ventriculography are the older techniques of visualizing the lateral ventricles. But nowadays MRI and CT scans have replaced the older methods.

Hydrocephalus

The hydrocephalus is accumulation of CSF in lateral ventricle, usually due to blockage of interventricular foramen of Monro.

Intraventricular Hemorrhage

The caudate nucleus is intimately related to the anterior horn and the central part and the inferior horn of the lateral ventricle. The hemorrhage in the caudate nucleus (usually due to hypertension) may break into the cavity of the lateral ventricle and cause intraventricular bleeding, which may be fatal.

101 Limbic System

The limbic system includes some parts of cerebrum, diencephalon and the midbrain. The numerous anatomical components and their numerous connections comprising the limbic system are the structural basis of the behavioral and emotional expression of the individual. The limbic system plays a role in feeling, feeding, fighting and fleeing activities. It is responsible for emotions necessary for sexual functions. It integrates the olfactory, visceral and somatic impulses through the hypothalamus. In addition to the above functions, the limbic system is an integral part of the processes involved in recent memory. The term limbus means a ring. The limbic structures are disposed along the edge of the hemisphere like a ring. The limbic system consists of cortical gray matter, subcortical gray matter and fiber tracts.

Cortical Gray Matter

a. Limbic lobe (cingulate gyrus, isthmus, parahippocampal gyrus and uncus) and orbitofrontal cortex
b. Hippocampal formation (hippocampus, dentate gyrus, gyrus fasciolaris and indusium griseum).

Since the cortical areas included in the limbic system are not totally agreed upon, many authorities include entorhinal area (anterior part of parahippocampal gyrus and uncus), septal area (which includes paraterminal and parolfactory gyri) and piriform lobe under this heading.

Subcortical Gray Matter

a. Dorsomedial (mediodorsal) nucleus of thalamus, which has reciprocal connections with entorhinal area, hypothalamus, prefrontal cortex and amygdaloid nucleus. It plays a role in affective behavior.
b. Anterior nucleus of thalamus, which is part of Papez circuit.
c. Amygdaloid complex
d. Hypothalamus including mamillary bodies
e. Septal nuclei
f. Interpeduncular nucleus
g. Habenular nuclei
h. Midbrain tegmental nuclei.

The interconnecting fibers tracts of limbic system include fornix, mamillothalamic tract (Vicq d' Azyr), stria terminalis, stria medullaris thalami, medial forebrain bundle, diagonal band of Broca, cingulum and fasciculus retroflexus.

Amygdaloid Nucleus (Fig. 99.1)

The amygdaloid nucleus is an almond-shaped collection of subcortical nuclear mass lying inside the uncus at the tip of the inferior horn of the lateral ventricle. It is continuous with the tail of caudate nucleus, claustrum and lentiform nucleus. Due to its wide-ranging connections, the amygdala occupies the central place in human being's emotional processing and hence functionally is an integral part of the limbic system.

Subcortical Connections of Amygdala

a. The stria terminalis originates in the amygdala and passes backwards in the roof of the inferior horn and then forwards in the floor of the central part of the lateral ventricle. It divides in three parts at the level of interventricular foramen. The supracommissural part ends in septal nuclei and septal area (paraterminal gyrus). The commissural part joins the anterior commissure to reach the opposite amygdaloid complex. The subcommissural part ends in preoptic and anterior nuclei of hypothalamus and the anterior perforated substance.

b. The ventral amygdalofugal fibers terminate in septal area anterior perforated substance, medial dorsal nucleus of thalamus, hypothalamic nuclei and basal nucleus of Meynert. There is connection with the midbrain and the corpus striatum also.

Cortical Connections of Amygdala

The amygdala is in connection with the entorhinal cortex, hippocampal formation, temporal and occipital cortices and the frontal, cingulate and insular cortices.

Hippocampal Formation

This consists of hippocampus, dentate gyrus, indusium griseum and medial and lateral longitudinal striae.

a. The hippocampus (Fig. 101.1) is part of cerebral cortex that resembles sea horse in appearance in its coronal section. It is also described as ram's horn or Ammon's horn. It forms a curved elevation in the floor of the inferior horn of lateral ventricle. Its anterior expanded end presents shallow grooves, which give it the appearance of the paw hence, called pes hippocampi. The hippocampus consists of three- layered cortex. The axons of the pyramidal neurons of the hippocampus form a white sheet called alveus that covers the ventricular aspect of the hippocampus under the ependyma. The alveus continues as the fimbriae, which continue backward as the crus of the fornix. The hippocampus receives connections from entorhinal area, septal area and cingulate gyrus. The structural layers of hippocampus are called CA1, CA2 and CA3 as shown in Figure 101.1 (CA stands for cornu ammonis). The pathologists recognize CA1 sector as Sommer's sector. The large pyramidal cells of this sector are very sensitive to hypoxia

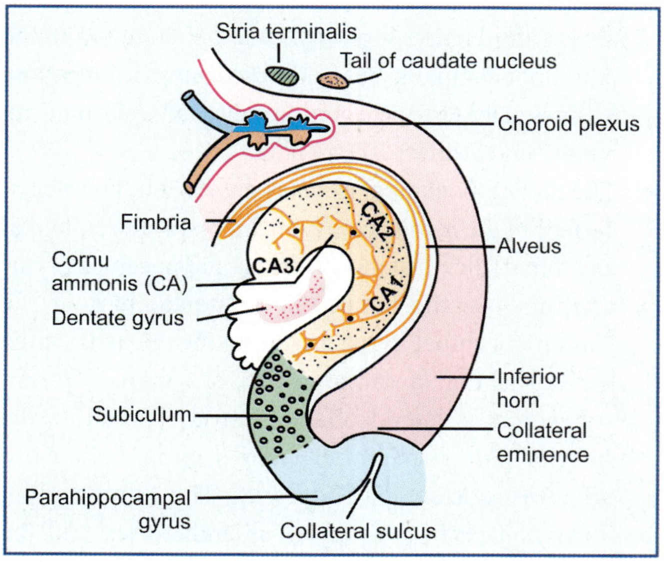

Fig. 101.1: Coronal section of hippocampus projecting in the inferior horn of lateral ventricle (Note that the choroid fissure between stria terminalis and fimbria is highly exaggerated)

b. The fornix forms the efferent pathway of hippocampus. It is a prominent bundle of projection fibers located on the medial surface of the cerebral hemisphere. It consists of a posterior part called crus, body and the anterior part called column. The crus is the continuation of fimbria. The two crura are united with each other by hippocampal commissure through which the right and left hippocampi are joined. The body of the fornix is the continuation of the crura and is connected to the corpus callosum by septum pellucidum. The body lies in contact with the superior surface of the thalamus and forms the superior boundary of the choroid fissure of the central part of the lateral ventricle. The anterior end of the body divides into right and left columns. Each column forms the anterior boundary of the interventricular foramen. The column divides in precommissural and postcommissural fibers. The precommissural fibers terminate in septal areas including the basal nucleus of Meynert, amygdaloid complex and anterior thalamus while the postcommissural fibers pass through the hypothalamus to terminate in the mamillary bodies from where the mamillothalamic tract connects it to anterior nucleus of thalamus.

Vestigeal Part of Hippocampal Formation

This includes the indusium griseum, gyrus fasciolaris, dentate gyrus and longitudinal striae. The indusium griseum is continuous anteriorly with the paraterminal gyrus while posteriorly it is continuous with gyrus fasciolaris and through it with the dentate gyrus, which is a longitudinal strip of gray matter in association with the hippocampus. The lateral margin of the dentate gyrus is fused with the hippocampus and its free medial margin is crenated giving it the appearance of teeth. Anteriorly the dentate gyrus ends in a tail, which runs across the inferior surface of uncus and terminates in it.

Papez Circuit (Fig. 101. 2)

It is a circular pathway that interconnects certain important structures in limbic system. It contains the following stations, the hippocampus projecting via the fornix to mamillary body, the mamillary nucleus projecting via the mamillothalamic tract to the anterior nucleus of thalamus, anterior nucleus of thalamus projecting to the cingulate gyrus and the cingulate gyrus projecting via the cingulum back to the hippocampus. Lesion in mamillary bodies results in Korsakoff' syndrome (amnestic confabulatory syndrome), in which there is severe impairment of memory.

Functional Importance of Hippocampus

It has been proved that hippocampus has no olfactory function. It plays important role in learning and recent memory and in the control of emotional behavior.

Clinical Highlights

a. Bilateral ablation of hippocampus leads to long-term memory loss.
b. In rabies, the lesion is found in the neurons of the hippocampus in the form of Negri bodies.
c. Bilateral ablation of amygdala and hippocampus (anterior temporal lobe) results in Kluver-Bucy syndrome (hyperphagia, docility and hypersexuality).

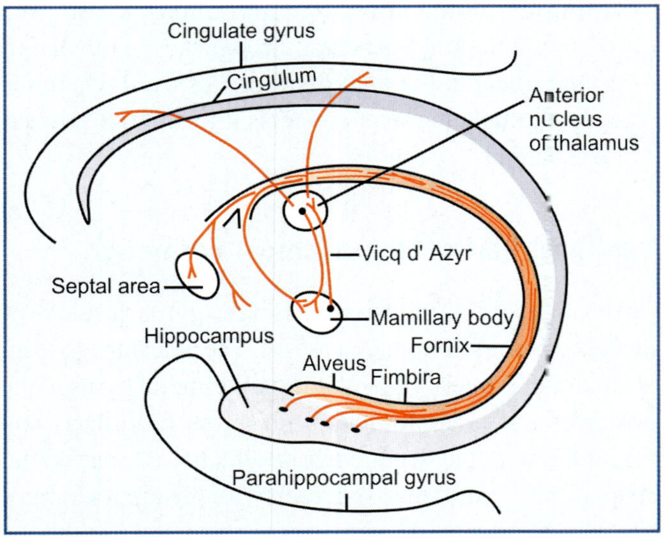

Fig. 101.2: Projection fibers of hippocampus and components of Papez circuit

Limbic Lobe

The limbic lobe consists of septal area, cingulate gyrus, isthmus and parahippocampal gyrus.

a. In human beings the septal area includes septum pellucidum and the paraterminal and subcallosal (parolfactory) gyri on the medial surface of the hemisphere. The septal nuclei are the sparse gray matter in the septum pellucidum and the subcortical gray matter in the septal region. The basal nucleus of Meynert can be included in septal nuclei since it is located in substantia innominata of basal forebrain between the globus pallidus and anterior perforated substance. The basal nucleus of Meynert projects via cholinergic fibers to the amygdala and the entire neocortex. It shows degeneration in Alzheimer's disease. The septal area has reciprocal connections with the hypothalamus via the median forebrain bundle and it projects via the stria medullaris thalami to the habenular nucleus.
b. The cingulate gyrus lies on the medial surface of the hemisphere starting below the rostrum of the corpus callosum. It follows the curve of the corpus callosum and continues round the splenium on the inferior surface, to merge with the parahippocampal gyrus through the narrow isthmus. The cingulate gyrus receives afferent connections from the anterior nucleus of thalamus (part of Papez circuit) and also from amygdaloid body. It projects via the cingulum to the parahippocampal gyrus and hippocampal formation. Lesions in the cingulate gyrus result in akinesia, mutism, apathy and indifference to pain.
c. The parahippocampal gyrus is present on the inferior surface of the hemisphere lying medial to the collateral and rhinal sulci. Anteriorly, the parahippocampal gyrus continues in the uncus. The anterior part of the parahippocampal gyrus including the uncus is called the entorhinal area (area 28). Its main afferent connection is lateral olfactory stria. Therefore, the anterior part of parahippocampal gyrus belongs to olfactory cortex (paleocortex). The hippocampal formation part of the gyrus is archicortex and the remaining part is neocortex.

102 Cerebrospinal Fluid

The cerebrospinal fluid is a clear, colorless, acellular fluid contained in the subarachnoid spaces, the ventricles of the brain and the central canal of the spinal cord. The CSF supports and cushions the brain and spinal cord against concussive injuries and removes metabolic waste products. Examination of CSF is necessary in the diagnosis of diseases like meningitis, for which the sample is obtained usually by lumbar puncture. Occasionally, cisternal puncture is performed to obtain CSF.

Site of Production

The choroid plexuses in the ventricles of brain secrete the CSF (choroid plexuses of lateral ventricles contribute maximum).

Characteristic Features of CSF

a. Daily production is around 1500 ml and the total volume of CSF is 140 to 150 ml. This suggests that entire volume of CSF is replaced several times a day.
b. The normal pressure in supine position in lumbar subarachnoid space is 50 to 200 mm of water and in sitting position 200 to 250 mm of water.
c. Its specific gravity ranges from 1.003 to 1.008
d. Glucose level is half of that of blood (40-60 mg%).
e. Protein content is very low compared to plasma proteins (20-40 mg%).
f. During lumbar puncture normally the rate of flow of CSF is one drop per second.

Circulation of CSF

The CSF flows from the ventricles to the subarachnoid space by passing successively through the lateral ventricles, interventricular foramina of Monro, third ventricle, cerebral aqueduct, fourth ventricle and through the lateral and median foramina in the roof of fourth ventricle into the subarachnoid space. The CSF in cranial subarachnoid space enters the spinal subarachnoid space. The movement of CSF is assisted by pulsations of the arteries in the subarachnoid space. CSF leaves the subarachnoid space mainly through the arachnoid villi and granulations projecting into the superior sagittal sinus and adjacent lacunae.

Queckenstedt's Test

This method tests the correlation between intracranial tension (ICT) and the rate of flow of CSF. Alternate compression of internal jugular veins results in rise in intracranial pressure. This is reflected in rise in intraspinal venous pressure provided the spinal subarachnoid space is patent. The increase in the intraspinal pressure is measurable by the manometer attached to the LP needle. In case of the block of the spinal subarachnoid space, there will not be a rise in intraspinal pressure in spite of rise in ICT.

Hydrocephalus

Hydrocephalus is the condition in which there is excess of CSF.

Types of Hydrocephalus

a. In external hydrocephalus the excess of CSF is in the subarachnoid space.
b. In internal hydrocephalus there is dilatation of ventricles. All the ventricles are dilated if the apertures in the roof of fourth ventricle are occluded. The third and lateral ventricles are dilated if the occlusion is located in the cerebral aqueduct. One lateral ventricle is enlarged if the obstruction is present at the level of interventricular foramen.

c. The communicating hydrocephalus is a combination of supratentorial internal hydrocephalus and subtentorial external hydrocephalus. The obstruction to the flow of CSF at the tentorial notch around the midbrain (due to herniation of the uncus) usually results in this type.

Blood-brain Barrier

The blood-brain barrier includes the tissues intervening between the blood in the capillaries and the neural tissue. There are tight junctions between the endothelial cells of the capillaries. So the barrier consists of endothelial cells with tight junctions, continuous basement membrane of the capillaries and the perivascular feet of the astrocytes. The blood-brain barrier protects the neural tissue from circulating toxic substances in the blood. It allows selective transport of substances and thereby provides the optimal microenvironment for the neurons. There are certain areas of brain, where blood-brain barrier is not present, the examples of which are, the median eminence of hypothalamus, the pituitary, choroid plexus, pineal gland and area postrema of fourth ventricle. The breakdown of blood-brain barrier occurs following brain damage due to ischemia or infection, which results in the entry of ions, fluid and proteins in the extracellular space. In newborn children the blood-brain barrier is not well-developed. In neonatal jaundice the bile pigments pass through the barrier and damage the basal ganglia producing kernicterus.

103 Overview of Autonomic Nervous System

The autonomic nervous system is concerned with the nerve supply of the smooth muscles, cardiac muscle and the glands of the body. Like the somatic system, it consists of efferent and afferent components. There is a basic difference in the somatic and autonomic efferent paths. In somatic system, the axons of lower motor neurons in the spinal cord or brainstem directly supply the voluntary muscles. In the case of the autonomic system, the axons of preganglionic neurons in the spinal cord or brainstem terminate in the ganglia outside the central nervous system and the axons of neurons in these ganglia (postganglionic fibers) supply the glands and involuntary musculature.

Subdivisions of Efferent Component

It has three subdivisions, sympathetic, parasympathetic and enteric. In general, most organs receive both sympathetic and parasympathetic innervation. The actions of the two systems appear to be antagonistic but are mutually complimentary. The sympathetic stimulation is increased in stress situations hence, it is required for fight, fright and flight responses, which result in increased heart rate and blood pressure. The parasympathetic stimulation causes reduction in heart rate and blood pressure and increase in digestion and absorption of food. Some examples of only sympathetic supply are, blood vessels, dilator pupillae, sweat glands and arrectorum pilorum muscles in skin. The end organs receiving only parasympathetic supply are, ciliaris and sphincter pupillae muscles of eyeball, majority of exocrine glands with the exception of the sweat glands.

Sympathetic Division (Thoracolumbar Outflow)

a. The preganglionic neurons of the sympathetic division are located in the intermediolateral column of all the thoracic and upper two lumbar segments of spinal cord. Thus, it is evident that the sympathetic part in CNS is confined to 14 segments of spinal cord. The preganglionic fibers (axons of preganglionic neurons) leave the spinal cord via the corresponding ventral roots. They are further carried from the spinal nerve by white rami communicantes (called white because they are myelinated) to the sympathetic chain, which is paravertebral in position. It is very important to understand that the number of white rami comminicantes is equivalent to the number of spinal segments containing preganglionic neurons. So the number of white rami communicantes is 14 only and they connect the spinal cord to the sympathetic chain.
b. The postganglionic neurons are located in two places, in the ganglia of sympathetic chains and in the collateral ganglia. The preganglionic fibers terminate on them and their axons become the postganglionic fibers, which supply the effector organs.

Sympathetic Chains or Trunks

The sympathetic chains are two ganglionated nerve trunks, which are paravertebral in location and extend from the base of cranium to the coccyx. The sympathetic ganglia contain the postganglionic neurons. The upper end of each trunk continues as internal carotid nerve, which forms sympathetic plexus around the internal carotid artery. At the lower end, the two chains join in front of the first piece of coccyx to form ganglion impar. Each trunk bears three cervical ganglia (superior, middle and inferior) 11 or 12 thoracic, 4 or 5 lumbar and 4 or 5 sacral ganglia. The superior cervical ganglion lies adjacent to second and third cervical vertebrae. The middle ganglion is found at the sixth cervical vertebral level. The stellate ganglion (when the inferior cervical ganglion fuses with the first thoracic ganglion) is in front of the neck of the first rib. The thoracic ganglia from second downwards lie on the heads of the ribs (except a few lower ones). The lowest two or three thoracic ganglia are lateral to the bodies of the corresponding thoracic vertebrae. The lumbar ganglia are on the anterior surface of the bodies of the lumbar vertebrae along the medial margin of the psoas major muscle. The pelvic part of the chain lies on the pelvic surface of the sacrum anterior to the anterior sacral foramina.

Collateral Ganglia

The collateral ganglia are located in the abdomen in front of the vertebral column. They include celiac ganglion, aorticorenal, superior and inferior mesenteric ganglia.

Modes of Termination of the Preganglionic Fibers

a. Some preganglionic fibers synapse in the cells of the corresponding sympathetic ganglia. A few fibers from the upper thoracic segments of spinal cord ascend in the sympathetic chain to synapse in the cervical ganglia.
b. A few fibers from the lower thoracic segments and upper two lumbar segments of spinal cord travel caudally in the sympathetic chain to synapse in the lumbar or sacral sympathetic ganglia.
c. Some preganglionic fibers pass through the thoracic sympathetic ganglia without relay. These myelinated preganglionic fibers leave the sympathetic trunk as the greater, lesser and least splanchnic nerves. The splanchnic nerves are composed of long preganglionic fibers. They terminate on the prevertebral ganglia and the suprarenal medulla.

Postganglionic Sympathetic Fibers

a. The postganglionic fibers from the ganglia join back to the corresponding spinal nerve by gray rami communicantes. It should be understood that the sympathetic chain is connected to each spinal nerve by a gray ramus communicans. Hence, there are 31 pairs of gray rami corresponding to the number of spinal nerves. In this way, sudomotor, vasomotor and pilomotor fibers are ensured in the territory of supply of each spinal nerve. Postganglionic fibers from the cervical ganglia supply the neck and thoracic viscera. The dilator pupillae muscle in the eyeball is unique in receiving its sympathetic innervation through a long route. The postganglionic fibers from thoracic ganglia supply thoracic viscera.
b. The postganglionic fibers from the collateral ganglia take part in plexuses, which supply the abdominal viscera. The postganglionic fibers from lumbar and sacral ganglia also form plexuses for abdominal and pelvic viscera (for details refer to Chapter 158).

Neurotransmitters at Sympathetic Synapses

The preganglionic sympathetic fibers are cholinergic. The postganglionic sympathetic fibers are adrenergic with the exception of sweat glands, which are supplied by cholinergic fibers.

Parasympathetic Division (Craniosacral Outflow)

The preganglionic neurons are located in the four cranial nerve nuclei in the brainstem and in the intermediomedial column of second to fourth sacral segments of spinal cord. The postganglionic neurons are located in peripheral parasympathetic ganglia

Cranial Outflow

a. Edinger-Westphall nucleus in the midbrain is part of oculomotor nucleus. The axons of this nucleus pass through the oculomotor nerve as preganglionic fibers and terminate on ciliary ganglion in the orbit. The postganglionic fibers from the ciliary ganglion supply ciliaris and sphincter pupillae muscles.

b. Superior salivatory nucleus in the pons sends its axons in the nervus intermedius of the facial nerve. The preganglionic fibers for lacrimal gland leave in greater petrosal branch of the facial nerve. The union of greater petrosal and deep petrosal nerves in the foramen lacerum forms the nerve of pterygoid canal (Vidian nerve) that carries the preganglionic fibers to the pterygopalatine ganglion. After the synapse in the ganglion the postganglionic fibers are carried to the lacrimal gland in the zygomatic branch of the maxillary nerve. The preganglionic fibers for submandibular and sublingual salivary glands leave in the chorda tympani branch of facial nerve. The chorda tympani nerve takes these fibers to the submandibular ganglion via the lingual nerve. After the synapse, the postganglionic fibers directly supply the submandibular and sublingual salivary glands.
c. Inferior salivatory nucleus in the upper medulla oblongata sends preganglionic fibers through the glossopharyngeal nerve. The tympanic branch of the glossopharyngeal nerve takes these fibers to the middle ear, where they form tympanic plexus. The lesser petrosal nerve arising from the tympanic plexus enters the infratemporal fossa to terminate on the otic ganglion. The postganglionic fibers join the auriculotemporal nerve, which takes them to the parotid gland.
d. Dorsal nucleus of vagus sends preganglionic fibers through the vagus nerve. These fibers leave the vagus in its various branches to reach the intramural ganglia, where they synapse. The intramural ganglia are located within or adjacent to the visceral organs. The short postganglionic fibers innervate viscera of thorax and abdomen as far as the junction of right two-thirds and left one-third of the transverse colon (derivatives of foregut and midgut).

Sacral Outflow

The preganglionic neurons in the second to fourth sacral segments of spinal cord leave along with the ventral roots of the second to fourth sacral nerves and separate out to form the pelvic splanchnic nerves or nervi erigentis. These nerves unite with the sympathetic plexuses in the pelvis and terminate on the intramural ganglia for synapse. The postganglionic fibers supply the pelvic viscera (detrusor muscle of urinary bladder, smooth muscle of genital organs) and the digestive tract beyond the territory of vagus nerve.

Neurotransmitter in Parasympathetic System

Both preganglionic and postganglionic fibers are cholinergic.

Enteric Nervous System

The enteric nervous system developed from neural crest, consists of intramural ganglia and plexuses (submucosal Meissner's and myenteric Aurbach's) in the wall of the gastrointestinal tract. The total number of neurons in the enteric plexuses is vast and a neuropil of the processes of glial cells and neurons surrounds them. The enteric nervous system is influenced by postganglionic adrenergic sympathetic input and preganglionic cholinergic parasympathetic input. It is essential for the normal functioning of gastrointestinal motility and secretion. The enteric nervous system is unusual in that it can function even after sympathetic and parasympathetic denervation.

Visceral Afferent or Autonomic Afferent Fibers

The general visceral afferent fibers travel to the CNS along with the sympathetic nerves or parasympathetic nerves. These fibers carry visceral pain and sensations for the autonomic reflexes. The afferent fibers accompanying the sympathetic nerves pass to the spinal nerve in the white ramus communicantes of T1 to L2 levels and reach the cell bodies in the spinal ganglion. The dorsal roots of the spinal nerves carry the sensations to CNS. General visceral afferents in the parasympathetic system follow the preganglionic and postganglionic fibers back to the brainstem and sacral spinal cord. Those carried in the facial, glossopharyngeal and vagus nerves have their cell bodies in corresponding sensory ganglia. The sacral fibers have their cell bodies in spinal ganglia S2-S4.

Higher Control of ANS

Hypothalamus is regarded as the head ganglion or master control of autonomic nervous system. The posterior part of hypothalamus controls sympathetic activity and its anterior part controls parasympathetic activity. The central autonomic pathways influence the preganglionic neurons in the brainstem and spinal cord.

Nerve Supply of Arteries of Upper Limb

The sympathetic nerves are vasomotor. The preganglionic sympathetic fibers arise from T2 to T5 or T6 segments of spinal cord and run up the sympathetic chain to synapse in stellate ganglion. The postganglionic fibers join the nerves that form brachial plexus for distribution to the arteries of upper limb. In vasospasm of upper limb, sometimes surgery is required, in which the sympathetic supply to the upper limb is severed by preganglionic cervicodorsal sympathectomy. The segment of the sympathetic chain below the origin of first white rami communicantes upto the T3 ganglion is removed after cutting the second and third rami communicantes. The nerve of Kuntz, if present, is also removed. The nerve of Kuntz is the gray ramus running upwards from the second thoracic ganglion to the first thoracic nerve. The T1 ventral ramus, first white ramus communicans and stellate ganglion are preserved since they contain preganglionic fibers for the eye and head including the face.

Nerve Supply of Arteries of Lower Limb

The preganglionic sympathetic fibers for lower limb arise from T10 to L3 spinal segments. They reach the lower thoracic and upper lumbar sympathetic ganglia through white rami. Some descend in the sympathetic chain to synapse in lumbar ganglia from where postganglionic fibers join the femoral nerve. Others descend to the upper 2 or 3 sacral ganglia from which postganglionic branches join the tibial part of sciatic nerve. The femoral and tibial nerves distribute sympathetic supply to the lower limb. The vasospasm and associated complications of the lower limb are at times treated surgically to improve the blood supply of the limb. In the procedure called lumbar sympathectomy lumbar second to fourth ganglia are removed. The first ganglion is preserved in males to avoid retrograde ejaculation and resultant sterility.

104 Clinicoanatomical Problems and Solutions

CASE 1

A 35-year-old man developed sudden and acute pain in the lumbar region after lifting a heavy suitcase. The pain radiated down to the outer side of the left leg. MRI of the vertebral column showed herniation of the disc in the posterolateral direction between L4 and L5 vertebrae.

Questions

a. Which nerve roots will be compressed if there is disc prolapse between L4 and L5 vertebrae.
b. In which area will there be sensory loss in disc prolapse at this level?
c. What is the difference between the spinal nerve root and the spinal nerve?
d. If the disc prolapse occurs in the midline in posterior direction at this level, which structure will be compressed?
e. Name the parts of the intervertebral disc giving the histological structure of its peripheral part.
f. Enumerate the functions of the disc and describe the diurnal variations in it.
g. Describe the development of the disc with the help of diagram.

Solutions

a. L5 nerve roots (Fig. 83.5).
b. There will be loss of sensation in the L5 dermatome on the left leg and foot (Fig. 1.5).
c. The spinal nerve roots (ventral and dorsal) are the filaments by which spinal nerves are attached to the spinal cord. The spinal nerve is formed by the union of ventral and dorsal nerve roots.
d. Cauda equina
e. The disc consists of inner nucleus pulposus and outer annulus fibrosus. The latter is made of white fibrocartilage.
f. The intervertebral discs provide elasticity and flexibility to the vertebral column. The discs act as shock absorbers. The discs show diurnal variation in size. During daytime when the vertebral column supports body weight the water content of the nucleus pulposus is reduced hence at night the disc is shortest. During rest in the night the water is absorbed in the nucleus therefore, in the morning the disc regains its original size.
g. The nucleus pulposus develops from notochord and the annulus fibrosus from the perichordal disc of the sclerotome (Fig. 83.1).

CASE 2

A 22-year-old woman with a history of birth of the first child with anencephaly wants to know whether this birth defect can recur in the next pregnancy and if it is preventable.

Questions

a. What are the features of anencephaly?
b. Give the embryological explanation of this defect.
c. What is the normal time of closure of anterior and posterior neuropores?
d. Name the methods of prenatal detection of open neural tube defects.
e. What is the therapeutic measure for prevention of open neural tube defects?

f. Explain the types of spina bifida with the help of diagrams.

Solutions

a. Anencephaly is a commonly found congenital anomaly of brain. There is absence of bones of the cranial vault causing exposure of the neural tissue. Anencephalic babies are stillborn (die before birth) or die shortly after birth.
b. The neural tube fails to close at its anterior end (anterior neuropore).
c. Anterior neuropore closes by 25th day and posterior neuropore by 27th day.
d. There is rise in AFP (alpha fetoproteins) in the amniotic fluid in this condition. So estimation of alpha-fetoproteins in amniotic fluid is one method. Other method is sonography.
e. Therapeutic measure to prevent occurrence of such defect consists of consumption of folic acid tablets by the mother around the time of fertilization.
f. Refer to Figure 88.3.

CASE 3

A person came to the hospital for a combination of motor and sensory symptoms. After neurological examination, he was diagnosed as a case of subacute combined degeneration of spinal cord. This disease is due to vitamin B_{12} deficiency.

Questions

a. Which anemia is associated with B_{12} deficiency?
b. What is the intrinsic factor of Castle and which cells produce it?
c. Draw a cross-section of the spinal cord to show the tracts.
d. Name the major tracts that undergo demyelination in this disease.
e. Give the clinical effects of the loss of function in these tracts.
f. What are the positional changes in the developing spinal cord?
g. Briefly describe the arterial supply of spinal cord.
h. What is conus medullaris? Name the cavity inside it.
i. Write short note on cauda equina.

Solutions

a. Pernicious anemia.
b. Intrinsic factor of Castle secreted by parietal cells of fundic glands of stomach helps in absorption of B_{12} from the small intestine.
c. Refer to Figure 84.6
d. The posterior columns, spinocerebellar and lateral corticospinal tracts undergo demyelination on both sides (usually in lumbosacral region).
e. Bilateral loss of position and vibratory sensations below the level of lesion, locomotor ataxia and spastic paraplegia (UMN).
f. During third month of intrauterine life, the length of the cord coincides with the length of the vertebral column. At birth, the lower end of the spinal cord coincides with the lower margin of L3 vertebra. In adult, the lower end of the cord ends at lower margin of L1 vertebra.
g. There are three longitudinal arterial channels on the surface of the spinal cord formed as follows: The two posterior spinal arteries and one anterior spinal artery (branches of vertebral arteries) are replenished at intervals by radicular arteries derived from the segmental arteries. The radicular artery on left side derived from lower posterior intercostal artery is especially large and takes the major share in supply of the lower part of the spinal cord. It is called arteria radicularis magna (artery of Adamkiewicz). The central branches of the anterior spinal artery supply the anterior two-thirds of the cross-sectional area and those of posterior spinal artery supply the posterior horns and posterior columns.
h. The lower tapering end of spinal cord is known as conus medullaris. The central canal expands slightly in the conus medullaris to form terminal ventricle.
i. Cauda equina consists of a leash of spinal nerve roots (resembling the tail of a horse) arising from the conus medullaris. It is located in the dilated part of the subarachnoid space known as lumbar cistern from L2 vertebra to S2 vertebra. It is composed of dorsal and ventral roots of lumbar, sacral and coccygeal nerves surrounding the filum terminale. The filum terminale, 5th sacral and coccygeal nerves pierce the dural sac to traverse the epidural space in the sacral canal. The

lumbar cistern is approached for drawing CSF sample or to inject anesthetic solution between spines of third and fourth lumbar vertebrae so as to avoid injuring the spinal cord. The nerves of the cauda equina are less likely to injure or if injured are capable of regeneration.

CASE 4

A patient was brought to the hospital with sudden onset of vertigo and nystagmus. The attending physician discovered that the patient had dysphagia, dysarthria and hoarseness of voice. On examination, it was found that the laryngeal and palatine muscles on left side were paralysed and there was loss of pain and temperature sensation on left half of face and on the body below the neck on the right side. The above signs and symptoms are indicative of a vascular lesion in the brainstem.

Questions

a. Name the parts of the brainstem and identify the syndrome.
b. Which artery is occluded in this syndrome and what is it a branch of?
c. Give reason for loss of pain and temperature on the left side of face.
d. Give reason for loss of pain and temperature sensations below the neck on the right side.
e. Lesion in which nucleus causes paralysis of laryngeal, pharyngeal and palatine muscles.
f. What is the reason for intact tactile sensation?

Solutions

a. The brainstem consists of midbrain, pons and medulla oblongata from above downwards. Lateral medullary syndrome.
b. Posterior inferior cerebellar artery (left side)—a branch of left vertebral artery.
c. Loss of pain and temperature sense on face on left side is due to lesion of left spinal tract of trigeminal nerve, which is an uncrossed tract.
d. The lateral spinothalamic tract carries sensation of pain and temperature from the body below the neck. Since this is a crossed tract the lesion of left side in medulla will cause effect below the neck on right side.
e. Nucleus ambiguus
f. The tactile sensation is spared because the fibers carrying touch sensation terminate in the main sensory nucleus in the pons.

CASE 5

An elderly woman with the history of hypertension developed paralysis of the left half of the body with increased muscle tone and increased tendon reflexes. The Babinski sign was positive on the affected side. There was altered sensation on the left half of the body. On CT scan a small lesion was noted inside the right hemisphere.

Questions

a. Is the paralysis in this case, of UMN or LMN type? Give reasons in support of your answer.
b. Name the parts of the internal capsule and mention the part in which the lesion was located.
c. Classify white matter of the cerebrum giving examples.
d. Draw a diagram of the internal capsule showing its fiber content.
e. Draw a diagram to show the arterial supply of the internal capsule.
f. Which arteries are called arteries of cerebral hemorrhage?

Solutions

a. Upper motor neuron type of paralysis. The typical features of this type are, increased muscle tone, increased tendon reflexes and positive Babinski sign.
b. The internal capsule consists of five parts: anterior limb, genu, posterior limb, sublentiform part and retrolentiform part. The lesion is likely to be located in anterior part of the posterior limb of internal capsule since the corticospinal fibers and superior thalamic radiations are crowded here.
c. The white matter of cerebrum is classified into three types: association, commissural and projection fibers. The association fibers remain confined to the same hemisphere as they connect different parts of the same hemisphere, example—cingulum. The commissural fibers connect the identical parts of the two hemispheres, example—corpus callosum. The projection fibers connect the cerebral cortex to other parts of CNS, example—corticospinal and corticonuclear fibers.

d. Refer to Figure 98.4
e. Refer to Figure 98.5
f. Lateral striate (lenticulostriate) branches of middle cerebral artery.

CASE 6

A 50-year-old man presented with mask like facies, poverty of movements, shuffling gait and pill rolling tremor at rest. On examination, it was observed that he lacked associated movements (no arm swinging during walking). These signs are typical of a neurodegenerative disease.

Questions

a. Identify the clinical condition giving the specific site, where neurons are affected.
b. What is the peculiarity of the cytoplasmic contents of these neurons?
c. Where do the axons of these neurons mainly project?
d. Deficiency of which neurotransmitter is found in this condition.
e. Give the components of corpus striatum.
f. Give the functional classification of corpus striatum.
g. Draw a horizontal section of the cerebral hemisphere to show the relations of the lentiform nucleus.

Solutions

a. Parkinson's syndrome. The neurons of substantia nigra of the midbrain show degeneration.
b. These neurons contain melanin pigment.
c. Nigrostriate fibers, which are the axons of these neurons project on corpus striatum (caudate nucleus and putamen).
d. Dopamine.
e. Corpus striatum consists of caudate nucleus and lentiform nucleus (lateral putamen and medial globus pallidus).
f. The corpus striatum has functionally two parts: paleostriatum (pallidum) and neostriatum (striatum). The globus pallidus is paleostriatum. The caudate nucleus and putamen are known as neostriatum.
g. Refer to Figure 99.1

CASE 7

A 68- year- old patient complained of difficulty in walking and altered sensation in his right lower limb He also complained of urinary incontinence. On examination, Babinski sign was positive on right side, there was motor weakness and impaired sensation in the right lower limb.

Questions

a. Is it a suprathalamic or infrathalamic lesion? Give reasons for your answer.
b. Identify the site and side of lesion.
c. Occlusion of which artery could be the cause of the lesion in the above mentioned site?
d. Describe the origin and course of this artery.
e. What is Heubner's artery a branch of? Give the effects of its occlusion.

Solutions

a. It is a suprathalamic lesion because the patient has impaired sensations in right lower limb (and not loss of sensations, which is characteristic of infrathalamic lesions).
b. The lesion is in the left paracentral lobule.
c. Occlusion of left anterior cerebral artery will cause infarction in the paracentral lobule.
d. Refer to Chapter 97 on Blood Supply of Brain.
e. Heubner's artery is the central branch of anterior cerebral artery. It is also described as medial striate artery. It pierces the anterior perforated substance to enter the hemisphere and supply the corpus striatum, anterior limb and part of genu of internal capsule. Its occlusion may manifest as contralateral spastic paresis of upper limb accompanied by facial weakness.

CASE 8

Give the effect of occlusion of left middle cerebral artery on the following functions in a patient:

a. Speech
b. Vision
c. Hearing
d. Voluntary movements of lower limbs
e. Ability to wrinkle forehead on right side
f. Sensations in right upper limb.

Solutions

a. Global aphasia
b. Deviation of eyes to left side.

c. No discernible effect since cochlea is represented bilaterally in the auditory cortex.
d. Normal
e. Preserved
f. Altered sensations in the right upper limb.

CASE 9

Neurological examination of a patient revealed following deficits:

a. Deviation of tongue to left side.
b. Loss of vibration sense and sense of conscious proprioception from right half of body.
c. Spastic hemiplegia on right side.

Questions

a. Name the syndrome and the artery occluded.
b. Name the structure involved to cause deviation of tongue to the left.
c. Name the structure involved to cause spastic paralysis of right half of body.
d. Sensory deficit on right side is due to injury to which structure?
e. Trace the path of conscious proprioception from upper limb with the help of diagram.

Solutions

a. Medial medullary syndrome (in which the medial region of the medulla oblongata including hypoglossal nucleus and nerve, pyramid and medial lemniscus are affected). Occlusion of anterior spinal artery is responsible for this syndrome.
b. Lesion of left hypoglossal nucleus or intramedullary part of left hypoglossal nerve causes deviation of tongue to the left (due to paralysis of left genioglossus muscle).
c. The lesion of corticospinal fibers in the left pyramid causes spastic paralysis in right half.
d. Medial lemniscus of left side
e. Refer to posterior column pathways of spinal cord in Chapter 84.

CASE 10

On neurological examination of a 50-year-old diabetic lady, it was noted that that she had weakness in the left half of the body. Examination of the eyes revealed dilated and fixed pupil and ptosis and laterally deviated right eye.

Questions

a. Identify the site of lesion giving reasons.
b. Name the syndrome.
c. Enumerate the functional components of the involved cranial nerve.
d. Give reason for weakness for left half of body.
e. Which examination will help you in deciding whether it is an UMN or LMN paralysis in the left half of body?
f. Trace the pyramidal tract from origin to termination.

Solutions

a. Dilated and fixed pupil, ptosis and lateral deviation of the eye confirm lesion of third nerve or nucleus. Therefore the lesion is in the right half of midbrain at the level of superior colliculus.
b. Weber's syndrome
c. The third nerve is composed of general visceral efferent and somatic efferent functional components.
d. The lesion of left crus cerebri will involve corticospinal fibers, which control the opposite half of the body.
e. This is a UMN paralysis because the patient will show exaggerated deep tendon reflexes, positive Babinski sign and spastic paralysis.
f. Refer to Chapter 98 on White Matter of Brain and to Chapter 84 on Spinal Cord.

SINGLE BEST RESPONSE TYPE MCQs

1. **Supramarginal gyrus is located in:**
   A. Superior temporal gyrus
   B. Inferior parietal lobule
   C. Inferior frontal gyrus
   D. Superior frontal gyrus
2. **Which is not a derivative of neural crest?**
   A. Oligodendroglia
   B. Schwann cells
   C. Spinal ganglia
   D. Suprarenal medulla

3. **Herniation of cerebellar tonsil through foramen magnum results in:**
   A. Dandy-Walker syndrome
   B. Arnold-Chiari syndrome
   C. Down syndrome
   D. Foster-Kennedy syndrome

4. **In occlusion of anterior spinal artery which of the following in the spinal cord is not affected?**
   A. Lateral corticospinal tract
   B. Dorsal spinocerebellar tracts
   C. Ventral spinocerebellar tract
   D. Tract of Gall and Burdach

5. **Injury to left paracentral lobule leads to paresis in:**
   A. Left side of face
   B. Right neck and scapular region
   C. Right leg
   D. Right upper limb

6. **The second order neurons of posterior column tracts carrying sensations from hand are located in:**
   A. Nucleus gracilis
   B. Nucleus cuneatus
   C. Nucleus dorsalis
   D. Accessory cuneate nucleus

7. **Which is not a branch of intracranial part of internal carotid artery?**
   A. Posterior communicating
   B. Carotico-tympanic
   C. Anterior cerebral
   D. Anterior choroidal

8. **The occlusion of intracranial part of anterior spinal artery does not affect:**
   A. Medial lemniscus
   B. Hypoglossal nucleus
   C. Dorsal nucleus of vagus
   D. Corticospinal fibers

9. **Following is the modification of pia mater:**
   A. Ependyma
   B. Septum pellucidum
   C. Linea splendens
   D. Superior medullary velum

10. **Occlusion of this artery in dominant hemisphere results in global aphasia:**
   A. Anterior choroidal
   B. Anterior cerebral
   C. Posterior cerebral
   D. Middle cerebral

11. **Which cranial nerve decussates in superior medullary velum?**
   A. Oculomotor
   B. Trochlear
   C. Trigeminal
   D. Abducent

12. **The temporal pole of the cerebrum receives blood from:**
   A. Cortical branch of anterior cerebral artery
   B. Recurrent branch of anterior cerebral artery
   C. Cortical branch of middle cerebral artery
   D. Cortical branch of posterior cerebral artery

13. **Most laterally located nucleus in the interior of cerebellum is:**
   A. Dentate
   B. Fastigii
   C. Emboliform
   D. Globose

14. **The spinothalamic tracts terminate on the following thalamic nucleus:**
   A. VPM
   B. VPL
   C. Pulvinar
   D. Ventral lateral

15. **The stria terminalis originates in:**
   A. Caudate nucleus
   B. Habenular nucleus
   C. Amygdalod body
   D. Mamillary body

16. **All the following structures are seen in interpeduncular fossa, *except:***
   A. Posterior perforated substance
   B. Anterior perforated substance
   C. Mamillary bodies
   D. Tuber cinereum

17. The axons of Purkinje cells terminate on:
- **A.** Granule cells
- **B.** Glomeruli
- **C.** Dentate nucleus
- **D.** Red nucleus

18. Which of the following is an example of association fibers:
- **A.** Corona radiata
- **B.** Tapetum
- **C.** Forceps minor
- **D.** Arcuate fasciculus

19. CN III passes between following arteries:
- **A.** Posterior cerebral and superior cerebellar
- **B.** Posterior cerebral and posterior choroidal
- **C.** Superior cerebellar and anterior inferior cerebellar
- **D.** Anterior inferior cerebellar and labyrinthine

20. Uncus is supplied by branches of following artery:
- **A.** Anterior choroidal
- **B.** Anterior cerebral
- **C.** Posterior cerebral
- **D.** Middle cerebral

Key to Single Best Response MCQs

1 B	2 A	3 B	4 D	5 C	6 B	7 B
8 C	9 C	10 D	11 B	12 C	13 A	14 B
15 C	16 B	17 C	18 D	19 A	20 C	

MULTIPLE RESPONSE MCQs WRITE TRUE(T) OR FALSE (F) AGAINST EACH STATEMENT

1. The cuneus:
- **A.** is part of frontal lobe
- **B.** is supplied by posterior cerebral artery
- **C.** stria of Generri is visible on its cut surface
- **D.** is located anterior to parieto-occipital sulcus

2. The MLF:
- **A.** connects para-abducent nucleus to contralateral oculomotor nucleus
- **B.** connects vestibular nucleus to nuclei of CN III, CN IV and CN VI
- **C.** is continuous with intersegmental tract of spinal cord inferiorly
- **D.** lies close to motor nucleus of CN V

3. The white commissure of spinal cord:
- **A.** its lesion produces unilateral effects
- **B.** anterior corticospinal tracts cross through it
- **C.** spinothalamic tracts cross through it
- **D.** is the site of cavitation in syringomyelia

4. The basis pedunculi:
- **A.** is dorsal part of midbrain
- **B.** is crossed by oculomotor nerve
- **C.** is pierced by trochlear nerve
- **D.** bounds the interpeduncular fossa postero-laterally

5. The lateral ventricle:
- **A.** its posterior horn contains choroid plexus
- **B.** stria terminalis courses in the roof of posterior horn
- **C.** floor of inferior horn is indented by collateral sulcus
- **D.** shape of its choroid fissure resembles anteriorly pointing "C"

6. Components of epithalamus:
- **A.** optic chiasma
- **B.** pineal gland
- **C.** mamillary body
- **D.** habenular nuclei

7. Contents of lateral sulcus:
- **A.** middle cerebral artery
- **B.** anterior perforated substance
- **C.** basal vein
- **D.** lesser wing of sphenoid

8. Regarding nucleus of Oluf:
- **A.** corresponds to Rexed lamina II
- **B.** confined to first and second sacral segments
- **C.** supplies striated muscles of perineum
- **D.** is part of sacral parasympathetic outflow

9. Regarding neurohypophysis:
- **A.** develops from mesencephalon
- **B.** secretes ADH and oxytocin
- **C.** contains Herring bodies
- **D.** is connected to hypothalamus by portal veins

10. Basivertebral veins:
- **A.** come out of the posterior surface of the vertebral bodies
- **B.** are large in size
- **C.** retrograde flow possible
- **D.** empty into internal vertebral venous plexus

105 Infratemporal Fossa

The infratemporal fossa is an irregular space below the temporal fossa. The knowledge of its bony boundaries (Fig. 105.1) is essential to understand the relations of the contents to each other and to understand the attachments of the pterygoid muscles. The roof is formed medially by the infratemporal surface of the greater wing of sphenoid. The roof separates the fossa from the middle cranial fossa. The features of the roof are, spine of sphenoid, foramen spinosum, foramen ovale and infratemporal crest. Sometimes, the roof may show emissary sphenoidal foramen (foramen of Vesalius) and foramen innominatum. Laterally, where the roof is deficient, the infratemporal fossa is in open communication with the temporal fossa behind the zygomatic arch. Medially, the fossa is bounded by lateral pterygoid plate of the sphenoid and pyramidal process of the palatine bone. The anterior boundary is the posterior surface of the body of maxilla (bearing maxillary tuberosity). Its medial and anterior walls meet below, but are separated above by pterygomaxillary fissure. The upper end of the pterygomaxillary fissure is continuous with the inferior orbital fissure. Medially, the fossa communicates with pterygopalatine fossa through the pterygomaxillary fissure and with the orbit through the inferior orbital fissure. Posteriorly, the temporomandibular joint, tympanic plate and the styloid process are seen. The fossa is open inferiorly.

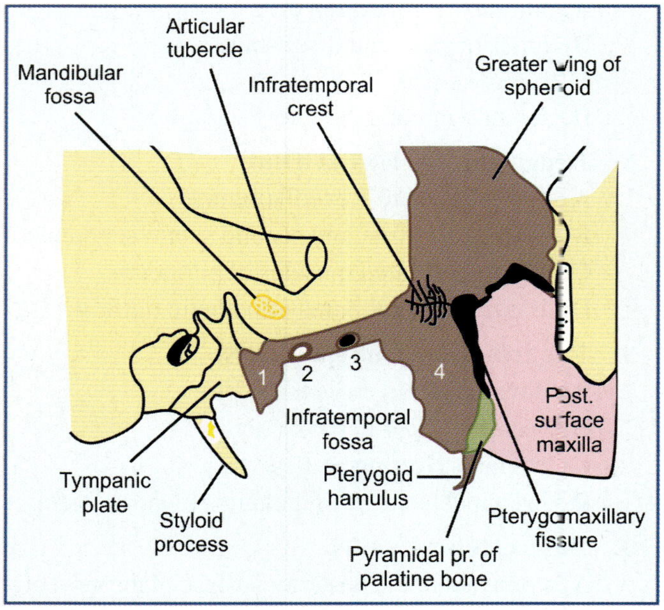

Fig. 105.1: Bony boundaries of infratemporal fossa: (1) Spine of sphenoid, (2) Foramen spinosum, (3) Foramen ovale, (4) Lateral pterygoid plate

Contents

The main contents are: the mandibular nerve and its branches, otic ganglion, chorda tympani nerve (for details of this nerve refer to facial nerve in Chapter 125), first and second parts of maxillary artery and their branches, pterygoid plexus of vein and maxillary vein, spheno-mandibular ligament, tendon of insertion of temporalis and medial and lateral pterygoid muscles (Fig. 108.5). Some authors include tensor veli palatini muscle in the list of contents.

Mandibular Nerve

This nerve is the largest of the three divisions of the trigeminal nerve. It consists of a large sensory root and a small motor root. The sensory root arises from the posterior end of the lateral surface of trigeminal ganglion in the middle cranial fossa. The motor root arises from the pons. It passes under the trigeminal ganglion (lying outside it). The two roots join each other in the foramen ovale or just outside the foramen and the trunk, thus formed enters the fossa to immediately terminate into anterior and posterior divisions.

Functional Components

a. The branchial efferent fibers supply muscles developed from the mesoderm of the first branchial arch.
b. The general somatic afferent fibers bring sensations from the skin of the face and head.

Extracranial Course (Fig. 105.2)

In the infratemporal fossa, the short trunk of the mandibular nerve passes between the lateral pterygoid and the tensor palati muscles and soon divides into anterior and posterior divisions.

Branches of Trunk

a. Meningeal branch (nervus spinosus) enters the middle cranial fossa through foramen spinosum to supply the dura mater of middle cranial fossa.
b. Nerve to medial pterygoid muscle supplies not only the medial pterygoid but also the tensor palati and tensor tympani muscles via its connection to the otic ganglion.

Branches of Anterior Division

a. Buccal branch is a large sensory nerve. It passes anteriorly between the two heads of the lateral pterygoid muscle to reach the buccinator muscle. It supplies the skin of the cheek and the mucous membrane lining the cheek in the oral cavity.

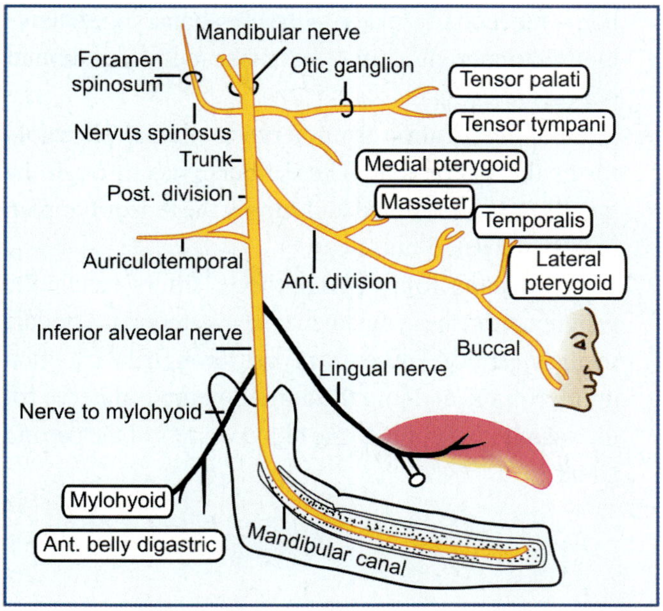

Fig. 105.2: Motor and sensory distribution of mandibular nerve

b. Nerve to lateral pterygoid enters the deep surface of the muscle.
c. Deep temporal nerves (two in number) for the temporalis pass superiorly to reach the temporal fossa, where they enter the deep surface of the muscle.
d. Nerve to masseter leaves the infratemporal fossa through the mandibular notch to enter the deep surface of the masseter.

Branches of Posterior Division

a. The auriculotemporal nerve arises by two sensory roots, which encircle the middle meningeal artery and unite behind it to form a single nerve. The auriculotemporal nerve receives postganglionic parasympathetic fibers from the otic ganglion for the secretomotor supply of the parotid gland. It leaves the fossa by passing posteriorly in relation to the lateral aspect of the spine of the sphenoid. It hooks round the back of the neck of the mandible and enters the parotid gland. The nerve leaves the gland at its upper end to enter the temporal region, where it supplies the sensory fibers to the pinna, external auditory meatus, tympanic membrane and the skin of the temple. The auriculotemporal nerve syndrome or Frey's syndrome is characterized by sweating in the skin (supplied by the nerve), whenever salivation is stimulated either by thought of food or by act of eating. The cause for the gustatory sweating, is, the faulty regeneration of fibers after injury to the auriculotemporal nerve (usually during parotid surgery), in which the secretomotor fibers are connected to the sympathetic fibers inside it. Occasionally, the secretomotor fibers are connected to the sympathetic fibers in the great auricular nerve, in which case, there will be sweating in the skin covering the parotid gland and the angle of the mandible during eating.
b. The inferior alveolar nerve passes vertically downward between the lateral and medial pterygoid muscles. After giving off the nerve to mylohyoid, it enters the mandibular foramen to travel in the substance of the mandible. Here, it supplies the mandibular teeth and gums and gives rise to the mental nerve, which leaves the mandible through the mental foramen to supply the skin of the chin and the lower lip. The inferior alveolar nerve block is used in dental practice. For this, the patient is asked to open the mouth to feel the

anterior margin of the ramus of the mandible and the sphenomandibular ligament. The injection is given in front of the lower end of the ligament.

c. The lingual nerve runs downward in anterior relation to the inferior alveolar nerve. It leaves the fossa by passing between the mandible and the mucous membrane covering it, just inferior to the last molar tooth. It travels in the submandibular region on the surface of the hyoglossus muscle, before entering the mouth. It supplies general sensory fibers to the anterior two-thirds of the tongue. The chorda tympani nerve enters the fossa through the petrotympanic fissure and joins the lingual nerve, which carries the chorda tympani in its substance (the chorda tympani consists of sensory fiber for taste sensations from the anterior two-third of tongue and preganglionic parasympathetic fibers to the submandibular ganglion). For details of chorda tympani nerve refer to submandibular salivary gland in Chapter 70, for nerve supply of tongue refer to Chapter 112 and for facial nerve refer to Chapter 125.

Otic Ganglion

This is a parasympathetic ganglion, which is a relay station on the secretomotor pathway of the parotid gland. It is located deep in the infratemporal fossa just below the foramen ovale. The ganglion lies between the trunk of mandibular nerve on lateral side and the tensor palati muscle on the medial side. The middle meningeal artery and the two roots of auriculotemporal nerve are very closely related to the ganglion.

Connections or Roots (Fig. 105.3)

a. The lesser petrosal nerve is the parasympathetic root of the ganglion. It brings preganglionic fibers, which make synaptic contacts with the neurons of the ganglion. The postganglionic fibers arising from the ganglion cells join the auriculotemporal nerve. The lesser petrosal nerve takes origin from the tympanic plexus in the middle ear. The tympanic branch of the glossopharyngeal nerve forms the tympanic plexus. The lesser patrosal nerve enters the middle cranial fossa, which it leaves via the foramen innominatum or the foramen ovale to enter the infratemporal fossa. Thus, it is the fibers of the glossopharyngeal nerve that are relayed in the otic ganglion. Hence otic ganglion is functionally related to the glossopharyngeal nerve though topographically it lies close to the mandibular nerve.

b. The communication from nerve to medial pterygoid forms the motor root. These fibers pass through the ganglion uninterrupted and supply the tensor tympani and tensor palati muscles.

c. The postganglionic sympathetic fibers reach the ganglion from the sympathetic plexus around the middle menigeal artery. These fibers pass through the ganglion uninterrupted and join the auriculotemporal nerve for the vasomotor supply to the blood vessels of the parotid gland.

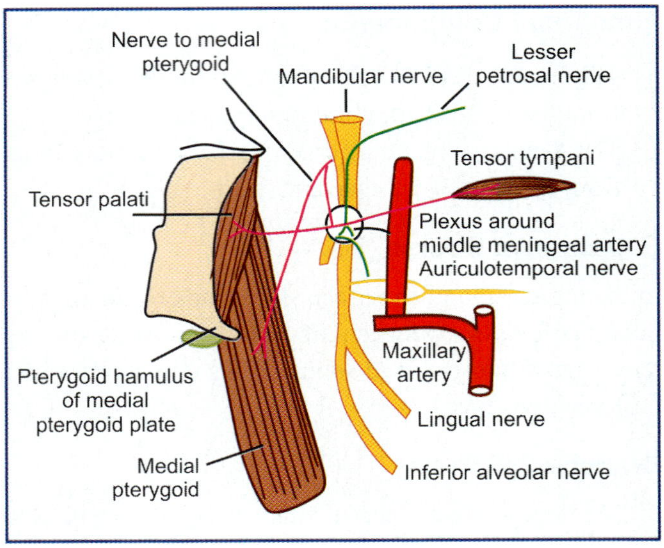

Fig. 105.3: Plan to show connections of otic ganglion. Motor root: Nerve to medial pterygoid. Parasympathetic root: Lesser petrosal nerve. Sympathetic root: Plexus around middle meningeal artery

106 Pterygopalatine Fossa

The pterygopalatine or sphenopalatine fossa is a small pyramidal space below the apex of the orbit. The root of the lateral pterygoid plate of the sphenoid and the adjoining part of the greater wing of the sphenoid limit the fossa posteriorly. The perpendicular plate of the palatine bone forms the medial boundary. The maxilla bounds the fossa anteriorly and laterally there is a pterygopalatine (pterygomaxillary) fissure.

Communications and Contents

The pterygopalatine fossa has a number of communications through which nerves and vessels leave or enter the fossa. The foramen rotundum transmits the maxillary nerve to the fossa from the middle cranial fossa. The pterygopalatine ganglion is suspended from the maxillary nerve. The nerve of the pterygoid canal (the motor root of the ganglion) reaches via the pterygoid canal, which connects the fossa to the foramen lacerum. The third part of maxillary artery enters the fossa via the pterygopalatine fissure from the infratemporal fossa. The nasopalatine nerves and vessels leave the fossa through the nasoplatine or sphenopalatine foramen to enter the nasal cavity. The palatinovaginal canal connects it to the nasopharynx and transmits the pharyngeal branch of the maxillary nerve. The greater palatine canal transmits the palatine nerves and vessels to the oral cavity. The inferior orbital fissure leads to the orbital floor and here the maxillary nerve continues as the infraorbital nerve.

Maxillary Nerve (Fig. 106.1)

The maxillary nerve is one of the three divisions of the trigeminal nerve. It is entirely sensory. It leaves the trigeminal ganglion between the ophthalmic and mandibular nerves in the middle cranial fossa and passes forwards in the lower part of the lateral wall of the cavernous sinus to reach the foramen rotundum, through which it enters the pterygopalatine fossa. In the cranial cavity, it gives meningeal branch to the dura mater of middle cranial fossa. From the posterior wall of the fossa, the maxillary nerve courses forwards in the upper part of the fossa and gives its ganglionic branches. The pterygopalatine ganglion is suspended from the maxillary nerve by its two ganglionic branches. The maxillary nerve turns sharply in the lateral direction in the inferior orbital fissure. About halfway between the orbital apex and the orbital rim, the nerve turns medially to enter the infraorbital groove and canal (in the floor of the orbit) to continue as the infraorbital nerve, which emerges on the face through the infraorbital foramen.

Branches of Trunk

a. The ganglionic branches pass through the pterygopalatine ganglion and supply the mucous membrane of the palate, nasopharynx and nasal cavity (see below).

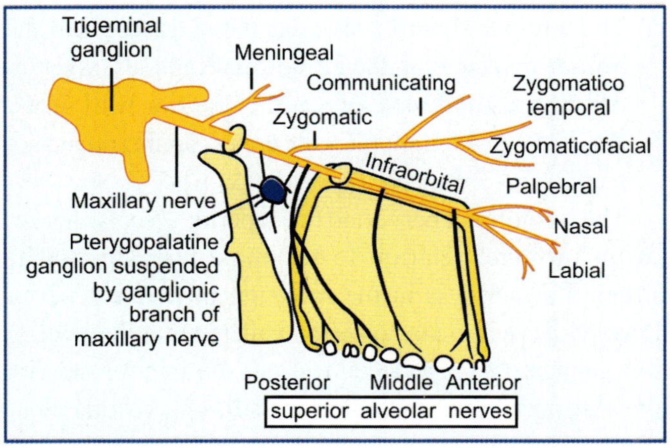

Fig. 106.1: Scheme depicting direct branches of maxillary nerve in middle cranial fossa and pterygopalatine fossa

b. The zygomatic nerve leaves the fossa through the inferior orbital fissure to enter the orbit. It travels forwards along the lateral wall of the orbit, where it divides into zygomaticotemporal and zygomaticofacial nerves. The zygomatic nerve usually carries the postganglionic parasympathetic fibers from the sphenopalatine ganglion to the lacrimal gland.

c. The posterior superior alveolar nerve supplies the upper molar teeth of its side.

Branches of Infraorbital Nerve

a. In the infraorbital canal, the infraorbital nerve gives rise to the middle superior alveolar and the anterior superior alveolar nerves.

b. After emerging on the face, the infraorbital nerve gives palpebral branches to lower eyelid, nasal branches to the side of the nose and the labial branches to the upper lip.

Superior Alveolar (Dental) Nerves

There are three superior alveolar nerves: posterior superior, middle superior and anterior superior alveolar nerves, which supply the upper gums and teeth.

a. The posterior superior alveolar nerve pierces the posterior surface of the maxilla and then descends under the mucosa of the maxillary sinus. It supplies the mucosa of the sinus and the molar teeth.

b. The middle superior alveolar nerve arises from the infraorbital nerve in the infraorbital canal. It passes downward and anteriorly in the lateral wall of the maxillary sinus. It supplies upper premolar teeth.

c. The anterior superior alveolar nerve arises from the infraorbital nerve in the infraorbital canal. It traverses downwards and medially in the anterior wall of the maxillary sinus. It supplies the upper canine and incisor teeth.

The infraorbital nerve and the superior alveolar nerves are in intimate relation to the maxillary sinus. The infraorbital nerve is in the roof, the posterior superior alveolar nerve is in the posterior wall, the middle superior alveolar nerve is in the lateral wall and the anterior superior alveolar nerve is in the anterior wall. Due to this close proximity, the inflammation in the maxillary sinus causes irritation of these nerves leading to pain in the maxillary teeth. So, a patient suffering from maxillary sinusitis may go to the doctor on account of toothache (a best example of correlation between anatomical relations and clinical presentation).

Pterygopalatine Ganglion

This ganglion is the largest of the peripheral parasympathetic ganglia. Though topographically it is related to the maxillary nerve, functionally it is related to the facial nerve.

Connections or Roots (Fig. 106.2)

a. The parasympathetic root is derived from the nerve of the pterygoid canal (Vidian nerve), which is formed by the union of the deep petrosal nerve and the greater petrosal nerve in the foramen lacerum. The greater petrosal nerve (a branch of facial nerve) carries preganglionic parasympathetic fibers for relay in the ganglion. The postganglionic fibers either join the zygomatic nerve or pass through the orbital branches of the ganglion to supply secretomotor fibers to the lacrimal gland. In addition, the nasal and palatine glands also receive secretomotor fibers through nasal and palatine nerves. Irritation of the nerve of pterygoid canal causes lacrimation and excessive secretion of nasal and palatine glands (typical features of allergic rhinitis or hay fever). Therefore, this nerve is called the "nerve of hay fever" (for the same reason the pterygopalatine ganglion is known as "hay fever ganglion)."

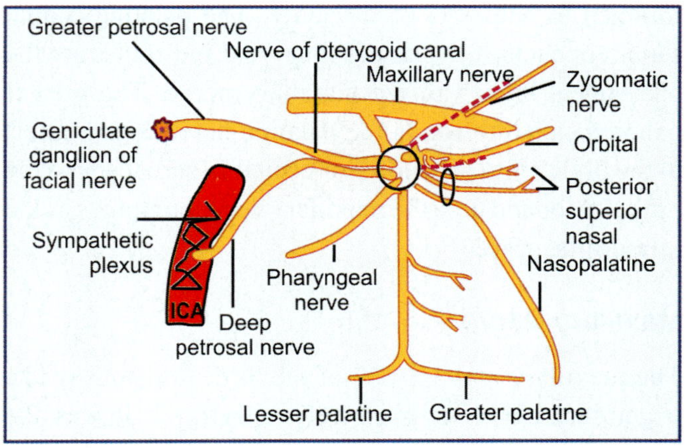

Fig. 106.2: Scheme to show connections of pterygopalatine ganglion (Note that sensory branches of ganglion are the indirect branches of maxillary nerve)

b. The sympathetic root is derived from the deep petrosal component of the nerve of pterygoid canal. The deep petrosal nerve arises from the sympathetic plexus around the internal carotid artery. This nerve brings postganglionic sympathetic fibers to the ganglion where they do not synapse. They leave through its orbital branches for the orbitalis muscle in the orbit and are vasomotor to nasal cavity and palate.
c. The sensory root is derived from the ganglionic branches of the maxillary nerve. These fibers of the maxillary nerve just pass through the ganglion and leave it through its following branches.

Sensory Branches

a. The branches to the palate include the greater and lesser palatine nerves, which enter the greater palatine canal and reach the oral cavity through the greater and lesser palatine foramina. They supply the mucous membrane and glands of the inferior surface of the palate.
b. The branches to the nasal cavity include a few posterior inferior nasal branches from greater palatine nerve to supply the mucosa covering the inferior nasal concha, inferior meatus and middle meatus in posteroinferior part of the lateral nasal wall. The nasal branches arise directly from the ganglion and pass through the sphenopalatine foramen to enter the nasal cavity. These are called posterior superior nasal nerves. They are divided in two sets. The nerves of the lateral set supply the nasal mucosa of the posterosuperior part of the lateral wall. The nerves of the medial set supply the roof and the posterior part of the nasal septum. One of the nerves of the medial set is long and is called the nasopalatine (sphenopalatine) nerve. It runs anteroinferiorly on the nasal septum lying in a groove and leaves the nasal cavity through the incisive foramen to enter the oral cavity, where it supplies the mucosa covering the anterior part of the hard palate.
c. The orbital branches enter the orbit through the inferior orbital fissure and supply the orbital periosteum.
d. The pharyngeal branch enters the palatinovaginal canal to enter the nasopharynx for the supply of the mucous membrane behind the opening of the auditory tube and the mucosa of the auditory tube.

107 Maxillary Artery

The maxillary artery is the larger of the two terminal branches of the external carotid artery. It begins behind the neck of the mandible in the substance of the parotid gland. It is divided in three parts. The first and second parts are in the infratemporal fossa while the third part lies in the pterygopalatine fossa. The maxillary artery supplies a wide area through its many branches.

Subdivisions (Fig. 108.7)

a. The first part (mandibular part) extends from the mandibular neck to the sphenomandibular ligament. It runs along the lower margin of the lateral pterygoid muscle. The first part alone is accompanied by maxillary vein. It gives off five branches.

b. The second part (pterygoid part) ascends obliquely forwards and upwards between the lower head of lateral pterygoid and the temporalis muscles. It then passes superficial or deep to the lower head of the lateral pterygoid. The pterygoid venous plexus surrounds this part. This part of the artery gives off four branches.

c. The third part (pterygopalatine part) passes between the two heads of the lateral pterygoid muscle and enters the pterygomaxillary fissure to reach the pterygopalatine fossa. Six branches arise from this part.

Branches in Infratemporal Fossa (Fig. 107.1)

First Part

a. The deep auricular artery ascends in the substance of the parotid gland and pierces the bony or cartilaginous part of the external acoustic meatus to supply the TMJ and external auditory meatus.

b. The anterior tympanic artery enters the tympanic cavity (middle ear) through the petrotympanic fissure.

c. The accessory meningeal artery enters the cranium through the foramen ovale and supplies the dura mater.

d. The inferior alveolar artery enters the mandibular foramen to travel in the mandibular canal located inside the body of the mandible. It gives lingual and mylohyoid branches before entry into the mandibular foramen. The lingual branch supplies the tongue and the mylohyoid branch accompanies the mylohyoid nerve in the mylohyoid groove. In the mandibular canal the inferior alveolar nerve gives branches to the lower teeth. Its named branch called mental artery comes out on the face through the mental foramen along with mental nerve.

e. The middle meningeal artery is a very important branch. It is described in detail in Chapter 86.

Second Part

a. The deep temporal branches (anterior and posterior) enter the temporal fossa to supply the temporalis muscle.

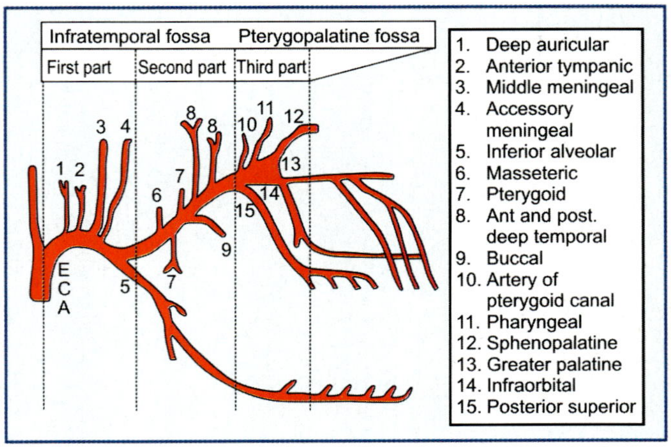

Fig. 107.1: Branches of maxillary artery in infratemporal and pterygopalatine fossae

b. Separate pterygoid branches for lateral and medial pterygoid muscles arise from this part.
c. The masseteric artery passes through the mandibular notch along with masseteric nerve to reach the deep surface of the muscle.
d. The buccal branch runs forward along with the buccal branch of mandibular nerve and supplies the external surface of the buccinator. It also provides blood to the buccal mucosa.

Branches in Pterygopalatine Fossa (Fig. 107.1)

Third Part

a. The posterior superior alveolar artery arises just as the maxillary artery enters the pterygomaxillary fissure and is spent in supplying the upper molar teeth.
b. The infraorbital artery may arise in common with posterior superior alveolar artery. It enters the orbit through the inferior orbital fissure and courses forwards in the infraorbital groove and canal in the floor of orbit. Along with the infraorbital nerve the artery appears on the face through the infraorbital foramen. In the infraorbital canal it gives rise to orbital branches for orbital contents and anterior superior and middle superior alveolar branches for the upper teeth.
c. The greater or descending palatine artery descends in the greater palatine canal and enters the oral cavity through the greater palatine foramen. It travels anteriorly on the surface of the hard palate to reach the incisive foramen through which some terminal branches enter the nasal cavity. The lesser palatine artery is a branch of the greater palatine artery as it lies in the palatine canal. These small arteries emerge through the lesser palatine foramina into the oral cavity.
d. The pharyngeal artery leaves through the palatino-vaginal canal and supplies the nasopharynx, auditory tube and sphenoidal sinus.
e. The artery of the pterygoid canal leaves through the pterygoid canal and supplies the nasopharynx, auditory tube and tympanic cavity.
f. The sphenopalatine artery is the continuation of the maxillary artery. It leaves through the sphenoplatine foramen to enter the nasal cavity.

Pterygoid Venous Plexus

The pterygoid venous plexus lies in the muscles of the infratemporal fossa. It continues as the maxillary vein, which accompanies only the first part of the maxillary artery. The pterygoid plexus receives the following veins, sphenopalatine, deep temporal, pterygoid and masseteric, buccal, alveolar (both superior and inferior), greater palatine, middle meningeal and a branch of inferior ophthalmic vein. The communications of the plexus are important in the spread of infection to the cavernous sinus. The deep facial vein connects the pterygoid plexus to the facial vein and the emissary vein connects it to the cavernous sinus. The dangerous area of face is thus brought in communication with the cavernous sinus. Any infection of this area of face may cause cavernous sinus thrombosis.

108 Temporomandibular Joint

The temporomandibular joint (TMJ) is the articulation between the cranium and the mandible. The right and left joints help in mastication and in opening and closing the mouth.

Special Features of TMJ

The unique feature of this articulation is that a single bone (mandible) articulates bilaterally with right and left mandibular fossae of temporal bone. Moreover, its cranial components are immobile while the lower component (mandible) alone is mobile. The right and left joints, though anatomically distinct, act as a single unit functionally. Each joint is completely divided into upper and lower compartments by an articular disc.

Type of Joint

TMJ is a bicondylar variety of synovial joint.

Articular Bones (Fig. 108.1)

The condyle or the head of the mandible forms a convex articular surface inferiorly. The mandibular fossa on inferior surface of squamous temporal bone and the adjacent articular tubercle at the root of zygoma form a concavoconvex articular surface superiorly. The articular surfaces are covered with fibrocartilage.

Fibrous Capsule

The upper attachment of the capsule is to the articular tubercle, periphery of the articular fossa and the squamotympanic fissure. The lower attachment is to the neck of the mandible just below the condyle. The fibrous capsule is loose above the articular disc but closely fitting below it.

Ligaments

a. The lateral or temporomandibular ligament extends from the tubercle of the root of the zygoma backward and downward to the posterior margin of the neck of the mandible. It is the thickening of the fibrous capsule. It is the strongest ligament of the joint that prevents posterior dislocation of the joint.
b. The sphenomandibular ligament is an accessory ligament of TMJ. It is situated on the medial aspect of the joint in the infratemporal fossa and extends from the spine of the sphenoid to the lingula of the mandible.
c. The stylomandibular ligament is an accessory ligament of TMJ. It extends from the styloid process of temporal bone to the angle of the mandible. It is the thickened part of cervical fascia.
d. The articular disc of the TMJ is a fibrocartilage. It is congruous with both the articular surfaces. Thus, its upper surface is concavoconvex and lower surface is

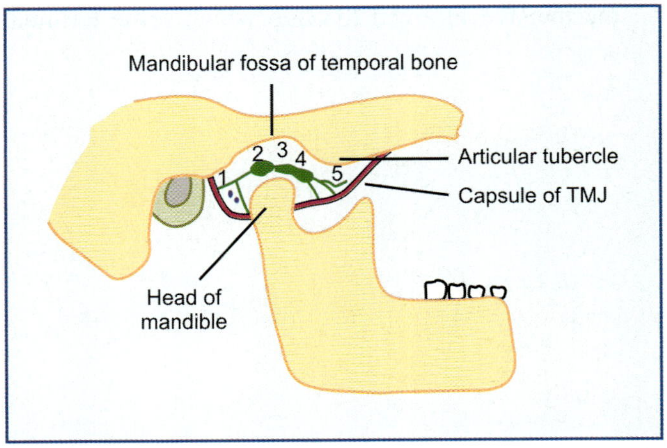

Fig. 108.1: Interior of TMJ showing parts of articular disc. (1) Bilaminar part with venous plexus, (2) Posterior thick band, (3) Intermediate zone, (4) Anterior thick band, (5) Anterior extension

concave. It divides the joint in upper meniscotemporal and lower meniscomandibular compartments. It is firmly attached to the fibrous capsule at its periphery. Anteriorly, it blends with the lateral pterygoid muscle at its insertion (the disc is regarded, morphologically a part of lateral pterygoid). It is firmly attached to the back of the neck of the mandible to ensure the movements of the mandibular head and the disc together in the upper compartment. The disc shows five different regions as follows: anterior extension, anterior thick band, intermediate zone, posterior thick band and bilaminar zone. The upper fibroelastic lamina of the bilaminar zone is attached to the mandibular fossa while the lower nonelastic lamina is attached to the back of the neck of the mandible. A venous plexus lies between the two laminae. When the articular disc is detached from the fibrous capsule, is known as derangement of the joint. It causes painful movements and clicking sound while opening and closing the mouth.

Synovial Membrane

The synovial membrane lines the fibrous capsule above and below the disc but does not line the disc. It also lines the nonarticular surfaces of the both the compartments.

Relations of TMJ

a. Anteriorly, it is related to the insertion of lateral pterygoid muscle. The masseteric nerve and vessels are related as they pass through the mandibular notch.
b. Laterally, the temporomandibular ligament is covered with parotid gland but the rest of the lateral aspect is subcutaneous being covered with fascia and skin. Therefore it is possible to feel the head of the mandible by a finger placed in front of the tragus.
c. Posteriorly, it is related to the glenoidal process of the parotid, which separates it from the bony part of external acoustic meatus (tympanic plate).
d. Medially, it is related to the maxillary artery and vein and the auriculotemporal nerve (structures in the infratemporal fossa).

Nerve Supply

The auriculotemporal nerve and the nerve to masseter, both branches of the mandibular nerve, supply the joint.

Movements (Fig. 108.2)

a. Depression or the downward movement of the mandible is responsible for opening the mouth.
b. Elevation or the upward movement of the depressed mandible brings about closure of the mouth.
c. Protraction (protrusion) means forward movement of the mandible.
d. Retraction means backward movement of the protracted mandible.
e. Side to side or grinding movements in right and left joints alternately are responsible for mastication.

The movements of elevation and depression take place around a mobile (dynamic) transverse axis in both the compartments of the joint. The protraction and retraction take place in the upper compartment around a transverse axis. The rotation of mandibular condyle takes place around a vertical axis in both the compartments in side-to-side movements.

Depression

The depression of mandible results in opening of the mouth. This movement takes place in three stages. At first, there is a forward rotation of the mandibular condyle in the lower compartment so that the condyle comes in contact with the intermediate area of the disc. The axis of this movement passes through the condyles of both mandibles. In the second stage, there is a forward movement of both the disc and the condyle in the upper

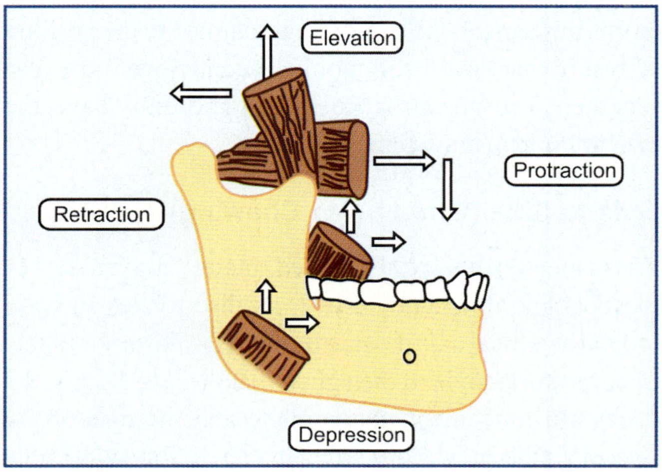

Fig. 108.2: Movements of mandible. Arrows indicate the direction of actions of muscles of mastication, which can be identified from the site of attachment of each

Section three

compartment around a mobile transverse axis. This movement ends when the upper lamina of the disc is stretched. At the end of this movement, the condyle lies below the anterior thick band of the disc. In the third stage, there is a forward and downward rotation of the condyle in the lower compartment, around a transverse axis passing through the mandibular foramina. At the end of this movement, the condyle comes to lie below the articular tubercle and the mouth is wide open. The lateral pterygoid muscles of both sides are active in this movement. The suprahyoid muscles (geniohyoid, anterior belly of digastric and mylohyoid) and the infrahyoid muscles help indirectly by keeping the hyoid bone steady. The gravity is also a factor in helping depression.

Elevation

In this movement, the stages in the rotation of condyle alone and condyle with disc as seen in depression are reversed. The masseter, temporalis and the medial pterygoid muscles of both sides contract to produce elevation.

Protraction or Protrusion

In this movement, the mandible is pulled forwards with the closed mouth. The condyle and the disc together slide forwards on the mandibular fossa of both sides in the upper compartment. The lateral pterygoid and the medial pterygoid muscles bring about protraction.

Retraction

In this movement, the mandible is returned to the position of rest by backward sliding of the condyle and the disc together. The posterior fibers of temporalis have the primary role in retraction.

Side to Side (Grinding or Chewing)

These movements are also called rotatory movements of mastication. One condyle with its disc rotates forward around a vertical axis passing through the posterior aspect of opposite condyle. It then glides backwards. During the backward movement, the condyle and the disc of the opposite side move forward. This alteration swings the mandible from side to side. The medial and lateral pterygoids of the two sides act alternately in grinding movements. Masseter and temporalis assist the pterygoid muscles.

Clinical Highlights (Fig. 108.3)

The anterior dislocation of the head of the mandible in the infratemporal fossa after opening the mouth widely, may occur due to sudden blow on the chin or due to spasm of lateral pterygoid muscles (as in sudden yawn). In this position the mouth cannot be closed. Reduction of the dislocated mandible is done as follows. The mandible is depressed posteriorly by exterting pressure on the lower molar teeth with the help of both the thumbs. Simultaneously the assistant elevates the chin. The first monoeuvre overcomes the muscular spasm and the second one pushes the condyle in the mandibular fossa.

Muscles of Mastication

There are four muscles of mastication (jaw muscles). Masseter lies external to the ramus of the mandible and is the most superficial of the four muscles. Temporalis lies partly in the temporal fossa and partly in infratemporal fossa. The lateral and medial pterygoid muscles lie in the infratemporal fossa. All the four muscles take origin from the cranium and insert in mandible, which they move at the TMJ. All the four muscles of mastication develop from the mesoderm of the first pharyngeal arch and

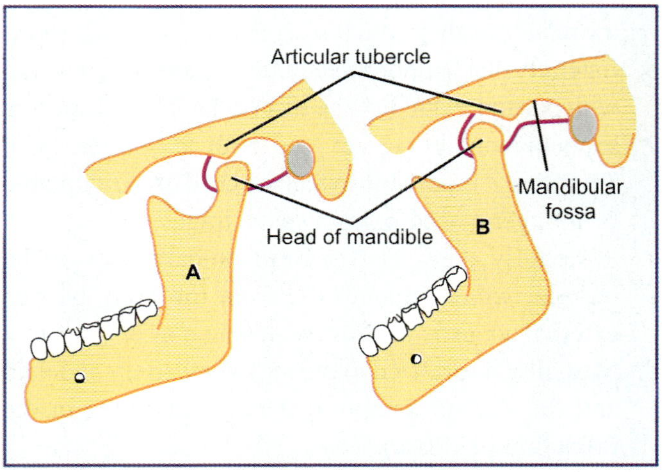

Fig. 108.3: Showing relation of mandibular head to articular tubercle. 'A' depicts widely open mouth, in which the head moves below the tubercle. 'B' depicts anterior dislocation of TMJ in which the head moves anterior to the tubercle

hence are supplied by the nerve of the first arch (mandibular nerve). The buccinator is regarded as the accessory muscle of mastication.

Masseter (Fig. 108.4)

It is quadrilateral shape. It can be palpated in the living on clenching the teeth. At its anteroinferior angle pulsations of the facial artery are felt.

Attachments

The masseter takes origin from the lower margin and deep aspect of the zygomatic arch and is inserted in the lateral aspect of ramus and coronoid process of mandible.

Relations

The parotid duct and branches of facial nerve cross the muscle superficially. The posterior part of its superficial surface is in contact with anteromedial surface of parotid gland. The buccal pad of fat separates its anterior border from the buccinator muscle. It is covered with parotideo-masseteric fascia, which is the extension of deep fascia of the neck in the face.

Nerve Supply

The anterior division of mandibular nerve supplies it.

Actions

The masseter elevates the mandible. Its superficial fibers help in protraction of mandible.

Temporalis

It is a fan-shaped muscle. It is covered with stiff temporal fascia, which is attached to the superior temporal line of parietal bone and to the medial and lateral margins of the zygomatic arch by two layers.

Attachments

The temporalis takes origin from the medial wall of temporal fossa and the temporal fascia and is inserted in the anterior margin of coronoid process and anterior margin of the ramus of mandible. The anterior fibers are vertical in direction while the middle fibers are obliquely placed and the posterior fibers are horizontally disposed.

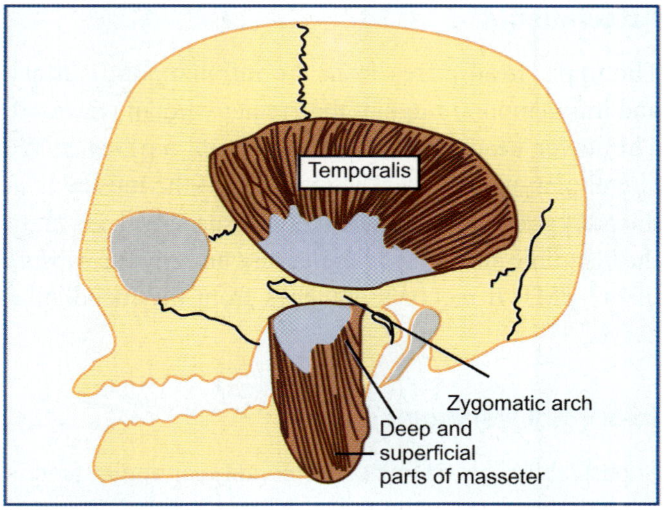

Fig. 108.4: Attachments of temporalis and masseter muscles

Actions

The anterior vertical fibers cause elevation. The posterior horizontal fibers are responsible for retraction. It also assists in side to side movements.

Nerve Supply

It is supplied by the deep temporal branches of the mandibular nerve.

Lateral Pterygoid (Fig. 108.5)

It is roughly triangular with base (origin) directed anteriorly and apex (insertion) posteriorly. It is a short muscle with two heads (upper and lower).

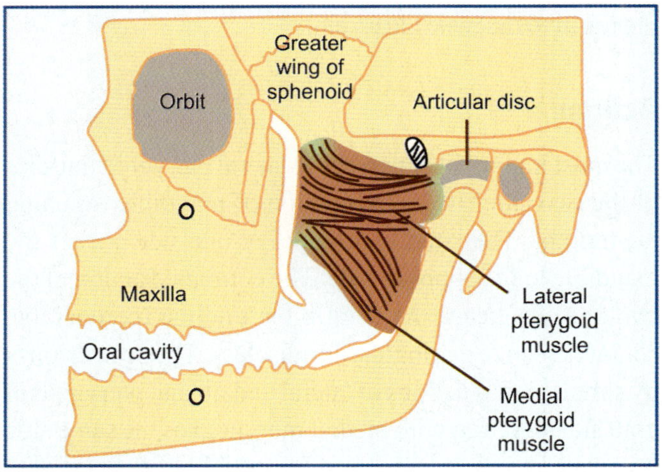

Fig. 108.5: Attachments of pterygoid muscles (Note that infratemporal fossa is exposed by removal of zygomatic arch and ramus of mandible)

Attachments

The upper head arises from the infratemporal surface and infratemporal ridge of the greater wing of sphenoid. The lower head arises from the lateral surface of the lateral pterygoid plate. The insertion of the muscle is in the pterygoid fovea on the anterior aspect of the neck of the mandible and in the articular disc and fibrous capsule of the TMJ. It receives branches from the mandibular nerve.

Important Relations (Fig. 108.7)

Superficially, it is related to the mandibular ramus, tendon of temporalis, masseter and the second part of maxillary artery (if it passes superficial to it). The medial pterygoid muscle, middle meningeal artery, second part of maxillary artery (if it passes deep to the lateral pterygoid), sphenomandibular ligament and the mandibular nerve are related to its deep aspect. Its upper border is related to the deep temporal nerves and masseteric nerve with accompanying vessels and its lower border is related to the lingual and inferior alveolar nerves, inferior alveolar vessels and the first part of maxillary artery (with its meningeal branches namely middle meningeal and accessory meningeal). In between the two heads of the muscle the buccal nerve emerges and maxillary artery enters to become the third part. The maxillary vein and pterygoid plexus of veins are intimately related to the lateral ptrygoid muscle. The contraction of the lateral pterygoid helps in propulsion of the blood in the pterygoid venous plexus in to the maxillary vein.

Actions

The most important action of the lateral pterygoid muscles of the two sides is the depression of mandible (opening the mouth). The lateral pterygoid of one side pushes the mandible to the opposite side. The combined action of the two muscles keeps the chin in the midline (comparable action is seen in genioglossus muscles). The protrusion is by simultaneous actions of lateral and medial pterygoid of both sides. Acting with medial pterygoid of the same side it causes lateral movement of mandible to the opposite side. When the same movement is followed in the opposite side, grinding or chewing of the food occurs.

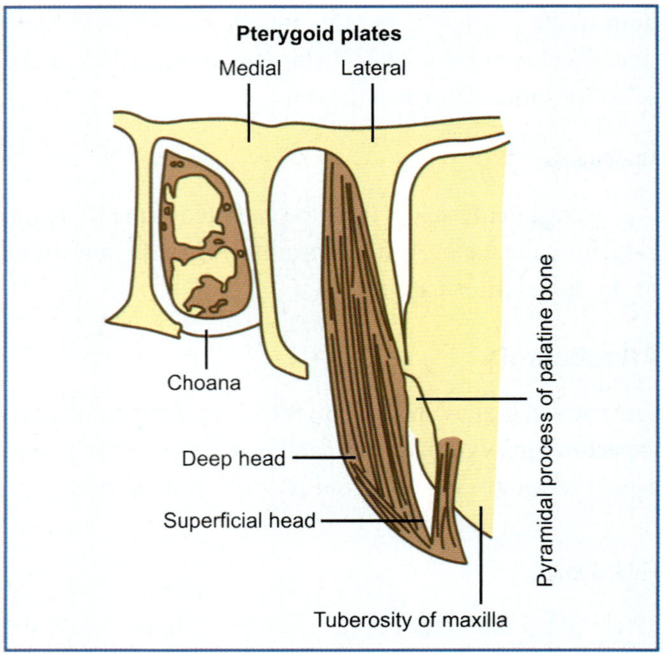

Fig. 108.6: Showing origin of medial pterygoid muscle

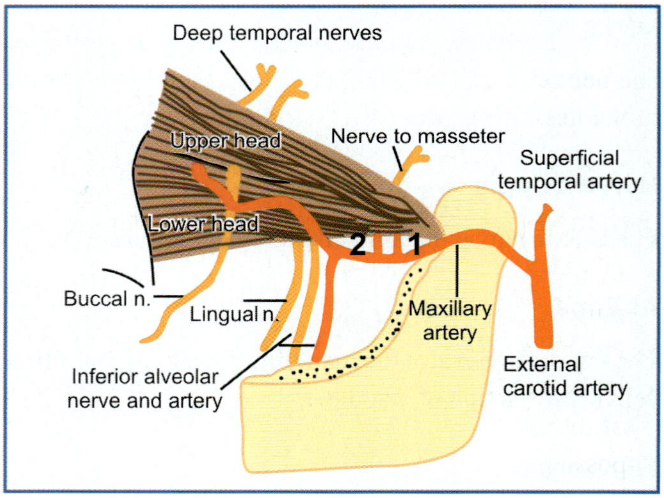

Fig. 108.7: Relations of lateral pterygoid muscle. 1-Middle meningeal artery, 2-Accessory meningeal artery

Nerve Supply

A branch from anterior division of mandibular nerve supplies lateral pterygoid.

Medial Pterygoid

This muscle is of quadrilateral shape. It has larger deep and smaller superficial heads, which embrace the lower head of the lateral pterygoid muscle.

Attachments (Figs 108.5 and 108.6)

The deep head arises from the medial surface of lateral pterygoid plate. The superficial head arises from the lateral surface of pyramidal process of palatine bone and from the maxillary tuberosity (it is worthy of note that medial pterygoid arises from three bones, sphenoid, palatine and maxilla). The two heads unite below the lower head of the lateral pterygoid muscle and are inserted on a roughened area on the medial surface of the ramus of mandible above the mylohyoid line.

Actions

The medial pterygoid muscles of both sides act to elevate the mandible (closure of mouth). The medial and lateral pterygoids of both sides act to protract the mandible. The medial and lateral pterygoid of one side act together to move the mandible in grinding movements and this is followed by similar movements in the opposite side.

Nerve Supply

The nerve to medial pterygoid arises from the trunk of mandibular nerve. For unusual features of the nerve to medial pterygoid, refer to otic ganglion.

Clinical Highlights

a. In tetanus, there is contraction of both masseter muscles (trismus), which causes locked jaw.
b. Paralysis and wasting of temporalis produce hollowing in the temple. Paralysis of masseter causes flattening of the angle of jaw and clenching of the teeth is not possible. Paralysis of the lateral pterygoid muscles causes the jaw to deviate towards the paralysed side on opening the mouth as a result of action of normal muscle (Fig. 108.8).

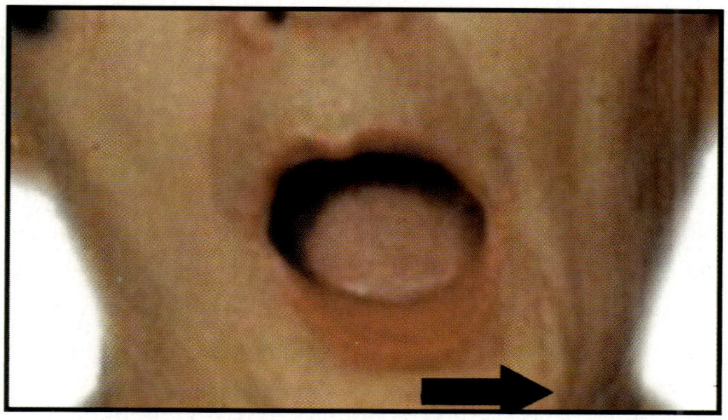

Fig. 108.8: Jaw deviation to the left due to paralysis of left lateral pterygoid muscle

Testing Muscle Function

The muscles of mastication are routinely tested in clinical assessment of trigeminal nerve.

a. A subject is asked to clench the teeth to test masseter and temporal muscles, which stand out in prominence equally on each side. This is checked by inspection and palpation of the muscles of both sides. There will be absence of contraction with unilateral paralysis of these muscles.
b. To test lateral pterygoid muscle, a subject is asked to open the mouth widely but slowly against resistance. The chin moves down in the midline in a normal case. Deviation of chin (lower jaw) to one side indicates paralysis of the lateral pterygoid of the side to which the chin deviates.

109 Orbit

The orbit is a pyramidal shaped bony cavity on the norma frontalis. It protects the delicate eyeball and other structures associated with it. The bony boundaries of the orbit are as follows:

a. The base, which is directed anteriorly, is formed by the orbital margin.
b. The narrow apex is located posteriorly.
c. The roof is formed by the orbital plate of the frontal bone. It separates the orbit from the anterior cranial fossa.
d. The floor is formed by the orbital plate of the maxilla. It separates the orbit from the maxillary air sinus.
e. The thick lateral wall consists of zygomatic bone in front and greater wing of sphenoid behind. At the junction of lateral wall and roof, there is a fossa for lacrimal gland.
f. The medial wall consists of four bones. From before backward they are, frontal process of maxilla, lacrimal bone, orbital plate of ethmoid and body of sphenoid. The orbital plate of ethmoid (lamina papyracea) is very thin and it separates the orbit from the middle and posterior ethmoidal sinuses. A deep lacrimal groove is present at the junction of maxilla and lacrimal bone for the lacrimal sac.

It is worthy of note that the medial walls of the right and left orbits are parallel to each other while the lateral walls meet each other at an angle of 90°.

The periorbita or orbital fascia is the periosteum that lines the orbit. It can be easily stripped off the bones. At the orbital margins the periorbita projects inside the eyelids as orbital septa, which are attached to the tarsal plates in the eyelids.

Communications

a. The supraorbital notch (foramen) located in the medial part of superior orbital margin transmits the supraorbital nerve and vessels from the orbit to the anterior quadrant of scalp.
b. The infraorbital groove and canal located in the orbital floor carries the infraorbital nerve to the infraorbital foramen through which it appears on the face.
c. The nasolacrimal canal connects the orbit to the inferior meatus of nasal cavity. It lodges the nasolacrimal duct.
d. The inferior orbital fissure is located posteriorly between the maxilla and the greater wing of sphenoid. It communicates the orbit to the pterygopalatine fossa and transmits the maxillary nerve, its zygomatic branch and inferior ophthalmic vein.
e. The superior orbital fissure is located posteriorly between the greater and lesser wings of sphenoid. It communicates with the middle cranial fossa and transmits a number of structures (Fig. 109.1), which are, the lacrimal, frontal and nasociliary (branches of ophthalmic nerve), the oculomotor, trochlear and abducent nerves in addition to superior ophthalmic vein.
f. The optic canal is located at the apex of the orbit, bounded by the lesser wing and the body of the sphenoid. It transmits the optic nerve and ophthalmic artery.
g. The anterior and posterior ethmoidal foramina are present on the medial wall for the passage of anterior and posterior ethmoidal nerves and vessels.
h. On the lateral wall, there are two foramina for the passage of zygomaticotemporal and zygomaticofacial nerves.

Contents

a. Eyeball is the most important content. It lies in the anterior part of orbit.
b. The nerves that are present inside the orbit are, the optic, oculomotor, trochlear and abducent nerves. In addition, the lacrimal, frontal and nasociliary branches of the ophthalmic division of the trigeminal nerve course through the orbit.

c. The ciliary ganglion (a peripheral parasympathetic ganglion) is present in topographical relation to the nasociliary nerve but in functional relation to the oculomotor nerve.
d. The ophthalmic artery with its branches and the superior and inferior ophthalmic veins are the blood vessels inside the orbit.
e. A group of six extraocular muscles are inserted into the sclera of the eyeball. In addition, levator palpebrae superioris passes closer to the roof to the orbit for insertion in the upper lid.
f. The lacrimal gland is located in relation to lateral wall and the lacrimal sac in relation to medial wall of the orbit.
g. The fascial sheath of the eyeball (fascia bulbi) and the orbital fat are the supporting tissue.

Extraocular Muscles (EOMs)

The extraocular muscles are so called because they lie outside the eyeball. However, they are inside the orbit hence called intraorbital muscles. They consist of a group of six muscles concerned with the movements of the eyeball and one concerned with the elevation of the upper eyelid. These muscles are divisible into two groups, voluntary and involuntary.

Voluntary Muscles

The voluntary muscles are named as, levator palpebrae superioris, superior and inferior recti, lateral and medial recti and superior and inferior oblique. Of the seven voluntary muscles the levator palpebrae elevates the upper eyelid while the four recti and two oblique muscles are responsible for the movements of the eyeball.

Involuntary Muscles

There are three involuntary or smooth muscles, the superior tarsal or Müller's muscle, inferior tarsal and orbitalis.

Special Features of Voluntary EOMs

The extraocular muscles have the smallest motor units among the skeletal muscles. The ratio of nerve fibre to muscle fibre is 1: 2 or 3 or 4 in extraocular muscles while it is 1: 125 in other skeletal muscles. The small motor units signify fine movements of eyeball by muscle contractions. These muscles are described as yoke muscles because simultaneous contraction of the muscles in the two eyes is necessary for conjugate movements of the eyes. For example, simultaneous contraction of right medial rectus and left lateral rectus muscles causes lateral conjugate movement of the eyes to the left.

Levator Palpebrae Superioris

This muscle has voluntary and involuntary parts. The involuntary part is known as Müller's muscle or superior tarsal muscle. It is the highest muscle in the orbit lying very close to the orbital roof.

Origin

The levator palpebrae superioris takes origin by a tendon from the inferior surface of the lesser wing of sphenoid at the apex of the orbit (Fig. 109.1). The muscle broadens as it passes forwards above the superior rectus and enters the upper lid as a wide aponeurosis, which splits in three laminae.

Insertion

The upper lamina is inserted in the anterior surface of superior tarsus and in the skin of upper eyelid. The middle lamina containing smooth muscle fibres of Müller's muscle is attached to the superior margin of superior tarsus and

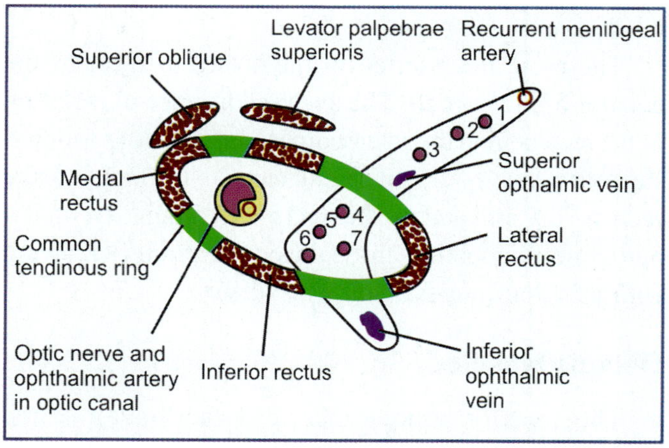

Fig. 109.1: Scheme to show common tendinous ring, optic canal and superior orbital fissure. (1) Lacrimal nerve, (2) Frontal nerve, (3) Trochlear nerve, (4) and (6) Upper and lower divisions of oculomotor nerve, (5) Nasociliary nerve, (7) Abducent nerve

Section three

the lower lamina gains attachment to the superior conjunctival fornix.

Nerve Supply

The voluntary part receives nerve supply from the upper division of oculomotor nerve. The involuntary part receives supply from the postganglionic sympathetic fibers from the superior cervical sympathetic ganglion (Fig. 4.2).

Actions

The levator palpebrae superioris elevates the upper eyelid. Therefore, it is antagonistic to orbicularis oculi.

Ptosis

Ptosis means drooping of the upper eyelid. Paralysis of levator palpebrae superioris due to injury to oculomotor nerve, results in complete ptosis. Paralysis of Müller's muscle occurs in Horner's syndrome. It is due to disruption of sympathetic nerve supply of the eye and results in partial ptosis.

Recti Muscles

The four recti muscles take origin from a common fibrous ring (tendon of Zinn), which encircles the optic foramen and adjacent part of the superior orbital fissure (Fig. 109.1). The superior, inferior, medial and lateral recti arise from the corresponding parts of the ring. The recti muscles run forward first encircling the optic nerve and then the eyeball, inside a muscular cone.

The recti are inserted in the sclera in front of the equator of the eyeball. The average distance of insertion of the recti behind the sclerocorneal junction is as follows, superior rectus—7.7 mm, lateral rectus—6.9 mm, inferior rectus—6.5 mm and medial rectus—5.5 mm. An imaginary line connecting these insertion points creates a configuration known as spiral of Tillaux.

Oblique Muscles (Fig. 109.2A)

a. The superior oblique muscle is the longest of the intraorbital muscles. It arises from the body of sphenoid just above and medial to the optic canal. It passes forward along the superomedial part of the orbit and ends in a tendon, which turns sharply in posterolateral direction by passing through the fibrocartilaginous trochlea on the frontal bone (trochlea is regarded as the functional origin of the muscle). The tendon passes inferior to the superior rectus muscle and is inserted in the posterosuperior quadrant of the sclera behind the equator of the eyeball.
b. The inferior oblique muscle is entirely separate from the other five muscles as far as its origin is concerned. It arises from the anteromedial part of the floor of the orbit, from the maxilla just lateral to the nasolacrimal groove. At first, it passes in posterolateral direction under the eyeball below the inferior rectus muscle. Then, it turns upward for insertion in the sclera close to that of superior oblique behind the equator of the eyeball.

Nerve Supply of EOMs

The lateral rectus muscle is supplied by abducent nerve and the superior oblique is supplied by trochlear nerve. The oculomotor nerve supplies superior rectus, medial

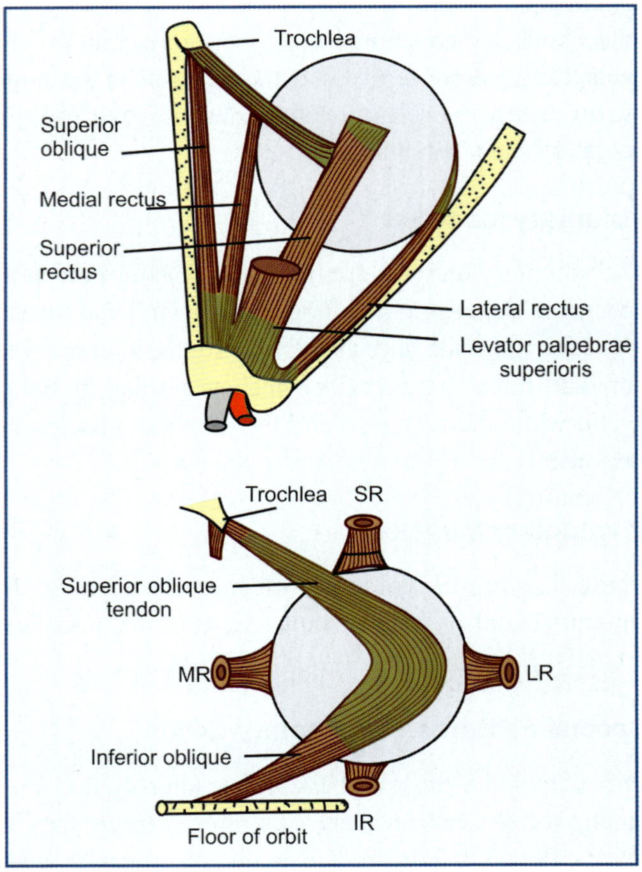

Fig. 109.2A: Showing attachments of extraocular muscles

rectus, inferior rectus and inferior oblique muscles. The nerve supply can be summed up by the formula- LR6, SO_4, rest 3.

Actions

The medial rotation (adduction) and lateral rotation (abduction) of the eyeball take place around a vertical axis passing through the equator. The elevation and depression take place around a transverse axis passing through the equator. Intorsion and extorsion (moving 12 o' clock position of cornea medially and laterally respectively) take place around the anteroposterior or visual axis.

Understanding the relationship of the visual axis and the line of the muscles is the basis of the actions of the extraocular muscles (Fig. 109.2B) and of testing the integrity of the nerves in clinical practice. The visual axis is the line that passes through the anterior and posterior poles of the eyeball. The superior and inferior recti are disposed at an angle of about 25° lateral to the visual axis in the primary position of the eyeball. Therefore, only in the abducted position of the eyeball the visual axis coincides with the axis of superior and inferior recti. The superior and inferior oblique muscles are disposed at an angle of about 51° medial to the visual axis in the primary position of the eyeball. Therefore, only in the adducted position of the eyeball the visual axis coincides with the axis of oblique muscles.

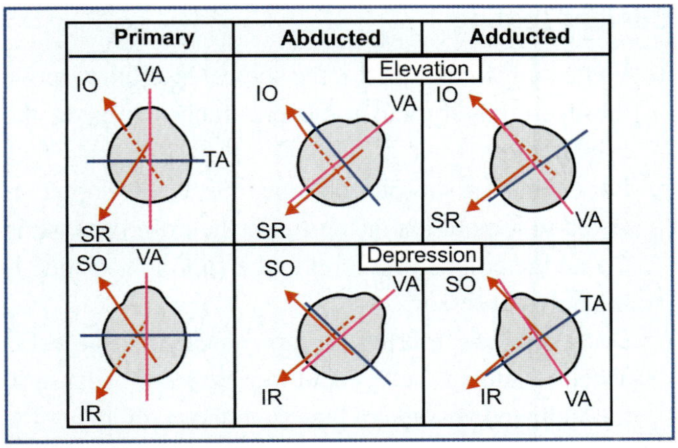

Fig. 109.2B: Showing effectiveness of an isolated muscle as elevator or depresser of eyeball with changing relationship to visual axis (VA: Visual axis, TA: Transverse axis, IO: Inferior oblique, SR: Superior rectus, SO: Superior oblique, IR: Inferior rectus)

Actions of Individual Muscles (Fig. 109.3)

a. The medial rectus causes adduction only while the lateral rectus causes abduction only.
b. The superior rectus causes elevation, adduction and intorsion in primary position of eyeball. It causes elevation only in the abducted position of the eyeball.
c. The inferior rectus causes depression, adduction and extorsion in the primary position while it causes depression only in the abducted position of the eyeball.
d. The superior oblique causes depression, abduction and intorsion in the primary position while it causes depression only in the adducted position of the eyeball.
e. The inferior oblique causes elevation, abduction and extorsion in the primary position while it causes elevation only in the adducted position of the eyeball.

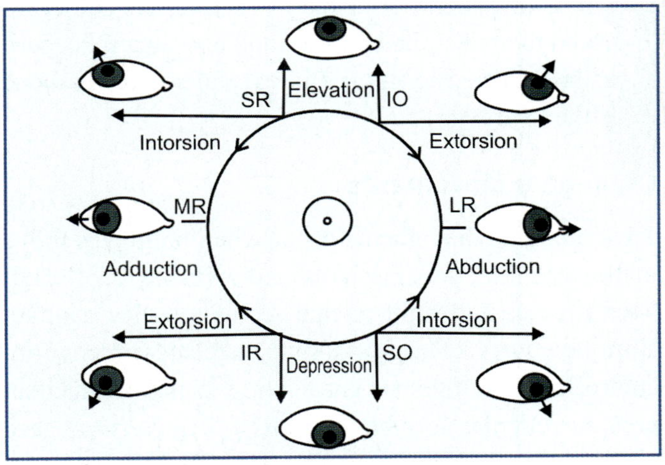

Fig. 109.3: Actions of extraocular muscles

Group Actions of Muscles

a. Adduction is the combined action of medial, superior and inferior recti.
b. Abduction is the combined action of lateral rectus and superior and inferior oblique muscles.
c. Pure elevation in the primary position is the combined action of superior rectus and inferior oblique muscles.
d. Pure depression in the primary position is the combined action of inferior rectus and superior oblique muscles.
e. Intorsion is the combined action of superior rectus and superior oblique muscles.
f. Extorsion is the combined action of inferior rectus and inferior oblique muscles.

Clinical Testing

a. For testing medial rectus, the subject is asked to move the eye medially and for lateral rectus to move the eye laterally.
b. For testing the superior oblique muscle, the subject is asked to look at his or her tip of the nose because in the adducted position of eye, the superior oblique is the only depressor.
c. For testing the inferior oblique muscle, the subject is asked to adduct the eye and look upward because in the adducted position of the eye, inferior oblique is the only elevator.
d. For testing the superior rectus muscle, the subject is asked to abduct the eye and then look upward because in the abducted position of the eye, superior rectus alone is the elevator.
e. For testing the inferior rectus muscle, the subject is asked to abduct the eye and look downward because in the abducted position of the eye, inferior rectus alone is the depressor.

Conjugate Movements

The conjugate movements occur when both eyes move in the same direction. For looking toward the left, the left lateral rectus and right medial rectus muscles contract simultaneously. The horizontal gaze movements are controlled by horizontal gaze centre in the paramedian pontine reticular formation (PPRF). The vertical gaze movements take place, when both eyes look up or down simultaneously and are controlled by vertical gaze centre in upper midbrain. Lesion in MLF alone or in MLF and PPRF in pons, can affect the horizontal movements of the eye as shown in Figure 90.10.

Clinical Highlights

Unilateral paralysis of a single muscle may produce strabismus or squint (deviation of the eye to the opposite side). This results in diplopia or double vision on looking towards the side of muscle action.

a. The paralysis of lateral rectus produces internal or medial squint and diplopia on turning the eye laterally. The paralysis of medial rectus causes external or lateral squint and diplopia on turning the eye medially.
b. The paralysis of superior rectus produces diplopia on looking up. The paralysis of inferior rectus produces diplopia on looking down.
c. In paralysis of superior oblique, there is no obvious squint but patient experiences diplopia on looking down for example while coming down the staircase. The paralysis of inferior oblique produces diplopia on looking up.
d. In cavernous sinus thrombosis, there may be ophthalmoplegia (paralysis of all extraocular muscles).

Ophthalmic Nerve (Fig. 109.4)

The ophthalmic nerve is one of the three divisions of the trigeminal nerve. It takes origin from the trigeminal ganglion and enters the lateral wall of the cavernous sinus. Here the nerve divides in three branches, lacrimal, frontal and nasociliary, which enter the orbit through the superior orbital fissure.

Lacrimal Nerve

It enters through the lateral part of the superior orbital fissure outside the tendinous ring. The lacrimal nerve passes forward along the upper border of lateral rectus muscle and receives a twig from the zygomatico-temporal nerve. This communication brings postganglionic parasympathetic fibres for the lacrimal gland from the pterygopalatine ganglion. The lacrimal nerve supplies the skin of the lateral part of the upper eyelid and conjunctiva.

Frontal Nerve

This nerve enters the orbit through the lateral part of the superior orbital fissure medial to the lacrimal nerve. After entering the orbit, the frontal nerve passes between the orbital roof and the levator palpebrae superioris. About halfway between the apex and the base of the orbit, the frontal nerve divides into supraorbital and supratrochlear nerves. The distribution of these nerves is mentioned in Chapter 57.

Nasociliary Nerve

This nerve enters the orbit through the common tendinous ring lying between the superior and inferior divisions of oculomotor nerve. Inside the orbit, the nasociliary nerve

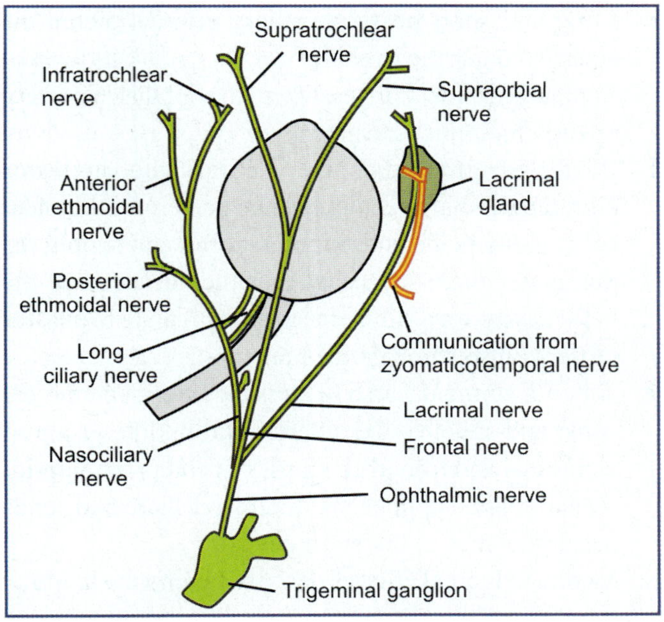

Fig. 109.4: Distribution of ophthalmic nerve on right side. (Note: The ciliary ganglion suspended from nasociliary nerve)

passes from lateral to medial side by crossing above the optic nerve. It continues as the anterior ethmoidal nerve after reaching the anterior ethmoidal foramen on the medial wall of the orbit.

Branches of Nasociliary Nerve

a. A communicating branch is given to the ciliary ganglion.
b. Two to three long ciliary nerves pierce the sclera around the attachment of optic nerve to the eyeball. They run forward in the space between the sclera and choroid and supply ciliary body, iris and cornea.
c. Infra-trochlear nerve emerges below the pulley of the superior oblique tendon. It supplies skin of both eyelids, adjoining part of the side of the nose, conjunctiva and lacrimal sac.
d. Anterior ethmoidal nerve is the continuation of nasociliary nerve. It has a very complex course. It leaves the orbit through the anterior ethmoidal foramen and canal to enter the anterior cranial fossa, where it lies on the cribriform plate of ethmoid bone. The nerve enters the slit by the side of the crista galli to enter the nasal cavity, where it divides into lateral and medial internal nasal branches. The lateral internal nasal branch emerges from the nose as the external nasal nerve to supply the skin of ala, vestibule and tip of the nose.
e. Posterior ethmoidal nerve is a slender branch that passes through the posterior ethmoidal foramen and supplies the ethmoidal and sphenoidal sinuses.

Ciliary Ganglion (Fig. 110.4)

This is a peripheral parasympathetic ganglion located in the posterior part of the orbit hung from the nasociliary nerve. It lies between the optic nerve and the origin of the lateral rectus muscle, the optic nerve being medial to it.

Connections

a. Motor or parasympathetic root is a branch from the nerve to inferior oblique. The motor root conveys the preganglionic fibres, which make synaptic contact with the ganglionic cells.
b. Sensory root is provided by connections to nasociliary nerve. This root contains sensory fibres from the eyeball and these fibres pass through the ganglion without relay.
c. Sympathetic root is derived from the plexus around the ophthalmic artery, carrying the postganglionic sympathetic fibres from the superior cervical ganglion. These fibres pass through the ganglion without relay and supply the dilator pupillae muscle.

Branches of Ciliary Ganglion

About 8 to 10 short ciliary nerves arise from the ganglion. These branches run anteriorly to pierce the sclera around the attachment of the optic nerve. The short ciliary nerves contain postganglionic parasympathetic, postganglionic sympathetic and sensory fibres. The postganglionic parasympathetic fibres supply the sphincter pupillae and ciliaris muscles.

Ophthalmic Artery (Fig. 109.5)

The ophthalmic artery is the sole supply of the contents of orbit including the eyeball. It arises from internal carotid artery after the latter's emergence from the roof of the cavernous sinus. The ophthalmic artery enters the orbit

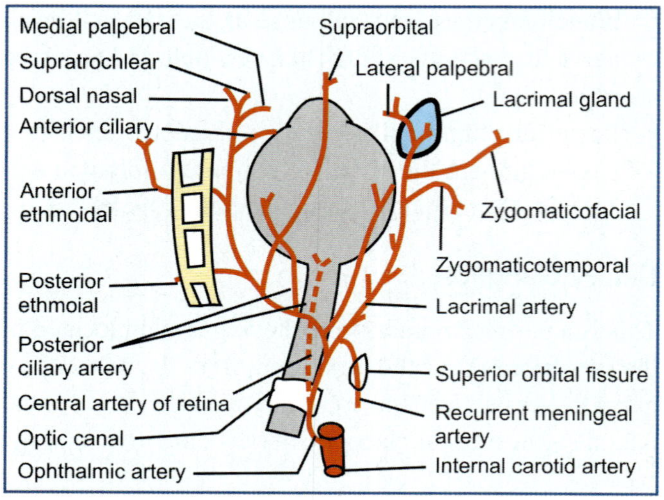

Fig. 109.5: Simplified plan to show branches of ophthalmic artery on right side

through the optic canal, where it lies below and lateral to the optic nerve. Inside the orbit, the ophthalmic artery runs forward lying lateral to the optic nerve and then crosses obliquely above the optic nerve to reach the medial wall of the orbit. The relations of the three structures crossing the optic nerve are the superior ophthalmic vein, the ophthalmic artery and the nasociliary nerve (VAN from before backward). At the medial end of the upper eyelid it divides in supratrochlear and dorsal nasal branches.

Branches

The ophthalmic artery gives rise to as many as ten branches.

a. Central artery of retina is the first branch, which enters the substance of the optic nerve.
b. Lacrimal artery supplies the lacrimal gland and ends by giving lateral palpebral branches to both the lids. A recurrent meningeal branch passes back via the lateral part of superior orbital fissure to anastomose with a branch of the middle meningeal artery. Sometimes, this anastomosis may replace the lacrimal artery.
c. Muscular branches (lateral and medial) are given to intraorbital muscles. These muscular branches give rise to anterior ciliary arteries, which travel with four recti to provide blood to the anterior segment of the eyeball.
d. Long and short posterior ciliary arteries pierce the sclera to enter the eyeball.
e. Supraorbital artery arises, where the ophthalmic artery crosses the optic nerve.
f. Posterior ethmoidal artery enters the posterior ethmoidal canal and supplies the posterior ethmoidal cells. It enters the anterior cranial fossa to supply the duramater there. Its nasal branches descend in the nasal cavity via a slit in the cribriform plate to anastomose with sphenopalatine branches.
g. Anterior ethmoidal artery enters the anterior ethmoidal canal and supplies the anterior and middle group of ethmoidal and frontal air sinuses. It enters the anterior cranial fossa, supplies the duramater there and sends nasal branches to the nasal cavity.
h. Medial palpebral arteries descend behind the lacrimal sac to enter the lids.
i. Supratrochlear artery is the terminal branch, which leaves the orbit superomedially.
j. Dorsal nasal artery is the other terminal branch. It emerges from the orbit and divides in two branches. One of the branches joins the terminal part of facial artery while the other runs along the dorsum of the nose joining the artery of the opposite side.

Ophthalmic Veins (Fig. 109.6)

a. The superior ophthalmic vein is formed posteromedial to the upper eyelid by the union of its two tributaries, which communicate with the facial and supraorbital

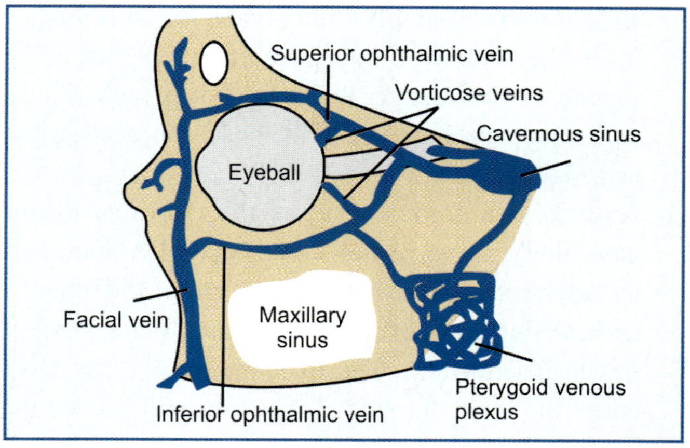

Fig. 109.6: Formation, course and termination of ophthalmic veins

veins. It travels backwards in the orbit along with the ophthalmic artery and leaves the orbit through the superior orbital fissure to terminate in the cavernous sinus. It receives venae vorticosae and the anterior ciliary veins from the eyeball.

b. The inferior ophthalmic vein begins near the anterior part of orbital floor in a network of veins and usually terminates in superior ophthalmic vein or may reach the cavernous sinus. It communicates with pterygoid venous plexus by way of small veins that pass through the inferior orbital fissure. The ophthalmic veins are potentially emissary veins since they connect the cavernous sinus to the veins in the face and thus become the route for the infection from face to spread to the cavernous sinus.

Fascia Bulbi or Tenon's Capsule

This is the fascial sheath of the eyeball. It extends from the optic nerve to the sclerocorneal junction. It provides the eyeball with a socket for free movements. The tendons of intraorbital muscles perforate the fascia bulbi, which sends the tubular sheaths around the tendons. The medial and lateral check ligaments are the extensions from the sheaths of the medial and lateral recti tendons to the orbital walls. The lateral check ligament is attached to the Whitnall's tubercle of the zygomatic bone. The medial check ligament is attached to the posterior lacrimal crest of the lacrimal bone. The suspensory ligament is the lower thick part of the fascia. The medial and lateral check ligaments and the suspensory ligament provide a hammock like support to the eyeball.

110 Eyeball

The eyeball is the peripheral organ of vision. It contains the refractive media, intraocular muscles and the photosensitive retina. The extraocular muscles are inserted in the sclera of the eyeball to give it mobility so that the visual axis remains under the neuromuscular control. This is essential in determining the spatial relationship of the two eyeballs to each other, which is needed for binocular vision and conjugate eye movements.

The eyeball is located in the anterior part of the orbital cavity embedded in the orbital fat and separated from it by a membranous envelope called fascia bulbi or Tenon's capsule. The eyeball is made up of the segments of two spheres of different sizes placed one in front of the other. The anterior segment is the transparent cornea and forms one-sixth of the eyeball. Its radius of curvature is about 8 mm. The posterior segment is the opaque sclera and forms five-sixth of the eyeball. Its radius of curvature is about 12 mm.

The anterior pole of the eyeball is the center of curvature of cornea and the posterior pole is the center of posterior curvature of the eyeball, which is located slightly lateral to the attachment of optic nerve. The geometric or optic axis is the line joining the two poles. The equator of the eyeball lies midway between the two poles. The visual axis is the line passing through the fovea centralis of retina. The visual axis lies lateral to the optic axis.

Development

The eyeball develops from neuroectoderm, surface ectoderm and the mesenchyme. During the fourth week of intrauterine life, bilateral optic vesicles project from the diencephalon (Fig. 88.4) and proceed laterally towards the surface ectoderm. The optic vesicle consists of the optic cup and the optic stalk (Fig. 110.1). Under the inductive influence of the optic vesicle, the overlying surface ectoderm becomes thickened to form the lens placode. The lens placode sinks below the surface ectoderm to become the lens vesicle by sixth week. The optic vesicle is invaginated to form the double-layered optic cup. The space between the inner and outer layers of the cup is called the intra-retinal space, which is gradually obliterated. The choroid fissure is the deficiency on the lower edge of the optic vesicle and of the optic stalk. Its function is to carry the hyaloid artery to the developing lens. By seventh week the choroidal fissure closes forming a narrow optic canal inside the optic stalk. Failure of the fissure to close completely results in coloboma. The pigment layer of retina develops from outer thinner layer of optic cup and its neural layer develops from the posterior four-fifth of the inner layer of optic cup. The retinal detachment takes place through the

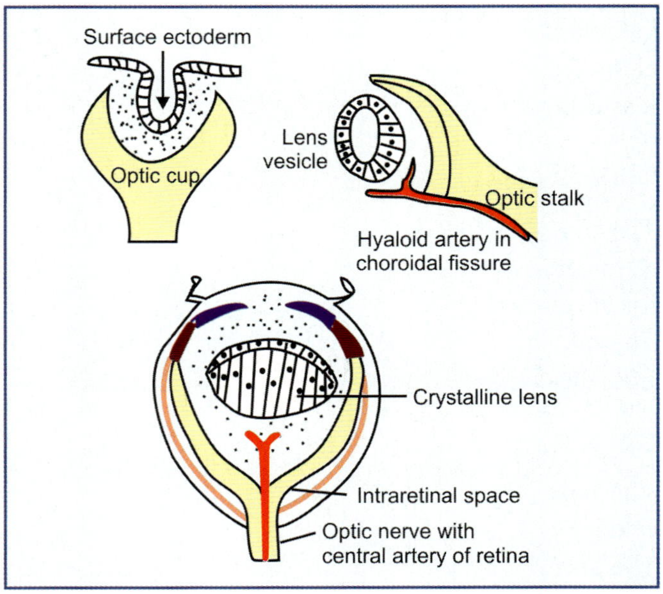

Fig. 110.1: Development of crystalline lens and retina

embryonic intra-retinal space. The optic stalk and the contained axons of the ganglion cells form the optic nerve. The myelination of the nerve fibers in optic nerve takes place after birth by oligodendroglia. The hyaloid vessels convert into central artery and vein of retina.

Crystalline Lens

The lens develops from the lens placode, which is a thickening of surface ectoderm formed under the inductive influence of the optic vesicle (in the absence of the inductive influence the lens fails to develop). The critical period in the development of the lens is fourth to the sixth weeks. Hence, if the mother is exposed to rubella virus (German measles) before seventh week of gestation the child may be born with congenital cataract. The lens placode invaginates to form the lens vesicle, which consists of anterior and posterior epithelial walls enclosing a cavity. The cells of the posterior wall rapidly elongate and are filled with crystallins, which make them transparent. These are known as primary lens fibers, which gradually obliterate the lens cavity. The mitotic division of the anterior epithelial cells at the equator forms the new lens fibers (secondary lens fibers) throughout life. The mesenchyme on the anterior surface of the developing lens condenses to form the pupillary membrane. At about eighth month of intrauterine life, the pupillary membrane begins to degenerate.

The developing lens is richly supplied through the vascular capsule fed by the hyaloid artery and the anterior choroidal artery. However, the vascular capsule of the lens disappears before birth.

Choroid, Ciliary Body and Iris (Uveal Tract)

The choroid and ciliary body develop from the condensation of mesenchyme surrounding the optic vesicle. The iris develops from both neuroectoderm and mesenchyme. The sphincter and dilator muscles of the iris are derived from the neuroectoderm while the ciliaris is mesodermal.

Cornea and Sclera

The corneal epithelium is derived from the surface ectoderm and the rest of the cornea from the mesenchyme. The sclera develops from condensation of the mesenchyme outside the optic cup.

Vitreous Body

The primary vitreous is derived from ectodermal cells of the developing lens and the neuroectoderm of the retinal layer of optic cup. The mesenchyme that enters the cup through the choroidal fissure also joins the primary vitreous. The branches of the hyaloid artery supply blood to the primary vitreous. The secondary vitreous develops from the retina and it pushes the primary vitreous behind the lens. The secondary vitreous is basically an extracellular matrix. When the hyaloid artery atrophies it leaves behind a hyaloid canal in the vitreous (Fig. 110.2).

Congenital Anomalies

a. Congenital cataract occurs during intrauterine life due to genetic factors, maternal rubella and malnutrition. Congenital cataract is more common in Down syndrome.
b. Congenital aphakia (absence of lens) is a rare anomaly, which is due to failure of the inductive influence of the optic vesicle on the surface ectoderm to form the lens placode.
c. Persistent pupillary membrane occurs when the central part of the pupillary membrane fails to disintegrate before birth.

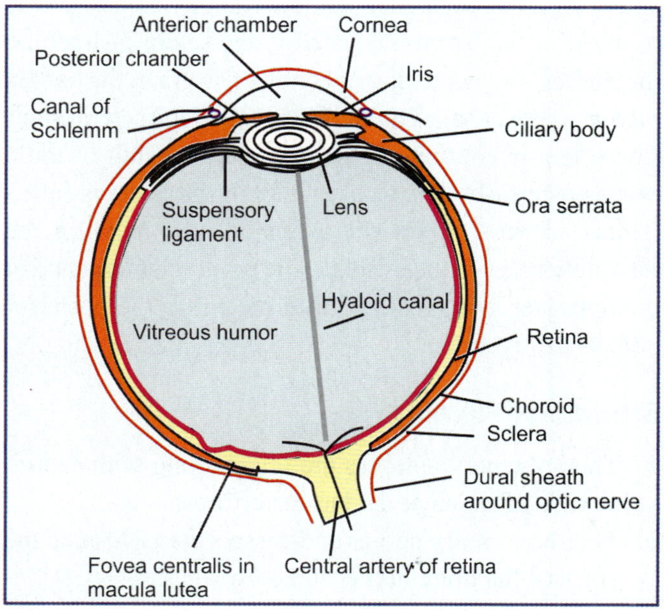

Fig. 110.2: Horizontal section through left eyeball showing its three coats and the interior

d. Coloboma is a notched defect in a part of iris, ciliary body, retina or choroid. It is caused by failure of the choroidal fissure to close. Coloboma iridis is a common abnormality of eye.

Coats of Eyeball (Fig. 110.2)

The eyeball consists of three layers, which from without inwards are, the fibrous layer, uveal tract (vascular and pigmented layer) and the neural layer.

Fibrous Layer

This layer consists of opaque and white sclera forming posterior five-sixth and transparent and colorless cornea forming anterior one-sixth.

Sclera

The sclera is a thick non-distensible membrane that maintains the shape of the eyeball. It helps in maintaining the normal intraocular pressure of about 15 to 20 mm of mercury. The external surface of the sclera is white and the internal surface is brown. The anterior part of sclera (known as the white of the eye) is covered with transparent conjunctiva. The rest of the sclera is covered with fascia bulbi and gives insertion to six extraocular muscles. The sclera is continuous with the cornea at the limbus anteriorly. A circular channel called sinus venosus sclerae or canal of Schlemm is located in the sclera just behind the limbus. A triangular projection of sclera in the cornea medial to the canal of Schlemm is called the scleral spur. The sclera is continuous with the dural sheath of optic nerve posteriorly. The weakest part of the sclera is called lamina cribrosa, where the axons of optic nerve pierce the sclera to leave the eyeball. The point of emergence of the optic nerve is located 3 mm medial to the posterior pole of the eyeball.

Structures Piercing

a. The optic nerve pierces the sclera along with central vessels of retina at the lamina cribrosa.
b. The short ciliary nerves and vessels pierce around the entry of the optic nerve.
c. The long ciliary nerves and vessels pierce the sclera in front of the short ciliary nerves and vessels.
d. The venae vorticosae pierce just behind the equator of the eyeball.
e. The anterior ciliary arteries from the muscular branches of recti enter at various points.
f. The aqueous veins, which drain the aqueous humor from the sinus venosus scleare in to the anterior ciliary veins pierce near the limbus.

Nerve Supply and Blood Supply

The sclera is richly supplied through the long and short ciliary nerves. Though sclera is relatively avascular, it receives blood through the anterior ciliary arteries (twigs from muscular branches of ophthalmic artery) and also from the long and short posterior ciliary arteries.

Cornea

The cornea is the transparent and avascular part of the fibrous layer. As the cornea is more convex than the sclera the sclerocorneal junction is indicated by a groove called the sulcus sclerae. The thickness of cornea is 1mm at the periphery and 0.5 mm at the center. The cornea is an important refractive medium of eye as the maximum refraction of light takes place from it.

Structure

a. The outer layer (corneal epithelium) is a stratified squamous non-keratinized type of epithelium.
b. Inner to the corneal epithelium is the anterior elastic lamina or Bowman's membrane.
c. The third layer called substantia propria contains lamellae of collagen fibers. The transparency of cornea is due to the parallel arrangement of collagen fibers and the chemical nature of the ground substance in this layer.
d. The fourth layer is the posterior elastic lamina or Descemet's membrane.
e. The innermost or endothelial layer consists of a single row of flat polygonal cells.

Nourishment

The cornea is avascular and devoid of lymphatic vessels. Therefore it is nourished by diffusion from capillaries at its edge and from aqueous humor at its internal surface. In addition to this, the central part of the cornea receives atmospheric oxygen dissolved in tear film. The avascularity of the cornea is of advantage in placing surgical incisions on it to approach the lens or the iris.

Nerve Supply

The cornea is richly innervated through the long ciliary branches of the nasociliary nerve.

Clinical Highlights

Inflammation of cornea is called keratitis, which may lead to the formation of corneal ulcers. Injuries to cornea can lead to corneal opacities resulting in blindness. It is possible to restore sight in such cases by corneal transplantation (keratoplasty). The corneal transplants are very readily accepted because the cornea is immunologically inert.

Corneal Reflex

The corneal reflex consists of touching the cornea with a wisp of cotton with resultant reflex closure of both eyes. The afferent limb is the ophthalmic division of the trigeminal nerve, the center of reflex is the motor nucleus of facial nerve and the efferent limb is the facial nerve.

Sclerocorneal Junction (SCJ)

The SCJ or the limbus is the site where cornea and sclera merge with each other. This is the region of the iridocorneal angle (Fig. 110.3). At the SCJ a circular venous sinus (canal of Schlemm) traverses the sclera. The pectinate ligaments of the iris or the fibrils of the Descemet's membrane of the cornea pass through the iridocorneal angle to get attached to the iris and give rise to the trabecular tissue in the angle. The trabecular tissue encloses endothelium lined spaces called spaces of Fontana, which communicate medially with anterior chamber and laterally with sinus venosus sclerae. The aqueous humor filters through the spaces of Fontana at the iridocorneal angle (filtration angle) and drains to the canal of Schlemm. Blockage of the filtration angle results in rise in intraocular pressure (glaucoma).

Uveal Tract

It is a vascular and pigmented layer consisting of from behind forwards, the choroid, the ciliary body and the iris. These parts are functionally different but form a continuous layer. Inflammation of the iris is called iritis and that of ciliary body, cyclitis. The combined inflammation of the iris and the ciliary body is called iridocyclitis.

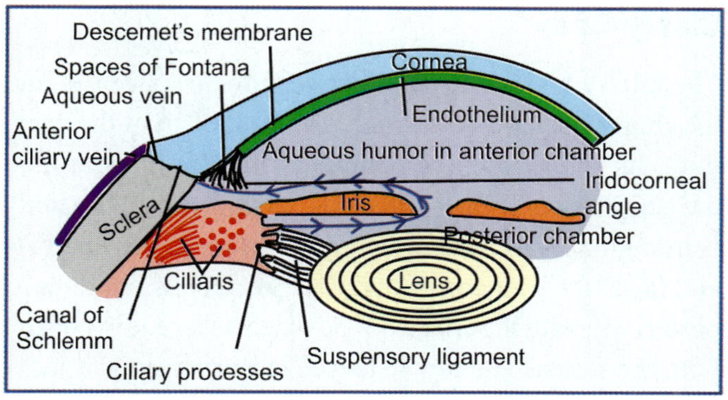

Fig. 110.3: Sclerocorneal junction (Note: The aqueous humor secreted by ciliary processes flows from the posterior to anterior chamber and onwards to spaces of Fontana, canal of Schlemm and aqueous vein to drain into anterior ciliary vein)

Choroid

The choroid is a brown coat situated inner to the sclera. It extends from the optic nerve posteriorly to the ciliary body anteriorly. Its inner surface is firmly attached to the pigment layer of retina. Its rough outer surface is separated from the sclera by a potential space called the perichoroidal space through which long posterior ciliary arteries and ciliary nerves (long and short) traverse.

Structure

The choroid is divided in four layers. The outer layer (in contact with sclera) is the supra-choroidal lamina, inner to which is the vascular layer of large and medium sized blood vessels with scattered melanocytes. Inner to this is the layer of choriocapillaries. Bruch's membrane, which is avascular, is believed to play a role in the passage of tissue fluid from the choriocapillaries to the retina. The choroid receives rich blood supply from the posterior ciliary arteries, which are the branches of the ophthalmic artery. The venous blood is drained by four or five vorticose veins, which pierce the sclera to join the ophthalmic veins. The choroid provides nutrition to outer layers of retina. The pigment cells in the choroid absorb excess light thus preventing reflection.

Ciliary Body

The ciliary body is located between the iris in front and the choroid behind. It is a highly vascular part of the uveal tract. Its shape is like a complete ring that runs around the periphery of the iris. On cross-section, the ciliary body is triangular. The base or anterior surface is very narrow and faces the iridocorneal angle. The apex is continuous posteriorly with the choroid. The outer surface is in contact with the sclera. The inner surface is curved since it faces the lens and the vitreous body and is covered with ciliary epithelium. It is this surface that sends ciliary processes to surround the iris. The inner surface is divisible in two parts, namely pars plicata or corona ciliaris in the anterior one-third and pars plana or orbicularis ciliaris or ciliary ring in the posterior two-thirds. The pars plicata presents ciliary processes, which are attached to the periphery of the iris. The ciliary processes project in the posterior chamber of the eyeball. The intervals in the adjacent ciliary processes give attachment to the fibers of the suspensory ligaments of lens. The pars plana, which is directed towards the vitreous humor ends at ora serrata. At this point the two layers of the epithelium of the non-nervous part of retina are continuous with the ciliary epithelium. The pars plana is devoid of ciliary processes.

Structure

The ciliary body is composed of ciliary epithelium, ciliary stroma and ciliary muscle.

a. The ciliary epithelium is bilaminar. Its deeper or inner layer is nonpigmented and secretory in function. The deep layer covering the pars plicata is responsible for the secretion of the aqueous humor. Similar cells lining the pars plana facing the vitreous humor are believed to secrete the vitreous body. The cells of the superficial layer of the ciliary epithelium are pigmented in nature. Both the layers are continuous with the retina at the ora serrata. They represent the pars ciliaris retinae and are continuous with the pars ciliaris iridis anteriorly.
b. The ciliary stroma consists of loose collagen fibers and supports the ciliaris muscle, long posterior ciliary arteries, anterior ciliary arteries, posterior short ciliary arteries and long and short ciliary nerves.
c. The ciliary muscle or ciliaris is the muscle of accommodation. The contraction of circular and meridional fibers relaxes the suspensory ligament of the lens thereby increasing the convexity of the lens. This in turn reduces the focal length of the lens, which helps in near vision (accommodation). The muscle receives parasympathetic nerve supply. The preganglionic fibers originate in the Edinger-Westphal nucleus in the midbrain (Fig. 110.4) and are carried in the oculomotor nerve to the ciliary ganglion, where the synapse takes place. The postganglionic fibers enter the short ciliary nerves, which pierce the sclera and reach the ciliary muscle along the perichoroidal space.

Iris

Iris means rainbow. The color of the iris varies from light blue to dark brown. The iris forms the circular diaphragm that is positioned between the lens behind and the cornea in front. It presents in its center an aperture called the pupil, through which the anterior and the posterior chambers of the eyeball communicate with each other. The main function of the iris is to regulate the amount of light that reaches the lens by regulating the size of the pupil.

Structure

The iris consists of the pigmented stroma containing the muscles of the iris, blood vessels and nerves. The stroma is lined posteriorly by a double-layered epithelium (the pars iridis retinae), which is deeply pigmented. The anterior surface of the iris is covered with epithelium of pupillary

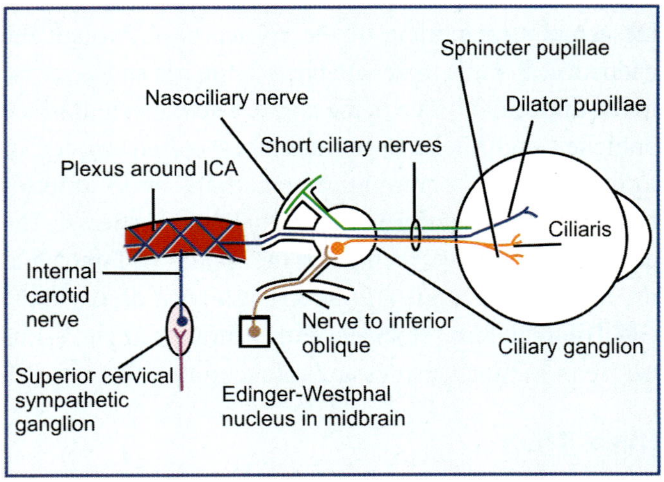

Fig. 110.4: Autonomic innervation of intraocular muscles (Note: Parasympathetic relay occurs in ciliary ganglion and sympathetic relay in superior cervical sympathetic ganglion)

membrane in fetal life, but by eighth month of intrauterine life, the membrane degenerates.

Muscles of Iris

a. The sphincter pupillae is a smooth muscle that encircles the pupil. When the muscle contracts the pupil is narrowed (miosis). The muscle receives nerve supply from the postganglionic parasympathetic fibers (Fig. 110.4). Parasympatholytic drugs like atropine relax the sphincter muscle thereby causing dilatation of the pupil.
b. The dilator pupillae is a thin smooth muscle. Its radially arranged fibers merge with those of the sphincter pupillae near the pupil. On contraction the muscle produces dilatation of the pupil (mydriasis). It receives sympathetic nerve supply as follows (Fig. 110.4). The long preganglionic fibers arise in intermediolateral horn of the T1-T2 segments of the spinal cord (ciliospinal center) and course upwards through the cervical sympathetic trunk to relay in the superior ganglion. The postganglionic fibers pass through the sympathetic plexus around the internal carotid artery to reach the dilator pupillae via the nerve plexus around the ophthalmic artery or via a communication with the nasociliary nerve. Injury to the sympathetic fibers in any location along this long course will give rise to Horner's syndrome in which the pupil is constricted.

Blood Vessels and Sensory Nerves

The major or greater arterial circle is present at the junction of the ciliary body and the iris. It is formed by the anastomosis between the long posterior ciliary arteries and the anterior ciliary arteries. Branches arise from this anastomosis and enter the iris to travel towards the pupil. These branches in turn anastomose close to the pupillary margin to form a minor or lesser arterial circle. Branches from both the circles supply the iris. The sensory nerves are derived from the long ciliary branches of ophthalmic nerve.

Retina

The retina is the photosensitive layer that is located innermost. The photoreceptors in the retina convert the light energy in to electrical impulses, which are processed in the retina and carried in the axons of ganglion cells contained in the optic nerve. The retina lies between the choroid externally and the hyaloid membrane of the vitreous body internally. Anteriorly it terminates at the ora serrata, where the nonnervous part of retina in the form of a bilaminar epithelium extends to line the deep surfaces of the ciliary body and the iris.

Parts

On ophthalmoscopic examination two areas of retina show distinguishable features. The macula lutea is the yellowish area near the center of the retina. It has a central depression called the fovea centralis, where the retina is thinnest. Because of high concentration of cone cells the visual acuity is greatest at fovea. The optic disc lies 3 mm nasal or medial to the macula lutea. At this point the optic nerve emerges from the retina. The central artery of the retina pierces the disc in the center. The disc is also called the blind spot because it is devoid of photoreceptors (rods and cones). Swelling of the disc (papilledema) occurs in optic neuritis and raised intracranial tension. Depression or cupping of the optic disc occurs in atrophy of the optic nerve and glaucoma.

Layers (Fig. 110.5)

There are ten layers of retina, which are numbered from outer to inner side. The first layer is adjacent to the choroid and the tenth layer is adjacent to the vitreous body.

a. Retinal pigment cells form a single layer of cubical cells. They contain melanin in their cytoplasm. The pigment cells absorb the excess light rays and prevent bouncing of light back in to the retina. Their defence role consists of phagocytosis of parts of rods and cones that are discarded. They also form an effective blood-retinal barrier between the retina and blood vessels of choroid.
b. The layer of rods and cones contains the outer segments of rod and cone cells, which are elongated photoreceptors. The rods are cylindrical in shape. They are larger in numbers compared to cones in the peripheral part of retina. They are absent at the fovea centralis. Their outer segments contain rhodopsin (visual purple), which senses low level of illumination and black and white colors. The cones are flask

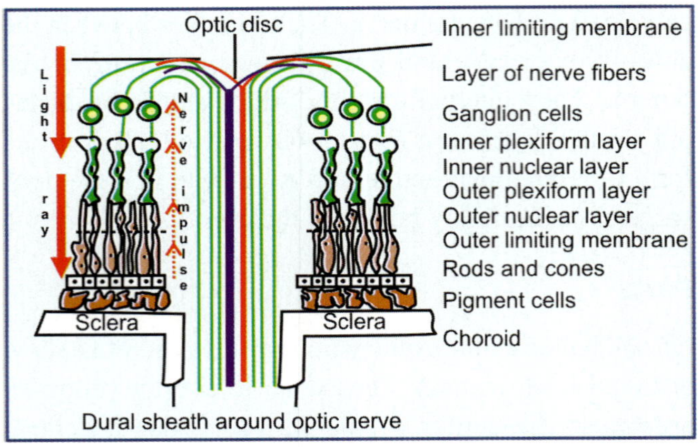

Fig. 110.5: Highly enlarged schematic diagram of retina, optic disc and the origin of optic nerve

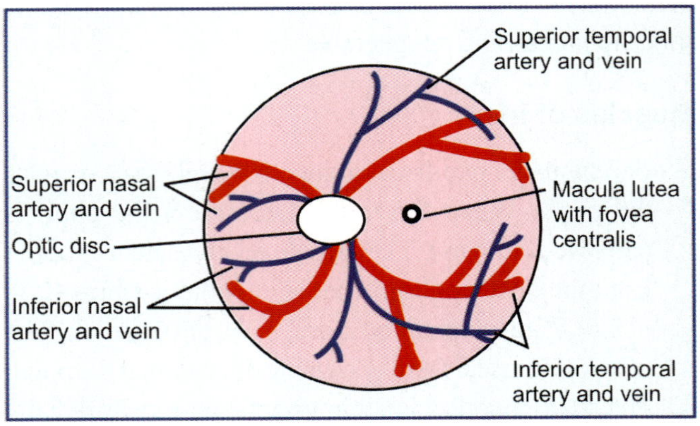

Fig. 110.6: Ophthalmoscopic view of retinal blood vessels (Note: That the arteries enter and veins leave the retina only at the optic disc)

shaped. Only cones are present in fovea centralis, where acuity is maximum. Their outer segments contain iodopsin, which senses bright light and colors.

c. External limiting layer is the junction between the retinoglial cells (Müller's cells) and the inner segments of the photoreceptors.
d. Outer nuclear layer consists of cell bodies of rods and cones and their nuclei.
e. Outer plexiform layer is made of synapses between the processes of rods and cones cells and the dendrites of bipolar cells and horizontal cells.
f. Inner nuclear layer is composed of cell bodies and nuclei of bipolar cells, amacrine cells, horizontal cells and the Müller's cells (retinal gliocytes). The bipolar cells are the first order neurons in the visual pathway. The amacrine and horizontal cells are the association neurons.
g. Inner plexiform layer is formed of numerous synapses between the axons of bipolar cells and amacrine cells and the dendrites of ganglion cells.
h. Ganglion cell layer contains the multipolar neurons, which are the second order neurons of the visual pathway.
i. Nerve fiber layer contains the unmyelinated axons of the ganglion cells. These axons aggregate at the optic disc to form the optic nerve
j. Internal limiting lamina is formed of the processes of retinal gliocytes. This layer separates the retina from the vitreous body.

Blood Supply (Fig. 110.6)

The outer layers of retina are nourished by diffusion from the choriocapillaries. The central artery of retina supplies the inner layers of the retina. This artery (a branch of ophthalmic artery) runs in the substance of optic nerve and enters the eyeball at the optic disc, where it divides in a superior and an inferior branch. Both these branches further divide in nasal and temporal branches. The superior nasal branch supplies the superior nasal quadrant and the superior temporal branch supplies the superior temporal quadrant of retina. Likewise, the inferior quadrants receive blood from the respective inferior branches. Beyond the optic disc, the central artery of retina is an end artery. Therefore, when this artery is blocked there is instant and total loss of vision. The veins follow the arteries. The arteries are placed superficial to the veins. The veins converge to form the central retinal vein, which opens in the cavernous sinus. The central vein is compressed as it passes through the subarachnoid space around the optic nerve in raised intracranial pressure. This results in papilledema and gradual loss of vision. The retina is the only place in the body, where the arteries can be examined directly with the help of the ophthalmoscope to note pathological changes in diseases like diabetes and hypertension.

Clinical Highlights

Detachment of retina is a very common clinical condition. The neural layer of retina or retina proper and the pigment layer, are normally in apposition to each other. However, there is a potential embryonic space between the two. When detachment of retina occurs due to any cause, the plane of separation is this potential space as is evident from the fact that in detachment, the pigment layer remains attached to the choroid while the rest of the retina is lifted towards the vitreous.

Refractive Media

The eyeball consists of four transparent media, the cornea, aqueous humor, crystalline lens and the vitreous body.

a. Cornea is exposed to the air hence maximum refraction of light takes place from its epithelium.
b. The aqueous humor is a thin watery fluid that fills the spaces in front of and behind the iris, namely anterior and posterior chambers of the eyeball. It is secreted by the epithelium of ciliary processes in the posterior chamber from where it reaches the anterior chamber through the pupil. It is absorbed in the sinus venosus sclerae at the iridocorneal angle (filtration angle). The aqueous fluid from this canal is drained in to the anterior ciliary veins via the aqueous veins in the sclera. The aqueous humor provides nourishment to the lens and cornea and maintains the intraocular pressure. It helps in refraction of the light. Blockage in the circulation of aqueous humor due to disease of the angle of filtration or due to blockage of the pupil (as a result of fusion of iris with the anterior surface of lens or posterior surface of cornea) results in rise of intraocular pressure. This is called glaucoma, which may lead to degeneration of retina and blindness.
c. The lens is avascular, transparent and biconvex in shape and is covered by a glassy elastic capsule. It is suspended from the ciliary body by the suspensory ligament. The lens is placed between the posterior chamber and the vitreous chamber. The equator separates the anterior and posterior surfaces. The curvature of its anterior surface can be adjusted by the action of the ciliaris muscle. This is useful for accommodation in near vision. The aqueous humor and vitreous body nourish the avascular lens.

   Common disorders of lens are as follows. Presbyopia is a condition caused by decreased elasticity of the lens in people over the age of forty. The lens loses power of accommodation. The cataract is the opacity of the lens. This may be present at birth due to maternal rubella or can develop in elderly due to age changes or due to systemic diseases like diabetes. The treatment consists of surgical removal of the lens. Intraocular lens implantation is nowadays a popular procedure to restore vision after cataract surgery.
d. The vitreous body occupies a large vitreous chamber, which is located behind the lens and the ciliary body and in front of the retina. The vitreous body is a jelly like material composed of water, hyaluronic acid and a meshwork of loose collagen fibrils. It is enveloped by hyaloid membrane, which separates it from the retina, ciliary body and lens. The posterior surface of the lens causes a depression in the hyaloid membrane called hyaloid fossa. A small passage called the hyaloid canal extending from the optic disc to the center of the posterior surface of the lens traverses the vitreous body. In fetal life, the canal contains the hyaloid artery, which later degenerates.

111 Oral Cavity

The oral cavity is divided into two parts. The vestibule is the anterior slit-like space bounded by the teeth and gums internally and the lips and cheeks externally. The parotid duct opens in the vestibule opposite the crown of second upper molar tooth (Fig. 111.1). The oral cavity proper lies behind the teeth. The palate forms its roof. The anterior two thirds of the tongue occupies its floor except in the anteriormost part. The oral cavity communicates with the oropharynx through oropharyngeal isthmus.

Dentition

There are two sets of teeth. The temporary (or milk or deciduous) teeth are twenty in number. Each jaw contains ten teeth of which five are present in each half of the jaw (two incisors, one canine and two molars). The milk teeth erupt in the following sequence, incisors (6-10 months), first molars (10-16 months), canines (16-20 months) and second molars (20-30 months). The permanent teeth are thirty-two in numbers. Each jaw has sixteen teeth of which eight are present in each half of the jaw (two incisors, one canine, two premolars and three molars). The permanent teeth erupt in the following sequence: first molars (6 years), incisors (7-9 years), premolars (10-12 years), canines (11-12 years), molar II (13-14 years) and molar III (17-22 years).

Development of Tooth

The enamel of the tooth develops from the ectoderm. It is the toughest tissue in the body. The pulp, dentine and cementum of the tooth develop from the mesoderm.

Jaw Necrosis After Tooth Extraction

After tooth extraction osteomyelitis of mandible is more common compared to that of maxilla. The reason for this

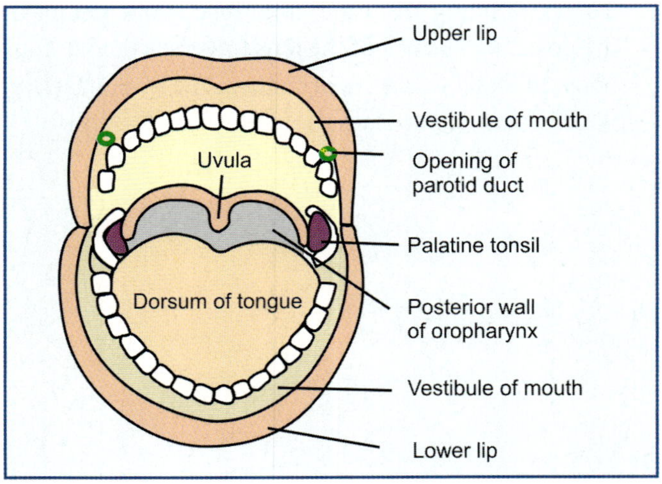

Fig. 111.1: Features of oral cavity and oropharynx on direct inspection

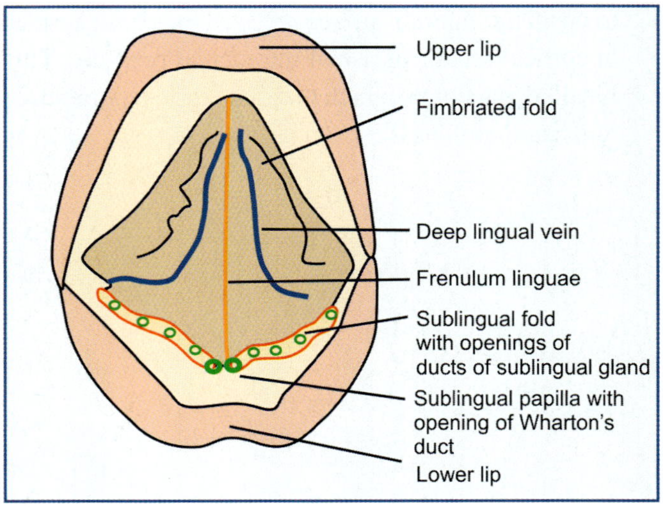

Fig. 111.2: Features on the floor of mouth and on ventral surface of tongue

lies in the difference in the arterial supply of the two bones. The mandible is supplied through inferior alveolar arteries only as against the maxilla, which receives branches through two sets of three superior alveolar arteries (anterior, middle and posterior superior alveolar). Infective thrombosis in a branch of the inferior alveolar artery during tooth extraction may result in bone necrosis, which is not the case if thrombosis takes place in any one artery supplying maxilla.

Floor of the Mouth (Fig. 111.2)

The frenulum linguae is a fold of mucous membrane connecting the undersurface of the anterior part of the tongue to the most anterior part of the floor of the mouth. The sublingual papillae are present on either side of the frenulum. On the summit of each papilla, the submandibular duct (Wharton's duct) opens. Numerous small ducts of sublingual salivary glands open on the sublingual fold on each side.

112 Tongue

The tongue is a mobile muscular organ located partly in the oral cavity and partly in the oropharynx. It is attached to the hyoid bone below, to the palate above, to the mandible in front and to the styloid process behind by means of muscles. It is a highly mobile organ. The tongue is the peculiar organ, where stratified squamous non-keratinized mucosa closely covers a mass of striated muscle fibers disposed in vertical, transverse and longitudinal directions. The substance of tongue is divided into two-halves by a median fibrous septum. The functions of the tongue include, tasting, masticating and swallowing the food besides its role in speech.

Parts of the Tongue

The tongue consists of a tip, a root, inferior surface and a curved dorsal surface.

The tip of the tongue is directed forwards and it remains in contact with the incisor teeth when the mouth is closed.

The root of the tongue lies in the floor of the mouth and is composed of genioglossus and hyoglossus muscles. Thus, the tongue is attached to the mandible and hyoid bones by its root. The inferior surface is covered with mucous membrane, which is continuous with the mucous membrane of the floor of the mouth. A midline mucosal fold called frenulum linguae connects the inferior surface to the floor of the mouth. The deep lingual vein is located on either side of the frenulum linguae. On both sides of the posterior end of frenulum there is a sublingual fold and papilla. The submandibular duct opens in the summit of this papilla. The curved dorsal surface or the dorsum of the tongue is its most important surface.

Gross Appearance of the Dorsum (Fig. 112.1)

The dorsum presents a V-shaped sulcus terminalis. The apex of the V is directed posteriorly and the limbs are directed forwards and laterally from the apex, which coincides with foramen caecum. The foramen cecum is a pit indicating the site of origin of embryonic thyroglossal duct, which develops in to thyroid gland. The sulcus terminalis divides the dorsum of the tongue into anterior two-third (presulcal or oral) and posterior one-third (postsulcal or pharyngeal). The mucous membrane covering the two parts differs in gross features, sensory innervation and development.

Anterior Two-third

The mucous membrane on this part of the tongue is characterised by the presence of lingual papillae, which are the projections of the mucosa. These papillae are responsible for the rough appearance to the dorsum. There are four types of papillae, filiform, fungiform, foliate and vallate or circumvallate.

a. The filiform papillae are conical in shape and cover most of the anterior two-third of dorsum. They are arranged in rows parallel to the sulcus terminalis on either side of the midline. The stratified squamous

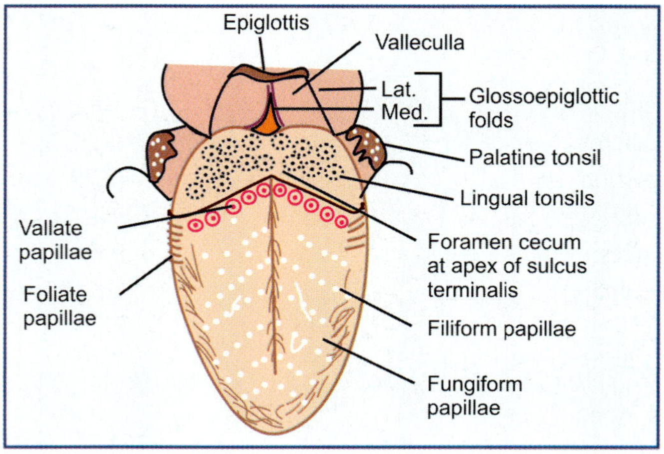

Fig. 112.1: Features on the dorsum of tongue

epithelium covering these papillae, is keratinized, hence the papillae appear whitish in color. The function of these papillae is to facilitate the friction between the tongue and the food. They are devoid of taste buds.

b. The fungiform papillae are found mainly on the margins of the tongue but a few are scattered on the dorsum. They are deep red in color due to absence of keratinized epithelium covering them. Each papilla usually bears taste bud at its apex.

c. The foliate papillae are present on the lateral margins of the tongue near the sulcus terminalis. They are red in color and appear as leaf-like mucosal ridges. They bear taste buds.

d. The vallate papillae are largest in size (number being ten to twelve). These papillae are located just in front of the sulcus terminalis. The shape of the vallate papilla is like that of an inverted cone with a narrow base and broad apex. Each papilla is 1 to 2 mm in diameter and lies in a well-marked depression or trench in the mucosa. Numerous taste buds are present on the walls of the papilla and the walls of the surrounding trench.

Posterior One-third

This part is located in the floor of oropharynx. The palatoglossal folds connect it to the palate. A median and two lateral glossoepiglottic folds attach the tongue to the epiglottis. The mucosa on the dorsum of this part is devoid of papillae, but the lingual tonsils give this part a characteristic cobblestone appearance. The lingual tonsils are the submucosal lymphatic nodules belonging to Waldeyer's lymphatic ring, the other components of the ring being, nasopharyngeal tonsil, tubal tonsils and palatine tonsils.

Muscles of Tongue

Each half of the tongue contains extrinsic and intrinsic muscles. The four pairs of extrinsic muscles alter the position and size of the tongue as they attach the tongue to neighboring bones on each side. The four pairs of intrinsic muscles located wholly within the tongue alter the shape of the tongue.

Extrinsic Muscles (Fig. 112.2)

a. The genioglossus muscle has a narrow tendinous origin from the upper genial tubercle of the mandible. It has

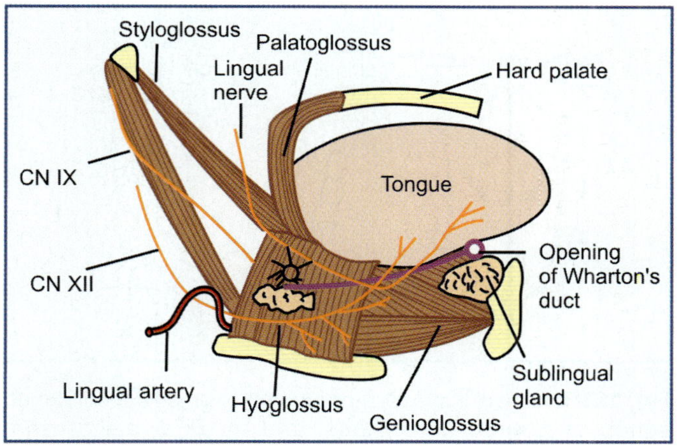

Fig. 112.2: Extrinsic muscles of tongue (Note: The glosso-pharyngeal nerve (CN IX) along stylopharyngeus muscle)

a wide insertion in the posterior aspect of tongue. The right and left genioglossi are very close to the midline. Acting together, the genioglossi pull the tongue forward to protrude the tip out of the mouth. The origin of the muscle is anterior in location compared to its insertion. On contraction, each muscle draws the posterior part of tongue forwards and medially. Because the medial pull of each muscle cancels out, protrusion of the tongue in the midline is the result. Unilateral action of the muscle pushes the tongue to the opposite side. This muscle is called the safety muscle of the tongue. The reason for this is that its attachment to the mandible prevents the tongue from falling back and obstructing the respiration. In unconscious patient, the mandible is manually pulled forward and retained in that position. In paralysis of one genioglossus, on protruding the tongue, its tip deviates to the affected side due to the medial pull of the normal muscle (Fig. 112.3).

b. The palatoglossus muscle is a common muscle of the tongue and palate. It takes origin from the palatine aponeurosis and is inserted in the side of the tongue. The muscle and the covering mucosa form the palatoglossal arch. The right and left muscles act together in bringing the two palatoglossal arches together thereby shutting the oral cavity from the oropharynx.

c. The styloglossus muscle arises from the anterolateral aspect of styloid process near its apex. It passes downwards and forwards to reach the tongue for insertion. It draws the tongue upwards and backwards.

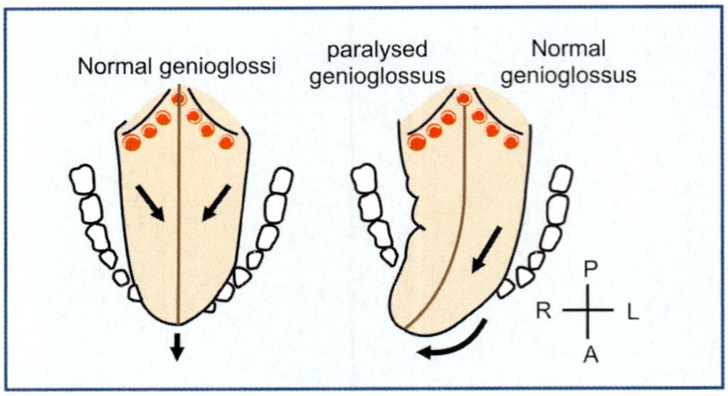

Fig. 112.3: Scheme to depict protrusion of tongue in combined action of normal genioglossi and in paralysis of right genioglossus

d. The hyoglossus muscle is quadrilateral in shape. It has very important relations (Fig. 112.2) hence it is regarded as the key muscle of the submandibular region. It arises from the greater cornua and the body of hyoid bone. The fibers pass upwards to insert in the side of the tongue. The hyoglossus of each side depresses the side of the tongue to make its dorsal surface more convex. The relations of the hyoglossus are as follows. Superficially, it is related from above downwards to, styloglossus, lingual nerve, submandibular ganglion, submandibular duct and the deep part of the submandibular gland. The lowest structure on this surface is the hypoglossal nerve. Three structures pass deep to the posterior margin of the muscle, glossopharyngeal nerve, stylohyoid ligament and lingual artery from above downwards. Anterior to the hyoglossus are placed the sublingual gland and geniohyoid muscle. Deep to the hyoglossus are found the same three structures that pass deep to its posterior margin and two muscles, namely, genioglossus and middle constrictor.

Intrinsic Muscles

a. The right and left superior longitudinal muscles arise from the posterior part of the medial fibrous septum of the tongue and are inserted in the respective sides of the tongue. On contraction, they make the dorsal surface concave from side to side.
b. The right and left inferior longitudinal muscles arise from the sides of the tongue and converge to the anterior part of the median septum for insertion. On contraction, they make the dorsal surface more convex.
c. The vertical muscles originate from the dorsum and descend through the fibers of genioglossus for insertion in the sides of tongue. On contraction, they increase the width of the tongue.
d. The transverse muscles originate in the septum and proceed transversely through the fibers of genioglossus, hyoglossus and vertical muscles to the margin of the tongue. On contraction, the two muscles narrow the tongue.

Motor Nerve Supply

All the muscles of the tongue except the palatoglossus are supplied by the hypoglossal nerve. The palatoglossus is the only one supplied by vago-accessory complex through pharyngeal plexus.

Sensory Nerve Supply

The sensory nerves of the tongue are divided in two groups:
a. Nerves carrying general sensations like pain, touch and temperature
b. Nerves carrying special sensation of taste.

Anterior Two-third

The lingual nerve carries the general sensations and the chorda tympani nerve carries the taste sensation from all taste buds except those on vallate papillae.

Posterior One-third

The glossopharyngeal nerve carries the general sensations as well as the taste sensation from the vallate papillae. The internal laryngeal nerve (a branch of vagus) supplies a small area adjacent to the epiglottis.

Correlation of Nerve Supply and Development (Fig. 112.4)

a. The muscles of the tongue and its mucosa develop from different sources. All the muscles of the tongue except the palatoglossus develop from occipital myotomes hence they are supplied by hypoglossal nerve. The palatoglossus develops from fourth arch mesoderm along with muscles of the palate hence it is supplied by the vago-accessory complex.
b. The mucosa of the anterior two-third develops from the fusion of three endodermal swellings in the floor of pharynx associated with the first arches (bilateral

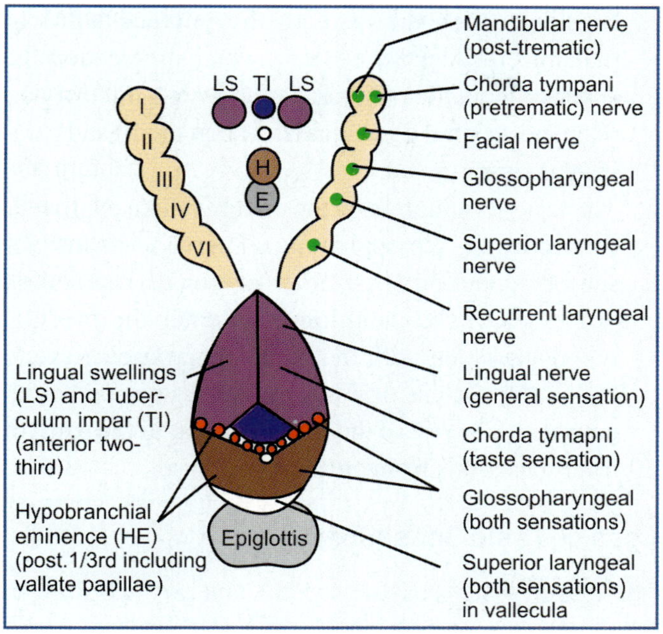

Fig. 112.4: Correlation of development with sensory nerve supply of tongue

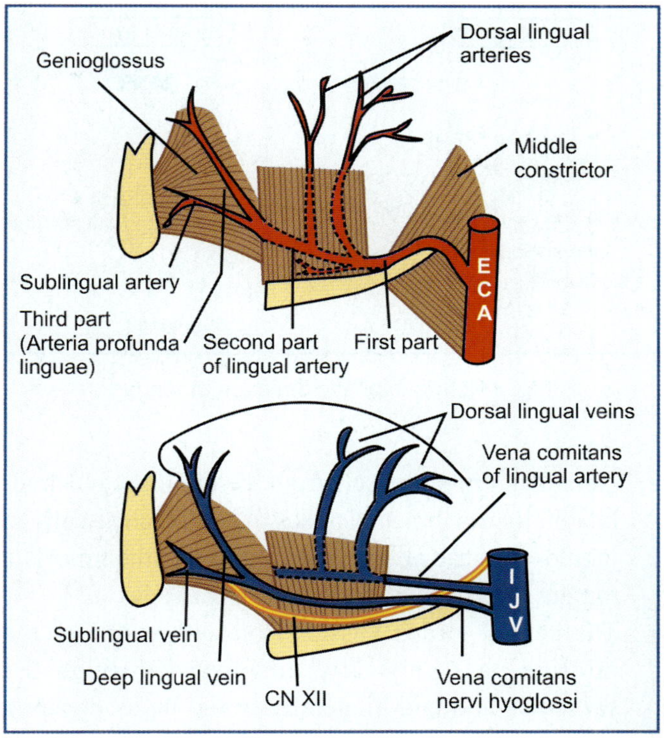

Fig. 112.5: Blood supply of tongue (Note that hyoglossus divides the lingual artery in three parts and is sandwiched between two sets of lingual veins)

lingual swellings and the midline tuberculum impar). This explains its general sensory innervation from the mandibular nerve (nerve of first arch) through its lingual branch. The pretrematic nerve of the first arch is the chorda tympani branch of facial nerve (nerve of second arch). Thus, the sensory supply to the taste buds of anterior two-third of the tongue by chorda tympani is justified.

c. The mucosa of the posterior one-third of the tongue develops from the cranial part of hypobranchial eminence, which is derived from the endoderm of third arches. Hence, the general and special sensory nerve of the posterior one-third is the glossopharyngeal nerve (the nerve of third arch). This nerve supplies the vallate papillae also because these papillae develop from hypobranchial eminence.
d. The mucosa of the vallecula develops from the fourth arch endoderm hence it is supplied by the internal laryngeal nerve (a branch of superior laryngeal nerve).

Arterial Supply (Fig. 112.5)

The lingual artery, a branch of external carotid artery, is the main arterial supply to the tongue through its dorsal and deep branches. The lingual branches of inferior alveolar artery also supply the tongue. The details of the lingual artery are described with branches of external carotid artery in Chapter 74.

Venous Drainage (Fig. 112.5)

The dorsal lingual veins drain the dorsum and sides of the tongue. They unite with the venae comitantes of the trunk of the lingual artery to form a lingual vein, which opens in the facial or internal jugular vein. The deep vein begins near the tip and travels on the inferior surface of the tongue. It joins the sublingual vein from the salivary glands to form the vena comitans of the hypoglossal nerve. This vein may drain in the lingual, the facial or the internal jugular vein.

Lymphatic Drainage (Fig. 112.6)

The lymphatic drainage of the tongue is of clinical importance because the cancer spreads via the lymphatics to the regional lymph nodes. The cancer of the tongue is very common in people habituated to tobacco chewing. The enlarged lymph nodes in this cancer are removed by block dissection of the neck along with total glossectomy or hemiglossectomy.

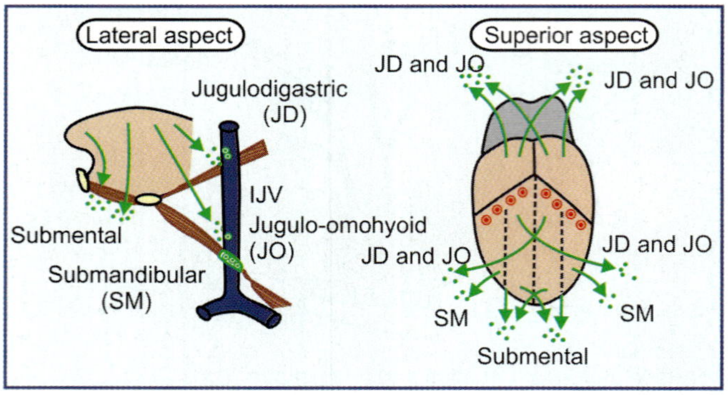

Fig. 112.6: Lymphatic drainage of tongue

a. Abundant lymph vessels from the tip of tongue drain bilaterally in submental nodes. A few reach directly to jugulo-digastric nodes. Thus, cancer of the tip of the tongue spreads to almost all cervical nodes.
b. The central lymph vessels from either side of the midline pass vertically downward through the substance and end bilaterally in the jugulodigastric nodes.
c. The lymphatics from the lateral part of the anterior two-thirds reach unilaterally to the submandibular nodes.
d. The lymphatics from the posterior one-third pass bilaterally to the jugulodigastric and jugulo-omohyoid nodes.

Gustatory or Taste Pathways

The taste pathways for the anterior two-third and the circumvallate papillae are different.

a. The taste sensations from the anterior two-third (fungiform and filiform papillae are carried in the chorda tympani nerve, which runs inside the lingual nerve upto the infratemporal fossa. The chorda tympani separates from the lingual nerve in the infratemporal fossa and enters the petrotympanic fissure to join the facial nerve 6 mm above the stylomastoid foramen. The taste fibers carried in the facial nerve are the dendrites or peripheral processes of the cells in the geniculate ganglion (first order neurons). The central processes of the ganglion cells join the nervus intermedius, through which the taste sensations reach the nucleus of tractus solitarius (second order neuron) in the medulla oblongata. The solitariothalamic path further carries the taste to the nucleus VPM of thalamus (third order neuron), which projects via the superior thalamic radiation to the antero-inferior part of the postcentral gyrus (parietal operculum) and para-insular cortex.
b. The taste sensation from the circumvallate papillae is carried by the glossopharyngeal nerve to its inferior sensory ganglion (first order neurons). The central processes of the ganglion cells enter the medulla oblongata along with the glossopharyngeal nerve to end in the nucleus of tractus solitarius (second order neurons). The rest of the path is similar to the path for taste sensations from anterior two-third.

Loss of Taste Sensations

The loss of taste sensations in the anterior two-third of the dorsum is seen in the lesion of the facial nerve proximal to the origin of the chorda tympani nerve or of the facial nucleus. The loss of taste from the vallate papillae is due to lesion of the glossopharyngeal nerve or its nucleus.

Clinical Highlights

a. The inspection of the dorsum of the tongue helps the clinician in diagnosis of not only the diseases of the tongue but also of the systemic diseases. The black hairy tongue is characteristic of AIDS. In inflammation of the tongue (glossitis) the tongue looks red. Apthous ulcer is a small painful ulcer usually on the tip, on the inferior surface or the sides of the anterior two-third of the tongue. Excessive furring of the dorsum can occur due to prolonged fever.
b. Congenital anomalies of the tongue include, lingual thyroid, which may present as a round and red swelling at the foramen caecum on the dorsum of the tongue or in the substance of the tongue. The other anomalies are, aglossia (congenital absence of tongue), ankylo-glossia or tongue-tie due to short frenulum and macroglossia or very large tongue, which is found in cretinism and Down's syndrome.
c. The inferior surface of tongue (Fig. 111.2) has deep lingual veins on it hence it is suitable for rapid absorption of medicines like, nitroglycerine, a coronary vasodilator (in angina pectoris), when kept sublingually.

113 Palate

The palate is composed of two parts. The hard palate forms the larger anterior part and the soft palate forms the posterior smaller part of the palate. The hard palate separates the oral cavity from the nasal cavity. The soft palate is a movable muscular curtain between the nasopharynx and the oropharynx.

Components of Hard Palate (Fig. 113.1)

The palatine processes of the maxillae and the horizontal plates of palatine bones unite by a cruciform suture to form the hard palate. A vascular groove extends from the greater palatine foramen along the lateral side of the inferior surface of the hard palate. It contains the greater palatine vessels. The epithelium lining the inferior or oral surface of hard palate is known as mucoperiosteum because it is fused with the periosteum of the hard palate. The palatine mucous glands are abundant on this surface.

Foramina in Hard Palate

a. Greater palatine foramen is located near the lateral palatal border behind the palatomaxillary suture.
b. Lesser palatine foramen is seen behind the greater foramen
c. Incisive fossa is situated anteriorly. It shows the openings of lateral incisive foramina.

Soft Palate

The soft palate is a muscular curtain that hangs from the posterior margin of the hard palate in a slightly downward and backward direction. Its free margin presents uvula in the midline. The soft palate is connected to the tongue by means of palatoglossal arches and to the pharyngeal wall by palatopharyngeal arches. Structurally, the soft palate is a fold of mucous membrane containing palatine aponeurosis, muscles, glands, blood vessels and nerves.

In the stretched position, the palate has an upper or nasopharyngeal surface and a lower or oropharyngeal surface. In the relaxed position, the upper surface becomes posterior and the lower surface becomes anterior.

Layers of Soft Palate

In relaxed position (from posterior to anterior), the layers of the soft palate are as follows:

a. Pseudostratified ciliated columnar epithelium
b. Layer of palatine glands and lymphoid tissue
c. Palatine aponeurosis for muscular attachment
d. Layer of palatine glands
e. Stratified squamous nonkeratinised epithelium on which taste buds are present.

The palatine aponeurosis strengthens the soft palate. It is attached to the posterior border of hard palate. It is the expanded tendon of tensor veli palatini muscles of both sides and it encloses the musculus uvulae near the midline. It provides attachment to other palatine muscles.

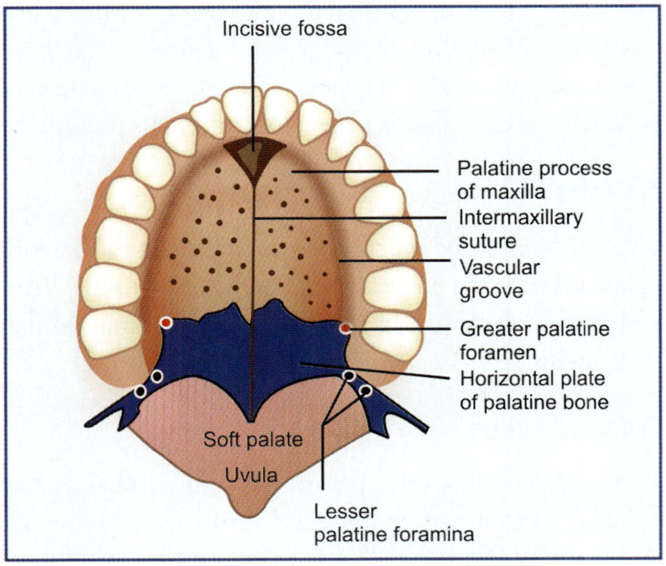

Fig. 113.1: Inferior view of bony and soft palates

Muscles of Soft Palate (Fig. 113.2)

There are five pairs of palatine muscles, tensor palati, levator palati, palatoglossus, palatopharyngeus and musculus uvulae.

Tensor Palati or Tensor Veli Palatini

This muscle takes origin from the scaphoid fossa at the base of medial pterygoid plate, lateral (membranous) wall of auditory tube and the spine of sphenoid (deep in the infratemporal fossa). It ends in a tendon, which winds round the pterygoid hamulus to turn medially towards the pharynx through the gap behind the tendinous band of origin of buccinator. It spreads out in the soft palate to become the palatine aponeurosis.

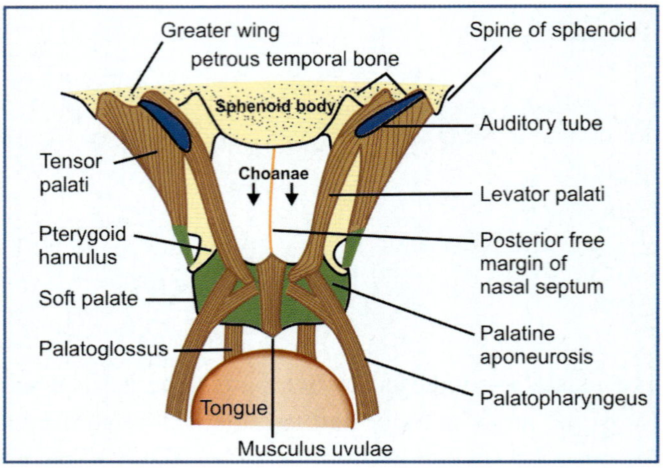

Fig. 113.2: Schematic representation of muscles of soft palate as seen in coronal section

Actions

The tensor palati is the tensor of the soft palate. It opens the auditory tube during deglutition and yawning to equalize the air pressure between the middle ear and the nasopharynx. Because of this function the fibers of tensor palati that take origin from the lateral wall of the tube are known as dilator tubae.

Levator Palati or Levator Veli Palatini

This muscle takes origin from the medial (cartilaginous) wall of the auditory tube and the part of petrous temporal bone in front of the lower opening of carotid canal. The levator palati follows the auditory tube over the free upper margin of superior constrictor muscle and enters the pharynx by piercing the pharyngobasilar fascia. It is inserted in the upper surface of palatine aponeurosis between the two strands of palatopharyngeus muscle.

Actions

The contraction of muscles both sides, raises the soft palate towards the posterior wall of the oropharynx. This action helps in closure of nasopharyngeal isthmus during swallowing.

Palatoglossus

This muscle takes origin from the oral surface of the palatine aponeurosis and extends forwards, downwards and laterally in front of the palatine tonsil to reach the side of the tongue. It is covered with mucosa of oropharynx and thus, forms the palatoglossal arch (anterior pillar of tonsillar fossa).

Actions

The contraction of the muscles of both sides elevates the base of the tongue and brings the two palatoglossal arches in approximation so as the close the oropharyngeal isthmus.

Palatopharyngeus

This muscle takes origin from the palate by two slips, the larger anterior slip from the posterior margin and adjacent upper surface of hard palate and the posterior slip from the posterior part of the upper surface of the palatine aponeurosis. The two slips are separated at origin by the insertion of levator palati. Both slips join to form a single muscle, which passes posterolaterally under cover of palatopharyngeal arch (posterior pillar of tonsillar fossa). The muscle travels through the pharyngeal wall for gaining attachment to the posterior border of the lamina of thyroid cartilage. Some fibers spread out in posterior direction to get attached to the pharyngeal raphe.

Actions

The muscle depresses the soft palate on the dorsum of the pharyngeal part of tongue. This prevents the soft palate being forced in the nasopharynx during blowing through the mouth against resistance.

The fibers of palatopharyngeus that arise from the hard palate pass horizontally backwards with the superior constrictor and meet each other to form a circular muscular ridge called Passavant's ridge. This muscular ridge is responsible for closure of the nasopharyngeal isthmus by approximating the pharyngeal wall to the raised soft palate.

Musculus Uvulae

These are the paired intrinsic muscles. Each takes origin from the posterior nasal spine of the hard palate and is inserted in the mucosa of the uvula. The palatine aponeurosis splits to enclose the musculus uvulae near the midline. The action of these muscles is to shorten and tense the uvula.

Motor Nerve Supply

a. The muscles of the soft palate are supplied by vago-accessory complex through the pharyngeal plexus except the tensor palati, which is supplied by mandibular nerve through its branch to medial pterygoid via otic ganglion. Paralysis of muscles of the soft palate may occur in injury to the vagus nerve or due to lesion of nucleus ambiguus in the medulla oblongata (lateral medullary syndrome). This results in nasal regurgitation of food and nasal voice.
b. The secretomotor supply to the palatine glands is by the postganglionic fibers of the sphenopalatine ganglion via the palatine nerves. The preganglionic fibers arise in the superior salivatory nucleus, travel in nervus intermedius, facial nerve, greater petrosal nerve and nerve of pterygoid canal to reach the sphenopalatine ganglion.

Sensory Nerve Supply

a. The general sensations like touch, pain and temperature are carried through the palatine nerves, nasopalatine nerve and glossopharyngeal nerve.
b. Taste sensation from the palate is carried in the lesser palatine nerves. After reaching the sphenopalatine ganglion the further course of the taste sensation is via the greater petrosal nerve, facial nerve, geniculate ganglion and nervus intermedius to end on nucleus of tractus solitarius. Some taste fibers reach the nucleus of tractus solitarius via the glossopharyngeal nerve.

Blood Supply

The greater palatine branch of maxillary artery supplies the palate. The ascending palatine branch of facial artery takes an unusual course. It first ascends to the upper limit of pharynx and then descends along the levator palati to reach the palate. The palatine branch of the ascending pharyngeal branch of external carotid artery also supplies the palate. The veins drain in the pterygoid and tonsillar venous plexuses.

Development (Fig. 113.3)

The part of the palate in front of the incisive fossa carrying the four incisor teeth develops from the frontonasal process (intermaxillary segment or premaxilla of the median nasal process). The rest of the palate develops from right and left palatal processes arising from the maxillary processes of respective side. Thus, the fusion of these three embryonic components by a Y-shaped suture forms the palate. The fusion takes place in antero-posterior direction. Membranous ossification occurs in the anterior part of the palate to give rise to the hard palate. The mesoderm of the pharyngeal arches migrates in the posterior part of the palate to give rise to musculature of the soft palate. Tensor palati alone develops from mesoderm of first arch hence it is supplied by the nerve of the first arch (mandibular nerve). The origin of the other muscles is believed to be from the fourth and sixth arches.

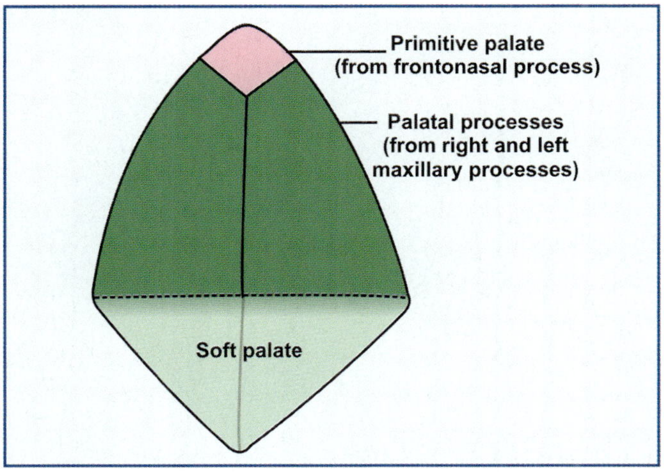

Fig. 113.3: Developmental sources of palate
(Note that in region of soft palate, mesoderm of pharyngeal arches migrates to give rise to palatal muscles)

Section three

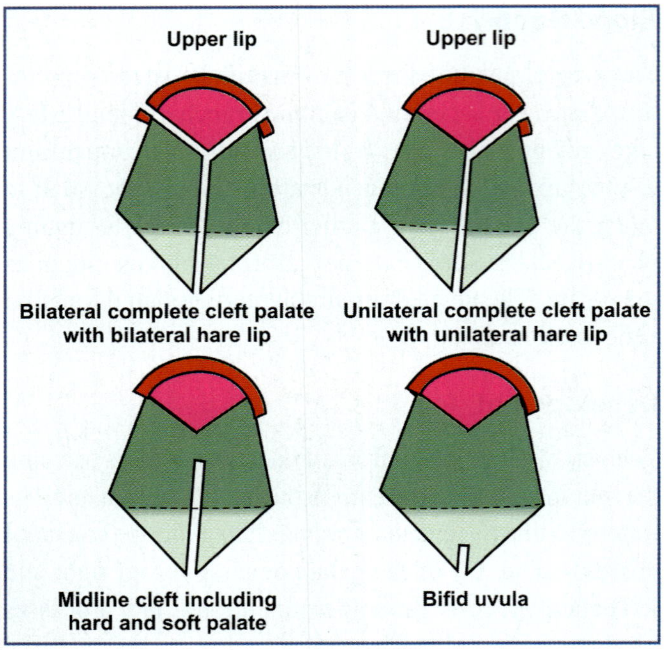

Fig. 113.4: Different types of cleft palate

Congenital Anomalies (Fig. 113.4)

Cleft palate may be associated with cleft upper lip. Different degrees of cleft palate occur depending on the complete or partial and unilateral or bilateral failure of fusion of the three embryonic elements forming the palate. The person has trouble in speech and swallowing unless surgical correction is carried out.

a. Bilateral complete cleft palate is due to complete failure of fusion of the Y-shaped suture. This is invariably associated with bilateral cleft upper lip.
b. Unilateral complete cleft palate is due to nonunion of palatine processes with each other and nonunion of palatal process and premaxilla on one side. This is invariably associated with unilateral cleft upper lip.
c. A midline cleft in both soft and hard palate is due to failure of fusion of the two palatine processes either fully or partially.
d. Cleft or bifid uvula occurs when there is failure of fusion in the posterior end of the two palatine processes.

114 Nasal Cavity

The nasal cavity is located between the two orbits and below the middle part of anterior cranial fossa. It is divided in right and left halves by a midline nasal septum. If the septum is deviated to one side the right and left halves are of unequal size. The nasal cavity opens on the face by two nostrils or anterior nasal apertures and it opens in the nasopharynx by two choanae or posterior nasal apertures (for boundaries of the choanae refer to Chapter 116 on Pharynx).

Each half of the cavity has four walls, floor and roof, lateral wall and medial wall. The vertical medial wall (septal wall) is common for the two halves.

Subdivisions

a. Each half of the nasal cavity is divided into nasal vestibule and nasal cavity proper. The vestibule forms the beginning of the nasal cavity hence it is located anteriorly. It is bounded laterally by the major alar cartilage and medially by the septal process of major alar cartilage. It is limited above and behind by limen nasi, which is a curved ridge, where the skin of vestibule is continuous with nasal mucosa of lateral wall. The vestibule is lined with skin and hence has sweat and sebaceous glands and coarse hairs called vibrissae.
b. Nasal cavity proper is subdivided in two functionally different areas, respiratory and olfactory (chemo-sensory). The respiratory area is large and covered by pseudostratified columnar ciliated epithelium supported by subjacent lamina propria containing numerous nasal glands and cavernous vascular plexuses. This mucosa covers major part of the lateral wall, septum, roof and floor. The olfactory area is limited to superior nasal concha, adjacent roof and upper part of septal wall.

Functions

a. The vibrissae in the vestibule trap the foreign bodies in the inspired air.
b. The respiratory mucosa is thick and spongy due to the presence of rich vascular plexuses. This helps in warming and humidification of the inspired air. The mucus secreted by the nasal glands traps the dust particles. Rhinitis is the inflammation of nasal mucosa, usually seen in common cold and hay fever. In rhinitis, the nasal mucosa becomes swollen due to rich vascularity and there is increased secretion of the nasal glands resulting in choked nose.
c. The olfactory mucosa occupies an area covering the postero-superior part of the lateral nasal wall (including the back of superior concha and the sphenoethmoidal recess), upper part of the perpendicular plate of ethmoid and the arching roof between the septum and the lateral wall. It is thicker than the respiratory epithelium and is yellowish brown in colour. It serves as an end organ of the sense of smell.

Communications

The nasal cavity communicates with the paranasal air sinuses. Besides, it shows following communications:

a. It communicates with anterior cranial fossa via cribriform plate of ethmoid bone. The cribriform plate carries the olfactory nerves to the cranium.
b. Close to the cribriform plate, there is canal for anterior ethmoidal nerve and vessels.
c. Occasionally, there is foramen caecum between crista galli and frontal bone. This foramen gives passage to the emissary vein connecting nasal veins with superior sagittal sinus.

d. The sphenopalatine foramen in the lateral wall, connects the nasal cavity with the pterygopalatine fossa. The structures passing through this foramen are, sphenopalatine artery, nasopalatine nerve and superior nasal branches of sphenopalatine ganglion.
e. Incisive canals in the incisive fossa in the hard palate, communicate the nasal cavity to the oral cavity. The nasal branches of greater palatine artery and palatine branches of nasopalatine nerve pass through these canals.
f. The nasolacrimal duct (carrying tears) communicates the nasal cavity with the lacrimal sac and through it with the conjunctival sac.

Boundaries of Nasal Cavity Proper (Fig. 114.1)

The nasal cavity proper presents floor, roof, lateral wall and medial wall or nasal septum. The floor is formed by the mucosa covering the superior surface of the hard palate.

Roof

The roof is the narrowest of the nasal walls and lies at the junction of lateral and medial walls. Its skeletal framework can be divisible into three parts as follows: The anterior sloping part is formed by the nasal cartilages, nasal and frontal bones. This is succeeded by the middle horizontal part formed by cribriform plate of ethmoid. The body of the sphenoid contributes to the posterior sloping part of the roof.

Clinical Highlights

a. It is important to note that the middle part of the roof separates the nasal cavity from the anterior cranial fossa. Therefore, in fracture of the cribriform plate of ethmoid CSF may leak in to the nasal cavity resulting in CSF rhinorrhea (dribbling of clear fluid (CSF) from the nose on bending or straining).
b. There is communication with subarachnoid space via the lymphatics from the nasal cavity forming a route for infection to spread into the cranial cavity.
c. The pituitary gland can be approached surgically via the posterior part of the roof (refer to Chapter 87).

Lateral Wall

The lateral wall of the nasal cavity is highly irregular as three bony shelf-like elevations project from the lateral wall. These elevations are due to superior, middle and inferior conchae or turbinates (Figs 114.1 and 114.2). The superior and middle conchae are parts of the ethmoid bone but inferior concha is a separate bone. The conchae divide the lateral wall into four spaces. They increase the surface area of the nasal cavity. Sometimes a fourth concha called concha suprema or highest nasal concha may be present.

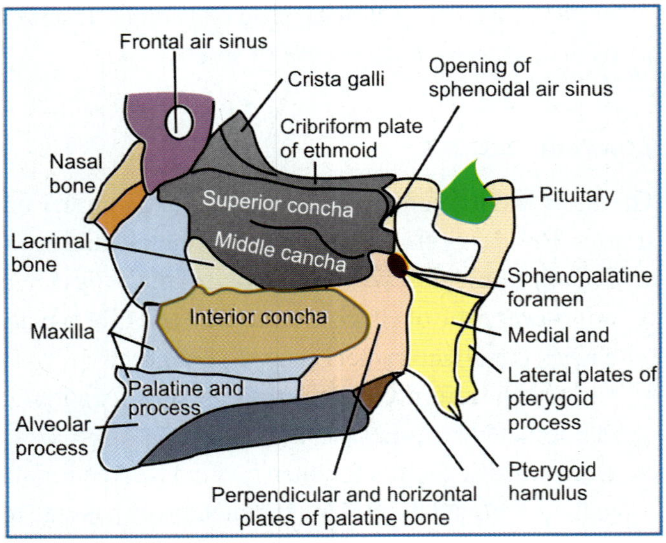

Fig. 114.1: Bony components of roof, lateral wall and floor of nasal cavity

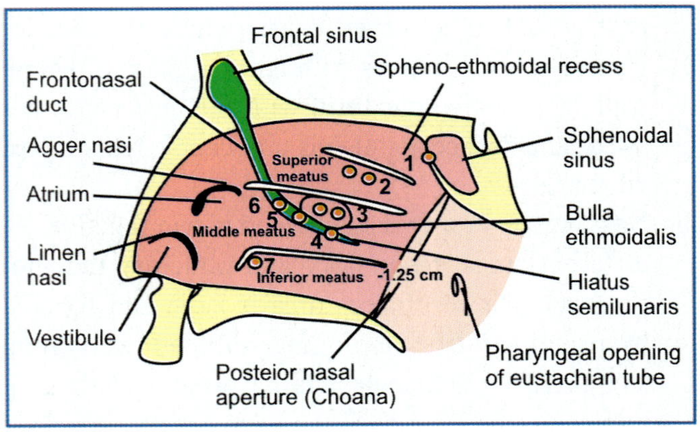

Fig. 114.2: Features of lateral wall of nasal cavity
Openings in lateral wall: (1) Sphenoidal sinus, (2) Posterior ethmoidal sinuses, (3) Middle ethmoidal sinuses, (4) Maxillary sinus, (5) Anterior ethmoidal sinus, (6) Frontal sinus, (7) Nasolacrimal duct

Meatuses

a. The inferior meatus lies between the nasal floor and the inferior concha. It runs along the entire length of the lateral wall and receives the opening of the nasolacrimal duct in its anterior part. The mucous membrane at this orifice is usually raised up as a lacrimal fold, which acts as a flap valve (of Hasner) preventing air and nasal secretions being blown up in the duct, when the intranasal pressure is raised. The inferior meatus provides an approach for draining out the pus in the maxillary sinus (Fig. 115.2).

b. The middle meatus is the space between the middle and inferior conchae. It runs in the posterior half of the lateral wall and receives openings of four paranasal sinuses. It is deeper in front than behind. It continues anteriorly in a space called atrium of the middle meatus. The atrium is limited above by agger nasi (which is produced by underlying ethmoidal crest in the lateral wall) and below by limen nasi.

   The prominent feature of the middle meatus is the presence of a rounded bulge called bulla ethmoidalis, which is produced by the middle ethmoidal cells. The middle ethmoidal sinus opens on or above it. The hiatus semilunaris is a curved cleft below and in front of the bulla. The hiatus leads into a funnel-shaped curved channel called ethmoidal infundibulum, the upper end of which may be continuous with the frontonasal duct by which the frontal sinus opens into the middle meatus. The anterior ethmoidal sinus opens in the anterior part of the ethmoidal infundibulum. The opening of the maxillary air sinus lies below the bulla ethmoidalis. This opening is reduced in size by four bones seen in the lateral wall namely, descending process of lacrimal bone in front, uncinate process of ethmoid bone above, inferior nasal concha below and perpendicular plate of palatine bone behind.

   The position of the opening of frontal sinus is at a higher level compared to that of the maxillary sinus. This favors the flow of fluid from the frontal to the maxillary opening for which reason maxillary sinus is considered the secondary reservoir of frontal sinus.

c. The superior meatus lies between the superior and middle conchae. It is limited to only the posterior third of the lateral wall. The posterior ethmoidal sinus opens into it.

d. The sphenoethmoidal recess lies above and behind the superior concha. It is very narrow and receives the opening of sphenoidal sinus.

Nasal Septum

The skeletal basis of the nasal septum is partly bony and partly cartilaginous (Fig. 114.3). The perpendicular plate of ethmoid bone forms the posterosuperior part of the septum and the vomer forms the posteroinferior part while the septal cartilage bridges the gap anteriorly. The other bones which make minor contributions to the periphery of the septum are, crest of nasal bones, nasal spine of frontal bone, rostrum of sphenoid, crests of palatine bones, and crest of maxilla. The posterior free margin of the septum is formed by the free margin of the vomer, which separates the two posterior nasal apertures or choanae. The free margin of the septum can be inspected through the nasopharynx by a procedure called posterior rhinoscopy (refer to "inspection of nasopharynx" in Chapter 116). The skeletal nasal septum is covered with mucoperichondrium and mucoperiosteum except where it forms the medial wall of the vestibule (this part being covered by skin). This part of the septum is mobile and is called the columellar septum.

Deviated Nasal Septum (DNS)

Deviated nasal septum is a common cause of nasal obstruction. The septum is deviated mostly at vomero-

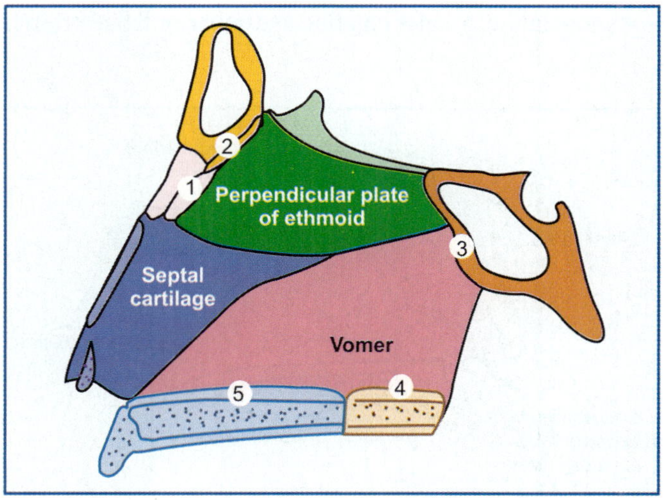

Fig. 114.3: Skeletal components of nasal septum
Note: Minor contributions around the edges: (1) Crest of nasal bone, (2) Nasal spine of frontal bone, (3) Rostrum of sphenoid, (4) Crest of palatine bone, (5) Crest of maxilla

Section three

ethmoidal suture. Trauma or error in development or unequal growth in the base of skull and palate may be the causes. Apart from nasal obstruction, DNS may give rise to headache, sinusitis, epistaxis, anosmia, and external deformity. Submucous resection is the operation of choice in adults. In this operation, the mucoperiosteum and mucoperichondrium are lifted after putting an incision in the epithelium of the septum. Then the deflected parts of the septum are removed and the mucosal flaps are repositioned.

Arterial Supply (Fig. 114.4)

The nasal cavity receives plenty of arterial supply from branches of internal and external carotid arteries.

Arterial Supply of Nasal Septum

Five arteries supply the septum. The anterior and posterior ethmoidal arteries are the branches of ophthalmic branch of internal carotid artery. The septal branches of superior labial branch of facial artery and the septal branches of the sphenopalatine and greater palatine branches of the maxillary artery belong to external carotid system. The greater palatine artery enters the nasal cavity via the incisive canal from the inferior aspect of hard palate.

Little's Area and Kiesselbach's Plexus

This is a vascular area in the antero-inferior part of the septum. The septal branches of the anterior ethmoidal, sphenopalatine, greater palatine and superior labial arteries

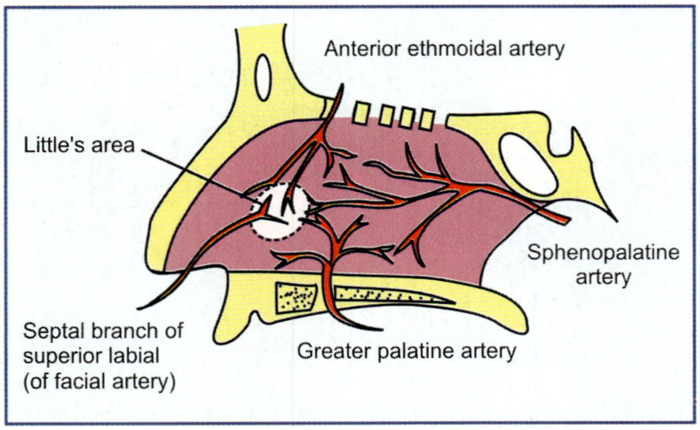

Fig. 114.4: Arterial supply of nasal septum
Note: The vascular plexus of Kiesselbach of Little's area, which is usual site of epistaxis (nasal bleeding)

and their corresponding veins form an anastomotic plexus (Kiesselbach's plexus) in this area. This area is the commonest site of epistaxis or nasal bleeding because it is exposed to fingernail trauma.

Arterial Supply of Lateral Wall

The lateral wall also receives blood from the same sources like that of the nasal septum except that instead of the septal branches of the superior labial branch of facial artery, the alar twigs from lateral nasal branch of facial artery supply the lateral wall.

Venous Drainage

The veins accompany the arteries and drain in the superior ophthalmic veins, pterygoid venous plexus and facial veins.

Nerve Supply (Fig. 114. 5)

a. The end organs of special sensation of smell in the olfactory zone are supplied by 10-20 olfactory nerves.
b. The nerves carrying general sensations supply the respiratory zone.
   i. The septum receives nerve supply from various sources. The posterior three fourth of the septum is supplied by branches of nasopalatine nerve and medial group of superior nasal branches of sphenopalatine ganglion. All these branches enter the nasal cavity via sphenopalatine foramen. The nasopalatine nerve produces a groove on the septum as it travels downwards and forwards to give branches to the septum and then to leave the nasal cavity through the incisive canal to enter the oral cavity. The branches of anterior ethmoidal nerve supply the upper and anterior part. Nasal branches of anterior superior alveolar nerve supply the skin of the vestibule and the anteroinferior part of the septum.
   ii. The lateral wall receives lateral group of posterior superior nasal branches from the sphenopalatine ganglion and nasal branches from greater palatine nerve. The anterior ethmoidal nerve supplies the anterosuperior part of the lateral wall.
c. The parasympathetic secretomotor fibers from the nerve of pterygoid canal (vidian nerve) supply the nasal glands after relay in the pterygopalatine

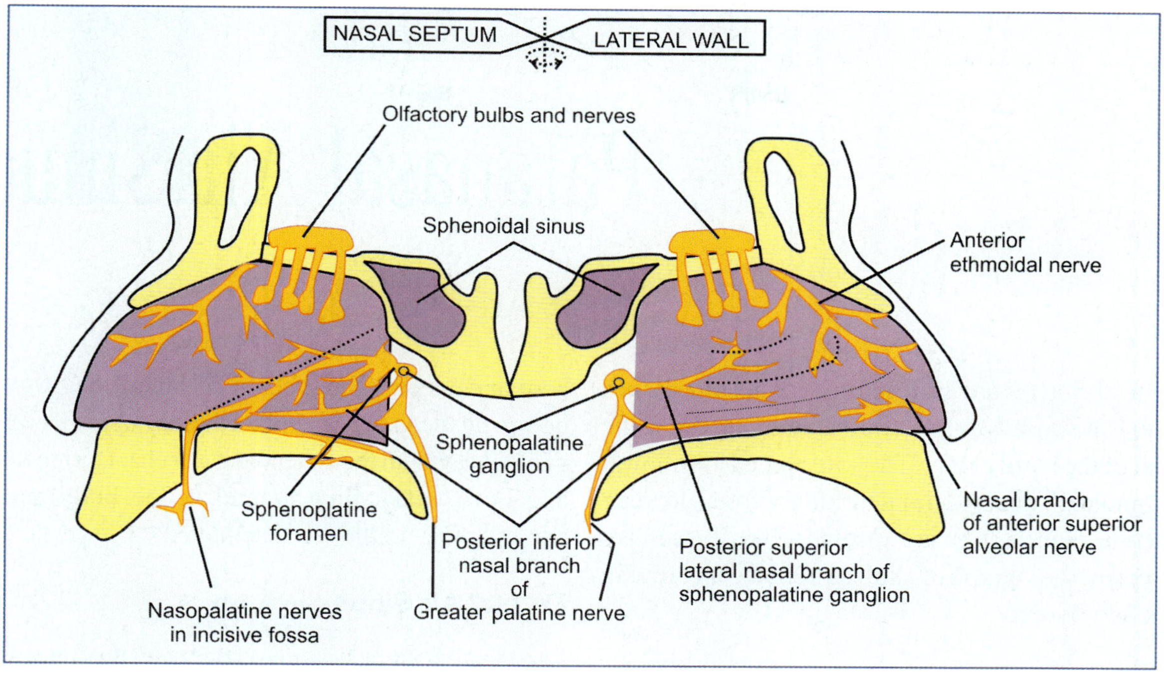

Fig. 114.5: Scheme to depict nerves of lateral and medial walls of nasal cavity (left side)

ganglion. The parasympathetic fibers are also vasodilators. The postganglionic sympathetic fibers carried in the vidian nerve supply the blood vessels. Irritation of the vidian nerve results in lacrimation and excessive secretion of nasal glands (typical features of allergic rhinitis or hay fever). Hence, this nerve is called nerve of hay fever. Uncontrollable secretion from the nasal glands can be controlled by surgical section of the vidian nerve.

Development of Nose and Nasal Cavity (Fig. 58.1)

The olfactory and the respiratory mucosa develop from the ectodermal olfactory (nasal) placode.

The development of nasal cavity from the olfactory placode takes place side by side with the development of face and palate. Initially the external nasal apertures are widely separated from each other due to the intervening median nasal process. Gradually these apertures come closer as the median nasal process becomes thinner. The nasal septum develops from the thinned out median nasal process. The nasal pits are cut off from the stomodeum by the formation of primitive palate from premaxilla. The deepened nasal pits are called the nasal sacs, which are separated from the stomodeum by bucconasal membrane or nasal fin. This membrane soon breaks down so that nasal sacs communicate with the stomodeum by an opening called posterior nasal aperture. The anterior part of the nasal septum is attached to the primitive palate but its posterior part has free lower edge after the disappearance of bucconasal membrane. During the formation of secondary palate from the fusion of palatal processes of the maxillary prominences, the lower edge of nasal septum fuses with the medial edges of the palatal processes. Thus, the oral cavity is completely shut off from the nasal cavity and the posterior nasal apertures shift backward to open into the nasopharynx. The lateral nasal processes (from frontonasal process) form the lateral wall of the nose.

115 Paranasal Air Sinuses

The paranasal sinuses are air filled spaces in some bones surrounding the nasal cavity. These sinuses open in the lateral wall of the nasal cavity. They are named as follows: frontal, ethmoidal, sphenoidal and maxillary corresponding to the bone in which they are located. The sinuses are visible on plain radiograph of skull as translucent areas in the respective bones.

General Characteristics

Developmentally, the paranasal sinuses are the extensions of the nasal cavity. Hence, they are lined with pseudo-stratified ciliated columnar epithelium with goblet cells. The secretions of the goblet cells are drained through the openings of the sinuses in to the nasal cavity. The main function of the paranasal sinuses is to warm and humidify the inspired air. They add to the resonance of voice and reduce the weight of skull. The sinuses are filled during expiration. The warmed and humidified air is released in the nasal cavity during inspiration.

Development

The paranasal sinuses develop as evagination or outpouching of the nasal epithelium into the bones surrounding the nasal cavity during the third to fourth month of intrauterine life. Therefore, the lining of the paranasal sinuses is ectodermal. The sinuses are not fully developed at the time of birth. The ethmoidal sinuses begin to develop before birth and a few cells are present at birth. The frontal sinuses are usually absent at birth. The maxillary sinuses are the first to develop. They appear as shallow grooves on the medial surface of each maxilla around third month of intrauterine life. At birth, the size of the maxillary sinus is around $7 \times 4 \times 4$ mm.The first spurt in the growth of the maxillary sinuses is during 6 to 7 years. They achieve adult size after the eruption of permanent teeth. The sphenoidal sinuses begin to develop before birth. At the time of birth, they appear as extension of nasal cavity in the sphenoidal concha. During the second and third years, they extend in the body and during adolescence, adult size is achieved.

Frontal Air Sinus (Figs 114.1 and 114.2)

Each frontal sinus is situated between the inner and outer tables of frontal bone above and deep to supra-orbital margin. The right and left sinuses are often asymmetrical as the septum between them is obliquely placed. The anterior wall of the sinus is thick and is related to the skin of the forehead. The posterior wall is thin and related to the meninges and frontal lobe of brain. Its inferior wall forms the roof of the orbit. The frontonasal duct begins in the opening of the sinus, which is located in the floor of the sinus. Usually the frontal sinus opens by this duct in the anterior end of the infundibulum of the middle meatus.

The frontal sinus is marked on the surface by drawing a triangle joining the following three points, nasion, a point 3 cm above nasion and a point at the junction of medial third and lateral two-third of the supraorbital margin.

The supraorbital nerve, a branch of frontal nerve, supplies the mucous membrane of the sinus.

Ethmoidal Sinuses (Fig. 115.1)

These sinuses are thin-walled air cells in the labyrinth of the ethmoid bone. They are located between the upper part of lateral nasal wall and the medial wall of orbit. Their roof is related to the meninges of the anterior cranial fossa. The lateral wall is formed by paper-like lamina of bone called lamina papyracea. This wall is extremely fragile hence, slightest injury to it can lead to spread of ethmoidal infection into the orbit. There are three groups of ethmoidal sinuses. The anterior group opens in the anterior part of infundibulum of middle meatus. The middle group projects into the middle meatus producing ethmoidal bulla. The middle group opens at the summit of the bulla. The posterior group opens in the superior meatus. The ethmoidal nerves (branches of nasociliary) and orbital branch of maxillary nerve supply the mucous membrane of the sinuses.

Sphenoidal Sinus (Figs 85.2 and 114.2)

These sinuses occupy the body of the sphenoid bone. The right and left sinuses are separated from each other by a deflected bony septum. The two sinuses are therefore asymmetrical in size. Each sinus opens in the spheno-ethmoidal recess of the lateral wall of the nasal cavity by an opening situated in the upper part of its anterior wall. Relations of the sinus are surgically important especially during trans-sphenoidal hypophysectomy. The anterior part of the roof is related to the optic chiasma while the posterior part of the roof is related to the pituitary gland. Each lateral wall is related to the cavernous sinus, internal carotid artery and oculomotor, trochlear, abducent and the three divisions of trigeminal nerve. The posterior ethmoidal nerves and orbital branches of maxillary nerve supply the mucous membrane of the sinuses.

Clinical Highlights

Due to the anatomical proximity of the sphenoidal sinus and the pituitary gland, the sinus is used as a route to approach the gland in a procedure called trans-nasal, trans-sphenoidal hypophysectomy. The mucoperiosteum of the nasal septum is elevated on both sides to reach the sphenoid bone via the roof of nasal cavity. The anterior wall of the sinus is opened and the septum between right and left sinuses is removed. Having gained entry inside the sinus, an incision is placed in the roof of the sphenoidal sinus (sella turcica) to approach the pituitary.

Maxillary Sinus (Fig. 115.1)

The maxillary sinus (antrum of Highmore) is the largest paranasal air sinus. It has the capacity of 15 ml in the adult. Each sinus occupies the body of the maxilla of its side. It is pyramid-shaped with base (its medial wall) directed towards the lateral wall of nasal cavity and apex pointing laterally towards the zygomatic bone.

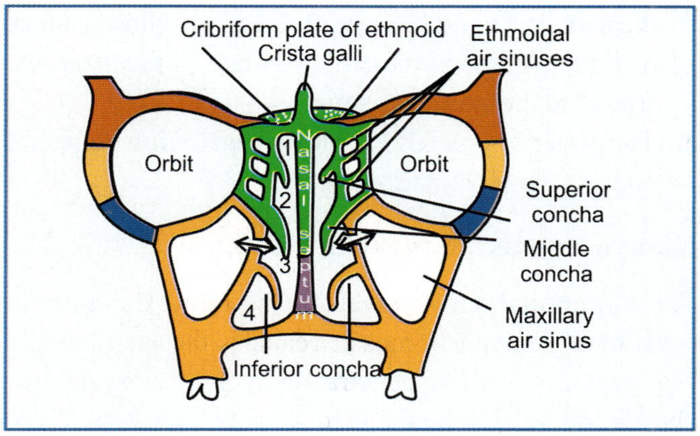

Fig. 115.1: Schematic coronal section showing relation of ethmoidal and maxillary sinuses to nasal cavity (Arrows indicate the openings of the maxillary sinuses. (1) Sphenoethmoidal recess, (2) Superior meatus, (3) Middle meatus, (4) Inferior meatus)

Relations of Walls of Sinus

a. The anterior wall is formed by the anterior surface of the maxilla covered by cheek.
b. The roof forms the floor of the orbit, through which travels the infraorbital nerve.
c. The floor is formed by the alveolar and palatine processes of the maxilla. It is located about 1 cm below the floor of nasal cavity (hard palate). The roots of the upper molar and premolar teeth almost project in the floor of the sinus since the bone is very thin here. Extraction of upper molar or premolar teeth may lead to a communication between the sinus and oral cavity. For the same reason infection from caries teeth is a common cause of maxillary sinusitis.
d. The medial wall is related to the lateral wall of the nasal cavity. The superior part of the medial wall bears the opening of the sinus in the middle meatus. The high position of the opening hinders the natural drainage of the sinus. This opening (maxillary hiatus) is reduced in size in the living state by following bony parts, the uncinate process of ethmoid from above, the descending process of lacrimal bone in front, perpendicular plate of palatine bone behind and the inferior nasal concha below (Fig. 114.1). The pus of frontal sinusitis may run via the hiatus semilunaris to

the maxillary sinus because the location of the openings of these sinuses favours the passage of pus from the frontal to the maxillary sinus.

e. The posterior wall is related to contents of infratemporal and pterygopalatine fossae.

Nerves Related to Maxillary Sinus (Fig. 106.1)

The infraorbital nerve travels in the roof. The anterior superior alveolar nerve runs in a canal in the anterior wall. The posterior wall is penetrated by posterior superior alveolar nerve. The pain due to sinusitis may be referred to the upper teeth and face. The same nerves supply the mucous membrane of the sinus.

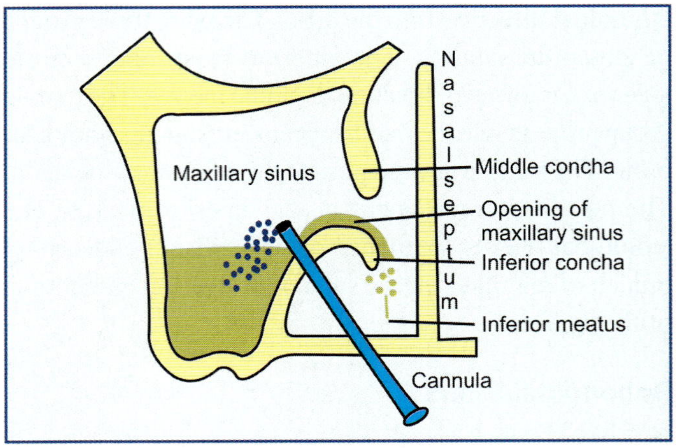

Fig. 115.2: Antral puncture through inferior meatus for irrigation of maxillary sinus

Clinical Highlights

a. This sinus is more prone to infections in chronic smokers because epithelium loses cilia, which hampers the drainage of sinus.

b. There are two surgical approaches to maxillary sinus. In intranasal antrostomy, an artificial opening is made in the lateral wall of inferior meatus of nasal cavity (Fig.115.2) This opening is closer to the floor of the sinus and hence facilitates drainage. In Caldwell-Luc operation the upper lip is retracted upwards and the angle of mouth is retracted laterally. An incision is placed in the mucous membrane and the periosteum covering the canine fossa. This exposes the anterior wall of the sinus closer to the floor. An artificial opening is created here to drain the pus.

c. Maxillary sinus is the common site of malignancy in paranasal sinuses. The cancer of maxillary sinus initially may present as symptoms of sinusitis. However, it easily spreads the neighboring regions because the walls of the sinus are very thin. The symptoms and signs depend on which anatomical structure near the sinus is involved. Invasion of the medial wall of the sinus causes obstruction to the nasal cavity and epistaxis. Involvement of the anterior wall gives rise to swelling of the cheek. The spread through floor results in dental pain, loosening of teeth, ulceration of gums and swelling of hard palate. Superior spread invades the orbit causing proptosis, ocular pain and epiphora (overflow of tears). Posterior spread in the sphenopalatine fossa may cause pain in the area of distribution of maxillary nerve. Spread in to infra-temporal fossa may lead to trismus.

d. Transillumination of maxillary sinus is performed in a darkened room. The torchlight is shown in the patient's mouth on one side of the hard palate. The light passes through the maxillary sinus and appears as a dull glow on the cheek. Absence of glow indicates infection, fluid or growth in the sinus.

116 Pharynx

The pharynx is the fibromuscular tube forming the upper part of the air and food passages. It is 12-14 cm long and extends from the base of skull to the lower border of cricoid cartilage (vertebral level C6), where it becomes continuous with esophagus. The shape of the pharynx is conical and hence its width at its roof is 3.5 cm and at its lower end (crico-esophageal junction) 1.5 cm. The anterior wall of pharynx has three deficiencies through which it opens into the nasal cavity, oral cavity and larynx, from above downwards.

Subdivisions (Fig. 116.1)

a. The nasopharynx or epipharynx performs respiratory function and communicates with nasal cavity.
b. The oropharynx is common to both respiratory and digestive tracts, which cross each other here.
c. The laryngopharynx or hypopharynx acts as a conduit of food from oropharynx to the esophagus. It also conducts air into the larynx via the laryngeal inlet.

Layers of Pharyngeal Wall

The wall of the pharynx consists of five layers. From within outward they are, the mucous membrane, submucosa, the pharyngeal aponeurosis or pharyngobasilar fascia, muscular coat and the buccopharyngeal fascia.

Mucosa

The mucous membrane lining the nasopharynx is continuous with that of pharyngotympanic tubes and nasal cavity. The nasopharynx is lined with respiratory epithelium which is pseudostratified ciliated columnar in

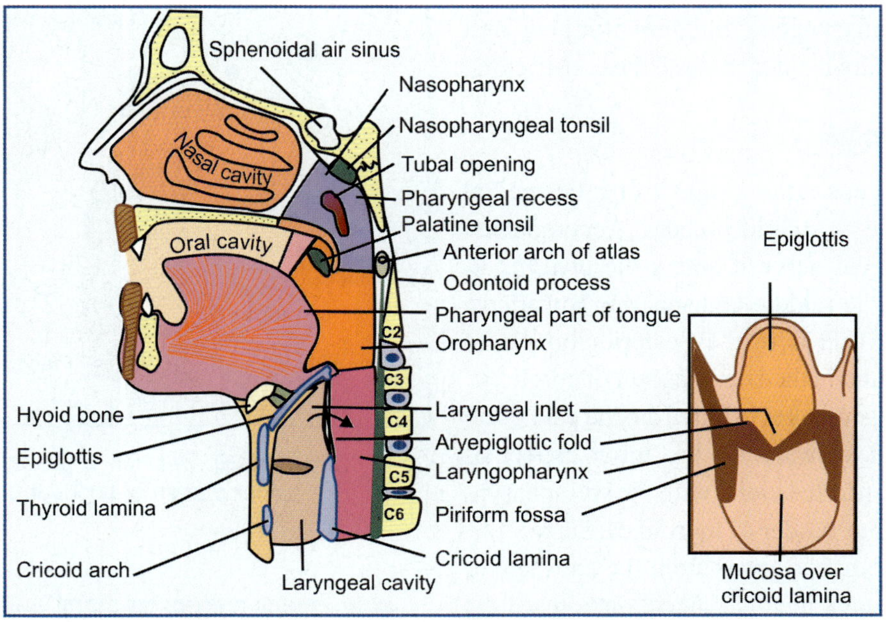

Fig. 116.1: Median section of head and neck showing subdivisions of pharynx. Insert shows features of laryngopharynx in posterior view

type. The mucous membrane of oropharynx is continuous with that of oral cavity and is of stratified squamous nonkeratinizing type. The mucosa of laryngopharynx is stratified squamous nonkeratinizing and is continuous with mucosa of larynx and that of esophagus.

Submucosa

The submucosa of the nasopharynx and oropharynx contains lymphatic aggregations, which are the constituent of a lymphatic ring called Waldeyer's ring located at the beginning of food and air passages.

Pharyngeal Aponeurosis (Pharyngobasilar Fascia)

This fascial layer lies outer to submucosa but inner to the muscular coat. The thick part of this fascia fills the gap (sinus of Morgagni) between the upper margin of superior constrictor and base of the cranium. Here, it is pierced by auditory tube, ascending palatine branch of facial artery, ascending pharyngeal artery and levator palati muscle (Fig. 116.2B).

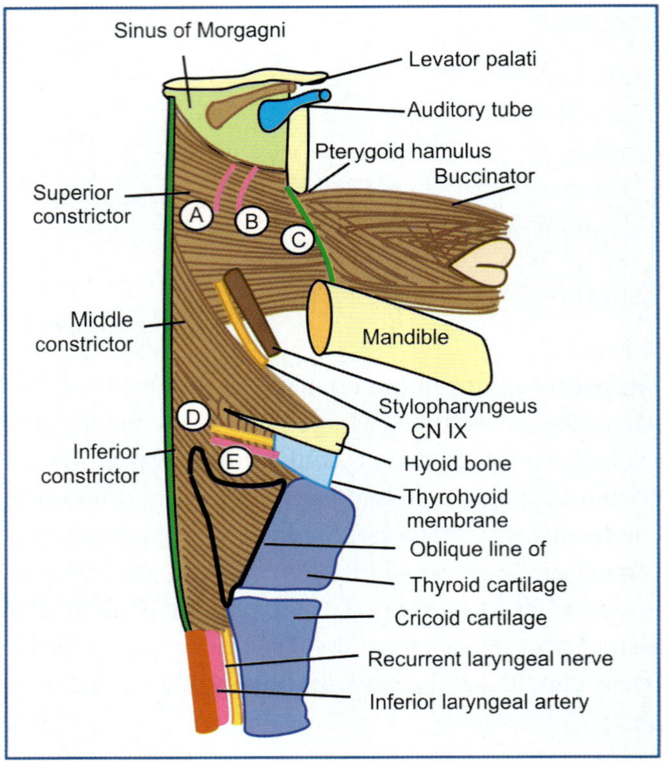

Fig. 116.2A: Simplified representation of constrictor of muscles of pharynx. (A) Palatine branch of ascending pharyngeal artery, (B) Ascending palatine branch of facial artery, (C) Pterygo-mandibular raphe, (D) Internal laryngeal nerve, (E) Superior laryngeal artery

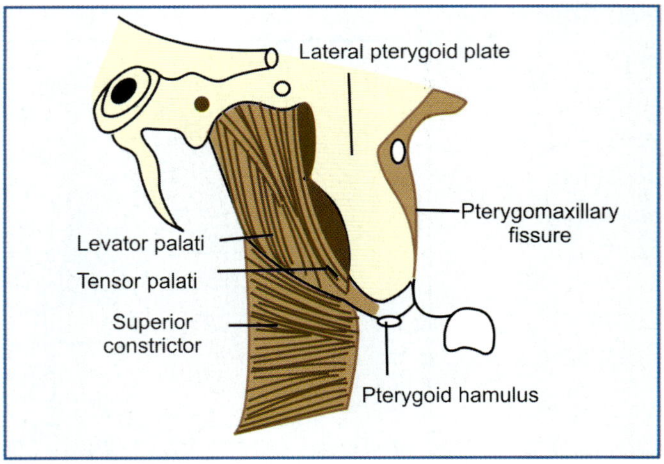

Fig. 116.2B: Relation of palatine muscles to upper margin of superior constrictor

Pharyngeal Muscles

The pharyngeal muscles consist of two groups, constrictors and longitudinal muscles. The constrictor muscles consist of superior, middle and inferior. The longitudinal muscles consist of salpingopharyngeus, palatopharyngeus and stylopharyngeus and are located inner to the constrictors.

Longitudinal Muscles

a. The stylopharyngeus takes origin from the medial aspect of the base of styloid process. Accompanied by glossopharyngeal nerve it enters the pharynx in the gap between the middle and superior constrictor muscles. Its insertion is in the posterior border of thyroid cartilage and in the lateral aspect of epiglottis.
b. The palatopharyngeus takes origin from the palate and runs vertically downward on the inner aspect of constrictors. It is inserted along with the stylopharyngeus in the posterior border of thyroid cartilage.
c. The salpingopharyngeus arises from the cartilage of the auditory tube near the pharyngeal opening of the tube. The fibers pass downward to blend with palatopharyngeus and insert along with it in the posterior border of thyroid cartilage.

Constrictors Muscles (Fig. 116.2A)

The three constrictor muscles lie in the posterior wall and sides of the pharynx. They overlap each other from below upwards. They are inserted into the median fibrous raphe, which extends from the pharyngeal tubercle at the base of cranium to the esophagus.

Superior Constrictor

This is a thin sheet of muscle lying in the wall of nasopharynx and oropharynx. It has a wide origin and according to the origin, it divided in four parts:

i. Pterygopharyngeal part originates from the posterior border of medial pterygoid lamina and pterygoid hamulus
ii. Buccopharyngeal part originates from the pterygomandibular raphe
iii. Mylopharyngeal part takes origin from posterior end of the mylohyoid line of mandible
iv. Glossopharyngeal part arises from the mucous membrane of the side of tongue.

From this wide origin, the superior constrictor is inserted in to the median fibrous raphe and superiorly in to the pharyngeal tubercle. This is the only constrictor muscle having attachment to the base of the skull.

Structures Piercing Superior Constrictor

This muscle forms the tonsillar bed in the lateral wall of oropharynx. A number of blood vessels and the lymphatic vessels of the tonsil pierce the muscle in this location (tonsillar branch of facial artery, tonsillar branches of ascending palatine and ascending pharyngeal arteries, paratonsillar or external palatine vein).

Passavant's Ridge or Palatopharyngeal Sphincter

Near its superior margin a few fibers of superior constrictor blend with a band of muscle fibers belonging to palatopharyngeus muscle. These fibers form a ring around the posterior and sidewalls of nasopharyngeal isthmus. When the soft palate is elevated the muscle band appears as a ridge known as Passavant's ridge. During the act of swallowing the Passavant's ridge and the soft palate are approximated by contraction of this sphincter and the levator palati. In this way, nasopharynx is shut off from oropharynx to prevent regurgitation of food in the nasopharynx and nasal cavity. The Passavant's ridge is hypertrophied in cases of complete cleft palate.

Middle Constrictor

This is a fan-shaped muscle with narrow origin and broad insertion. It takes origin from the lower part of stylohyoid ligament, lesser cornu and upper border of greater cornu of hyoid bone. The fibers fan out and are inserted in the median fibrous raphe.

Inferior Constrictor

This is the thickest of the three constrictors. The inferior constrictor is related to the medial surface of the lateral lobe of thyroid gland and it is part of the floor of the carotid triangle of neck.

According to the origin, the muscle is divisible into thyropharyngeus and cricopharyngeus parts, which function paradoxically. When thyropharyngeus muscle contracts the cricopharyngeus relaxes and vice versa.

i. The thyropharyngeus arises from oblique line of thyroid cartilage, the tendinous band stretching between the inferior thyroid tubercle and cricoid cartilage and from the inferior cornu of thyroid cartilage. Its fibers are obliquely disposed as they curve to reach the median fibrous raphe for insertion.
ii. The cricopharyngeus arises from the side of cricoid cartilage and its fibers are transversely disposed. At the lower end, cricopharyngeus is continuous with circular muscle coat of esophagus. The muscles of the two sides form a sphincter at the pharyngo-esophageal junction. The function of this sphincter is to prevent the entry of air in to the esophagus in the interval between acts of swallowing. So, this sphincter relaxes during the act of swallowing but contracts in between the acts of swallowing.

Important Relations of Constrictor Muscles (Fig. 116.2A)

a. The interval between the free superior border of superior constrictor and the cranium (sinus of Morgagni) is closed by the pharyngobasilar fascia and buccopharyngeal fascia. The superior border of the muscle is related to eustachian tube and the tensor palati and levator palati muscles (Fig. 116.2B). The levator palati pierces the fasciae to enter the oropharynx while the tensor palati hooks round the pterygoid hamulus to enter the oropharynx deep to tendinous origin of buccinator.

b. The inferior margin of the superior constrictor overlaps the superior margin of middle constrictor. The stylopharyngeus muscle and glossopharyngeal nerve enter the pharynx between these two muscles.
c. The internal laryngeal nerve and superior laryngeal artery pierce the thyrohyoid membrane to enter the laryngopharynx through the gap between the lower margin of middle constrictor and the upper margin of inferior constrictor muscles.
d. The recurrent laryngeal nerve and inferior laryngeal artery pass deep to the lower margin of the inferior constrictor in the tracheo-esophageal groove. The external laryngeal nerve pierces the inferior constrictor on way to the cricothyroid.

Killian's Dehiscence

It is a potential gap between the thyropharyngeus and cricopharyngeus parts of the inferior constrictor muscle. It is indicated by a dimple in the lining mucosa of the pharynx and is the weak area of the pharyngeal wall. Pharyngeal diverticulum (Zenker's diverticulum) develops if the cricopharyngeus fails to relax during swallowing due to neuromuscular incordination. The raised intra-pharyngeal pressure forces the mucosa and submucosa posteriorly through the Killian's dehiscence. The diverticulum so formed gradually enlarges in downward direction usually on the left side. Perforation can occur at this site during passage of esophagoscope.

Buccopharyngeal Fascia

This fascia covers the pharynx externally. It derives its name from the fact that it covers pharyngeal muscles as well as the buccinator muscle. Posteriorly, the bucco-pharyngeal fascia is in contact with prevertebral muscles and cervical vertebral column. The pharyngeal plexus of nerves lies in the fascia, where it covers the middle constrictor.

Pharyngeal Plexus of Nerves

The following nerves take part in the formation of the pharyngeal plexus:

i. The pharyngeal branch of vagus, (which carries cranial part of accessory nerve) is motor to muscles of soft palate except tensor palati and to the muscles of pharynx, except stylopharyngeus.
ii. Pharyngeal branch of glossopharyngeal nerve is sensory to mucosa of oropharynx and nasopharynx.
iii. Sympathetic nerves from superior cervical ganglion are vasomotor in function.

Nerve Supply of Pharyngeal Muscles

The pharyngeal plexus of nerves (via vago-accessory complex) supplies all the pharyngeal muscles except the stylopharyngeus, which is supplied by glossopharyngeal nerve. The inferior constrictor receives additional supply from the recurrent laryngeal and external laryngeal nerves.

Actions of Pharyngeal Muscles

The successive contraction of the constrictor muscles (except the cricopharyngeus) from above downwards, propels the food down in the esophagus. During this phase, the longitudinal muscles are relaxed. After the food reaches the esophagus, the longitudinal muscles contract to pull the pharynx up to bring it back to its original position.

Nasopharynx (Fig. 116.1)

Being the uppermost part of pharynx it is called epipharynx. It communicates anteriorly with nasal cavities. It communicates with oropharynx through nasopharyngeal isthmus and with middle ear through the auditory tubes. The nasopharynx is always kept patent unlike the other two subdivisions of pharynx. It has important role in hearing. It supplies atmospheric air to the middle ear, thus equalizing air pressure on lateral and medial aspects of tympanic membrane.

Walls

The nasopharynx has roof, posterior wall, lateral walls, floor and anterior wall. The roof and posterior wall form a continuous sloping surface. The roof consists of a small area of the base of the cranium extending from the pharyngeal tubercle to the line joining the roots of the medial pterygoid plates. It includes part of the body of sphenoid and the basiocciput. The pharyngobasilar fascia and superior constrictor muscle supported by the anterior arch of atlas (on posterior aspect) are the components of the posterior wall.

Features of Roof

a. The nasopharyngeal or pharyngeal tonsil is a lymphoid collection that projects in the nasopharynx from the junction of roof and posterior wall. It is the mucosa related lymphatic tissue (MALT). It increases in size up to the age of six years and then gradually atrophies. Hypertrophy of nasopharyngeal tonsil is called adenoids. Sometimes, in children the adenoids may obstruct the nasopharynx completely resulting in mouth breathing.
b. A midline pharyngeal bursa is present in this tonsil. This bursa denotes the site of attachment of the notochord to the endoderm of primitive pharynx. It is an epithelium-lined recess extending posteriorly right up to the roof. Infection of this bursa is called pharyngeal bursitis. An abscess in the bursa presents as a cystic swelling on the posterior wall of nasopharynx.
c. A dimple in the mucosa above the nasopharyngeal tonsil denotes the site of the path of the embryonic Rathke's pouch. Sometimes, the remnant cells of the Rathke's pouch may give rise to pharyngeal hypophysis, which may turn malignant (craniopharyngioma).

Features of Lateral Wall

a. The tubal orifice, which is the medial opening of the pharyngotympanic tube is situated 10-12 mm behind and slightly below the posterior end of inferior nasal concha. The tubal orifice is bounded above and posteriorly by tubal elevation (torus tubaris) produced by the prominent cartilage of the pharyngeal end of the tube. The tubal elevation is a landmark that helps in locating the tubal orifice during passage of catheter in the tube.
b. The salpingopharyngeal fold is a mucous fold passing vertically downward from the tubal elevation.
c. The tubal tonsil is the collection of submucous lymphoid tissue (MALT) lying on the tubal elevation. The pharyngeal recess or Rosenmuller's fossa is a depression behind the tubal elevation. This is the commonest site of carcinoma of nasopharynx.

Posterior Nasal Apertures (Choanae)

Anteriorly the nasopharynx communicates with the nasal cavity through two large and oval apertures called choanae. These apertures are 2.5 cm in length and 1.25 cm in width. Their bony boundaries are, posterior free margin of vomer medially, inferior surface of the body of sphenoid superiorly, medial edge of medial pterygoid plate laterally and posterior margin of hard palate inferiorly.

Features of Floor

Anterior part of the floor is formed by the soft palate. Posterior to the soft palate, the floor shows the deficiency (nasopharyngeal or pharyngeal isthmus). The boundaries of this isthmus are, the posterior surface and free margin of soft palate anteriorly, the Passavant's ridge posteriorly and the palatopharyngeal arch on each side.

Sensory Supply of Nasopharynx

The glossopharyngeal nerve through the pharyngeal plexus and the pharyngeal branch of maxillary nerve near the tubal orifice, supply the mucosa.

Inspection of Nasopharynx

The nasopharynx is inspected by a procedure called posterior rhinoscopy. The tongue of the patient is depressed with a tongue depressor and then the rhinoscopic mirror is introduced until it reaches the posterior one-third of the tongue. The light from the head mirror is focused on the rhinoscopic mirror to illuminate the nasopharynx. By tilting the mirror in different directions, one can see the reflection of the interior of the nasopharynx.

Clinical Highlights

Carcinoma in the nasopharynx arises usually in the pharyngeal recess (fossa of Rosenmuller). The malignant growth has a tendency to infiltrate the neighboring structures resulting in diverse symptoms and signs. Due to proximity of the nasopharynx to the cranial base, the cranial nerves are involved by direct spread or by intracranial extension through various foramina (foramen lacerum, carotid canal, jugular foramen, foramen spinosum and ovale). Direct spread in the soft palate may cause elevation and immobility of soft palate of the same side. Direct spread to the auditory tube may result in conduction/conductive deafness. The extension of cancer in the nasal cavity may cause epistaxis. Retropharyngeal and cervical lymph nodes may enlarge due to lymphatic spread.

Oropharynx

The oropharynx lies behind the oral cavity, below the nasopharynx and above the laryngopharynx. It communicates with the oral cavity through the oropharyngeal isthmus and with the nasopharynx through the pharyngeal isthmus. At its lower end, it continues as laryngopharynx at the level of upper border of epiglottis.

Walls of Oropharynx

a. The roof is formed by undersurface of soft palate in anterior part and is deficient in posterior part due to presence of pharyngeal isthmus.
b. The floor is formed by posterior third of the tongue and the valleculae. The dorsum of the posterior third of tongue is characterized by subepithelial lymphatic collection (MALT) known as lingual tonsils. The tongue is connected to the epiglottis by three mucosal folds, one median and two lateral glossoepiglottic folds. The vallecula is the space bounded by median and lateral glosso-epiglottic folds on each side.
c. The anterior wall is deficient due to presence of oropharyngeal isthmus. The boundaries of the oropharyngeal isthmus are the soft palate superiorly, dorsal surface of posterior third of tongue inferiorly and the palatoglossal arch on each side.
d. The posterior wall is supported by the body of second cervical vertebra (axis) and upper part of body of third cervical vertebra.
e. The lateral walls present palatoglossal and palatopharyngeal arches enclosing tonsillar fossa for the palatine tonsils.

Palatine Tonsil (Faucial Tonsil)

The palatine tonsils are the collections of lymphoid tissues in the submucosa of oropharynx. They belong to MALT or mocosa-associated lymphoid tissue. The palatine tonsils are the common site of infection producing sore throat and fever. They are placed one on each side in the tonsillar fossa or sinus in the lateral wall of oropharynx. The tonsils are of large size during early childhood but diminish in size after puberty.

Surface Marking

An almond-shaped area over the lower part of masseter muscle, a little above and in front of the angle of mandible marks the tonsil on the surface.

Boundaries of Tonsillar Fossa or Fauces

a. Anterior boundary (also known as anterior pillar of fauces) is the palatoglossal arch, which is the mucosal fold containing the palatoglossus muscle.
b. Posterior boundary (also known as posterior pillar of fauces) is the palatopharyngeal arch, which is the mucosal fold containing palatopharyngeus muscle.
c. Lateral wall (Fig. 116.3) forms the tonsillar bed, which consists of pharyngobasilar fascia, superior constrictor (along with few fibers of longitudinal muscles of pharynx), and glossopharyngeal nerve. It has important relations (vide infra). The internal carotid artery lies about 25 mm lateral and behind the tonsil.

Parts of Tonsil and Relations

The tonsil has two poles (upper and lower), two borders (anterior and posterior) and two surfaces (lateral or deep and medial or free).

a. The upper pole of the tonsil extends into the soft palate. A semilunar fold in newborn covers the medial aspect of the upper pole. It is the remnant of embryonic mucosal fold and is replaced by lymphatic tissue after birth.
b. The lower pole extends into the tongue. A triangular fold of mucosa, which is a remnant of embryonic fold from the palatoglossal arch, covers the lower pole in newborn, but it soon obliterates.
c. The medial or free surface (Fig. 116.3) faces the oropharynx and is covered with nonkeratinizing stratified squamous epithelium, which dips in its substance as tonsillar crypts. About 15 to 20 crypts open on the surface giving it a pitted appearance. One of the crypts

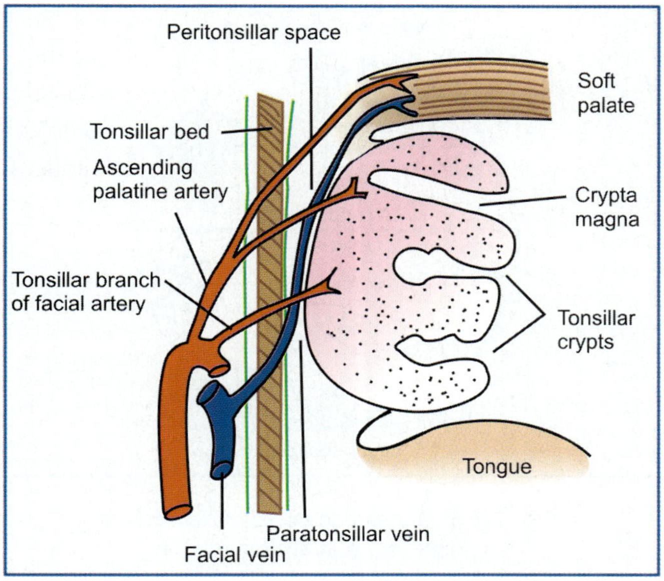

Fig. 116.3: Schematic diagram showing blood vessels passing through tonsillar bed (Note that the tonsillar bed consists of superior constrictor muscle flanked medially by pharyngobasilar fascia and laterally by buccopharyngeal fascia)

located near the upper pole is very deep and hence called intratonsillar cleft or crypta magna. It is the remnant of embryonic second pharyngeal pouch. The crypts branch within the substance of the tonsil so that there is an intimate association of the epithelial cells and the lymphocytes in the tonsil, which is referred to as lymphoepithelial symbiosis. This facilitates direct transport of the antigen from the external environment to the tonsillar lymphoid tissue.

d. The lateral or deep surface is covered with a well-defined hemicapsule. Lateral to the capsule, the submucosa (peritonsillar space) contains loose areolar tissue and paratonsillar vein. This space is the plane of dissection during tonsillectomy. The paratonsillar vein that passes through this space is often a source of postoperative bleeding. Accumulation of pus in this space in chronic tonsillitis gives rise to peritonsillar abscess or quinsy.

The tonsillar bed is related to certain arteries, which are in jeopardy during tonsillectomy. These arteries are the loop of the facial artery and its ascending palatine branch, ascending pharyngeal artery and the internal carotid artery. Styloglossus muscle, stylopharyngeus muscle and glossopharyngeal nerve are the other relations of this surface.

Blood Supply (Fig. 116.4)

The tonsil is supplied by five sets of arteries, the dorsal lingual branch of lingual artery, the ascending palatine branch of facial artery, descending palatine branch of ascending pharyngeal artery, the tonsillar branch of facial artery (main tonsillar artery) and the greater palatine branch of maxillary artery. The venous plexus around the tonsil drains by tonsillar veins, which accompany the tonsillar branch of facial artery. They open in common facial vein. Some veins drain into the paratonsillar vein, which opens in pharyngeal venous plexus or in the common facial vein.

Nerve Supply

The lesser palatine branches of maxillary nerve and the tonsillar branches of glossopharyngeal nerve form a plexus called circulus tonsillaris. This plexus supplies the tonsil, soft palate and oropharyngeal isthmus. The pain of tonsillitis is referred to the ear due to common innervation by glossopharyngeal nerve.

Lymphatic Drainage

The lymphatics draining the tonsil pierce the superior constrictor muscle to reach the upper deep cervical nodes, mainly, the jugulodigastric nodes. These nodes are called tonsillar nodes since they are enlarged in tonsillitis and are palpable below the angle of mandible.

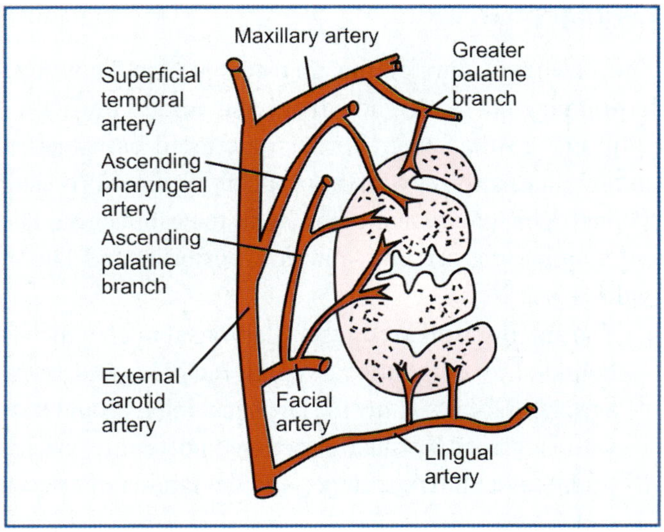

Fig. 116.4: Sources of arterial supply of palatine tonsil

Inspection of Oropharynx

The oropharynx (including the tonsils) is directly visible when the patient opens the mouth wide. To test the movements of the soft palate, the patient is asked to say 'Aa.' The posterior one-third of the tongue is examined by digital palpation and by indirect laryngoscopy.

Waldeyer's Ring (Fig. 116.5)

This is a ring of lymphatic tissue at the beginning of food and air passages (in the nasopharynx and oropharynx). It is much enlarged in early childhood. This ring is composed of mucosa associated lymphatic tissue (MALT). The characteristic feature of MALT is the close approximation of epithelium and the lymphatic tissue. The Waldeyer's ring consists of the faucial or palatine tonsils on both sides, nasopharyngeal tonsil on the posterior wall of nasopharynx, the tubal tonsils on the lateral walls of nasopharynx and the lingual tonsils on the dorsum of posterior one-third of tongue in the floor of oropharynx. The lymphatic follicles produce B and T lymphocytes. When the epithelium comes in contact with the antigen (microorganism) its cells sample the antigen and pass it on to the lymphatic follicles. In response to the sampling, the B and T-lymphocytes produce appropriate antibodies. Thus, the Waldeyer's ring offers not only the local defense but also produces lymphocytes for sending to other lymph nodes via the efferent lymph vessels.

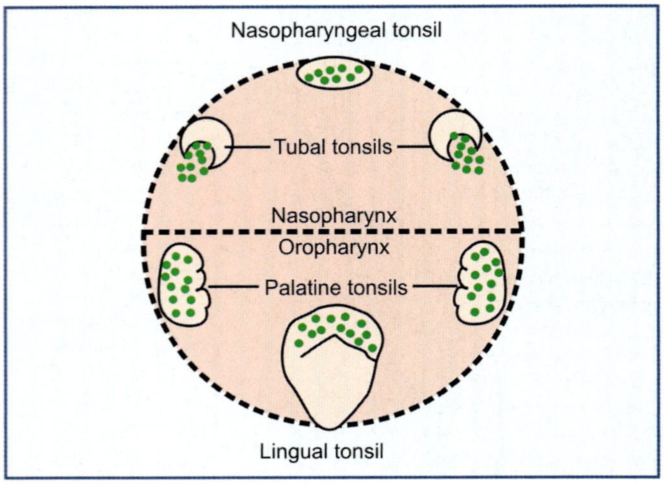

Fig. 116.5: Scheme to depict collections of lymphoid tissue in Waldeyer's ring

Laryngopharynx

The laryngeal part of the pharynx is also known as hypopharynx. It extends from the upper border of epiglottis to the lower border of cricoid cartilage. It communicates above with the oropharynx, anteriorly with the laryngeal cavity and below with the esophagus. The laryngopharynx presents anterior, posterior and lateral walls (Fig. 116.1).

a. The anterior wall presents the laryngeal inlet, which is bounded by epiglottis, aryepiglottic folds and interarytenoid folds. Below the laryngeal inlet, the anterior wall is formed by mucosa-covered posterior surfaces of the arytenoids cartilages and the lamina of cricoid cartilage.
b. The posterior wall consists of constrictor muscles supported by prevertebral muscles and third to sixth cervical vertebrae.
c. The lateral wall is characterized by piriform fossa (recess) on either side of the laryngeal inlet. These recesses form the lateral channels for food on each side. The boundaries of the fossa are: medially, aryepiglottic fold and laterally, the mucosa covering the inner surface of the thyrohyoid membrane and the lamina of thyroid cartilage. The internal laryngeal nerve pierces the thryrohyoid membrane and traverses under the mucosa of the piriform recess from lateral to medial side to enter the laryngeal cavity. So, the internal laryngeal nerve is intimately related to the piriform fossa. The foreign bodies like fish bone may get impacted in the fossa. During removal of the foreign body, the internal laryngeal nerve may be injured if the instrument pierces the mucosa. In the carcinoma of piriform fossa, pain is referred to ear due to common innervation by vagus. The piriform fossa is colloquially given a fancy name of "smuggler's fossa" since it is used by the smugglers to hide precious gems.

Nerve Supply

The internal laryngeal nerve supplies the mucosa of the laryngopharynx.

Inspection of Laryngopharynx

In indirect laryngoscopy, the patient is asked to protrude the tongue, which is held by the examiner between thumb and index finger. The laryngeal mirror is then introduced and held firmly against soft palate. Light is focused on the laryngeal mirror to inspect the laryngopharynx and posterior one-third of the tongue. Direct laryngoscopy is performed under general anesthsia. The laryngoscope is introduced through the oral cavity and the oropharynx into the laryngopharynx.

117 Larynx

Larynx is the upper part of respiratory tract. Its main function is to protect the lower respiratory tract so that foreign bodies do not enter the trachea. If a foreign body touches the mucosa of the larynx, it reflexly gives rise to violent coughing until the foreign body is expelled. Thus, larynx is correctly described as a watchdog of the lungs. Another function of the larynx is production of the voice, hence the name voice box. The framework of the larynx is composed of cartilages and membranes. The laryngeal muscles primarily move the cartilages and through them, the vocal cords during respiration and phonation.

Location

The larynx is located in front of the neck opposite the third to sixth cervical vertebrae in adult. It moves vertically up and down during swallowing and phonation. The larynx extends from the upper border of epiglottis to the lower margin of cricoid cartilage. It opens in the laryngopharynx through the laryngeal inlet and is continuous with trachea below. Its anterior aspect is covered with skin, fasciae and strap muscles (omohyoid, sternothyroid, sternohyoid) and its posterior aspect projects in the laryngopharynx.

Differences in Male and Female

Until puberty, the larynx of male differs very little from that of female. After puberty, the male larynx grows rapidly due to the increase in the size of laryngeal cartilages. The laryngeal prominence (Adam's apple) becomes prominent in males. The laryngeal prominence is produced due to decrease in the thyroid angle, which is 90° in males and 120° in females. The length of vocal cords is approximately 24 mm in males and 16 mm in females. Because of these differences, the voice is low pitch in males and high pitch in females.

Differences in Adult and Infant

a. Infant larynx is smaller, funnel shaped and narrower than that of the adult (about one-third the size of adult).
b. The laryngeal cartilages are softer and collapse easily in infant.
c. The larynx is placed at a higher level in infants. Its upper margin at rest is at the level of axis vertebra and that of the elevated larynx it is at the level of median atlanto-axial joint.
d. The epiglottis is longer and deeply grooved, which is more suited to protect the air passage during suckling.
e. The submucosa in infant's larynx is thicker and becomes edematous faster after irritation. Therefore, the obstruction of the airway takes place faster in infants.
f. The neonatal subglottic cavity extends posteriorly as well as inferiorly. This point is to be noted during passage of endotracheal tube in infants.

Laryngeal Cartilages (Fig. 117.1)

The skeleton of larynx consists of three unpaired and three paired cartilages. The unpaired cartilages are, the epiglottis, the thyroid and the cricoid. The paired cartilages are: the arytenoid, cuneiform and the corniculate.

a. The epiglottis is a leaf-shaped elastic cartilage. It forms the anterior wall of the laryngeal inlet. Its upper end projects upwards and backwards behind the hyoid bone (Fig. 117.2) and the base of tongue. Its upper end is free and broad and lower end is narrow and pointed. It has anterior and posterior surfaces and two lateral margins. The upper part of anterior surface is covered with stratified squamous epithelium and is connected to the tongue by three mucosal folds, the median and lateral glosso-epiglottic folds. The lower part of

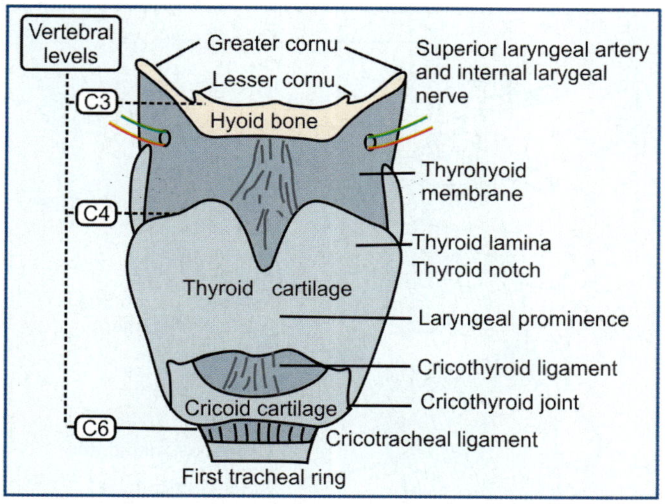

Fig. 117.1: Anterior view of the framework of larynx

anterior surface, which is devoid of mucosa, is connected to hyoid bone by hyoepiglottic ligament. Below this attachment, the anterior surface is separated from the thyrohyoid membrane by a space called pre-epiglottic space, which is filled with fat. Each lateral margin provides attachment to the aryepiglottic fold in its lower part. The lower end is attached to inner surface of thyroid angle by thyro-epiglottic ligament. The mucosa on the posterior surface of epiglottis is of respiratory type in the lower part and stratified squamous type in the upper part and is pitted by small mucous glands. The branches of internal laryngeal nerve pierce the mucosa on this surface.

b. The thyroid cartilage is the largest of the laryngeal cartilages. It is made of hyaline cartilage hence it tends to calcify and ossify as age advances. Its interesting feature is that it gives attachments to nine pairs of muscles (three on the posterior margin, three on the oblique line, two on the internal surface and one on the inferior margin). The thyroid cartilage consists of two quadrilateral laminae, which meet in the midline anteriorly at the thyroid angle but leave the thyroid notch between them above. The thyroid angle (laryngeal prominence) is called Adam's apple in males. It is subcutaneous and hence easily palpable. Internally, the thyroid angle is covered with mucosa of larynx and gives attachment in the midline to thyroepoglottic ligament, bilateral vestibular ligaments and bilateral vocal ligaments from above downwards. Lateral to the vocal ligament it gives attachments to thyroarytenoid and thyroepigotticus muscles from medial to lateral side. The oblique line on the external surface of each lamina gives attachment to three muscles (sternohyoid, thyrohyoid and inferior constrictor of pharynx). The upper pole of the lateral lobe of thyroid gland is related to this surface as far as the oblique line. The internal surface of the lamina (covered with mucosa) forms the lateral boundary of piriform fossa of laryngopharynx. The superior border corresponds to C4 vertebra. It gives attachment to thyrohyoid membrane, which is attached above to the upper border of the hyoid bone, a bursa intervening between the two. The inferior border corresponds to C5 vertebra. Its anterior part is attached to arch of cricoid by conus elasticus. Rest of the inferior border gives attachment to cricothyroid muscle. The two posterior borders are free. Each receives the common insertion of stylopharyngeus, palatopharyngeus and salpingopharyngeus muscles. The posterior border extends upward as superior horn, which is connected to the tip of greater cornu of hyoid bone by lateral thyrohyoid ligament. The posterior border extends below as inferior horn, which bears an articular facet for the cricoid cartilage at the cricothyroid joint.

c. The cricoid cartilage is the only cartilage of larynx that forms a complete ring around the cavity of larynx. Its shape is like that of a signet ring. Its broad lamina is posterior and narrow arch is anterior to the laryngeal cavity. The cricoid cartilage is of hyaline variety and hence prone to calcification and ossification with age. The cricoid cartilage is a landmark for following events: (i) Its arch can be felt in the midline below the thyroid cartilage and corresponds to C6 vertebra. (ii). At this level pharynx ends and oesophagus begins and larynx ends and trachea begins. (iii) It is the only laryngeal cartilage that articulates with thyroid and arytenoid cartilages to form bilateral synovial joints. Therefore, the cricoid cartilage is crucial for the movements of the vocal cords. (iv) It denotes the level of middle cervical sympathetic ganglion. (v) The inferior thyroid artery enters the thyroid gland at this level. (vi) The recurrent laryngeal nerve enters the larynx behind the cricothyroid joint.

The external surface of the cricoid arch gives attachments to cricothyroid muscle and to the inferior constrictor of pharynx (cricopharyngeus part). The inferior border gives attachment to cricotracheal ligament. The superior border gives attachment to median cricothyroid ligament (conus elasticus) in the midline and lateral cricothyroid ligament on either side.

The posterior surface of the cricoid lamina shows median ridge for the attachment to the upper end of longitudinal fasciculi of the oesophageal muscle. On either side of the median ridge, the posterior cricoarytenoid muscle is attached. Posterior to these muscular attachments, the cricoid lamina is covered with mucosa of the laryngopharynx, as this aspect of the lamina forms the anterior wall of the laryngopharynx. The internal surface of both the arch and lamina is covered with mucosa of infraglottic larynx.

d. The arytenoid cartilage is a three- sided pyramid (Fig. 117.2). It has base and apex, two processes (vocal and muscular) and three surfaces (posterior, medial and anterolateral). The apex articulates with corniculate cartilage and gives attachment to aryepiglottic fold with its contained aryepiglotticus muscle. The base articulates with the superior aspect of lamina of cricoid to form the cricoarytenoid joint. The muscular process projects laterally and gives attachment to both lateral and posterior cricoarytenoid muscles. The vocal process projects anteriorly and it gives attachment to vocal ligament. The anterolateral surface gives attachment to thyroarytenoid and vocalis muscles. The vestibular ligament is attached just above the vocal ligament. The medial surface is covered with laryngeal mucosa and forms the interarytenoid (intercartilaginous) part of rima glottis along with opposite medial surface. Except the apex and vocal process, which are made of elastic cartilage, the rest of the arytenoid cartilage is hyaline in microstructure.
e. The cuneiform is the nodular elastic cartilage within the posterior end of the aryepiglottic fold.
f. The corniculate is the rod-shaped elastic cartilage the lies anterior to the cuneiform.

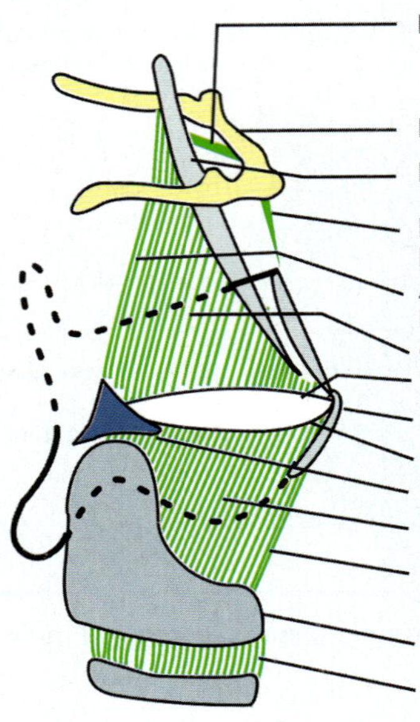

Fig. 117.2: Intrinsic membranes and ligaments of larynx in lateral view. The dotted line indicates outline of thyroid lamina, which has been removed to expose the interior

Both cuneiform and corniculate cartilages support the aryepiglottic fold of their side.

Membranes and Ligaments of Larynx

The extrinsic membranes of the larynx lie external to the cavity of the larynx.

a. The thyrohyoid membrane (Fig. 117.1) stretches between the upper border of thyroid cartilage and the upper border of the body and greater cornua of hyoid bone. It is separated from the body of hyoid bone by a bursa, which facilitates ascent of larynx during swallowing. The internal laryngeal nerve and superior laryngeal vessels pierce it. Its median thick part is called median thyrohyoid ligament. Its posterior margin is thickest and called lateral thyrohyoid ligaments, which connects the ends of greater horns to the upper horns of thyroid cartilage.
b. The extrinsic ligaments are, cricotracheal ligament between lower margin of cricoid and the first tracheal ring, median (anterior) cricothyroid ligament in the midline of neck and hyoepiglottic ligament between the hyoid bone and epiglottis.

The intrinsic membranes are covered on the inner aspect with laryngeal mucosa (Fig. 117.2).

a. The quadrangular or quadrate membrane is a fibroelastic membrane stretching between the epiglottis, thyroid angle and arytenoid cartilage. Its free upper margin is in the aryepiglottic fold while its free lower margin forms the vestibular ligament stretching between the thyroid angle and vocal process of arytenoids above the attachment of the vocal ligament.
b. The cricovocal membrane is a triangular fibroelastic membrane that stretches between the cricoid, arytenoid and thyroid cartilages. Its upper free margin extending between the middle of the thyroid angle and the tip of vocal process of arytenoid is called vocal ligament. Its lower margin is attached to the arch of cricoid cartilage. The cricovocal membranes of the two sides are continuous across the midline and form the conus elasticus.

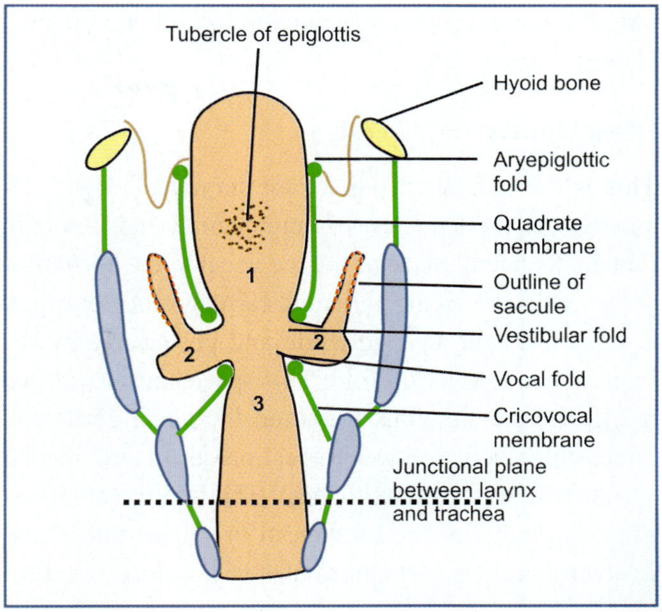

Fig. 117.3: Posterior view of diagrammatic coronal section showing subdivisions of laryngeal cavity: (1) Supraglottic part (vestibule), (2) Right and left ventricle (sinus), (3) Infraglottic part

Subdivisions of Cavity of Larynx (Fig. 117.3)

The laryngeal cavity extends from the laryngeal inlet to the lower margin of cricoid cartilage. The inlet of the larynx is an oblique opening bounded anteriorly by the free margin of upper end of epiglottis, on the sides by free margins of aryepiglottic folds and posteriorly by interarytenoid fold. Two pairs of mucosal folds (upper vestibular and lower vocal) project inside the cavity and divide it into three parts, the vestibule above the vestibular folds, the sinus or ventricle of larynx between the vestibular and vocal folds and the infraglottic or subglottic part below the vocal folds.

Sinus or Ventricle of Larynx

It is a deep space between the vestibular and vocal folds and extends for a short distance above and lateral to vestibular folds. A mucous diverticulum called saccule extends upwards blindly from the anterior part of the sinus on each side. The secretion of the mucous glands contained in the saccule lubricates the vocal folds. When the saccule is abnormally enlarged and distended it forms the laryngocele, which is an air containing sac presenting in the neck.

The vestibular folds are called false vocal cords because they do not take part in phonation. They are flaccid folds covered by respiratory epithelium. Each vestibular fold contains vestibular ligament and submucosa with capillaries and mucous glands. The vestibular folds appear pink on laryngoscopy due to the presence of capillaries in the submucosa. The space enclosed between the right and left vestibular folds is called rima vestibuli.

The vocal folds are called true vocal cords since their movements are responsible for phonation. Each vocal fold contains vocal ligament and vocalis muscle. Due to absence of submucosa, the stratified squamous non-keratinised epithelium tightly covers it. Lack of blood capillaries and the type of covering epithelium give the vocal cords a characteristic pearly white appearance. The cords are nourished and lubricated by mucous secretion of the glands in the saccule (which is aptly called the oil can of larynx). A narrow slit like space enclosed by the vocal folds is called rima glottis or glottidis. Reinke's space is a potential space under the epithelium of the vocal folds. Accumulation of fluid here causes fusiform swelling of the folds (Reinke's edema). Vocal nodules (singers or screamers nodes) appear on the free edges of both cords at the junction of anterior one-third and posterior two-third. This area shows maximum vibration of the cords.

Vocal nodules are the occupational hazards for singers, teachers, actors, etc.

Rima Glottis (Fig. 117.4)

This is the narrowest part of the laryngeal cavity. Its anteroposterior diameter is 24 mm in male and 17 mm in female. Its lateral margins are the vocal folds, vocal processes and bases of the arytenoid cartilages. Anteriorly it is limited by the thyroid angle and posteriorly by the interarytenoid mucosal fold. This space consists of two parts, intermembranous (between the vocal cords and intercartilaginous (between vocal processes and medial surfaces of arytenoid cartilages). The intermembranous part contributes to anterior three-fifth (or two-thirds) and intercartilaginous part contributes to posterior two-fifth (or one-third). The shape of rima glottis undergoes changes due to movements of vocal folds during respiration and phonation.

a. During quiet respiration (position of rest), the intermembranous part is triangular and intercartilaginous part is rectangular. The cords are gently abducted and lie about 7 mm from the midline.
b. During forced inspiration, the vocal cords are fully abducted and hence the rima assumes rhomboid or diamond shape, where both parts of rima are triangular in shape. The cords lie 9.5 mm from the midline.
c. In preparation of the phonation, both the parts of the rima glottis are closed due to approximation of vocal cords and arytenoid cartilages. The expired air forces open the cords, so that the air is released as small puffs, which vibrate the vocal cords. The rima appears as a small linear chink at the beginning of speech. The cords are in midline. Simultaneously the vocal cords tense by increasing the length to alter the pitch of voice.
d. During whispering, the intermembranous part is narrowed due to adduction of the vocal folds but the intercartilaginous part remains widely open to allow air to escape. The shape of rima glottis is described as inverted funnel.
e. In the cadaveric position of the vocal cords, the rima glottis is moderately wide as the vocal cords are in intermediate position between adduction and abduction. The cords are about 3.5 mm from the midline. This is also described as neutral or intermediate position.

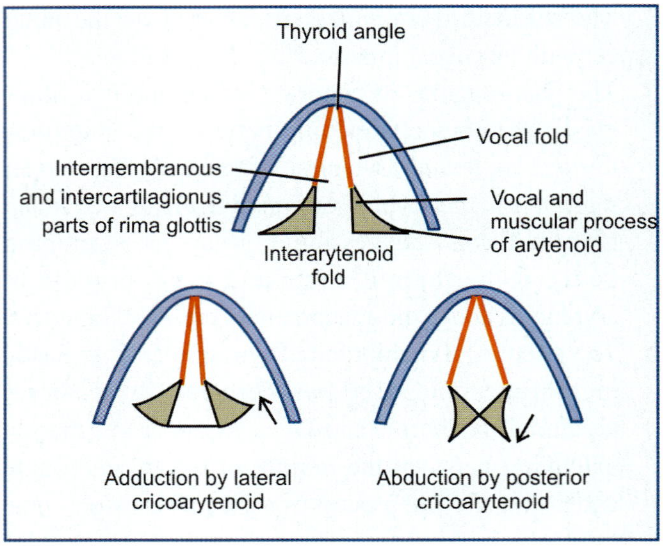

Fig. 117.4: Rima glottis and changes in its shape in adduction and abduction of vocal folds (Note: The inverted funnel shape in adduction and diamond shape in abduction)

Mucosa of Laryngeal Cavity

The laryngeal mucosa is respiratory type (pseudostratified ciliated columnar) except in two locations, upper part of the posterior surface of epiglottis and on the vocal cords, where it is wear and tear type (stratified squamous non-keratinised). The mucosa is loosely attached everywhere (except over the vocal cords) due to the presence of submucosa. There are plenty of mucous glands in the submucosa.

Sensory Nerve Supply and Blood Supply

The internal laryngeal nerve supplies the mucosa above the level of vocal folds while the recurrent laryngeal nerve supplies below this level. The vocal folds in all probability receive innervation from both sources. The laryngeal branches of superior and inferior thyroid arteries supply the larynx. Above the vocal folds, the superior laryngeal branch of superior thyroid artery while below the vocal folds, the inferior laryngeal branch of inferior thyroid artery are the sources of blood.

Lymphatic Drainage

Above the vocal folds, the laryngeal mucosa is drained by lymphatics, which pierce the thyrohyoid membrane and go to upper deep cervical lymph nodes. The infraglottic larynx is drained by lymphatics, which pierce the cricothyroid membrane and go to pretracheal and prelaryngeal nodes and then to lower deep cervical and mediastinal nodes. Carcinoma of larynx spreads by lymphatic route to regional lymph nodes.

Laryngoscopic Examination

The interior of larynx can be inspected by indirect and direct laryngoscopy. In the indirect method, the subject is asked to protrude the tongue and the laryngeal mirror is passed through the mouth and held against soft palate. The light is focused on the laryngeal mirror and the reflexion of the epiglottis, aryepiglottic folds, arytenoids, vestibular and vocal folds and the interior of larynx can be seen in the mirror. The movements of the vocal folds can also be observed. The direct laryngoscopy is performed with the help of special instrument under general anaesthesia. The laryngoscope is introduced in the mouth using left hand along one side of tongue. When the posterior third is reached, the laryngoscope is moved to the midline and then advanced behind the epiglottis into the laryngeal cavity.

Laryngeal Muscles (Fig. 117.5)

The laryngeal muscles are subdivided in intrinsic and extrinsic groups. The intrinsic muscles are confined to the larynx in their attachments. There are seven paired muscles and one unpaired muscle in this group. The extrinsic muscles connect the laryngeal cartilages to neighboring structures. They are responsible for vertical movement of the larynx during phonation and swallowing. They are grouped as elevators and depressors of larynx. Inferior constrictor is the only muscle, which falls in the category of extrinsic laryngeal muscles (by above definition) but does not move the larynx.

The extrinsic muscles are divided into elevators and depressors of larynx.

The elevators of the larynx are divided into primary and secondary elevators.

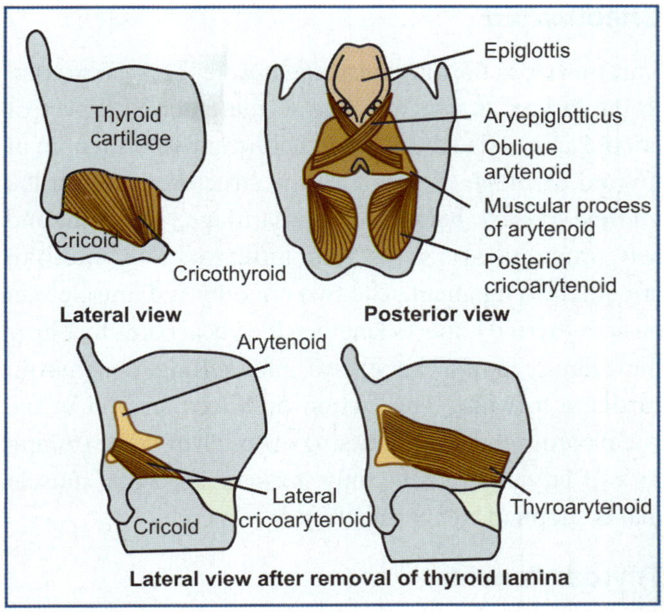

Fig. 117.5: Intrinsic muscles of the larynx

The primary elevators are attached to the thyroid cartilage from above. They consist of stylopharyngeus, palatopharyngeus, salpingopharyngeus and thyrohyoid muscles.The secondary elevators are attached to the to hyoid bone from above. They consist of mylohyoid, geniohyoid, stylohyoid and digastric muscles. The depressors of the larynx are attached to the thyroid cartilage or hyoid bone from below. They consist of sterno-hyoid, sternothyroid and omohyoid muscles.

Classification of Intrinsic Muscles

a. Muscles that increase or decrease the length of the vocal cords:
   i. Cricothyroid (increases the length)
   ii. Posterior cricoarytenoid (increases the length)
   iii. Thyroarytenoid (decreases the length)
   iv. Vocalis.
b. Muscles that abduct or adduct the vocal cords:
   i. Posterior cricoarytnoid (abductor)
   ii. Lateral cricoarytenoid (adductor)
   iii. Transverse arytenoids (adductors).
c. Muscles that open or close the laryngeal inlet:
   i. Thyroepiglottic (open)
   ii. Aryepiglottic (close)
   iii. Oblique part of interarytenoids (close).

Cricothyroid

This muscle is the only intrinsic muscle that lies external to the larynx as it is attached to the external aspect of cricoid arch and to the inferior margin and inferior horn of thyroid cartilage. It is one of the structures seen in the midline of neck below thyroid cartilage. The right and left muscles are separated anteriorly by median cricothyroid ligament. The two cricothyroid muscles act on cricothyroid joints to lengthen the vocal cords by tilting the cricoid lamina backward and pulling the thyroid cartilage forward. This action produces tension in the vocal cords required for raising the pitch of voice (tuning fork of larynx). It is the only intrinsic laryngeal muscle that is supplied by external laryngeal nerve.

Thyroarytenoid, Thyroepiglottic and Vocalis

The thyroarytenoid muscle arises from the posterior surface of the thyroid angle just lateral to the attachment of vocal cords. It is inserted posteriorly into the antero-lateral surface of arytenoid cartilage. Some of the deeper fibres (known as vocalis) originate from the vocal ligament and pass for attachment to the lateral surface of vocal process of arytenoid cartilage. The vocalis has no attachment to thyroid cartilage. The upper lateral fibres of thyroarytenoid turn upward towards epiglottis to form thyroepiglottic muscle. The action of thyroarytenoid muscles is to pull the vocal processes forward thereby slackening or shortening the vocal cords. The vocalis slackens or decreases the length of the posterior part of the vocal cord while the anterior part is kept tense. This action is essential for raising the pitch. The recurrent laryngeal nerve supplies these muscles.

Posterior Cricoarytenoid

It is the most important muscle of larynx. Each muscle arises from the posterior surface of the lamina of cricoid on either side of midline. It is inserted on the back of muscular process of arytenoid cartilage of its side. The muscle acts on the cricoarytenoid joint to rotate the arytenoid with its vocal process laterally so that the muscular process turns posteriorly. In this way, abduction of the vocal cords and widening of rima glottis takes place. It is the sole abductor of vocal cords and bilateral paralysis may lead to the adduction of vocal cords and suffocation. Hence, the posterior cricoarytenoids are called safety muscles of larynx. Another action of the muscle is to assist the cricothyroid muscle in lengthening the vocal cords by pulling the arytenoids backwards. The posterior cricoarytenoid receives branches from recurrent laryngeal nerve.

Lateral Cricoarytenoid

It is attached anteriorly to the arch of cricoid and passes in posterosuperior direction to insert in the front of muscular process of arytenoids cartilage. Its action is to pull the muscular process forward and rotate the arytenoids so that its vocal process turns medially. The simultaneous actions of the right and left muscles result in adduction of the intermembranous parts of vocal cords thereby closing the glottis. The recurrent laryngeal nerve supplies the muscle.

Transverse Arytenoid

It is the only laryngeal muscle that is unpaired. It passes from the back of the arytenoid of one side to the back of the arytenoid of opposite side. Its contraction causes the adduction of vocal processes and consequent closure of the intercartilaginous part of rima glottis. It receives twigs from both recurrent laryngeal nerves.

Oblique Arytenoid and Aryepiglottic

The oblique arytenoid muscles are superficial to the transverse muscle. Each muscle passes from the back of muscular process of one arytenoid cartilage to the apex of opposite one, thus crossing each other above the lamina of cricoid. Some fibres of the oblique muscle run in the aryepiglottic mucous fold to form aryepiglottic muscle. These two muscles close the laryngeal inlet by bringing the aryepiglottic folds together and approximating the arytenoid cartilages to the tubercle of epiglottis. The muscles receive supply from recurrent laryngeal nerve.

Clinical Highlights

a. Since laryngeal cavity is very narrow and it opens in to the laryngopharynx, accidental swallowing of food particle or foreign body into it may lead to acute laryngeal obstruction. This can cause choking due to blockage of air entry in the lungs. It is an acute emergency and unless promptly treated is fatal. Foreign bodies like, buttons, dentures or fish bones may get stuck in the laryngeal cavity. The symptoms of obstruction are stridor (noisy breathing), aphonia and dyspnea. Cyanosis may set in. The tracheostomy is life-saving.

b. The laryngeal mucosa is supplied by bilateral internal laryngeal nerves (branches of superior laryngeal nerve from vagus) and recurrent laryngeal nerves (branches of vagus). The muscles of larynx are supplied by recurrent laryngeal nerves and external laryngeal nerve (a branch of superior laryngeal nerve). Injury may occur to any of these branches causing specific effects.

   i. Unilateral recurrent laryngeal nerve injury results in ipsilateral paralysis of all the intrinsic muscles except the cricothyroid and transverse arytenoid (cricothyroid is supplied by external laryngeal nerve and transverse arytenoid receives bilateral nerve supply). The paralysed vocal cord assumes median or paramedian position and is motionless. This does not give rise to respiratory symptoms and the speech is not affected much because the healthy cord compensates by crossing the midline to meet the paralysed cord. Due to unilateral loss of cough reflex the patient cannot cough clearly (bovine cough).

   ii. Bilateral recurrent laryngeal nerve injury is also called bilateral abductor paralysis. The vocal cords lie in the median or paramedian position. This causes symptoms like dyspnea (difficulty in breathing), inspiratory stridor but no loss of phonation. There is loss of cough reflex.

   iii. Unilateral superior laryngeal nerve injury causes paralysis of the cricothyroid muscle (supplied through external laryngeal branch) and ipsilateral anaesthesia above the vocal folds. The voice becomes weak and pitch cannot be raised. There is ipsilateral shortening of the vocal cord.

   iv. Bilateral superior laryngeal nerve injury results in weak and husky voice. The loss of sensations above the vocal cords gives rise to increased chances of aspiration of fluid in the larynx. Both vocal cords are shortened.

118 Mechanism of Deglutition

The deglutition or act of swallowing is an integrated process depending on neuromuscular coordination. During deglutition there are orderly movements of lips, tongue, soft palate, pharynx and larynx and reflex closure of oropharyngeal, nasopharyngeal and laryngeal openings. The sequence of deglutition can be best understood only with the sound knowledge of the anatomy of the muscles of the lips, tongue, soft palate, pharynx and larynx. Several cranial nerves control the three phases of deglutition.

Oral Phase

The oral phase is under voluntary control. The mouth is held shut by the action of the orbicularis oris (controlled by facial nerve). The muscles of mastication (controlled by mandibular nerve) chew the food. The tongue is elevated against the hard palate by the mylohyoid and digastric muscles (mandibular nerve). Then the intrinsic lingual muscles (controlled by hypoglossal nerve) press the tip of tongue against the hard palate to squeeze the bolus backwards and to push it through the oropharyngeal isthmus in to the oropharynx. In summary, the first phase is controlled by the trigeminal, facial and hypoglossal nerves.

Pharyngeal Phase

In this phase, the oropharyngeal isthmus is closed so that food does not regurgitate into the oral cavity. This is achieved by reflex contraction of palatoglossi in response to the arrival of food in oropharynx. Then the nasopharyngeal isthmus is closed by reflex contraction of Passavant's ridge and elevation of soft palate by levator palati and tensor palati. This act prevents the regurgitation of food into the nasal cavity through the nasopharynx. This is followed by closure of the inlet of larynx before the food enters the laryngopharynx to prevent entry of food in the airway. For closure of laryngeal inlet, the larynx is elevated with the help of extrinsic muscles of larynx (direct and indirect elevators of larynx). In the raised larynx, the epiglottis assumes a more horizontal position so as to close the laryngeal inlet and the aryepiglottic muscles contract to pull the arytenoids in contact with tubercle of epiglottis. After this, the sequential contraction of superior and middle constrictor muscles and thyropharyngeus part of inferior constrictor muscle propels the food through the piriform fossae on either side of larynx. This phase is controlled by the fifth, ninth, tenth and cranial accessory nerves.

Esophageal Phase

It is an involuntary phase. The cricopharyngeus part of inferior constrictor muscle relaxes as the food is propelled from the laryngopharynx in the esophagus. The peristalsis of the esophagus moves the food further down. The relaxation of lingual and palatal and pharyngeal muscles opens the oropharyngeal and nasopharyngeal seals. The infrahyoid muscles (depressors of larynx) contract to restore the larynx to its normal position so that the laryngeal inlet opens. The cricopharyngeus contracts to act as sphincter at the lower end of pharynx so that air does not enter the esophagus in between the acts of swallowing. The vagus and cranial part of accessory nerve control the third phase.

119 Development of Ear

It is essential to have a general orientation about the subdivisions and functions of the ear (Fig.119.1). The ear consists of three parts: external, middle and internal. The external ear is separated from the middle ear by tympanic membrane. The middle ear is separated from the internal ear by a bony wall. The function of the external ear is to collect sound waves, which cause vibrations of the tympanic membrane. The middle ear is the air-filled cavity, which receives air from the nasopharynx via the auditory tube. It contains three ear ossicles, which conduct the vibrations of the tympanic membrane to the perilymph of the inner ear. The internal ear contains the peripheral receptor organs of sound and equilibrium, namely semicircular ducts and cochlear duct inside the bony labyrinth. The neural impulses from the receptors are carried by the cochlear and vestibular nerves to the brainstem.

External Ear

a. The auricle develops from the fusion of six tubercles that appear around the dorsal end of first branchial cleft at the sixth week of embryonic life. Three tubercles are cranial to the first branchial cleft while three are on the cranial edge of the second arch. The first tubercle develops in the tragus. The remaining tubercles form the other parts of the auricle. Initially, the auricles are located in the lower neck region but with the development of mandible, they ascend to the side of cranium to the level of eyes.
b. The external acoustic meatus develops from the ectoderm of the first branchial cleft (Fig. 72.1).

Congenital Anomalies of Auricle

a. Preauricular sinus or cyst is present between tragus and crus of helix and is due to incomplete fusion of first tubercle with the rest.
b. Preauricular appendage (accessory auricle) is a skin-covered tag containing cartilage, which may lie on the line from the tragus to the angle of mouth. The tag may be single or multiple.
c. Anotia is complete absence of auricle.
d. Microtia is small size of auricle. It is one of the features of Down syndrome facies.
e. Low set auricles are due to failure of the developing auricles to ascend.

Congenital Anomalies of Meatus

a. Atresia of the meatus is due to failure of canalization of the ectodermal plug that fills the first branchial cleft until the seventh month of intrauterine life. The atresia may be the cause of congenital deafness.
b. A fistula may be present with one opening in the external meatus and the other opening in the neck just below the angle of mandible. It represents the first branchial cleft.

Tympanic Membrane

The tympanic membrane is unique in that is the only structure in the body developed from all the three germ

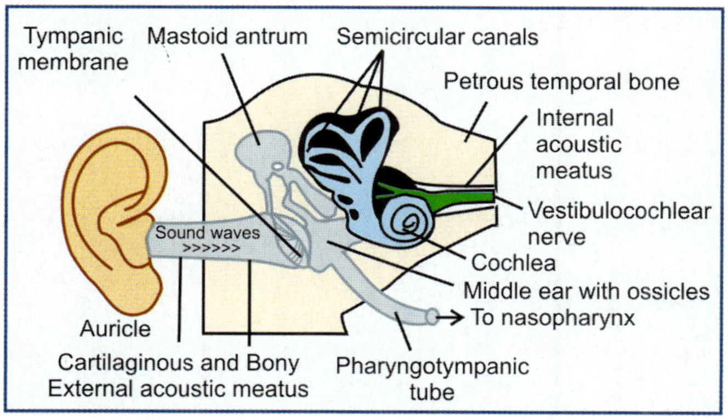

Fig. 119.1: Orientation scheme to depict external, middle and internal ear

layers since it develops from the first cleft membrane (Fig. 72.1). The outer cuticular layer develops from ectoderm, the middle fibrous layer from mesoderm and the inner mucosal layer from endoderm.

Middle Ear (Fig. 72.4)

The middle ear develops from the endoderm of tubotympanic recess, which gives rise (besides middle ear) to pharyngotympanic tube, mastoid antrum and mastoid air cells. The middle ear is of adult size at birth.

Ear Ossicles

The malleus and incus develop in Meckel's cartilage of first branchial arch while stapes develops from Reichert's cartilage of second arch. All the three ossicles ossify in cartilage. The ossification centre appears in each ossicle by fourth month of intrauterine life. The ossicles are of adult size in newborn.

Membranous Labyrinth (Inner Ear)

The ectodermal thickening in the region of hindbrain (in the vicinity of future first branchial cleft) forms the auditory or otic placode in the fourth week of intrauterine life. The placode sinks beneath the surface to form otocyst or auditory vesicle, from which different parts of membranous labyrinth develop. The inner ear achieves adult size by the sixteenth week of fetal life.

Congenital Anomalies of Inner Ear

a. Michel aplasia is complete absence of inner ear.
b. Maternal infection with rubella (German measles) during the sixth to ninth weeks of gestation may lead to congenital deaf-mutism due to destruction of organ of Corti. Drugs like streptomycin, thalidomide and chloroquine given to the pregnant woman during early pregnancy may cross the placental barrier and damage the cochlea.

120 External Ear

The external ear consists of auricle (pinna) and external acoustic meatus or ear canal, which is closed medially by the tympanic membrane. The auricle collects the sound waves and the external meatus conducts them to the tympanic membrane.

Auricle (Pinna)

The auricle consists of an irregularly curved elastic cartilage covered with skin. The various elevations and depressions on the cartilage give the auricle its characteristic appearance. The auricle has lateral (outer) and medial (cranial or inner) surfaces. It is attached to side of the cranium by ligaments and muscles. There are rudimentary intrinsic and extrinsic auricular muscles in human being. They are supplied by the facial nerve.

Features of Lateral Surface (Fig. 120.1)

The helix is the peripheral prominent ridge curving around anterior, superior and posterior margins of pinna. The antihelix lies parallel and anterior to the posterior part of helix. It divides above in two branches, which enclose triangular fossa between them. The scaphoid fossa is the space between helix and antihelix. The concha of the auricle is a deep space, which is encircled by the antihelix and is continuous with the external acoustic meatus. The crus or anterior end of helix projects into the concha. The conchal area above the crus is called cymba conchae, which is the surface landmark for the suprameatal triangle. The tragus is the curved projection below the crus. There is no cartilage between the crus and tragus. The antitragus lies opposite the tragus but separated by intertragic notch. The lobule lies below the tragus and antitragus. It is devoid of cartilage and is the only soft part of the ear.

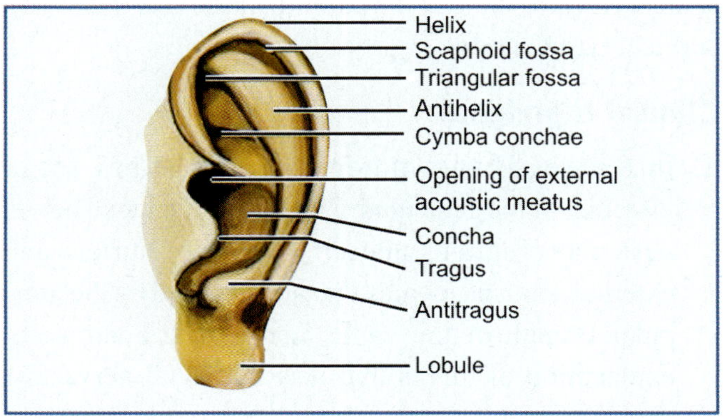

Fig. 120.1: Features of lateral surface of left pinna

Nerve Supply (Fig. 120.2)

a. The lateral surface receives twigs from three sources: The great auricular nerve (from cervical plexus) supplies the posterior part of this surface including the lobule. The auriculotemporal nerve (from mandibular nerve) supplies the anterior part of this surface excluding the lobule. The auricular branch of the vagus supplies the concha.
b. The medial or cranial surface receives twigs from three sources: The lesser occipital nerve (from cervical plexus) supplies its upper part. The great auricular nerve supplies the larger lower area including the lobule. The auricular branch of the vagus supplies a small part of the eminentia (prominence on cranial aspect corresponding to concha on lateral aspect). It should be noted that great auricular nerve supplies the lobule on both sides.

External Acoustic Meatus

The external meatus extends from the bottom of the concha to the lateral surface of tympanic membrane. In

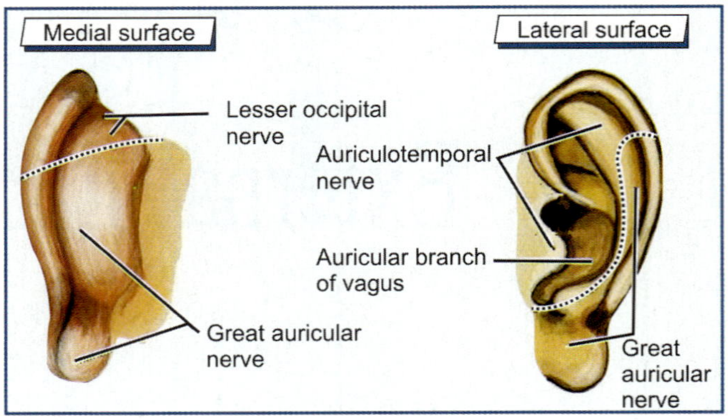

Fig. 120.2: Showing areas of supply of sensory nerves of pinna (Note that great auricular nerve supplies both surfaces of lobule)

adult, the length of the meatus is 24 to 25 mm. It has two parts, lateral (outer) cartilaginous and medial (inner) bony. The length of its anterior wall and floor is more than that of posterior wall and roof, because the tympanic membrane is set at an angle of 55° with its floor. The shape of the meatus is sinuous due to two curves. The outer part is directed upward, backward and medially while its inner part is directed downward, forward and medially. In the newborn, the external meatus is short and straight. It lacks bony part and has no constrictions.

Parts of the Meatus

a. The cartilaginous part is 8 mm long. It is continuous with auricular cartilage laterally but medially it is attached to the rim of the bony part of the meatus by fibrous tissue. Its anterior wall has two or three deficiencies known as fissures of Santorini through which infections from parotid gland can enter the meatus. The lining skin has thick subcutaneous tissue containing ceruminous glands, which are modified sweat glands. The glands secrete cerumen or earwax. The meatal hair and cerumen protect the ear from insects. The cerumen prevents the maceration of meatal skin by trapped water.
b. The inner bony part is 16 mm long. The tympanic plate of temporal bone forms its anterior wall, inferior wall and most of the posterior wall. The squamous part of temporal bone forms the remaining walls. The bony part presents a foramen of Huschke in its floor in children up to the age of four to five years and in some adults. Its skin is thin and devoid of hair and ceruminous glands.

Constrictions

a. At the junction of cartilaginous and bony parts, the meatus is narrow. This fact should be borne in mind while removing foreign body from the external meatus. The speculum should not be inserted beyond this constriction.
b. Isthmus, which is located in the bony part, is 6 mm lateral to the tympanic membrane. It is the narrowest part of meatus.

Relations

Superiorly the bony meatus is related to the middle cranial fossa. Anteriorly the cartilaginous meatus is related to the temporomandibular joint. A blow on the chin may cause the posterior dislocation of the condyle of mandible into the meatus. A part of parotid gland intervenes between the condyle and the meatus. Posteriorly the meatus is related to the mastoid air cells.

Nerve Supply

The auriculotemporal nerve supplies the anterior and superior walls and the auricular branch of vagus supplies the posterior and inferior walls.

Arterial Supply

The posterior auricular artery, deep auricular artery and the auricular branches of superficial temporal artery supply the meatus and the auricle.

Lymphatic Drainage

The lymph vessels from the auricle and the external acoustic meatus drain in the parotid, mastoid and the deep cervical lymph nodes.

Clinical Highlights

a. In Ramsey-Hunt syndrome, due to herpes zoster infection of the geniculate ganglion of the facial nerve, vesicular eruptions appear in parts of auricle and external acoustic meatus that are supplied by the auricular branch of the vagus nerve. The anatomical explanation of this is that it is the facial nerve that supplies cutaneous branches to the auricle through a communication with the auricular branch of the vagus (Alderman's nerve) in the petrous temporal bone.

b. Localized acute otitis externa is due to furuncle, which is the inflammed hair follicle in the cartilaginous part of the meatus. This causes severe pain because the meatal skin is tightly adherent to the perichondrium.
c. Impacted wax is the condition in which excess wax is deposited as a plug in the meatus. The impacted wax may dry up and cause a sense of blocked ear, tinnitus and giddiness. Stimulation of auricular branch of vagus by impacted wax or during syringing the ear canal may give rise to reflex coughing (ear cough). Vomiting may occur in children after syringing.
d. If there is irritation of lingual nerve as in carcinoma tongue or inferior alveolar nerve as in caries of lower teeth, it will cause reflex pain in ear canal. This is because, the lingual, inferior alveolar and auriculo-temporal nerves are branches of the mandibular nerve.

121 Middle Ear

The middle ear is an air-filled space in the petrous temporal bone. The middle ear receives atmospheric air from the nasopharynx via the pharyngotympanic tube.

Subdivisions

The middle ear cavity is divisible in the tympanic cavity proper (opposite the tympanic membrane) and the epitympanic recess or attic above the level of tympanic membrane.

Shape and Measurements

The middle ear resembles in shape the RBC (biconcave). Its vertical and anteroposterior diameters are each 15 mm. The transverse diameter varies at three levels because the medial and lateral walls of middle ear bulge inside the cavity. At the upper limit of the cavity, the transverse diameter is 6 mm, at the central part, it is 2 mm and at the lower limit, it is 4 mm.

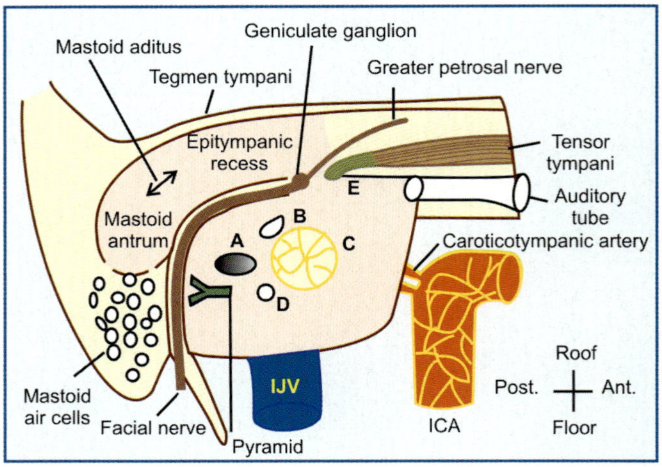

Fig. 121.1: Features on the walls of middle ear
(Note the canal of the facial nerve on the medial and posterior walls: (A) Sinus tympani, (B) Fenestra vestibuli, (C) Promontory with tympanic plexus, (D) Fenestra cochleae, (E) Processus trochleariformis)

Walls of Middle Ear (Fig. 121.1)

The walls of the middle ear are, the roof, floor, lateral wall, anterior wall, medial wall and the posterior wall. Each wall has important features and relations.

Roof or Tegmental Wall

The tegmen tympani, which is a thin plate of petrous temporal bone roofs the middle ear. It separates the middle ear from the middle cranial fossa and temporal lobe of cerebrum. The greater petrosal and lesser petrosal nerves pierce the roof to enter the middle cranial fossa.

Floor or Jugular Wall

The jugular fossa forms the floor, which separates the middle ear from the internal jugular vein. When the bony floor has multiple tiny deficiencies the mucosa of the middle ear forms the floor at these sites. The medial wall of jugular fossa shows an aperture for tympanic branch of glossopharyngeal nerve (Jacobson's nerve), which enters the middle ear to form tympanic plexus on the promontory of its medial wall.

Lateral Wall (Fig. 121.2)

The lateral wall separates the middle ear from the external acoustic meatus. The tympanic membrane is the main constituent with a small peripheral contribution by the tympanic sulcus, which presents a notch in its superior part. The tympanic membrane is thickened circumferentially except at its superior part, which corresponds to the notch in the tympanic sulcus. The thickened peripheral rim of the membrane is called fibrocartilaginous ring, which fits into the tympanic sulcus. From the margins of the

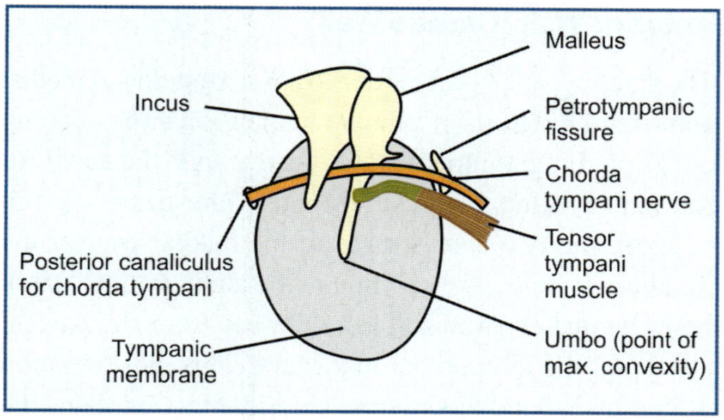

Fig. 121.2: Medial surface of tympanic membrane as seen through the middle ear

notch, anterior and posterior malleolar (mallear) folds pass to the lateral process of malleus. The posterior canaliculus for chorda tympani nerve is present near the posterior end of the notch. It is the upper opening of the bony canal of chorda tympani nerve, through which the nerve enters the substance of tympanic membrane. The nerve leaves the tympanic membrane through the anterior canaliculus at the anterior end of the notch.

Structure of Tympanic Membrane

Tympanic membrane consists of three layers (derived from the three germ layers). The outer cuticular layer is continuous with the skin of the external acoustic meatus. The middle layer consists of fibrous tissue. The inner mucosal layer is continuous with the mucosa of middle ear. The chorda tympani nerve passes between the fibrous and mucosal layers in the upper part. The handle of malleus passes between the mucosal layer and fibrous layer from the umbo upwards.

Parts of Tympanic Membrane (Fig. 121.3)

a. Pars flaccida is a small triangular area of tympanic membrane situated between the malleolar folds. This part is lax because of the absence of the middle fibrous layer.
b. Pars tensa is the larger part and kept tense by its firm attachment to the tympanic sulcus.

Quadrants of Tympanic Membrane

The lateral surface of the tympanic membrane faces the meatus and is concave. It can be divided in four quadrants by two imaginary lines. The first line passes through the handle of malleus and the second passing through the umbo is at right angles to the first. The medial surface is convex. The point of maximum convexity on the medial surface, where the tip of the handle of malleus is attached, is called umbo.

Speculum Examination (Fig. 121.3)

On inspection through the speculum introduced through the external acoustic meatus, the tympanic membrane looks pearly gray and semitransparent. It is obliquely set at an angle of 55° to the meatal floor. Hence, its lateral surface faces forwards, laterally and downwards. In the newborn, since there is no bony meatus the tympanic membrane lies horizontally and is very close to the surface. Some structures of the middle ear can be seen through the membrane. The handle of malleus looks like a reddish-yellow streak extending from the umbo upwards. The lateral process of the malleus is seen as a white round prominence at the upper end of the handle of malleus near the roof. The long process of incus is seen behind and parallel to the upper part of handle of malleus. A bright cone of light is seen in the anteroinferior quadrant. This is due to concavity of the lateral surface. The cone of light is lost if the membrane bulges laterally due to any cause.

Blood Supply and Nerve Supply

The lateral surface of the tympanic membrane shares its blood and nerve supply with that of external acoustic

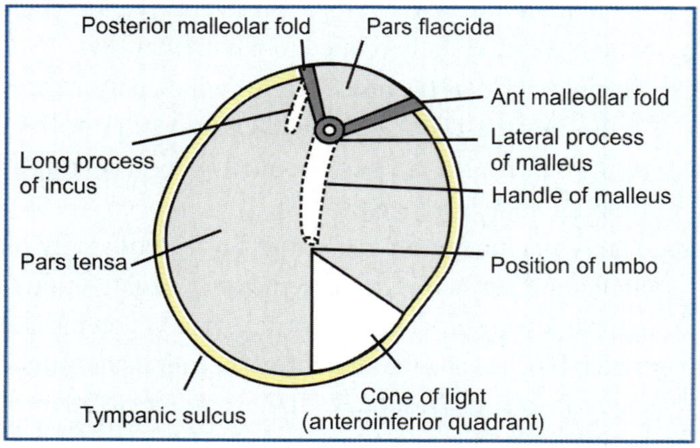

Fig. 121.3: Lateral surface of right tympanic membrane as seen through a speculum

meatus while the medial surface shares with that of middle ear.

Lateral Surface

a. Arterial supply is by the deep auricular branch of maxillary artery.
b. Veins drain into external jugular vein.
c. The main nerve supply is by the auriculotemporal nerve and a small area by auricular branch of vagus nerve.

Medial Surface

a. Arterial supply is by tympanic branch of maxillary artery and stylomastoid artery (derived either from posterior auricular artery or from occipital artery).
b. The veins drain into transverse sinus and in the venous plexus around pharyngotympanic tube.
c. The nerve supply is by the glossopharyngeal nerve through tympanic plexus.

Clinical Highlights

a. The arterial supply reaches the membrane from the periphery towards the center. Hence, the central part of the membrane (umbo) has poor blood supply. Thus, the central part is in danger of perforation when the arteries at the periphery are thrombosed in inflammatory disease of the middle ear.
b. Myringotomy is the procedure by which a surgical incision is placed in the tympanic membrane to drain the fluid in the middle ear or to inject air into the middle ear in case of blocked pharyngotympanic tube. The incision is placed in the postero-inferior quadrant to avoid injury to chorda tympani nerve and ear ossicles, which are intimately related to the membrane.
c. Myringoplasty is the procedure by which perforations in the pars tensa are closed with the use of graft from temporal fascia or perichondrium of the tragus (immunologically inert tissues).
d. The tympanic membrane retracts or its concavity on the lateral surface is increased due to negative intra-tympanic pressure. This occurs if the pharyngotympanic tube is blocked and the already existing air in the middle ear is absorbed. The cone of light is absent in retracted membrane. The membrane bulges if there is excess fluid in the middle ear.

Anterior Wall (Carotid Wall)

The anterior wall is narrow due to approximation of medial and lateral walls. Its prominent feature is a large opening of the pharyngotympanic tube. Above this, the canal for the tensor tympani muscle opens. The bony septum between the two canals turns to the medial wall of the middle ear. Below the opening of the auditory tube, a thin bony lamina separates the middle ear from the carotid canal and the internal carotid artery. This close relation of middle ear and the internal carotid artery explains the swishing tinnitus (noise in the ear) experienced by the patient in carotid aneurysm. The caroticotympanic branches of the internal carotid artery and the nerves of the same name from the sympathetic plexus around the artery enter the middle ear by piercing the bony lamina.

Medial Wall (Labyrinthine Wall)

The features of the medial wall are shown in Figure 121.1.

a. The promontory, which is the rounded elevation in the middle of the medial wall, is produced by the basal turn of cochlea in the internal ear. The tympanic plexus of nerves is located on its surface.
b. Posterior to the promontory, there is a depression called sinus tympani.
c. Above the sinus tympani, there is an opening called fenestra vestibuli or the oval window, which is closed by footplate of stapes and the annular ligament. The footplate separates the air of the middle ear from the perilymph in scala vestibuli.
d. The fenestra cochleae or round window is present below the sinus tympani and is closed by secondary tympanic membrane. The perilymph in scala tympani is separated by the secondary tympanic membrane from the air in the middle ear. The secondary tympanic membrane consists of inner cochlear lining, middle fibrous tissue and outer mucosal lining of middle ear.
e. The canal for the facial nerve passes in anteroposterior direction just above the fenestra vestibuli. Occasionally, the bone may be deficient in the facial bony canal. In such cases, the facial nerve is exposed to the middle ear.
f. Another feature of the medial wall is the presence of a hook-like process called processus trochleariformis (cochleariformis) in front of the oval window. It is

formed by the bony septum between the canal for tensor tympani and bony part of auditory tube. It acts as a pulley for the tendon of tensor tympani to take a sharp turn in lateral direction and reach the neck of malleus for insertion.

Posterior Wall (Mastoid Wall)

The aditus to the mastoid antrum is a large opening in the upper part of posterior wall, which leads from the epitympanic recess into the mastoid antrum. The facial nerve in its bony canal runs down in the medial part of posterior wall. Pyramid is a hollow projection from the canal of facial nerve into the middle ear cavity towards the promontory. It contains stapedius muscle. The tendon of stapedius enters the middle ear through a tiny aperture at the apex of pyramid for insertion in the neck of stapes. The nerve to stapedius (branch of facial nerve) travels through the connection between the canal of facial nerve and the pyramid, which houses the stapedius. Fossa incudis is present lateral to the aditus. Short process of incus is attached to the fossa incudis by ligaments. The chorda tympani nerve enters the substance of tympanic membrane through the posterior canaliculus, which is located at the junction of lateral and posterior walls.

Contents of Middle Ear

The air is the real content. The other contents like three ear ossicles; two muscles, blood vessels and nerves are covered with mucosa of the middle ear. Therefore, these structures lie outside the mucosa-lined cavity. The mucosa (mucoperiosteum) is continuous with that of nasopharynx through the pharyngotympanic tube and with that of mastoid antrum and air cells. The middle ear is lined by ciliated columnar epithelium except over the posterior part of the medial wall, posterior wall and parts of the medial surface of tympanic membrane, where it is cuboidal. The epitympanic cavity is lined by flat epithelium.

Nerve Supply

The tympanic plexus provides sensory supply to the mucosa. The tympanic plexus is formed by tympanic branch of the glossopharyngeal nerve and carotico-tympanic nerves from the sympathetic plexus around internal carotid artery.

Blood Supply

The middle ear receives rich arterial supply through several sources, anterior tympanic branch of maxillary artery, stylomastoid branch of occipital or posterior auricular artery, petrosal branch of middle meningeal artery, a branch from ascending pharyngeal artery, a branch from artery to the pterygoid canal and caroticotympanic branches of internal carotid artery. The veins drain into pterygoid venous plexus and the superior petrosal sinus.

Lymphatic Drainage

The lymphatics from the middle ear drain in the parotid group and upper deep cervical nodes. A few reach the retropharyngeal nodes.

Clinical Highlights

a. Fracture of the roof of middle ear (tegmen tympani) may cause rupture of the tympanic membrane and escape of blood and CSF from the ear.
b. Otitis media is common because the infection easily reaches the middle ear cavity through nasopharynx. The tympanic membrane may perforate if the pus accumulates in the cavity. The chronic otitis media may lead to hearing loss.
c. Serious complications of chronic suppurative otitis media (CSOM) are meningitis, mastoiditis, sigmoid sinus thrombosis, internal jugular vein thrombosis and brain abscess.
d. Chronic bone disease in the medial wall of tympanic cavity (due to chronic otitis media) may cause injury to facial nerve with resultant facial paralysis.

Ear or Auditory Ossicles

There are three ear ossicles: malleus, incus and stapes.

a. The malleus is the largest and derives its name from resemblance to mallet meaning hammer. It has head, handle and the neck, which is the constriction between head and handle. The anterior and lateral processes arise just below the neck. The head lies in the epitympanic recess and articulates with the body of incus at the saddle type of synovial articulation called incudomalleolar joint. The neck gives attachment to tensor tympani tendon. The lateral process provides attachment to anterior and posterior malleolar folds. The anterior ligament of malleus is attached to the anterior process.

b. The incus derives its name from resemblance to anvil though actually its shape is more like a premolar tooth. It has body and two processes, long and short. Its body and short process are confined to epitympanic recess. The body articulates with head of malleus. The short process is attached to fossa of incudis in posterior wall of middle ear. The long process goes down parallel to handle of malleus. Its lower end articulates with the head of stapes to form incudo-stapedial joint, which is ball and socket type of synovial joint.

c. The stapes resembles a stirrup. It is the smallest bone in the body. It has head, neck and two limbs of unequal lengths, which are joined to an oval plate called base or footplate. The neck receives insertion of stapedius. The footplate is attached to the margins of fenestra vestibuli by annular ligament. In otosclerosis, there is fixation of stapes leading to conduction deafness. Removing the stapes (stapedectomy) and putting an implant between the incus and fenestra vestibuli is the surgical treatment for restoring the hearing in otosclerosis.

Intratympanic Muscles

a. The tensor tympani muscle takes origin from the cartilaginous part of the pharyngotympanic tube and the adjacent greater wing of the sphenoid. It enters the anterior wall of middle ear via its bony canal and then its tendon takes a sharp turn around the processus cochleariformis of the medial wall of middle ear. It is inserted in the neck of malleus. The tensor tympani muscle receives its nerve supply from the mandibular nerve because it develops from the mesoderm of the first arch. The nerve supplying the tensor tympani reaches it by an indirect route (via the otic ganglion from the branch to the medial pterygoid muscle in the infratemporal fossa).

b. The stapedius muscle is entirely intratympanic in location. It takes origin from within the pyramid on the posterior wall of middle ear. Its tendon emerges from the aperture at the apex of pyramid and is inserted in neck of stapes. The stapedius is supplied by the facial nerve as it develops from the mesoderm of the second branchial arch.

Actions of Intratympanic Muscles

The tensor tympani and stapedius muscles contract simultaneously in response to loud sounds. They restrict the vibrations of the tympanic membrane and the ossicles. The tensor tympani muscle tenses the tympanic membrane thereby damping down the vibrations of the malleus. The stapedius pulls the neck of the stapes to damp down its vibrations. The muscles, thus, protect the inner ear from noise trauma. Paralysis of stapedius produces hyperacusis in which normal sounds appear too loud.

122 Auditory Tube

The auditory tube (pharyngotympanic tube or Eustachian tube) connects the nasopharynx to the middle ear. The function of the tube is to replenish atmospheric air in the middle ear so that both surfaces of the tympanic membrane are subjected to equal pressure. Through the middle ear, the tube supplies air to the mastoid antrum and air cells. The tube opens during deglutition, yawning and sneezing. Otherwise, it remains closed. The length of the tube in the adult is 36 mm.

From the anterior wall of the middle ear, the tube passes downwards, medially and forwards to reach the lateral wall of nasopharynx by passing through the pharyngobasilar fascia above the free margin of the superior constrictor.

Parts of the Auditory Tube

The auditory tube consists of lateral (outer) bony and medial (inner) cartilaginous parts and the isthmus, which is the junction between the two parts. The diameter of the tube is greatest at its pharyngeal opening, least at the isthmus and again increases towards the middle ear.

a. The length of the bony part is 12 mm and it is located within petrous temporal bone. It extends from anterior wall of middle ear to the junction between the squamous and petrous parts of temporal bone, where it ends in a jagged margin for attachment to the cartilaginous part. Its epithelium is thin and of ciliated columnar type and is continuous with that of middle ear.
b. The length of the cartilaginous part is 24 mm. The cartilage is of elastic type. This part is fixed to the base of the cranium in a groove (sulcus tubae) bounded by petrous temporal bone and greater wing of sphenoid. Its wall is composed mainly of cartilage but partly of fibrous tissue. A triangular plate of cartilage is bent on itself to form a broad medial lamina and narrow lateral lamina. This forms the posteromedial wall of the tube. Inferolateral wall is made of fibrous tissue. The epithelium is ciliated columnar but thickened due to presence of subjacent mucous glands. The cartilage projects at the pharyngeal orifice to give rise to tubal elevation (torus tubaris) behind the orifice. This elevation serves as a landmark during the passage of catheter in the tubal orifice. The pharyngeal opening is the widest part of the tube and is located 1 to 1.25 cm behind the posterior end of inferior nasal concha.

Muscles Attached to Auditory Tube

a. Salpingopharyngeus is attached to the medial lamina of cartilage near the pharyngeal opening (Fig. 122.1).
b. Levator palati arises from the medial lamina of the cartilage.

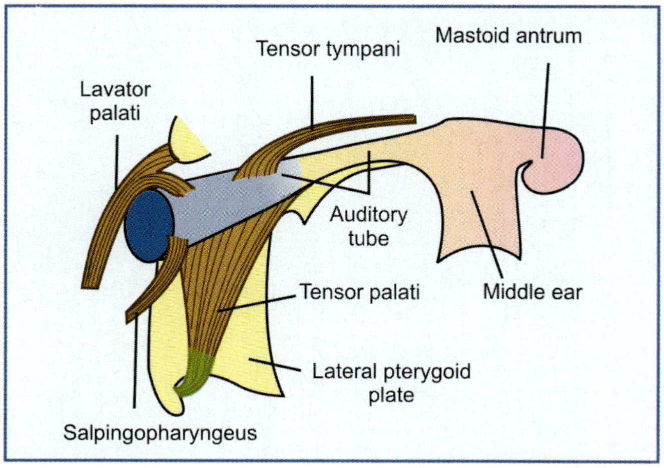

Fig. 122.1: Schematic diagram depicting muscles attached to cartilaginous part of auditory tube

c. Tensor palati arises from the lateral lamina of cartilage and the membranous wall of the tube. The fibers of tensor palati attached to the membranous wall are called dilator tubae.
   The functional role of these muscles is uncertain. The salpingopharyngeus and dilator tubae (whose existence is questioned by some authorities) probably open the tube during deglutition. Levator palati raises the cartilage of the tube thereby releasing tension on the tube and assisting passively to open it.
d. The tensor tympani takes origin from the medial lamina of the cartilage.

Blood Supply

The arterial supply of the auditory is from the ascending pharyngeal artery, middle meningeal artery and artery of pterygoid canal. The veins drain in pharyngeal plexus and pterygoid venous plexus.

Nerve Supply

The glossopharyngeal nerve through the tympanic plexus in the middle ear supplies the lateral part of the tube. The pharyngeal branch of the sphenopalatine ganglion (indirect branch of maxillary nerve) supplies the pharyngeal end of the tube.

Lymphatic Drainage

The lymphatics drain in retropharyngeal and upper deep cervical nodes.

Development

Along with middle ear, the auditory tube develops from the endoderm of tubotympanic recess. The tube is half the length of the adult in the newborn. Its direction is horizontal thus facilitating spread of infection from the nasopharynx to the middle ear in infants. Its bony part is wider. Its narrow pharyngeal opening is at the level of palate and is without tubal elevation (torus tubaris). Hence, it is difficult to locate the tubal orifice during the procedure of passing a catheter in the tube in infants. Fossa of Rosenmuller may be mistakenly entered.

Clinical Highlights

If the auditory tube is blocked completely, negative pressure is created in the middle ear due to absorption of the already existing air. Long-term obstruction of the auditory tube results in secretory otitis media or glue ear, which leads to conduction deafness especially in school-going children. The causes of tubal block are, enlarged tubal tonsils, chronic pharyngitis, chronic tonsillitis and nasopharyngeal carcinoma.

123 Mastoid Antrum

The mastoid antrum (tympanic antrum) is an air-filled space in the petrous temporal bone. It is in communication with the epitympanic recess of middle ear anteriorly and with mastoid air cells inferiorly (Fig. 121.1). Its capacity is about 1 ml. The mastoid antrum and air cells develop from the endoderm of tubotympanic recess. The mastoid antrum is of adult size but the mastoid process is absent at birth. The mastoid process begins to grow as a small projection at the end of first year and mastoid air cells invade it at puberty.

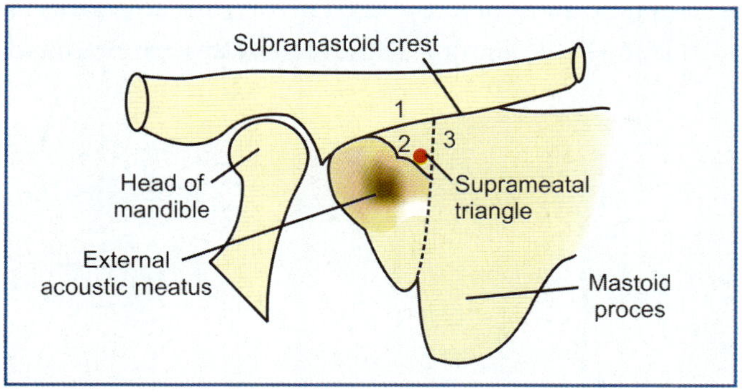

Fig. 123.1: Boundaries of McEwen's suprameatal triangle (1) Supramastoid crest above, (2) Posterosuperior margin of external meatus in front, (3) Vertical tangent to posterior margin of meatus behind

Boundaries

Its anterior wall presents aditus, which leads into the epitympanic recess of the middle ear. The tegmen tympani roofs the antrum and separates it from the middle cranial fossa and the temporal lobe of the cerebrum. Inferiorly, it is continuous with mastoid air cells in the mastoid process. Posteriorly, it is related to the sigmoid sinus and the cerebellum in the posterior cranial fossa. Medially, it is related to lateral semicircular canal of inner ear. The lateral wall corresponds to the suprameatal triangle of McEwen. This wall is only 2 mm thick at birth but increases at the rate of 1 mm per year to attain final thickness of 12-15 mm. The suprameatal triangle is bounded superiorly by the supramastoid crest of the squamous temporal bone, anteriorly by the posterosuperior margin of the external acoustic meatus and posteriorly by a vertical tangent to the posterior margin of external meatus (Fig. 123.1). The surface marking of the suprameatal triangle is the cymba conchae of auricle. Therefore, for aspiration of pus from the antrum, the needle is inserted 2 mm deep in infants and about 12 to15 mm deep in adults through the cymba conchae.

Mastoid Air Cells

The air cells inside the mastoid process look like a honeycomb. Their number varies considerably. Depending on the development of air cells there are three types of mastoid process, well-pneumatised or cellular type with plenty of air cells, diploetic with marrow spaces but few air cells and sclerotic or acellular with no air cells or marrow spaces.

Extramastoidal Sites of Air Cells

The mastoid air cells may be present in surrounding bones as follows, zygomatic air cells in the root of zygoma, tegmen air cells in the tegmen tympani, perilabyrinthine air cells around inner ear, peritubal cells around auditory tube, tip cells at the tip of mastoid process, squamosal cells in the squamous temporal bone and in the occipital bone. The importance of the extramastoidal air cells is that they can become sites of infection.

Clinical Highlights

a. Mastoiditis is a common complication of otitis media. The infection in the mastoid epithelium spreads to the bone causing its destruction. The mastoid air cells are also infected. There is production of copious pus, which may break through the bone forming subperiosteal abscess or discharging fistula. This causes swelling over the mastoid, which pushes the pinna forward and downward.

b. Complications of mastoiditis involve the structures in relation to the antrum. These include abscesses around the mastoid process, labyrinthitis (inflammation of internal ear), facial paralysis, intracranial abscesses, meningitis and sigmoid sinus thrombosis.

c. Bezold abscess is formed if the pus breaks through the tip of mastoid process in the fascial sheath of the sternomastoid muscle and Citelli's abscess is formed if the pus travels along the posterior belly of digastric and appears as a swelling in the digastric triangle. Formation of Bezold abscess and Citelli’s abscess has anatomical basis (sternomastoid and posterior belly of digastric are attached to mastoid process).

124 Internal Ear

The internal ear or labyrinth is located medial to the middle ear in the petrous temporal bone. It has a very complex structure. Broadly, it consists of two parts, the outer bony labyrinth and the inner membranous labyrinth. The bony labyrinth contains the perilymph. The membranous labyrinth contains the endolymph and houses the receptors of hearing and equilibrium.

Bony or Osseous Labyrinth (Fig. 124.1)

The bony labyrinth consists of three interconnecting parts, cochlea, vestibule and semicircular canals.

Bony Cochlea

The bony cochlea is a conical structure resembling the shape of the shell of a snail. It consists of a spiral cochlear canal around a central modiolus, which has a broad base and a narrow apex. The cochlear canal takes two and three fourth turns around the modiolus. The basal turn produces the bulge of promontory on the medial wall of middle ear. The base of the modiolus is directed towards the bottom of internal acoustic meatus (sieve-like tractus spiralis foraminosus) through which fibers of cochlear nerve pass. An osseous spiral lamina is a shelf-like projection from the modiolus into the cochlear canal. The modiolus is traversed by linear minute canals for the passage of the fibers of cochlear nerve. The linear canals turn laterally to enter the spiral canal of modiolus. The spiral canal (Rosenthal's canal) runs in the base of osseous spiral lamina and lodges the spiral ganglion of cochlear nerve. The free edge of spiral lamina presents a C-shaped sulcus, which divides the free edge into vestibular and tympanic lips. The upper surface of vestibular lip gives attachment to vestibular ligament and its tip to the tectorial membrane. The tip of the tympanic lip gives attachment to basilar membrane. The cochlear canal contains three spaces, cochlear duct (scala media) in the

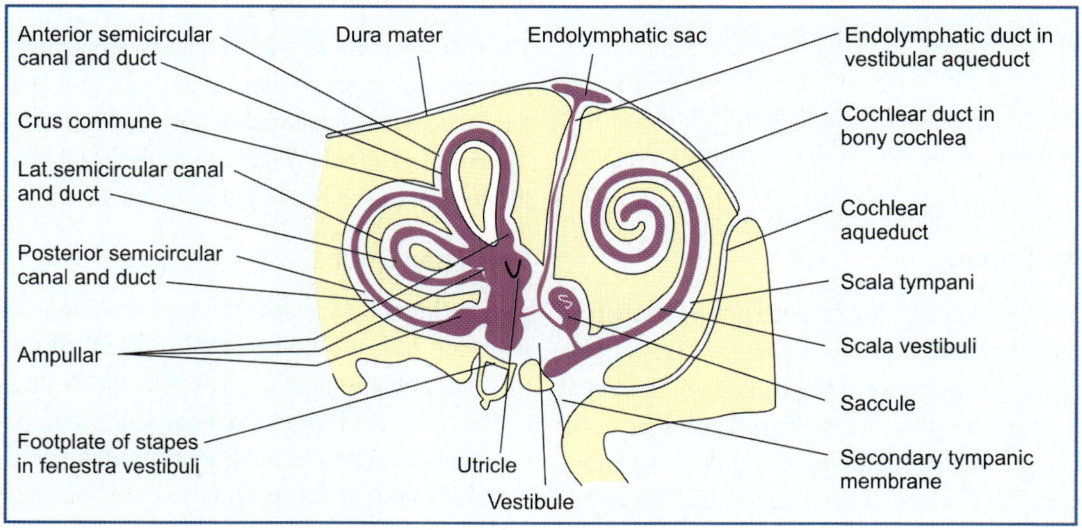

Fig. 124.1: Scheme to depict parts of bony and membranous labyrinth

middle, scala tympani below and scala vestibuli above. The scala media is filled with endolymph but the scala tympani and scala vestibuli are filled with perilymph. The scala tympani and scala vestibuli communicate with each other at the apex of cochlea, through an opening called helicotrema. At the base of cochlea, the opening of scala tympani (fenestra cochleae) is closed by secondary tympanic membrane but the scala vestibuli continues into the vestibule. The scala tympani is connected to the subarachnoid space by aqueduct of cochlea or perilymphatic duct or cochlear canaliculus, which is a minute bony canal opening in the subarachnoid space at the inferior surface of the petrous temporal bone in the jugular fossa.

Vestibule

The vestibule is the central part of the bony labyrinth. It lies medial to the tympanic cavity behind the cochlea and in front of semicircular canals. Its contents are the utricle and saccule of membranous labyrinth.

The anterior wall of the vestibule shows an opening leading into the scala vestibuli of cochlear canal. The lateral wall presents fenestra vestibuli on the medial wall of middle ear. It is closed by footplate of stapes and annular ligament. The posterior wall bears five openings of three semicircular canals. The inner surface of medial wall shows two recesses. The spherical recess lodges the saccule and the fibers of vestibular nerve reach the saccule through the floor of the recess. The elliptical recess lodges the utricle and the fibers of the vestibular nerve reach the utricle through the floor of this recess. The opening of the bony canal called aqueduct of vestibule (for passage of endolymphatic duct) is located below the elliptical recess. The aqueduct of vestibule reaches the epidural space on the posterior surface of petrous temporal bone.

Semicircular Canals

The three semicircular canals are situated postero-superior to the vestibule. The canals are named, anterior (superior), lateral (horizontal) and posterior. They contain semicircular ducts and lie in planes that are at right angles to each other. Each canal has an ampullated or dilated end and a non-ampullated end. The non-ampullated ends of posterior and anterior canals unite to form crus commune. In this way, the semicircular canals open in the vestibule by five openings. The anterior (superior) semicircular canal produces arcuate eminence in the anterior surface of petrous temporal bone in the middle cranial fossa. The lateral semicircular canal is in relation to the medial wall of middle ear, medial wall of mastoid antrum and its aditus. The right and left lateral semicircular canals are in the same plane but the anterior canal of one side is parallel to the posterior canal of the opposite side.

Perilymph

The source, circulation and absorption of perilymph are yet, not fully known. The perilymph contains high sodium, low potassium and high protein. The cochlear canaliculus (perilymphatic duct or aqueduct of cochlea) carries the perilymph into the subarachnoid space at the roof of the jugular foramen. So probably, the perilymph is partly derived from CSF and partly from the blood vessels surrounding perilymphatic spaces of the bony labyrinth. The movements of the perilymph follow a definite sequence. The medial movement of the footplate of stapes in fenestra vestibuli produces pressure waves in the perilymph of the vestibule and of the scala vestibuli. The waves are passed on to the perilymph of scala tympani at helicotrema. After producing movements of basilar membrane, the waves cause a compensatory bulge of the secondary tympanic membrane in the middle ear. Thus, the wave is generated at fenestra vestibuli and terminated at fenestra cochleae.

Membranous Labyrinth (Fig. 124.2)

The membranous labyrinth consists of cochlear duct, utricle and saccule, three semicircular ducts and endolymphatic duct and sac, which together form endolymph filled closed system of channels. The membranous labyrinth contains the receptors for hearing and balance.

Cochlear Duct

The cochlear duct or membranous cochlea or scala media is coiled like the bony cochlea. It is blind at the apex (lagena) but is connected to the saccule by ductus reuniens at the base. It is located near the outer part of bony cochlear canal between the scala tympani below and scala vestibuli above. Its boundaries are, basilar membrane inferiorly (which separates it from the scala tympani), the vestibular or Reissner's membrane superomedially

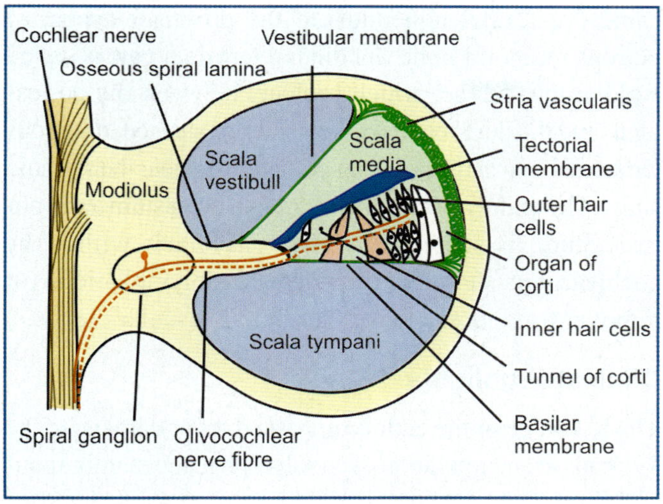

Fig. 124.2: Scheme to depict spiral organ of Corti in a section through a turn of cochlea

(which separates it from the scala vestibuli) and stria vascularis laterally. The width of the basilar membrane increases from the basal to the apical region of the cochlear duct because the width of the osseous spiral lamina decreases from below upwards. The receptors of hearing, spiral organ of Corti, is located inside the cochlear duct.

Spiral Organ of Corti

The spiral organ is composed of a special type of sensory epithelium and the tectorial membrane. The epithelium consists of sensory hair cells and different types of supporting cells, which are arranged on the basilar membrane. The pillar cells rest on the basilar membrane by broad bases. The outer and inner pillar cells enclose a central triangular space (tunnel of Corti). This tunnel contains cortilymph, which nourishes the sensory epithelium. Internal to the inner pillar cells there is a single row of inner hair cells. External to the outer pillar cells there are three or four rows of outer hair cells. The tectorial membrane is a stiff gelatinous plate containing glycoproteins (tectorins). It is attached to the vestibular lip of the spiral lamina. It overlies the apical aspect of the sensory epithelium. The hair or stereocilia of outer hair cells are embedded in it. The vibrations of basilar membrane cause the shearing forces between the tectorial membrane and hair cells. These forces stimulate the outer and inner hair cells, which transduce sound energy into electrical impulse. The nerve fibers supplying the hair cells (peripheral processes of the bipolar neurons of spiral ganglion) carry the nerve impulse to the cochlear nerve. The hair cells also receive efferent olivocochlear fibers from the superior olivary nucleus via the Oort's anastomosis. These fibers are believed to modulate the function of inner hair cells through inhibitory influence of outer hair cells.

Clinical Highlights

a. Inflammation of labyrinth is called labyrinthitis.
b. Noise trauma can lead to hearing loss. Degenerative changes in organ of Corti may occur in people exposed to continuous loud sounds over a period. Boilermakers, coppersmiths, ironsmiths and artillerymen are susceptible to this condition. Sudden loud sound (loud explosion, gunfire or a powerful cracker) may damage hair cells in organ of Corti or rupture the vestibular membrane.
c. Presbycusis is the physiological hearing loss associated with aging process. This may be due to degeneration of organ of Corti or of cells in spiral ganglion or of stria vascularis or of basilar membrane.
d. Cochlear implants are the electronic devices that are used for totally nonfunctioning cochlea. They convert sound energy into electrical impulse, which stimulates the cochlear nerve. During the operation of implantation, the electrode (for stimulating the cochlear nerve) is placed on the promontory or scala tympani or cochlear nerve in the modiolus.

Utricle and Saccule

The utricle is an irregular sac that occupies the elliptical recess of bony vestibule. It receives five openings of the semicircular ducts. The saccule is a globular sac lying in the spherical recess of the bony vestibule. It is connected to the cochlear duct by the ductus reuniens. Y-shaped utriculo-saccular duct connects the saccule and utricle to each other. The vertical limb of the Y continues as the endolymphatic duct. The macula is the sensory epithelium of the utricle and saccule. It consists of large number of hair cells. The cilia of the hair cells project in the gelatinous cap called statoconial or otolithic membrane containing crystals of calcium carbonate (otoliths). The hair cells respond to orientation of head with respect to gravity hence the maculae of utricle and saccule are known as static labyrinth. The peripheral processes of the neurons of vestibular ganglion supply sensory fibers to hair cells of maculae. Excessive stimulation of utricle and saccule is responsible for motion sickness, in which the person experiences vertigo, nausea and vomiting. Deaf-mutes do not experience motion sickness because of the absence of labyrinth.

Semicircular Ducts

The semicircular ducts are much smaller in diameter than the semicircular canals of bony labyrinth. The anterior, lateral and posterior ducts open by five openings in the utricle. The ampullary end of each duct bears a raised crest (crista ampullaris), which projects in the lumen. Each ampullary crest carries specialized hair cells. The stereocilia and one kinocilium from the hair cell are inserted in a vertical plate of gelatinous material called cupula. The angular acceleration and deceleration movements of head bring about movements of endolymph in semicircular ducts, which results in deflecting of cupula and stimulation of the hair cells of crest. The peripheral processes of the bipolar neurons of vestibular ganglion provide sensory supply to these hair cells. The ampullary cristae are also known as kinetic labyrinth on account of their function.

Endolymphatic Duct and Sac

The endolymphatic duct continues from the junction of Y-shaped utriculosaccular duct. It is carried in a bony canal (vestibular aqueduct) to the posterior aspect of petrous temporal bone. Its dilated terminal part is called endolymphatic sac, which projects between the periosteum and the dura mater on the posterior surface of petrous temporal bone in the posterior cranial fossa near the sigmoid sinus. The endolymph, which is rich in potassium and poor in sodium, is secreted by stria vascularis within the cochlear duct. It enters the ductus endolymphaticus for removal from its sac in the extradural vascular plexus.

Clinical Highlights

The blockage of the endolymphatic duct or damage to the sac leads to accumulation of endolymph in the membranous labyrinth. This condition is called endolymphatic hydrops or Meniere's disease. It is characterized by vertigo, hearing loss and tinnitus.

Blood Supply of Labyrinth

The labyrinthine artery, more frequently a branch from anterior inferior cerebellar artery (instead of the basilar artery) enters the inner ear via internal acoustic meatus. At the bottom of the meatus, it divides into cochlear and vestibular branches, of which the cochlear branch enters the modiolus. The stylomastoid branch of either the occipital or the posterior auricular artery may also give additional supply to the labyrinth. The venous drainage is by the labyrinthine vein, which drains into the superior petrosal sinus.

125 Cranial Nerves

Olfactory Nerve and Pathway

The olfactory nerves are the first pair of cranial nerves. They begin in the olfactory mucosa of the nasal cavity, which consists of bipolar olfactory receptor cells (first order neurons of the olfactory path). The unique feature of these neurons is that they develop from the surface ectoderm and not the neuroectoderm. The long axons of the bipolar cells collect together to form about 20 bundles of each olfactory nerve. They pass through the cribriform plate of the ethmoid to enter the anterior cranial fossa, where they terminate in the olfactory bulb. The bundles of olfactory nerve are surrounded by all the three meninges at the cribriform plate. This provides a communication between the subarachnoid space and the lymphatics of the nasal mucosa and a route for the infection from nose to the meninges.

Olfactory Bulb (Fig. 96.2)

This is situated in the anterior cranial fossa, below the olfactory sulcus on the orbital surface of the frontal lobe of cerebrum. The main neurons of the olfactory bulb are the mitral and tufted cells with which the nerve fibers in the olfactory nerve make synaptic contacts in the glomeruli. These neurons are the second order neurons in the olfactory path.

Olfactory Tract

The axons of the mitral and tufted neurons form the olfactory tract on each side. The olfactory tract runs backwards and widens in olfactory trigone at the anterior aspect of anterior perforated substance. The lateral and medial olfactory striae extend from the angles of this trigone on either side of the anterior perforated substance. If a third stria, called intermediate stria is present, it terminates in the anterior perforated substance. The medial stria covered with a thin sheet of gray matter (medial olfactory gyrus) terminates in paraterminal gyrus in front of the lamina terminalis. The lateral olfactory stria covered with a thin layer of gray matter, (lateral olfactory gyrus) terminates in the primary olfactory cortex.

Olfactory Cortex

The primary olfactory cortex consists of anterior perforated substance, lateral olfactory gyrus, gyrus ambiens and part of amygdaloid body. From the primary cortex the fibers are projected to the secondary olfactory cortex constituted by entorhinal area (area 28). This area includes the uncus and the adjacent anterior part of parahippocampal gyrus. The sense of smell is perceived in both primary and secondary olfactory cortices.

Nervi Terminalis

This is variously described as zero cranial nerve or thirteenth cranial nerve or mysterious nerve. Its existence in man is doubtful. It is postulated that it may be an additional chemosensory path for olfaction. It is also postulated that this nerve contains fibers belonging to luteinizing hormone releasing hormone (LHRH) carrying neurons and associated ganglia. Thus, it might be a remnant of embryonic migrating path of these neurons from the olfactory placode to the hypothalamus.

Optic Nerve and Visual Pathway (Fig. 125.1)

The visual or the optic pathway conveys visual (light) impulses from the retina to the visual cortex in the occipital lobe of the cerebrum. The visual impulse is generated in the rod and cone cells of the retina. In fact, these photoreceptor cells act as transducers converting light

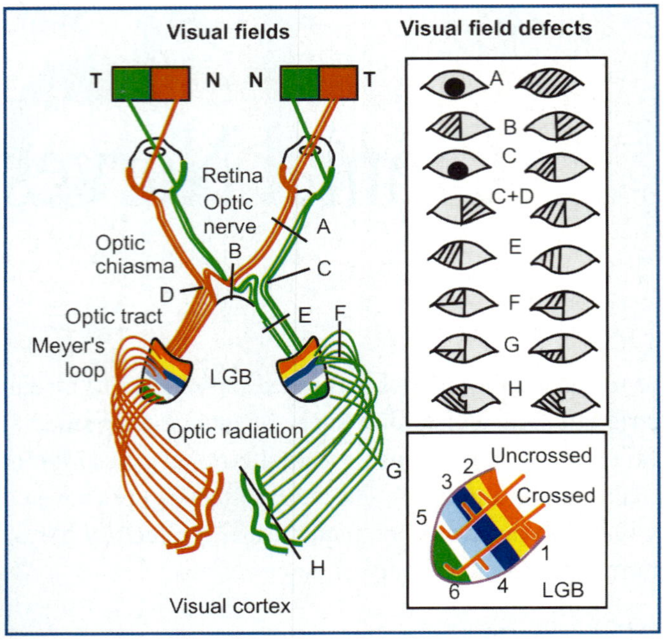

Fig. 125.1: Components of visual pathway and effects of lesion at various sites
A–Total blindness right eye, B–Bitemporal hemianopia, C–Right nasal hemianopia, C + D. Binasal hemianopia E and LGB–Left homonymous hemianopia, F–Left homonymous superior qudrantanopia, G–Left homonymous inferior qudrantanopia, H–Left homonymous hemianopia with macular sparing

signals into electrical signals. These signals are processed in the bipolar cells (first order neurons) and then in the ganglion cells (second order neurons). The axons of the ganglion cells collect to form the optic nerve, which carries the impulse through the optic chiasma and optic tract to the lateral geniculate body (LGB). The neurons of LGB are third order neurons, which give origin to the optic radiation, which finally terminates on the visual cortex.

Optic Nerve

The optic nerve emerges from the retina at the optic disc and is composed of axons of the ganglion cells of retina. It travels backward in the orbit, which it leaves via the optic foramen to enter the cranial cavity, where two optic nerves unite to form optic chiasma. The optic nerve is about 4 cm in length. Developmentally, it is the extension of the diencephalon of the brain and hence is covered with three meninges, like the brain. The subarachnoid space extends around the optic nerve inside the orbit. This fact has clinical bearing because rise in the intracranial tension slows the venous return from the central vein of the retina causing papilledema. Being a part of CNS, its axons are myelinated by oligodendroglia. The disadvantage of this is the inability to regenerate on injury, unlike the peripheral nerve, where cells of Schwann are capable of regenerating the nerve.

Parts

The optic nerve is subdivided into intraorbital, canalicular and intracranial parts.

a. The intraorbital part, about 2.5 cm, is surrounded by the extraocular muscles. The central retinal artery enters the substance of the nerve on its inferomedial aspect about 1.2 cm behind the eyeball. The optic nerve is crossed superiorly by three structures (nasociliary nerve, ophthalmic artery and superior ophthalmic vein) from lateral to medial side.
b. The canalicular part passing through the optic canal is about 0.5 cm in length. Here, it is very closely related to the ophthalmic artery.
c. The intracranial part is 1 cm in length. Above, it is related to the gyrus rectus of the inferior surface of the frontal lobe, olfactory tract and anterior cerebral artery and laterally to the internal carotid artery. Below, it rests on the tuberculum sellae and the diaphragm sellae.

Arterial Supply

The superior hypophyseal artery supplies the intracranial part, the branches of the ophthalmic artery supply the canalicular part and the posterior ciliary artery and the central artery of retina supply the intraorbital part.

Arrangement of Nerve Fibers

The fibers that arise from the four quadrants of the retina are arranged in the same relative positions in the optic nerve. The papillomacular fibers occupy the lateral part of the nerve nearer the eyeball but shift in the central part behind the point of entry of the central vessels.

Fields of Vision and Retinal Quadrants

The temporal hemiretina receives image input from the nasal visual field while the nasal hemiretina receives image input from the temporal visual field. The upper retinal quadrants receive images from the lower visual field while the lower retinal quadrants receive images from the upper visual field.

Optic Chiasma

The optic chiasma (Figs 87.5 and 125.1) is a midline structure in the middle cranial fossa. It is formed by partial decussation of the fibers of the optic nerve. The fibers of the optic nerve from the nasal halves of the retinae decussate in the central part of the chiasma while the fibers from the temporal half of retina of same side occupy the lateral part of the chiasma. The macular fibers cross in the posteroinferior margin of the chiasma. One peculiar feature that is observed regarding inferonasal fibers is that after crossing they project for a distance of about 4 mm in the adjacent optic nerve (of opposite side) before turning back posteriorly in the chiasma. This bend of nasal fibers is known as Willibrandt's knee. However, the existence of this loop is not universally accepted.

Relations of Chiasma

a. Superiorly, the chiasma is related to the floor of the third ventricle.
b. Laterally, it is related to the bifurcation of internal carotid artery and the anterior perforated substance.
c. Anteriorly, the lamina terminalis extends from it to the paraterminal gyrus. The anterior communicating artery is related on this aspect.
d. Posteriorly, it is related to infundibulum, tuber cinereum and mammillary bodies.
e. The pituitary gland is its posteroinferior relation.
   In pathology of these neighboring structures there is compression of the optic chiasma, producing typical defects in the visual field.

Arterial Supply

The optic chiasma receives ample supply from the branches of anterior cerebral, internal carotid, posterior communicating and middle cerebral arteries.

Optic Tract

The right and the left optic tracts continue from the posterolateral ends of the optic chiasma. Each optic tract is composed of ipsilateral temporal fibers and contralateral nasal fibers. The optic tract courses along the anterolateral boundary of the interpeduncular fossa and after crossing the cerebral peduncle majority of its fibers end in the lateral geniculate body of its side. A few end in the superior colliculus via superior brachium.

Arterial Supply

The optic tract receives twigs from the anterior choroidal artery, middle cerebral and posterior communicating arteries. The anterior choroidal artery crosses the tract twice, hence it is called the satellite artery of the optic tract.

Lateral Geniculate Body (LGB)

LGB is a thalamic relay station for visual impulses. It receives fibers from ipsilateral temporal retina and contralateral nasal retina. The neurons are arranged in six laminae. The contralateral fibers terminate in neurons of layers 1, 4 and 6 while ipsilateral fibers end on neurons in layers 2, 3 and 5. A few fibers involved in visual reflexes leave the LGB without interruption via the superior brachium to make synaptic contacts with neurons of the pretectal nucleus and of the superior colliculus. The medial part of LGB receives fibers from the upper half of retina and its lateral part receives fibers from the lower half of the retina. The peripheral part of retina is represented in the anterior part while the macular fibers terminate in larger central and posterior area. The axons of the neurons in LGB give rise to the geniculocalcarine tract or optic radiation, which terminates in the visual cortex.

Arterial Supply

The central branches of posterior cerebral artery and branches of posterior choroidal arteries supply the lateral geniculate body.

Optic Radiation

The optic radiation (geniculocalcarine tract) passes through the retrolentiform part of the internal capsule to reach the visual cortex. The upper fibers of the optic radiation sweep directly backwards and end in the cuneus in the upper lip of the calcarine sulcus. These fibers carry impulses from the superior retinal quadrants, representing inferior visual field. The lower fibers of the optic radiation form a loop

(Meyer's loop) by first turning anteriorly in the temporal lobe. This loop is in close relation to the inferior horn of the lateral ventricle (Fig. 100.1). After this, the fibers turn posteriorly to terminate in the lingual gyrus in the lower lip of the calcarine sulcus. These fibers carry impulses from the inferior retinal quadrants representing superior visual fields.

Arterial Supply

a. The perforating branch of anterior choroidal artery supplies the anterior part of radiation, where it passes laterally superior to the inferior horn of lateral ventricle.
b. The deep optic artery (central branch of middle cerebral artery) supplies the posterior part of radiation, where it passes lateral to the posterior horn of lateral ventricle.
c. The terminal part of the radiation near the visual cortex receives supply from perforating cortical branches from calcarine branch of posterior cerebral artery and from middle cerebral artery.

Visual Cortex

The visual cortex is also known as the striate cortex (area 17). The area includes cuneus and lingual gyri and the calcarine sulcus. The visual cortex receives impulses from the retinal halves of the same side (opposite half of field of vision) via the LGB. The upper quadrants of retina are projected on the upper lip of the calcarine sulcus and the lower quadrants on the lower lip. The macular fibers terminate very close to the occipital pole.

Arterial Supply

The calcarine branches of the posterior cerebral artery supply the major part of the visual cortex. However, a small area near the occipital pole receives twigs from the middle cerebral artery also.

Clinical Highlights (Fig. 125.1)

Depending on the site of the lesion, the symptoms and signs vary.

Optic Nerve

a. Compression of optic nerve results in optic atrophy and eventually in ipsilateral total blindness (anopia).
b. Foster Kennedy syndrome is characterized by ipsilateral optic atrophy, ipsilateral anosmia and contralateral papilledema. A tumor of the orbital surface of the frontal lobe or the meningioma in the floor of the anterior cranial fossa near the optic canal, may give rise to this syndrome by compressing the optic nerve and the olfactory tract. The contralateral papilledema is due to rise in the intracranial pressure because of the tumor.

Optic Chiasma

a. Compression of central portion of chiasma by, for example, an expanding pituitary tumor results in bitemporal hemianopia. In this defect, the patient is able to see the objects placed in the nasal halves of the visual fields only. There is loss of peripheral vision and retention of central vision in both eyes (tunnel vision).
b. If the optic chiasma in compressed at its lateral angle on one side only, it causes ipsilateral nasal hemianopia. Bilateral lesion of lateral angles of optic chiasma results in binasal hemianopia as may occur in bilateral internal carotid artery calcification or aneurysm.

Optic Tract

Lesion of the right optic tract results in left homonymous hemianopia and vice versa. The pupillary light reflex is absent in the blind half of each retina.

Lateral Geniculate Body

The destruction of the right LGB results in left homonymous hemianopia and vice versa. The pupillary light reflex is retained as the fibers for superior colliculus have already gone out of the tract.

Optic Radiation

a. The lesion of the upper part of the optic radiations (usually due to parietal lobe pathology) results in contralateral inferior homonymous quadrantanopia (quadrantic hemianopia).
b. The lesion of the lower fibers including the looping fibers (Meyer's loop) results in contralateral superior homonymous quadrantanopia (quadrantic hemianopia). The temporal lobe pathology may be the cause of lesion in Meyer's loop.

Visual Cortex

In occlusion of posterior cerebral artery there is contralateral homonymous hemianopia with sparing of the macular vision (macula being supplied by middle cerebral artery also).

Occipital Pole

This being an exclusively macular area, lesion here causes loss of half macular vision. Right occipital pole lesion will cause loss of left half of macular vision.

Pupillary Light Reflexes

a. The direct pupillary reflex consists of reflex constriction of the pupil in response to bright light shone in the eye.
b. The consensual light reflex consists of reflex constriction in pupil of the opposite eye in response to light shone in one eye.

In both the direct and consensual light reflexes the optic nerve is the afferent limb, pretectal nucleus is the center and the oculomotor nerve is the efferent limb.

Accommodation Reflex

For viewing near objects the eyes converge, the ciliaris muscles contract to modify the shape of the lens and the pupils constrict to increase the depth of the focus (it is to be noted that the path for pupillary constriction in accommodation is different from that of papillary constriction in response to the light). The afferent limb of accommodation reflex consists of optic nerve, optic tract, lateral geniculate body and optic radiation. The center of the reflex is the cortical visual area. The efferent limb consists of corticotectal fibers, tectobulbar fibers, Edinger-Westphal nucleus and the oculomotor nerve.

Argyll-Robertson Pupil

If there is lesion in papillary reflex center (pretectal nucleus in midbrain) the path of light reflex is disrupted but the path of accommodation reflex remains intact. As a consequence, the pupillary constriction in response to light is lost but in response to accommodation is retained. Such a pupil is known as Argyll-Robertson pupil (aid to memorize—ARP = **A**ccommodation **R**eflex **P**resent and PRA= **P**upillary **R**eflex **A**bsent).

Oculomotor Nerve

This is the third cranial nerve. It is a motor nerve that supplies five extraocular muscles and two intraocular muscles.

Functional Components

It consists of general somatic efferent (GSE) and general visceral efferent (GVE) types of fibers.

Nuclei of Origin

The oculomotor nucleus lies in the periaqueductal gray in the midbrain at the level of superior colliculi, anterior to the cerebral aqueduct and posterior to the medial longitudinal bundle. It consists of somatic component (main oculomotor nucleus) and autonomic component (Edinger-Westphal nucleus). The somatic component is subdivided into different groups, which supply the individual extraocular muscles. The Edinger-Westphal nucleus gives parasympathetic supply to the intraocular muscles (ciliaris and sphincter pupillae).

Connections

The corticonuclear fibers from the opposite cortex are connected to the oculomotor nucleus. There are connections with superior colliculi and the pretectal nucleus. The vestibular nuclei are connected through the medial longitudinal bundle. The rostral interstitial nucleus of MLF and the interstitial nucleus of Cajal, associated with vertical eye movements project on the somatic cell groups of oculomotor complex. The MLF connects the nucleus for medial rectus muscle to the contralateral PPRF or horizontal gaze center and para-abducent nucleus in the pons.

Course through Midbrain

The axons of the neurons of the oculomotor nucleus travel in the midbrain forwards through the red nucleus and the medial part of the substantia nigra (Fig. 90.8).

Point of Emergence (Fig. 90.1)

The oculomotor nerve emerges from the ventral aspect of midbrain by piercing the medial aspect of cerebral peduncle. It appears in the posterior part of the interpeduncular fossa.

Intracranial Course

In its subarachnoid course, the oculomotor nerve lies between the posterior cerebral and the superior cerebellar arteries and in close relation to the posterior communicating artery. It passes through the tentorial notch (Fig. 85.1) and then enters the lateral wall of the cavernous sinus, where it lies in the most superior position. The oculomotor nerve is in danger of compression at the tentorial notch as a result of herniation of uncus and in cavernous sinus thrombosis.

Exit from Cranium

The nerve leaves the middle cranial fossa to enter the orbit through the superior orbital fissure (Fig. 109.1). Before entering the fissure it divides into superior and inferior divisions. Both the divisions are enclosed in the common tendinous ring along with the nasociliary and abducent nerves.

Intraorbital Course and Distribution

The superior division passes forwards and upwards lateral to the optic nerve and supplies the superior rectus and levator palpebrae superioris muscles. The inferior division gives three branches for the supply of medial rectus, inferior rectus and inferior oblique muscles. The branch to inferior oblique muscle provides a communicating twig to the ciliary ganglion. The communicating twig contains preganglionic parasympathetic fibers from the Edinger-Westphal nucleus.

Ciliary Ganglion (Fig. 110.4)

This is a peripheral parasympathetic ganglion located in the posterior part of the orbit. The preganglionic fibers originate in the Edinger-Westphal nucleus and travel in the oculomotor nerve. They leave the oculomotor nerve through its branch to inferior oblique. The preganglionic fibers pass via a connection of this branch to the ganglion and synapse with the ganglion cells. The postganglionic fibers leave through short ciliary nerves, which arise from the ganglion. These branches run anteriorly to pierce the sclera around the attachment of the optic nerve to enter the eyeball and supply the sphincter pupillae and ciliaris muscles (for details of the connections of the ganglion refer to Chapter 109).

Clinical Highlights

The effects of lesion of oculomotor nerve are as follows:

a. Ptosis is due to paralysis of levator palpebrae superioris.
b. External strabismus in affected eye is due to unopposed action of lateral rectus and superior oblique muscles (with paralysis of medial rectus, inferior rectus and superior rectus and inferior oblique muscles).
c. Diplopia or double vision is present on looking medially, inferiorly and superiorly.
d. Dilated and fixed pupil is due to loss of parasympathetic supply to sphincter pupillae and ciliaris muscles.
e. Cycloplegia (paralysis of accommodation) is due to loss of parasympathetic supply to ciliaris.

To sum up, ptosis and external strabismus with large pupil and absence of accommodation are the hallmarks of oculomotor injury.

Trochlear Nerve

The trochlear nerve is the fourth cranial nerve.

Unique Features

a. It is the most slender of all the cranial nerve.
b. It is the only cranial nerve to emerge from the dorsal aspect of the brainstem.
c. It is the only cranial nerve that shows decussation of fibers before emerging from the midbrain so that the left trochlear nerve contains fibers originating in right trochlear nucleus.
d. Its nucleus receives only the ipsilateral corticonuclear fibers.

Functional Component

The trochlear nerve contains only one functional component, general somatic efferent (GSE).

Nucleus of Origin (Fig. 90.7)

The trochlear nucleus lies immediately caudal to the oculomotor nucleus in the periaqueductal gray matter at the level of inferior colliculus. The axons curve round the periaqueductal gray in backward direction and decussate with the axons from the opposite nucleus in the superior medullary velum.

Point of Emergence

The trochlear nerve emerges from the posterior aspect of midbrain just below the inferior colliculus on each side of the frenulum veli.

Intracranial Course

Each trochlear nerve winds round the cerebral peduncle to reach the front of the midbrain. While crossing the cerebral peduncle it lies between the posterior cerebral and superior cerebellar arteries. The trochlear nerve pierces the dura mater just below the free margin of tentorium cerebelli and enters the lateral wall of the cavernous sinus. Here, it is located between the oculomotor nerve above and the ophthalmic nerve below.

Exit from Cranium

It leaves the middle cranial fossa through the lateral part of the superior orbital fissure lying outside the tendinous ring (Fig. 109.1) and enters the orbit.

Intraorbital Course

The trochlear nerve travels anteromedially above the superior rectus muscle to enter the superior oblique muscle, which it supplies.

Clinical Highlights

In injury to trochlear nerve the eyeball turns medially and there is diplopia on looking laterally, when the eyeball is depressed (for example, while descending the steps). Reason for this is as follows: The depression is the combined action of superior oblique and inferior rectus muscles. Therefore, even if superior oblique is paralyzed the patient can depress the eyeball. The eye is adducted in the absence of abduction action of superior oblique. This produces medial squint and diplopia on looking laterally in a depressed eyeball.

Trigeminal Nerve and Related Sensory Pathways

The trigeminal nerve is the fifth cranial nerve and is largest of the cranial nerves. It has a large sensory root and small motor root. Its sensory ganglion is known as trigeminal or Gasserian ganglion. Besides the sensory ganglion, the branches of the main subdivisions of the trigeminal nerve are related to four peripheral parasympathetic ganglia, namely, the otic, ciliary, submandibular and sphenopalatine.

Functional Components

The motor nucleus of the trigeminal nerve belongs to the branchial efferent group and the sensory nuclei belong to the general somatic afferent group.

Nuclei of Origin

There is one motor nucleus and three sensory nuclei in the brainstem.

a. The motor nucleus is located in the upper pons (Fig. 90.6).
b. The long sensory nucleus extends the entire length of the brainstem and is divided into three parts (Fig. 125.2).
    i. The principal or chief sensory nucleus is present in the pons lateral to the motor nucleus.
    ii. The nucleus of spinal tract of trigeminal nerve begins in the principal nucleus and goes down beyond the lower end of the medulla oblongata, where it is continuous with the substantia gelatinosa upto the C2 segment of the spinal cord.
    iii. The mesencephalic nucleus lies in the midbrain but it is continuous inferiorly with the principal nucleus.

Each of these nuclei has different function. The mesencephalic nucleus is concerned with proprioception

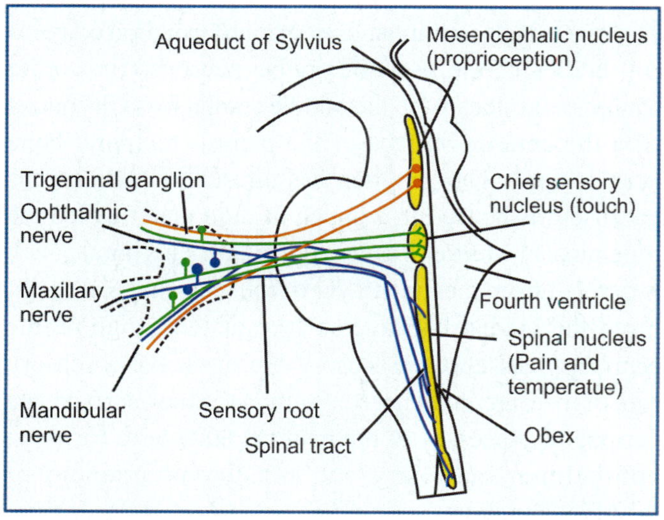

Fig. 125.2: Simplified scheme to show the termination of sensory fibers of trigeminal nerve on its sensory nuclei
Color code for fibers: Red–Proprioception. Green–Touch sensation. Blue–Pain and temperature

from muscles of face, orbit and mastication. It is equivalent to the sensory ganglion as it contains pseudounipolar neurons. The principal sensory nucleus receives fibers subserving discriminative touch from face and head and the nucleus of spinal tract is concerned with pain, temperature and light touch from the face and head. The spinal nucleus is divisible into three parts, pars rostralis above followed by pars interpolaris and pars caudalis. Within the spinal nucleus and the spinal tract there is orderly arrangement of the fibers of the three divisions of trigeminal nerve. The ophthalmic fibers lie ventrolaterally and terminate in pars caudalis. The mandibular fibers reach upto the obex and lying dorsomedially in the tract, terminate in pars rostralis. The maxillary fibers terminate in pars interpolaris and extend upto the lower end of the medulla oblongata. At its lower end, the spinal nucleus is continuous with the substantia gelatinosa of the posterior gray horn and the spinal tract is continuous with the tract of Lissauer in the spinal cord.

Point of Emergence (Fig. 90.1)

The motor and sensory roots of the trigeminal nerve emerge from the ventrolateral aspect of the pons at its junction with the middle cerebellar peduncle. The motor and sensory roots pass anteriorly in the cisterna pontis. The sensory root bears the trigeminal ganglion.

Trigeminal Ganglion

The trigeminal (semilunar or gasserian) ganglion contains cell bodies of the pseudounipolar neurons (first order neurons). It is located in the middle cranial fossa in contact with the anterior surface of the petrous temporal bone near its apex. The ganglion has unusual dural relations because it is housed in a pouch of dura mater called the trigeminal or Meckel's cave (Fig. 125.3). This dural pouch is derived from the inner layer of the tentorium cerebelli. From the medial concave surface of the ganglion, the central processes of the sensory neurons leave as sensory root of the trigeminal nerve. From its convex surface, the peripheral processes of the neurons emerge to form the ophthalmic, maxillary and sensory component of mandibular nerves.

Intracranial Course of Ophthalmic Nerve

This is a purely sensory nerve. It arises from the antero-medial aspect of trigeminal ganglion and pierces the dura mater of the trigeminal cave to enter the lateral wall of cavernous sinus, where it lies below the trochlear nerve. It divides in nasociliary, lacrimal and frontal branches in the lateral wall of the sinus. All the three branches enter the orbit through the superior orbital fissure.

Intracranial Course of Maxillary Nerve

This is a purely sensory nerve. It arises from the middle of the convex surface of the trigeminal ganglion and pierces the dura mater of the trigeminal cave to enter the lateral wall of the cavernous sinus, where it occupies the lowest position. It gives a meningeal branch to the dura mater of middle cranial fossa and enters the pterygopalatine fossa via the foramen rotundum.

Intracranial Course of Mandibular Nerve

This is the largest of the three divisions and is a mixed nerve containing both sensory and motor fibers. Its sensory root arises from the trigeminal ganglion in the middle cranial fossa. The motor root originates from the motor nucleus in the pons and passes deep to the trigeminal ganglion to join the sensory root at or just below the foramen ovale to form a short trunk of the mandibular nerve. It leaves the cranium via the foramen ovale to enter the infratemporal fossa.

Motor Distribution of Mandibular Nerve

The trunk of the mandibular nerve after entering the infratemporal fossa gives a branch to medial pterygoid muscle (which also supplies the tensor tympani and tensor

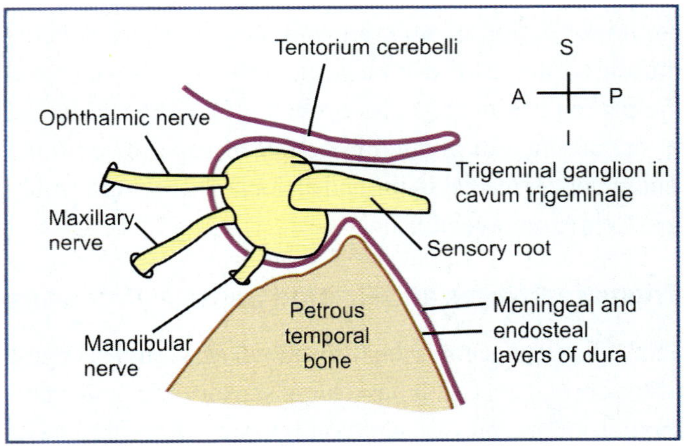

Fig. 125.3: Dural relations of trigeminal ganglion
(Note: The outpouching of the meningeal layer of dura to form cavum trigeminale)

palati muscles via otic ganglion). The anterior division of mandibular nerve supplies masseter, temporalis and lateral pterygoid muscles. The posterior division gives a branch called inferior alveolar nerve. This branch sends mylohyoid nerve that supplies mylohyoid muscle and anterior belly of digastric.

Summary of Sensory Distribution of Trigeminal Nerve

a. The area of the mandibular nerve, supplied through its sensory branches is as follows:

   The nervus spinosus supplies the dura mater of the middle cranial fossa. The buccal nerve supplies the skin over the buccinator and the buccal mucous membrane. The auriculotemporal nerve supplies to auricle, external acoustic meatus, lateral aspect of tympanic membrane and the skin of the temple. The lingual nerve is sensory to the mucosa of the anterior two-thirds of the dorsum of the tongue and the inferior alveolar nerve is sensory to the lower teeth and gums. The mental branch of the inferior alveolar nerve supplies the skin of the lower lip and chin.

b. The sensory area of the maxillary nerve is as follows.

   Its meningeal branch supplies the dura mater of the middle and anterior cranial fossae. The zygomatic branches supply the skin of the prominence of the face and of temple. The superior alveolar branches are for the upper teeth and gums. The infraorbital nerve supplies the lower eyelid, side of nose and upper lip. The palatine branches supply to the mucosa of the palate. The nasopalatine branches supply the mucosa of nasal cavity, palate and maxillary sinus. The pharyngeal branch is sensory to the Eustachian tube and mucosa of nasopharynx. The orbital branches supply the periosteum of orbit, sphenoidal and ethmoidal sinuses.

c. After giving its recurrent tentorial branch (which supplies the tentorium cerebelli) the ophthalmic nerve divides into lacrimal, frontal and nasociliary branches.
   i. The lacrimal nerve is sensory to the upper eyelid and conjunctiva.
   ii. The frontal nerve divides into supratrochlear and supraorbital nerves. The supratrochlear nerve supplies the upper eyelid, conjunctiva and forehead near the midline. The supraorbital nerve supplies the upper eyelid, conjunctiva, forehead and scalp upto the vertex and the frontal sinus.
   iii. The following are the branches of nasociliary nerve: The anterior ethmoidal nerve supplies the nasal cavity and skin of the tip of nose while the posterior ethmoidal nerve supplies the ethmoidal and sphenoidal sinuses. The infratrochlear nerve supplies the nose above the medial canthus of eye, conjunctiva, upper eyelid, lacrimal sac and lacrimal caruncle. The long ciliary nerves supply the ciliary body, iris and cornea.

Trigeminal Sensory Pathways

The mandibular, maxillary and ophthalmic nerves carry general sensations of touch, pain and temperature to the trigeminal ganglion, from where the sensations reach the brainstem. The trigeminal sensory tracts pass through three orders of neurons before reaching the face area of the postcentral gyrus.

(From some parts of external ear, cutaneous sensations do not follow the trigeminal nerve. Instead, they are carried in the general somatic afferent fibers of vagus and facial nerves. These sensory fibers are the peripheral processes of the neurons of the geniculate ganglion of facial nerve. The central processes of these first order neurons terminate on the spinal nucleus of trigeminal nerve. In their further course they merge with the trigemino-thalamic tracts).

The trigeminal sensory paths begin in the first order neurons in the trigeminal ganglion. The central processes of these neurons form the sensory root of the trigeminal nerve, which enters the pons to terminate on the second order neurons in the sensory nuclei of the trigeminal nerve (Fig. 125.3). The fibers that terminate on the chief sensory nucleus convey discriminative touch and pressure sensations. The fibers that terminate on the nucleus of spinal tract convey the sensations of pain and temperature. The fibers in the spinal tract show definite arrangement. The ophthalmic fibers are ventrolateral in location and descend to upper two or three cervical segments of spinal cord. The maxillary fibers are posterior to the ophthalmic and descend to the lower limit of medulla oblongata. The mandibular fibers are dorsomedial in position and descend upto the mid-medullary level (obex). The second order neurons give rise to ascending trigeminal tracts as follows:

The axons of the neurons in the nucleus of spinal tract gradually cross to the opposite side to form ventral trigeminal tract, which also receives few axons from the ventral part of the contralateral chief sensory nucleus. The axons from the dorsal part of the chief nucleus ascend in the same side as dorsal trigeminal tract. The ventral and dorsal trigeminal tracts join to form trigeminal lemniscus, which is well-defined in the upper part of the pons. The trigeminal lemniscus ascends through the midbrain to terminate on the third order neurons in the VPM nucleus of the thalamus, which projects via the superior thalamic radiation to the postcentral gyrus in the face area.

Role of Mesencephalic Nucleus

The mesencephalic nucleus is equivalent to the sensory ganglion as its neurons are pseudounipolar. It receives proprioceptive fibers directly from the peripheral receptors (muscle spindles, pressure and joint receptors) from muscles of mastication, extraocular muscles, facial muscles and temporomandibular joints. It projects to the trigeminal motor nucleus of both sides to mediate jaw jerk reflex. This is the only supraspinal monosynaptic reflex. Through the afferent limb of the reflex proprioceptive impulses reach the mesencephalic nucleus, which is connected to the motor nucleus (reflex center). The efferent limb originates in this nucleus and supplies the masseter muscles. Thus both afferent and efferent limbs are contained in sensory and motor parts of mandibular nerve. To elicit the reflex the patient opens the mouth slightly and then the examiner places the index finger on the middle of patient's chin and gently taps it. This results in bilateral contraction of masseter muscles.

Clinical Highlights

The trigeminal neuralgia or tic douloureux is characterized by paroxysms of acute pain in the sensory area of one of the branches of trigeminal nerve on one side. The treatment consists of injecting the trigeminal ganglion with phenol via foramen ovale. In this procedure, there is total sensory loss in the entire trigeminal area. An alternate method is section of the spinal tract, which cuts the fibers carrying pain and temperature but preserves the discriminative touch. This selective tractotomy is possible due to specific arrangement of fibers of the three divisions in the spinal tract.

Abducent Nerve

The abducent nerve is the sixth cranial nerve. It has a long course in the subarachnoid space. Its unique feature is that it is the only cranial nerve, whose nucleus of origin contains two types of neurons (motor and interneurons). The axons of the motor neurons leave the brainstem as the abducent nerve while that of interneurons remain confined to the brainstem. The lesion of the abducent nucleus and that of abducent nerve do not produce same effects.

Functional Component

The abducent nerve contains general somatic efferent type of fibers.

Nucleus of Origin (Fig. 90.5)

The abducent nucleus is located in the lower part of the pons immediately deep to the pontine part of the floor of the fourth ventricle. Its position is indicated by the facial colliculus, produced by the internal genu of the facial nerve. There are two types of neurons in the abducent nucleus (large motor neurons and small para-abducent neurons). The axons of the large typical motor neurons pass in the abducent nerve and supply the lateral rectus muscle of the same side. The axons of the small neurons, which are variously called interneurons or internuclear or para-abducent neurons cross the midline, ascend in the contralateral MLF and terminate upon cells in the oculomotor nucleus, which supply the medial rectus muscle of the opposite side. The abducent nucleus is controlled by PPRF or horizontal gaze center, which almost coexists with it. This is to ensure the simultaneous contraction of the ipsilateral lateral rectus and the contralateral medial rectus muscles. The other connections of the abducent nucleus are the corticonuclear fibers and the MLF.

Intrapontine Course

The axons of the abducent neurons pass anteriorly through the substance of pons lying close to the midline.

Point of Emergence (Fig. 90.1)

The abducent nerve emerges at the pontomedullary junction cranial to the pyramid.

Intracranial Course

The abducent nerve runs upwards, forwards and laterally to pierce the dura mater lateral to the dorsum sellae of the sphenoid. Having reached the upper border of petrous temporal bone, it takes a sharp bend to enter the middle cranial fossa. At the apex of the petrous temporal bone it enters a fibro-osseous canal (Dorello's canal) formed by the apex of petrous temporal and petrosphenoid ligament. Then it enters the cavernous sinus, where it lies close to the floor of the sinus in lateral relation to internal carotid artery (Fig. 85.3). The abducent nerve is vulnerable to compression in conditions of raised intracranial tension due to its long intracranial course and its sharp bend over the petrous temporal bone.

Exit from Cranium

The abducent nerve passes through the medial part of the superior orbital fissure enclosed in the tendinous ring. Here it lies between the two divisions of oculomotor nerve and inferolateral to the nasociliary nerve (Fig 109.1).

Intraorbital Course

Its intraorbital course is very simple as the nerve travels forwards towards the lateral side to enter the ocular surface of the lateral rectus muscle.

Clinical Highlights

a. In unilateral lesion of the abducent nerve or its fibers in the pons, the affected eye is adducted (turned towards the nose) due to paralysis of lateral rectus muscle.
b. Internuclear ophthalmoplegia (or MLF syndrome) results from the lesion of MLF. It causes ipsilateral medial rectus weakness. So, on attempted lateral movement towards the normal side there is weak adduction in the adducting eye and nystagmus in the abducting eye despite the normal lateral rectus muscle (Fig. 90.10).
c. In the lesion of abducent nucleus and adjacent PPRF, there is paralysis of lateral rectus on the side of the lesion accompanied by weakness of contralateral medial rectus. This results in paralysis of horizontal gaze on the side of the lesion.

Facial Nerve

The facial nerve is the seventh cranial nerve. It is the nerve of second branchial arch; hence supplies all the muscles that develop from the mesoderm of the second arch. It is a mixed nerve with a large motor root and a small sensory root (nervus intermedius). The sensory root carries taste sensations from anterior two-third of tongue and cutaneous sensations from the external ear. It also carries secretomotor fibers for submandibular and sublingual salivary glands and the lacrimal gland. So, the sensory root is not purely sensory but a mixed root. A sensory ganglion called geniculate ganglion is located on the trunk of the intrapetrous part of facial nerve.

Functional Components

The facial nerve is mainly composed of four types of fibers.

a. The fibers that take origin from the motor nucleus are called special visceral efferent.
b. The fibers that originate in the superior salivatory nucleus are general visceral efferent.
c. The fibers that terminate on the nucleus of the tractus solitarius are special visceral afferent.
d. A few cutaneous fibers that terminate on the spinal nucleus of trigeminal nerve are general somatic afferent.

Nuclei of Origin (Fig. 90.5)

a. Motor nucleus of facial nerve lies in the lower part of pons medial to the spinal nucleus of trigeminal nerve. Its corticonuclear connections are unique. The neurons in the dorsal group, which innervate muscles in scalp and upper face, receive bilateral corticonuclear fibers. The neurons in the ventral group, which supply muscles of lower face, receive contralateral corticonuclear fibers. Thus, UMN lesions of facial nerve cause contralateral paralysis of lower face, while LMN lesions cause complete ipsilateral facial palsy (Fig. 125.4).
b. Superior salivatory nucleus is divisible into salivatory and lacrimatory nuclei. The axons of the salivatory component of the nucleus are the preganglionic parasympathetic fibers for the submandibular and sublingual salivary glands while those of lacrimatory nucleus are for the lacrimal gland. They leave the pons along with the nervus intermedius.

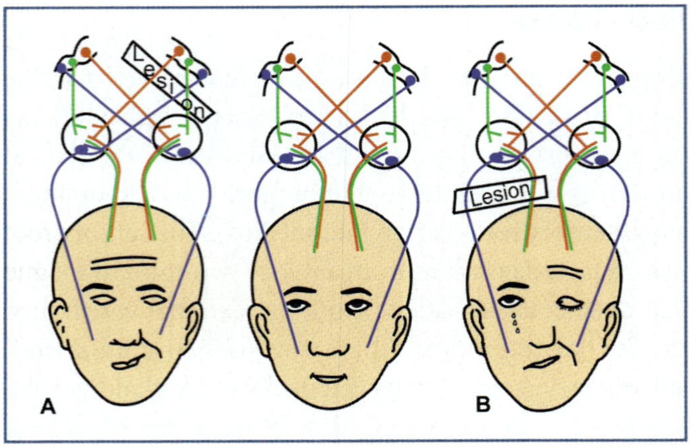

Fig. 125.4: Corticonuclear connections of motor nucleus of facial nerve and effects of UMN and LMN lesions
The central figure depicts that muscles of upper face have bilateral cortical control as against contralateral cortical control of lower face. Figure A depicts UMN lesion resulting in paralysis of lower face on contralateral side. Figure B depicts LMN lesion resulting in paralysis of entire face on ipsilateral side

c. Nucleus of tractus solitarius receives taste fibers from the anterior two-third of tongue.
d. Nucleus of the spinal tract of trigeminal nerve receives a few cutaneous fibers from the external ear.

Intrapontine Course (Fig. 90.5)

The fibers from the motor nucleus pursue an unusual course through the pons. These fibers first turn posteromedially to reach the medial aspect of abducent nucleus. Then the fibers wind round the cranial aspect of the abducent nucleus and bend in infero-lateral direction. The sharp bend around the abducent nucleus is called internal genu of facial nerve and it is indicated on the floor of fourth ventricle by a surface elevation known as facial colliculus. The fibers of the motor nucleus leave the pons by passing in anterior direction between the nucleus of spinal tract of trigeminal nerve and the facial nucleus.

Point of Emergence (Fig. 90.1)

The sensory and motor roots emerge from the lateral aspect of pontomedullary junction. The motor root is larger than the sensory root, which is located in between the auditory nerve and the motor root of facial nerve.

Course through Posterior Cranial Fossa

From the superficial attachment to the brainstem to the opening of internal acoustic meatus, the two roots of the facial nerve pass laterally and forwards in the cerebellopontine angle along with vestibulocochlear nerve and labyrinthine artery. These structures together enter the internal acoustic meatus.

Intrapetrous Course (Fig. 125.5)

The intrapetrous course can be divided into two parts, meatal and in the facial canal. The meatal part is in the internal acoustic meatus, where the motor root is lodged in a groove on the anteroinferior surface of the auditory nerve but the sensory root separates them. At the bottom of the internal acoustic meatus, the two roots unite to form the trunk of facial nerve, which then enters the facial canal. The course of the nerve in the facial canal is subdivided into three segments.

i. The first or labyrinthine segment passes laterally above the vestibule of the inner ear to reach the anterior end of the medial wall of the middle ear near the processus trochleariformis. Here it bends backwards at a sharp turn called external genu of the facial nerve, which has geniculate or sensory ganglion on it.
ii. The second or tympanic segment passes backwards in the medial wall of the middle ear till it reaches the posterior end of this wall. The second segment is also known as horizontal part.

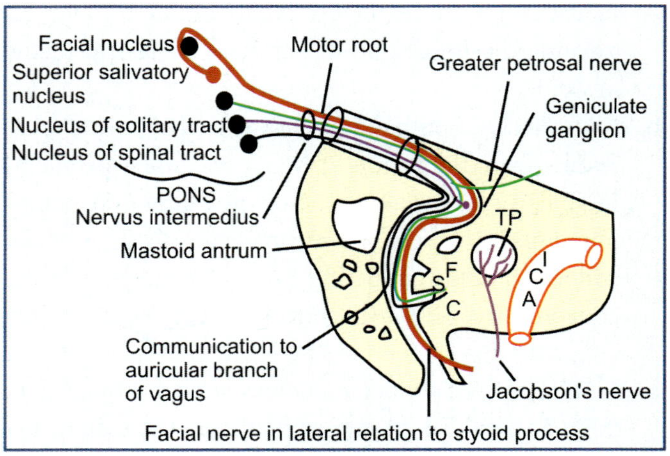

Fig. 125.5: A plan of intrapetrous course, branches and communications of facial nerve (TP–Tympanic plexus, F–Fenestra vestibuli, S–Stapedius, C–Chorda tympani)

iii. The third or mastoid segment begins at the posterior end of the medial wall and passes downwards in relation to the posterior wall of middle ear to reach the stylomastoid foramen. The third segment is known as the vertical segment of the facial nerve.

During its course through the bony facial canal the facial nerve changes direction twice, first at the junction of labyrinthine and tympanic segments (external genu) and second at the junction of tympanic and mastoid segments.

Exit from Cranium

The facial nerve leaves the cranium through stylomastoid foramen, which is located at the base of cranium between the base of styloid process and the mastoid process. Since the mastoid process is absent at birth, the stylomastoid foramen is very close to the skin compared to the adult. The foramen lies at the depth of about 2 cm from the midpoint of anterior border of mastoid process. Hence, facial nerve is vulnerable to injury in newborn.

Extracranial Course (Fig. 60.2)

The extracranial course of the facial nerve is described in Chapter 60.

Branches of Facial Nerve

Location	*Branches of distribution*	*Branches of communication*
Geniculate ganglion		1. Connected to pterygopalatine ganglion by greater petrosal nerve 2. Connected to sympathetic plexus around middle meningeal artery via external petrosal nerve
Facial nerve in facial canal	1. Nerve to stapedius 2. Chorda tympani	To auricular branch of vagus
Just outside stylomastoid foramen	1. Posterior auricular nerve 2. To posterior belly of digastric 3. To stylohyoid muscle	To IX and X cranial nerves
On face	1. Temporal 2. Zygomatic 3. Buccal 4. Marginal mandibular 5. Cervical	To branches of three divisions of trigeminal nerve

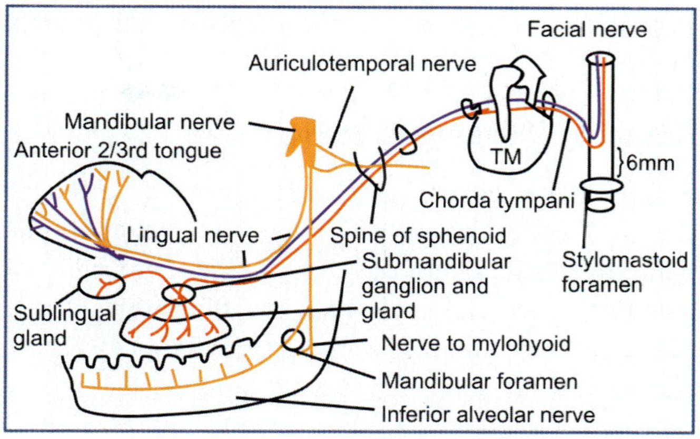

Fig. 125.6: Plan to show course and distribution of chorda tympani nerve (Note: The nerves related to spine of sphenoid)

Chorda Tympani Nerve (Fig. 125.6)

This branch of the facial nerve carries taste sensations from the anterior two-third of the tongue and carries preganglionic secretomotor fibers. The sensory fibers that carry taste sensations are the peripheral processes of the neurons in the geniculate ganglion. The preganglionic fibers are the axons of the neurons in the superior salivary nucleus. Thus, chorda tympani is a mixed nerve. It arises from the vertical segment of the facial nerve about 6 mm above the stylomastoid foramen.

Intrapetrous Course of Chorda Tympani

At first, the nerve ascends in the bony canal to reach the posterior canaliculus, through which it enters the substance of the tympanic membrane. As it proceeds anteriorly, it crosses the incus and the handle of malleus. At the anterior margin of the tympanic membrane, it enters another bony canal called anterior canaliculus, which opens at the medial end of the petrotympanic suture.

Exit from Petrous Temporal Bone

The chorda tympani nerve gains entry into the infratemporal fossa via the medial end of the petrotympanic fissure.

Course through Infratemporal Fossa

At first, the nerve descends lying very close to the medial surface of the spine of the sphenoid bone. Then, it joins the posterior aspect of the lingual nerve at an acute angle. It is very essential to understand that after joining the lingual nerve the chorda tympani loses its independent existence.

Course inside Lingual Nerve

The lingual nerve carries the chorda tympani nerve through the submandibular region, where its preganglionic parasympathetic fibers leave to join the submandibular ganglion. After relay in the ganglion, the postganglionic fibers supply submandibular and sublingual salivary glands. As the lingual nerve reaches the tongue, the chorda tympani supplies the taste buds on the anterior two-thirds of the tongue.

Clinical Highlights

The facial paralysis is a very common clinical condition. It is seen in supranuclear, nuclear and infranuclear lesions.

a. The most common cause of supranuclear lesion (upper motor neuron paralysis) is hemorrhage in the internal capsule (stroke) involving corticonuclear fibers. This results in paralysis of lower part of face and hemiplegia on the contralateral side.
b. The most common cause of the nuclear lesion of the facial nerve is the vascular accident in the pons. This usually involves the adjacent abducent nucleus also. The effects are, ipsilateral lower motor neuron facial paralysis (affecting both upper and lower parts of face), accompanied by internal strabismus. When the pontine lesion includes corticospinal fibers and facial nucleus, it gives rise to Millard-Gubler syndrome (contralateral hemiplegia and ipsilateral facial paralysis).
c. The infranuclear lesion is the one that involves the facial nerve beyond its emergence from the pons. This causes complete facial palsy on the side of the lesion. The infranuclear palsy produces different signs and symptoms depending on the site of lesion.
   i. A lesion in cerebellopontine angle or internal acoustic meatus produces facial paralysis with tinnitus and imbalance due to lesion of vestibulocochlear nerve.
   ii. A lesion at the external genu produces facial paralysis associated with reduced lacrimation, decreased salivary secretion (of submandibular and sublingual glands), loss of taste sensations on the anterior two-thirds of tongue and hyperacusis on the ipsilateral side. Herpes zoster infection of the geniculate ganglion causes Ramsey-Hunt syndrome, which results in facial paralysis accompanied by painful vesicles on external ear.
   iii. A lesion in the medial wall of the middle ear results in ipsilateral facial paralysis accompanied by loss of taste sensation on the anterior two-thirds of tongue and hyperacusis.
   iv. A lesion in the vertical segment of the facial canal causes facial palsy and the loss of taste in anterior two-thirds of tongue on the ipsilateral side.
   v. A lesion at the stylomastoid foramen results in ipsilateral facial paralysis. The term Bell's palsy is synonymous with idiopathic facial palsy (Fig. 125.7). It may be caused by sudden exposure to cold. In Bell's palsy there is loss of horizontal wrinkles on the forehead, inability to close the eye, epiphora, loss of corneal reflex, absence of nasolabial fold, inability to show the teeth. While smiling the angle of mouth on the affected side remains motionless and that of the normal side moves upwards and laterally. All these defects occur due to paralysis of muscles of facial expression.

Vestibulocochlear Nerve

This is the eighth cranial nerve, which is composed of the cochlear and vestibular nerves. Both nerves carry special somatic afferent fibers from the internal ear. The unique feature about the sensory ganglia related to these two nerves is that they contain bipolar neurons unlike the sensory ganglia elsewhere.

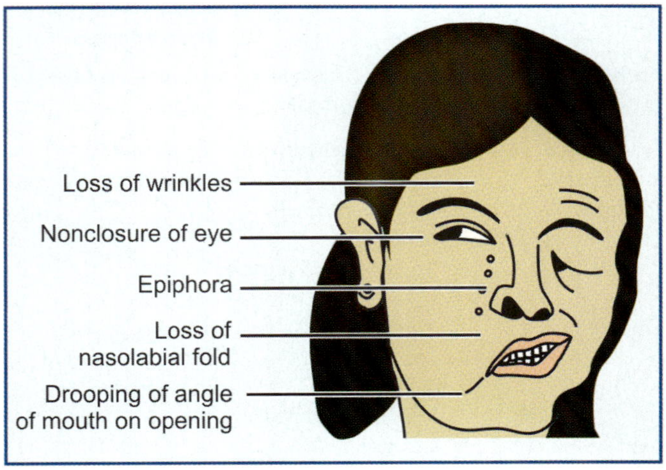

Fig. 125.7: Bell's palsy (right side)

Vestibular Nerve

The vestibular nerve carries sensation of position and movements of head in space from the maculae (static labyrinth) and the cristae (kinetic labyrinth) of the inner ear. The sensory ganglion related to the vestibular nerve is called vestibular or Scarpa's ganglion.

Origin and Intrapetrous Course

The nerve begins in the vestibular ganglion at the lateral end of internal acoustic meatus. The peripheral processes of the bipolar neurons group as three distinct branches namely, superior and inferior divisions and singular nerve. These branches pass through the foramina in the medial end of the internal meatus and supply the ampullary cristae and the maculae. The central processes of the ganglion cells collect to form the trunk of vestibular nerve. In the internal meatus, the vestibular nerve is in close relation to the cochlear nerve, facial nerve and the labyrinthine vessels.

Course through Posterior Cranial Fossa

The vestibular nerve enters the posterior cranial fossa and passes through the cerebellopontine angle to reach the brainstem. It is attached to the brainstem at the pontomedullary junction slightly lateral and posterior to the facial nerve.

Nuclei of Termination

The vestibular nuclear complex consists of superior, inferior, lateral and medial subdivisions. These nuclei occupy the vestibular area in the lateral part of the floor of fourth ventricle. Hence, they are seen in lower part of pons and upper part of medulla. Apart from the vestibular nerve, the nuclei receive cerebellovestibular fibers from flocculus and nodule, spinovestibular fibers and reticulovestibular fibers.

Efferent Connections of Vestibular Nuclei

a. The vestibulocerebellar fibers enter the cerebellum via inferior cerebellar peduncle.
b. The medial longitudinal fasciculus connects the vestibular nuclei to the motor nuclei of third, fourth and sixth cranial nerves. It is through these connections that vestibulo-ocular reflexes are mediated. The anterior horn cells of the cervical spinal cord receive vestibular input from medial vestibular nucleus via medial longitudinal fasciculus for coordination of head, neck and eye muscles.
c. The vestibulospinal tract contains fibers from ipsilateral lateral vestibular nucleus for anterior horn cells of the entire spinal cord. This connection is responsible for extensor muscle tone in antigravity muscles required for maintaining upright posture.

Central Vestibular Path

A few ascending vestibular fibers in the MLF terminate in the VPI (ventral-postero-inferior) and VPL (ventralis posterolateralis) nuclei of thalamus and possibly to pulvinar. The thalamocortical projection is believed to be on the parietal lobe at the junction between intraparietal and postcentral sulci or in the superior temporal gyrus.

Clinical Highlights

Lesion of vestibular nerve results in disequilibrium, vertigo and nystagmus. Vertigo is a feeling of giddiness with a sense of rotation of head. It may occur due to excessive stimulation of semicircular canals and is associated with nystagmus (involuntary and in-coordinated eye movements).

Cochlear Nerve and Auditory Pathway (Fig. 125.8)

The cochlear nerve carries the sound impulses to the cochlear nuclei in brainstem from where the central auditory pathway carries the impulses to the auditory cortex. The cochlear nerve also contains efferent fibers from the superior olivary nucleus to the hair cells of the organ of Corti.

Origin and Intrapetrous Course

The cochlear nerve begins in the spiral ganglion, which is located in spiral canal in the bony modiolus of internal ear. The central processes of the bipolar neurons pass through the tractus spiralis foraminosus at the medial end of the internal acoustic meatus, where they assemble to form the cochlear nerve. Its further course in the internal meatus is similar to that of the vestibular nerve. The dendrites of the bipolar neurons arrange in three groups (inner radial for inner hair cells, basilar for outer hair cells

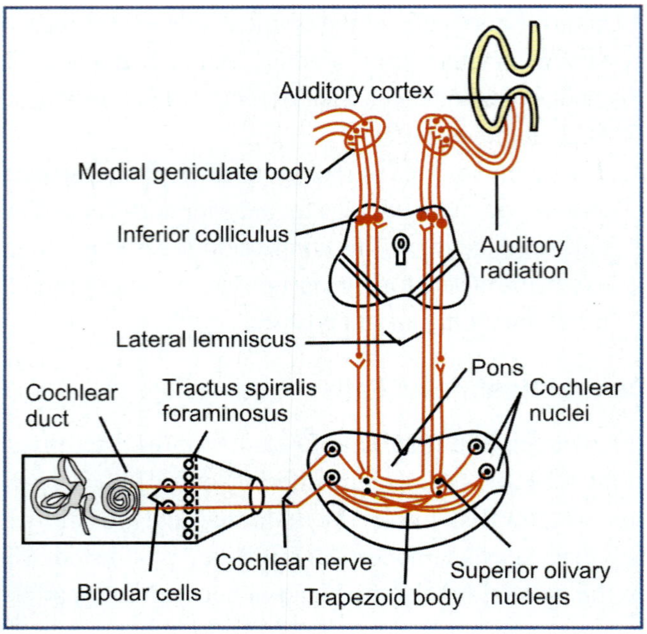

Fig. 125.8: Scheme to show the path of auditory impulse

and outer spiral for outer hair cells). The outer spiral group also contains efferent fibers called olivocochlear fibers from the superior olivary nucleus of both sides (olivocochlear fibers join the cochlear nerve through the anastomosis of Oort with the vestibular nerve in the internal meatus).

Course in Posterior Cranial Fossa

The cochlear nerve (along with the vestibular and facial nerves) passes through the pontocerebellar angle to reach the lateral aspect of pontomedullary junction. It enters the pons and divides into ascending and descending fibers, which terminate in ventral and dorsal nuclei in the floor of the fourth ventricle.

Auditory Pathway

This pathway is unique in having more than three neurons in its course. The bipolar cells of spiral ganglion are the first order neurons. The neurons in the cochlear nuclei are the second order neurons. The superior olivary nucleus (dorsal trapezoid and nucleus of lateral lemniscus) and inferior colliculus contain the third order neurons and the medial geniculate body contains the fourth order neurons.

A large number of axons from the ventral cochlear nuclei decussate with those of the other side to give rise to trapezoid body in the lower pons. The trapezoid body has some scattered nuclei, where a few axons relay. Others terminate in contralateral superior olivary nuclei for relay. A few other axons that do not relay in superior olivary nuclei do so in the nuclei of lateral lemniscus. The uncrossed axons synapse in ipsilateral superior olivary nuclei and then ascend in the lateral lemniscus of the same side. Some axons from ventral cochlear neurons pass dorsally to reach the opposite side as intermediate acoustic striae. In their further course, they probably join contralateral lateral lemniscus. Axons from dorsal cochlear nucleus turn dorsomedially across the midline as dorsal acoustic striae. They ascend in contralateral lateral lemniscus (bypassing superior olivary nuclei) and probably relay in the nuclei of lateral lemniscus. The neurons of the superior olivary complex, trapezoid nuclei, lateral lemniscus nuclei and some neurons of inferior colliculi are regarded as the third order neurons in the auditory path.

Lateral Lemniscus

This fiber tract is the main ascending tract of this pathway. It extends from superior olivary nucleus to the inferior colliculus. It is composed of both crossed and uncrossed fibers, which belong to second and third order neurons. It is connected to the contralateral lateral lemniscus via commissural fibers, through which it receives fibers from the contralateral superior olivary nuclei. A minority of fibers in lateral lemniscus terminates in the inferior colliculus for relay. But the majority passes through the colliculus without relay.

Inferior Colliculus

The inferior colliculi receive auditory input from lateral lemniscus. It is also connected to opposite colliculus. Both relayed and non-relayed fibers project to medial geniculate body through the brachium of inferior colliculus. The structural arrangement of neurons suggests a tonotopic organization between the neuronal layers and cochlear turns. The inferior colliculus is concerned with localization of the source of sound and is the center of auditory reflexes.

Medial Geniculate Body

The medial geniculate body is a part of metathalamus. The neurons show laminar organization. The brachium of inferior colliculus ends in medial geniculate body, which is the highest order neuron to project to the auditory cortex. The higher frequency sound impulses are received medially and the low frequency impulses are received laterally.

Auditory Radiation

The auditory radiation is composed of axons of the neurons of medial geniculate body. It passes through the sublentiform part of internal capsule to reach the auditory cortex.

Auditory Cortex

The primary auditory area is located on transverse temporal gyri of Heschl on the superior aspect of superior temporal gyrus. It is area 41 and 42. It projects to the auditory association area or area 22 on the lateral aspect of superior temporal gyrus. The auditory area receives auditory impulses from both cochlea because auditory fibers travel via ipsilateral and contralateral routes with multiple decussations. Therefore, lesion in auditory cortex of one side (as in thrombosis of middle cerebral artery) will not cause hearing loss.

Glossopharyngeal Nerve

The glossopharyngeal nerve (Fig. 125.9) is the ninth cranial nerve. Developmentally, it is the nerve of the third branchial arch. It contains motor, secretomotor and sensory fibers. Its sensory component is larger than the motor.

Nuclei of Origin

a. Nucleus ambiguus belongs to branchial efferent or special visceral efferent group that supplies the stylopharyngeus muscle.
b. Inferior salivatory nucleus belongs to general visceral efferent group for the secretomotor supply of parotid gland.
c. Nucleus of solitary tract and nucleus of spinal tract of trigeminal nerve receive general visceral afferent fibers from tongue, pharynx, palate, ear and auditory tube.
d. Nucleus of solitary tract also receives special visceral afferent fibers from the taste buds on circumvallate papillae.

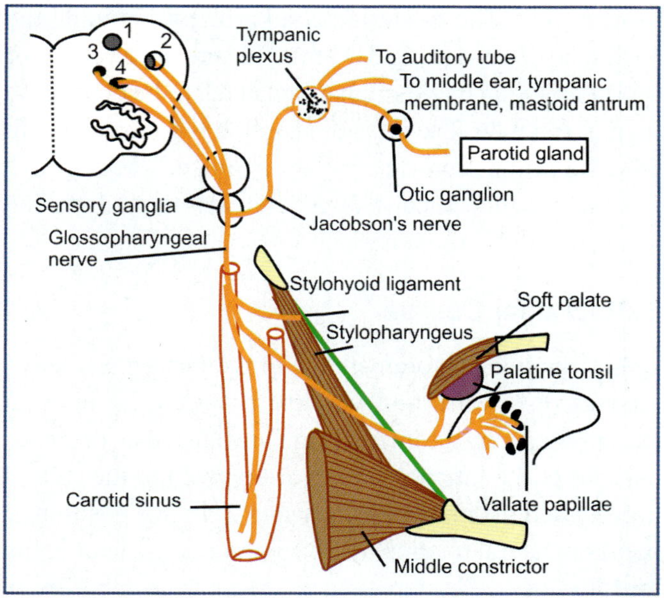

Fig. 125.9: Plan of origin, course and distribution of glossopharyngeal nerve.
(Note: The route of tympanic, muscular, carotid, pharyngeal, lingual and tonsillar branches. 1–Nucleus of tractus solitarius, 2–Spinal nucleus of trigeminal nerve, 3–Inferior salivatory nucleus, 4–Nucleus ambiguus)

Point of Emergence (Fig. 90.1)

The nerve emerges by 4 to 5 rootlets from the medulla oblongata at the upper part of the groove between the olive and inferior cerebellar peduncle.

Course in Posterior Cranial Fossa

From the medulla oblongata, the nerve passes laterally and anteriorly towards the inferior surface of petrous temporal bone. It comes in contact with the jugular tubercle of occipital bone and then turns abruptly down to enter the jugular foramen.

Exit from Cranium

The glossopharyngeal nerve passes through the central part of jugular foramen lying in front of vagus and accessory nerves but in a separate dural sheath.

Relations in Jugular Foramen

The jugular foramen is divided into three compartments. The anterior compartment gives passage to inferior petrosal sinus. The central compartment contains ninth, tenth and eleventh cranial nerves in that order from anterior to posterior. The posterior compartment contains the beginning of internal jugular vein. The superior and inferior sensory ganglia of glossopharyngeal nerve lie on it in the jugular foramen. The inferior ganglion is concerned with taste sensation from the vallate papillae. The superior ganglion is concerned with general sensations from the areas of supply of the nerve.

Extracranial Course

Below the jugular foramen, the glossopharyngeal nerve courses downward and forward between the internal carotid artery and the internal jugular vein. It then descends anterior to the internal carotid artery deep to the styloid process and the muscles attached to it. In this position, it comes in lateral relation of the superior constrictor at the tonsillar fossa. The nerve reaches the posterior border of stylopharyngeus muscle and then follows the muscle on its anterior aspect. The two structures enter the pharynx in the gap between the superior and middle constrictor muscles.

Branches (Fig. 125.9)

a. Tympanic nerve (Jacobson's nerve) is the first branch and leaves the inferior ganglion in the jugular foramen. It is a mixed nerve carrying parasympathetic preganglionic fibers and the general sensory fibers. The tympanic nerve enters a small foramen in the jugular fossa leading into a canal called tympanic canaliculus. Through this canal the tympanic nerve travels in the substance of the petrous temporal bone to reach the middle ear. It forms a tympanic plexus on the surface of promontory of middle ear. The plexus supplies sensory branches to middle ear, lateral part of auditory tube and mastoid antrum and air cells. It gives off a lesser petrosal nerve, which carries the preganglionic fibers. This nerve enters the middle cranial fossa, from where it enters the infratemporal fossa to reach otic ganglion for relay. The postganglionic fibers supply the parotid gland.
b. Carotid branches arise just below the inferior ganglion for the supply to the carotid body and carotid sinus. The carotid body contains chemoreceptors that monitor CO_2, O_2 concentration in blood and the carotid sinus contains baroreceptors that monitor arterial blood pressure.
c. Pharyngeal branches arise in the pharyngeal wall. These filaments form a pharyngeal plexus (in the buccopharyngeal fascia covering the middle constrictor) by uniting with pharyngeal branch of vagus and pharyngeal branch of the sympathetic chain. The sensory supply to the pharyngeal mucosa is provided through the plexus.
d. Muscular branch supplies the stylopharyngeus muscle.
e. Tonsillar branches supply the tonsil, fauces and soft palate.
f. Lingual branches supply the vallate papillae and the mucosa of posterior third of the tongue.

Clinical Highlights

a. For assessing the function of glossopharyngeal nerve it is not possible to test the stylopharyngeus muscle individually. Hence, the general sensations at the posterior wall of pharynx, soft palate and faucial tonsils are tested.
b. The gag reflex or the pharyngeal reflex is elicited by applying stimulus to the posterior pharyngeal wall or soft palate or tonsillar fossa. This results in elevation of pharynx, elevation of palate and retraction of tongue. The afferent limb of this reflex is the glossopharyngeal nerve while efferent limb is the vagus nerve. Thus, gag reflex is lost in lesion of either the ninth or tenth cranial nerve.
c. Glossopharyngeal neuralgia is characterized by intractable episodic pain precipitated by swallowing and felt in throat, behind the angle of jaw and in the ear. Surgical sectioning of the glossopharyngeal nerve (neurectomy) or nerve block relieves the symptoms. The nerve is approached through the tonsillar fossa for this purpose.
d. Injury to glossopharyngeal nerve results in ipsilateral loss of gag reflex, ipsilateral loss of taste from vallate papillae, ipsilateral loss of general sensations in pharynx, soft palate, fauces and posterior third of tongue and ipsilateral loss of salivation from parotid gland. Isolated injury to glossopharyngeal nerve is rare. It is often involved with vagus and accessory nerves in conditions

like, pseudobulbar palsy, bulbar palsy, lateral medullary syndrome and jugular foramen syndrome.

Vagus and Cranial Accessory Nerves

The vagus nerve is the tenth cranial nerve. It is the longest and the most widely distributed cranial nerve. This is a mixed nerve containing both motor and sensory fibers. It has two sensory ganglia (superior or jugular and inferior or nodosum) on its trunk. It is the only cranial nerve that has the thoracic and abdominal distribution. Another interesting feature of the vagus nerve is that it carries the cranial part of accessory nerve in its substance for peripheral distribution. The cranial part of accessory nerve takes origin from the nucleus ambiguus and leaves the medulla oblongata below the vagal roots. It joins the spinal part of the same nerve in the jugular foramen to form the accessory nerve, which divides in spinal and cranial parts just outside the jugular foramen. The cranial part merges with the vagus nerve immediately and is distributed through the vago-accessory complex via the pharyngeal and recurrent laryngeal branches of vagus.

Functional Components

a. The vagus nerve contains branchial efferent or special visceral efferent fibers for the muscles of the soft palate (except tensor palati), pharynx (except stylopharyngeus) and larynx.
b. Its general visceral efferent fibers supply the cardiac muscle, smooth muscle and glands of the digestive tract upto the junction of right two-third and left one-third of transverse colon and smooth muscle and glands of the respiratory tract.
c. It carries general visceral fibers from the viscera.
d. It carries special visceral afferent fibers from the vallecula.
e. It carries general somatic afferent fibers from the skin of the external ear.

Nuclei of Origin

a. Dorsal nucleus of vagus lies below the floor of fourth ventricle in the vagal trigone. It is a mixed nucleus containing both general visceral efferent and general visceral afferent neurons. Its GVE part gives origin to preganglionic parasympathetic fibers, which end on the postganglionic neurons located in the intramural ganglia of the concerned viscera. The GVA part of the dorsal nucleus receives visceral sensations from digestive and respiratory tracts as well as from heart via the central processes of the neurons of its inferior ganglion.
b. Nucleus ambiguus lies deep in the medulla oblongata. It belongs to the special visceral efferent column. It supplies the voluntary muscles developed from fourth and sixth pharyngeal arches. The palatal (except the tensor palati) pharyngeal (except the stylopharyngeus) and laryngeal muscles are supplied by this nucleus. It also supplies the striated muscle of the upper third of esophagus.
c. Nucleus of tractus solitarius receives afferent gustatory fibers from the valleculae of oropharynx and epiglottis via the central processes of the neurons in the inferior ganglion. It belongs to the special visceral afferent column.
d. Nucleus of spinal tract of trigeminal nerve belongs to the general somatic afferent functional column and receives cutaneous sensations from the external ear carried through auricular branch of vagus to the superior ganglion of the vagus nerve. The central processes of the ganglion cells terminate on the spinal nucleus.

Point of Emergence

The vagus nerve emerges from the medulla oblongata by 10-12 roots is series with the cranial part of accessory nerve and glossopharyngeal nerve in the sulcus between the olive and inferior cerebellar peduncle.

Course through Posterior Cranial Fossa

The vagal roots unite to form a flat nerve trunk, which passes below the flocculus of cerebellum along with the cranial accessory nerve towards the jugular foramen. The tenth and eleventh cranial nerves are inside the common dural and arachnoid sheath.

Exit from Cranium

The vagus nerve leaves through the jugular foramen in the intermediate compartment. The relations of the structures in jugular foramen from before backwards are, inferior petrosal sinus, glossopharyngeal nerve, vagus and accessory nerves and internal jugular vein.

Sensory Ganglia

The vagus nerve bears a pair of ganglia on its trunk. The superior or jugular ganglion is located in the jugular foramen. The inferior or nodose ganglion lies just below the jugular foramen. The afferent fibers carried in the vagus nerve, terminate on the pseudounipolar neurons in these ganglia.

Superior Ganglion

a. The auricular branch of vagus, which arises from the superior ganglion, brings general somatic sensations from the external ear to the ganglion cells. The central processes of the ganglion cells end on nucleus of spinal tract of trigeminal nerve. The auricular branch is known as Alderman's nerve. It gives a few twigs to the cranial surface of the auricle, the external acoustic meatus and the posteroinferior part of the lateral surface of the tympanic membrane. Stimulation of auricular branch of vagus, for example, while syringing the ear or by earwax, may cause ear cough, vomiting and giddiness. This branch may receive cutaneous fibers from the facial nerve in the mastoid canaliculus. In such situations, the herpes zoster of geniculate ganglion of facial nerve will give rise to blisters in the cutaneous area of vagus nerve.
b. Meningeal branches arise from superior ganglion and enter the posterior cranial fossa. They supply somatic sensory fibers (C1 and C2 spinal nerves) and sympathetic fibers to the dura mater of posterior cranial fossa. C1 and C2 fibers reach the ganglia through communicating branches to the upper two cervical nerves.

Inferior Ganglion

The general visceral afferent fibers from heart, respiratory tract and lungs, digestive tract from pharynx upto the junction of right two-third and left one-third of transverse colon are the peripheral processes of the neurons in the inferior ganglion. The central processes of these neurons end in dorsal nucleus of vagus. The taste fibers from vallecula and epiglottis also are the peripheral processes of the neurons in the ganglion. The central processes of these neurons end on nucleus of tractus solitarius.

Extracranial Course

The extracranial course is divided into three parts, cervical, thoracic and abdominal.

Cervical Course

The vagus nerve descends vertically in the carotid sheath. It lies between the internal carotid artery and internal jugular vein but on a slightly posterior plane upto the level of superior margin of thyroid cartilage. Below this level it lies between the common carotid artery and the internal jugular vein. At the root of the neck, it comes out of the carotid sheath.

Branches of Cervical Part

a. Pharyngeal branch is the first to arise just below the inferior ganglion. It carries cranial accessory fibers in it. It takes part in pharyngeal plexus, through which it supplies the pharyngeal muscles (except stylopharyngeus) and palatine muscles (except tensor palati).
b. Superior laryngeal nerve arises just below the pharyngeal branch. It soon divides in internal and external laryngeal nerves. The external laryngeal nerve supplies the cricothyroid and inferior constrictor of pharynx. The internal laryngeal nerve is sensory to the mucosa of larynx above the vocal folds.
c. A small twig supplies the carotid body.
d. Superior and inferior cervical cardiac branches enter the thorax through the thoracic inlet. The inferior cervical cardiac branch of left vagus takes part in superficial cardiac plexus while the other three cervical cardiac branches end in the deep cardiac plexus.
e. Right recurrent laryngeal nerve originates from the right vagus anterior to the first part of subclavian artery. It winds round the artery to occupy the groove between the trachea and esophagus. The recurrent laryngeal nerve is in close relation to the medial surface of thyroid gland. Its relation to inferior thyroid artery is of surgical importance. The recurrent laryngeal nerve supplies all the intrinsic laryngeal muscles except cricothyroid. It sends motor twigs to the inferior constrictor muscle and cardiac filaments to deep cardiac plexus. It is sensory to laryngeal mucosa below the vocal folds. The nonrecurrent right recurrent laryngeal nerve is a variation in, which the right recurrent laryngeal nerve arises from the right vagus higher up near the thyroid

cartilage. This results from developmental anomaly of the right subclavian artery called aberrant right subclavian artery. In this anomaly, the right subclavian artery is a branch of the arch of aorta.

Entry in Thorax

The vagus nerves enter the thorax by passing through the thoracic inlet. The right vagus nerve crosses in front of the first part of subclavian artery but behind the internal jugular vein. The left vagus nerve enters the thorax between the left subclavian and left common carotid arteries but behind the left brachiocephalic vein.

Relations of Right Vagus Nerve in Thorax

The right vagus nerve courses first through the superior mediastinum. It passes downwards posterior to the right brachiocephalic vein and the superior vena cava and in contact with the right surface of trachea. The mediastinal surface of right lung and pleura are lateral to it. At the level of sternal angle, the azygos vein lies laterally. To enter the posterior mediastinum, the nerve passes behind the right principal bronchus and reaches the posterior aspect of right pulmonary hilum, where it breaks up to form posterior pulmonary plexus by uniting with the sympathetic fibers from upper thoracic ganglia. At the lower end of the pulmonary hilum, 2-3 branches arise from the plexus to reach the posterior aspect of esophagus. Here these branches of right side meet a branch from left vagus to form posterior esophageal plexus. The posterior vagal trunk arising from the oesophageal plexus descends posterior to the esophagus to enter the abdomen through the esophageal opening in diaphragm.

Branches of Right Vagus Nerve in Thorax

a. Cardiac branches take part in deep cardiac plexus.
b. Pulmonary branches supply lung, trachea and bronchial tree through the pulmonary plexus.
c. Esophageal branches supply esophagus through the plexuses.

Relations of Left Vagus Nerve in Thorax

The left vagus nerve passes through the superior mediastinum lying between the left subclavian artery and left common carotid artery. It is crossed anteriorly from lateral to medial side by the left phrenic nerve. It is in relation to the left surface of the arch of aorta. At the posterior aspect of the hilum of the left lung, the vagus nerve divides into branches, which take part in the formation of left posterior pulmonary plexus along with the sympathetic fibers from upper thoracic ganglia. Two branches descend from the lower end of the pulmonary plexus and unite with a branch from right vagus nerve on the anterior aspect of the esophagus to form anterior esophageal plexus. The anterior vagal trunk originates from the esophageal plexus and it travels on the anterior surface of esophagus to enter the abdomen through the esophageal opening of diaphragm.

Branches of Left Vagus Nerve in Thorax

a. Left recurrent laryngeal nerve is longer than the right since it takes origin in the thorax as the left vagus crosses the left side of the arch of aorta. It winds round the ligamentum arteriosum near the inferior aspect of arch of aorta. It ascends in relation to right and posterior surface of arch of aorta lying in a groove between the trachea and esophagus. Its cervical course and distribution are similar to that of right side. The left recurrent laryngeal nerve is liable for damage in thorax if compressed by aneurysm of aorta or enlarged left atrium or bronchogenic carcinoma.
b. The vagus nerve gives the cardiac, pulmonary and esophageal branches.

Abdominal Course

The anterior vagal trunk travels in contact with the muscular wall of abdominal esophagus, whereas the posterior vagal trunk lies in loose tissue a little behind the esophagus. The anterior trunk may be double but the posterior one is rarely so. The anterior trunk contains mostly the fibers of left vagus while the posterior trunk contains the fibers of right vagus.

a. The first branch of the anterior vagal trunk is the hepatic branch, which supplies the liver, biliary apparatus and duodenum through the hepatic plexus along the hepatic artery. Then the main trunk (now called anterior nerve of Latarjet) passes parallel to lesser curvature (at a distance of 1 cm) into the lesser omentum. Gastric branches leave the nerve of Latarjet at right angles to it and enter the stomach to supply its anterosuperior surface. At the incisura, the main trunk terminates as a cluster of branches called the crow's foot to supply the pyloric antrum and pylorus (Fig. 133.7).

b. The posterior trunk sends major branch to the celiac plexus, which supplies the digestive tract upto the junction of right two-thirds and left one-third of transverse colon and other viscera of the abdomen like kidneys, pancreas, etc. Another important branch arising high up (known as criminal nerve of Grasse) is for the fundus of stomach. This branch may arise in thorax and enter the abdomen along with the main nerve. Failure to recognize and divide this branch may lead to incomplete vagotomy during the operation of parietal cell vagotomy. The main continuation of the posterior vagal trunk after the origin of celiac branch is called the posterior nerve of Latarjet. It runs along the lesser curvature and supplies gastric branches to the posteroinferior surface of stomach.

Clinical Highlights

Effects of unilateral complete section of vagus nerve are as follows:

a. Unilateral paralysis of soft palate muscles (except tensor palati) results in lowering of the palate on affected side and on phonation the palate fails to elevate. The uvula moves to the normal side. There is unilateral loss of palatal reflex (normally touching the palate evokes its elevation). There is nasal voice and nasal regurgitation of food.
b. Unilateral paralysis of pharyngeal muscles leads to deviation of the posterior pharyngeal wall, on phonation, to the normal side. The paralyzed side moves like a sliding curtain towards the normal side and this is referred to as "curtain effect".
c. There is ipsilateral loss of gag reflex (normally, touching one side of the pharyngeal wall with a swab stick evokes its contraction and elevation of the posterior one-third of the tongue resulting in a feeling to vomit).
d. There is unilateral loss of sensations in the pharyngeal mucosa.
e. All laryngeal muscles are paralyzed. The vocal cord on the affected side lies in cadaveric position. There is ipsilateral loss of sensations in the laryngeal mucosa.

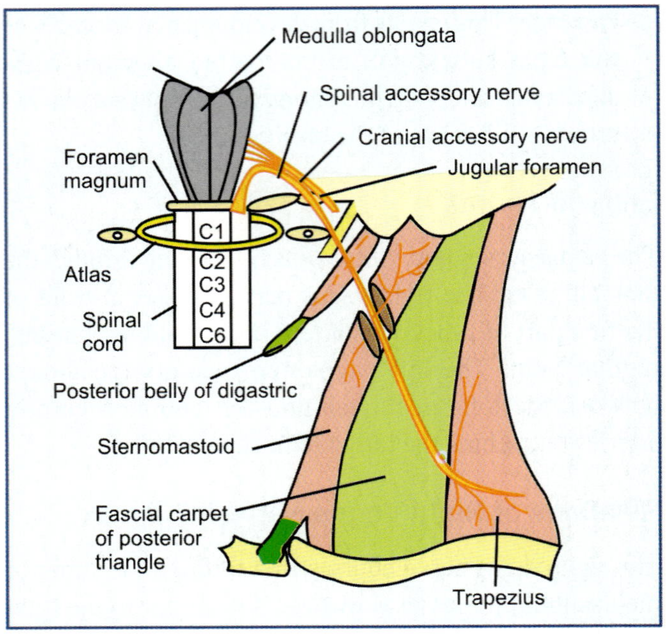

Fig. 125.10: A plan of origin, course and distribution of spinal accessory nerve (Note that after exit from cranium spinal accessory nerve crosses in front of transverse process of atlas and behind styloid process and posterior belly of digastric. The lesser occipital nerve hooks round the spinal accessory in posterior triangle

Spinal Accessory Nerve (Fig. 125.10)

The spinal accessory nerve arises from ventral horns of C1 to C5 segments of the spinal cord by separate rootlets midway between the attachments of the cervical ventral and dorsal rootlets. The rootlets join to form the nerve, which ascends in the cervical vertebral canal and enters the cranium through the foramen magnum. In the posterior cranial fossa, the spinal accessory nerve joins the cranial root to form the trunk of the accessory nerve near the jugular foramen. The nerve trunk leaves through the middle compartment of the jugular foramen to immediately divide into the spinal and cranial parts at the base of the cranium.

Extracranial Course

At first, the spinal accessory nerve travels in posterolateral direction to come in anterior relation to the tip of the transverse process of the atlas. From here the nerve descends in posterior direction deep to the styloid process, stylohyoid muscle and posterior belly of digastric. It passes through the upper part of the carotid triangle and then enters the substance of the sternomastoid muscle, to which it gives branches. The nerve enters the posterior triangle around the midpoint of the posterior margin of the sternomastoid. At this point, the lesser occipital nerve hooks round the accessory nerve to turn in the upward direction and the accessory nerve is surrounded by superficial cervical lymph nodes. The spinal accessory nerve descends in the posterior triangle from medial to lateral side between the fascial floor and roof, but lying adherent to the roof. It enters the trapezius about 5 cm above the clavicle and travels towards the back lying plastered to the deep surface of the trapezius and along with the superficial branch of the transverse cervical artery. It gives branches to the trapezius.

Surface Marking

The first point is marked in front of the tragus. The second point lies midway between the mastoid process and the angle of mandible. The third point is at the midpoint of the posterior margin of sternomastoid. The fourth point is on the anterior margin of trapezius about 5 cm above the clavicle. A line joining the four points represents the extracranial part of accessory nerve.

Clinical Highlights

a. The spinal accessory nerve may be injured during operations on the neck or in penetrating injury to the neck. It results in the paralysis of the trapezius and sternomastoid muscles.
b. The functions of trapezius and sternomastoid muscles are tested to assess the integrity of this nerve.

Hypoglossal Nerve (Fig. 125.11)

The hypoglossal nerve is the twelfth cranial nerve. It is a purely motor nerve. It has only one functional component (general somatic efferent). It supplies the lingual muscles developed from occipital myotomes (all intrinsic muscles and all extrinsic muscles of tongue except palatoglossus).

Nucleus of Origin

The hypoglossal nucleus lies in the inferior half of the floor of fourth ventricle subjacent to the hypoglossal trigone (Fig. 92.3). It receives contralateral corticonucler connections.

Intramedullary Course

After emerging from the nucleus, the hypoglossal fibers traverse anteriorly in the reticular formation of medulla oblongata lying in lateral relation to the medial lemniscus. Near the anterior end of medial lemniscus, the nerve fibers turn laterally between the pyramid and inferior olivary nucleus.

Point of Emergence (Fig. 90.1)

The hypoglossal nerve emerges as a series of rootlets from the sulcus between the pyramid and olive.

Course inside Posterior Cranial Fossa

The rootlets of the hypoglossal nerve run laterally posterior to the vertebral artery and collect in two bundles, which perforate the dura mater separately near the anterior condylar or hypoglossal canal in the occipital bone.

Exit from Cranium

The two bundles unite in the anterior condylar canal and leave the posterior cranial fossa through it.

Extracranial Course

a. At the base of cranium the hypoglossal nerve lies medial to the internal carotid artery and to the structures

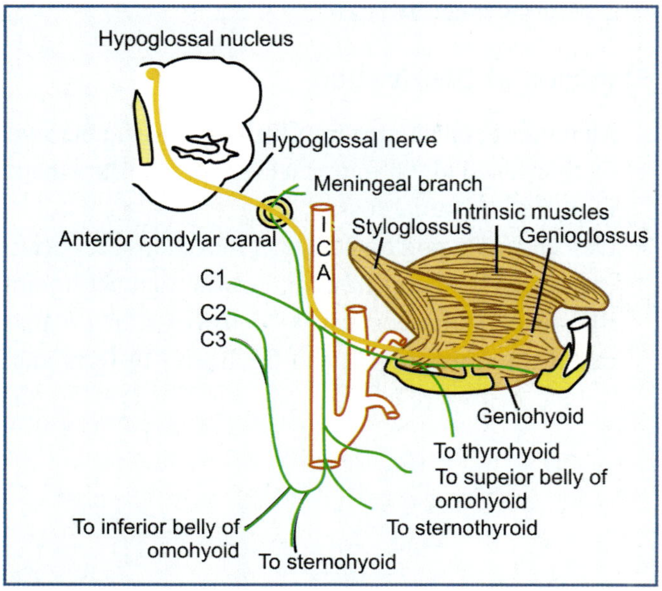

Fig. 125.11: Plan of origin, course, communications and distribution of hypoglossal nerve (Note: The formation of ansa cervicalis from C1 to C3 nerves)

passing through the jugular foramen. It inclines laterally to pass behind the internal carotid artery and the ninth and tenth cranial nerves. It spirals around the lateral aspect of inferior ganglion of the vagus to lie in front of the vagus nerve (outside the carotid sheath). Then it passes vertically downward medial to the posterior belly of digastric. At the level of angle of mandible it passes deep to the posterior belly of digastric and turns forward to enter the carotid triangle.

b. In the carotid triangle it crosses first the internal carotid artery and then the external carotid artery. It crosses the loop of the lingual artery just above the tip of greater cornua of hyoid bone. Here the hypoglossal nerve is quite superficial. It enters the digastric triangle by passing deep to intermediate tendon of digastric and stylohyoid muscle.

c. In the digastric triangle (submandibular region) the nerve crosses the hyoglossus muscle on its superficial aspect (Fig. 112.2). Here the hypoglossal nerve lies below the submandibular duct and the deep part of submandibular gland and then passes deep to mylohyoid to pierce the genioglossus and enter the substance of the tongue.

Branches of Communication

It receives a large communication from the ventral ramus of first cervical nerve.

Branches of Distribution

a. Meningeal branch carrying C1 fibers arises at the level of anterior condylar foramen to supply the dura mater of posterior cranial fossa.

b. Descendens hypoglossi or upper root of ansa cervicalis (carrying C1 fibers) arises in carotid triangle. It joins the descendens cervicalis or lower root of ansa cervicalis (carrying C2 and C3 fibers) to form ansa cervicalis, which supplies the sternohyoid, sternothyroid and the two bellies of the omohyoid muscles.

c. Nerve to thyrohyoid carrying C1 fibers.

d. Nerve to geniohyoid carrying C1 fibers.

e. Terminal branches supply all intrinsic muscles and the three extrinsic muscles (styloglossus, hyoglossus and genioglossus).

Clinical Highlights

a. To test the integrity of hypoglossal nerve the function of genioglossi is assessed. The subject is asked to protrude the tongue. If the hypoglossal nerves are intact the protruded tongue lies in the midline.

b. Unilateral lower motor neuron lesion of hypoglossal nucleus or of the nerve causes unilateral paralysis of tongue. The protruded tongue deviates to the side of the lesion.

c. In bilateral lesion of hypoglossal nerve, the tongue lies motionless causing difficulty in speech and swallowing.

d. In upper motor neuron lesion of hypoglossal nerve (lesion of corticonuclear fibers in the genu of internal capsule), the nucleus is normal but there is paralysis of the muscles of the side opposite to that of the lesion. Hence, on protrusion the tongue deviates opposite to side of the lesion.

e. Medial medullary syndrome consists of unilateral lesion of hypoglossal nucleus, medial lemniscus and pyramid. It is characterized by ipsilateral paralysis of the tongue, contralateral hemiplegia and contralateral loss of conscious proprioception.

f. Lesser's triangle is the triangular space bounded by hypoglossal nerve and anterior and posterior bellies of digastric muscles. The lingual artery lies deep to this space. This is the preferred site to ligate the artery by removing fibers of hyoglossus from the hyoid bone during hemiglossectomy or hemimandibulectomy.

126 Clinicoanatomical Problems and Solutions

CASE 1

A patient presented with a red, swollen and painful right eye accompanied by high temperature. Because the movements of the right eye were painful, the doctor could not test the muscles of that eye. The pupil in the right eye was fixed and dilated. CT scan showed thrombosis in cavernous sinus.

Questions

a. What is the location of the cavernous sinus?
b. Draw a diagram to show the nerves in relation to the cavernous sinus.
c. Draw a diagram to show the communication of this sinus with the dangerous area of the face.
d. Name the dural venous sinuses, which are the tributaries of the cavernous sinus and which are the draining channels.
e. Name the cerebral vein, which is a direct tributary of the cavernous sinus.
f. Dilated and fixed pupil is suggestive of involvement of which cranial nerve.
g. Describe the nuclei of origin, course and distribution of this nerve to the extraocular and intraocular muscles.
h. Name the condition of this sinus, which results in pulsatile exophthalmos.

Solutions

a. The cavernous sinus is located in the middle cranial fossa on either side of the body of the sphenoid.
b. Refer to Figure 85.3
c. Refer to Figure 85.4
d. Sphenoparietal sinus and middle meningeal sinus are the tributaries. The superior and inferior petrosal sinuses are the draining channels.
e. Superficial middle cerebral vein is the direct tributary of the sinus.
f. Dilated and fixed pupil is suggestive of involvement of oculomotor nerve.
g. Refer to oculomotor nerve in Chapter 125.
h. Arteriovenous fistula or carotid-cavernous fistula.

CASE 2

On ophthalmoscopic examination it was noted that a 47-year-old man was having edema of both optic discs (papilledema) and congestion of retinal veins. CT scan of head showed a large intracranial tumor.

Questions

a. Explain the presence of papilledema in this case.
b. Give the development of retina and optic nerve.
c. Give the length of optic nerve, its parts and arterial supply.
d. Draw a diagram of the visual pathway.
e. Write a brief note on optic disc.
f. Draw a diagram of the microscopic structure of retina.
g. Name the neurons in the retina.

Solutions

a. Since the optic nerve is surrounded by the pia mater, arachnoid mater and dura mater the intracranial subarachnoid space also surrounds it upto its entry in to the eyeball. Rise in intracranial pressure due to intracranial tumor will compress the optic nerve and the central retinal vein as it enters the subarachnoid space. This is the cause of venous congestion and papilledema.

b. The retina develops from optic cup and the optic nerve from optic stalk of the optic cup (derived from diencephalon).
c. Optic nerve is 4 cm in length. It consists of intraorbital part (supplied by posterior ciliary artery and central artery of retina), canalicular part (supplied by ophthalmic artery) and intracranial part (supplied by superior hypophyseal artery).
d. Refer to optic nerve in Chapter 125.
e. Optic disc is a circular pale area visible on the retina on ophthalmoscopic (fundus) examination. It is situated medial and superior to the posterior pole of the eyeball. The optic nerve begins at the optic disc. It is devoid of rods and cones hence it is called the blind spot of the eye. The disc presents a depression in the centre called physiological cup. The central artery of retina enters the retina at the centre of the disc and the central vein emerges at the same point. The edema of the disc is known as choked disc or papilledema. It occurs in raised intracranial tension, in which central vein of retina undergoes compression.
f. Refer to Chapter 110 on Eyeball.
g. The neurons in the retina are bipolar cells, ganglion cells, amacrine and horizontal cells.

CASE 3

A 52-year-old man and a chronic smoker came to the ENT consultant with complaints of recurrent sinusitis, weight loss and severe pain in upper teeth and right half of face. On examination, it was noted that the right cheek was swollen and there was proptosis of right eye. Transillumination test of maxillary sinus showed opacity. CT scan confirmed presence of growth in the sinus.

Questions

a. What is the probable diagnosis?
b. Name the regions invaded if the growth in the maxillary sinus spreads anteriorly, medially, posteriorly and upwards.
c. Draw a labelled diagram to show the nerves closely related to the sinus.
d. Comment on the opening of the maxillary air sinus.
e. Which route is used for antral puncture for drainage of pus from this sinus?
f. Draw a diagram of lateral wall of nasal cavity to show the location of openings of all the paranasal sinuses.
g. Which paranasal air sinus is not present at birth?

Solutions

a. Carcinoma of maxillary air sinus.
b. If the growth spreads anteriorly, it will invade the soft tissues of the cheek. If it spreads medially, it will invade the nasal cavity. Posterior spread leads to infiltration into infratemporal and sphenopalatine fossae and upward spread leads to infiltration into orbit.
c. Refer to Chapter 106.
d. The maxillary sinus opens in the hiatus semilunaris of the middle meatus of the nasal cavity by an opening that is located high up on its medial wall. So, it does not favor natural drainage. Moreover, the position of the opening of maxillary sinus in hiatus semilunaris compared to opening of the frontal sinus favors drainage from the frontal to the maxillary sinus. This is the reason maxillary sinus is described as reservoir of frontal sinus.
e. Accumulation of pus in the maxillary sinus is drained by a method called antral puncture, which is done through the inferior meatus.
f. Refer to Chapter 114 on Nasal Cavity.
g. Frontal air sinus is not present at birth.

CASE 4

A man developed painful vesicles in the area of distribution of ophthalmic division of the trigeminal nerve due to herpes zoster (shingles).

Questions

a. Which neurons show inflammation in herpes zoster of ophthalmic nerve?
b. Where does the ophthalmic nerve begin?
c. Where does the ophthalmic nerve divide? Name its terminal branches.
d. Draw a diagram of the superior orbital fissure to show the location of the three terminal branches.

e. Which of the terminal branches of the ophthalmic nerve crosses the optic nerve in the orbit?
f. Describe the course and distribution of this terminal branch.
g. Which nerves supply the tip of nose?
h. Give the nerve supply of the cornea.

Solutions

a. Pseudounipolar neurons in the trigeminal ganglion are involved in herpes zoster.
b. The ophthalmic nerve begins in the trigeminal ganglion in the middle cranial fossa.
c. The ophthalmic nerve courses in the lateral wall of the cavernous sinus, where it divides into nasociliary, frontal and lacrimal nerves.
d. Refer to Chapter 109 (Fig. 109.1)
e. Nasociliary nerve crosses the optic nerve in the orbit.
f. Refer to Chapter 109.
g. External nasal branches of anterior ethmoidal nerves.
h. The cornea receives rich supply from long ciliary branches of nasociliary nerve.

CASE 5

On speculum examination, it was noted that the external acoustic meatus (ear canal) was full of wax in a patient. While syringing the ear to remove the wax, the patient felt giddiness. His pulse rate was low.

Questions

a. Name the glands that secrete earwax.
b. Name the parts and the length of the external acoustic meatus.
c. Give the nerve supply of the auricle and of the external acoustic meatus
d. Correlate bradycardia with syringing of meatus.
e. Mention the developmental source of the external meatus.

Solutions

a. Ceruminous glands of external meatus are modified sweat glands.
b. The parts of external acoustic meatus are, lateral cartilaginous and medial bony. Its total length is 24 mm, out of which cartilaginous is 8 mm and bony is 16 mm in length.
c. The lateral surface of the auricle receives nerve supply from great auricular nerve, auriculotemporal nerve and a small area in the concha by auricular branch of vagus nerve. The cranial surface receives nerve supply from the great auricular and lesser occipital nerve.

   The external acoustic meatus receives branches from auriculotemporal nerve and from auricular branch of vagus.
d. Syringing the external meatus stimulates the auricular branch of the vagus (Alderman's nerve) and vagus is cardioinhibitory
f. The ectoderm of the first cleft of pharyngeal arches gives rise to external meatus.

CASE 6

A 10-year-old boy came to the hospital with a history of recurrent attacks of sore throat. On inspection of the oropharynx, the palatine tonsils almost touched each other in the midline.

Questions

a. What is crypta magna and its developmental significance?
b. Name the main structures forming tonsillar bed.
c. Draw a diagram of the arterial supply of the tonsil
d. Which is the tonsillar lymph node?
e. Draw a diagram of Waldeyer's ring.
f. Why is the medial surface of the tonsil pitted?
g. Write briefly on peritonsillar space.

Solutions

a. A deep tonsillar crypt located near the upper pole is known as crypta magna or intratonsillar cleft. It is the remnant of second pharyngeal pouch.
b. The pharyngobasilar fascia, superior constrictor muscle and the buccopharyngeal fascia form the bed of the tonsil.
c. Refer to Figure 116.4.
d. The jugulo-digastric lymph nodes are called tonsillar nodes.
e. Refer to Figure 116.5.
g. The epithelium of the medial surface dips in the substance of the tonsil as tonsillar crypts. The openings

of about 15 to 20 crypts on the medial surface are responsible for pitted appearance.

h. The submucosa in relation to the lateral surface of tonsil is known as peritonsillar space since it is filled with loose areolar tissue. It separates the tonsillar hemicapsule from the tonsillar bed. Paratonsillar vein passes through this space. Since this space provides a plane of dissection during tonsillectomy (surgical removal of tonsil) the paratonsillar vein is likely to be injured causing postoperative bleeding. Pus accumulates in this space in chronic tonsillitis resulting in abscess formation, which is known as peritonsillar abscess or quinsy.

CASE 7

A student yawned widely during afternoon anatomy lecture class. To his dismay he could not close it. His jaw was stuck.

Questions

a. Name the joint that is dislocated.
b. Give the type of this joint and name the bones taking part in it.
b. Which bone is mobile in this articulation?
c. Name the parts of the articular disc and the muscle attached to the disc.
d. Name the movements of the joint and the muscles responsible for them.
e. Which part of the ear is a close relation of the joint?
f. How is the anterior dislocation of the TMJ reduced?

Solutions

a. Temporomandibular joint
b. Bicondylar type of synovial joint. Bones taking part in it are the condyle of the mandible and the mandibular fossa of squamous temporal bone.
c. Mandible is mobile
d. From anterior to posterior the parts are, anterior extension, anterior thick band, intermediate zone, posterior thick band and bilaminar zone. The lateral pterygoid muscle is inserted in to it.
d. Elevation and depression (opening the mouth), protraction and retraction and chewing or side-to-side movements. For muscles refer to Chapter 108.
e. Bony part of external acoustic meatus.
f. The mandible is depressed posteriorly by exerting pressure on lower molar teeth with the help of both thumbs. This will overcome the spasm of pterygoid muscles. Simultaneously the assistant elevates the chin so that head of mandible is pushed in the fossa.

CASE 8

A 4-year-old-child swallowed a shirt button. Since the child began to suffocate she was rushed to the hospital, where on X-ray examination, impaction of foreign body in the larynx was confirmed.

Questions

a. Which is the narrowest part of laryngeal cavity?
b. Give the attachments and contents of the vocal folds.
c. What is the color of the vocal folds?
d. Name the parts of rima glottis.
e. Which muscle is called the safety muscle of larynx and why?
f. Enumerate the differences in the adult and infant larynx.
g. Name the emergency operation for restoring the airway in case of blocked glottis.
h. Which anatomical layers in the midline of neck are encountered during surgical approach to trachea?

Solutions

a. Rima glottis is the narrowest part of laryngeal cavity.
b. The vocal folds extend from the vocal process of arytenoid to inner surface of the middle of thyroid angle. Each fold contains vocal ligament and vocalis muscle.
c. The color of the vocal folds is pearly white.
d. The parts of rima glottis are, anterior three-fifth, intermembranous and posterior two-fifth, intercartilaginous.
e. Posterior cricoarytenoid muscle is the safety muscle of the larynx. It is so called because being the only abductor of the vocal folds it keeps the rima glottis open to allow air to enter the lungs.
f. Refer to Chapter 117.
g. Tracheostomy
h. Skin, superficial fascia with platysma, investing layer of deep fascia, infrahyoid group of strap muscles and

pretracheal fascia are encountered in succession from superficial to deep.

CASE 9

An ENT surgeon performed an operation of radical mastoidectomy on right side in a patient. Postoperatively the patient complained of inability to close the right eye, drooling of saliva from right angle of mouth, excessive tears in right eye and loss of taste sensation.

Examination revealed loss of horizontal wrinkles on right half of forehead on raising the eyebrow, loss of right nasolabial fold, deviation of angle of mouth to left on talking, loss of taste sensation on anterior 2/3rd of tongue, presence of epiphora and no hyperacusis.

Questions

a. Name the nerve that is injured giving approximate site of injury.
b. Mention whether it is LMN or a UMN lesion with reason.
c. Name the nuclei of this nerve giving their functional classification.
d. How does this nerve leave the cranium?
e. Mention its intracranial branches.
f. Identify the intracranial branch that is involved giving reason for identification.
g. What is the reason for loss of wrinkles on forehead?
h. Paralysis of which muscle results in inability to close right eye?
i. Describe the extracranial course and distribution of the affected nerve.

Solutions

a. Facial nerve in intrapetrous course just proximal to the origin of chorda tympani branch.
b. It is lower motor neuron lesion (LMN) because there is paralysis of entire face on the side of the lesion.
c. For nuclei, refer to facial nerve in Chapter 125.
d. Facial nerve leaves the cranium via stylomastoid foramen.
e. During its intrapetrous course, the facial nerve gives off greater petrosal nerve from the geniculate ganglion, nerve to stapedius and chorda tympani from its vertical segment.
f. Chorda tympani branch is affected because there is loss of taste sensation from anterior two-thirds of tongue.
g. Loss of wrinkles on forehead is due to paralysis of frontalis muscle.
h. Paralysis of right orbicularis oculi
i. For extracranial course and distribution of facial nerve refer to Chapter 60 on muscles of facial expression and Figure 60.2.

CASE 10

An old woman involved in road traffic accident was brought to the casualty of a hospital. On examination, she was found to be conscious. On testing the movements of the right eyeball, it was noticed that she could not look towards the tip of her nose and she experienced diplopia (double vision) on looking down and to the right. There was no ptosis in the eyes.

Questions

a. Which muscle is tested in this patient when asked to look at the tip of her nose?
b. Name the nerve supplying this muscle.
c. How does it enter the orbit?
d. Name two peculiarities of this nerve.
e. Which extraocular muscle does not take origin from the apex of the orbit?
f. Which muscle is the only elevator in the abducted position of the eyeball?
g. Describe the origin, insertion and nerve supply of levator palpebrae superioris.

Solutions

a. Right superior oblique
b. Trochlear nerve
c. The trochlear nerve enters the orbit through the superior orbital fissure (Fig. 109.1).
d. This is the only cranial nerve that is attached to dorsal surface of the brainstem (it leaves the midbrain below the inferior colliculus). It is the only cranial nerve that decussates before leaving the brainstem (it decussates in superior medullary velum). The importance of

knowing this is that when right trochlear nucleus is affected it is the left nerve that shows the effects.

e. Inferior oblique
f. Superior rectus
g. Refer to Chapter 109.

SINGLE BEST RESPONSE MCQs

1. **The safety muscle of the tongue is:**
   A. Intrinsic B. Hyoglossus
   C. Genioglossus D. Styloglossus
2. **Which of the following laryngeal cartilages forms a complete ring?**
   A. Epiglottis B. Thyroid
   C. Arytenoid D. Cricoid
3. **Effect of injury to the right optic tract causes:**
   A. Bitemporal hemianopia
   B. Right homonymous hemianopia
   C. Left homonymous hemianopia
   D. Amblyopia
4. **Which of the following is a branch of geniculate ganglion?**
   A. Lesser petrosal B. Deep petrosal
   C. External petrosal D. Greater petrosal
5. **Cornea lacks all, *except:***
   A. Nerve supply B. Blood supply
   C. Color D. Lymphatic vessels
6. **The following structures pass through the sinus of Morgagni, *except:***
   A. Ascending palatine artery
   B. Tensor palati
   C. Auditory tube
   D. Levator palati
7. **The medial pterygoid muscle takes origin from all bones, *except:***
   A. Sphenoid B. Palatine
   C. Maxilla D. Zygomatic
8. **Which of the following cells in the retina is not a neuron?**
   A. Bipolar
   B. Müller's
   C. Horizontal
   D. Amacrine
9. **The muscles attached to pterygomandibular raphe are supplied by following nerve pair.**
   A. Facial and vagus
   B. Facial and glossopharyngeal
   C. Mandibular and facial
   D. Glossopharyngeal and mandibular
10. **The chorda tympani nerve arises at the following distance from the stylomastoid foramen:**
    A. 6 cm above B. 6 mm above
    C. 6 mm below D. 6 cm below
11. **Tympanic membrane develops from following cleft membrane:**
    A. Fourth
    B. Third
    C. Second
    D. First
12. **A lesion of left hypoglossal nerve causes:**
    A. Deviation of the tongue to the right on protrusion
    B. Total inability to protrude the tongue
    C. Deviation of the tongue to the left on protrusion
    D. Loss of taste sensations on the left half of posterior one-third
13. **Piriform fossa is located in:**
    A. Laryngeal inlet B. Laryngopharynx
    C. Oropharynx D. Nasopharynx
14. **Lateral wall of mastoid antrum is formed by:**
    A. Tympanic plate B. Tegmen tympani
    C. Suprameatal triangle D. Mastoid process
15. **What is true about nasopharynx?**
    A. Is always patent
    B. Is located below the soft palate
    C. Choanae open in its posterior wall
    D. Is connected to the inner ear
16. **The following parts are of adult size in newborn, *except:***
    A. Auditory ossicles
    B. Mastoid antrum
    C. Bony and membranous labyrinths
    D. Auditory tube

17. The circumvallate papillae develop from:
- **A.** Hypobranchial eminence
- **B.** Lingual swellings
- **C.** Tuberculum impar
- **D.** Both B and C

18. The pinna of the ear receives sensory fibers from all nerves, *except:*
- **A.** Great auricular
- **B.** Lesser occipital
- **C.** Posterior auricular
- **D.** Auriculotemporal

19. Which is the second order neuron in the path way for touch from head and face?
- **A.** Trigeminal ganglion
- **B.** Principal sensory nucleus
- **C.** Mesencephalic nucleus of CN V
- **D.** Nucleus of spinal tract

20. The scala media and scala vestibuli are separated by:
- **A.** Basilar membrane
- **B.** Tectorial membrane
- **C.** Vestibular membrane
- **D.** Stria vascularis

Key to Single Best Response MCQs

1 C	2 D	3 C	4 D	5 A	6 B	7 D
8 B	9 A	10 B	11 D	12 C	13 B	14 C
15 A	16 D	17 A	18 C	19 B	20 C	

MULTIPLE RESPONSE MCQ—WRITE TRUE (T) OR FALSE (F) AGAINST EACH RESPONSE

1. Constriction of pupil occurs due to lesion of:
- **A.** Ciliary ganglion
- **B.** Internal carotid nerve
- **C.** Superior cervical sympathetic ganglion
- **D.** Middle cervical sympathetic ganglion

2. Medial wall of the middle ear shows:
- **A.** Pyramid
- **B.** Fenestra vestibuli
- **C.** Canal for tensor tympani
- **D.** Canal for chorda tympani

3. Hypoglossal nerve:
- **A.** Carries fibers from C2 ventral ramus
- **B.** Supplies all muscles of the tongue
- **C.** In LMN lesion the tongue deviates to the side of the lesion
- **D.** In UMN lesion the tongue deviates to the opposite side of the lesion

4. Tensor palati:
- **A.** Originates from scaphoid fossa
- **B.** Is seen in infratemporal fossa
- **C.** Receives nerve supply through geniculate ganglion
- **D.** Develops from first arch mesoderm

5. The spine of sphenoid:
- **A.** Is related medially to auriculotemporal nerve
- **B.** Is present in the roof of infratemporal fossa
- **C.** Its necrosis leads to loss of secretion in submandibular gland
- **D.** Its necrosis leads to loss of taste in posterior one-third of tongue

6. Inferior oblique muscle of eyeball:
- **A.** Originates from maxilla
- **B.** Inserted into the sclera into front of the equator of the eyeball
- **C.** Its axis coincides with visual axis in laterally rotated eyeball
- **D.** It is the only elevator in medially rotated eyeball

7. Chorda tympani:
- **A.** Is purely sensory
- **B.** Carries special sensory fibers from posterior one-third of tongue
- **C.** Carries preganglionic parasympathetic fibers for sublingual salivary gland
- **D.** Is a branch of lingual nerve

8. Branches of glossopharyngeal nerve:
- **A.** Tympanic branch pierces the floor of middle-ear
- **B.** Pharyngeal branch supplies stylopharyngeus
- **C.** Tympanic branch is sensory to medial end of auditory tube
- **D.** Carotid branch supplies carotid sinus

9. Regarding larynx:
- **A.** All laryngeal cartilages are of elastic type
- **B.** Laryngeal prominence refers to cricoid cartilage
- **C.** Laryngeal inlet is the narrowest part
- **D.** Cricothyroid is the tuning fork of larynx

10. Parts of retina:
- **A.** Ora serrata is non-neural
- **B.** Optic disc is a blind spot
- **C.** Macula lutea has bright red color
- **D.** Fovea centralis lacks rods

Annexure: Radiographs of Head and Neck

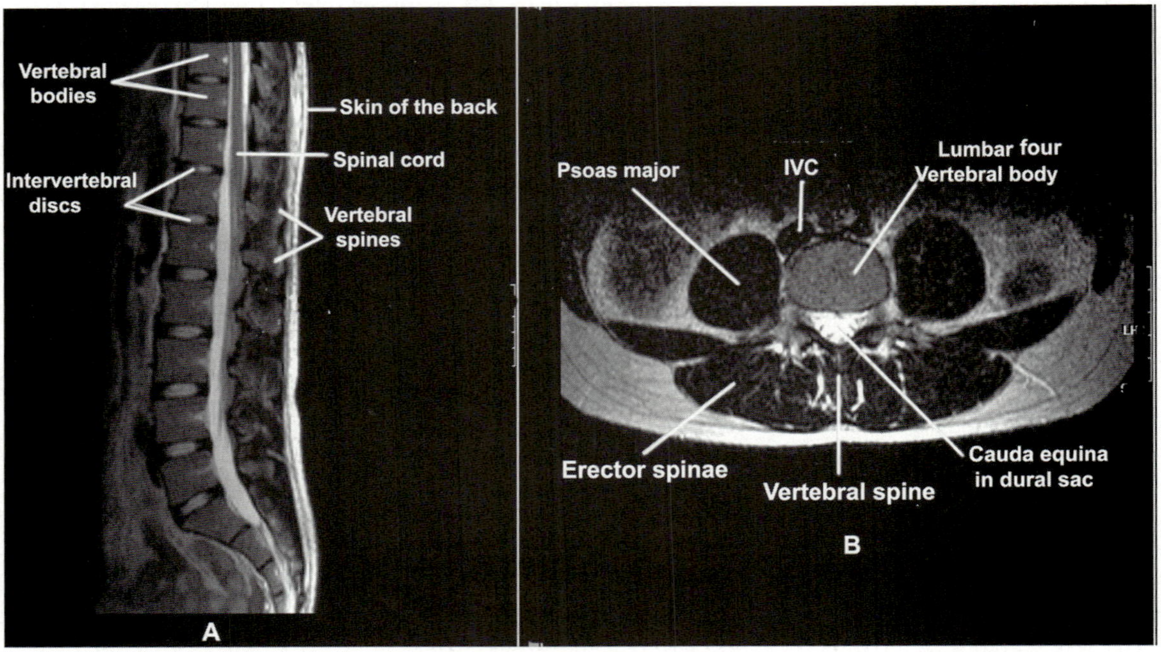

HN-R1: MRI images of sagittal (A) and transverse (B) sections of vertebral column

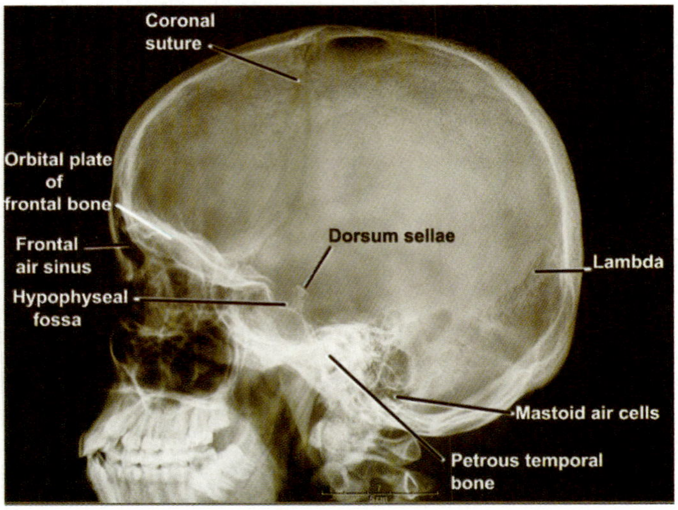

HN-R2: Radiograph of lateral view of skull

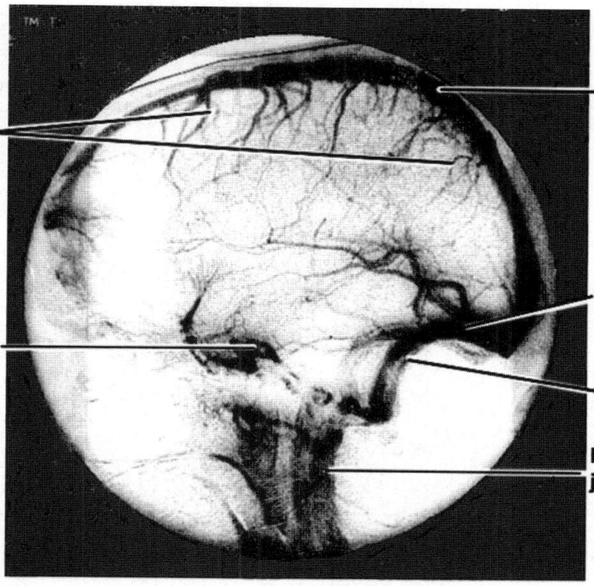

HN-R3: Venogram to show dural sinuses

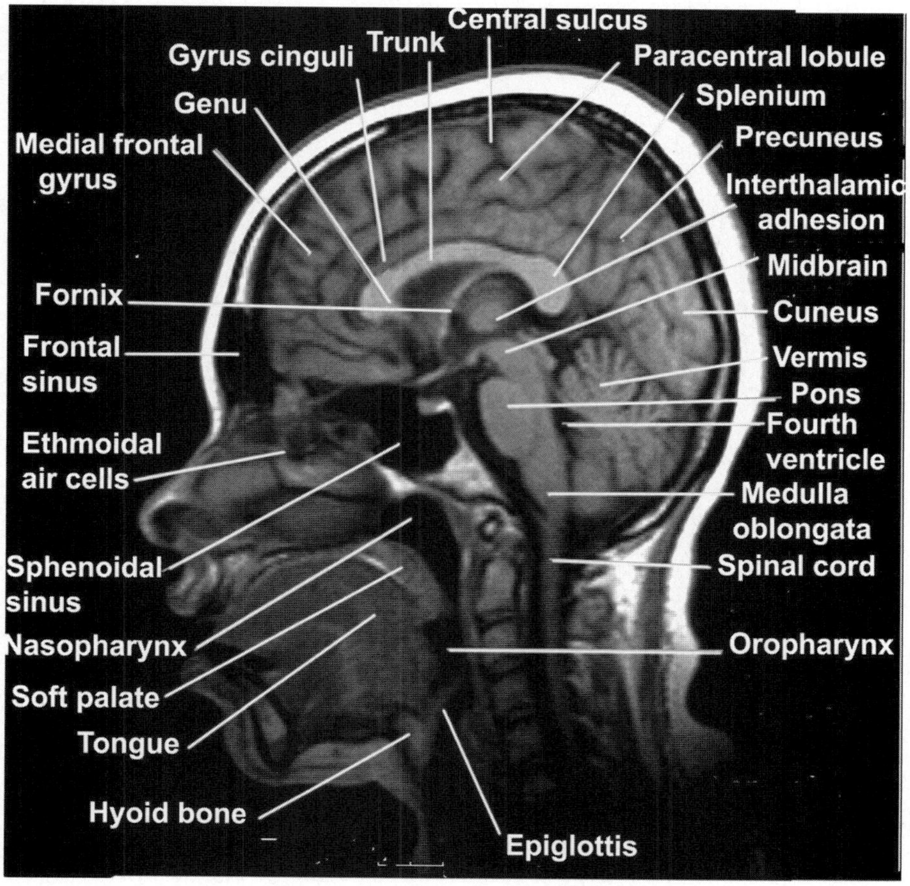

HN-R4: Anatomical structures visualized in MRI of sagittal section of head and neck

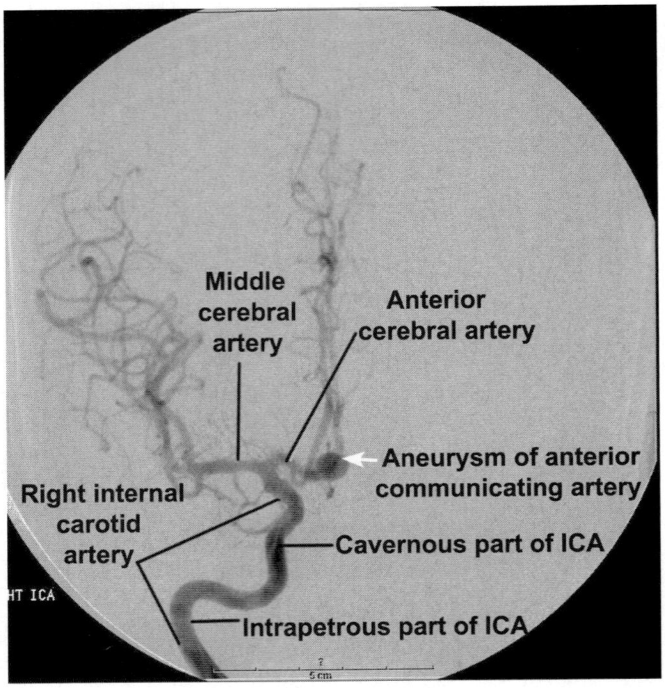

HN-R5: Right internal carotid arteriogram showing carotid siphon and aneurysm of communicating artery

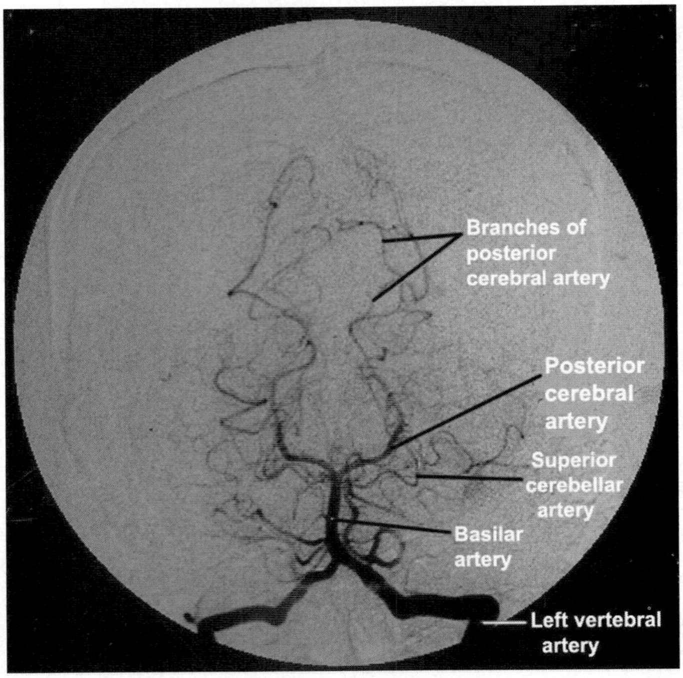

HN-R6: Digital subtraction angiogram of left vertebral artery

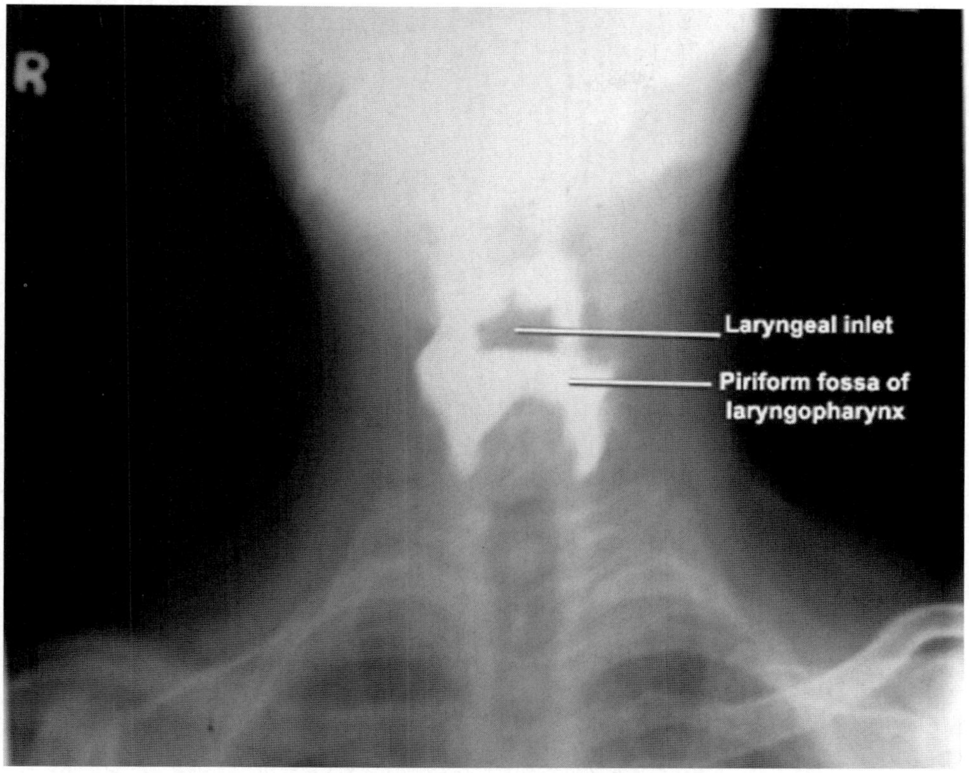

HN-R7: Barium swallow radiograph showing piriform fossa of laryngopharynx (Courtesy: Department of ENT, Dr SMCSI Medical College, Karakonam)

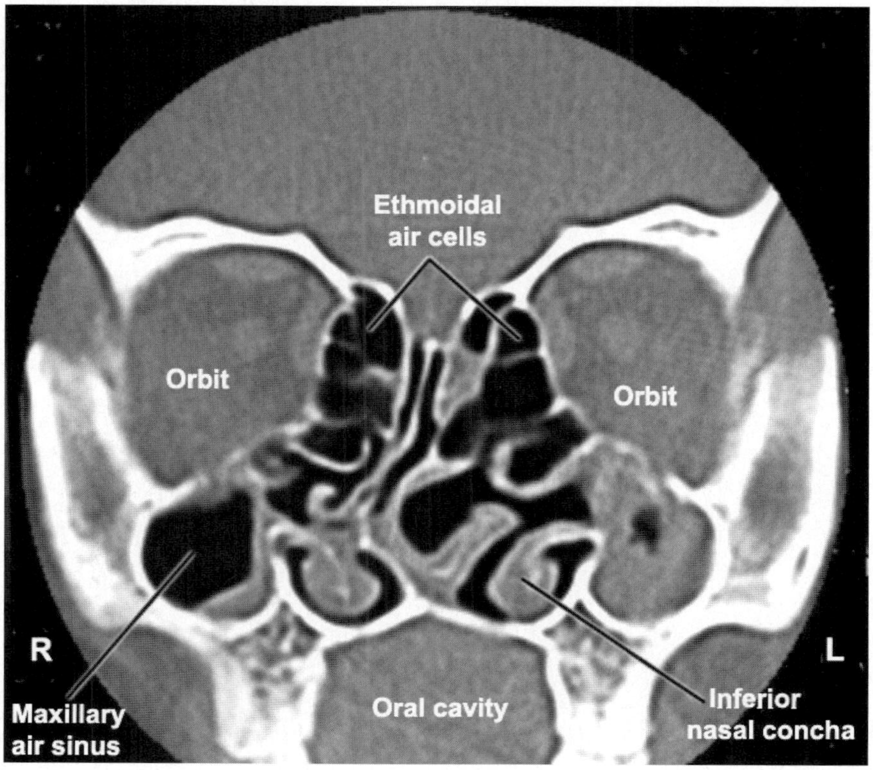

HN-R8: CT scan of coronal section of face showing deviation of nasal septum and lesion in left maxillary sinus

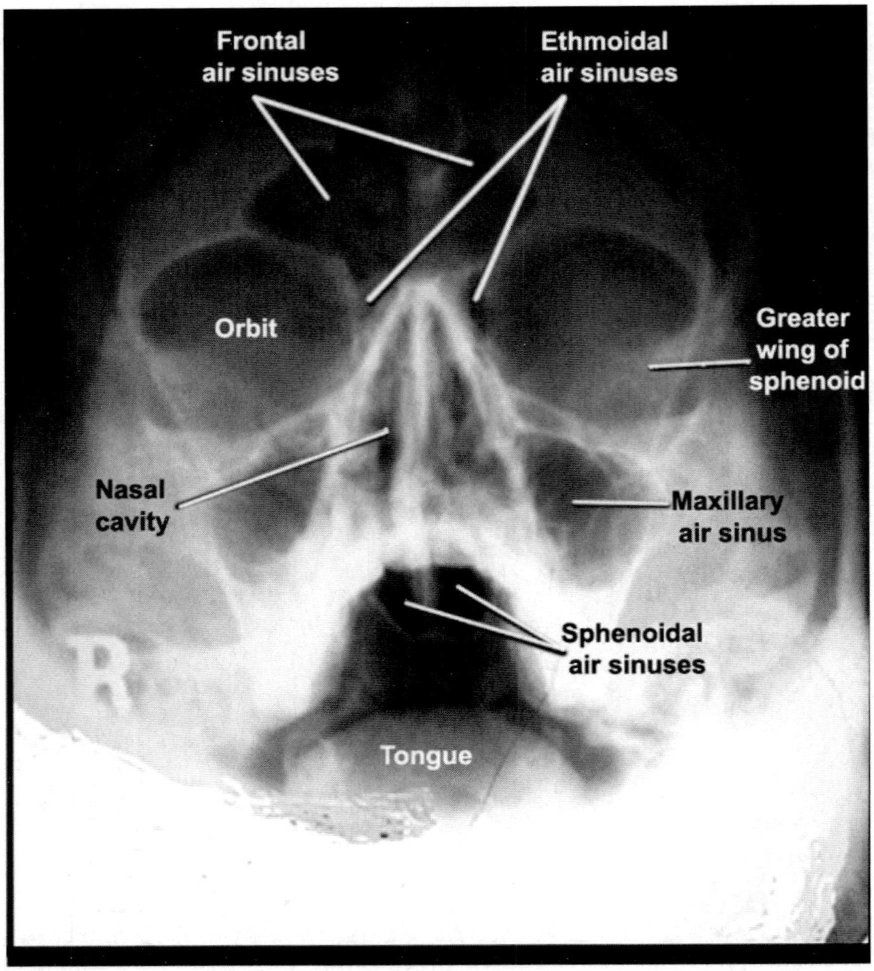

HN-R9: Radiograph of skull (modified Water's view) showing paranasal air sinuses

SECTION FOUR

Abdomen, Pelvis and Perineum

127 Anterior Abdominal Wall

Abdomen

Abdomen is part of the trunk extending from the thoracic diaphragm to the pelvic diaphragm. Its cavity consists of two parts, abdomen proper and lesser pelvis (pelvic cavity or true pelvis). The two cavities are continuous with each other at the plane of pelvic inlet (Fig. 127.1).

Boundaries of Abdomen Proper

The lower part of the thoracic cage forms the upper part of the anterior abdominal wall. Below this, the wall is musculoaponeurotic. Nearer the midline, the wall consists of rectus abdominis and pyramidalis inside the rectus sheath, which is formed by the aponeuroses of external oblique, internal oblique and transversus abdominis muscles. Laterally, the wall consists of fleshy parts of the three flat muscles. The lumbar vertebrae, diaphragmatic crurae, psoas major and quadratus lumborum muscles constitute the posterior wall of the abdomen. The diaphragm is the superior boundary of abdominal cavity. The upper abdominal organs, which fill the concavity of the diaphragm, lie internal to the lower part of the thoracic cage, pleura and lungs. This overlapping of the upper abdominal cavity by the lower thorax has clinical importance because the penetrating wounds of the lower thorax may injure the abdominal viscera. Inferiorly, the abdominal cavity is in continuity with the true pelvis through the pelvic inlet, which is an oblique plane passing through the sacral promontory and linea terminalis on either side. Each linea terminalis includes the arcuate line, iliopectineal line and pubic crest.

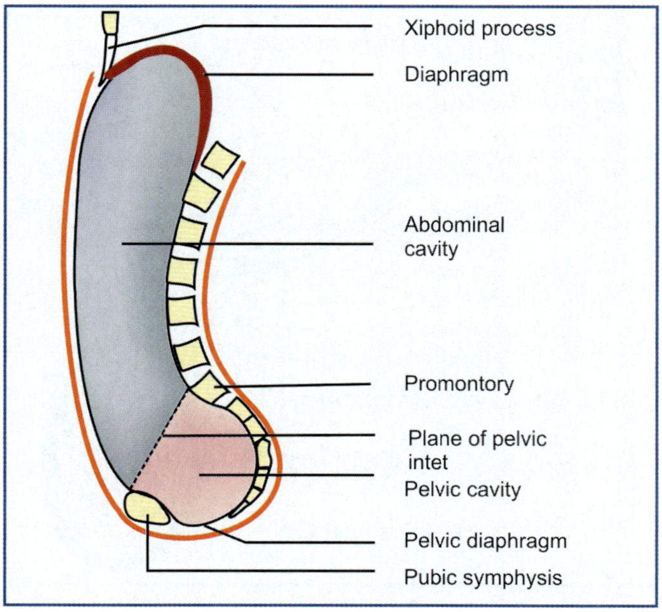

Fig. 127.1: Sagittal section showing abdominopelvic cavity

Anterior Abdominal Wall

The anterior abdominal wall extends from the anterior aspects of the lower rib cage and xiphoid process to the pubic symphysis, inguinal ligament and iliac crest. It is divided into 9 regions by 2 vertical and 2 horizontal lines.

a. The transpyloric plane passes through the midpoint between jugular notch and the symphysis pubis. It corresponds to the lower border of first lumbar vertebra.
b. The transtubercular plane passes through the tubercles of iliac crests and corresponds to upper border of fifth lumbar vertebra.
c. The vertical right and left lateral planes pass through the midpoint of the line joining the anterior superior iliac spine and the pubic symphysis (midinguinal point).

Thus, the anterior abdominal wall is divided into 3 midline and 3 left and right regions (Fig. 127.2). From above downward, the midline regions are, epigastrium, umbilical and hypogastrium (pubic). From above downward, the lateral regions are, hypochondrium, lumbar (lateral) and iliac (inguinal). These regions are of use to the clinician, while describing the site of pain felt by the patient or areas of swelling in the abdomen or for locating the internal organs. In addition, the following reference planes are useful clinically.

a. The subcostal plane passes through the lowest part of the costal margin (10th rib) and corresponds to the L3 vertebra.
b. The supracristal plane passes through the highest point of iliac crest and corresponds to the spine of L4 vertebra.
c. The interspinous plane passes through the anterior superior iliac spines and corresponds to the lumbosacral disc or the sacral promontory depending on the extent of lumbar lordosis or the sacral curvature.

Surface Features

Umbilicus is a prominent landmark but not reliable due to its inconstant position especially in obese persons. The linea alba is a median groove. The umbilicus lies below the midpoint of linea alba. The linea semilunaris indicates the lateral margin of rectus sheath. It extends from the pubic tubercle and reaches the costal margin at the tip of the ninth costal cartilage. The tendinous intersections of the rectus abdominis muscle are visible through the skin as three grooves crossing the rectus muscle between the xiphoid process and the umbilicus. The midinguinal or femoral point is the point between the pubic symphysis and the anterior superior iliac spine. It marks the position of femoral pulse, which is felt immediately below it.

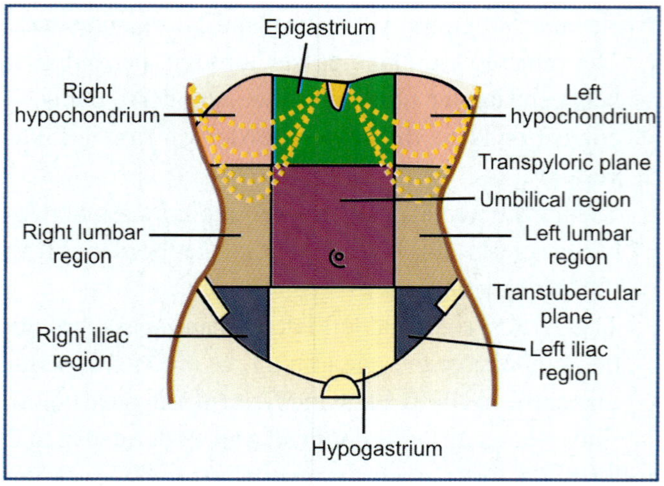

Fig. 127.2: Regions of abdomen

Layers of Anterior Abdominal Wall (Fig. 127.3)

From outer to inner aspect, the anterior abdominal wall has 8 layers, namely, the skin, superficial fascia, external oblique abdominis, internal oblique abdominis, transversus abdominis, fascia transversalis, extraperitoneal tissue and parietal peritoneum. It is to be noted that the deep fascia is lacking on the anterior abdominal wall. There is continuity between the layers of abdominal wall, coverings of spermatic cord and coverings of testis inside the scrotum.

Skin

a. The skin shows the umbilicus in the linea alba, indicating the site of attachment of the umbilical cord to the anterior abdominal wall of fetus. In a healthy lean and young adult, the umbilicus is located at the level of lower border of third lumbar vertebra, but its position tends to change with deposition of fat in the anterior abdominal wall. The midline pigmentation and striae gravidarum in the lower part are the signs of previous pregnancy in female.
b. The superficial fascia in the infraumbilical abdominal wall is composed of two layers, the superficial fatty layer or Camper's fascia and the deep membranous

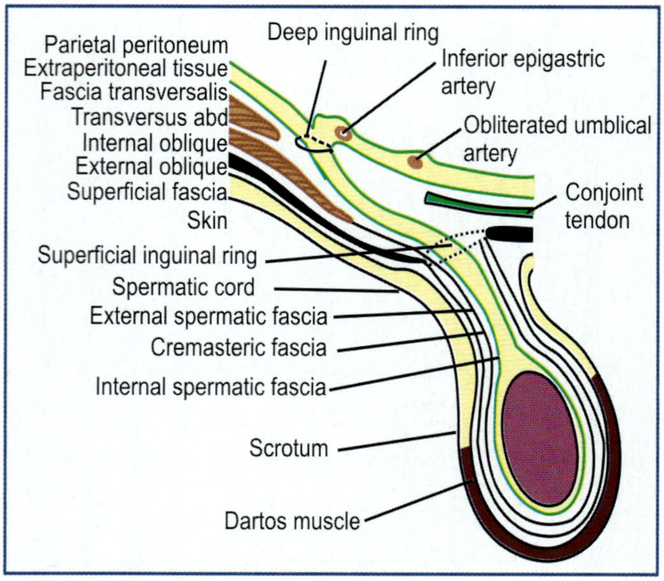

Fig. 127.3: Scheme to depict layers of anterior abdominal wall and their continuity with coverings of spermatic cord and scrotal layers

layer or Scarpa's fascia. The fatty layer is continuous below with the superficial fascia of the perineum and thighs. The membranous layer is continuous with the superficial fascia of thorax above. Laterally, it is continuous with superficial fascia of the back. Inferiorly, it passes in front of the inguinal ligament into the thigh to become continuous with the membranous layer of superficial fascia of the upper part of thigh. In the midline inferiorly it passes in front of the pubis and is continuous with the membranous layer of superficial fascia in the perineum. Thus, the potential space between the membranous layer and the external oblique aponeurosis is continuous with the superficial perineal pouch. In case of rupture of male urethra, the extravasated urine enters this potential space but cannot enter the thigh because of the fusion of the membranous layer of superficial fascia of upper thigh with the fascia lata along Holden's line (Fig. 177.1).

c. The cutaneous nerves and the dermatomes of the anterior abdominal wall are clinically important. The lower 5 intercostal (T7 to T11), subcostal (T12) and the iliohypogastric (L1) nerves supply the skin (Fig. 127.4). The anterior cutaneous branches of the lower 5 intercostal and subcostal nerves pierce the anterior wall of rectus sheath a little away from the median plane. The anterior cutaneous branch of iliohypogastric nerve pierces the skin outside the rectus sheath above the superficial inguinal ring to supply the skin on the pubic symphysis. The lateral cutaneous branches of the lower 5 intercostal nerves supply the skin of antero-lateral abdominal wall. Thus, the skin of the anterior abdominal wall is segmentally innervated (Fig. 1.5). There are 7 consecutive dermatomes starting from T7 to L1 on the anterior abdominal wall. T7 dermatome is located over the xiphoid process; T10 dermatome overlies the band of skin at the level of the umbilicus and L1 lies on the pubic symphysis and inguinal ligament. The pain of appendicitis is referred to T10 dermatome (around the umbilicus) and the pain of renal colic is referred from T10 to L1 dermatomes.

d. The arteries accompanying the lateral cutaneous branches of intercostal nerves arise from the posterior intercostal arteries of corresponding spaces. The arteries, which accompany the anterior cutaneous

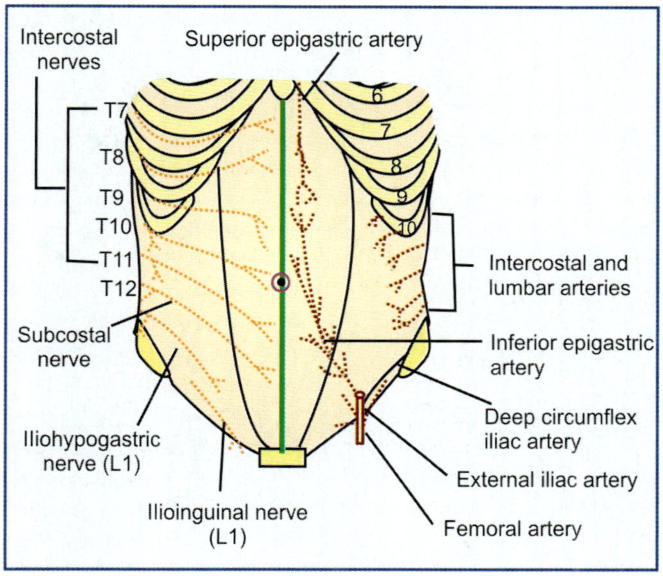

Fig. 127.4: Scheme to depict nerves and arteries of anterior abdominal wall. Note ant. and lat. cutaneous branches of lower intercostal, subcostal and iliohypogastric nerves on right side and corresponding cutaneous arteries on the left side

nerves, arise from the superior and inferior epigastric arteries (Fig. 127.4). The infraumbilical skin and superficial fascia are supplied by three branches of femoral artery namely, superficial epigastric, superficial circumflex iliac and superficial external pudendal.

e. The venous drainage of supraumbilical part of the abdominal wall is as follows (Fig. 127.5). The superficial veins drain in superior epigastric veins closer to the midline. On the lateral sides, the venous network drains in axillary vein via the lateral thoracic vein. The thoracoepigastric vein is a connecting link between lateral thoracic vein and the superficial epigastric venous network. Thus, the veins of the supraumbilical abdominal wall drain into superior vena cava while the veins of the infraumbilical abdominal wall drain finally into inferior vena cava. The superficial veins closer to the midline, drain in inferior epigastric vein. On the lateral side, the venous network drains via the superficial epigastric, superficial circumflex iliac and superficial external pudendal veins into the great saphenous vein. In the obstruction of either the superior vena cava or the inferior vena cava, the thoraco-epigastric veins, along the anterolateral abdominal wall, enlarge and become tortuous. On the other hand, in

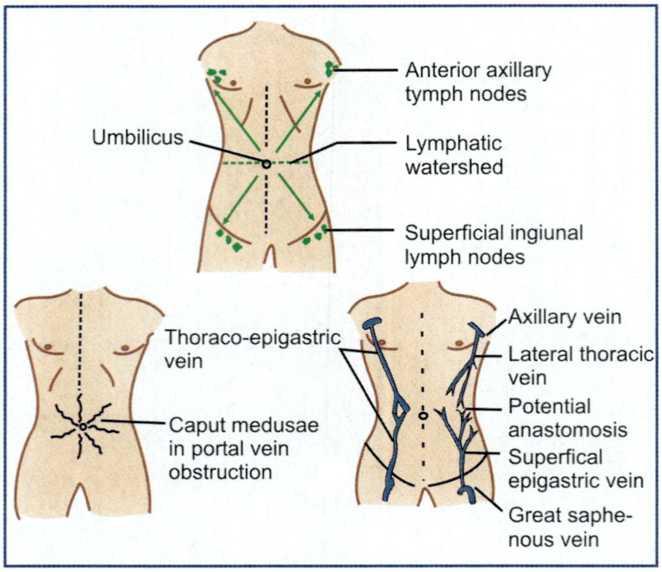

Fig. 127.5: Showing lymph vessels and venous connections of anterior abdominal wall (Note: Dilated thoraco-epigastric vein in systemic venous obstruction)

the case of portal vein obstruction, the potential portosystemic anastomosis opens up around the umbilicus producing a typical pattern of dilated and tortuous veins radiating from the umbilicus. This pattern of veins is called caput medusae (Fig. 127.5) because of its fancied resemblance to the head of Greek mythological character, Medusa, who has snakes on her head in place of hair.

f. The umbilicus is the lymphatic watershed on the anterior abdominal wall because the lymph vessels above the level of umbilicus drain into the anterior or pectoral group of axillary lymph nodes while those below it drain in the inguinal lymph nodes (Fig. 127.5). Therefore, an inflammation or cancer of the umbilicus can spread bilaterally to both the axillary and inguinal lymph nodes.

Anterolateral Muscles

The anterolateral muscles of anterior abdominal wall are disposed as three flat muscles. They are, external oblique abdominis, internal oblique abdominis and transversus abdominis. These muscles are fleshy in the lateral part but become aponeurotic medially, where all the three take part in the formation of rectus sheath.

External Oblique Abdominis (Fig. 127.6)

This muscle takes origin from the outer surfaces of the 5 to 12 ribs by fleshy slips. It has a wide insertion. The fleshy fibers from the 11 and 12 ribs form a free posterior border and are inserted in the anterior two-thirds of the outer lip of the iliac crest. The fleshy fibers from the 5 to 10 ribs end in a wide aponeurosis. The upper margin of this aponeurosis is attached to xiphoid process. Succeeding part of the aponeurosis is attached to linea alba and its lower part has bony attachment to the pubic crest and tubercle. The aponeurosis has an inrolled free margin called the inguinal ligament between the anterior superior iliac spine and the pubic tubercle.

Nerve Supply

The lower 5 intercostal nerves and the subcostal nerve supply the external oblique muscle.

Modifications of External Oblique Aponeurosis

a. The inguinal ligament (Fig. 127.7) is located at the junction between the anterior abdominal wall and the front of the thigh. It is attached medially to the pubic tubercle and laterally to anterior superior iliac spine.

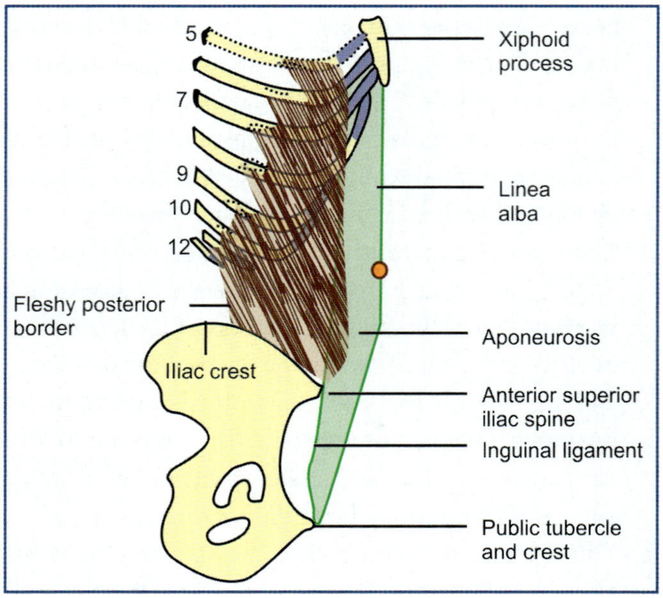

Fig. 127.6: To show attachments of obliquus externus abdominis

Its length in the adult is about 12-14 cm. The fascia lata is attached to its lower surface and hence, exerts a downward pull on the ligament. The medial half of the ligament forms the floor of the inguinal canal.

i. The internal oblique originates from lateral two-thirds of the inguinal ligament and the transversus from the lateral one-third.
ii. The structures that enter the thigh behind the inguinal ligament are, the femoral nerve, lateral cutaneous nerve of thigh, femoral branch of genitofemoral nerve, femoral vessels and iliopsoas muscle. The lateral cutaneous nerve of thigh may enter the thigh by piercing the lateral end of the inguinal ligament. The compression of the nerve in this location causes pain, numbness and paresthesia in the lateral aspect of thigh. This is known as meralgia paresthetica. To relieve the symptoms, it may be necessary to cut the deeper fibers of the inguinal ligament, at this site.

b. The lacunar ligament or the pectineal part of inguinal ligament is the extension of inguinal ligament from its medial end. It is triangular and has an apex and a base. The apex is at the pubic tubercle. The base or free margin is directed laterally and forms the medial margin of femoral ring. Anteriorly, the lacunar ligament is continuous with the inguinal ligament and posteriorly, it is attached to the medial part of pecten pubis. Its upper surface forms part of the floor of the inguinal canal. Its concave free margin bounds the femoral ring medially. Hence it is of importance to the surgeon, who operates on strangulated femoral hernia. The surgeon cuts the free margin of the ligament, to increase the size of the femoral ring so as to facilitate reduction of the hernia. While incising the ligament care should be taken not to injure the abnormal obturator artery, which is in relation to it in some percentage of population (Fig. 178.3). The pectineal ligament of Astley-Cooper extends from the lacunar ligament along the pecten pubis.
c. The reflected part of the inguinal ligament (reflex inguinal ligament) is an expansion from the lateral crus of superficial ring upwards and medially behind the external oblique but in front of the conjoint tendon. The right and left ligaments decussate in the linea alba.

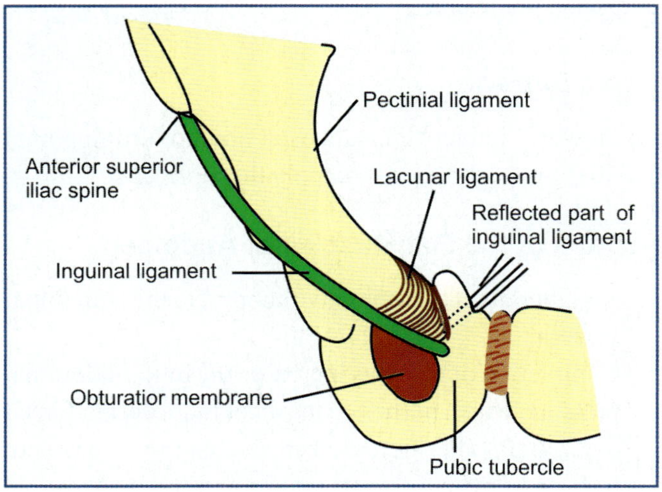

Fig. 127.7: Inguinal ligament and its extensions

Superficial Inguinal Ring

This is an opening in the aponeurosis of the external oblique muscle just above the pubic crest. It is triangular in shape. It has two margins called the crura. The lateral crus is stronger and formed by fibers of inguinal ligament attached to pubic tubercle. The medial crus is attached to the front of pubic symphysis. The inter-crural fibers arch (criss-cross) above the apex of the ring and help in holding the crura together (inter-crural fibers are derived from the fascial covering of the external oblique muscle and are at right angles to the fibers in the aponeurosis). The aponeurosis of external oblique prolongs around the spermatic cord from the margins of the superficial ring as the external spermatic fascia. The structures that pass through the ring are described with inguinal canal.

Internal Oblique Muscle (Fig. 127.8)

This muscle takes origin from the lateral two-thirds of the upper surface of inguinal ligament, anterior two-thirds of the iliac crest and lateral fused margin of the three layers of thoracolumbar fascia. It has wide insertion as follows:

a. The fibers taking origin from the thoracolumbar fascia and the posterior part of iliac crest have fleshy insertion in the lower borders of the 10, 11 and 12 ribs.
b. The fibers arising from the rest of the iliac crest and the lateral part of inguinal ligament end in a wide aponeurosis, which is attached to the costal cartilages of the 7, 8 and 9 ribs at the costal margin and the

entire length of linea alba. The aponeurosis splits in two laminae at the lateral margin of rectus muscle. The anterior lamina fuses with the aponeurosis of external oblique and the posterior lamina fuses with the aponeurosis of transversus muscle. The fused laminae enclose the rectus muscle and insert in the linea alba. Below the level of anterior superior iliac spine, the aponeurosis of internal oblique does not split but passes in front of the rectus along with the other two muscles.

c. The fibers taking origin from middle third of inguinal ligament arch over the inguinal canal and become tendinous in the posterior wall of the canal, where they fuse with tendinous fibers of transversus muscle to form the conjoint tendon or falx inguinalis. Thus, through the conjoint tendon, the internal oblique is attached to the pubic crest and pecten pubis.

Nerve Supply

The lower 5 intercostal, subcostal, iliohypogastric and ilioinguinal nerves supply the internal oblique muscle.

Cremaster Muscle and Fascia

The internal oblique contributes a thin musculofascial covering to the spermatic cord as it passes under the arched fibers of the muscle in the inguinal canal. This covering is known as cremaster muscle and fascia. The cremaster is attached to the middle third of the upper surface of inguinal ligament, the pubic tubercle and crest and the conjoint tendon. The muscle fibers form a series of loops around the cord. The contraction of the muscle pulls the testis up towards the superficial ring, which may help in plugging the ring. The other possible role is in the control of the temperature of the testis. The genital branch of genito-femoral nerve (L1, L2) supplies the cremaster muscle (the cremaster muscle in female consists of a few non-functional muscle fibers around the round ligament of uterus).

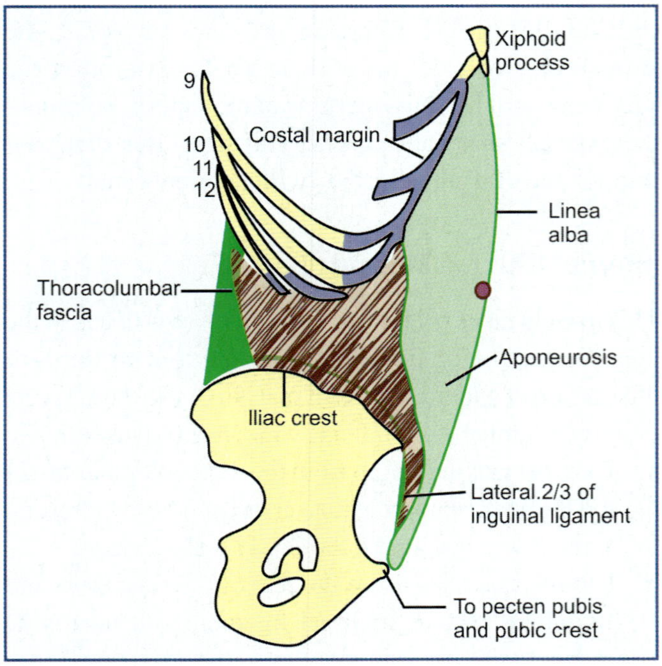

Fig. 127.8: To show attachments of obliquus internus abdominis

Cremasteric Reflex

Stroking the skin of the medial side of the upper thigh results in elevation of the testis and scrotum on the stimulated side. The afferent limb of the reflex is the femoral nerve, the reflex center is in the L1 and L2 segments of the spinal cord and the efferent limb is the genitofemoral nerve.

Transversus Abdominis (Fig. 127.9)

The transversus muscle takes origin from the inner aspect of lower 6 costal cartilages near the costal margin, thoracolumbar fascia, anterior two-thirds of the iliac crest and the lateral one-third of the upper surface of inguinal ligament. It is inserted into the linea alba. The inguinal fibers arch over the inguinal canal and then end in the aponeurosis, which fuses with that of internal oblique to form conjoint tendon through which it is attached to pecten pubis and pubic crest.

Nerve Supply

The lower 5 intercostal, subcostal and both ilioinguinal and iliohypogastric nerves supply the muscle.

Actions of the Flat Muscles of Abdomen

a. The abdominal muscles give support to the abdominal viscera.
b. Contraction of muscles increases the intra-abdominal pressure, which pushes up the diaphragm during forced expiration. The increased intra-abdominal pressure helps in expulsive processes like vomiting, defaecation, micturition and parturition.

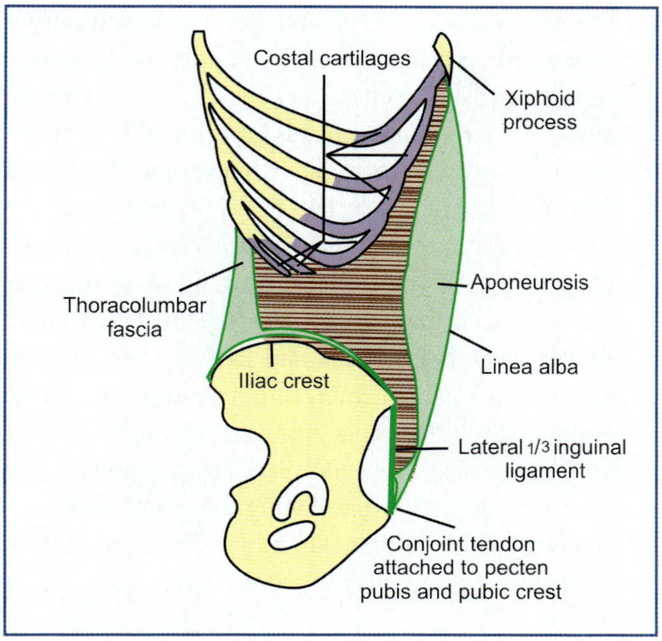

Fig. 127.9: To show the attachments of transversus abdominis muscle

c. The muscles cause flexion of vertebral column and rotation of trunk to right by left external oblique acting with right internal oblique and rotation to left by right external oblique acting with left internal oblique.

Conjoint Tendon or Falx Inguinalis

The lower arched fibers of the internal oblique and transversus muscles end in the aponeurosis behind the medial end of the inguinal ligament. The fusion of the two aponeuroses forms the conjoint tendon, which is attached to the pubic crest and pecten pubis. The conjoint tendon forms the medial half of the posterior wall of the inguinal canal. It strengthens this wall opposite the deficiency (superficial ring) in the anterior wall. Medially, it blends with the anterior wall of rectus sheath. Laterally, it may extend occasionally as interfoveolar ligament, which is medial to deep ring as it passes to be attached to the inguinal ligament and superior ramus of pubis. The conjoint tendon may weaken in old age due to decreased tone of the muscles of the anterior abdominal wall. It weakens if there is injury to iliohypogastric and ilioinguinal nerves. The weakened conjoint tendon predisposes to direct inguinal hernia.

Rectus Sheath (Fig. 127.10)

The rectus sheath is an aponeurotic covering for the rectus abdominis and pyramidalis muscles on either side of the linea alba. Its aponeurotic anterior wall covers the muscles from end to end while the aponeurotic posterior wall is deficient above and below. The anterior wall fuses with the rectus muscle at intervals but the posterior wall is free. The rectus sheath extends laterally upto the linea semilunaris. Its formation varies at three levels as follows:

Formation of Rectus Sheath

a. Above the level of costal margin:
   i. Anterior wall is formed by the aponeurosis of the external oblique muscle only.
   ii. Posterior wall is deficient hence, the rectus muscle rests directly on the fifth, sixth and seventh costal cartilages.
b. From the costal margin to midway between umbilicus and pubic symphysis:
   i. Anterior wall is formed by fusion of aponeurosis of external oblique with the anterior lamina of the aponeurosis of internal oblique.

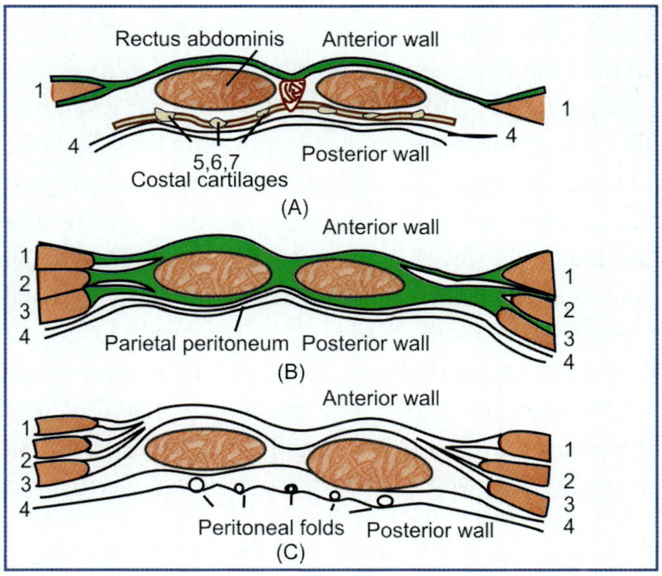

Fig. 127.10: Scheme showing formation of rectus sheath. (A) above the level of costal margin, (B) between costal margin and midway between umbilicus and symphysis pubis, (C) below the point midway between umbilicus and symphysis pubis. 1. External oblique, 2. Internal oblique, 3. Transversus abdominis, 4. Fascia transversalis

ii. Posterior wall is formed by fusion of posterior lamina of internal oblique aponeurosis with the aponeurosis of transversus abdominis. The lower margin of the aponeurotic posterior wall is called arcuate line or linea semilunaris of Douglas. It lies at the level of anterior superior iliac spine. The inferior epigastric artery enters the rectus sheath at the arcuate line.

c. Below the level of the point midway between umbilicus and pubic symphysis:
   i. Anterior wall is formed by fusion of the aponeuroses of the three muscles.
   ii. Posterior wall is deficient hence the rectus muscle rests directly on fascia transversalis.

Recent View of Formation of Rectus Sheath

Each flat muscle has a bilaminar aponeurosis. Of the 6 laminae on each side 3 pass in front of the rectus muscle and 3 behind. The laminae do not terminate into linea alba but decussate with other laminae and continue as the laminae of the contralateral muscle. This arrangement, sort of, joins the bilateral oblique and transversus muscles in pairs thus converting them into digastric muscles. According to this concept, the anterior wall of rectus sheath between the costal margin and umbilicus has trilaminar architecture consisting of 2 laminae of external oblique and the anterior lamina of internal oblique. The criss-cross pattern of the fibers in these laminae resembles the cross-grain of plywood. The posterior wall likewise consists of posterior lamina of internal oblique and two laminae of transversus abdominis. Below the umbilicus, the layers change their superficial to deep sequence and near the pubis they are modified by the presence of conjoint tendon. It is apparent that recent view does not subscribe to the view that at the arcuate line the aponeurotic posterior wall abruptly ends. The fibers of posterior wall gradually hand over the fibers to the anterior wall as well as to the fascia transversalis to make it stronger.

Contents of Rectus Sheath

The rectus sheath contains 2 muscles (rectus abdominis and pyramidalis), 2 vessels (superior and inferior epigastric) and 6 nerves (lower 5 intercostal nerves and subcostal nerve).

a. The rectus abdominis muscle derives its name from its straight vertical course. The right and left muscles are separated by the linea alba (Fig. 127.11). The rectus arises by 2 tendinous heads, the medial from the anterior surface of symphysis pubis and the lateral from the pubic crest. It has fleshy insertion into the xiphoid process and the 5, 6 and 7 costal cartilages. This muscle is characterized by 3 tendinous intersections, which are located at the tip of the xiphoid process, at the umbilicus and midway between the previous two. Each intersection is attached to the anterior wall of the rectus sheath but not to the posterior wall. This arrangement allows the superior and inferior epigastric vessels to pass along the posterior aspect of rectus muscle without hindrance. The intersections divide the long muscle into shorter segments for better action
   The lower 5 intercostal and the subcostal nerves supply the rectus muscle.
   The rectus abdominis is the flexor of the vertebral column and it supports the abdominal viscera.
   For testing the function of the rectus the subject is asked to raise the head and shoulder from the bed against resistance. The contraction of the normal muscle can be seen and felt.

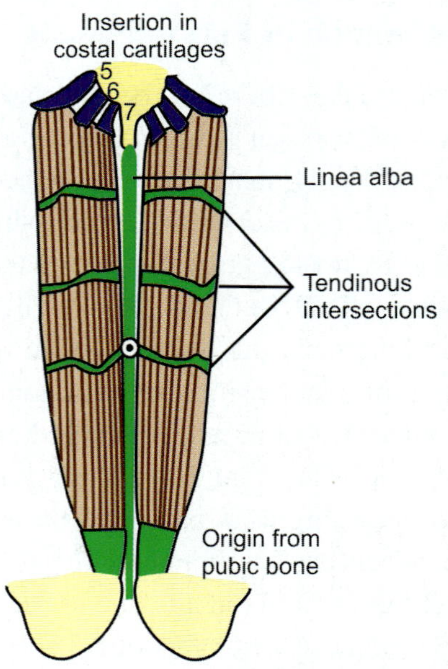

Fig. 127.11: Scheme showing attachments of rectus abdominis muscles

b. The pyramidalis is a small muscle situated in front of the lower part of the rectus muscle. It takes origin from the anterior surface of the body of pubis by a rounded tendon and is inserted into the linea alba. The subcostal nerve supplies it. It is supposed to be the tensor of the linea alba.

Linea Alba

It is a tendinous raphe extending from the xiphoid process to the pubic symphysis and is formed by the ducussation of the fibers in the aponeurosis of the flat muscles of the two sides. Therefore, linea alba can be regarded as a common insertion of the right and left oblique and transversus muscles. The pyramidalis muscles are inserted in its lower part. The umbilicus is located just below its midpoint. Its infraumbilical part is narrower compared to the supraumbilical part, where due to divergence of recti the linea alba is relatively broader.

Clinical Highlights

In divarication (separation) of recti the upper abdominal viscera bulge through widened linea alba while in standing position or during straining. It is usually seen in elderly multiparous women with weak abdominal muscles. Herniation through the upper part of linea alba is called epigastric hernia. Surgical incisions in the avascular linea alba are sometimes preferred to approach the abdominal organs.

Fascia Transversalis

It is a thin layer of connective tissue lying between the transversus muscle and extraperitoneal connective tissue. It is continuous with diaphragmatic fascia above. Posteriorly, it is continuous with anterior layer of the renal fascia. Inferiorly, its attachments are as follows. It is attached to the whole length of iliac crest between the origins of transversus and iliacus muscles. Between the anterior superior iliac spine and femoral vessels, it is attached to the posterior margin of inguinal ligament. Along this attachment, it fuses with iliac fascia. In the region of the femoral vessels, the transversalis fascia passes over the vessels for a distance of 3 to 4 cm and forms the anterior wall of the femoral sheath. Medial to femoral vessels, it is attached to the pecten pubis and conjoint tendon. The deep inguinal ring is the deficiency in the fascia transversalis and the internal spermatic fascia is a prolongation of the transversalis fascia on the spermatic cord at the deep ring.

Nerves of Anterior Abdominal Wall

a. The thoraco-abdominal nerves are the lower 5 intercostal nerves (T7 to T11). These nerves are distributed to both the thoracic and abdominal walls. In their thoracic course, the nerves travel in the neurovascular plane of the thoracic wall (between the internal intercostal and intercostalis intimus muscles) to reach the anterior ends of the respective intercostal spaces. They supply the motor branches to the intercostal muscles and sensory branches to the parietal pleura and periosteum of the ribs of their respective spaces. The T7 and T8 intercostal nerves enter the abdominal wall between the digitations of transversus abdominis and then curve superomedially across the deep costal surface to reach the deep aspect of posterior lamina of the internal oblique aponeurosis. Thus, these 2 nerves immediately enter the rectus sheath by piercing its posterior wall. The T9 to T11 intercostal nerves enter the abdominal wall by passing through the gap between digitations of diaphragm and transversus abdominis muscle. These nerves travel in the neurovascular plane of the anterior abdominal wall between internal oblique and transversus muscles and pierce the lateral margin of the rectus sheath. The collateral branches of all the thoraco-abdominal nerves supply the three flat muscles of the anterior abdominal wall. Inside the rectus sheath, the main nerves supply the rectus abdominis. The cutaneous branches of the main nerves pierce the rectus abdominis and the anterior wall of the rectus sheath. Inwardly directed branches of the intercostal nerves are sensory to the parietal peritoneum.

b. The subcostal nerve is the ventral ramus of the twelfth thoracic nerve. In its thoracic course it passes along the inferior border of the twelfth rib accompanied by subcostal artery (a branch of descending thoracic aorta) and vein. It leaves the thorax by passing behind the lateral arcuate ligament to enter the lumbar region of the posterior abdominal wall, where it lies between the posterior surface of the kidney and the anterior surface of quadratus lumborum muscle. In the lumbar region, it supplies the serratus posterior inferior muscle along with T9, T10 and T11 intercostal nerves and the quadratus lumborum muscle along with lumbar ventral rami. It perforates the aponeurotic origin of transversus muscle at the lateral margin of the thoracolumbar fascia to gain entry in the neurovascular plane of anterior abdominal wall. Finally, it enters the rectus sheath. The subcostal nerve supplies the three flat muscles of the anterior abdominal wall. Inside the rectus sheath, it supplies the rectus abdominis and the pyramidalis muscles. Its lateral cutaneous branch crosses the iliac crest to distribute branches to the skin of the upper lateral part of the gluteal region. Its anterior cutaneous branches supply the infraumbilical skin of anterior abdominal wall.

c. The iliohypogastric and ilioinguinal nerves are the branches of the lumbar plexus, the root value of each being L1.The iliohypogastric nerve is located higher and it is larger in size compared to the ilioinguinal nerve.

   The iliohypogastric nerve comes out from the lateral margin of the psoas major muscle on the posterior abdominal wall and runs laterally in the lumbar region lying in front of the anterior layer of lumbar fascia and behind the kidney. Then, it enters the neurovascular plane of abdominal wall by piercing the aponeurotic origin of transversalis muscle from the lumbar fascia. After giving its lateral cutaneous branch a little behind the iliac tubercle, it pierces the internal oblique muscle to course downwards and medially between the external aponeurosis and internal oblique. Just above the superficial inguinal ring, it pierces the aponeurosis of external oblique and terminates as anterior cutaneous branch, which supplies the skin above the pubis. Its lateral cutaneous branch supplies the skin of the gluteal region. The motor branches supply the internal oblique and transversus muscles.

The course of the ilioinguinal nerve in the posterior abdominal wall is similar to that of iliohypogastric nerve. This nerve is smaller in size and lies at a little lower level compared to the iliohypogastric nerve. It pierces the transversus abdominis near the anterior end of the iliac crest and runs downward and medially to pierce the arched fibers of the internal oblique and enter the inguinal canal. It accompanies the spermatic cord (or the round ligament of uterus) and comes out through the superficial ring. The nerve gives motor branches to the internal oblique and transversus muscles. It has no lateral cutaneous branch. It supplies the skin of the upper part of the medial surface of the thigh and the skin covering the root of penis and upper part of scrotum in the male or that covering the mons pubis and adjacent labium majus in the female. Like the thoraco-abdominal and subcostal nerves, the iliohypogastric and ilioinguinal nerves give sensory branches to parietal peritoneum.

Clinical Highlights

The segmental nerves of the anterior abdominal wall give innervation to skin, the muscles and the parietal peritoneum lining the anterior abdominal wall. The inflammation of parietal peritoneum causes severe pain in the skin. Local reflexes involving the same nerves bring about protective increase in the tone of the muscles of the anterior abdominal wall. The increased tone and reflex rigidity is known as muscle guarding. It is to be noted that inflammation of parietal pleura (pleurisy) may also give rise to similar symptoms and signs in the abdominal wall.

Arteries of Anterior Abdominal Wall

a. The branches of internal thoracic artery, the superior epigastric and musculophrenic arteries enter the abdominal wall from above. The superior epigastric artery is the medial terminal branch of the internal mammary artery. It enters the rectus sheath by passing through the gap between the sternal and costal origins of the diaphragm. The artery lies deep to the rectus abdominis muscle resting on the posterior wall of the sheath and ends by anastomosing with the inferior epigastric artery at the level of umbilicus. The musculophrenic artery begins in the sixth intercostal space as the lateral terminal branch of the internal mammary artery. It passes inferiorly behind the seventh to the ninth costal cartilages and gives a pair of anterior intercostal arteries, to the seventh, eighth and ninth intercostal spaces. It pierces the diaphragm between the costal slips of origin to enter the anterior abdominal wall.

b. The branches of thoracic aorta, the lower 2 posterior intercostal arteries (tenth and eleventh) and the subcostal artery enter along with the corresponding nerves. The tenth and eleventh intercostal spaces are open at their anterior ends and do not have anterior intercostal arteries. Therefore, the tenth and eleventh posterior intercostal arteries enter the neurovascular plane of the abdominal wall along with the corresponding nerves. The subcostal artery accompanies the subcostal nerve. These branches of the thoracic aorta anastomose with the lumbar branches of abdominal aorta and with branches of musculophrenic and epigastric arteries.
c. Two branches of the external iliac artery enter the abdominal wall from below.
   i. The inferior epigastric artery is a branch of the external iliac artery. Its surface marking corresponds to a line joining the midinguinal point to a point about one fingerbreadth from the midline at the level of anterior superior iliac spine. The artery lies medial to the deep inguinal ring and ascends in the extraperitoneal tissue towards the rectus sheath. When it reaches the lateral margin of rectus sheath it pierces the transversalis fascia to enter inside the sheath by crossing the arcuate line and gives muscular and cutaneous branches inside the sheath. The inferior epigastric artery gives two named branches outside the rectus sheath, the cremasteric and the pubic. The cremasteric branch enters the spermatic cord and the pubic branch passes medially in close relation to the lacunar ligament and anastomoses with the pubic branch of the obturator artery. When the pubic branch of inferior epigastric artery is large, it is called abnormal obturator artery. This artery is often called "artery of death" by surgeons since it may be injured while cutting the lacunar ligament (during the operation for strangulated femoral hernia) resulting in life-threatening hemorrhage.
   ii. The deep circumflex iliac artery is a branch of the external iliac artery. It courses laterally along the inguinal ligament towards the anterior superior iliac spine. Here, it gives a large ascending branch, which travels in the neurovascular plane. The main trunk runs backwards along the inner lip of the iliac crest. At the midpoint of the iliac crest it pierces the transversus muscle to enter the neurovascular plane and terminates by anastomosing with the iliolumbar and superior gluteal arteries.
   iii. The lumbar arteries (the dorsal branches of abdominal aorta) enter the abdominal wall from the side.

Umbilicus

This area of the abdomen is very important clinically and embryologically.

Clinical Highlights

The umbilicus lies in the linea alba in a skin depression which, has a puckered appearance. It denotes the site of attachment of umbilical cord to the ventral body wall of the fetus.

a. T10 dermatome overlies the band of skin surrounding the umbilicus. This is the reason why visceral pain of appendicitis is referred to the umbilicus.
b. The umbilicus is the lymphatic watershed because the abdominal wall above it drains into the anterior axillary nodes and below it into the superficial inguinal nodes.
c. Caput Medusae is a characteristic clinical sign of portal hypertension, in which dilated and tortuous superficial veins radiate from the umbilicus.
d. For clinical testing of the muscles of the abdominal wall, the movement of the umbilicus is watched as follows. Ask the supine patient to lift the head and shoulder from the bed against light resistance. If the abdominal muscles contract normally, the umbilicus remain stationary. If the abdominal muscles in the infraumbilical part are paralyzed, the umbilicus moves straight upwards by active contraction of the supraumbilical part of the muscles. This is called Beevor's sign and is positive in lesion of the spinal cord at T10 level.
e. Umbilical hernia may be congenital or acquired. The acquired hernia occurs due to weakness of the anterior abdominal wall, as for example, in long standing ascites.

Embryological Importance

During the 5th to 10th weeks of intrauterine life, the midgut loop herniates into the umbilical cord. This physiological umbilical hernia returns to the abdominal cavity during 10th to 12th weeks. Two endodermal tubes (allantois and vitellointestinal duct) project into the umbilical cord. The allantois is a diverticulum from endodermal cloaca (part of it gives rise to urinary bladder) and vitellointestinal duct is a diverticulum from the midgut. Three umbilical blood vessels (two arteries and one vein) are present inside the umbilical cord. After birth, when the cord is severed, these structures are cut at the root of umbilical cord. The fate of the intra-abdominal parts of the contents of the umbilical cord after birth is as follows. The allantois becomes the urachus, which becomes the median umbilical ligament. The vitellointestinal duct completely obliterates normally. Left umbilical vein becomes the round ligament of liver. The right and left umbilical arteries become the fibrous medial umbilical ligaments and the superior vesical arteries.

Congenital Anomalies

a. Failure of vitellointestinal duct to obliterate completely, results in fecal fistula at the umbilicus.
b. Patent urachus results in urinary fistula at the umbilicus.
c. Exomphalos or omphalocele is due to failure of the midgut hernia to return to the abdominal cavity during 10th to 12th weeks of intrauterine life. The umbilical swelling is covered with amnion. The congenital umbilical hernia is due to weakness of umbilicus, through which intestines protrude. Such a swelling is covered with peritoneum.

128

Surgical Incisions on the Anterior Abdominal Wall

Surgeries on the abdominal and pelvic organs are very common. The principles observed while placing the surgical incision on the anterior abdominal wall to open the abdominal cavity, are to protect nerves and blood vessels of the wall and to cut the muscles in the direction of their fibers to promote healing with minimum scar tissue formation. Depending on the preference of the surgeon and the organ to be operated upon, different types of incisions are used (Fig. 128.1). All incisions have anatomical basis.

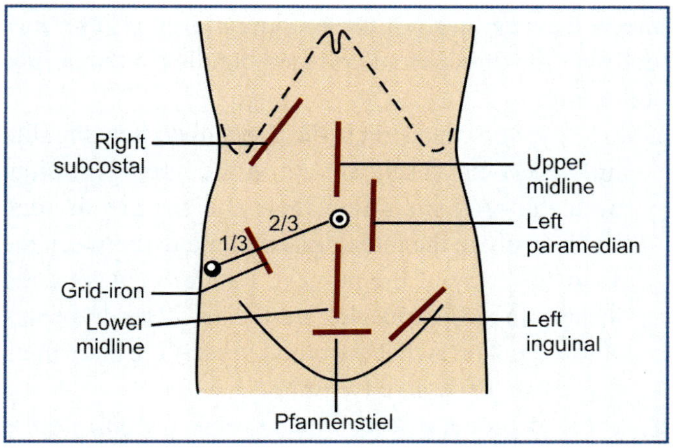

Fig. 128.1: Locations of surgical incisions on anterior abdominal wall

Midline Incisions

This incision is placed on the linea alba. The advantage of this incision is that it gives a bloodless exposure (linea alba being avascular). No muscle is cut as the incision passes through the skin, superficial fascia, linea alba, transversalis fascia and parietal peritoneum. The disadvantage of this incisiion is that healing is delayed hence there is more scar tissue.

Incisions Related to Rectus Sheath

a. Paramedian incision is placed 2.5 cm lateral and parallel to the midline. At first, the skin, superficial fascia and anterior wall of rectus sheath are incised. Then, the tendinous intersections are divided to free the rectus muscle from the anterior wall and the muscle is retracted laterally to preserve the nerves entering the muscle from the lateral side. The posterior wall of the sheath is incised followed by transversalis fascia and parietal peritoneum. This is the most preferred incision.
b. Pararectal incision is placed over the lateral part of rectus sheath just medial to the linea semilunaris. The skin, fascia and anterior wall of rectus sheath are cut along the line of incision. The rectus muscle is retracted medially to expose the posterior wall. The nerves entering the posterior wall are also retracted before incising the posterior wall.
c. Transrectal muscle splitting incision is placed 3 to 4 cm lateral and parallel to the midline. The skin, superficial fascia and the anterior wall of rectus sheath are cut and then the rectus muscle is cut vertically and finally the posterior wall of the sheath. In this incision, the rectus is not freed from the anterior wall of its sheath. The only disadvantage is that the medial part of the muscle loses its nerve supply.

Gridiron Muscle Splitting Incision

This incision is usually used for conventional appendicectomy. An oblique incision is placed at the McBurney's point right angles to the right spinoumbilical line. The skin, 2 layers of superficial fascia and the external oblique aponeurosis are incised along the line of incision. The fleshy fibers of the internal oblique and of transversus are split along their directions. The muscles are retracted to expose the fascia transversalis and the parietal peritoneum. If the iliohypogastric nerve is damaged in this location, the conjoint tendon will be weakened. Unless carefully identified there is likelihood of injuring the ascending branch of the deep circumflex iliac artery, which travels vertically upwards from the anterior superior iliac spine.

Transverse Incisions

The transverse incisions heal quickly and have better cosmetic value since the incisions lie along the Langer's lines (cleavage lines) of the abdominal skin. These lines represent the direction of collagen bundles in the dermis of the skin.

a. In a transverse incision in the upper abdomen, the skin and superficial fascia are cut in the line of incision. Both the recti including their sheaths are divided transversely in the intersegmental plane (between the points of entry of the nerves). Laterally, beyond the sheath, three flat muscles are incised. The drawback of this incision is that the blood vessels are cut, which may cause excessive bleeding.
b. Some surgeons prefer a transverse or skin crease incision of Lanz for appendicectomy. This is placed 2 cm below the umbilicus on either side of the line passing through the right vertical plane.
c. The transverse incision in the lower abdomen (Pfannenstiel's incision) is commonly used for approaching the pelvic organs, especially in surgeries related to uterus and ovaries. The incision is placed just above the symphysis pubis. It cuts through the skin, 2 layers of superficial fascia and the anterior wall of the rectus sheath. The right and left recti and pyramidalis muscles are separated to expose the transversalis fascia and the parietal peritoneum (the posterior wall of the rectus sheath is deficient here), which are incised for intraperitoneal approach to the uterus and ovaries. To gain the extraperitoneal approach to the urinary bladder, these last mentioned layers are pushed upwards.

Paracentesis of Abdomen (Fig. 128.2)

The paracentesis means tapping or withdrawing the excessive fluid from the serous cavities. Accumulation of fluid in the peritoneal cavity is called ascites. It is essential to first make sure that patient has passed urine. In the infraumbilical midline approach, the needle passes in succession the skin, superficial fascia, linea alba, fascia transversalis, extraperitoneal fatty tissue and parietal peritoneum. In the lateral approach, the needle is inserted lateral to the inferior epigastric artery. The needle passes through the skin, superficial fascia, aponeurosis of external oblique, internal oblique muscle, transversus muscle, transversalis fascia, extraperitoneal fatty tissue and the parietal peritoneum.

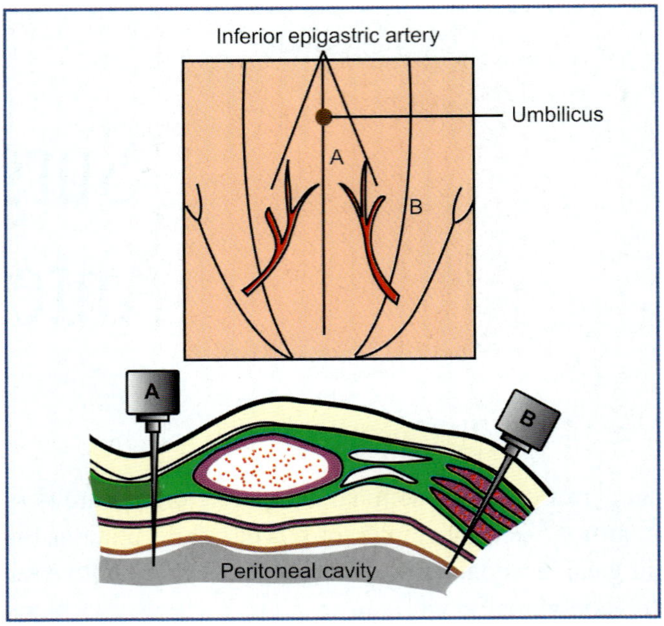

Fig. 128.2: Points on the abdominal wall for aspiration of fluid from the peritoneal cavity (Note: The layers of the wall pierced by the needle at point 'A' and point 'B')

Laparoscopy

Nowadays, instead of the conventional open surgery, minimum access surgery using laparoscope is preferred by some surgeons. The laparoscopic surgery is less disabling and disfiguring compared to open surgery. In this technique, an endoscope is introduced through small keyhole ports in the anterior abdominal wall, into the peritoneal cavity (which is already inflated by CO_2). Thus, the trauma of a long incision and of exposure of internal organs to atmosphere is reduced.

129 Inguinal Canal

The inguinal herniae are very common in all age groups. The inguinal herniae are treated by surgical repair. Therefore, to diagnose and treat inguinal hernia a thorough knowledge of the anatomy of inguinal region is essential.

The inguinal canal is about 4 cm long oblique intermuscular passage in the lower part of the anterior abdominal wall. It is located just above the medial half of the inguinal ligament. It begins at the deep inguinal ring in the fascia transversalis and courses in the anterior, inferior and medial direction to end at the superficial inguinal ring in the external oblique aponeurosis. Thus, its lateral end is the deep ring and its medial end is the superficial ring.

Surface Marking (Fig. 129.1)

The canal is marked by drawing two parallel lines (which are 1 cm apart and 4 cm long) just above the medial half of inguinal ligament. The deep ring is drawn at the lateral end of these lines 1 cm above the midinguinal point. The superficial ring is drawn at the medial end of the parallel lines just above the pubic tubercle. The relationship of the inferior epigastric artery to the deep ring is shown in Figure 129.1. This artery extends from the midinguinal point, passes medial to the deep ring to reach a point 1 fingerbreadth lateral to the midline at the level of anterior superior iliac spine.

Development of Inguinal Canal

The inguinal canal is created in the intrauterine life during the descent of the gonads (Fig. 160.1). In the male, the testes (pleural of testis) are pulled down from the abdominal cavity into the scrotum via the passage in the lower abdominal wall. In the female, ovaries are inside the pelvic cavity, nonetheless, they are pulled down from higher position by the same mechanism. By the end of fourth month of fetal life, a fibrous strand called gubernaculum testis or ovarii extends from the lower pole of the gonad, which develops in the lumbar region of the posterior abdominal wall of the embryo, to the labioscrotal swelling (future site of scrotum or labium majus). A peritoneal pouch called the processus vaginalis evaginates through the abdominal wall, following the course of the gubernaculum. Therefore, the inguinal canal is formed by the passage of the gubernaculum and the processus vaginalis, which drag the layers of the abdominal wall after their passage through the canal. After the testis reaches the scrotum, the gubernaculum is reduced in size (represented by scrotal ligament) and the inguinal canal is occupied by the spermatic cord. The caudal part of the processus vaginalis forms the tunica vaginalis (a serous covering of the testis) and the part between the tunica vaginalis and the general peritoneal cavity is reduced to a

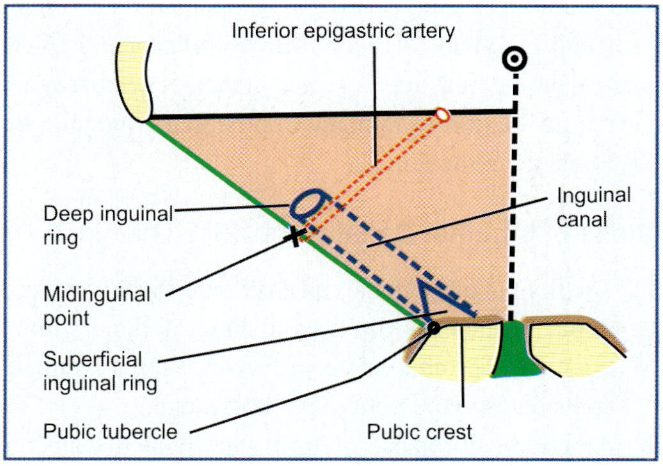

Fig. 129.1: Surface marking of inguinal canal (Note: The surface markings of the inferior epigastric artery and its medial relation to deep ring)

fibrous remnant. In the female, the ovary is retained in the pelvic cavity. Therefore, the gubernaculum ovarii remains long and becomes the ligament of ovary (between the ovary and the uterus) and the round ligament of uterus (between the uterus and labium majus). Thus, it is the round ligament of uterus, which comes to occupy the inguinal canal in female. The entire processus vaginalis is reduced to a fibrous remnant in female.

Contents of Inguinal Canal in Male

The spermatic cord and the ilioinguinal nerve are the main contents. As shown in Figure 161.2, the spermatic cord consists of vas deferens (ductus deferens), testicular artery, pampiniform plexus of veins, artery to ductus deferens, cremasteric artery, fibrous remnant of processus vaginalis, lymphatics, genital branch of genitofemoral nerve and autonomic nerve plexuses. The coverings of the cord from inside out, are internal spermatic fascia (derived from transversalis fascia), cremasteric muscle and fascia (derived from internal oblique muscle and external spermatic fascia (derived from external oblique aponeurosis. Figure 127.3 depicts the continuity of the layers of anterior abdominal wall with those of spermatic cord and scrotum.

The ilioinguinal nerve (L1) enters the inguinal canal by piercing its roof.

Contents of Inguinal Canal in Female

The round ligament of uterus accompanied by an artery to round ligament (a branch of the inferior epigastric artery), ilioinguinal nerve, genital branch of genitifemoral nerve and the fibrous remnant of processus vaginalis are the contents in the female.

Walls of Inguinal Canal (Figs 129.2 and129.3)

a. The floor of the inguinal canal is formed by the grooved upper surface of the medial half of the inguinal ligament. The abdominal surface of lacunar ligament contributes to the floor at its medial end.
b. Anterior wall consists of, from superficial to deep, the skin and superficial fascia, external oblique aponeurosis in the entire extent and the inguinal fibers of internal oblique muscle in the lateral third.

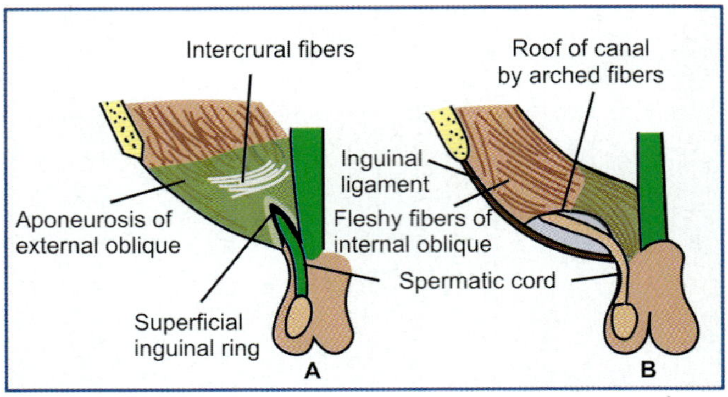

Fig. 129.2: Anterior wall of inguinal canal: (A) shows entire extent of anterior wall and (B) shows lateral 1/3rd of this wall

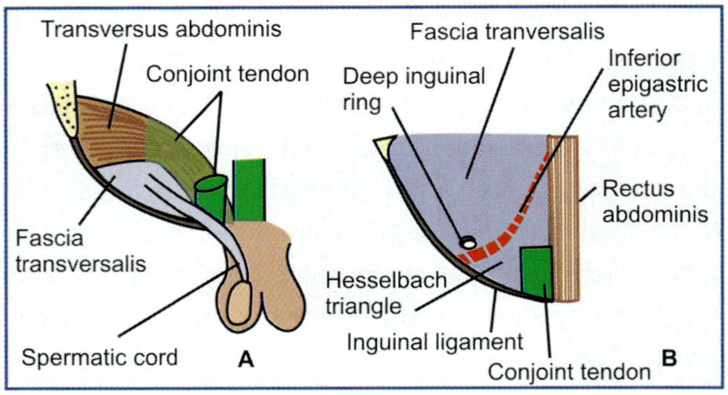

Fig. 129.3: Posterior wall of inguinal canal: (A) shows medial half of the posterior wall and (B) shows the entire posterior wall

The superficial inguinal ring is the deficiency in the anterior wall.

c. The roof consists of the arched fibers of internal oblique muscle. Above the internal oblique, the inguinal fibers of transversus abdominis also arch over the roof of the canal.
The ilioinguinal nerve enters the canal by piercing the arched fibers of the internal oblique muscle.
d. The posterior wall consists of the transversalis fascia in the entire extent. The conjoint tendon (formed by fusion of aponeuroses of internal oblique and transversus muscles) is present in the medial half of posterior wall (in front of the fascial wall). The reflected part of inguinal ligament forms the medialmost part of the posterior wall (in front of the conjoint tendon).

The deep inguinal ring is a deficiency in the posterior wall. Hesselbach's triangle (inguinal triangle) is an area of surgical importance on the posterior wall. It is bounded laterally by inferior epigastric artery, medially by lateral margin of rectus abdominis and inferiorly by medial part of inguinal ligament. The triangle is divided into lateral and medial parts by the ligamentous remnant of obliterated umbilical artery. The hernia protruding through its medial part is called the medial direct hernia and the one protruding through its lateral part is called the lateral direct hernia.

Deep (Internal) Inguinal Ring

The deep ring is a circular opening in the fascia transversalis. It lies 1.25 cm above the midinguinal point. Internal spermatic fascia is the extension of the fascia transversalis from the margins of the deep ring. In the male, the structures passing through the deep ring are, ductus deferens, testicular artery, artery to cremaster, artery to vas deferens, testicular veins, genital branch of genitofemoral nerve, autonomic plexuses and lymphatics. In the female, the round ligament of uterus and genital branch of genitofemoral nerve pass through the deep ring. The inferior epigastric artery is medial relation of the deep ring and the oblique or indirect inguinal hernia enters the canal through it.

Superficial (External) Inguinal Ring

This is a triangular opening in the aponeurosis of external oblique muscle. It lies just above the pubic crest and the pubic tubercle. The pubic crest forms the base of the ring. The margins of the ring are called lateral and medial crura, which are held together by intercrural fibers. The stronger lateral crus formed by fibers of inguinal ligament is attached to the pubic tubercle. The weaker medial crus is attached to the front of the pubic symphysis. The lateral crus is curved in male because it supports the heavy spermatic cord. From the margins of the ring, aponeurosis of external oblique prolongs as external spermatic fascia. The structures passing through the ring in male, are, ductus deferens, testicular artery, pampiniform plexus, artery to vas and cremasteric artery, genital branch of genitofemoral and ilioinguinal nerves, autonomic nerve plexuses, lymphatics and two fascial layers (cremaster muscle and fascia and internal spermatic fascia). In the female, the structures passing through the small sized ring are, round ligament of uterus, ilioinguinal nerve, genital branch of genitofemoral nerve and a few lymphatics. Both direct and indirect inguinal herniae come out through the superficial ring.

Examination of Superficial Ring in Male

It is easy palpate the ring in a supine patient. The skin of the bottom of the scrotum is invaginated with a finger, in superolateral direction until the pubic tubercle is felt. The finger is then rotated and pushed further up to enter the ring, where the crura of the ring can be felt.

Protection of Inguinal Canal

The inguinal canal is the weak part of the anterior abdominal wall because it is constantly subjected to the weight of the abdominal contents in the erect position. Therefore, the abdominal contents tend to herniate through the canal. To counteract this tendency there are some inherent protective devices.

a. Obliquity of the inguinal canal facilitates its closure during rise in intra-abdominal pressure by approximation of its anterior and posterior walls.
b. The fleshy fibers of the internal oblique muscle in the anterior wall compensate the weakness in the posterior wall (deep ring). Similarly, the strong conjoint tendon in the posterior wall compensates the weakness in the anterior wall (superficial ring).
c. The internal oblique muscle surrounds the canal from front, above and behind (triple relation). Hence, its contraction obliterates the canal by bringing the roof in contact with the floor, whenever there is rise in intra-abdominal pressure. This is described as the shutter mechanism of the inguinal canal.
d. The contraction of cremaster provides an effective plug for the superficial inguinal ring in the male.
e. The intercrural fibers hold the crura of the superficial ring together whenever pressure rises in the abdomen.

Clinical Highlights

A hernia is a protrusion of the peritoneal sac with or without a contained viscus through any weakness in the abdominal wall. The inguinal canal is a common site of herniation, since; it is a weakness in the anterior abdominal wall. A hernia in the inguinal canal is known as inguinal hernia. There are two types of inguinal herniae, oblique (or indirect) and direct. The indirect hernia enters the inguinal canal through the deep ring and the direct hernia enters through the posterior wall. The inguinal hernia is more common in males for obvious reasons.

The inguinal hernia usually presents as a swelling in, the inguinal region (groin). On coughing, the swelling increases in size. It is possible to reduce the hernia manually by pushing it upwards or the hernial swelling may disappear automatically in supine position.

Ring occlusion test is performed to distinguish the indirect from the direct hernia. After reducing the hernia, the deep ring is occluded with thumb and then the patient is asked to cough. If the swelling appears medial to the thumb it is a direct hernia. If the swelling does not appear it is an indirect hernia.

The relation of the hernia to the pubic tubercle differentiates inguinal from the femoral hernia. The inguinal hernia lies above the pubic tubercle as against the femoral hernia, which lies below and lateral to the pubic tubercle.

Indirect or Oblique Inguinal Hernia

It is more common in children and younger age boys as the predisposing congenital factor for this type of hernia is the complete or partial patency of the processus vaginalis. The hernia enters the canal via the deep inguinal

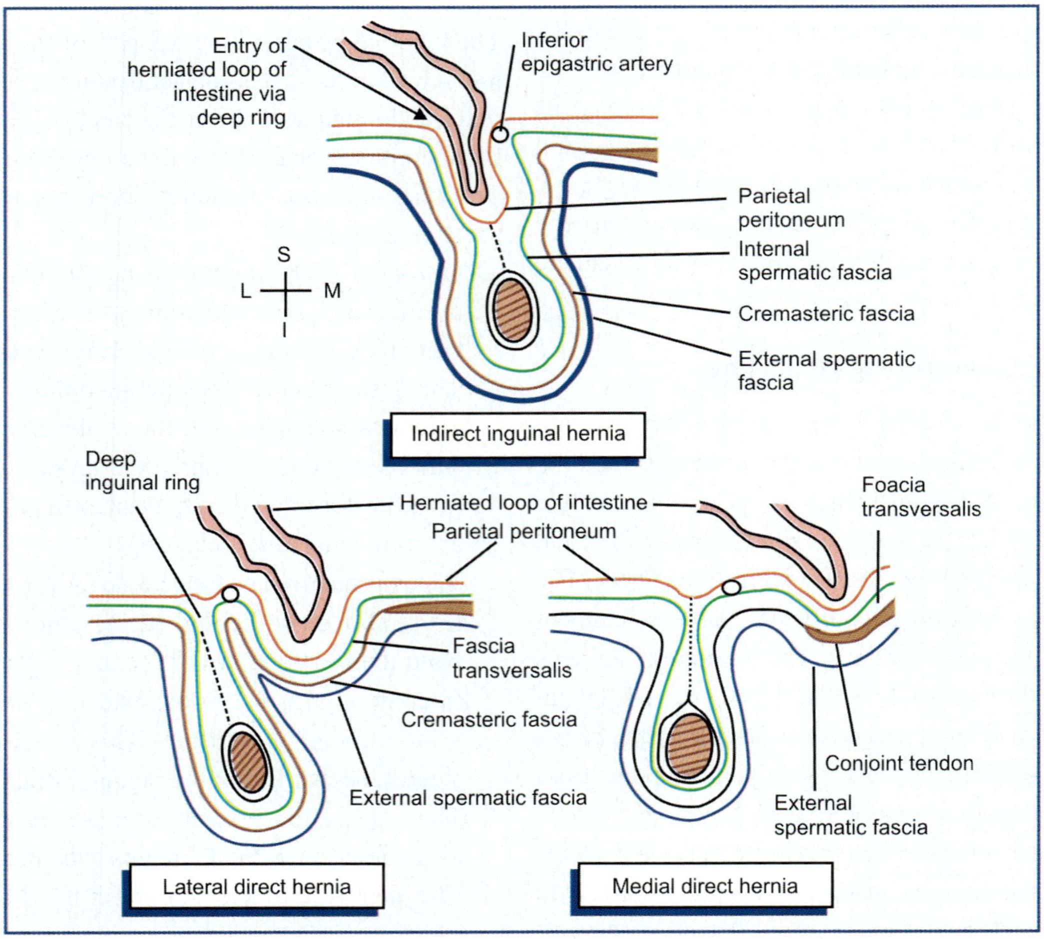

Fig. 129.4: Simplified scheme to depict coverings of indirect and direct inguinal herniae

ring and then passes through the entire inguinal canal to come out through the superficial inguinal ring. It is inside the coverings of spermatic cord hence enters the scrotum. The neck of hernial sac is lateral to the inferior epigastric artery.

Direct Inguinal Hernia

It is more common in old age. The predisposing factor in old age is weakness of abdominal muscles. Other causes are, chronic rise in intra-abdominal pressure, chronic constipation, chronic cough and lifting heavy weights. This hernia enters the inguinal canal through the medial part of the posterior wall (Hesselbach's triangle). It may enter the medial part of the canal by pushing the conjoint tendon (medial direct hernia) or by pushing the fascia transversalis (lateral direct hernia). The hernia comes out via the superficial ring. It lies outside the spermatic cord. The neck of hernial sac is medial to the inferior epigastric artery.

Coverings of Inguinal Herniae (Fig. 129.4)

a. The indirect hernia is covered in succession with, parietal peritoneum, extraperitoneal tissue, internal spermatic fascia, cremaster muscle and fascia, external spermatic fascia and skin.
b. The lateral direct hernia is covered with parietal peritoneum, extraperitoneal tissue, fascia transversalis, cremaster muscle and fascia, external spermatic fascia and skin.
c. The medial direct hernia is covered with parietal peritoneum, extraperitoneal tissue, fascia transversalis, conjoint tendon, external spermatic fascia and skin.

130 Development of Gut and Peritoneum

There is an intimate association between the gut and the peritoneum right from the embryonic stage. Therefore, the knowledge of the development of gut or digestive tract is an essential prerequisite for understanding the complex peritoneal relations and the definitive positions of the various parts of gut in the abdominopelvic cavity.

Primitive Gut

The primitive gut is formed from the endodermal germ layer and part of the yolk sac during the folding of the embryonic disc. It is divisible in three parts (Fig. 130.1). The foregut is enclosed in the head fold and the hindgut in the tail fold of the embryo. The midgut inside the lateral folds, however, is in open communication with the definitive yolk sac by means of the vitellointestinal duct. The foregut meets the ectodermal stomodeum at the buccopharyngeal membrane, which ruptures at the end of fourth week. The hindgut meets the ectodermal proctodeum at the cloacal membrane, which ruptures at end of seventh or eighth week. In this way, the primitive gut establishes communication with the exterior at both ends. Thus, the lining epithelium of the gut is endodermal. The rest of the gut wall (smooth musculature, connective tissue and visceral peritoneum) is derived from the splanchnopleuric mesoderm. The primitive peritoneal cavity is derived from the intraembryonic coelom inferior to the diaphragm. The splanchnopleuric mesoderm surrounding the gut forms the visceral peritoneum and the somatopleuric mesoderm lining the body wall forms the parietal peritoneum.

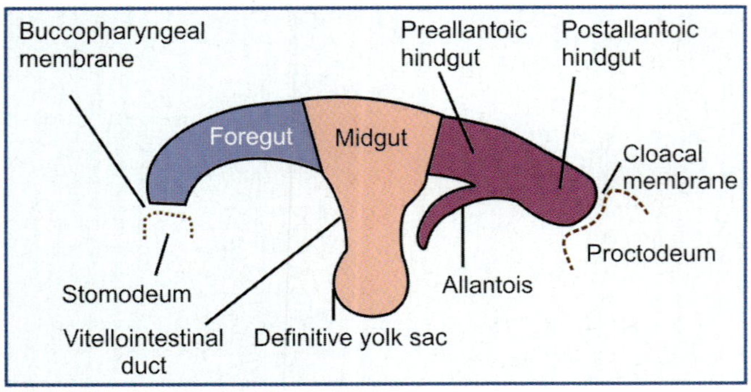

Fig. 130.1: Parts of primitive gut

Formation of Embryonic Mesenteries

The ventral and dorsal mesenteries (peritoneal folds) suspend the gut from the ventral and dorsal body walls respectively. However, the ventral mesentery (septum transversum) degenerates except in the region of the foregut. The dorsal mesentery is important since it carries blood vessels and nerve plexuses to the gut. The artery of the foregut is the coeliac trunk, that of midgut is the superior mesenteric artery, and that of hindgut is the inferior mesenteric artery. These arteries supply the derivatives of the respective parts of the gut. The derivatives of foregut and midgut receive parasympathetic supply from the vagus and those of the hindgut from the sacral parasympathetic nerves.

Derivatives of Abdominal Part of Foregut

The abdominal part of foregut develops into the stomach, first part of duodenum and second part of the duodenum proximal to the opening of common bile duct, liver, biliary apparatus (consisting of gallbladder, cystic duct, hepatic ducts and common bile duct) and the pancreas. The detailed account of the development of these organs is found along with the description of the individual organ.

Fate of Mesenteries of Foregut

a. The ventral mesentery of the foregut is called the ventral mesogastrium, which is a part of the septum transversum. The development of liver in the ventral mesogastrium alters its original position and splits it into the lesser omentum, falciform ligament and the right and left triangular and coronary ligaments.

b. The dorsal mesentery of the foregut is called the dorsal mesogastrium. The changes in position, size and shape of the stomach due to the development of lesser sac and the development of spleen in the dorsal mesogastrium, totally modify the dorsal mesogastrium. The gastrophrenic ligament, gastrosplenic ligament, lienorenal ligament and the greater omentum, are the 4 peritoneal folds derived from the dorsal mesogastrium. The part that gives rise to greater omentum becomes an enormously elongated and double-folded in which the cavity of lesser sac extends.

Derivatives of Midgut

The midgut gives rise to the duodenum beyond the opening of common bile duct, jejunum, ileum, caecum and appendix, ascending colon and right two-thirds of transverse colon.

Formation of Midgut Loop and its Herniation (Fig. 130.2)

The midgut elongates rapidly and forms a U- shaped loop known as primary intestinal loop, which has cranial and caudal limbs. The dorsal mesentery elongates to lie between the two limbs and the superior mesenteric artery runs through the mesentery to distribute branches to the

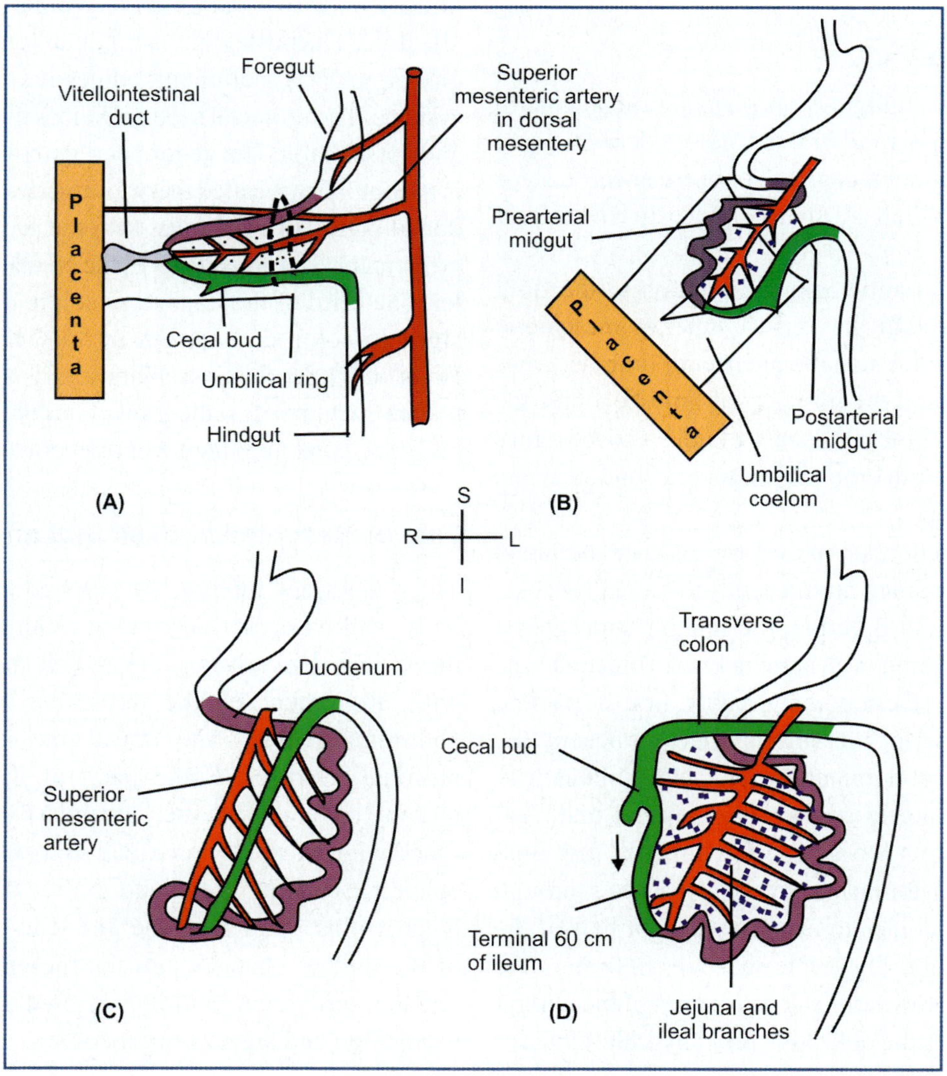

Fig. 130.2: Stages in the rotation of gut: (A) Physiological herniation of midgut loop in umbilical coelom, (B) Anticlockwise rotation through 90°, (C) Reduction of prearterial segment with further rotation through 180°, (D) Reduction of postarterial segment through 180° rotation

two limbs. Hence, the cranial limb becomes the prearterial and the caudal limb the postarterial. At the junction of the limbs, the vitellointestinal duct is attached. This duct connects the midgut to the definitive yolk sac in the umbilical cord and normally degenerates by 5 to 6 weeks.

Physiological Herniation

Due to the large size of liver at this stage of embryo, the space in the abdominal cavity is insufficient for the rapidly elongating intestinal loop. Hence, the midgut loop undergoes herniation in the umbilical cord during the fifth week. This is known as physiological umbilical herniation. The migut loop remains in the umbilical cord till tenth week.

Rotation of Midgut

The rotation of the midgut loop plays a crucial role in attaining the final position of the different derivatives of the gut in the abdominal cavity. There are specific steps in this process, which must take place in an orderly sequence:

a. At first, there is anticlockwise rotation to the right through 90° around the axis of superior mesenteric artery because of which the prearterial limb becomes the right limb and the postarterial limb becomes the left. The right limb elongates rapidly and becomes coiled and the left limb shows a cecal bud near the apex of the loop.
b. Next, there is reduction of the physiological hernia in a sequential manner during tenth to twelfth weeks. During reduction of hernia, the midgut undergoes a further 180° rotation in an anticlockwise direction. The right limb enters the abdominal cavity, first, by passing behind the superior mesenteric artery to occupy the left half of the abdominal cavity. This explains why superior mesenteric artery gives jejunal and ileal branches from its left side. After this, the left limb returns to the abdominal cavity. It also rotates through 180° before it comes to occupy the right half of the abdominal cavity. The left limb passes in front of the superior mesenteric artery. The rotation of the midgut loop determines the definitive relation of the superior mesenteric artery to the third part of duodenum and the transverse colon.
c. After the return of hernia, the caecum is in the subhepatic position and the ascending colon is not distinguishable. The final step of rotation consists of descent of the caecum and development of ascending colon. The details of this process are described with caecum and appendix in Chapter 137.

Derivatives of Hindgut

The hindgut lies in the tail fold of the embryo. From its ventral aspect, it sends a diverticulum called the allantois, towards the umbilical opening. The allantois divides the hindgut into two parts, namely preallantoic and post-allantoic. The postallantoic hindgut is called endodermal cloaca, which is common to digestive and genitourinary systems. The urorectal septum divides the cloaca in ventral and dorsal parts. The ventral part with which the allantois is in continuity is called the primitive urogenital sinus. The dorsal part is in continuity with the preallantoic hindgut proximally. The derivatives of the preallantoic hindgut are, left one-third of the transverse colon, descending colon, sigmoid colon and rectum up to the middle valve of Houston. The derivatives of the dorsal part of postallantoic gut are, rectum below the level of middle valve of Houston and anal canal upto the level of pectinate line.

Fate of Mesenteries of Midgut and Hindgut

The midgut and hindgut are suspended from the dorsal body wall by dorsal mesentery. With differentiation of the various derivatives of the midgut and the hindgut and with attainment of the definitive positions in the abdominal cavity, the dorsal mesentery undergoes profound changes. Some parts of the gut lose their mesentery and become secondarily retroperitoneal (duodenum except the proximal 2 cm, caecum, ascending colon, descending colon and the rectum). This process is known as fixation of the gut. The dorsal mesentery of the midgut changes into the mesentery (attached to jejunum and ileum) and that of hindgut into transverse mesocolon and sigmoid mesocolon.

Congenital Anomalies

a. The exomphalos or omphalocele results due to failure of the reduction of physiological hernia. In this anomaly, the intestines remain inside the umbilical sac, which is covered with amnion.
b. In congenital umbilical hernia, the intestinal loop herniates through the imperfectly closed umbilicus. Therefore, the hernial sac is covered with peritoneum.
c. Failure of rotation of the midgut or non-rotation results in location of small intestine on right side and caecum and ascending colon on left side.
d. Reverse rotation gives rise to an anomaly in which the superior mesenteric artery goes behind the third part of the duodenum and the transverse colon is behind the superior mesenteric artery.
e. Failure of fixation results in excessive mobility of different parts of the gut, which predisposes to complications like volvulus or torsion of the gut.
f. Meckel's diverticulum or ileal diverticulum is the persistent proximal part of vitellointestinal duct. It is five cm (2 inches) long and is present in about 2 percent of population. It is situated on the antimesenteric border of the ileum about 60 cm (2 feet) proximal to the ileocecal junction (Rule of 2's). Sometimes, acid secreting-oxyntic cells of stomach or pancreatic cells are seen in the mucosa of the diverticulum. This may produce peptic ulceration and perforation. The inflammtion of the diverticulum (ileal diverticulitis) gives rise to symptoms, which are indistinguishable from appendicitis.
g. If the vitellointestinal duct leaves behind a fibrous remnant connecting the ileum to the umbilicus, a loop of small bowel may revolve around this remnant and cause intestinal twisting. This may lead to intestinal obstruction or occlusion of blood vessels.
h. In complete patency of the vitellointestinal duct, ileum communicates with the exterior at umbilicus (umbilical fistula). If the duct is fibrosed at its intestinal and umbilical ends but remains cystic in the mid-portion, it gives rise to enterocystoma and if it persists at its distal end, it may give rise to raspberry red tumor at the umbilicus.

131 Abdominopelvic Cavity

The abdominopelvic cavity is the largest cavity in the body. It is completely filled with viscera. The outline of the cavity is described as kidney-shaped. This is due to the forward bulging of the lumbar vertebral column and the backward protrusion of the pelvic cavity. The abdominal and pelvic cavities, though continuous, are not in the same plane (Fig. 127.1).

CONTENTS

Peritoneal cavity, which is the largest and most complexly arranged serous sac, is present inside the abdominopelvic cavity. It is a potential space between the parietal and visceral layers of peritoneum. The parietal layer lines the inner surfaces of the walls of the abdomen and pelvis. The visceral layer either completely or partially covers the abdominal viscera. The visceral and parietal layers are continuous with each other along the lines of reflection of the peritoneum on the abdominal and pelvic walls. Along these lines, the visceral peritoneum leaves as two layers of the peritoneal fold, which reaches the particular viscera to become continuous with the visceral peritoneum surrounding the same viscera. The purpose of such peritoneal folds is to carry blood vessels and nerves to the viscera from the major vessels located behind the parietal peritoneum on the posterior abdominal wall.

General Disposition of Viscera

a. The liver occupies the right hypochondrium, extends in the epigastrium and also in the left hypochondrium. It is almost completely covered with peritoneum except for some non-peritoneal areas. The liver gives attachments to five peritoneal folds. The falciform ligament extends from the anterior abdominal wall to the anterior surface of the liver. The right and left triangular and coronary ligaments connect the liver to the diaphragm. The lesser omentum connects the liver to the lesser curvature of stomach. The major part of gallbladder lies hidden under the inferior surface of liver. However, its fundus projects below the inferior margin of the liver at the tip of right ninth costal cartilage.
b. The spleen is located deep in the left hypochondrium posterior to the stomach and anterior to the upper part of left kidney. The gastrosplenic ligament connects it to the greater curvature of stomach and the lienorenal ligament to the posterior abdominal wall.
c. The stomach lies obliquely in the epigastrium and the left hypochondrium. The liver, diaphragm and the anterior abdominal wall cover the greater part of the stomach. The stomach gives attachments to four peritoneal folds. The lesser omentum passes from the lesser curvature of stomach to the liver, carrying in its free margin the triad of portal vein, common bile duct and the hepatic artery. The greater omentum is the longest and four-layered peritoneal fold connecting the greater curvature of stomach to the posterior abdominal wall. The gastrosplenic ligament carries the branches of splenic vessels to the stomach. The gastrophrenic ligament connects the stomach to the diaphragm.
d. The C-shaped duodenum is the first part of the small intestine. It is divided into four parts. Except the proximal two cm of the first part, the rest of the duodenum is retroperitoneal. The duodenum is located to the right of the midline except the duodenojejunal junction, which lies to the left of midline just below the level of transpyloric plane. Being retroperitoneal, it lies hidden under the liver, gallbladder and the transverse colon.
e. The pancreas is a large gland. It is located across the

132 Peritoneum

The peritoneum is a thin but firm serous membrane. The surface area of the peritoneum is very vast, almost equaling to that of the skin covering the entire body. The epithelial lining of the peritoneum is called the mesothelium, which is a single layer of flattened squamous cells supported by submesothelial connective tissue containing lymphocytes, macrophages and adipocytes (fat cells). The walls of the abdominopelvic cavity are lined with parietal peritoneum. The viscera in the cavity are covered completely or partially with visceral peritoneum. The parietal and visceral layers of the peritoneum are continuous with each other along the lines of peritoneal reflection. Thus, the folds of visceral peritoneum suspend the viscera from the posterior abdominal wall. Such double-layered peritoneal folds are described as omenta, mesenteries, mesocolons and ligaments in different situations. The terms, mesentery, omenta and epiploic mean pertaining to peritoneum.

Functions of Peritoneum

The peritoneal fluid secreted by the lining epithelium (mesothelium) keeps the surfaces moist and prevents friction between adjacent viscera. The presence of the antibody producing cells in its submesothelial tissue helps in resisting infections. The peritoneal fluid is rapidly absorbed from the thin and vacsularized serous membrane.

Subdivisions of Peritoneal Cavity (Fig. 132.1)

There are two subdivisions of the peritoneal cavity, the larger, greater sac and smaller, lesser sac. These sacs are in communication with each other only at the epiploic foramen. The greater sac is further divided into supracolic and infracolic compartments. The supracolic space occupies the upper anterior part of the abdominal cavity. The infracolic space occupies the entire abdominopelvic cavity below the transverse colon. The lesser sac lies hidden behind the lesser omentum and the stomach but infront of the pancreas and transverse mesocolon. In childhood, the lesser sac extends in the double layers of greater omentum but in the adult, this part of the sac is obliterated.

Vertical Disposition of Peritoneum

Prior knowledge of peritoneal relations of the liver is essential to trace the continuity of the peritoneum in its vertical extent. The liver is connected to the diaphragm, anterior and posterior abdominal walls and the stomach by different peritoneal folds. The lines of attachments of

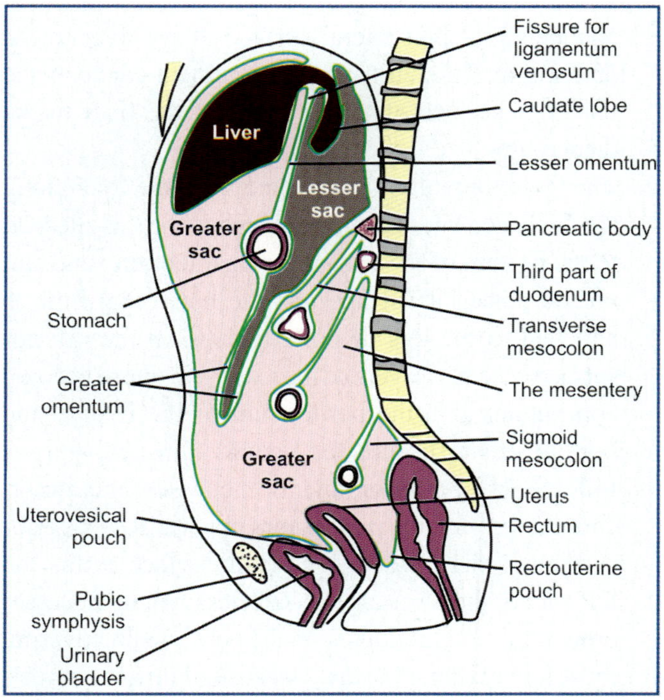

Fig. 132.1: Sagittal section through abdomen and pelvis showing peritoneal sacs, folds and pouches

these peritoneal folds, though present at different places on the liver, are continuous with each other.

a. The falciform ligament leaves the supraumbilical part of the anterior abdominal wall as two layers, which enclose the ligamentum teres of the liver in its free margin. It reaches the anterior surface of the liver, where its layers become continuous with the peritoneum covering the anterior surfaces of the right and the left lobes of the liver. The line of attachment of this ligament to the anterior surface of the liver demarcates the right and left lobes.

b. The coronary, left triangular and right triangular ligaments connect the diaphragm and the liver. The coronary and right triangular ligaments connect the right lobe of the liver to the diaphragm as follows. The superior layer of the coronary ligament reflects from the posterior surface of the right lobe to the diaphragm. The inferior layer of the coronary ligament reflects from the posterior surface of the right lobe on to the posterior abdominal wall in the region of right kidney. However, the superior and inferior layers of coronary ligaments are separated from each other to enclose the triangular bare area of liver on the posterior surface. These two layers meet each other at the apex of the bare area to form the right triangular ligament, which connects the right lateral surface of the liver to the diaphragm. The left triangular ligament connects the posterior surface of the left lobe of the liver to the diaphragm.

c. The lesser omentum is reflected from the liver along the L-shaped line. The vertical limb of the L is attached to the bottom of the fissure for ligamentum venosum on the posterior surface and the horizontal limb is attached to the lips of porta hepatis on the inferior surface. The two layers of the lesser omentum become continuous with the peritoneum of the liver at the bottom of the fissure for ligamentum venosum as follows. The posterior layer of the lesser omentum is continuous with the peritoneum covering the anterior surface of the caudate lobe (this surface forms the left wall of the fissure). The anterior layer of the lesser omentum is continuous with the peritoneum covering the left wall of the fissure. Because of this, the fissure contains four layers of peritoneum inside it. The anterior and posterior layers of the vertical limb are in continuity with the attachments of the horizontal limb at the margins of the porta hepatis. From this L-shaped line of reflection the lesser omentum runs towards stomach as two layers, which are continuous with each other around the right free margin of the lesser omentum. This margin carries portal vein and hepatic artery to the liver and the common bile duct from the liver to the duodenum. At the lesser curvature of the stomach, the anterior and posterior layers of the lesser omentum separate to cover the anterosuperior and postero-anterior surfaces of stomach respectively and again meet at the greater curvature to form the greater omentum.

d. The greater omentum extends from the greater curvature of the stomach to the posterior abdominal wall, where it is attached along the anterior surface of the head and the anterior margin of the body of pancreas. The greater omentum is composed of four layers of peritoneum. Its anterior two layers leave at the greater curvature of the stomach and descend to a variable distance before doubling to form its posterior two layers. These layers are continuous with each other at the sides. The posterior layers ascend in front of the transverse colon and its mesocolon to reach the pancreas. They usually fuse with the anterior surface of the transverse colon and its mesocolon, which gives an impression that the greater omentum extends from the greater curvature of stomach to the transverse colon (hence the term gastrocolic ligament for the greater omentum). Due to the doubling of the greater omentum on itself, its first layer becomes the fourth and the second layer becomes the third. After reaching the anterior aspect of the pancreas the third layer of the greater omentum becomes continuous with the peritoneum lining the posterior abdominal wall of the supracolic compartment. On reaching the medial side of the cardiac end of the esophagus, the peritoneum covers the diaphragm and then is reflected on the liver at the upper margin of caudate lobe.

e. From the anterior margin of the body of pancreas, the fourth layer of the greater omentum is reflected downwards as the upper layer of transverse mesocolon, which encloses the transverse colon and returns back to the anterior margin of pancreas, as the lower layer of transverse mesocolon. The upper layer of transverse mesocolon and the fourth layer of greater omentum are adherent but separable from each other.

f. The lower layer of the transverse mesocolon becomes continuous with the parietal peritoneum on the inferior surface of the body of pancreas. Below this, it is continuous with the peritoneum on the posterior abdominal wall, from where it is reflected as the right layer of the root of the mesentery. This covers the jejunum and ileum and returns to the posterior abdominal wall as the left layer of the mesentery. The line of reflection of the mesentery runs obliquely on the posterior wall dividing the infracolic compartment into right superior and left inferior regions. From the root of the mesentery, its left layer can be traced as the parietal peritoneum covering the left inferior region of the infracolic compartment, from where it crosses the pelvic brim to become the pelvic peritoneum.

g. Once inside the pelvis, the parietal peritoneum is reflected on the left side as the anterior layer of pelvic mesocolon, which encloses the sigmoid colon and returns to the pelvic wall as its posterior layer. The root of the pelvic mesocolon is inverted V-shaped. Its left limb is attached to the left pelvic brim and the right limb extends upto the third sacral vertebra, the apex of the V being near the division of left common iliac vessels. The pelvic peritoneum descends on the anterior surface and sides of the upper third and the front of the middle third of the rectum.

h. The pelvic peritoneum in the male, can be traced further as follows. The peritoneum leaves the anterior surface of the rectum at the junction of its middle and lower thirds and passes forward along the superior surface of the seminal vesicle to the superior surface of the urinary bladder, forming the rectovesical peritoneal pouch. The bottom of this pouch lies 7.5 cm above the anal orifice. This is the lowest limit of the peritoneal cavity in male. From the superior surface of urinary bladder, the peritoneum is reflected on the anterior abdominal wall, where it becomes continuous with the parietal peritoneum. Lateral to the rectum and the urinary bladder the peritoneum can be traced along the superior surface of pelvic diaphragm until it becomes continuous with the parietal peritoneum on the lateral pelvic walls. The peritoneal cavity in the male is described as a closed space.

i. The pelvic peritoneum in female (Fig. 132.1) can be traced further as follows. The peritoneum leaves the anterior surface of the rectum at junction of its middle and lower thirds and passes forwards to cover the posterior fornix of vagina. It ascends to cover the posterior surface of uterus. The peritoneal pouch between the rectum and the uterus is called the rectouterine pouch of Douglas. The bottom of this pouch is the lowest part of the peritoneal cavity in female and lies 5.5 cm above the anal orifice. After covering the fundus of the uterus, the peritoneum covers the anterior surface as far as the junction of the body and cervix of the uterus. From here, it is reflected on the superior surface of the urinary bladder forming a shallow uterovesical pouch. From the urinary bladder, the visceral peritoneum is reflected on the anterior abdominal wall. Laterally, the peritoneum leaves the uterus as the two layers of broad ligament, which connects the uterus to the lateral walls of the pelvic cavity. The broad ligament consists of anteroinferior and posterosuperior layers, which are continuous with each other at the free margin of the broad ligament. The fallopian tube is enclosed in the free margin. The part of the broad ligament continuous with the germinal epithelium of ovary is called the mesovarium. The ovum liberated in the peritoneal cavity at the time of ovulation, is picked up by the tubal ostium with the help of fimbriae at the lateral end of the fallopian tube. In this way, through the tubal ostium and the tube the peritoneal cavity is in communication with the uterine cavity (through it with the exterior via the vaginal orifice). Hence, the peritoneal cavity in the female is described as open unlike in the male.

Transverse Disposition of Peritoneum

Tracing the continuity of the peritoneum in a transverse plane at the level of epiploic foramen in the supracolic compartment can be understood from the Figure 132.2.

Epiploic Foramen

The epiploic foramen (Omental foramen or foramen of Winslow) is located at the level of the T12 vertebra. It is the only site, where the peritoneum of the greater and lesser sacs is in continuity with each other. The boundaries of epiploic foramen are depicted in Figure 132.4. The free margin of the lesser omentum with its three contents namely portal vein, bile duct and hepatic artery are present anteriorly. The inferior vena cava is the posterior relation. The caudate process of the liver forms the superior boundary and the first part of the duodenum, the inferior boundary. The applied importance of the foramen is described below.

Lesser Sac (Figs 132.1 to 132.3)

The lesser sac (or omental bursa) is a recess of the peritoneal cavity that is hidden behind the lesser omentum and the posterior surface of stomach. The lesser sac communicates with the greater sac only through the epiploic foramen. It is called omental bursa because it acts as a bursa for the stomach allowing for its expansion and mobility. The lesser sac has two walls, four margins, three recesses and one opening. Since its margins are not straight lines, the shape of lesser sac is irregular.

Boundaries

a. The anterior wall of the lesser sac (from above downward) consists of posterior layer of the lesser omentum, peritoneum covering the posterior surface of stomach and the anterior two layers of greater omentum.
b. The posterior wall of the lesser sac (from below upward) consists of posterior two layers of the greater omentum and the parietal peritoneum covering the stomach bed in the supracolic compartment.
c. The upper margin is the peritoneal continuity from the caudate lobe of the liver to the diaphragm (on right side) and the gastrophrenic ligament (on the left of the caudate lobe.
d. The blind lower margin is the line of continuity of the two anterior layers of the greater omentum with its two posterior layers.
e. The left margin (from below upward) in the infracolic compartment, is formed by the left margin of the greater omentum and the lienorenal and gastrosplenic ligaments in the supracolic compartment.
f. The right margin is complicated and is formed (from below upward) in the infracolic compartment by the right margin of greater omentum and by the reflection of peritoneum from the pancreas to the posterior aspect of the proximal part of the duodenum. The cross-section of the peritoneal cavity at the level of L1 vertebra depicts the right margin of the lesser sac at this level (Fig. 132.3). Immediately above the first part of the duodenum, the right margin is deficient (this site being called the epiploic foramen). Above this level, the right margin is formed by the peritoneum covering the caudate lobe, at the upper end of which it becomes continuous with the superior margin.

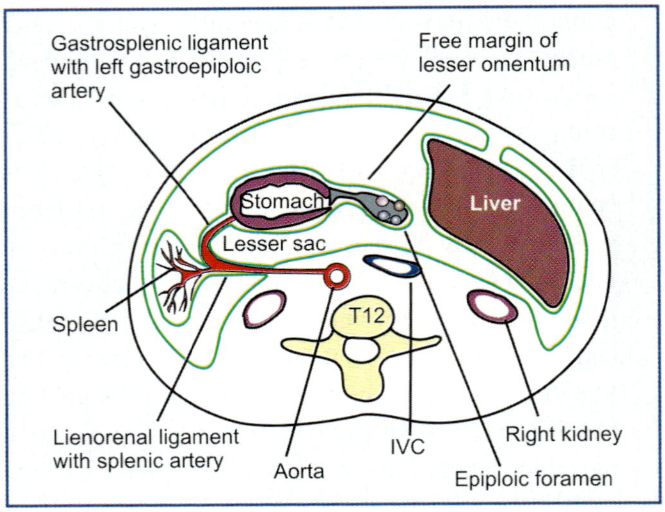

Fig. 132.2: Transverse section through the abdomen at the level of epiploic foramen

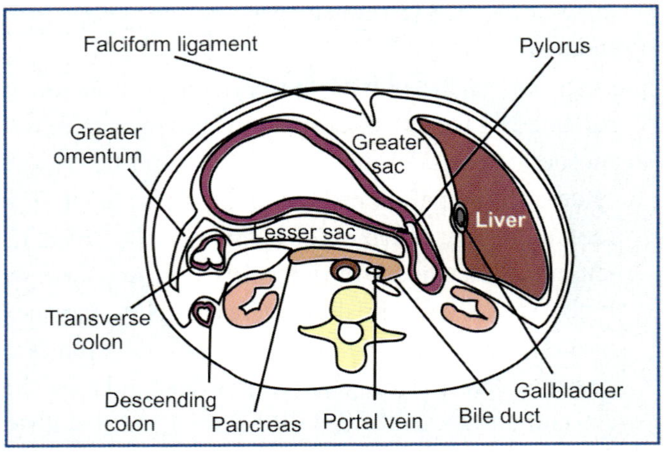

Fig. 132.3: Transverse section of the abdomen at the level of pylorus

Subdivisions of Lesser Sac

The lesser sac is divided into five parts, vestibule, body and three recesses (superior, splenic and inferior).

a. The vestibule is the part of the lesser sac immediately to the left of epiploic foramen. Superiorly, it leads in the superior recess of the lesser sac. To the left, the vestibule leads into the space (foramen bursae omenti majoris) between the right and left gastropancreatic folds of peritoneum, which are produced by the common hepatic and left gastric arteries respectively.

b. The body of the omental bursa lies posterior to the lesser omentum and stomach.
c. The splenic recess is the extension of the body to the hilum of spleen in between the gastrosplenic and lienorenal ligaments.
d. The inferior recess is the part extending in the greater omentum. The inferior recess is normally obliterated in adult stage due to fusion of the layers of greater omentum.
e. The superior recess extends upwards above the epiploic foramen posterior to the caudate lobe of liver.

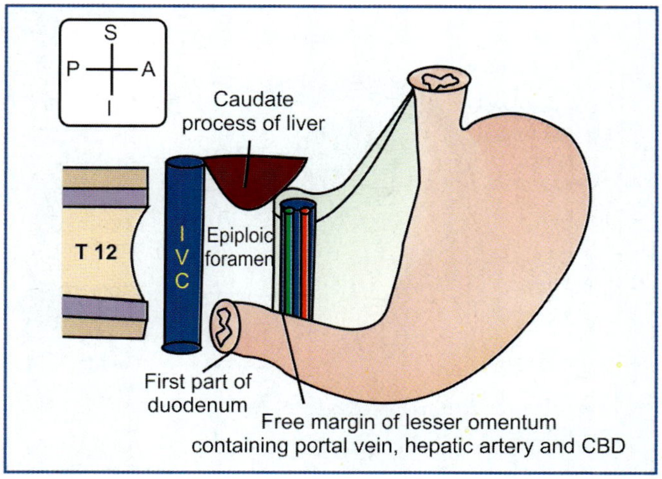

Fig. 132.4: Scheme depicting boundaries and vertebral level of epiploic foramen

Clinical Highlights

a. In internal herniation, a loop of intestine herniates through the epiploic foramen into the omental bursa. If the herniated loop is strangulated the reduction is not possible through the epiploic foramen because of its important relations. The alternate approach is through the posterior wall of the lesser sac by dissection along the plane of cleavage between the greater omentum and transverse mesocolon. The omental bursa is approached through the separated greater omentum. This is a bloodless plane between the gastroepiploic vessels in the greater omentum and the middle colic vessels in the transverse mesocolon. After the aspiration of the swollen intestinal loop, it is possible to reduce the intestine back to the greater sac through epiploic foramen.
b. The collection of inflammatory fluid in the omental bursa may occur due to perforation of the gastric ulcer located on the posterior wall of stomach or from the postoperative collection of fluid in the hepatorenal pouch via the epiploic foramen. The collection of fluid in the space due to pancreatitis is known as pseudo-pancreatic cyst.

Subphrenic Spaces (Fig. 132.5)

These spaces are in close proximity to the liver. They are described by a common term, subphrenic spaces, which consist of four intraperitoneal and two extraperitoneal spaces. The knowledge of the location, boundaries and communications of these spaces helps in understanding the direction of flow of peritoneal fluid. It is also helpful in the diagnosis of subphrenic abscess in case any one of the spaces becomes infected and cut off from the peritoneal cavity. The subphrenic spaces are divided into right and left spaces.

Right Subphrenic Spaces

a. Right anterior intraperitoneal space (right subdiaphragmatic)
b. Right posterior intraperitoneal space (right subhepatic or Morison's hepatorenal pouch)
c. Right extraperitoneal space (bare area of liver).

Left Subphrenic Spaces

a. Left anterior intraperitoneal space (left subdiaphragmatic)
b. Left posterior intraperitoneal space (lesser sac)
c. Left extraperitoneal space.

Right Anterior Intraperitoneal Space

The boundaries of this space are as follows:
Superior—superior layer of coronary ligament
Anterior—anterior abdominal wall
Posterior—anterior and superior surfaces of the right lobe of liver

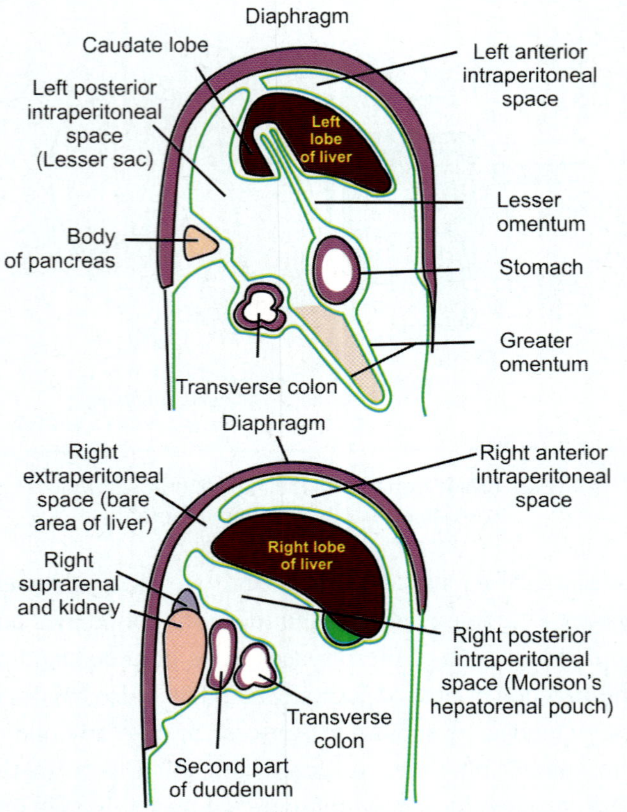

Fig. 132.5: Subphrenic spaces related to liver

Left—falciform ligament.
Inferiorly and to the right the space is open.

Left Anterior Intraperitoneal Space

This space has the following boundaries:
Superior—anterior layer of the left triangular ligament
Anterior—anterior abdominal wall
Posterior—anterior surface of the left lobe of the liver
Right—falciform ligament.
Inferiorly and to the left the space is open.

Right Posterior Intraperitoneal Space

It is known as the Morison's hepatorenal pouch.
Superior—inferior layer of coronary ligament
Anterior—visceral surface of right lobe of liver
Posterior—Parietal peritoneum, covering right suprarenal, and right kidney.

The space opens in the right paracolic gutter, through which it communicates with the pelvic cavity. To the left, the space is in communication with the lesser sac via the epiploic foramen.

Left Posterior Intraperitoneal Space

The other name of this space is the lesser sac (for boundaries, refer to lesser sac).

Right Extraperitoneal Space

The boundaries of this space coincide with those of the bare area of liver:
Superior—superior layer of coronary ligament
Inferior—inferior layer of coronary ligament
Anterior—bare area of the liver
Posterior—diaphragm
Left—groove for inferior vena cava
Right—right triangular ligament.

Left Extraperitoneal Space

This space is located behind the bare area of stomach and in front of the diaphragm, left suprarenal and upper part of left kidney.

Clinical Highlights

The subphrenic abscess forms if any one of the subphrenic spaces, harbors infection and gets loculated. Such abscesses are inaccessible to clinical examination. Hence, diagnosis often poses a problem. The amoebic abscess in the right extraperitoneal space may rupture into the right pleural cavity through the diaphragm. Morison's pouch is the commonest site of abscess formation, postoperatively, because it is the dependent space in the supine position. The abscess may form here secondary to appendicitis, cholecystitis, perforated duodenal ulcer or upper abdominal surgery. The abscess formation in the pelvis is because the pelvis is the most dependent part of the peritoneal cavity in the erect position and is in continuity with right paracolic gutter and hepatorenal pouch.

Spaces of Infracolic Compartment

There are right and left lateral paracolic gutters and right and left medial paracolic gutters. These spaces are the dependent parts of the peritoneal cavity in supine position.

The right lateral gutter is in continuity with Morison's hepatorenal pouch above and with pelvic cavity below. The left lateral gutter is separated from the supracolic compartment by the phrenico-colic ligament but is in free communication with the pelvic cavity.

Peritoneal Recesses or Fossae

At the transition sites, where the embryonic intraperitoneal gut loses its mesentery to become retroperitoneal, small peritoneal folds may persist. Such folds occur at the duodenojejunal junction, ileocecal junction and at the root of the pelvic mesocolon. The locations of the recesses, their surgical importance and important vascular relations are described with the fourth part of duodenum, caecum and pelvic mesocolon.

Blood Supply and Nerve Supply of Peritoneum

a. The parietal peritoneum is sensitive to touch, pain and temperature. The phrenic nerves supply the central part of diaphragmatic peritoneum and the intercostal nerves supply its peripheral part. Irritation of the central part of diaphragmatic peritoneum will give rise to pain in the C4 dermatome (shoulder pain). The lower five intercostal, subcostal and first lumbar nerves supply the rest of the peritoneum. Irritation of the peritoneum in these areas will cause muscle rigidity and referred pain in the anterior abdominal wall.
b. The visceral peritoneum receives autonomic innervation like the viscera. It is pain insensitive. Stretching the viscera due to acute distention or ischemia of the visceral musculature causes diffuse pain, which may be referred to the skin corresponding to the segmental level of autonomic innervation.

Clinical Highlights

a. Ascites is accumulation of fluid in the peritoneal cavity. A few causes of ascites include, congestive cardiac failure (CCF), cirrhosis of liver, abdominal malignancy and renal diseases. Since the peritoneal cavity is very capacious the accumulation of fluid cannot be detected clinically until about 1500 ml of fluid is collected. The removal of fluid (by tapping or abdominal paracentesis) is necessary to relieve the distress to the patient. While choosing the site for puncture care is taken to avoid inferior epigastric vessels.
b. The peritoneal dialysis is a method by which waste products like urea are removed from the blood in patients of renal failure. The peritoneum offers a large surface area with rapid absorptive properties, which is utilized for removal of the waste products of the blood. The peritoneal dialysis is practised in many centers because it is cheaper compared to the newer method called hemodialysis.
c. Peritonitis is the inflammation of the peritoneum, which may be localized or generalized. The generalized peritonitis is a much-feared complication after abdominal and pelvic surgery. The other causes of peritonitis include bacterial infection, perforation of the gastric ulcer or appendix or fallopian tube.
d. Hemoperitoneum is accumulation of blood in the peritoneal cavity. Some causes of hemoperitoneum include injury to the artery during surgery, rupture of the fallopian tube in ectopic pregnancy and traumatic rupture of any viscera.
e. Pneumoperitoneum is accumulation of air in the peritoneal cavity. This is usually due to perforation of intestine. Presence of air under the right side of diaphragm in a plain radiograph of abdomen is the early sign of pneumoperitoneum.

133 Stomach

The stomach (gaster) is the most dilated and distensible part of the digestive tube. It is obliquely placed in upper part of abdominal cavity, where it occupies epigastrium and left hypogastrium and extends to a variable extent into the umbilical region.

Functions

The stomach is a reservoir of food. Its capacity in an adult is 1000-1500 ml and in a newborn, 30-50 ml. It is a seat of digestion of food, which is achieved by mechanical and chemical actions. The musculature of the stomach contracts to break down the food particles and brings about thorough mixing of the food and the gastric juices. The gastric juice consists of pepsin (secreted by chief cells of gastric glands), HCl and Castle's intrinsic factor (secreted by parietal cells of gastric glands) and mucin (secreted by mucous neck cells of gastric glands). Hydrochloric acid has bactericidal action. Castle's intrinsic factor helps in absorption of vitamin B_{12} in the small intestine.

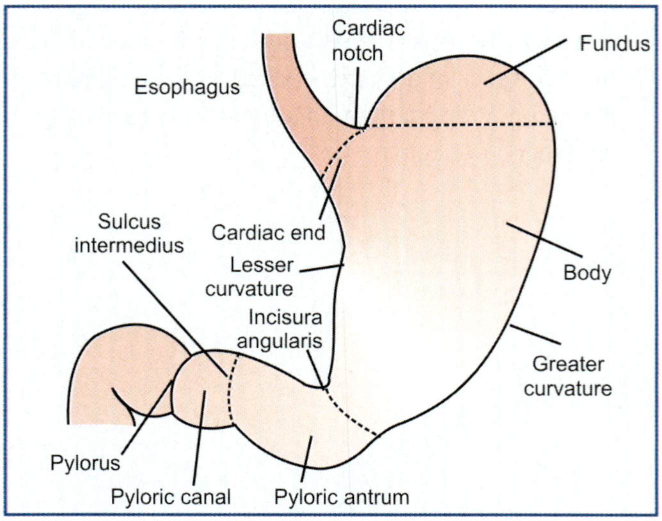

Fig. 133.1: Parts of stomach

Development of Stomach

The stomach is first recognized as a midline fusiform dilatation of the caudal part of foregut, suspended from the body wall by ventral and dorsal mesogastrium. Then, it undergoes rotation to right through 90° around the longitudinal, transverse and anteroposterior axes so that its right and left surfaces, upper and lower ends and anterior and posterior borders acquire definitive shapes and orientation. Concomitant development of omental bursa also contributes to the definitive shape of the stomach.

Parts of Stomach (Fig. 133.1)

The stomach consists of the fundus, body and pyloric part. The body of the stomach has two surfaces (anterosuperior and posteroinferior), two orifices (cardiac and pyloric) and two borders (greater and lesser curvatures). The fundus lies above the level of cardiac orifice. The body constitutes the major part of the stomach. A line passing through the incisura angularis of the lesser curvature indicates the demarcation of body and pyloric part. The pyloric part consists of pyloric antrum, pyloric canal and pylorus.

Surface Marking

Since the position and size of the stomach are variable its surface projection is also variable. The approximate outline of an empty stomach in supine position is easy to draw if its orifices are drawn first.

a. The cardiac orifice is about 2 cm in width. Its midpoint coincides with a point on the seventh left costal cartilage 2.5 cm from the median plane.
b. The pyloric orifice is 2 cm wide and presents left upper margin and right lower margin. Its midpoint coincides

with a point 1.2 cm to the right of midline on the transpyloric plane (at the level of the tip of 9th costal cartilage).

c. The fundus is represented by a line, which shows upward convexity and joins the right and left ends of the cardiac orifice. The upper limit of this convex line coincides with the left fifth intercostal space below the nipple.

d. The greater curvature begins at the left margin of the cardiac orifice, where the fundus ends. It coincides with a convex line starting at the left end of cardiac orifice and turning downwards and medially to meet the lower right margin of the pyloric orifice.

e. The lesser curvature is marked by a line that connects the right margin of the cardiac orifice to the left margin of the pyloric orifice. This line is concave upwards and its lowest point of concavity (corresponding to the incisura angularis) reaches slightly below the transpyloric plane.

Gastric Orifices

a. The cardiac orifice is the junction between lower end of the esophagus and stomach. It is located 10 cm deep to the anterior abdominal wall and 40 cm from the incisor teeth.

b. The pyloric orifice is the junction between the pyloric end of the stomach and the first part of the duodenum. The prepyloric vein of Mayo on the anterior surface of the pyloric orifice serves as its identification mark during surgery. A true sphincter composed of thick circular muscle layer surrounds the pyloric orifice. At the site of the sphincter, on palpation, one can feel a firm lump. The sphincter regulates the entry of stomach contents into the duodenum. The pyloric end is thicker, more superficial and more mobile compared to the cardiac end of the stomach.

Gastric Curvatures

a. The lesser curvature is the right margin of the stomach. It is concave towards the right side. A notch called incisura angularis marks its most dependent part. The lesser curvature gives attachment to the lesser omentum.

b. The greater curvature is four or five times longer than the lesser curvature. Opposite the incisura angularis of lesser curvature, there is a bulge on the greater curvature. A line passing through the angular incisure and the corresponding bulge on the greater curvature is the left limit of the pyloric antrum. The greater curvature gives attachments to greater omentum, gastrosplenic ligament and gastrophrenic ligament.

Peritoneal Relations (Fig. 133.2)

The stomach is completely covered with peritoneum, except a small area called the bare area of stomach near the cardiac orifice, where the gastrophrenic ligament is attached.

a. The lesser omentum extends between the lesser curvature of the stomach and the liver. It has a right free margin forming the anterior boundary of the epiploic foramen. The contents of the right free margin are the portal vein, the common bile duct and the hepatic artery. The gastric vessels located close to the lesser curvature, are the right and left gastric vessels. Besides these, the extraperitoneal tissue, lymphatics, lymph nodes and the gastric nerves are the other contents of the lesser omentum.

b. The greater omentum extends from the greater curvature of the stomach and is the longest peritoneal fold consisting of 4 layers. Its layers fuse with each

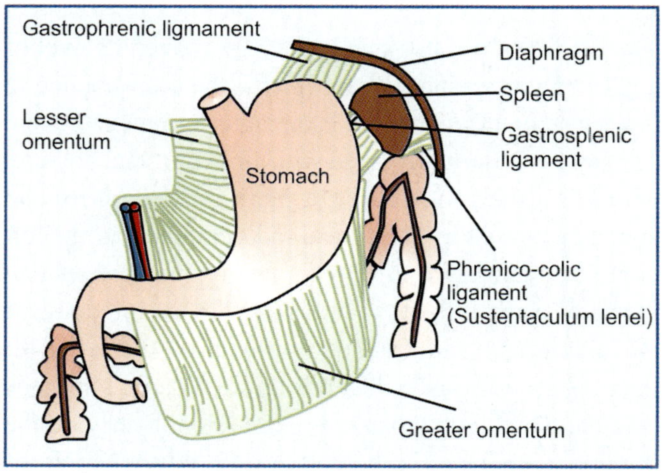

Fig. 133.2: Schematic diagram of peritoneal folds attached to stomach. Note: Structures in free margin of lesser omentum (portal v., hepatic a. and CBD). Note that the spleen rests on phrenico-colic ligament, which is not a peritoneal fold of stomach

other and contain variable amount of fat depending on the nutritional status of the individual. The 2 posterior layers ascend in front of the transverse colon and mesocolon to reach the posterior abdominal wall. The plane between the transverse mesocolon and the greater omentum is an embryological plane of adhesion; hence, it can be opened up without blood loss (plane passes between the omental vessels and the mesocolic vessels). About a fingerbreadth below the greater curvature, the 2 anterior layers of the greater omentum contain the arcade formed by right and left gastroepiploic arteries. The other contents of the greater omentum are lymph nodes and lymphatics, fat, extraperitoneal tissue and aggregations of free macrophages (milky spots). The greater omentum acts as a storehouse of fat. It is called the policeman of the abdominal cavity because of its defensive functions. It wraps an inflamed organ thereby localizing the infection and the macrophages in the milky spots help in combating the infection.

c. The gastrosplenic ligament connects the upper end of the greater curvature to the spleen near the hilum. It contains short gastric vessels and left gastroepiploic vessels.

d. The gastrophrenic ligament connects the cardiac end of the stomach to the diaphragm. It encloses a small bare area of stomach between its layers.

Fundus of Stomach

The fundus of the stomach is the part above the level of angle of His or cardiac notch, which is the deep angulation between the left margin of esophagus and the stomach. The fundus is normally filled with air in the erect posture, which is usually visible in a plain radiograph of the abdomen as well as in Ba meal radiograph under the left dome of diaphragm. Inferiorly, the fundus continues in the body. Superiorly, the fundus touches the left dome of the diaphragm and reaches the level of the left fifth intercostal space just below the nipple. Traube's space is an area, which is tympanic to percussion, overlying the fundus of stomach. Its boundaries are lower margin of the resonance of left lung, lateral margin of spleen, lower margin of left lobe of liver and left costal margin. This space is obliterated in pleural effusion on left side and in hypertrophy of spleen and liver.

Relations of Gastric Surfaces

a. The anterosuperior surface on the right side is related to the gastric impression of the left lobe of liver and nearer the pylorus to the quadrate lobe of liver. The left half this surface is in contact with the diaphragm and rib cage. The lower part of the anterior surface is in direct contact with anterior abdominal wall. This area is described as gastric triangle, which is bounded by lower margin of liver, left costal margin and transverse colon. The clinical usefulness of this triangle is not universally accepted but it is the site for insertion of a gastrostomy tube.

b. The posteroinferior surface is related to a number of structures on the posterior abdominal wall, which collectively are called stomach bed (Fig. 133.3). The lesser sac intervenes between the stomach and its bed, which consists of the following, posterosuperior part of diaphragm, left suprarenal gland, left kidney, splenic artery, anterior surface of pancreas, transverse mesocolon and left colic flexure. From the above definition of the stomach bed, the spleen should be excluded since it is separated from the stomach by greater sac and comes in contact with the backward facing anterior surface on the left end. However, all authorities do not agree on this point.

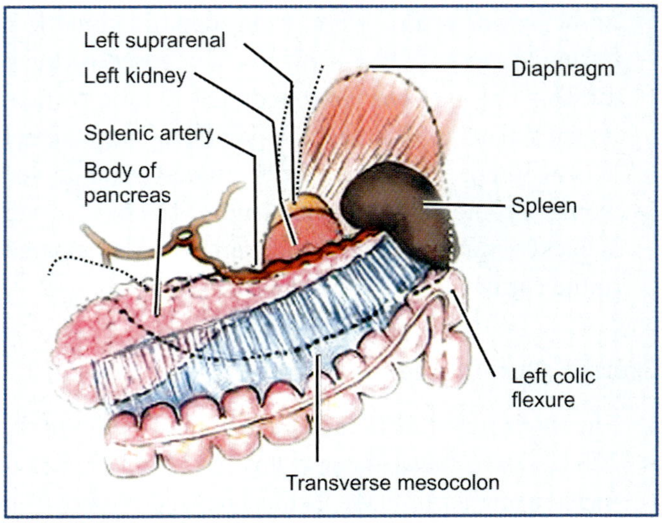

Fig. 133.3: Schematic diagram depicting structures forming stomach bed (Note that outline of stomach is shown in dotted line in the foreground for reference)

Pyloric Part

The pyloric part lies below or to the right of the incisura angularis. It consists of 3 parts in succession, pyloric antrum, and pyloric canal and pyloric orifice (pylorus). The pyloric antrum is the dilated part between the sulcus intermedius, (which is a slight groove on the pyloric part) on the right and the line joining the incisura angularis and the corresponding bulge on the greater curvature, on the left. The pyloric canal (2 to 3 cm long) begins at the sulcus intermedius and ends at the pyloric orifice.

Clinical Highlights

a. Pylorospasm is the condition in which the pyoric sphincter fails to relax normally. In such cases, the gastric emptying is slow and the food tends to accumulate in the stomach. It is usually seen in newborn. The infant vomits frequently to relieve the high intragastric pressure. Pylorospasm is treated with drugs that relax the sphincter.
b. Congenital hypertrophic pyloric stenosis is due to hypertrophy of the circular muscle layer in the region of pyloric orifice resulting in narrowing of the pyloric orifice. It is found more in firstborn male children with O blood group. The characteristic symptom is the projectile vomiting in which there is spraying of the vomitus some distance away from the infant. The hypertrophied sphincter can be palpated per abdomen as a lump. During surgery, it is identified by the presence of prepyloric vein of Mayo. Ramstedt's operation is the treatment of choice. In this procedure, the circular muscle is cut through by blunt dissection to widen the orifice.

Radiological Appearance

The radiological examination by barium meal is done to assess the size, shape and position of the stomach. The following radiological types of stomach are encountered, typical J-shaped stomach, steer-horn stomach (horizontally oriented and resembling the shape of the bull's horn) and intermediate type.

Interior (Fig. 133.4)

The direct inspection of the interior of stomach is possible through a gastroscope. The internal surface of the stomach

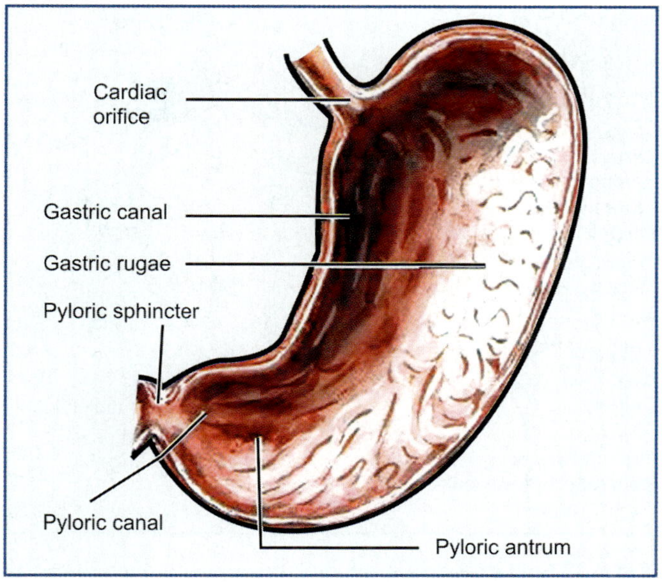

Fig. 133.4: Interior of stomach

presents longitudinal foldings of gastric mucosa called rugae, which are more marked along the greater curvature. The gastric canal (magenstrasse), which extends along the lesser curvature from the cardiac orifice to incisura angularis, forms during swallowing. The canal is bounded by longitudinal gastric folds and is apparent here due to the absence of oblique muscle layer along the lesser curvature. The saliva and fluids pass towards the pylorus along the gastric canal. Therefore, the mucous membrane of the gastric canal is prone to injury by irritant liquids.

Arterial Supply (Fig. 133.5)

A total of five arteries supply the stomach. The left gastric artery, a branch of coeliac trunk and the right gastric artery, a branch of the common hepatic artery, form an arterial arcade close to the lesser curvature in the lesser omentum. The left gastroepiploic artery, a branch of splenic artery and right gastroepiploic artery, a branch gastroduodenal artery, form an arterial arcade in the greater omentum a little away from the greater curvature. The short gastric arteries from the splenic artery reach the fundus via the gastrosplenic ligament. The arterial branches enter the stomach wall at right angles to its long axis and form extensive submucosal plexuses. The mucosal arteries arising from these plexuses end in spirally running capillaries. This complex arrangement is to ensure adequate blood supply to the mucosa. However, the mucosa along the lesser curvature receives blood from

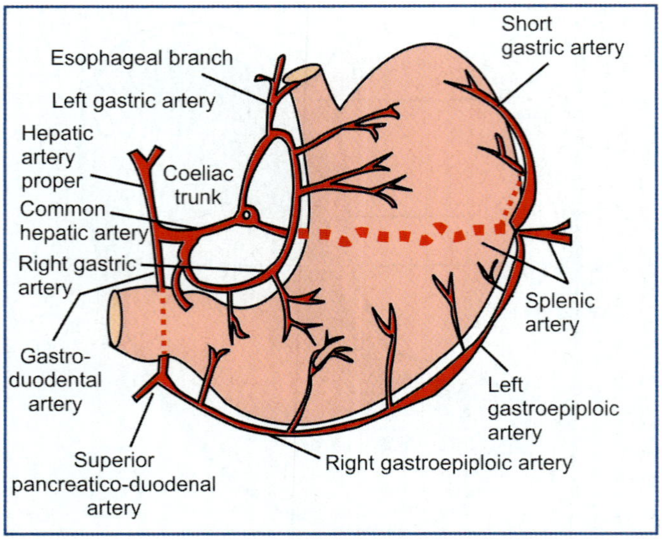

Fig. 133.5: Depicting the arterial supply of stomach through branches of coeliac trunk

the long parallel arteries with minimum anastomoses. Therefore, occlusion of these arteries is likely to result in ischemia and ulceration.

Venous Drainage

The right and left gastric veins are the tributaries of portal vein. The short gastric and left gastroepiploic veins open into the splenic vein. The right gastroepiploic vein opens in superior mesenteric vein. The gastroesophageal junction is the site of portosystemic anastomosis between the tributaries of the left gastric vein and esophageal tributaries of hemiazygos vein. This anastomosis opens and dilates in portal hypertension. Such dilated veins in the submucosa may burst causing vomiting of frank blood (hematemesis).

Lymphatic Drainage (Fig. 133.6)

For descriptive purposes, the stomach is divided into 4 areas or zones. The fundus and left half of the body drain into the pancreaticosplenic nodes, which lie near the hilum of spleen. The upper part of the right half of body drains into the left gastric nodes located in lesser omentum. The lower part of the right half of body drains into the right gastroepiploic nodes and the pyloric region drains in pyloric, hepatic and left gastric nodes. The lymph from these regional nodes passes ultimately to coeliac group of pre-aortic nodes. Carcinoma stomach spreads through the lymph vessels to these nodes.

Nerve Supply (Fig. 133.7)

The stomach possesses both intrinsic and extrinsic nerve supply. The intrinsic nerves are present in the myenteric plexus of Aurbach and submucosal plexus of Meissner. The extrinsic nerves consist of branches of sympathetic and parasympathetic. Sympathetic branches reach through the coeliac plexus. The efferent sympathetic fibers are vasomotor and the afferent fibers carry pain to the spinal cord. Hence referred pain from the stomach is felt in the epigastrium in the dermatomal areas of T7 to T9. The parasympathetic supply is derived from the vagus nerves. Vagal simulation increases acid and enzymatic secretion, decreases sphincter tone and increases gastric motility. The left vagus nerve becomes the anterior gastric nerve and the right vagus nerve becomes the posterior gastric nerve after entering the abdomen.

a. The anterior gastric nerve enters the lesser omentum and gives off hepatic branches towards the right. Then, it travels down giving gastric branches from its left aspect. Beyond the origin of gastric branches, it is called nerve of Latarjet, which breaks in a handful of antral branches in crow's foot fashion.
b. The posterior gastric nerve enters the lesser omentum and gives off its coeliac branches. It gives off criminal nerve of Grassi for the supply of fundus. Then, it supplies gastric branches to the posterior surface of stomach. Beyond the origin of gastric branches, the nerve is called posterior nerve of Latarjet, which breaks in handful of antral branches like the corresponding anterior nerve.

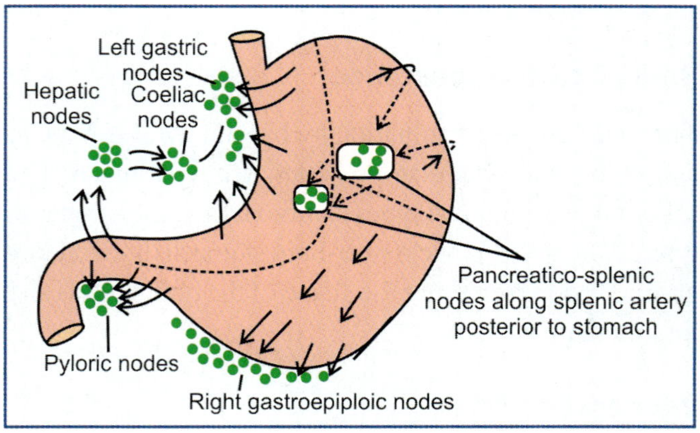

Fig. 133.6: Plan of lymphatic drainage of various zones of stomach

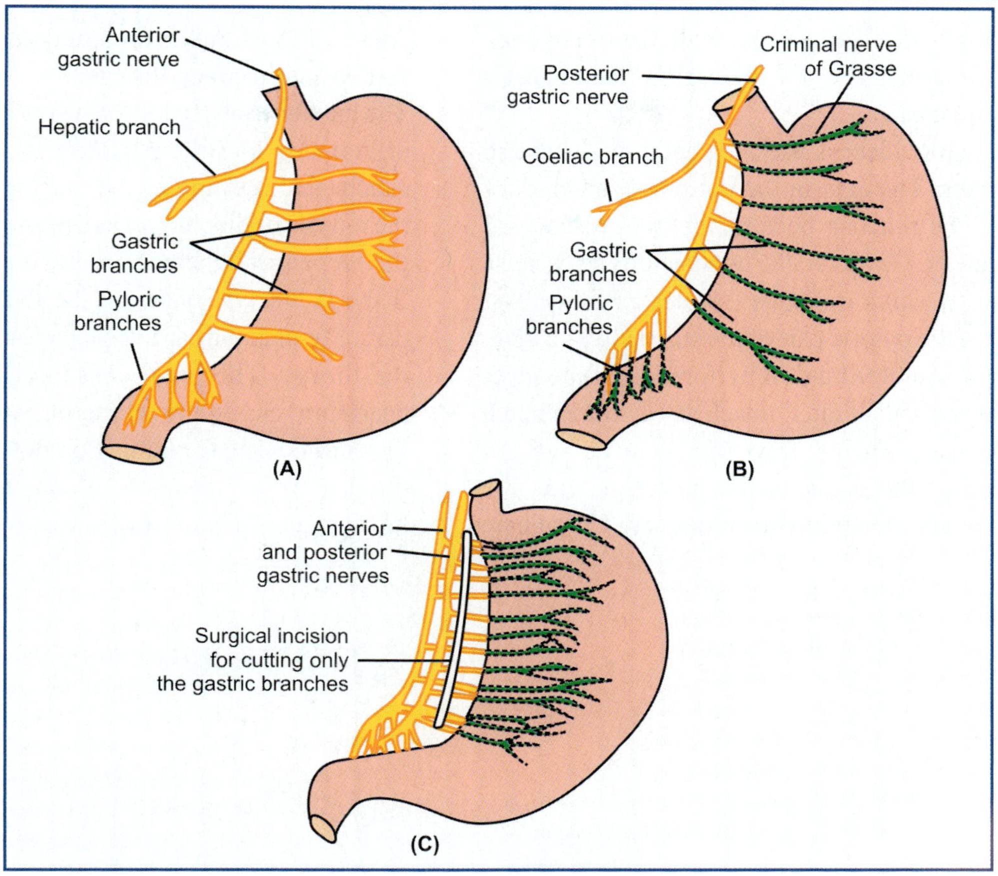

Fig. 133.7: Depicting nerve supply of stomach in (A), (B) and highly selective vagotomy in (C). Note the pyloric branches (supplying the sphincter) are presserved in (C)

Vagotomy

Vagotomy means cutting the vagus nerves. There are three different types of vagotomy operations:

a. In truncal vagotomy, the trunks of both gastric nerves are divided at the lower end of esophagus.

b. In selective vagotomy, the hepatic and coeliac branches are preserved but the main trunks of gastric nerves including the nerves of Laterjet are cut to denervate the stomach and pylorus.

   The disadvantage of both truncal and selective vagotomy, is that pyloric antrum is denervated as a result of which gastric emptying is affected.

c. In highly selective vagotomy, only the parietal cells of the stomach are denervated. So, the gastric branches alone are cut along the lesser curvature. The nerve of Grassi is carefully dissected and cut. If this nerve is missed the fundic glands will remain functional. The advantage of highly selective vagotomy is that it preserves the nerves of Latarjet and their antral branches (thus gastric emptying remains normal).

Clinical Highlights

a. The gastric cancer spreads by lymph vessels to the lymph nodes depicted in Figure 133.6. Sometimes, the enlarged and palpable left supraclavicular node (Trosier's sign) may be the first sign of gastric cancer. Therefore, clinicians make it a point to palpate left supraclavicular lymph nodes, whenever gastric cancer is suspected. In the operation of partial gastrectomy for gastric cancer part of the stomach is removed along with all the lymph nodes of the stomach. Occasionally, the cancer cells penetrate the muscle layer and serosa to reach the liver, pancreas or colon. The metastasis into the peritoneum leads to ascites. The ovaries may be the sites of transcoelomic spread (Krukenberg's tumor). In advanced stage, the malignant cells may reach the umbilicus, where they give rise to Sister Joseph's nodules.

b. The term peptic ulcer is used for both duodenal and gastric ulcers. The acid in the normal stomach does not injure the mucosa because of the presence of mucous barrier. However, the hyperacidity may cause gastric ulcers, which are usually located near the lesser curvature in the pyloric part of the stomach. The ulcer causes pain and bleeding. In perforation of the ulcer on the anterior wall of the stomach, the acidic stomach contents are emptied into the greater sac. In perforation of the ulcer on the posterior wall, the stomach contents enter into the lesser sac. The splenic artery in the stomach bed may get eroded, causing serious internal hemorrhage.

c. The hiatal hernia (Fig. 40.4 B) is a protrusion of a part of stomach into the posterior mediastinum via the esophageal opening of the diaphragm. Weakness of the muscle of diaphragm and consequent widening of the esophageal opening are the predisposing factors. In the sliding type of hernia, the abdominal esophagus, part of fundus and cardioesophageal junction slide into the thorax. This may cause symptoms like pain, heartburn, etc. In the rolling or paraesophageal type, the cardioesophageal junction does not shift upward but a part of stomach slides into the posterior mediastinum. This variety is usually symptomless.

134 Duodenum

The duodenum is a Latin word, derived from "Do-deka-dactalos", which means width of twelve fingers. Since the length of duodenum is equal to the width of twelve fingers put together, (25 cm) it is given the name duodenum. It is the first part of the small intestine and is the shortest, widest and the most fixed part. It is retroperitoneal except the proximal 2 to 2.5 cm. The fixation of the duodenum is necessary because a mobile duodenum will cause twisting and kinking of the common bile duct and pancreatic duct, which open into it. The main function of the duodenum is digestion. The chyme is mixed with bile and pancreatic enzymes here. The arrival of the chyme stimulates the duodenal mucosa to produce cholecystokinin and secretin. The former stimulates the pancreatic enzymes and the bile and the latter stimulates bicarbonate ions to flow into the duodenum.

Development

The duodenum above the level of entry of bile duct is derived from endoderm of the foregut and below this level from the endoderm of midgut. Therefore, the first part of the duodenum develops from the foregut. The second part develops from both foregut and midgut. The third and fourth parts develop from the midgut. The duodenum becomes retroperitoneal as follows. Because of rotation of stomach to the right, the duodenal loop falls to the right. Its dorsal mesentery fuses with the parietal peritoneum of dorsal abdominal wall. During 8th week, the lumen of duodenum is obliterated by proliferation of lining cells. However, by the end of 3rd month the lumen is recanalized.

Congenital Anomalies

a. Duodenal stenosis (narrowing of lumen) is due to incomplete recanalization.
b. Duodenal atresia is due to failure of recanalization, usually, in its second part beyond the opening of bile duct. Due to total obstruction in this part, there is distention of the first part and the stomach. The newborn vomits from birth and the vomitus is bile stained. On plain X-ray or ultrasound scan, one can see the characteristic double bubble sign (air bubble in fundus and in first part of duodenum). Duodenal atresia is accompanied by polyhydramnios (excessive amniotic fluid) and is more common in Down syndrome babies.
c. Obstruction to second part may occur due to a ring shaped pancreatic tissue surrounding it (as seen in a congenital anomaly called annular pancreas).

Gross Features

The duodenum is 25 cm long. It is C-shaped and begins at the pyloric orifice and ends at the duodeno-jejunal flexure. It is C shaped. The C of the duodenum is open to the left and clasps the head of pancreas.

Parts of Duodenum (Fig. 134.1)

The duodenum has two bends in its course, superior and inferior flexures, which divide the duodenum into four parts for descriptive purposes. The first or superior part passes upward, backward and to the right, from the pylorus in the transpyloric plane at the level of L1vertebra. It is 5 cm long and ends at the superior flexure near the neck of the gallbladder. From here, the second or descending part goes downward to the level of L3 vertebra at the inferior flexure. The second part is 8 cm long. The third or horizontal part is about 10 cm long and passes from the right to the left. It crosses the midline at the level of L3 vertebra. The fourth or ascending part is 2 cm long. It

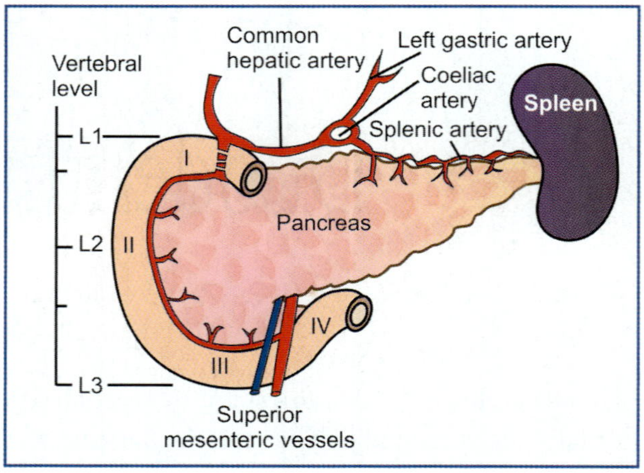

Fig. 134.1: Showing the shape, parts and vertebral level of duodenum (Note that the 'C' of duodenum clasps the head of pancreas. Parts: I–Superior, II–Descending, III–Horizontal, IV–Ascending)

turns upward and to the left and ends by joining the jejunum at the level of L2 vertebra.

Surface Marking

The duodenum is above the level of the umbilicus. The pyloric orifice (denoted by a point 1.2 cm to the right of the median plane on the transpyloric plane) is joined to the superior duodenal flexure (denoted by a point 2.5 cm to the right of previous point just below the right costal margin) by two parallel lines about 2.5 to 3 cm wide. The second part begins at the termination of the first part and goes down for a distance of 7.5 cm. The outline of the second part is 2.5 cm wide and its outer line coincides with the right lateral line. The third part is a 10 cm long and 2.5 cm broad line starting from the end of second part and reaching the midline on the subcostal plane just above the umbilicus. The fourth part begins at the end of the third part and reaches the duodeno-jejunal flexure, which is represented by a point 2.5 cm to the left of median plane and 1cm below the transpyloric plane.

Relations of First Part (Fig. 134.2)

The proximal 2 cm of the first part is intraperitoneal. It gives attachment to both greater and lesser omenta. The part of the lesser omentum extending between the liver and the proximal 2 cm is called hepatoduodenal ligament. The distal 3 cm of the first part is covered with peritoneum only on anterior aspect.

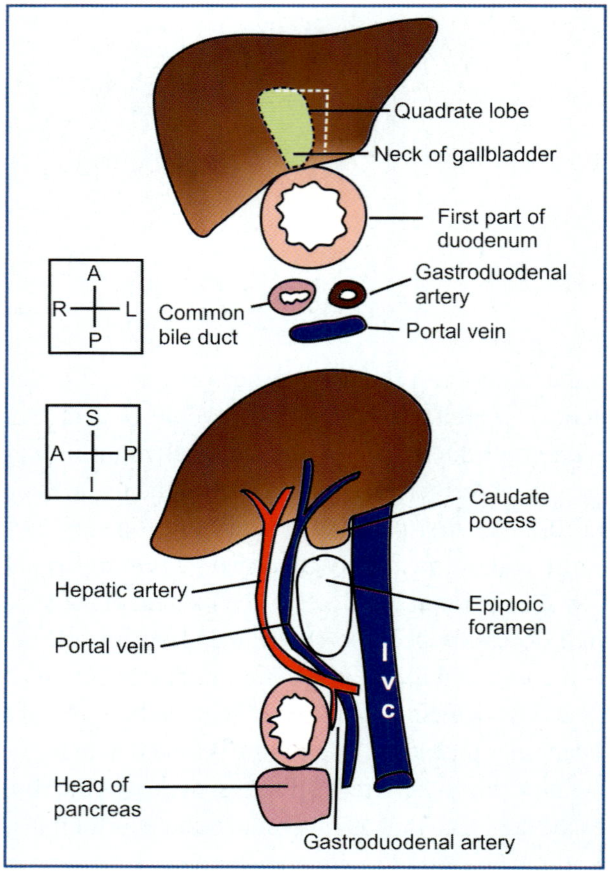

Fig. 134.2: Highly simplified plan showing relations of first part of duodenum

a. Anteriorly, the first part is related to the quadrate lobe of liver and neck and body of the gallbladder. The clinical importance of this relation is that a large gallstone may erode through the anterior wall of the duodenum to enter its cavity.
b. Posterior relations are the gastroduodenal artery, portal vein and the common bile duct.
c. Superior relations are the horizontal part of hepatic artery and the epiploic foramen.
d. Inferior relations are the head and neck of pancreas.

Special Features of First Part

a. It is the most movable part of duodenum being enclosed in lesser and greater omenta.
b. It is the only part of duodenum that is related to the lesser sac.
c. It has sparse blood supply (less blood supply) compared to the rest of the duodenum because its arteries are end arteries.

d. Due to absence of circular folds of mucous membrane, it shows a characteristic smooth appearance in contrast radiographs. Duodenal cap (bulb) is visible on barium meal because the first part is kept patent by protrusion of the pylorus in its proximal part while the rest of the duodenum remains collapsed.
e. Peptic ulceration is very common here because the acid contents of the stomach first come in contact with the mucosa of the first part. One major complication of an ulcer is perforation of the duodenal wall. If the ulcer perforates the inferior wall, it may penetrate the pancreas causing pain in the back. Perforation of the anterior wall leads to acidic contents entering the hepatorenal pouch. An ulcer on the posterior wall may erode the gastroduodenal artery leading to serious internal bleeding. Therefore, the gastroduodenal artery is called the "artery of duodenal hemorrhage."

Relations of Second Part

The relations of the second part are very important.

a. Anterior relations are the 3 structures, which from above downward are, gallbladder, transverse colon, and coils of jejunum (Fig. 134.3). The proximity to gallbladder may be the cause of erosion of duodenal wall in cases of gallstones leading to entry of gallstones in the duodenum.
b. Posterior relations are the anterior surface of right kidney, structures at the hilum of the kidney, IVC and right psoas major muscle (Fig. 134.4).
c. On its right, it is related to the right colic flexure.
d. On its left, it is related to the head of pancreas. The common bile duct and pancreatic duct enter its medial wall.

Interior of Second Part

The hepatopancreatic ampulla (of Vater) passes through the medial wall of the second part (Figs 134.4 and 134.6). Normally, the common bile duct and the main pancreatic duct unite to form the hepaticopancreatic ampulla, but variations are common. The hepatico-pancreatic sphincter of Oddi surrounds the ampulla. The accessory pancreatic duct if present also passes through the medial wall. The interior of the second part presents mucosal folds, duodenal papillae and the openings of bile and pancreatic ducts.

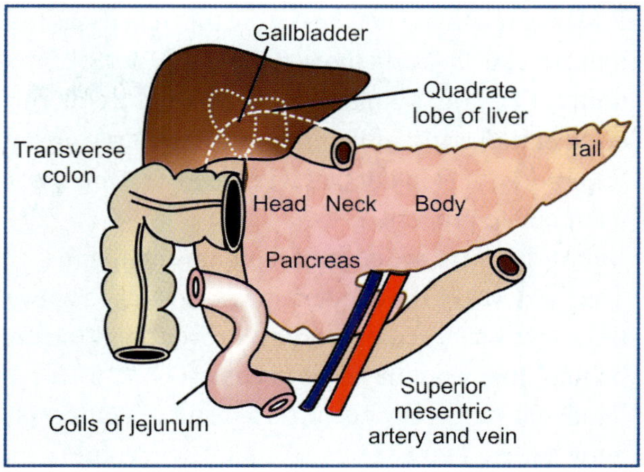

Fig. 134.3: Anterior relations of first, second and third parts of duodenum

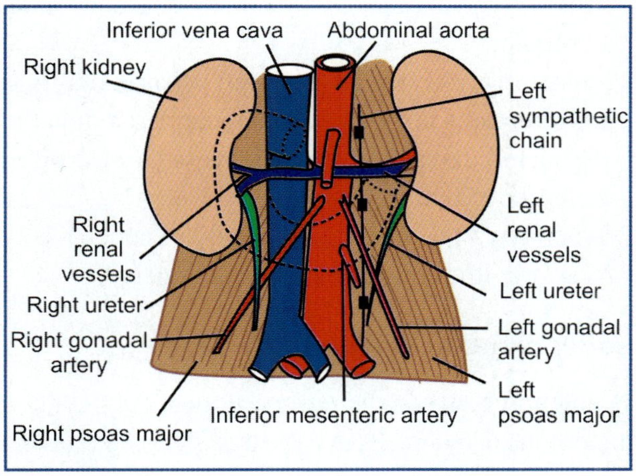

Fig. 134.4: Posterior relations of second, third and fourth parts of duodenum (Note that the outline of duodenum is shown in the foreground for reference)

The circular mucosal folds are numerous and increase the surface area. There is one prominent longitudinal fold on the medial wall and the major duodenal papilla lies at the proximal end of this fold. The major duodenal papilla is an elevation of the mucosa on which the ampulla of Vater opens. The accessory pancreatic duct opens at the minor duodenal papilla, which is located proximal to the major papilla. The distance of the major papilla from the pyloric orifice is 10 cm while that of the minor papilla is 7 to 8 cm.

Relations of Third Part

a. Anteriorly, it is related to the superior mesenteric vessels (Fig. 134.3) in the root of the mesentery.

b. Posterior relations (Fig. 134.4) are the right psoas major muscle and the structures lying on it namely, right ureter, IVC, right gonadal vessels and the abdominal aorta at the origin of the inferior mesenteric artery.
c. Superiorly, it is in contact with head of pancreas and its uncinate process.
d. Inferiorly, there are coils of jejunum and ileum. The third part of the duodenum is sandwiched between the superior mesenteric artery in front and the aorta behind, like a nut in the nutcracker (Fig. 134.5). The duodenal stasis may occur, as a result of compression between the two arteries (Wilkie's syndrome).

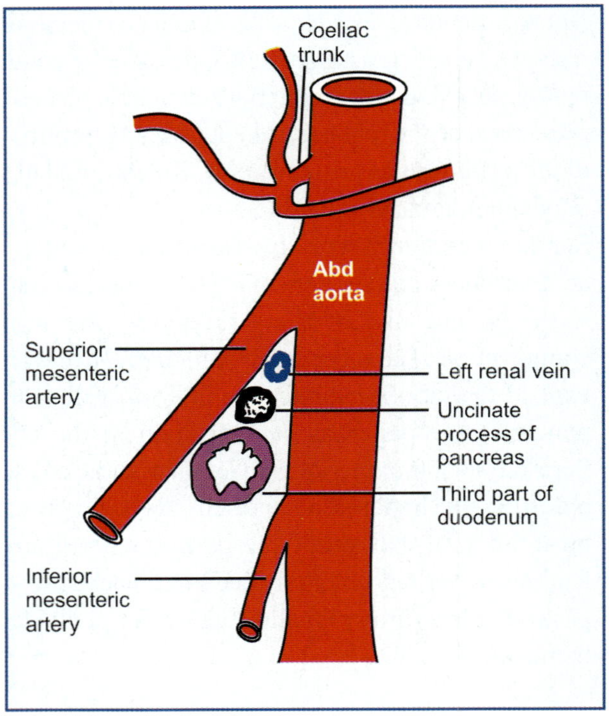

Fig. 134.5: Showing vascular relations of third part of duodenum (Note: The vascular nutcracker formed by superior mesenteric artery and aorta)

Relations of Fourth Part

a. Anteriorly, it is related to the transverse colon and its mesocolon.
b. Posteriorly, it is related to the left psoas major muscle and structures in front of it, namely, left sympathetic chain, left renal and gonadal vessels and inferior mesenteric vein.
c. Superiorly, it is related to the body of pancreas.
d. Inferiorly, the coils of intestine are related.

Duodenojejunal Flexure

The junction between the retroperitoneal duodenum and intraperitoneal jejunum is marked by a sharp forward bend. It is located on the left of the midline, its vertebral level being L2. It is held in position by the suspensory muscle of the duodenum (ligament of Treitz), which is a fibromuscular band attached to the duodenojejunal flexure and right crus of diaphragm close to the esophageal opening. There are 2 components of this muscle. The upper part has striated muscle (from the diaphragm) and the lower part has smooth muscle (from the duodenum). These two parts are joined by fibrous tissue, which surrounds the coeliac trunk. The striated part is innervated by phrenic nerve and the smooth muscle has autonomic innervation. The function of this muscle is to augment the duodenojejunal flexure so that it can act as its valve.

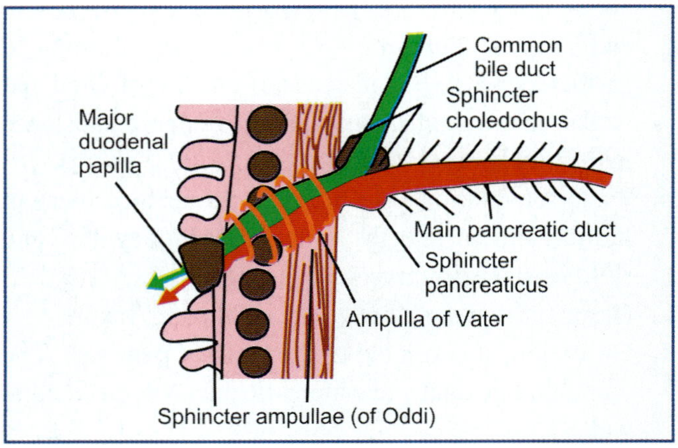

Fig. 134.6: Scheme to show ampulla of Vater and related sphincters in the wall of second part of duodenum

Arterial Supply (Fig. 134.7)

The arterial supply of duodenum reflects its development. The parts derived from foregut receive blood from the branches of coeliac artery and parts from midgut from the branches of superior mesenteric artery.

a. The first part receives blood from 3 arteries. The supraduodenal artery of Wilkie is a branch of gastroduodenal or right gastric or hepatic artery. In 30 percent of cases, it is absent. The infraduodenal artery is a branch of right gastroepiploic artery and the retroduodenal artery is a branch of gastroduodenal artery. These arteries are practically end arteries. This is the reason for less arterial supply to the first part of duodenum and its vulnerability to ischemia.

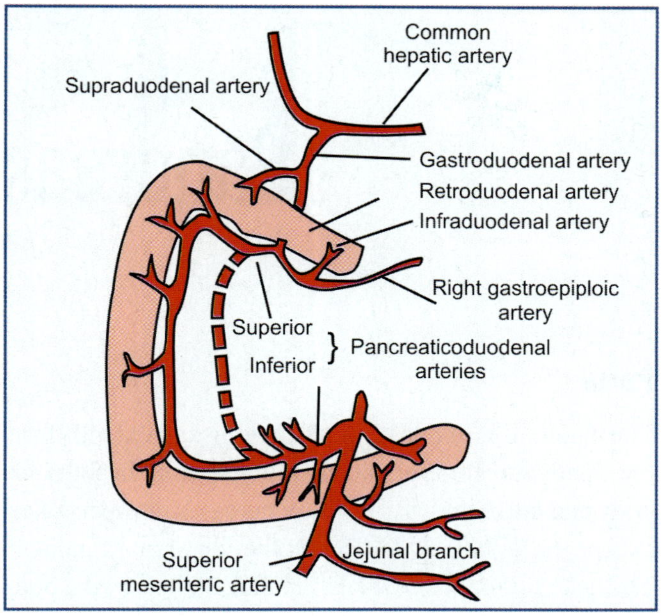

Fig. 134.7: Depicting arterial supply of duodenum through branches of coeliac and superior mesenteric arteries

b. The second part receives ample blood supply from branches of both coeliac and superior mesenteric arteries. The superior pancreatico-duodenal artery divides into anterior and posterior branches, which run in front of and behind the pancreatic head respectively. They supply the second part of duodenum and head of pancreas and anastomose with branches of the inferior pancreatico-duodenal arteries from the superior mesenteric artery.
c. The third and fourth parts receive branches from the anastomotic ring formed by the branches of the inferior pancreaticoduodenal artery.

Venous Drainage

The veins correspond to the arteries and terminate in the splenic and superior mesenteric veins. Some veins may end directly into the portal vein.

Lymphatic Drainage

The lymph vessels drain into pancreatoduodenal as well as pyloric groups of lymph nodes. From here, the lymph flows to the coeliac nodes.

Nerve Supply

Sympathetic supply comes from coeliac and superior mesenteric plexuses. The segmental innervation is T6 to T8. The parasympathetic supply comes from both vagus nerves.

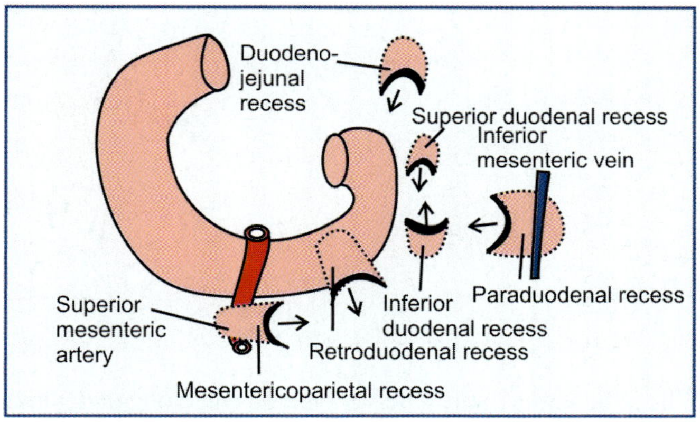

Fig. 134.8: Peritoneal recesses around duodenum

Peritoneal Recesses in Relation to Duodenum (Fig. 134.8)

A number of peritoneal recesses are encountered near the fourth part of duodenum. The reason for this is that the retroperitoneal duodenum suddenly changes to an intraperitoneal jejunum. Occasionally, these recesses trap a loop of intestine, which may strangulate and produce acute symptoms of strangulated internal hernia leading to intestinal obstruction. Depending on the site of the peritoneal folds, the recesses are named, the superior duodenal recess, inferior duodenal recess, paraduodenal recess, retroduodenal recess and the duodenojejunal recess. The paraduodenal recess is the only one bounded by a vascular fold carrying the inferior mesenteric vein in it.

Contrast X-ray of Duodenum

The barium meal shows the proximal part of the first part of duodenum as a homogenous triangular shadow called duodenal cap. The duodenal cap has a well-demarcated base towards the pylorus and a less distinct apex. The remaining parts of the duodenum show feathery shadow. The reason for this difference is that the first part has no circular folds of mucosa and its lumen is kept patent by the pylorus, which protrudes into the proximal duodenum. The rest of the duodenum possesses circular folds of mucosa and being retroperitoneal its lumen remains in a collapsed state. Any filling defect in the duodenal cap is an indication of a duodenal ulcer.

135 Pancreas

The pancreas is a soft, finely lobulated and elongated gland. It is located behind the peritoneum on the posterior abdominal wall, more or less in transpyloric plane. Due to its deep position, the pancreas is not easily accessible for direct clinical examination. Therefore, the diagnosis of pancreatic diseases is largely dependent on ultrasound scan, CT scan, endoscopic retrograde cholangio-pancreatography (ERCP), etc. apart from clinical symptoms and biochemical tests.

FUNCTIONS

Functionally, the pancreas consists of two parts, exocrine and endocrine. In response to a meal, the exocrine pancreas secretes digestive enzymes in a bicarbonate rich fluid. The daily secretion of pancreatic juice amounts to one liter. The exocrine cells secrete lipase, amylase and trypsinogen while the epithelium of the ducts secretes bicarbonate, which protects the duodenum from gastric acid and ensures optimum pH for activity of digestive enzymes. The endocrine cells of the pancreas (islets of Langerhans) secrete insulin and glucagon, which control blood glucose level. They also secrete pancreatic gastrin and somatostatin.

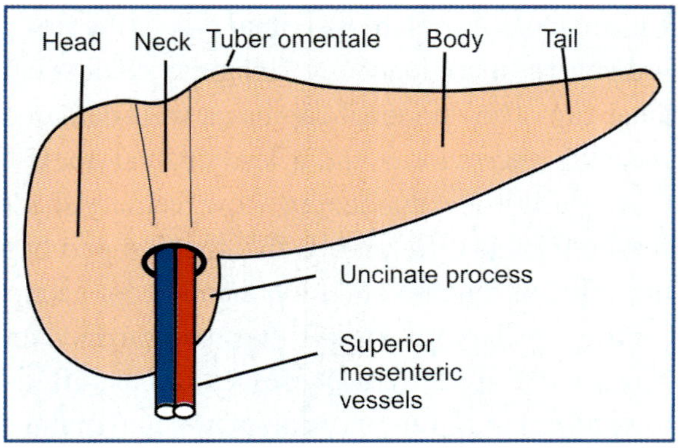

Fig. 135.1: Parts of pancreas

Parts

The pancreas is about 12 to 15 cm long and extends from the duodenum to the spleen. It consists of head, neck, body and tail (Fig. 135.1). The pancreas is retroperitoneal except for its tail, which lies in the lienorenal ligament. The head lies opposite the L1 and L2 vertebrae, the body lies more or less in transpyloric plane and the tail is at the level of T12 vertebra.

Development (Fig. 135.2)

The pancreas develops from the dorsal and ventral endodermal pancreatic buds, which originate from the caudal end of the foregut, during the fourth week of intrauterine life. The ventral bud arises in common with hepatic bud, but the dorsal bud arises singly. The pancreatic buds fall to the right with the rotation of the duodenal loop to the right. The axial rotation of the second part of duodenum shifts the ventral bud across the posterior aspect of the duodenum to meet the dorsal bud. The fusion of the buds takes place in the seventh week. The dorsal bud gives rise to the acini and ductules of tail, body, neck and upper part of the head. The ventral bud gives rise to acini and ductules of lower part of head and uncinate process. The pancreatic ducts develop as follows. An anastomotic communication is established between the ducts of ventral and dorsal buds. The main pancreatic duct develops from the distal part of the duct of dorsal bud, anastomotic channel and the duct of ventral bud. The accessory pancreatic duct develops from the proximal part of the duct of the dorsal bud. The islet cells develop during third month of intrauterine life from the acinar cells, which are detached from the acini. These detached cells form separate cell masses and are surrounded by sinusoids.

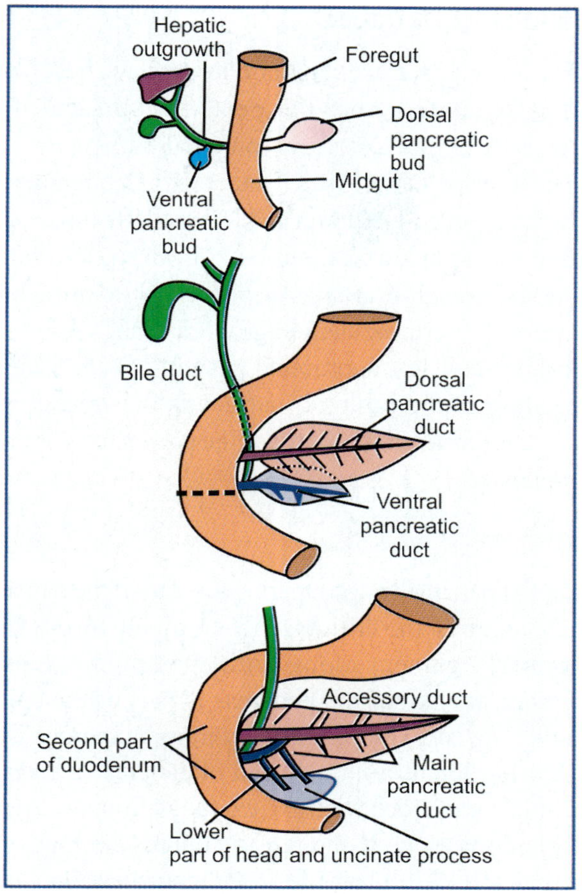

Fig. 135.2: Stages in development of pancreas

Congenital Anomalies

a. Annular pancreas occurs if the ventral pancreatic bud splits into two parts of which one part remains posterior to and the other goes anterior to the duodenum, to meet the dorsal bud. The ring of pancreatic tissue thus formed around the second part of duodenum usually causes its obstruction. For signs and symptoms of the obstruction of doudenum, refer to congenital anomalies of duodenum in Chapter 134.
b. Pancreas divisum is a condition in which the duct of the ventral bud does not fuse with duct of the dorsal bud or the ventral and dorsal pancreatic buds do not fuse. The body and tail of pancreas drain through minor duodenal papilla by duct of dorsal bud and the head drains through major duodenal papilla by duct of ventral bud.
c. Sometimes, the pancreatic tissue is spilled in ectopic locations, such as, the greater omentum or Meckel's diverticulum. Digestive enzymes in ectopic pancreas may destroy normal tissue resulting in ulceration and perforation.

Surface Marking

The surface marking of the duodenal curve marks the head of pancreas. For the body of the pancreas, 2 lines, approximately 2.5 to 3 cm apart are drawn from the head towards the left for a distance of about 10 cm on the transpyloric plane, with an upward slant. These lines meet at the left end above the transpyloric plane and their meeting point represents the tail.

Relations of Head (Fig. 135.3)

The head of the pancreas lies in the C-shaped concavity of the duodenum. A blunt uncinate process arises from the lower part of the head and turns to the left behind the superior mesenteric vessels.

a. The anterior relations of the head from above downwards are, first part of duodenum, transverse colon and coils of jejunum.
b. Posteriorly, the common bile duct is intimately related, as it is almost embedded in the posterior aspect of head. The other posterior relations are, IVC and the termination of the right and left renal veins into it.
c. Above, below and to the right, the head is in close relation to the duodenum. The pancreaticoduodenal

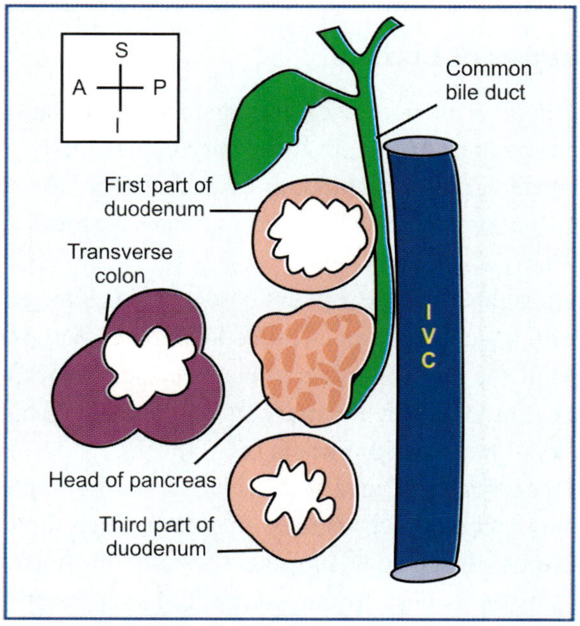

Fig. 135.3: Relations of the head of pancreas

anastomotic arcades lie in the groove between the duodenum and head of pancreas.

d. The uncinate process is related anteriorly to superior mesenteric vessels and posteriorly to the abdominal aorta. This vascular relationship is described in 2 ways, the uncinate process is sandwiched between the superior mesenteric vessels in front and abdominal aorta behind or it is compressed in a vascular nutcracker formed by the abdominal aorta and its superior mesenteric branch (as shown in Fig. 134.5).

Relations of Neck

a. Anteriorly, it is related in the upper part to the gastroduodenal artery and to the pylorus of stomach, from which it is separated by lesser sac.
b. Posteriorly, it is in relation to the portal vein, which is formed behind the neck by the union of splenic and superior mesenteric veins.

Relations of Body

The body of pancreas is triangular with 3 borders and 3 surfaces. The anterior surface lies between the anterior and superior borders. The inferior surface lies between the anterior and inferior borders. The posterior surface is between the superior and inferior borders.

Relations of Borders

a. The anterior border gives attachment to transverse mesocolon. In fact, in the embryological stage, this border gives attachments to 2 posterior layers of greater omentum and 2 layers of transverse mesocolon (Fig.132.1).
b. The right end of the superior border, which is in contact with lesser omentum, is called tuber omentale. At this point, the superior border is related to the coeliac trunk. The tortuous splenic artery runs to the left along the rest of the superior margin (Fig. 134.1).
c. The inferior border is in relation to the superior mesenteric vessels as they emerge through the head to cross the uncinate process. The inferior mesenteric vein passes deep to this margin to reach the splenic vein.

Relations of Surfaces

a. The anterior surface is part of the stomach bed, hence, it is separated from the posterior surface of the stomach by the lesser sac (omental bursa).
b. The inferior surface is in contact with duodenojejunal flexure, coils of jejunum and left colic flexure.
c. The posterior surface is related from right to left, to the abdominal aorta at the origin of superior mesenteric artery, left crus of diaphragm, left renal vessels, left kidney and left suprarenal gland. A very intimate relation of the posterior surface is the splenic vein, which runs from the hilum of the spleen to the neck of pancreas.

Tail

The tail of pancreas is the tapering left end of the pancreas, which reaches the hilum of the spleen through the lienorenal ligament along with the splenic vessels. Therefore, the tail of the pancreas is part of the splenic pedicle. The islet cells are usually more numerous in the tail. During splenectomy, the tail of pancreas is likely to be injured unless identified and excluded from the ligature for splenic vessels. If the tail is injured, the pancreatic enzymes will leak out and destroy the surrounding tissues leading to chemical peritonitis or pancreatic fistula.

Pancreatic Ducts (Fig. 135.4)

a. The main pancreatic duct or duct of Wirsung runs in the entire length of the gland. It begins in the tail and gradually increases in size as it gathers more and more tributaries, which are arranged in herringbone pattern. In the body of pancreas, the duct lies nearer the posterior surface. At the junction of head and neck, the duct turns sharply in inferior direction and then to the right to enter the second part of duodenum. It usually joins the common bile duct just outside or inside the duodenal wall. These ducts unite to form a hepatopancreatic ampulla just before opening on the major duodenal papilla. The sphincter of Oddi surrounds the ampulla. The pancreatic and biliary ducts may open separately on the major duodenal papilla, which is 8 to 10 cm distal to pylorus.
b. The accessory pancreatic duct or the duct of Santorini starts in the lower part of the head and then, travels up crossing in front of the main duct. It opens in the

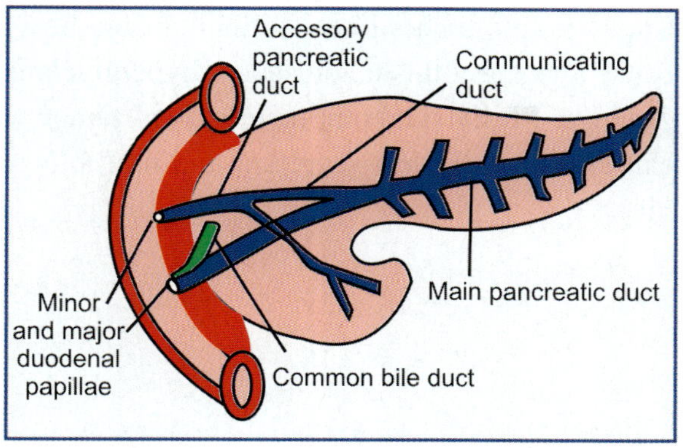

Fig. 135.4: Scheme to depict pancreatic ducts

second part of the duodenum at the summit of minor duodenal papilla, 2 cm proximal to the major duodenal papilla. It communicates with the main duct while crossing it.

Radiological Examination of Ducts

To visualize the duct system a special investigation called endoscopic retrograde cholangiopancreatography (ERCP) is performed, in which a contrast medium (dye) is injected into the ampulla of Vater, through an endoscope introduced through the stomach and duodenum. The dye outlines the pancreatic duct system and the common bile duct.

Microscopic Structure of Pancreas

The parenchyma of the gland consists mainly of the acini and ducts interspersed with islets of Langerhans. The acinar cells show characteristic bipolar staining (infranuclear basophilic cytoplasm and supranuclear acidophilic cytoplasm). The basal cytoplasm contains numerous rough endoplasmic reticulum and the supranuclear cytoplasm contains the membrane bound zymogen granules. The narrow intercalated ducts lined by centroacinar cells begin inside the acini. The simple cuboidal or columnar epithelium lines the larger ducts. The islets are present as clusters of small, scattered and pale cells. Islet cells are of three types, A (alpha) cells secrete glucagon, B (beta) cells secrete insulin and D (delta) cells secrete pancreatic gastrin and somatostatin.

Arterial Supply (Figs 134.1 and 134.7)

a. The head receives blood from the anterior and posterior anastomotic arcades between the branches of superior and inferior pancreaticoduodenal arteries.
b. The pancreatic branches of splenic artery supply numerous branches to the neck, body and tail of pancreas. The arteria pancreatica magna and arteria caudae pancreatic are the named pancreatic branches of the splenic artery.

Venous Drainage

The veins from the pancreas drain into splenic, superior mesenteric and portal veins.

Lymphatic Drainage

The head and body drain into pyloric and pancreatico-splenic nodes, which ultimately drain into pre-aortic nodes. The tail drains into the splenic nodes.

Nerve Supply

The coeliac plexus supplies both sympathetic and parasympathetic nerves to the pancreas. The visceral afferent fibers travel in the greater and lesser splanchnic nerves. The segmental level of innervation is T7 to T11. The searing pancreatic pain typically radiates to the middle of the back and is due to irritation of the parietal peritoneum covering the pancreas.

Clinical Highlights

a. Inflammation of pancreas is called pancreatitis. It may occur as a complication of mumps. The symptoms of pancreatitis include loss of appetite, nausea, typical pancreatic backache and fever. These are usually accompanied with bulky and fat filled stools. Acute pancreatitis is characterized by rise in serum amylase level four times its normal value. Recurrent pancreatitis predisposes to stasis of pancreatic juice in the ducts leading to calculi formation in the pancreas.
b. The omental bursa (lesser sac) is anteriorly related to the anterior surface of the body of pancreas. Therefore, inflammatory fluid collects in the omental bursa in pancreatitis. Such a swelling gives a false impression of a cyst arising from pancreas hence, the name, pancreatic pseudocyst.
c. Carcinoma of the head of pancreas produces symptoms related to compression of the surrounding

structures. The compression of common bile duct results in obstructive jaundice, that of the portal vein in ascites and that of second part of duodenum in intestinal obstruction.

d. The islet cell tumors like insulinoma from beta cells cause hyperinsulinism and severe hyperglycemia. In Zollinger-Ellison syndrome there is G-cell tumor, which causes excess gastrin secretion and multiple peptic ulcers.

136 Jejunum and Ileum

The jejunum and ileum are highly coiled parts of the small intestine. Together they measure about 6 meters in length, of which upper two-fifth is jejunum and lower three-fifth is ileum. The coils of small intestine are packed in the infracolic compartment of the greater sac. The greater omentum normally covers the anterior aspect of the coils of small intestine and separates them from the anterior abdominal wall. Being a highly mobile part of the digestive tract, it is often herniated and found in the sacs of the inguinal, femoral or umbilical herniae.

Extent

The jejunum starts at the duodenojejunal junction at the left of midline and the ileum terminates at the ileocaecal junction in the right iliac fossa.

The Mesentery

The mesentery of the small intestine suspends the jejunum and ileum from the posterior abdominal wall. It has the root (attached margin) and the free margin (intestinal margin). The root is roughly 15 cm long and contains the superior mesenteric vessels. The free margin is about 6 meters long and contains the intestine inside it. The mesentery is highly folded due to the difference between the lengths of its two margins. The root of the mesentery is obliquely attached to the posterior abdominal wall from the left side of second lumbar vertebra to the right sacroiliac joint. It crosses the following structures from above downward, third part of the duodenum, abdominal aorta, inferior vena cava, right gonadal vessels and right ureter on the anterior surface of right psoas major muscle.

Contents

The mesentery contains the coils of jejunum and ileum, jejunal and ileal branches of superior mesenteric vessels, ileal branches of ileocolic vessels, large numbers of mesenteric lymph nodes, intestinal lymph vessels, nerve plexuses and the extraperitoneal loose connective tissue laden with variable amount of fat.

Surface Marking (Fig. 136.1)

The point representing the duodenojejunal flexure is 2.5 cm to the left of the midline and 1 cm below the transpyloric plane. The point of intersection of right lateral and transtubercular lines represents the ileocecal junction. An oblique line joining the above two points is the surface marking of the root of mesentery.

Clinical Highlights

The mesentery is a site of cystic swelling, which commonly arises from the mesenteric lymph nodes. The cyst presents clinically, as a painless fluctuant swelling near the

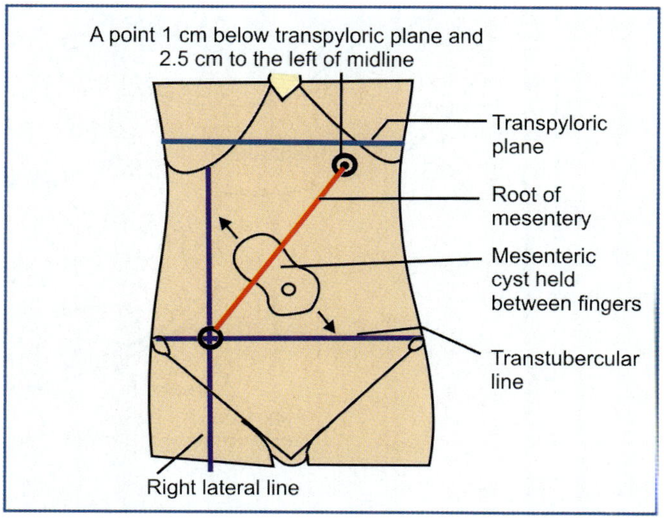

Fig. 136.1: Surface marking of root of the mesentery and its clinical importance (Note that the cyst is mobile in the direction at right angles to the line representing the root of mesentery)

umbilicus. The characteristic feature of the swelling is that it is more mobile in the direction at right angles to the line of attachment of the mesentery but very little along the line of attachment.

Distinguishing Features (Fig. 136.2)

a. The diameter and thickness of the wall of the jejunum are greater than that of ileum.
b. The arterial arches in the mesentery of the jejunum are less in number hence, the vasa recta are longer. In the case of ileum, the arterial arches are more and hence, the vasa recta are short.
c. There are transparent windows in the mesentery of jejunum due to absence of fat while in the case of the ileum, there are opaque windows due to the presence of fat.

Arterial Supply

Several (about 12-20) jejunal and ileal branches arise from the left side of the superior mesenteric artery and enter the mesentery to reach the intestine. The only part not supplied by the ileal branches of superior mesenteric artery, is the terminal part of the ileum, which is supplied by the ileal branches of ileocolic branch of superior mesenteric artery. As soon as the jejunal and ileal branches enter the mesentery, they divide into smaller branches that anastomose with each other to form a series of arterial arcades. From the terminal arcades, vasa recta (straight vessels) are given off, which enter the gut wall. Since the arcades are fewer in jejunum compared to the ileum, the length of the vasa recta is longer in jejunum and shorter in ileum. The fat in the mesentery of the ileum is present right up to the wall of the gut but in the case of the jejunal mesentery, the fat is lacking nearer the gut. The spaces between the long vasa recta in the jejunal part of the mesentery, present the appearance of transparent windows when held against light. On the contrary, the spaces between the short vasa recta in the ileal part of the mesentery present the appearance of opaque windows. This feature may be helpful in identifying the gut loop at the time of surgery. The functional importance of arterial arcades is that they provide abundant collateral circulation.

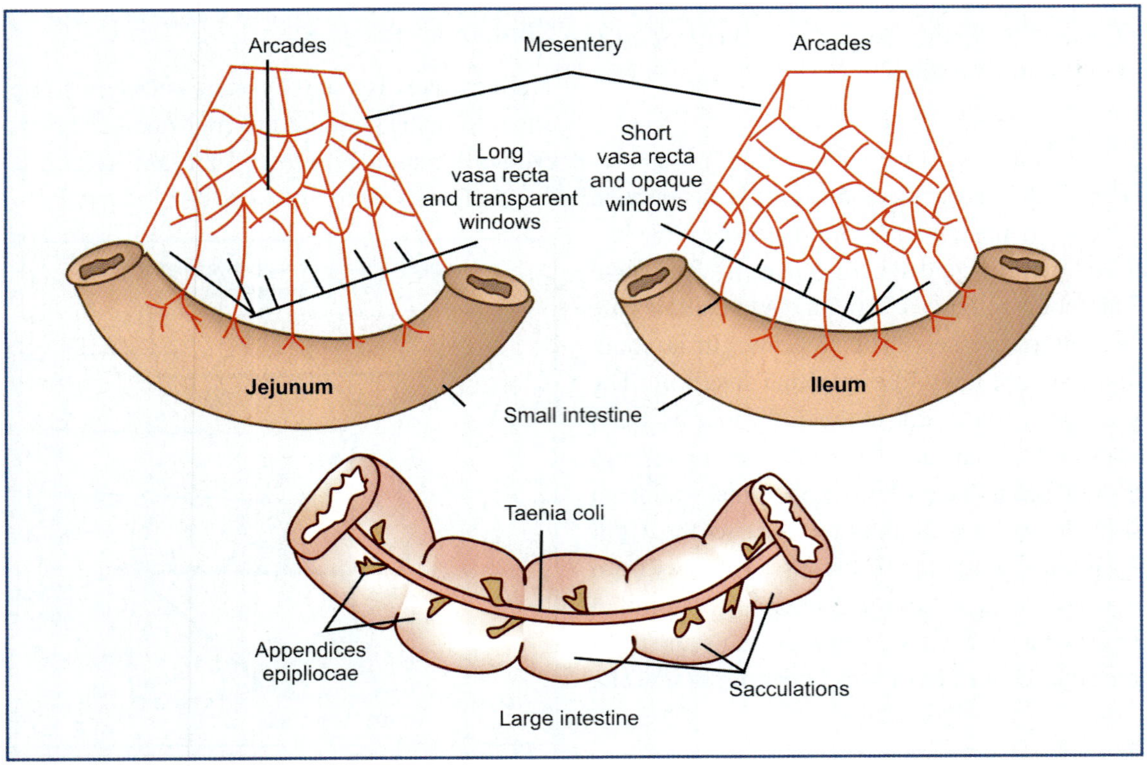

Fig. 136.2: Depicting contrasting features of jejunal and ileal mesentery and those between small and large intestines

This is of particular importance during peristaltic movements, when some of the vasa recta may be constricted.

Venous Drainage

The veins follow the arteries and empty into the superior mesenteric vein. They carry the products of digestion of proteins and carbohydrates to the portal circulation.

Lymphatic Drainage

The lymph vessels in the small intestine assume more importance because they carry products of fat digestion to the thoracic duct, in addition to the lymph from the gut. Each villus in the mucosa of the jejunum and ileum carries a central lymph vessel called lacteal. The lymph from the lacteals drains in the lymph plexuses of the wall of the gut and then to the lymphatics in the attached border of the gut. Having reached the mesentery, the lymph passes through lymph nodes in the mesentery and ultimately drains in the preaortic nodes.

Nerve Supply

Parasympathetic supply is by vagus nerves through the superior mesenteric plexus. The stimulation of vagus promotes peristalsis. The sympathetic supply is by lesser splanchnic nerve (T10-T11) through the superior mesenteric plexus. The pain sensation is carried by sympathetic fibers in lesser splanchnic nerve to the thoracic sympathetic chain and then to the T10 and T11 segments of the spinal cord. The pain from the jejunum and ileum is referred to umbilical region.

Clinical Highlights

a. The Peyer's patches can be felt through the anti-mesenteric margin of the ileum. They may ulcerate in typhoid fever and give rise to characteristic vertically oriented ulcers in the intestinal mucosa. In typhoid fever, the bacteria, ingested through contaminated food, cause enteritis (inflammation of small intestine). As a generalized immune response of the body, not only the Peyer's patches but also the mesenteric lymph nodes and the spleen are enlarged in typhoid fever. After healing, the typhoid ulcers do not cause intestinal obstruction unlike the tuberculous ulcers, which are circularly oriented and hence after healing by fibrous tissue, may constrict the lumen.
b. The parasitic infestations like roundworm, hookworm are commonly seen in small intestine, especially in children. The roundworms may cause obstruction of intestine while hookworms are notorious for absorbing the products of digestion from the intestine thus depriving the host of the nutrition. Hookworm infestation is the important cause of anemia in India.
c. Intussusception is the invagination or telescoping of a segment of intestine into the lumen of preceding or succeeding part. The common site is the terminal ileum at the ileocaecal junction.
d. Meckel's diverticulum is the persistent proximal part of the embryonic vitellointestinal duct. It is found in 2 percent of population. It is about 5 to 6 cm long and is attached to the antimesenteric border of the ileum 60 cm proximal to the ileocaecal junction. Its dimension is similar to that of the ileum and its wall has the same layers as that of the ileum. When inflamed its symptoms are similar to that of acute appendicitis. Therefore, the dictum is that in a case clinically diagnosed as appendicitis, if a healthy appendix is found during operation: look for Meckel's diverticulum. If the diverticulum has ectopic gastric or pancreatic tissue, its thin wall may perforate and mimic acute abdomen.

137 Large Intestine

The large intestine extends from the ileocecal junction to the anus in the perineum. It is one and half meters in length. The different parts of the large intestine (Fig. 137.1) are the caecum and appendix, ascending colon, transverse colon, descending colon, sigmoid colon, rectum and anal canal.

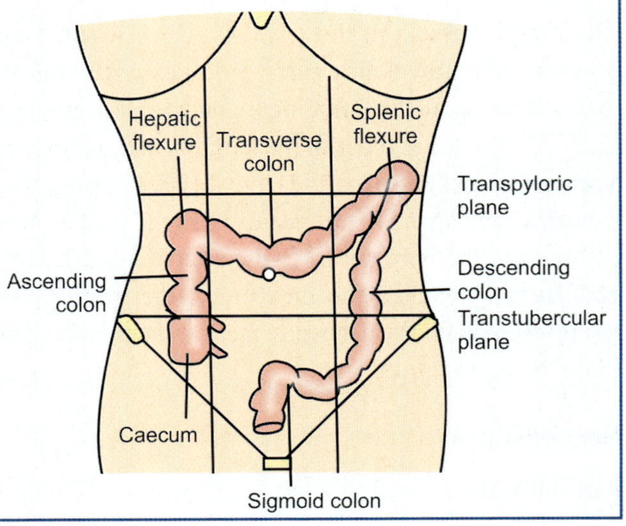

Fig. 137.1: Surface projection of caecum and various parts of colon

Functions

The main function of large intestine is absorption of water from the fluid contents of large intestine and help in formation, storage and expulsion of feces. Besides this, the large intestine manufactures vitamin B complex with the help of natural bacterial flora of intestine.

Distinguishing Features (Fig. 136.3)

a. The longitudinal muscle layer is disposed as three bands instead of as a uniform layer. The bands are called taeniae coli, which are present on all parts of colon and caecum.
b. The haustrations or sacculations are the dilated parts in between the taeniae. They are responsible for the characteristic puckered appearance of the large intestine.
c. The appendices epiploicae are the fat filled bags of visceral peritoneum attached to the taeniae of the large intestine.

Development

The caecum, appendix, ascending colon and right two-thirds of transverse colon develop from midgut and hence, supplied by branches of superior mesenteric artery. The left one-third of transverse colon, descending colon, sigmoid colon, rectum and anal canal above the level of pectinate line, develop from hindgut and hence, are supplied by branches of inferior mesenteric artery.

Development of Caecum and Appendix

After the return of the herniated midgut into the abdominal cavity, the cecal bud is in the subhepatic position. Then, it gradually descends to reach the right iliac fossa. Arrest of descent may lead to ectopic locations of caecum and appendix (Fig. 137.2). At birth, the caecum is conical with tubular appendix attached to its tip. Later, differential growth of the walls of caecum is essential to acquire definitive shape and for the shift in the position of the appendix. Arrest of growth during this stage leads to variation in the shapes of caecum. The infantile or infundibular caecum is conical in shape with appendix attached to its apex. The taeniae coli are equidistant from each other. In the quadrate type, the saccules of equal size are present on either side of anterior taeniae coli and the appendix is attached in between the saccules. In the ampullary type the right saccule grows more rapidly and

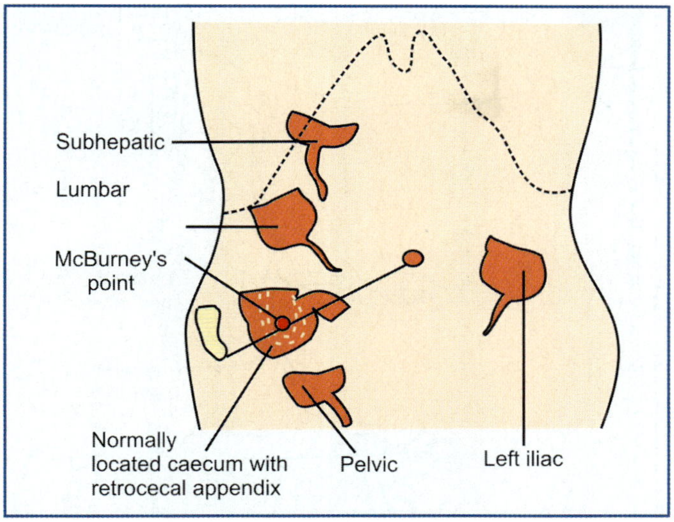

Fig. 137.2: Schematic diagram depicting abnormal locations of caecum and appendix with reference to normal location

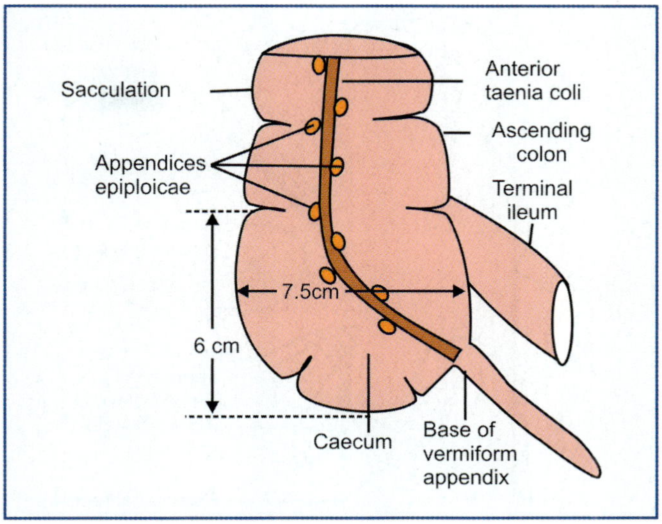

Fig. 137.3: Measurements and external features of caecum

forms the base of the caecum thus pushing the appendix towards ileocecal junction. This is the commonest type found in adults.

Caecum (Fig. 137.3)

The meaning of the word caecum, in Latin, is blind. The caecum is the blind end of the large intestine below the level of ileal opening. Its peculiarity is that its length (6 cm) is smaller than the breadth (7.5 cm). The caecum is located in the right iliac fossa just above the lateral half of the inguinal ligament. It is continuous above the level of ileocecal opening with the ascending colon. It has an inferior convex wall, a lateral wall and a medial wall showing openings of ileum and appendix. The vermiform appendix is attached to its posteromedial wall below the ileocecal junction. There are three taeniae coli, anterior, posteromedial and posterolateral, which converge towards the base of appendix to merge with the uniform longitudinal muscle coat of the appendix. This is the basis of locating the appendix during surgery by tracing the anterior taeniae coli to the appendicular base.

Surface Marking (Fig. 137.1)

The point of intersection of transtubercular and right lateral planes indicates the position of ileocecal opening. A 6 cm long line from this point drawn vertically downwards marks the left margin. A 6 cm long parallel line, which is 7.5 cm to the right of the previous line, marks the right margin. Joining the lower ends of the above two lines by a line that is convex downwards indicates the lower margin of the caecum.

Relations

The caecum is almost entirely covered with peritoneum on all sides though it has no mesentery. This gives freedom of movement to the caecum. When distended the caecum comes in contact with the anterior abdominal wall in the right iliac fossa but when empty the coils of small intestine lie in front of its anterior surface. Posterioly, it is related to the iliacus and psoas major muscles, femoral nerve and lateral cutaneous nerve of thigh.

Peritoneal Recesses (Fig. 137.4)

At the ileocecal junction, peritoneal recesses called ileocecal recesses are frequently present. The superior ileocecal recess is present above the terminal ileum. Its anterior boundary is by a vascular peritoneal fold containing the anterior cecal vessels. The inferior ileocecal recess is present below the terminal ileum. The bloodless fold of Treves forms its anterior boundary. The retrocecal recess is present behind the caecum. It is related anteriorly to the caecum and posteriorly to the parietal peritoneum in the right iliac fossa. Usually, the retrocecal vermiform appendix occupies this recess.

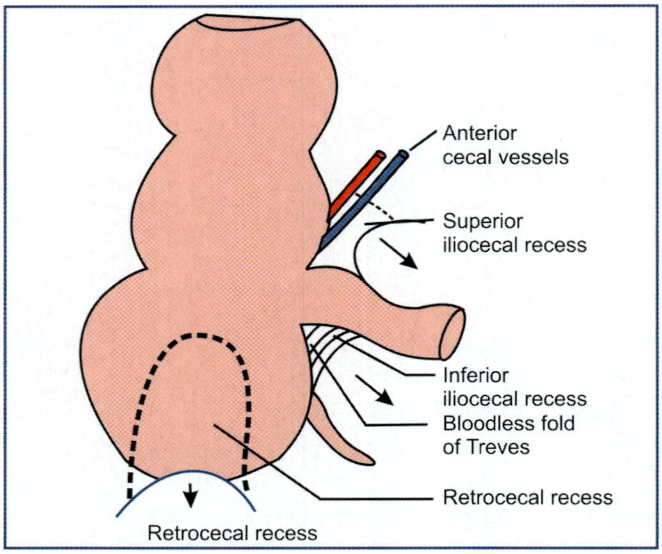

Fig. 137.4: Peritoneal recesses around caecum

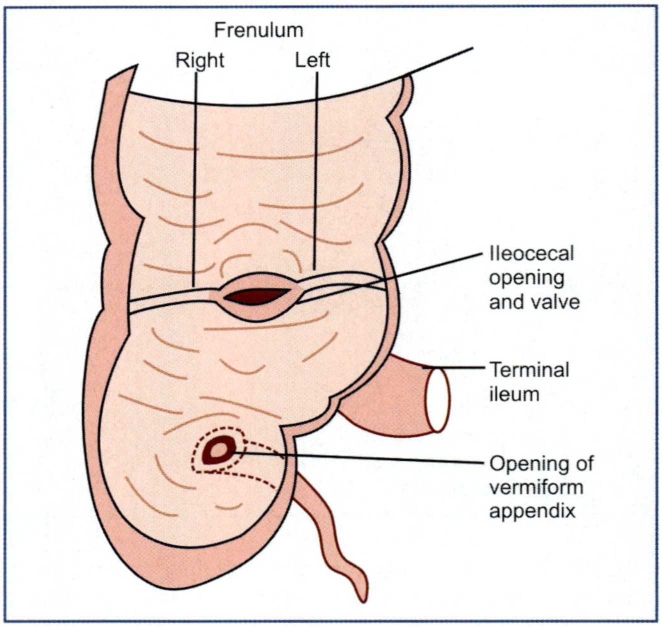

Fig. 137.5: Highly magnified view of the interior of caecum

Interior of the Caecum (Fig. 137.5)

The interior of the caecum shows two openings:

a. The ileocecal orifice is the prominent feature of the interior of caecum. The terminal segment of the ileum projects in the posteromedial wall of the caecum. This forces the mucosa, submucosa and the circular muscle of the ileal wall into the lumen of caecum surrounding the ileocecal orifice. The protrusion raises two parallel transverse folds called upper and lower lips of the ileocecal valve. These folds extend as single lines called frenula of the valve on either side of the orifice. The ileocecal valve regulates the flow of ileal contents into the caecum. However, tightening of the frenula prevents the reflux of the cecal contents into the ileum, by drawing the lips of the valve closer in distended caecum.

b. A small appendicular opening is situated 1 to 2 cm below the ileocecal orifice on the posteromedial wall of the caecum. An insignificant valve (of Gerlach) guards this opening.

Blood Supply (Fig. 137.6)

The anterior and posterior cecal branches of ileocolic branch of the superior mesenteric artery supply the caecum. The veins of the caecum follow the arteries and drain in the portal venous system.

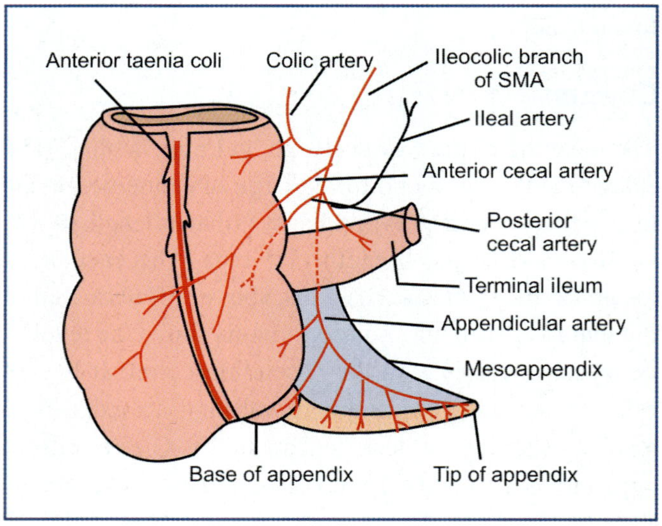

Fig. 137.6: Arterial supply of caecum and appendix through ileocolic branch of superior mesenteric artery

Lymphatic Drainage

The lymph vessels from the caecum drain into ileocolic lymph nodes and finally in the superior mesenteric nodes.

Clinical Highlights

The ileocecal area is the site of pathologic lesions of caecum giving rise to a swelling or mass in right iliac fossa.

The ileocecal intussusception (telescoping of terminal ileum into the caecum) is common in children. The tuberculosis of caecum and adjacent ileum, carcinoma of caecum and amebiasis of the caecum are other causes of cecal pathology. The amebiasis of caecum may spread to the right lobe of liver due to channeling of blood flow in the portal vein. The inflammation of caecum is known as typhlitis.

Vermiform Appendix

The vermiform appendix is worm like in appearance. Its length is variable, the average being 8 to 9 cm. The wall of the appendix contains large aggregations of lymphatic tissue hence, the appendix has been termed the abdominal tonsil.

Parts

a. It has a base, which is attached to the caecum, 2 cm or less, below the ileocecal junction. The position of the base is constant. The taeniae coli of the caecum become continuous with the complete longitudinal coat of the appendix at the base. The appendix opens into the posteromedial wall of the caecum by its base.
b. The apex of the appendix is free and its position is variable.
c. The lumen is very narrow. If the lumen is blocked, a small mass of intestinal contents gets isolated in it, which predisposes to inflammation.

Peritoneal Relation

The appendix is intraperitoneal organ. Its mesentery is called the mesoappendix, which is part of the mesentery of the terminal part of the ileum. It is very transparent in childhood. The appendicular artery runs through the mesoappendix.

McBurney's Point

McBurney's point lies at the junction of the lateral third and medial two-thirds of the spinoumbilical line from the anterior superior iliac spine to umbilicus on the right side (Fig. 137.1). It is the area of maximum tenderness in acute appendicitis and it is the site for placing gridiron incision for classical appendicectomy.

Surface Marking

The base of the appendix is constant in position hence only the base can be represented on the anterior abdominal wall by a point, which is 2 cm or less below the ileocecal junction (a point of intersection of transtubercular and right lateral lines). In this connection, it is worthy of note that this point and the McBurney's point do not exactly coincide anatomically though they are in close topographical proximity. This may be the reason for equating the surface marking of the base of appendix to the McBurney's point for practical purposes (described as "useful surgical approximation" in 38th edition of Grey's Anatomy).

Positions of the Tip of Appendix (Fig. 137.7)

The various positions of the appendix are, retrocecal (60%), pelvic (30%), subcecal (2%), paracecal (1%), promontoric (1%), preileal (1%) and postileal (5%).

Retrocecal Appendix

This is the most common position. The retrocecal appendix is related anteriorly to the caecum and its posterior relations are the psoas major and iliacus muscles. The psoas test depends on this anatomical relationship (psoas sign is positive in retrocecal appendicitis). The irritation of the psoas muscle gives rise to pain, when the patient's right thigh is extended from the flexed position. This happens because psoas major is the flexor of hip joint and when the thigh is extended, it is put to stretch.

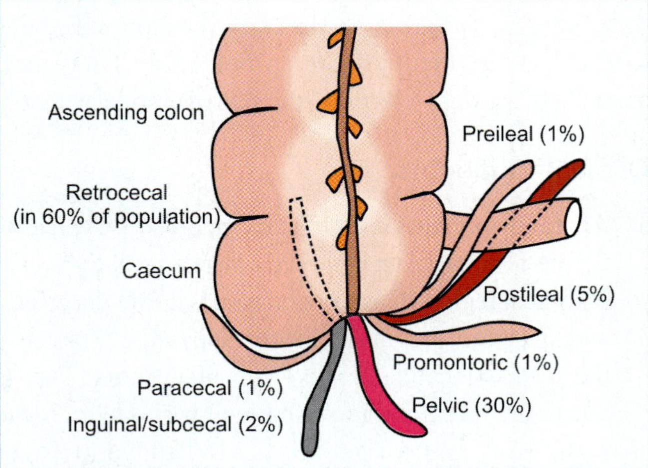

Fig. 137.7: Different positions of the appendix with percentage of their occurrance in population

Pelvic Appendix

In the pelvic position, the tip of the appendix crosses the pelvic brim and comes in close relation to the pelvic viscera. In female, the vicinity to right ovary and right fallopian tube may pose problems in differentiating the inflammation of ovary or the fallopian tube from appendicitis. A case of appendicitis may be missed, thinking it to be a disease of pelvic organs. The pelvic appendix is related to obturator internus muscle and this relationship is the basis of obturator test, which is positive in pelvic appendicitis. Passive medial rotation of flexed thigh elicits pain (the inflamed pelvic appendix irritates the obturator internus).

Blood Supply

A single appendicular artery, a branch of inferior division of ileocolic artery, supplies the appendix. The appendicular artery passes behind the terminal ileum to enter the mesoappendix and travels in it to reach the tip of the appendix (which is the least vascular part). Moreover, the mesoappendix is so short towards the tip that the artery comes to rest on the appendicular wall. In inflammation of appendix, this part of the artery is affected and thrombosed first so that tip becomes gangrenous and may perforate. The appendicular vein drains in the portal venous system.

Nerve Supply

Sympathetic afferent fibers in lesser splanchnic nerve via the superior mesenteric plexus carry the pain sensations to the T10 segment of the spinal cord. Therefore, appendicular pain is referred to the skin of umbilical region.

Clinical Highlights

a. Acute appendicitis is a surgical emergency. Typically, the pain of acute appendicitis is felt initially in the umbilical region. This visceral pain is due to distension and spasm of the muscle of the appendix. Gradually the pain is localized to the right iliac fossa. This is due to the inflammation of parietal peritoneum in the right iliac fossa. Usually, vomiting and fever accompany the pain. On palpation of the abdominal wall, an area of maximum tenderness is found at the McBurney's point. Irritation of the parietal peritoneum also gives rise to abdominal rigidity and muscle guarding. Some complications of appendicitis include perforation, gangrene and appendicular abscess. Atypical presentation like the appendicitis mimicking the symptoms of acute cholecystitis is due to inflammation of subhepatic appendix.
b. Incisions for appendicectomy are based on anatomy of anterior abdominal wall (Fig. 128.1). A gridiron (shape of a cross beam) skin incision is placed at right angles to the McBurney's point in the plane of cleavage lines. The three flat muscles are identified and split along the direction of their fibres. Branches of deep circumflex iliac artery and iliohypogastric nerve are identified in the plane between the transversus and internal oblique to avoid injury. The transversalis fascia and parietal peritoneum are incised together. The caecum is identified by presence of taeniae coli and is withdrawn from its bed. By tracing anterior taeniae coli, the base of appendix is located. The appendicular artery is ligated in the mesoappendix. The appendix is cut at its base and removed. Some surgeons prefer Lanz's transverse incision, which is placed 2 cm below the umbilicus (instead of gridiron incision). Its center lies along a vertical line passing through the mid-inguinal point. Nowadays, laparoscopic appendicectomy is in vogue.

Ascending Colon

The average length of the ascending colon is 15 cm. It begins from the caecum at the level of ileocecal orifice and reaches the hepatic flexure of the colon below the liver, where the ascending colon becomes the transverse colon. The ascending colon lies in the right lumbar and iliac regions in the retroperitoneal position.

External Features

The ascending colon has all the three characteristics of the large intestine. The taeniae are anterior, posteromedial and posterolateral in position.

Relations

Anterior to the ascending colon, there are coils of small intestine and greater omentum. The posterior relations can be divided in two parts. Above the iliac crest, the transversus abdominis and quadratus lumborum muscles and iliohypogastric and ilioinguinal nerves are the posterior relations. The lower pole of the right kidney is also related posteriorly. Below the iliac crest, the iliacus muscle and lateral cutaneous nerve of thigh come in posterior aspect.

Transverse Colon

The transverse colon extends from the hepatic flexure to the splenic flexure of colon, where it continues as the descending colon. The average length of the transverse colon is 50 cm. Its right end, which is below the level of transpyloric plane, is fixed. Its left end is above the transpyloric plane in the left hypochondrium and is fixed. The intervening part of the transverse colon is suspended from the posterior abdominal wall by the transverse mesocolon. The intermediate mobile part usually extends to the level of umbilicus, but it may reach down as far as the pelvis. Thus, the transverse colon is shaped like a U with limbs of unequal lengths. The anterior surface of transverse colon is closely related to the anterior abdominal wall. This makes the exposure of this part of the colon simple for the surgeon who wants to perform transverse colostomy (making an opening into the transverse colon).

External Features

Since the transverse colon is suspended by a mesentery the position of the taeniae is different. It has anterior, superior and posterior taeniae.

Relations

The posterior surface of its right extremity is devoid of peritoneum and hence is fused to the anterior surface of the second part of duodenum and the head of pancreas. The other posterior relations are the upper end of the mesentery, the duodenojejunal flexure and the coils of jejunum and ileum. Anteriorly, the transverse colon is related to the greater omentum with which it is fused. The greater omentum separates it from anterior abdominal wall. Superiorly, it is related to the liver, gallbladder, greater curvature of stomach and the lateral end of spleen from the right to the left.

Transverse Mesocolon

The transverse mesocolon is attached by two layers of peritoneum to the anterior border of the body of pancreas. The anterior surfaces of the transverse colon and the mesocolon are fused with the posterior layers of greater omentum. This gives an impression of two peritoneal folds being attached to the transverse colon, the mesocolon to its upper border and the greater omentum to its lower border. The contents of transverse mesocolon are, the transverse colon, middle colic vessels, ascending branches of left colic vessels, marginal artery, lymph nodes, lymphatics and nerve plexuses embedded in loose areolar tissue with variable amount of fat.

Comparative Features of Hepatic and Splenic Flexures

a. The hepatic flexure is located in the right lumbar region and the splenic flexure is deep in the left hypochondrium.
b. The hepatic flexure is below the transpyloric plane while the splenic flexure is above.
c. The vertebral level of the hepatic flexure is L2 and that of splenic flexure is T12.
d. The angulation of the hepatic flexure is wider compared to that of the splenic, which is acute.
e. The splenic flexure is attached to the diaphragm by phrenicocolic ligament.
f. The vagus supplies the hepatic flexure but the pelvic splanchnic nerve supplies the splenic flexure.
g. The hepatic flexure being a derivative of midgut receives arterial supply from the right colic branch of superior mesenteric artery. The splenic flexure develops from the hindgut. It receives blood supply from the marginal artery formed by the left colic branch of the inferior mesenteric artery and the middle colic branch of superior mesenteric artery. Therefore, the splenic flexure is at the junction of the territories of the superior and inferior mesenteric arteries and hence is more prone to ischemia.

Descending Colon

The descending colon is longer, narrower and more deeply placed than the ascending colon. It starts at the splenic flexure in the left hypochondrium and descends through the left lumbar and iliac regions to become continuous with the sigmoid colon at the medial margin of left psoas major in front of the left external iliac vessels at the left pelvic brim. Its average length is 25 cm. It is retroperitoneal.

Surface Marking

The descending colon is represented by two parallel lines, which are 2.5 to 3 cm apart and start from the left eighth costal cartilage and course downwards vertically to the inguinal ligament.

Relations

a. Anteriorly, its upper part is covered with the terminal part of transverse colon and the coils of intestine. The lower part of the descending colon is in the left iliac fossa; so it is related anteriorly to the anterior abdominal wall when distended with gas or feces and can be palpated above the inguinal ligament.
b. Posteriorly, the upper part of the descending colon is related to the anterior surface of the lower lateral part of left kidney. Below the level of iliac crest, the posterior relations are, the iliacus and psoas major muscles, lateral cutaneous nerve of thigh, femoral and genitofemoral nerves, external iliac artery and testicular vessels in male. The loaded descending colon may compress the left testicular vein. This is one of the predisposing factors for the causation of varicocele (enlarged and dilated pampiniform plexus) on left side.

Sigmoid Colon

The sigmoid colon is also called the pelvic colon. It begins at the left brim of the true pelvis and forms a loop of variable length, which normally lies within the true pelvis. It ends at rectosigmoid junction where it becomes the rectum, level with third sacral vertebra. The sigmoid colon first descends in contact with the left pelvic wall, and then crosses the pelvis between the rectum and urinary bladder in male, and between rectum and uterus in female. The average length of the sigmoid colon is 40 cm. It is suspended from the posterior pelvic wall by a mesentery called the pelvic mesocolon.

Pelvic Mesocolon

The pelvic mesocolon is attached to the posterior pelvic wall by an inverted V- shaped root. The left limb of the root is attached along the left brim of the pelvis medial to the left psoas major muscle. The right limb is attached to the pelvic surface of sacrum and it ends in the midline on the third piece of sacrum. The apex of the root is located in front of the bifurcation of the left common iliac artery. An intersigmoid peritoneal recess is often found at the apex (its important relation is the left ureter). The pelvic mesocolon contains the sigmoid colon, superior rectal vessels in the right limb, sigmoid branches of inferior mesenteric artery in the left limb, marginal artery, lymph nodes, lymph vessels, nerve plexuses in the loose areolar tissue and variable amount of fat.

Relations of Sigmoid Colon

On the left side, it is related to structures on the left pelvic wall, namely, external iliac vessels, obturator nerve, and ovary in female and vas deferens in male. On the posterior side, it is related to left internal iliac vessels, sacralplexus, left ureter and piriformis muscle. Inferiorly, it rests on urinary bladder in male and uterus and urinary bladder in female. On the right side, it is related to coils of small intestine.

Blood Supply of Colon

a. The ileocolic artery supplies the lower smaller part and the right colic artery supplies the larger part of ascending colon.
b. The right two-thirds of transverse colon receives branches from the middle colic branch of superior mesenteric artery and its left third from the left colic branch of inferior mesenteric artery.
c. The left colic artery supplies the descending colon including the splenic flexure.
d. The sigmoid colon receives branches from the sigmoid branches of inferior mesenteric artery as well as from the superior rectal artery.

Marginal Artery (Fig. 137.8)

This is known as the marginal artery of Drummond. It is located very close to the margin of the colon. The marginal

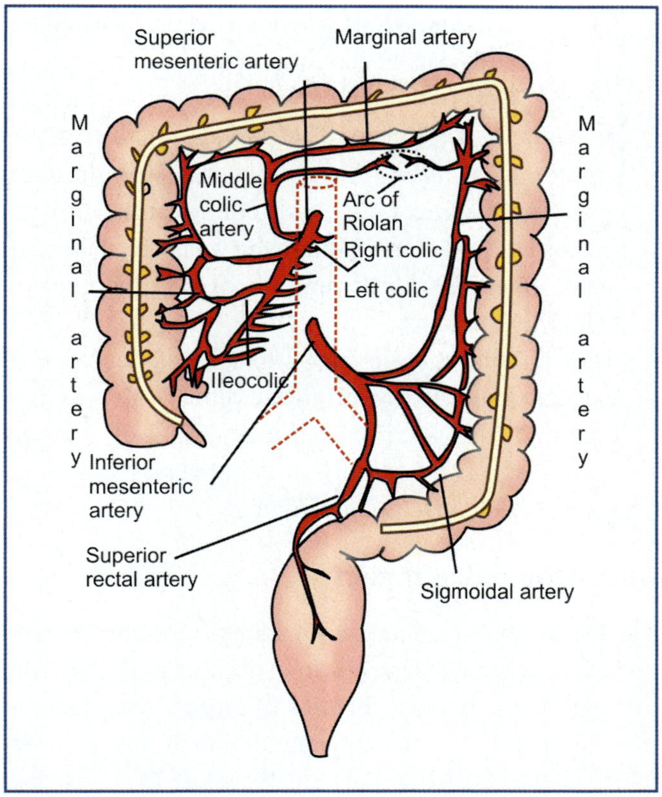

Fig. 137.8: Schematic diagram of arterial supply of large intestine through branches of superior and inferior mesenteric arteries

artery is a circumferential arterial channel extending from the ileocecal junction to the rectosigmoid junction. It supplies vasa longa and vasa brevia to the wall of the colon. The marginal artery is an anastomotic channel formed by the colic branches of the superior and inferior mesenteric arteries. In the event of a block in the inferior mesenteric artery, the blood reaches the left side of the colon through the marginal artery. If the superior mesenteric artery is occluded, the marginal artery becomes enormously dilated since it supplies the entire small intestine through the connection between the ileal branches of ileocolic and ileal branches of superior mesenteric artery. It is observed that at the junctional area of the supply of the superior and inferior mesenteric arteries, the anastomosis may not be sufficient. This area is the splenic flexure, where the ascending branch of left colic artery may fail to communicate with the left branch of middle colic artery (at the level of marginal artery). There is another anastomosis connecting the trunk of middle colic artery with the ascending branch of left colic artery. This anastomosis is called arc of Riolan. If by any chance, this anastomosis is not well-developed then the arterial supply of the splenic flexure is endangered, in case of obstruction of any one of the two parent arteries. This explains the relative frequency of ischemic lesions in the region of splenic flexure. Therefore, the critical point on the gut is said to exist at the splenic flexure.

Venous Drainage

The veins accompanying the ileocolic, right colic and middle colic arteries join the superior mesenteric vein while the veins accompanying the branches of inferior mesenteric artery join the inferior mesenteric vein. Both the veins ultimately drain in portal circulation.

Lymphatic Drainage

The lymphatic drainage of colon is important since carcinoma of colon spreads by lymphatic route. There are numerous colic lymph nodes collecting the lymph from the colon, which are arranged in four groups. The epicolic nodes are minute nodules on the colonic wall. The paracolic nodes lie very close to the marginal arterial anastomosis. The intermediate colic nodes lie along the right, middle and left colic arteries and the preterminal nodes lie along the trunks of superior and inferior mesenteric arteries.

Nerve Supply

The superior and inferior mesenteric nerve plexuses supply the colon.

a. The parasympathetic supply is derived from two sources. The vagus supplies the part of colon that develops from the midgut (ascending colon and right two-thirds of transverse colon). The pelvic splanchnic nerve or nervi erigentes (S2, S3, and S4) supplies the colon that develops from the hindgut (left one-third of transverse colon, descending colon and the sigmoid colon). Hirschsprung's disease or congenital megacolon is a condition in which there is congenital absence of parasympathetic neurons in a segment of the colon. This results in absent peristalsis in that particular segment with resultant obstruction of the large bowel. The colon proximal to the obstruction undergoes dilatation due to accumulation of feces.

b. The visceral pain sensation from the ascending colon and the transverse colon travels through the lesser splanchnic nerve to the T10 and T11 segments of the spinal cord hence pain is referred to the umbilical and hypogastric regions. The pain from the descending and sigmoid colon is carried in the lumbar splanchnic nerves to L1 and L2 segments of spinal cord hence pain from these parts is referred to inguinal region and thigh.

Clinical Highlights

a. The barium enema is used for visualizing the colon to study its interior. The typical pattern of colon due to sacculations is very clearly seen. The endoscopic examination of the colon is done with the help of colonoscope. For sigmoid colon, sigmoidoscope is used.
b. The carcinoma of colon is a slow growing tumor, which produces constriction of the colon. Initially, the tumor spreads by lymphatics but in advanced cases, it spreads to the liver via the portal circulation. If diagnosed early, hemicolectomy (partial removal of colon) and resection of all the lymph nodes of the colon are the effective measures. To overcome the obstruction in the colon (in inoperable cases), an artificial opening is made in the transverse colon (colostomy) and it is brought to the surface of the abdomen to drain out the fecal matter.
c. The diverticulosis is common in sigmoid colon. The small vessels perforate the wall of colon to reach the appendices epiploicae. The passage of the vessels creates weak areas. In cases where intraluminal pressure is quite high, (chronic constipation) the mucosa may herniate through the weak areas forming small diverticula. Inflammation of the diverticula is called diverticulitis.
d. The sigmoid colon is prone to volvulus because of extreme mobility of its mesocolon. Volvulus is a condition in which the peritoneal fold of a viscus rotates and twists around it endangering the blood supply of the viscus concerned.

Rectosigmoid Junction

The rectosigmoid junction corresponds to the third sacral vertebra, where the pelvic mesocolon ends. All the distinguishing external features of large bowel cease to exist here. There is an acute angulation at this junction, which causes difficulty during passage of an endoscope. The rectosigmoid junction lies at the distance of 15 to 17 cm from the anal orifice. The perforation of bowel at this site may occur during sigmoidoscopy unless care is exercised while negotiating the instrument at this junction.

138 Rectum

The rectum is the part of large intestine, which lies between the rectosigmoid and anorectal junctions. It is about 12 to 15 cm long and its diameter is similar to that of the sigmoid colon. The anorectal junction lies about three cm in front of and just below the tip of the coccyx.

Curvatures

Though the meaning of the word rectum is straight, it is curved in sagittal and coronal (lateral) planes. The upper and lower ends of the rectum are in the midline. The sagittal curvatures are the sacral and perineal. The sacral curvature is the one by which the rectum is moulded to the concavity of sacrum. The perineal curvature is present at the anorectal junction, which is encircled by the puborectalis muscle and shows an acute angulation (120°) with forward convexity. The three coronal curvatures are the upper with convexity to the right, middle with convexity to left and the lower with convexity to the right.

Interior (Fig. 138.1)

Corresponding to the coronal curves, three folds (valves of Houston) project in the interior of the rectum. These valves are semilunar transverse folds containing mucosa, submucosa and circular muscle of the rectal wall. Being permanent folds, they do not disappear after rectal distension. The upper valve lies near the beginning of rectum. The middle valve is the largest and most constant. It projects from the anterior and right wall. The lowest valve is inconstant and on the left side. The part of the rectum below the level of middle valve is called the ampulla. It has been suggested that the middle valve divides the rectum in two functionally different parts.

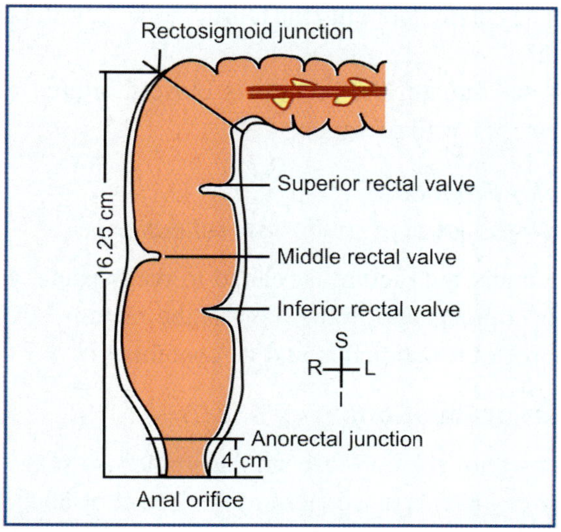

Fig. 138.1: Interior of rectum

Above the level of the middle valve, the rectum stores feces and can freely expand in the peritoneal cavity. The part below the middle valve is normally empty (except during defecation) since it has no space to expand.

Peritoneal Relations

The upper third of the rectum is covered with peritoneum on the front and sides. The middle third is covered only on the front and the lower third is devoid of peritoneal covering. The peritoneum is reflected from the junction of middle and lower third of rectum to the urinary bladder in the male to form rectovesical pouch (Fig. 154.2). In the female, the peritoneum is reflected from the same level to the posterior fornix of vagina to form a deeper rectouterine pouch (Fig.154.5). The coils of small intestine and the sigmoid colon are the usual contents of the peritoneal pouches in both the sexes.

Anterior Relations
(below the level of peritoneal reflection)

a. In the male, the rectovesical fascia (Denonvillier's fascia) separates the rectum from the following structures, base of the urinary bladder, seminal vesicles, vasa deferentia, prostate and terminal parts of ureters (Fig. 154.2). The rectovesical fascia represents the obliterated part of rectovesical peritoneal pouch, which in the males extends right upto the pelvic floor upto the fourth month of intrauterine life.
b. In the female, the rectum is closely related to the posterior wall of vagina.

Anterior Relations
(above the level of peritoneal reflection)

In the male, the rectum is related to rectovesical pouch and its contents and in the female, the rectum is related to the rectouterine pouch and its contents.

Posterior Relations (Fig. 138.2)

The posterior relations are similar in the two sexes. The rectum is attached to the sacrum and coccyx by connective tissue (fascia of Waldeyer) enclosing the lymph nodes, lymphatics and perirectal fat. There are different structures posteriorly in the midline and on lateral sides (right and left).

a. The midline structures are, the lower three pieces of sacrum and coccyx, ganglion impar (formed by the union of the lower ends of the sympathetic trunks) and median sacral artery.
b. On the lateral side, there are three muscles (piriformis, coccygeus and levator ani), sympathetic chain, sacral plexus, coccygeal nerve, pelvic splanchnic nerve (nervi erigentes), branches of superior rectal artery and the lower lateral sacral vessels.

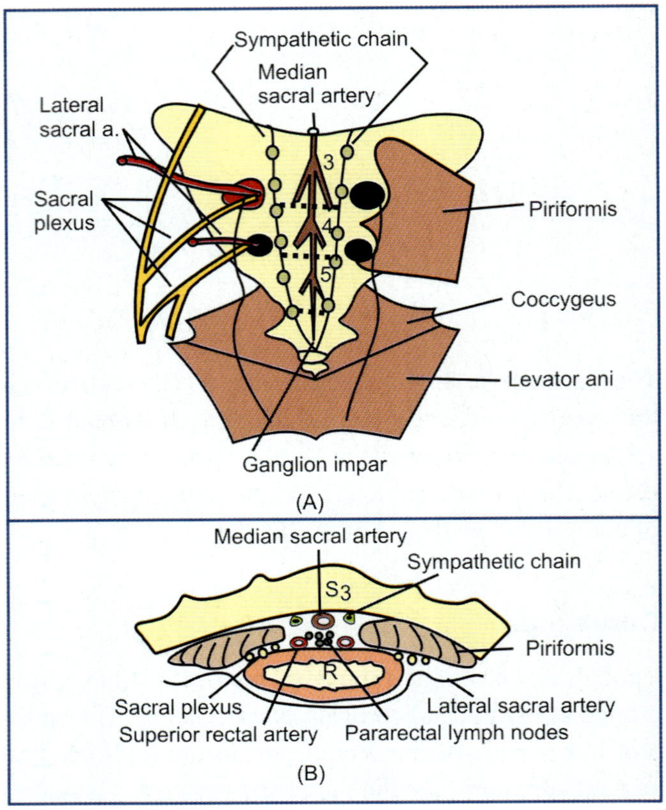

Fig. 138.2: Posterior relations of rectum depicted in (A) where outline of rectum is seen in foreground, (B) depicts posterior relations of upper third in transverse section

Lateral Relations

Muscles of the pelvic diaphragm, namely, levator ani and coccygeus, intimately surround the lower part of the rectum to provide support.

Fascial Relations

The pelvic fascia around the rectum is thicker in consistency and is organized in different parts, which collectively can be grouped as rectal supports. These fascial supports of the rectum have surgical importance since they need to be divided during surgery to mobilize the rectum. The fascia of Waldeyer is a strong condensation in posterior relation, which connects the lower part of anterior surface of the sacrum to the anorectal junction. The lateral rectal ligament is the fascial thickening around the middle rectal vessels. It extends from the lateral pelvic wall to the rectum.

Rectal Supports

The puborectalis sling maintains the angulation at the anorectal junction. The pelvic diaphragm and the fascial supports are important in maintaining the position of the rectum. The weakness of the supports predisposes to rectal prolapse.

Blood Supply of Rectum (Fig. 138.3)

The arterial supply is separate for the mucosa and for the wall of the rectum.

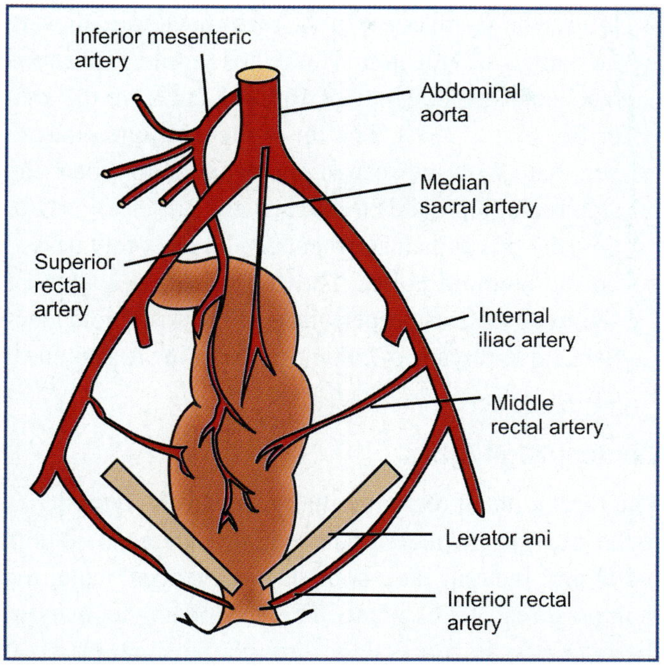

Fig. 138.3: Arterial supply of rectum

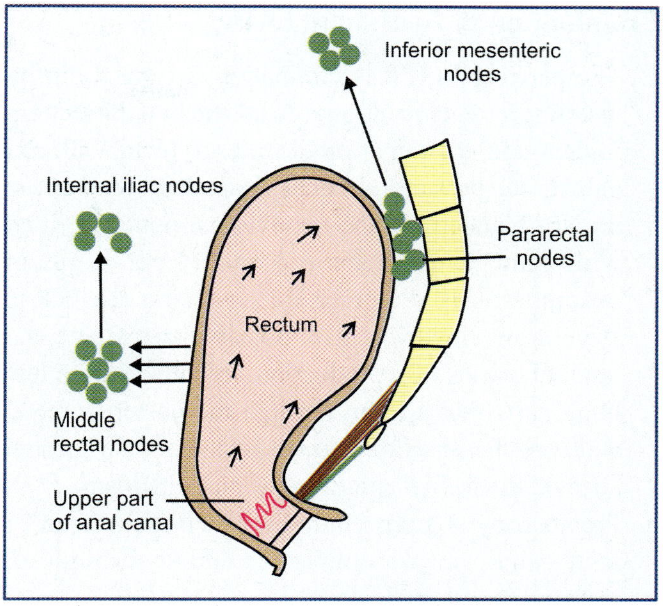

Fig. 138.4: Lymphatic drainage of rectum

a. The arterial supply of the mucosa of the rectum is by the superior rectal artery, which is a continuation of inferior mesenteric artery. The superior rectal artery courses behind the rectum and divides into right and left branches at the level of third piece of sacrum. Their further branches pierce the rectal wall at various points and supply the entire mucosa of the rectum via the submucous plexuses.
b. The arterial supply of the wall of the rectum is from three sources. The branches of superior rectal artery supply the upper part. The branches of the middle rectal artery (a branch of the anterior division of the internal iliac artery) supply the wall of the lower part. The median sacral artery (a branch of abdominal aorta) supplies the back of the anorectal junction.
c. The veins in the rectal mucosa form internal rectal venous plexuses, which drain via the superior rectal vein into the portal vein. The veins of the wall of the rectum form external rectal venous plexus, which drains into the internal iliac vein via the middle rectal veins or the inferior rectal veins.

Lymphatic Drainage (Fig. 138.4)

The lymph vessels along the superior rectal vessels reach the superior rectal lymph nodes (pararectal nodes of Gerota), which lie in close contact with the posterior wall of the rectum. The pararectal nodes drain into the inferior mesenteric nodes. The lymph vessels along the middle rectal vessels end in middle rectal nodes, from which the lymph drains in the internal iliac nodes.

Nerve Supply

The rectum receives both sympathetic and parasympathetic innervation.

Development and Anomalies

The rectal mucosa is endodermal in origin. Its upper part until the middle valve of Houston is derived from preallantoic hindgut and below that level from postallantoic hindgut. The rectal wall develops from the splanchnic mesoderm. The rectal fistula is the condition in which the rectum is in communication with the viscus in front of it. This is due to defect in the formation of urorectal septum. If the rectum communicates with urinary bladder it is called rectovesical fistula. If the lower part of rectum communicates with urethra in the male, it is called rectourethral fistula and if it communicates with vagina in the female, the rectovaginal fistula is the result.

Examination of Rectum in Living

a. The per rectum (PR) examination is carried out by inserting a finger in the anal canal and into the rectum. In the male, the finger in the anterior rectal wall can palpate the prostate, seminal vesicle and base of the urinary bladder and the rectovesical pouch if filled with fluid. In the female normally per vaginum examination is preferred for assessing the pelvic structures. However, it is possible to palpate the internal organs of reproduction. In both sexes, a few bony parts that are felt through the posterior rectal wall are the anterior surface of lower sacrum and coccyx, the ischial spine and ischial tuberosity.
b. Proctoscopy is a procedure by which the interior of anal canal and rectum is inspected through an instrument called proctoscope.
c. The sigmoidoscope is used to inspect the interior of the upper part of rectum and the sigmoid colon. The patient lies in the left lateral position. The instrument is passed through the anal canal in the direction of the umbilicus to ensure that it lies in the long axis of the anal canal. After a distance of 4 cm, the instrument enters the ampulla of rectum. At this point, the tip of the instrument is directed posteriorly in the midline to follow the sacral curve of the rectum without injuring the valves of Houston. The rectosigmoid junction is reached at the distance of 16 to 17 cm from the anal orifice (Fig. 138.1). The tip of the instrument has to negotiate with the rectosigmoid junction, where the sigmoid colon bends to the left and anteriorly. After this, the tip of the instrument can be smoothly passed up the sigmoid colon. The serious complication of sigmoidoscopy is the perforation of rectosigmoid junction and the escape of colonic contents in the peritoneal cavity.

Clinical Highlights

The carcinoma of rectum initially spreads by lymphatics to the local lymph nodes of the rectum (pararectal, middle rectal and internal iliac nodes). In advanced stage, the venous spread takes place. The secondary deposits to the liver pass in succession, through the superior rectal vein, inferior mesenteric vein, splenic vein and the portal vain. The cancer may spreads to the surrounding structures by direct invasion. Extension of the cancer in the sacral plexus may give rise to severe pain in the lower extremity. Extension of cancer in anterior direction may cause recto-vesical fistula in the male, or rectovaginal fistula, in the female.

139 Anal Canal

The anal canal is the terminal part of the large intestine. It extends from the anorectal junction to the anal orifice. The anorectal junction lies in the pelvic cavity but the anal canal lies below the pelvic diaphragm in the anal triangle of the perineum. The anal canal is about four cm long and is directed backwards and downwards from the anorectal junction. It remains closed except during defecation. The muscular junction between the rectum and the anal canal is the anorectal ring, which can be felt as a thickened ridge by digital examination.

Relations

Posteriorly, the anal canal is in contact with anococcygeal ligament. Anteriorly, the perineal body separates the anal canal from the lower part of the vagina, in the female and from the penile bulb and membranous urethra, in the male. On each side, the anal canal is related to the ischiorectal fossa (Fig. 168.1).

Internal Appearance (Fig. 139.1)

The anal canal is divided in three parts. The upper part is 15 mm in length, the middle part (pecten) is 15 mm in length and the lower part is 8 to 10 mm in length.

Upper Fifteen mm

The mucous membrane in this part is like that of the rectum (simple columnar epithelium). It is reddish in color and shows following features:

a. There are 6-10 longitudinal folds of mucous membrane called columns of Morgagni. Each column contains the terminal radicles of the superior rectal artery and vein. These terminal radicles are well-developed in the left lateral, right posterior and right anterior positions hence piles are more common at these three sites.
b. Anal valves are transverse folds of mucous membrane uniting the lower ends of anal columns. They may show presence of small anal papillae, which are the remnants of anal membrane of embryonic life. The passage of hard stools may injure the anal valves thereby causing anal fissure.
c. Anal sinus is the space above each anal valve and the anal glands open in the sinus. The opening of the glands is called anal crypt. The anal sinuses on the posterior wall are deepest and hence are prone to infection due to fecal matter being retained there. This may give lead to abscess formation.
d. Pectinate line is a transverse line, which runs all round the anal canal along the lower limit of the anal valves. It is the dividing line between the endodermally derived and ectodermally derived anal canal. The pectinate line is called the watershed line because it

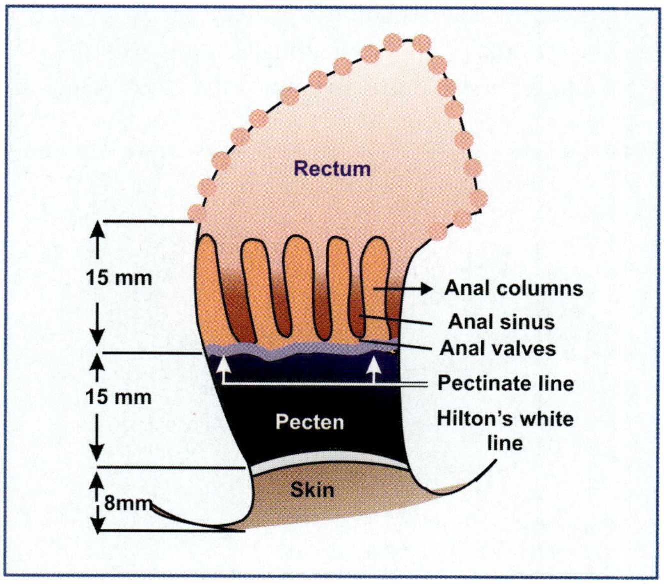

Fig. 139.1: Subdivisions and internal features of anal canal

separates the two entirely different parts of the anal canal (in terms of development, nerve supply, blood supply and lymphatic drainage).

Pecten

This part of the anal canal is lined by stratified squamous epithelium. The mucosa is less mobile here compared to the upper part. This region is referred to as a transitional zone. It is bluish in color because of the presence of rich venous plexus underneath it. The white line of Hilton denotes the lower limit of the pecten. Its appearance is whitish compared to the bluish appearance of the pecten and corresponds to the intersphincteric groove in the wall of the anal canal.

The Lowest 8 to 10 mm

It is the shortest part of the anal canal and is lined by true skin with sweat and sebaceous glands.

Anal Musculature (Fig. 139.2)

The musculature of the anal canal is divided in four groups (internal sphincter, external sphincter, anorectal ring and longitudinal muscle layer).

a. The internal sphincter (sphincter ani internus) is the thickened circular smooth muscle, which surrounds the upper three-quarters of the anal canal. It extends from the anorectal junction to the intersphincteric groove. It receives autonomic nerves.
b. The external sphincter (sphincter ani externus) is a voluntary muscle that surrounds the entire length of the anal canal. It is divisible in, deep, superficial and subcutaneous parts.
   i. The deep part surrounds part of the internal sphincter. It has no bony attachment, but a few fibers are attached posteriorly to the anococcygeal raphe.
   ii. The superficial part lies below the deep part and extends up to the intersphincteric groove, which lies between the subcutaneous part of external sphincter and lower border of internal sphincter. It is elliptical in shape. It is the only part of the external sphincter having bony attachment. It takes origin posteriorly from the last piece of coccyx and is inserted anteriorly into the perineal body.
   From these attachments, it is clear that this muscle fails to support the wall the anal canal posteriorly. This factor could be responsible for the frequent occurence of fissures in the midline on the posterior wall (Fig. 139.7).
   iii. The subcutaneous part encircles the lowest part of anal canal below the intersphincteric groove and has no bony attachments.
   The inferior rectal nerve, a branch of pudendal nerve and the perineal branch of fourth sacral nerve supply the external sphincter.
c. The anorectal ring is a muscular band composed of puborectalis part of levator ani, fibers of the deep part of external sphincter and part of internal sphincter. This muscular ring forms a sling from the pubic bones. On contraction of puborectalis, the anorectal junction is pulled forward thereby increasing the angulation between the rectum and the anal canal. Injury to the anorectal ring results in rectal incontinence.
d. The longitudinal muscle of the anal canal (Fig. 168.1) separates the internal and external sphincters. It is the continuation of the longitudinal layer of rectum with a small contribution from the puborectalis muscle. This layer becomes progressively fibroelastic and breaks in a number of fibrous strands nearer the lower end of the anal canal. A large number of the fibrous strands pass through the subcutaneous anal sphincter and attach to the dermis of the skin around the anus. These connections are responsible for puckering of the perianal skin. Some strands pass laterally between the subcutaneous and superficial parts of external sphincter to reach the ischiorectal fossa. Most medial strands pass medially through the intersphincteric groove to terminate in the anal mucosa at that level.

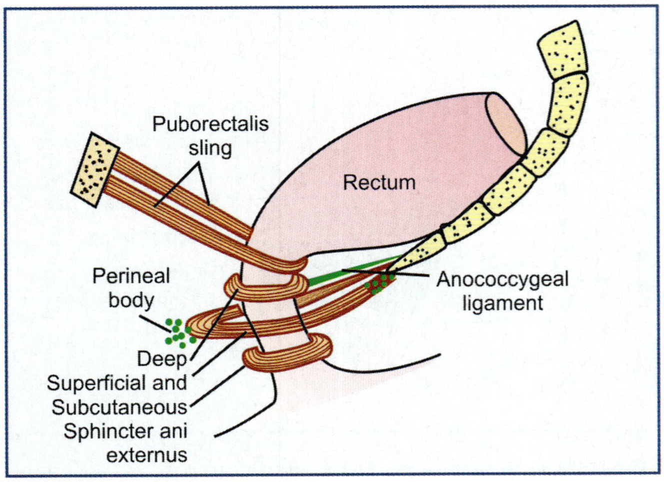

Fig. 139.2: Highly schematic depiction of voluntary sphincters of anal canal

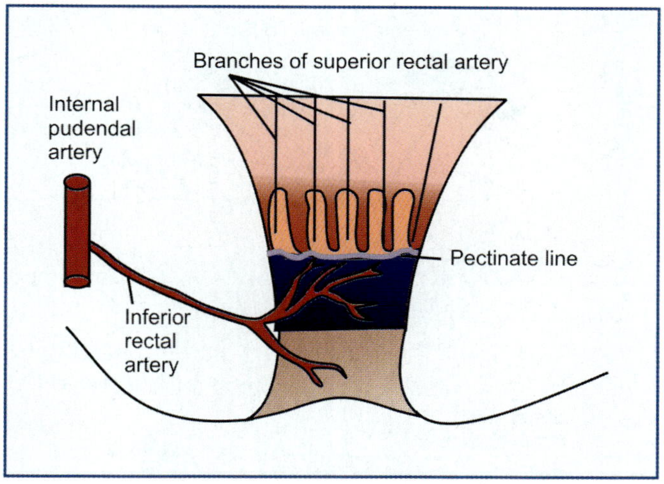

Fig. 139.3: Arterial supply of anal canal (Note that pectinate line is a watershed between superior and inferior rectal supply)

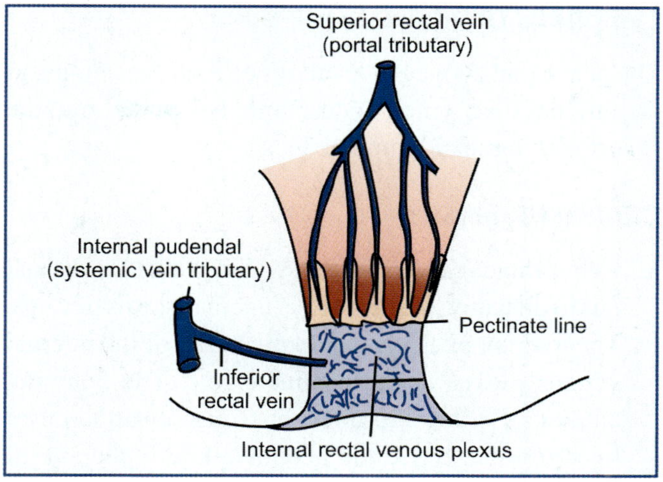

Fig. 139.4: Venous drainage of anal canal (Note that pectinate line is a site of portosystemic anastomosis)

Development of Anal Canal

The anal canal develops from dual sources. The part above the pectinate line is endodermal (postallantoic hindgut) while the part below the pectinate line is ectodermal (proctodeum). The pectinate line indicates the position of intervening anal membrane, which ruptures by 7th or 8th week of intrauterine life. The imperforate anus is very common. The common cause of imperforate anus is the persistence of the anal membrane. The other causes are the congenital atresia of lower part of rectum or the rectal fistulae.

Arterial Supply (Fig. 139.3)

The arterial supply of the anal canal is from two sources.

a. The submucosal plexuses of the superior rectal artery extend into the anal canal as terminal radicles in the anal columns and supply blood to the mucosa of the anal canal above the level of pectinate line.
b. The mucosa of the anal canal below the level of pectinate line receives blood from the inferior rectal artery, which is a branch of internal pudendal artery.

Venous Drainage (Fig. 139.4)

a. The anal canal above the level of pectinate line is drained through the internal rectal venous plexus into the superior rectal vein. The blood from the superior rectal vein drains ultimately in the portal circulation.

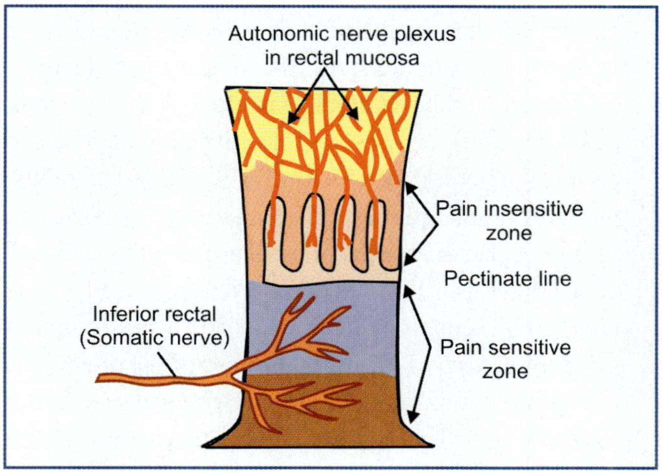

Fig. 139.5: Nerve supply of anal mucosa

b. The venous plexus below the level of pectinate line drains in the inferior rectal vein, a tributary of systemic vein.

Nerve Supply of Anal Mucosa (Fig. 139.5)

The anal canal above the pectinate line, is insensitive to pain because the mucosa receives autonomic nerves. Therefore, the internal piles remain asymptomatic for a long time till they become big enough to rupture and cause painless bleeding per rectum. Contrary to this, the mucosa below the pectinate line is supplied by the inferior rectal nerve, which carries somatic sensations hence the mucosa at this level is pain sensitive and any pathology including a small external pile may give rise to intense pain.

Lymphatic Drainage (Fig. 139.6)

The anal canal above the level of pectinate line drains in the internal iliac lymph nodes while below that into the superficial inguinal lymph nodes.

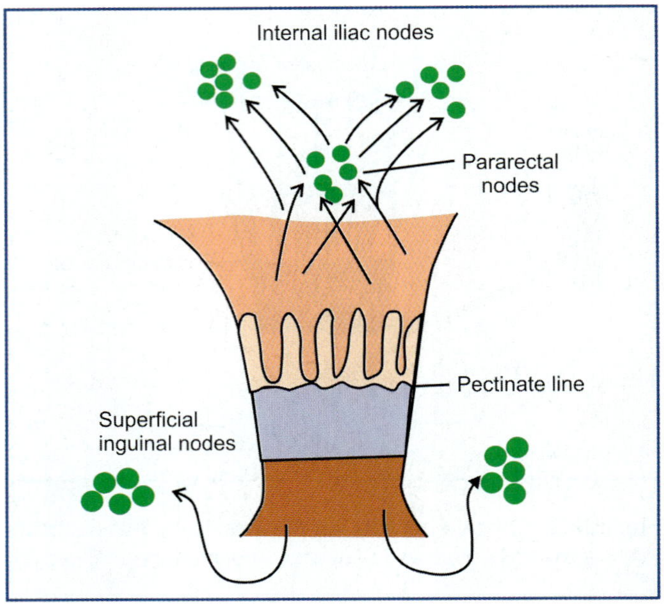

Fig. 139.6: Lymphatic drainage of anal canal

Clinical Highlights

a. Hemorrhoids or piles are the swellings in the anal canal due to dilatation of submucous internal plexus of veins. The internal piles are due to dilatation of the internal venous plexus at the pectinate line. The common causes of piles include constipation and portal hypertension. Since the pectinate line is the site of portosystemic anastomosis, in portal hypertension this anastomosis dilates to form internal piles (internal hemorrhoids). The venous radicles in right anterior, right posterior and left lateral positions are particularly large and hence are the frequent sites of primary piles. With reference to the clock, the primary internal piles are located at the 3 o' clock, 7 o' clock and 11 o' clock positions (Fig. 139.7A). The internal piles cause painless bleeding per rectum. The dilatation of the internal venous plexus below the level of pectinate line gives rise to external piles. This part of the internal venous plexus is drained by inferior rectal vein and is covered by sensitive mucosa and skin. One treatment of piles consists of injecting the base of the pile with a sclerosing agent. The precaution to be observed during injection is to inject above the pectinate line, where the mucosa is insensitive to pain.

b. Painful conditions of anal canal such as, fissures, abscesses and fistulae are very common. The susceptibility of anal canal to these conditions is due to trauma during passage of hard stools and exposure to infection.
   i. Fissure is a tear in the mucosa at the anal valves with extension into the pecten (Fig. 139.7B). Being extremely painful the fissure produces reflex spasm of the external sphincter.
   ii. Infection of the anal sinus due to impaction of fecal particle may result is abscess in the wall of anal canal.
   iii. The abscess may find its way in the ischiorectal fossa and thence to the perianal skin. This gives rise to a fistula, an abnormal tract connecting the anal canal to the perianal skin. Presence of multiple external openings of the anal fistulae gives to a typical appearance of watering can perineum.

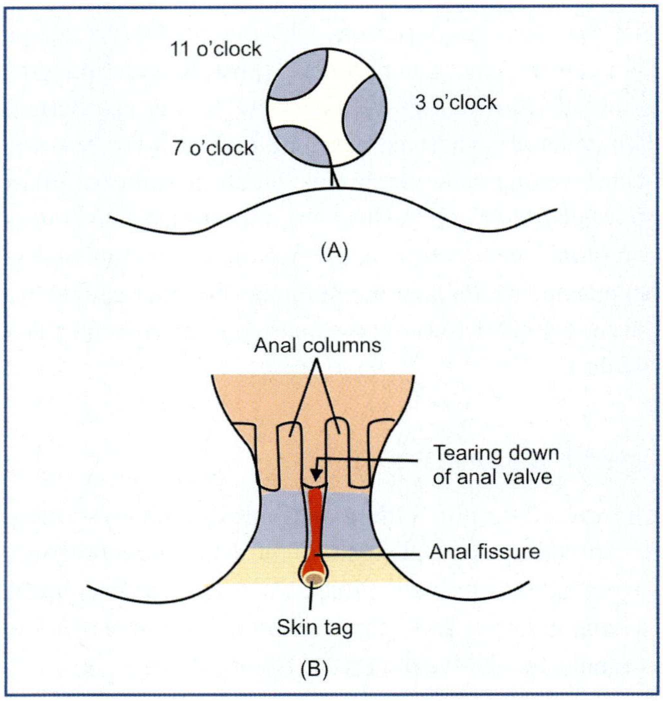

Fig. 139.7: Anatomical basis of clinical conditions of anal canal (A) depicts common position of internal piles as seen through proctoscope, (B) shows a midline anal fissure on posterior wall

140 Liver

The liver is the largest gland associated with the digestive system. It is situated below the diaphragm mainly in the right hypochondrium, extending across the epigastrium to the left hypochondrium. The liver descends with inspiration and ascends with expiration. It is an extremely vascular organ, which makes it a soft, reddish-brown and friable organ in the living state. The liver is wedge-shaped and the heaviest organ. Its weight in adult is 1200 to 1500 gm.

Development

The hepatic bud (hepatic outgrowth) arises from the endoderm of the caudal end of the foregut closer to the origin of ventral pancreatic bud (Fig. 135.2). The hepatic bud divides into two parts. The larger cranial part (pars hepatica) invades the septum transversum and rapidly enlarges to give rise to the right and left lobes of the liver. The smaller part (pars cystica) gives rise to the gallbladder and the cystic duct. The part of the bud proximal to pars cystica develops into common bile duct.

The septum transversum gives rise to the Glisson's capsule and the sinusoids of the liver. Hemopoesis begins in the liver at about the sixth week. The hepatocytes start secreting bile at about twelfth week. The bile enters the intestine and imparts a dark green color to the intestinal contents (meconeum), in the fetus.

Surfaces and Borders

The liver has five surfaces, superior, posterior, right lateral, anterior and inferior (visceral). The anterior, posterior, superior and right lateral surfaces are round and continuous with each other without a definite margin. These four surfaces together make a large diaphragmatic surface. The inferior surface is demarcated by sharp inferior margin from the anterior surface. The inferior margin is palpated while examining the liver in a patient.

Surface Marking

a. To draw the inferior margin of the liver following five points are marked. The first point corresponds to the right tenth costal cartilage in the midaxillary line. The second point is at the tip of right ninth costal cartilage. The third point lies in the median plane, where the transpyloric plane cuts it. The fourth point corresponds to the tip of left eighth costal cartilage and the fifth point lies on the left fifth rib at the midclavicular line.
b. The superior margin is indicated by a line that joins a point on the left fifth rib at midclavicular line to a corresponding point on the right side. The superior margin is concave in its central part and crosses behind the xiphisternal joint.
c. The right margin is convex to the right and is indicated by a line that joins the right ends of the superior and inferior margins.

Palpation

The inferior margin of the liver is hidden under cover of right costal margin. The direction of enlargement of liver is vertically downwards towards the right iliac fossa. Therefore, the palpation of the liver is begun from the right iliac fossa towards the right costal margin.

Relations

a. The superior surface has convexities on the right and left lobes for close fitting in the respective domes of the diaphragm. A depressed area between the two convexities is related to the central tendon of diaphragm and is known as the cardiac impression. The superior surface is covered with peritoneum except for the area of cardiac impression, where the layers of the falciform ligament separate. The cardiac impression is related to base of right lung, pericardium and part of the base of left lung.

b. The anterior surface (Fig. 140.1) gives attachment of the two layers of falciform ligament. The anterior surface of right lobe is related to the right anterior intraperitoneal space. The anterior surface of the left lobe is related to the left anterior intraperitoneal space. A part of this surface in the middle area is in relation to anterior abdominal wall in the infrasternal region.

c. The right lateral surface is covered with peritoneum and extends from the seventh rib above to the eleventh rib below (Fig. 140.2). It is related to the diaphragm and through it, to the right lung and pleura in the upper one-third, the right costodiaphragmatic recess in the middle third and the tenth and eleventh ribs in the lower third. For taking biopsy, the liver is approached at the midaxillary line in the ninth or tenth intercostal space.

d. The posterior surface is largely devoid of peritoneum. The features of this surface, from right to left are, the bare area of liver, groove for inferior vena cava (caval groove), the caudate lobe, fissure for ligamentum venosum and a shallow impression for esophagus and stomach fundus.

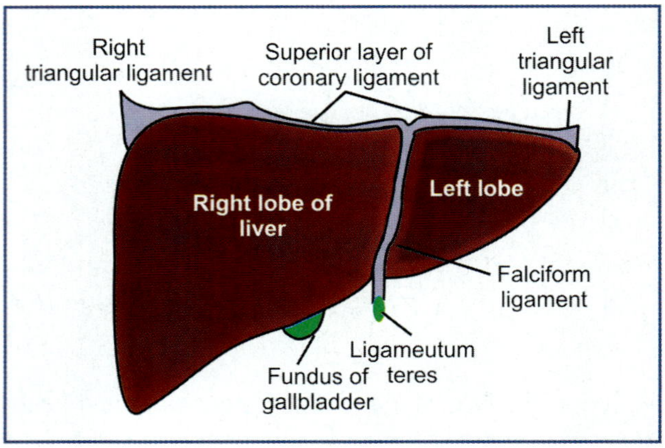

Fig. 140.1: Features of liver as seen from anterior aspect

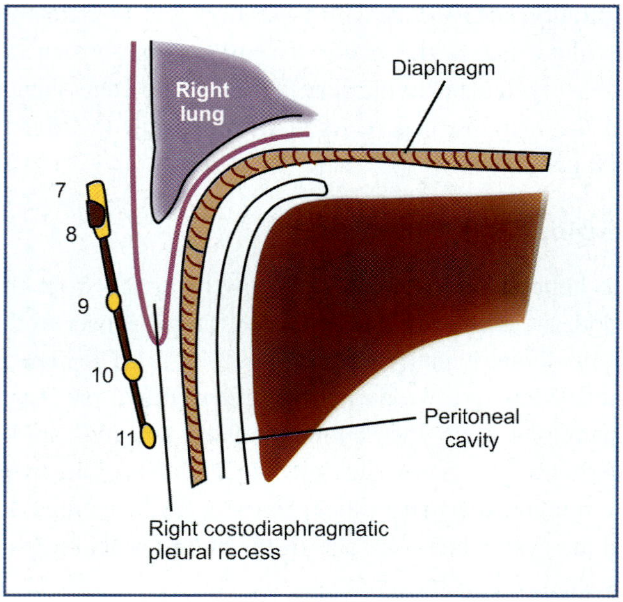

Fig. 140.2: Relations of right lateral surface of liver

Details of Posterior Surface (Fig. 140.3)

a. The bare area of liver is triangular. Its boundaries are, base formed by groove for IVC, the apex by the right triangular ligament, upper margin by the superior layer of coronary ligament and the lower margin by the inferior layer of the coronary ligament. The bare area is in direct contact with the diaphragm. The right suprarenal gland is related to its inferomedial part. The bare area of liver is surgically important as it encloses the right extraperitoneal space. In amebic hepatitis, the pus may collect in this space and form an abscess, which may burst through the diaphragm in to the right pleural cavity.

b. The inferior vena cava grooves the posterior surface of the liver. The floor of this groove is devoid of peritoneum. The hepatic veins pierce the floor of the groove to open in the IVC.

c. The caudate lobe belongs to the right lobe of the liver. Its boundaries are, the groove for IVC on the right, fissure for ligamentum venosum on the left, porta hepatis inferiorly and the indefinite margin (between superior and posterior surfaces) superiorly. The caudate lobe has two processes, the papillary process arises from the left side and the caudate process connects it to the rest of the right lobe. The caudate lobe is unique because it is the only part of the liver that is covered by peritoneum of the lesser sac

(Fig. 132.1). In fact, the caudate lobe projects in the superior recess of the lesser sac.

d. The fissure for the ligamentum venosum is a deep cleft on the posterior surface of the liver, having a floor and right and left walls. Its floor is in contact with the ligamentum venosum, which is a fibrous remnant of the ductus venosus of fetal circulation. This fissure has unusual peritoneal relations because four layers of peritoneum (Fig. 132.1) are present inside it. The vertical limb of the lesser omentum extends to the floor of the fissure from where its anterior layer is reflected on the left wall and the posterior layer on the right wall of the fissure.

e. The abdominal part of esophagus is related to posterior surface of left lobe on the left side of the upper end of the fissure for ligamentum venosum. The fundus of stomach is related to the left lobe just to the left of the esophageal groove.

Inferior or Visceral Surface (Fig. 140.3)

The fissure for the ligamentum teres extends from the notch on the inferior border of liver to the left end of porta hepatis. The fissure lodges the ligamentum teres, which is a fibrous remnant of the left umbilical vein. It demarcates the left and right lobes on the inferior surface.

Inferior Surface of Left Lobe

a. The gastric impression is a large area in contact with anterosuperior surface of stomach and it is in continuity with the esophageal impression on the posterior surface of the left lobe.

b. The tuber omentale is a slight elevation of the left lobe near the left side of the lower end of fissure for ligamentum venosum. It comes in contact with the lesser omentum and hence the name.

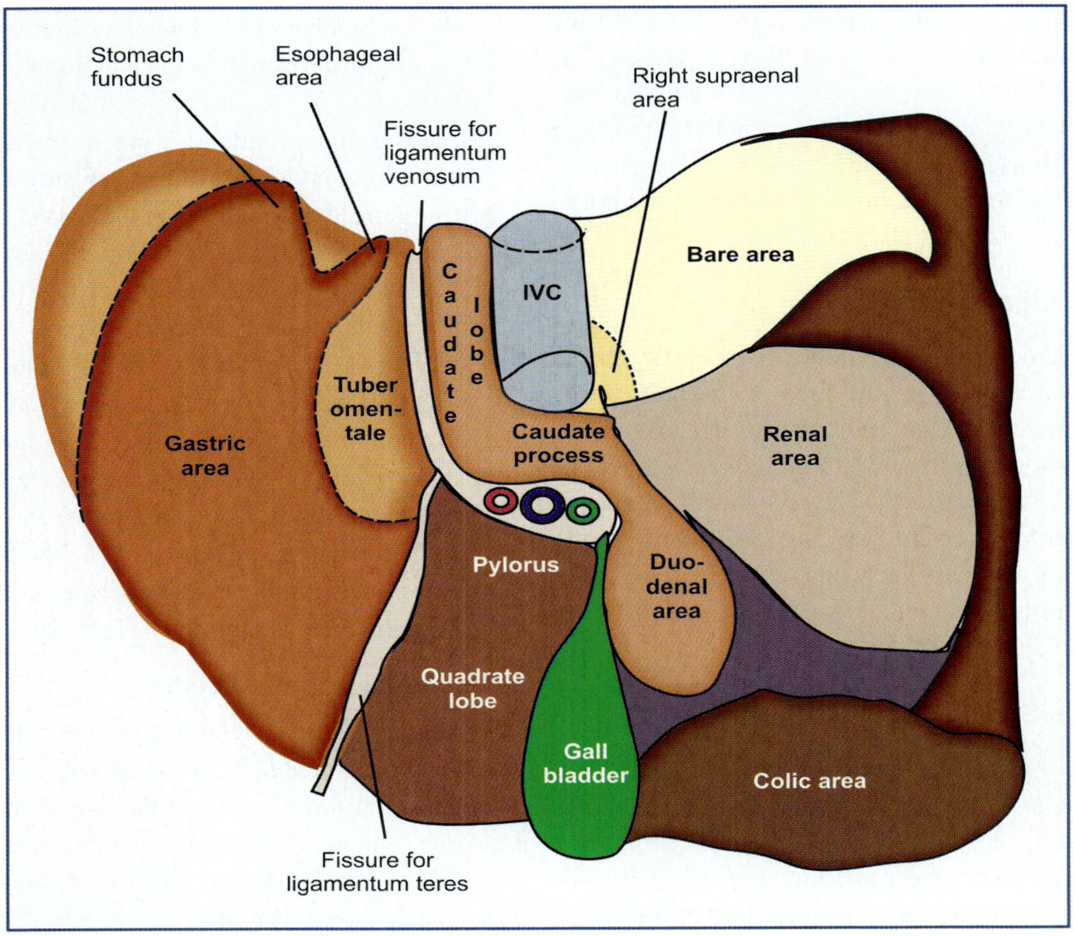

Fig. 140.3: Relations of visceral and posterior surfaces of liver

Inferior Surface of Right Lobe

The prominent features on this surface are the quadrate lobe and the fossa for gallbladder.

a. The boundaries of the quadrate lobe are fossa for gallbladder to the right, fissure for ligamentum teres to the left, the porta hepatis above and the inferior margin of liver below. The quadrate lobe is related to pyloric end of stomach and the first part of duodenum.
b. The fossa for gallbladder occupies a large part and is nonperitoneal.
c. Colic impression for right colic flexure is closer to inferior margin and to the right of the gallbladder.
d. Posterior to the colic area, the inferior surface bears a large renal impression for the right kidney.
e. The duodenal impression (for the junction of its first and second parts) is to the right of the upper part of the gallbladder behind the colic impression.
f. The porta hepatis (gateway of liver) lies between the posterior limit of the quadrate lobe and the caudate process. The structures entering the porta are the hepatic artery, portal vein and nerve plexuses. The structures leaving the porta are, right and left hepatic ducts and the lymph vessels. The arrangement of these structures is as follows. The hepatic ducts are anterior. The hepatic artery lies in the middle and the portal vein and its branches are posterior.

Peritoneal Ligaments

The liver is covered with peritoneum except at certain nonperitoneal areas. The bare area of the liver on its posterior surface is the largest nonperitoneal area. A few other nonperitoneal sites are, porta hepatis, groove for IVC and fossa for gallbladder. The peritoneum is reflected from the liver via the peritoneal ligaments, namely, the lesser omentum, coronary ligament, right and left triangular ligaments and falciform ligament. These ligaments are described in Chapter 132.

Subphrenic Spaces (Fig. 132.5)

Out of the five surgically important subphrenic spaces in close relation to liver, four are intraperitoneal and one is extraperitoneal.

a. Right subphrenic or right anterior intraperitoneal space is related to anterior, superior and right lateral surfaces of the right lobe.
b. Left subphrenic or left anterior intraperitoneal space is related to anterior and superior surfaces of left lobe.
c. Right subhepatic or right posterior intraperitoneal space of Morison's is related to right half of visceral surface.
d. Part of left subhepatic space (superior recess of the omental bursa) is related to the caudate lobe.
e. Right extraperitoneal space or bare area of liver is related to the posterior surface of the right lobe.

Blood Supply

The blood supply of the liver is unique because it consists of arterial supply, portal venous supply and venous drainage.

a. The hepatic artery proper enters the liver through the porta hepatis and divides into right and left branches, which supply the respective lobes of the liver. The interlobular branches open into hepatic sinusoids. The quadrate lobe receives a branch from the left subdivision of the hepatic artery while the caudate lobe receives branches from both the subdivisions.
b. The portal vein brings blood, which contains products of digestion of proteins and carbohydrates, from the intestine and products of erythrocyte breakdown (bilirubin and iron) from the spleen. Its tributaries open in the hepatic sinusoids. The intrahepatic ramifications of the portal vein closely follow the arterial pattern. The caudate lobe receives tributaries from both the right and left branches of portal vein.
c. The venous ends of the liver sinusoids join the central veins (belonging to systemic veins), which unite to form sublobular veins. Ultimately, three large-sized hepatic veins (right, middle and left) emerge from liver by piercing the floor of the groove for IVC. Since, they immediately open in the IVC, the hepatic veins do not have extrahepatic existence. In Budd-Chiari syndrome there is thrombosis in hepatic veins.

Anatomical Lobes of Liver

The plane dividing the liver into a large right and a small left lobe passes through the line of attachment of falciform ligament on the anterior surface, the fissure for ligamentum teres on the inferior surface and the fissure for ligamentum venosum on the posterior surface. According to this subdivision, the caudate and quadrate lobes belong to right lobe of liver.

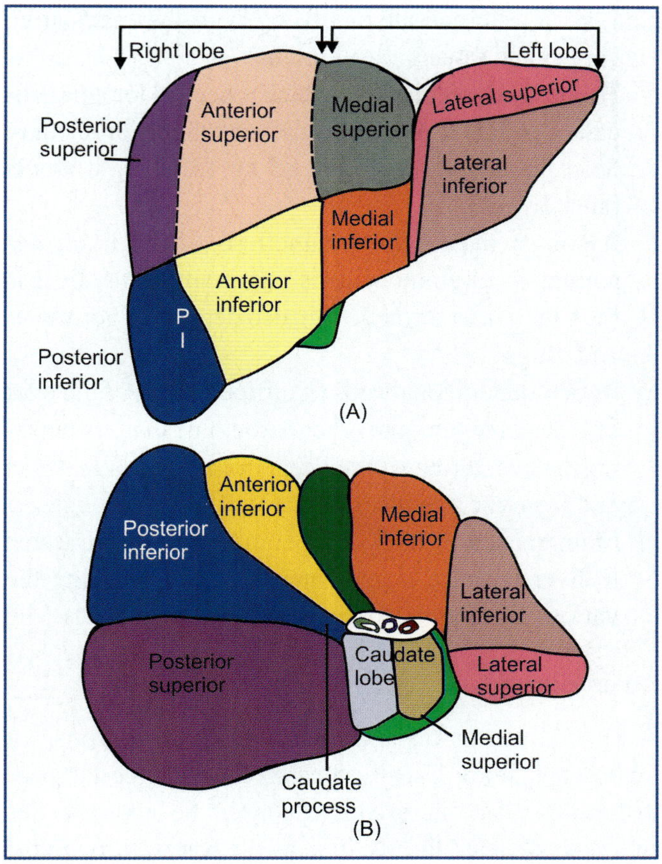

Fig. 140.4: Depiction of functional segments of liver on (A) anterior surface and (B) visceral surface

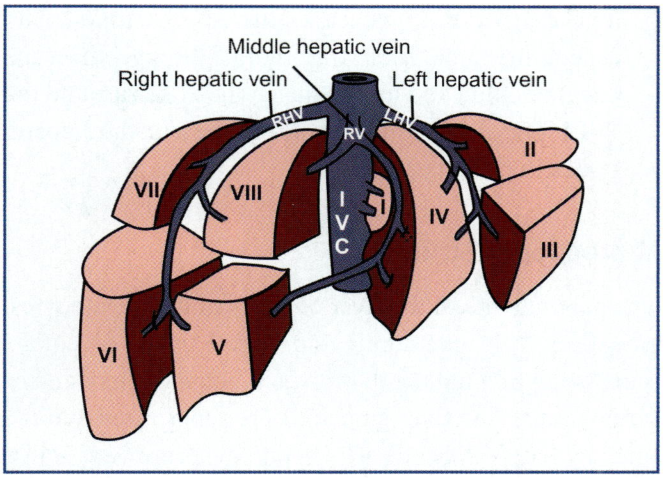

Fig. 140.5: Depiction of functional segments (I to VIII) of liver named after Couinaud (Note that each segment is independently provided with a tributary of hepatic vein and a branch of hepatic artery, portal vein and bile duct)

Functional Lobes of Liver

The functional or physiological subdivision of liver into right and left lobes is based on the area of drainage of bile by the right and left hepatic ducts. The line of demarcation passes through middle of the fossa for gallbladder and the left side of the groove for IVC. This plane (Cantlie's line) roughly falls along the middle hepatic vein. According to this subdivision, the quadrate lobe belongs to the left lobe of the liver and the caudate lobe belongs to both right and left lobes.

Segmental Anatomy of Liver

Based on the branching pattern of the biliary system, arterial pattern and of portal tributaries, the liver is divided into nine hepatobiliary segments as per the old nomenclature (Fig. 140.4). The segmental anatomy is of importance during segmental resection of the liver.

Couinaud's Hepatic Segmentation (Fig. 140.5)

According to the nomenclature of Couinaud, the liver is divided into eight segments numbered I to VIII. Each segment has independent artery, bile duct, tributary of hepatic vein and the portal tributary. The right hemiliver is divided into V to VIII segments. The left hemiliver is divided into I to IV segments. The segment- I or posterior segment is the caudate lobe, which is unique because it receives blood from right and left branches of hepatic artery and portal vein and it drains into both right and left biliary ducts and directly into the IVC. The hepatic veins are intersegmental in position. So, during segmental resection of liver, intraoperative ultrasound is used to detect the intersegmental planes.

Lymphatic Drainage

A large volume of lymph from the liver reaches the thoracic duct. The lymphatic vessels of the liver begin as blind sacs in the space of Mall around the vessels and ducts in the portal canals.

a. The superficial lymph vessels emerge from all over the liver and join the retrosternal, phrenic and mediastinal lymph nodes. Some parts of liver drain in hepatic lymph nodes in the porta hepatis. The posterior surface of the left lobe drains in paracardiac nodes near the lower end of esophagus. A few lymph vessels from right lobe drain directly in celiac nodes.

b. The deep lymph vessels form two trunks. The ascending trunk enters the thorax through the vena caval opening and terminates in the nodes around the IVC. The descending trunk empties in the hepatic nodes in porta hepatis.

Microscopic Structure

The parenchyma of the liver consists of the hepatocytes, sinusoids, bile canaliculi and portal triads or canals (consisting of a radicle of bile duct, hepatic artery and of portal vein). The liver sinusoids are fenestrated and are lined by Kupffer's cells. The hepatocytes are very active cells and possess a remarkable capacity to regenerate. The space of Disse is present between the sinusoids and the hepatocytes. It contains reticulin fibers and Ito cells (perisinusoidal cells), which secrete collagen for the repair and maintenance of hepatic laminae and they store vitamin A. The spaces of Disse are continuous with spaces of Mall situated in the portal canals at the periphery of the hepatic lobule. The hepatic lobule is the liver parenchyma arranged around the central vein. The hepatocytes are arranged in radiating and anastomosing laminae. The portal triads or canals are located at the periphery of the hepatic lobule. The portal lobule is the parenchyma bounded by the central veins at the periphery with the portal triad in the center. The portal lobule collects bile from the adjacent hepatic lobules. The portal acinus is the parenchyma between the two central veins and supplied by preterminal branch of hepatic arteriole and corresponding portal vein radicle. The portal acinus shows three zonations depending on oxygen supply of the parenchyma. The zone next to artery has rich oxygen supply while the zone close to central vein has least oxygen supply.

Functions

a. The liver is a seat of metabolism of carbohydrtes, proteins and fats.
b. Most serum proteins except the immunoglobulins are synthesized in liver. Decrease in albumin level because of liver disease may be a cause of edema and ascites.
c. Blood clotting depends on production of prothrombin and fibrinogen by the liver. Liver failure results in defective clotting leading to bleeding tendencies.
d. Liver is a storage site for glycogen, triglycerides, iron, copper and fat-soluble vitamins.
e. Hepatocytes secrete bile, which is needed for emulsification of fats. Lack of bile affects digestion of fatty food leading to excretion of fat filled light stools (steatorrhea).
f. Amongst the catabolic functions of the liver, deamination of aminoacids is important. Thus, liver is the site of urea formation. It also detoxifies hormones and drugs.
g. Reticuloendothelial cells (Kupffer's cells) of the liver kill the pathogens and other particulate matters reaching the liver through portal vein from the intestinal tract and from the hepatic artery.
h. Maintenance of body temperature is also attributed to liver because it generates lot of heat during the various metabolic reactions.

Liver Biopsy

A bit of liver tissue is drawn out for the purpose of microscopic study. Usually, the right ninth intercostal space in the midaxillary line is chosen to insert the biopsy needle. After the skin and fasciae, the needle passes through the external oblique and the intercostal muscles. It then passes through the right costodiaphragmatic recess, diaphragm and the peritoneal cavity in relation to the right lateral surface of liver (right anterior subphrenic space). Thus, to reach the liver the needle passes through two serous cavities.

Clinical Highlights

a. The displacement of liver in downward direction may occur if the abdominal muscles are weak. The liver is retained in normal position by the attachment of the hepatic veins to the IVC. The coronary and triangular ligaments and muscular tone of anterior abdominal wall contribute to a certain extent.
b. The liver may be ruptured by a broken rib or by a stab injury. Due its vascularity, the liver bleeds profusely, when ruptured. During laparotomy, the surgeon at first uses a simple pincer technique called Pringle's maneuver (in which the hepatic artery in the free margin of lesser omentum is pressed between the thumb and forefinger) to control bleeding.

c. Cirrhosis of liver is the scarring or fibrosis of liver parenchyma due to toxic effects of ingested substances or drugs. Alcohol is the most common cause of cirrhosis. In congestive cardiac failure the pressure in hepatic veins is raised, which leads to venous congestion in liver and cardiac cirrhosis. Another type of cirrhosis, called biliary cirrhosis results due to prolonged obstruction to the biliary ducts. Cirrhosis leads to portal hypertension.

d. Hepatic carcinoma is the primary malignancy of liver parenchyma. The secondary malignancy of liver occurs due to spread from primary cancer in the gastrointestinal tract via the portal vein. Malignant cells from breast, lung or pelvic organs also reach the liver.

e. Viral hepatitis is a common inflammatory disease of liver, which manifests by appearance of jaundice. The hepatitis A virus enters the body through contaminated water and Hepatitis B virus enters through the contaminated needles from the blood of the infected person or after blood transfusion from an infected person.

f. Blockage of hepatic artery may not always lead to necrosis of liver. Reason for this is that, oxygen requirements of liver are partly met by portal vein. If the portal vein is thrombosed, then the liver is entirely dependent on hepatic artery. Occlusion of common hepatic artery proximal to origin of right gastric artery allows collateral circulation via gastric and gastroepiploic arteries. In occlusion of hepatic artery proper, there is no collateral circulation.

141 Biliary Apparatus

The biliary apparatus consists of intrahepatic and extrahepatic parts. The function of the intrahepatic component is to drain bile secreted by the hepatocytes outside the liver and that of extrahepatic component is to store the bile in the gallbladder and carry it to the second part of the duodenum as and when necessary.

Intrahepatic Part

This consists of a series of bile canaliculi, bile ductules and interlobular bile ducts. The interlobular ducts of right and left lobes of the liver unite to form the right and left hepatic ducts respectively.

Extrahepatic Part (Fig. 141.1)

The extrahepatic biliary apparatus consists of the right and left hepatic ducts, common hepatic duct, gallbladder, cystic duct and the common bile duct. It collects bile from the liver, stores it in the gallbladder and transmits it to the second part of the duodenum.

Right and Left Hepatic Ducts

The right and left hepatic ducts emerge from the porta hepatis, where the arrangement of structures from behind forwards is, branches of portal vein, branches of hepatic artery and hepatic ducts.

Common Hepatic Duct

The common hepatic duct (about 3.5 cm long) is formed by the union of right and left hepatic ducts at the right end of the porta hepatis. It unites with the cystic duct (from gallbladder) at an acute angle after descending a about 2 cm or so to form the common bile duct. Its function is to carry the bile to the cystic duct for storage in the gallbladder.

Gallbladder

The gallbladder is the reservoir of bile. It is a pear-shaped organ having a slate blue color. It is 7 to 10 cm long and 3 cm broad at its widest part. It is capable of considerable distension. Its functions are the storage of the bile and concentration of the bile to about ten times. The simple columnar epithelium of the gallbladder is adapted for absorption of a considerable amount of water and electrolytes.

Capacity

The normal capacity of gallbladder is 30 to 50 ml.

Location

The gallbladder is normally located in the shallow fossa on the inferior surface of the right lobe of liver. It extends from the right end of the porta hepatis to the inferior margin of the right lobe of the liver.

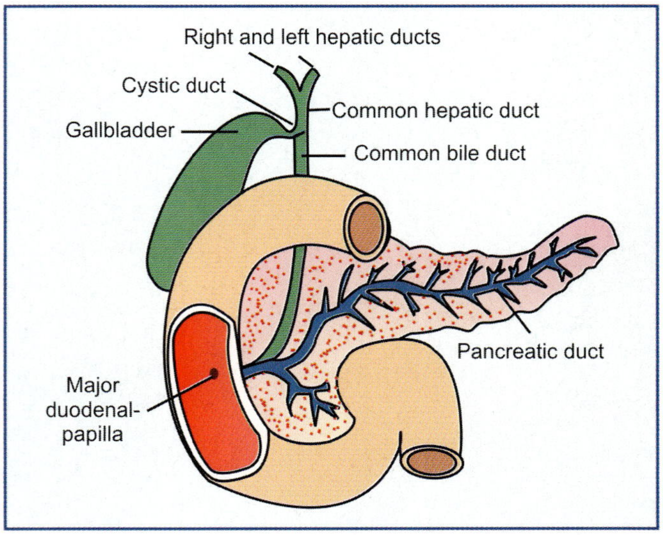

Fig. 141.1: Parts of extrahepatic biliary apparatus

Parts

The gallbladder consists of three parts, fundus, body and neck.

Fundus of Gallbladder

The fundus is the most anterior and expanded part of the gallbladder, which projects beyond the inferior margin of the liver. It is related anteriorly to the anterior abdominal wall. Its surface marking is important. The fundus corresponds to the tip of the right ninth costal cartilage (point of intersection of the right linea semilunaris and the transpyloric plane). The pressure on the tip of the right ninth costal cartilage (with patient in sitting position and while taking deep breath) gives sharp pain in cholecystitis. This is known as Murphy's sign.

Body of Gallbladder

The body of gallbladder is in contact with the inferior surface of the liver at the fossa for gallbladder. The body continues as the neck near the right end of the porta hepatis. Its superior surface is in contact with the liver. Its inferior surface is related to the transverse colon, second part of duodenum and the first part of duodenum from before backwards (Fig. 141.2). This relationship is important because sometimes the stones in the gallbladder ulcerate through its wall into the duodenum or the transverse colon.

Neck of Gallbladder

The neck is the narrow part of the gallbladder, which continues from the body. At first, it curves upwards and forwards and then abruptly backwards and downwards to become the cystic duct. Inferiorly, the neck is related to the first part of duodenum. The lumen of the neck has spiral valve. The neck shows a small projection from its right side called Hartman's pouch or infundibulum. Gallstones lodged in the pouch may cause adhesions with duodenum and perforation.

Peritoneal Relations

The superior surface of gallbladder is nonperitoneal and is connected to the inferior surface of right lobe of liver by connective tissue. The inferior surface is covered with

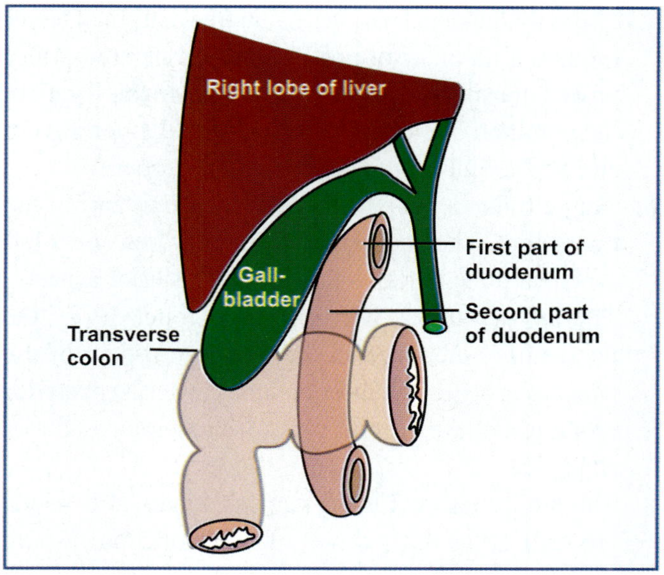

Fig. 141.2: Inferior relations of body of gallbladder

peritoneum. The fundus of gallbladder is completely covered with peritoneum.

Cystic Duct

The cystic duct is described as S-shaped. It is three to four cm long. It begins in the neck of the gallbladder and passes backwards, downwards and to the left to join the common hepatic duct to form common bile duct. Its lumen shows mucous folds, which form the spiral valve like that of the neck of gallbladder. The cystic duct is a two-way passage. The gallbladder receives bile through the cystic duct from the common hepatic duct and sends bile out through the cystic duct to the common bile duct.

Common Bile Duct (CBD)

The common bile duct (also known as bile duct) is usually 7.5 to 8 cm long and less than 6 to 7 mm in diameter. The cystic duct unites with common hepatic duct to form the common bile duct. It descends in the free margin of the lesser omentum and then passes behind the first part of the duodenum. On its way to the second part of the duodenum, it passes posterior to the head of pancreas.

Subdivisions

Its course is divided into four parts, supraduodenal, retroduodenal, and infraduodenal and intraduodenal (intramural).

a. The supraduodenal part lies in the free margin of lesser omentum along with portal vein and hepatic artery proper, constituting the hepatic pedicle. In this location, the common bile duct lies anterior to the portal vein and to the right of the hepatic artery proper.
b. The retroduodenal part is behind the first part of the duodenum. The gastroduodenal artery lies on its left aspect and the portal vein is on its posterior aspect.
c. The infraduodenal part lies in the concavity of the duodenum embedded in the posterior aspect of the pancreatic head. The inferior vena cava is its posterior relation and the second part of duodenum is on its right side.
d. The intramural part is the narrowest part. It is inside the wall of the second part of the duodenum, where the bile duct is in close relation to the main pancreatic duct. The two ducts unite to form hepatopancreatic ampulla in the wall of the duodenum very close to the summit of the major duodenal papilla. The ampulla is surrounded by sphincter of Oddi (Fig. 134.6), which is also called the hepatopancreatic sphincter. The sphincter is composed of circular muscle around the terminal part of the common bile duct, including the ampulla and the terminal part of pancreatic duct. The release of bile from the gallbladder is under hormonal control. The arrival of acid or fat in the second part of duodenum causes liberation of cholecystokinin (CCK) in the blood. The muscle of the gallbladder contracts under the influence of CCK. There is rise in pressure in the gallbladder. This is a stimulus for the sphincter of Oddi to relax. The bile now can flow in the second part of duodenum.

Arterial Supply (Fig. 141.3)

a. The gallbladder receives blood from the cystic artery, which arises from the right branch of hepatic artery. A few small arterial twigs from the liver through the fossa for gallbladder form an additional source.
b. The arterial supply of the common bile duct is clinically important. Its upper part receives twigs from the descending branches of cystic artery and its lower part from the ascending branches of the superior pancreaticoduodenal artery. If the anastomosis between the superior and inferior pancreaticoduodenal arteries is poor the ligation of the superior pancreaticoduodenal artery during surgery, may cause stricture or gangrene of the common bile duct (postoperative complication).
c. Hepatic artery proper or its right branch forms a minor source to the middle part of CBD.

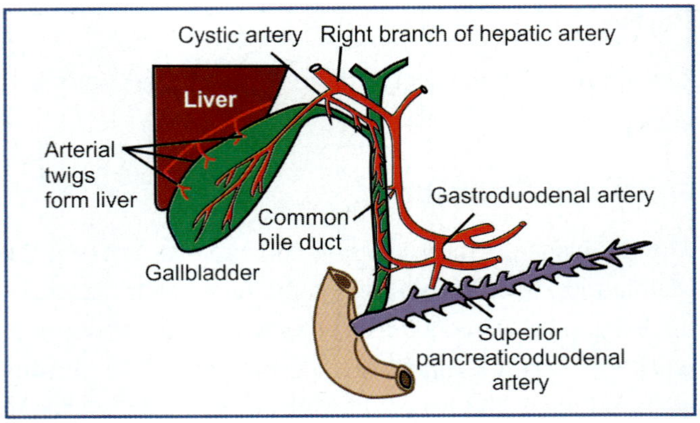

Fig. 141.3: Arterial supply of extrahepatic biliary apparatus (Note that CBD is supplied by branches descending from cystic artery and ascending from superior pancreaticoduodenal artery)

Cystic Artery

The cystic artery usually takes origin from right branch of hepatic artery and passes behind the common hepatic duct and the cystic duct in the Calot's triangle to reach the superior aspect of the neck of the gallbladder.
b. The cystic artery may be a branch of hepatic artery proper, of the gastroduodenal artery or of right gastric artery.
c. Occasionally, the accessory cystic artery arises from the gastroduodenal artery.
d. The cystic artery is very short, when the hepatic artery and its right branch take a tortuous course (Moynihan's hump or caterpillar turn shown in Figure 141.4. In such cases, clamping the artery during the gallbladder surgery poses problem to the surgeon.

Venous Drainage

The cystic veins draining the gallbladder vary in their mode of termination. Those coming out of the superior surface of the gallbladder directly enter the liver substance and open into the hepatic veins. The remaining veins from the gallbladder join to form one or two cystic veins, which usually enter the liver directly. A few veins, which

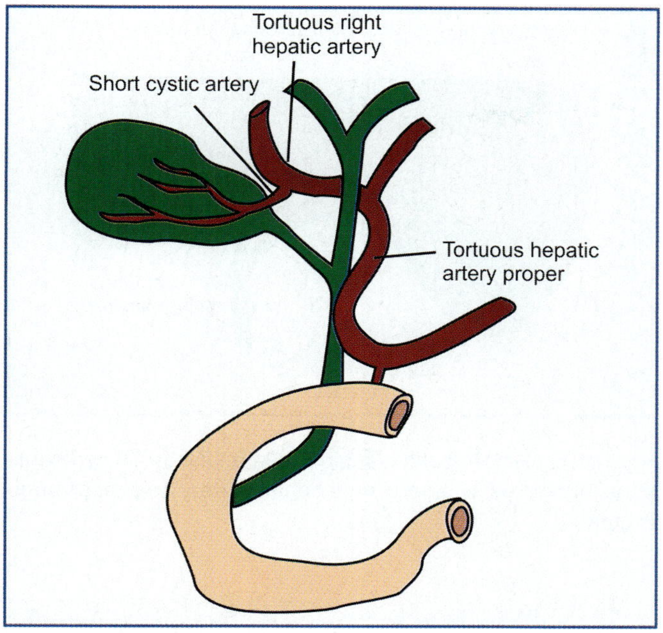

Fig. 143.4: Moynihan's hump. Tortuosity of hepatic artery and its right branch is also known as caterpillar turn

accompany the cystic artery, open in the right branch of the portal vein. Thus, the gallbladder drains into both the systemic and portal veins.

Lymphatic Drainage

The lymphatic vessels originate in the rich lymphatic plexuses in the subserosal and submucosal locations in the gallbladder. Majority of these vessels end in cystic node of Lund located in Calot's triangle. Efferent vessels from this node end in the hepatic group. A few vessels on the superior surface of gallbladder make connections with the subcapsular lymph channels of the liver. The common bile duct drains in the hepatic nodes and pancreaticosplenic nodes.

Nerve Supply

The gallbladder receives both sympathetic and parasympathetic nerves from the celiac plexuses. Fibers from the right phrenic nerve reach the gallbladder through communications between the phrenic plexus and celiac plexus. This is the explanation of referred pain to the right shoulder in gallbladder inflammation. The sympathetic supply is from T7 to T9 segments. This explains why gallbladder pain is referred to inferior angle of right scapula.

Radiology of Biliary Apparatus

a. Cholecystography consists of the contrast radiography of biliary apparatus after ingestion of contrast medium. In the preparation of the patient for this method, in order to empty the gallbladder completely, fat filled meal is given on the previous day. The contrast medium is given by mouth with water and after nine hours the radiographs are taken. A fatty meal is then given to stimulate gallbladder contraction and another X-ray is taken. Nowadays, this investigation is not preferred. In its place, intravenous cholecystography is practiced.
b. Ultrasonography is a non-invasive method to inspect the gallbladder and other components of the biliary apparatus.
c. Endoscopic retrograde cholangiopancreatography (ERCP) is the procedure in which the fiberoptic duodenoscope is used to inspect the duodenal opening of the hepatopancreatic ampulla. Then the ampulla is cannulated and the bile and pancreatic ducts are visualized, after injecting water-soluble contrast.

Congenital Anomalies of Gallbladder

a. Floating gallbladder is the one with a mesentery.
b. Phrygian cap is a radiologically seen anomaly of the shape of the gallbladder. The gallbladder resembles the cap worn by people of Phrygia (an ancient country of Asia Minor), due to a constriction between the fundus and the body.
c. Sessile gallbladder is a condition in which the cystic duct is absent.

Clinical Highlights

a. Gallstones or cholelithiasis is a very common clinical condition. Gallstones may cause biliary colic as a result of impaction of stone in the cystic duct. The biliary pain is referred to T6 to T8 dermatomes and typically radiates to the angle of scapula. The pain of peritoneal irritation is felt over the right shoulder.

b. The obstruction of CBD is usually due to impaction of gallstones, pancreatic carcinoma, cancer of bile duct, enlarged neoplastic hepatic lymph nodes or congenital biliary atresia. The obstruction to bile flow results in jaundice, which is called obstructive or surgical jaundice. The treatment consists of the surgical removal of the obstruction.
c. Courvoisier's law states that if the gallbladder is palpable and distended, the jaundice is more likely to be due to obstruction of CBD (for example due to carcinoma of pancreatic head). On the contrary, if the gallbladder is contracted, the jaundice is due to cholelithiasis (gallstones). Thus, this law helps in finding the cause of jaundice.
d. Calot's triangle or cystohepatic triangle is an arbitrary triangle, which a surgeon must identify during surgery on gallbladder. The boundaries of Calot's triangle are the cystic duct inferiorly, the common hepatic duct medially and the inferior surface of liver above (Fig. 141.5). The right hepatic artery, cystic artery and the cystic lymph node of Lund are the contents. During cholecystectomy (removal of gallbladder) the surgeon identifies the cystic artery with the help of the lymph node as the artery is routinely found behind the node.

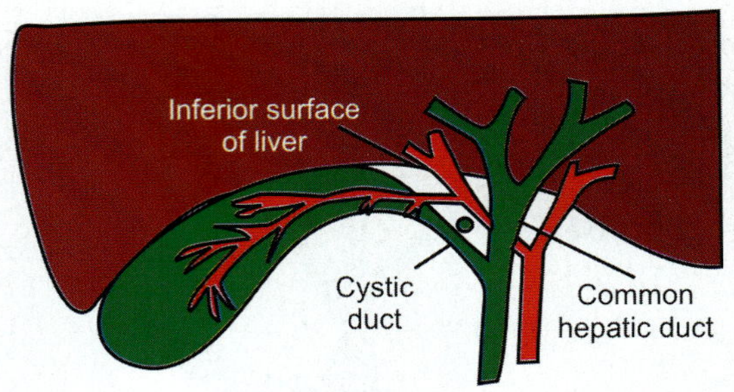

Fig. 141.5: Cystohepatic triangle (of Calot) (Note: The contents of the triangle cystic artery, right hepatic artery and lymph node of Lund)

The gallbladder surgery is very intricate because the ductal and arterial variations are very common in this region. Severe bleeding due to injury to cystic artery is the most feared complication. The simplest method to control the bleeding is to compress the hepatic artery proper between the finger and thumb, where it lies in the free margin of the lesser omentum. This is known as Pringle's maneuver.

142 Spleen

The spleen is a large hemolymphoid organ consisting of vascular and lymphatic tissue. It has friable texture similar to that of liver on account of the rich vascularity. Direct trauma to the overlying ribs can rupture the spleen and cause bleeding into the peritoneal cavity.

Development

The spleen develops in the dorsal mesogastrium as several condensations of the mesenchymal cells. These separate masses (splenules) fuse to form the spleen. Failure of the fusion of the splenic masses results in accessory spleens called splenunculi in the peritoneal ligaments of the spleen or in the greater omentum.

Location

The spleen is located in the left hypogastrium between the fundus of the stomach and the diaphragm, opposite the ninth to eleventh ribs. Its long axis lies parallel to the long axis of the left tenth rib. The spleen moves with respiration.

Size and Measurements

The size of the spleen roughly corresponds to the cupped hand or fist of the subject. In the adult, the spleen is 12 cm long, 7 cm broad and 3 cm thick and its weight varies from 80 to 150 gm.

Surfaces, Borders and Poles

The spleen has diaphragmatic and visceral surfaces, the superior and inferior borders and anterior (lateral) and posterior (medial) ends or poles (Fig. 142.1).

a. The posterior (medial) end is rounded and lies four cm from the midline at the level of the spine of tenth thoracic vertebra.
b. The anterior (lateral) end is broad lies between the anterior basal and posterior basal angles. The anterior basal angle is the junction of superior border and the anterior or lateral end. This angle lies in the midaxillary line on the tenth rib.
c. The superior border separates the diaphragmatic surface from the visceral surface. It is sharp and bears two or three notches near its lateral end. The developmental importance of the notches is that they are indicative of the fact that the spleen develops by fusion of separate masses. Its clinical importance is that in an enlarged spleen the notching is exaggerated. This feature distinguishes the splenic swelling from other swellings in the abdominal cavity.
d. The inferior border separates the diaphragmatic and the visceral surfaces. It is more rounded than the superior border and corresponds in position to the lower margin of the eleventh rib.

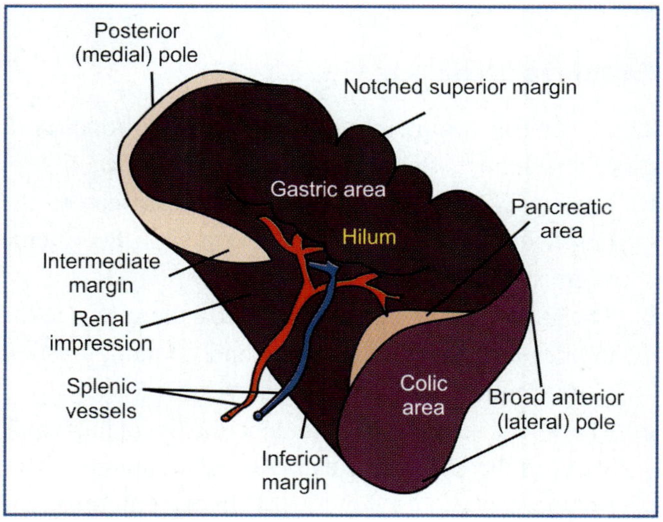

Fig. 142.1: Showing morphological features and relations of visceral surface of spleen

e. The diaphragmatic surface is convex and faces posterosuperiorly and to the left. It lies in contact with the inferior surface of diaphragm, which separates it from the left lung and left costodiaphragmatic recess (Fig. 142.2).
f. The visceral surface bears the hilum of the spleen, through which splenic vessels and nerve plexuses enter or leave the spleen. The lienorenal and gastrosplenic ligaments are attached to the hilum. The area between the superior border and the hilum is the gastric area. The part between the inferior border and the hilum is related to the anterior surface of the left kidney. There is a raised margin separating the gastric and renal areas. The colic impression (left colic flexure) is below the hilum. The tail of pancreas is related to the hilum just above the colic impression.

Surface Marking

The outline of the spleen can be drawn on the lower posterior thoracic wall on the left side. A point about four to five cm away from the midline at the level of the spine of tenth thoracic vertebra represents the upper or posterior or medial end. A point on the tenth rib in the midaxillary line represents the anterior basal angle of the lateral end. The superior border is indicated by joining the two points by a convex line along the upper border of ninth rib. The inferior border is indicated joining the same points by a line, which passes along the lower margin of the eleventh rib.

Peritoneal Relations (Fig. 142.3)

The spleen is completely covered with peritoneum. It gives attachments to two peritoneal folds.

a. The lienorenal ligament connects the spleen to the posterior abdominal wall and contains the splenic vessels and the tail of pancreas.
b. The gastrosplenic ligament connects the spleen to the greater curvature of stomach and contains the left gastroepiploic and short gastric vessels.
c. The spleen rests on the phrenicocolic ligament, which attaches the left colic flexure to the diaphragm. This ligament prevents downward displacement of the spleen. Based on this function the ligament is given the name, sustentaculum lienei.

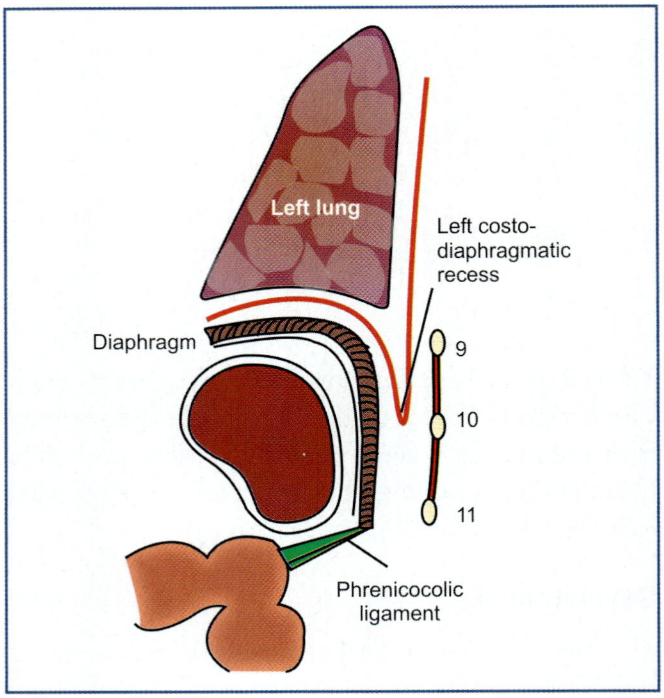

Fig. 142.2: Relations of diaphragmatic surface of spleen

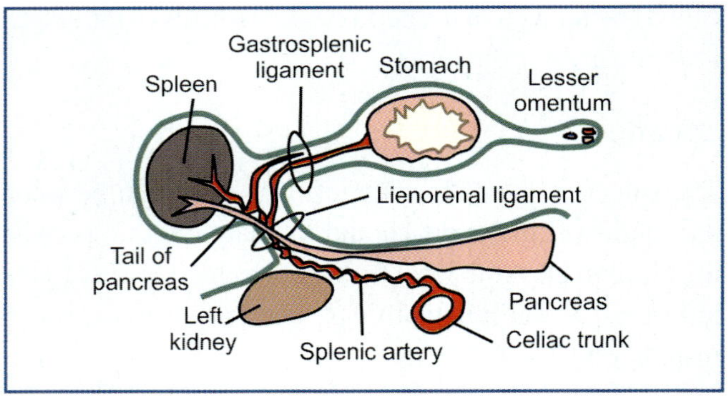

Fig. 142.3: Peritoneal ligaments of spleen

Blood Supply

The highly tortuous splenic artery enters the hilum of the spleen and breaks up into four or five branches, which travel along the splenic trabeculae. The splenic vein emerges out of the hilum and joins the superior mesenteric vein behind the neck of the pancreas to form the portal vein.

Lymphatic Drainage

As the spleen filters blood and not the lymph, it receives no afferent lymphatic vessels. However, the efferent vessels from the stroma and capsule terminate in pancreaticosplenic lymph nodes. The cancer cells rarely spread to the spleen because it lacks afferent lymph vessels and its microenvironment does not favor implantation and growth of malignant cells.

Splenic Circulation

The splenic artery divides into 5 or 6 segmental branches in the lienorenal ligament. The segmental arteries enter the hilum of spleen and follow the trabeculae to ramify throughout the substance of the spleen. Once these arteries narrow to the arteriolar dimensions, they enter the white pulp of spleen, where the arterioles lose their connective tissue adventitia and acquire the periarterial lymphatic sheath. At places, this sheath is enlarged to form lymphatic follicles called Malpighian follicles. Inside the lymphatic follicle the arteriole is typically in eccentric position. The periarterial lymphatic sheath and the Malpighian follicles constitute the white pulp of the spleen. The arteriole comes out of the white pulp to enter the red pulp, where it abruptly divides into three to five straight penicillar arterioles. A sheath of macrophages called ellipsoid surrounds the terminal part of each penicillar arteriole. These sheathed arterioles terminate in arterial capillaries. Beyond this, the venous side of splenic circulation starts. In close theory of splenic circulation, the arterial capillaries communicate with venous sinusoids by direct arteriovenous connections. In open theory of splenic circulation, the arterial capillaries discharge their blood in the spaces of red pulp and thence to the venous sinusoids. The components of the red pulp are the cords of Billroth (made of macrophages and reticulocytes) and the splenic sinusoids, which are lined by reticuloendothelial cells. The venous sinusoids congregate to form venules, which join to form trabecular veins. The smaller trabecular veins join to form larger trabecular veins, which approach the hilum of the spleen and unite at or just outside the hilum to form the splenic vein. Since the periarterial lymphatic sheath is B-cell dominant and Malpighian corpuscles are T-cell dominant areas, the main function of the white pulp is to produce lymphocytes and plasma cells. In inflammatory conditions, the white pulp is antigenically stimulated. As a result, the lymphatic follicles develop germinal centers and become big in size causing increase in the size of the spleen. The functions of the red pulp are as follows. The worn out and damaged erythrocytes are brought to the red pulp for catabolism. Similarly, the granulocytes, platelets, bacterial pathogens, particulate matter and parasites (for example malarial parasite) also reach the red pulp for phagocytosis. The red blood corpuscles are broken down in two components, namely heme and globin. The heme contains iron and bilirubin. The iron is sent to bone marrow for reutilization or to liver for storage. Amino acids from hydrolysis of globin are returned to the amino acid pool of the body. The end product of hemoglobin breakdown (bilirubin) enters the liver via the splenic and portal veins. The hepatocytes process the bilirubin and add it to the bile.

Clinical Highlights

a. A normal spleen is not palpable. Only when enlarged almost twice its normal size, the spleen becomes clinically palpable under the left costal margin. The spleen does not enlarge in a vertically downward direction due to the presence of phenicocolic ligament. It enlarges along the spinoumbilical line, which extends from the right anterior superior iliac spine to the umbilicus. In massive enlargement the spleen may reach the right iliac fossa. Therefore, palpation of the spleen follows the spinoumbilical line towards the left costal margin.
b. Splenomegaly is the term used for enlarged spleen. A few causes of splenomegaly include, portal hypertension due to any cause, malaria, typhoid fever, hemolytic anemia and leukemia.
c. The splenic pulp pressure reflects the portal venous pressure. Therefore, splenic puncture is done in the left tenth intercostal space in the midaxillary line to record the portal venous pressure.
d. Surgical removal of spleen is called splenectomy. The gastrosplenic and lienorenal ligaments with the contained vessels form the two pedicles of the spleen. During splenectomy, both the pedicles are dissected carefully to isolate and tie the blood vessels and preserve the tail of the pancreas.

143 Portal Vein

The portal vein is an important venous channel that collects blood from the abdominal and pelvic parts of digestive tract (excluding lower part of anal canal), pancreas, spleen and gallbladder. It carries products of digestion of carbohydrates and proteins and other nutrients from the intestines and also products of hemoglobin catabolism from the spleen to the liver sinusoids. The portal vein begins like a vein in the capillary bed and terminates in the hepatic sinusoids like an artery. Since it passes through two sets of exchange vessels, the portal pressure is higher than systemic venous pressure. The normal portal pressure is 5 to 15 mm of Hg. The portal vein and its tributaries are valveless. The portal vein and its tributaries act as reservoir of blood since they contain up to one-third of the total volume of blood in the body.

Formation

The portal vein is formed posterior to the neck of pancreas by the union of superior mesenteric and splenic veins at the level of L2 vertebra. It has extrahepatic and intrahepatic parts (vide infra).

Termination

The portal vein terminates into right and left branches at the right end of porta hepatis.

Development

The portal vein and its terminal branches develop from the right and left vitelline veins of the embryo. Three intervitelline anastomoses form a "figure of 8" anastomosis around the developing duodenum (Fig.143.1). The anastomoses are named as caudal ventral duodenal, intermediate dorsal duodenal and cranial ventral duodenal. Some parts of this vascular configuration disappear to give rise to the portal vein and its two branches as follows:

a. The trunk of the portal vein develops from a small part of left vitelline adjacent to the dorsal anastomosis, the entire dorsal anastomosis and the right vitelline vein up to the cranial ventral anastomosis.
b. The right branch of the portal vein develops from the right vitelline vein cranial to the cranial ventral anastomosis.
c. The left branch of the portal vein develops from the cranial ventral anastomosis and left vitelline vein cranial to it.

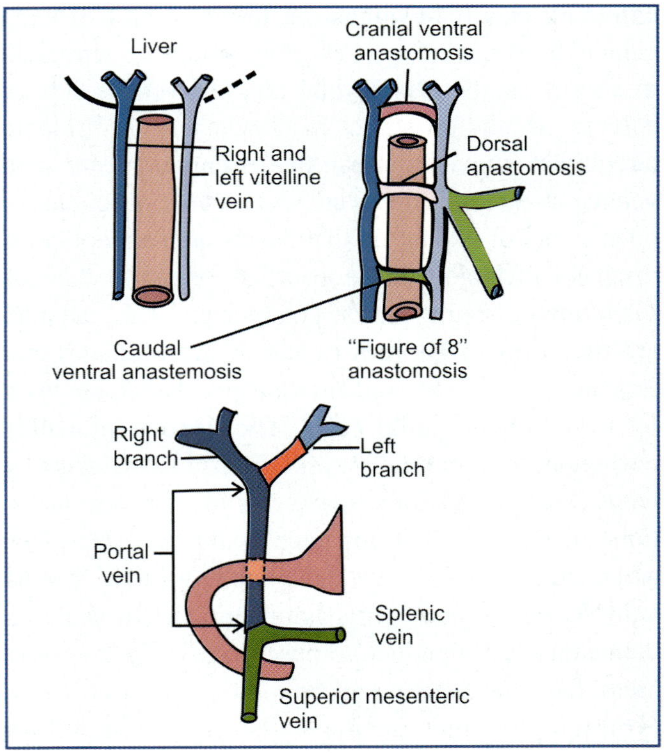

Fig. 143.1: Stages in the development of portal vein and its branches (Note: The color code relates to the developmental sources of the vessels)

Extrahepatic Part

The extrahepatic part, about 8 to 10 cm long, is divided into three parts, infraduodenal, retroduodenal and supraduodenal.

a. The infraduodenal part lies below the first part of the duodenum. It is related anteriorly, to the neck of pancreas, posteriorly to the inferior vena cava and on its right to common bile duct.
b. The retroduodenal part lies posterior to the first part of duodenum. It is related anteriorly to the first part of duodenum, with common bile duct and gastroduodenal artery separating the two. Posteriorly, it is in relation to inferior vena cava.
c. The supraduodenal part is located in the free margin of lesser omentum. The common bile duct and hepatic artery proper lie anterior to it in the omentum, the artery being medial to the duct. Posteriorly, the epiploic foramen intervenes between the portal vein and the inferior vena cava.

Intrahepatic Part

At the right edge of porta hepatis the portal vein divides into two terminal branches. The right branch is shorter and wider and may receive a cystic vein before entering the right lobe of liver. The longer left branch enters the left lobe. Three structures join the left branch inside the liver (ligamentum teres, ligamentum venosum and paraumbilical veins).

Blood Flow in Portal Vein (Fig. 143.2)

The portal vein contains two sluggish streams of blood probably due to the wide angle of union between the superior mesenteric and splenic veins. The right stream carries blood from the superior mesenteric vein and the left stream carries blood from the splenic vein. The right branch of the portal vein distributes blood to the right lobe of liver from the intestine upto the right two-thirds of the transverse colon. The left branch of the portal vein distributes blood to the left lobe of liver (including the caudate and quadrate lobes), from the stomach, spleen, pancreas and the large intestine distal from the left one-third of transverse colon, rectum and anal canal upto the pectinate line. Therefore, primary cancer or infective emboli from the sigmoid colon deposit in the left lobe and that from the caecum in the right lobe of liver.

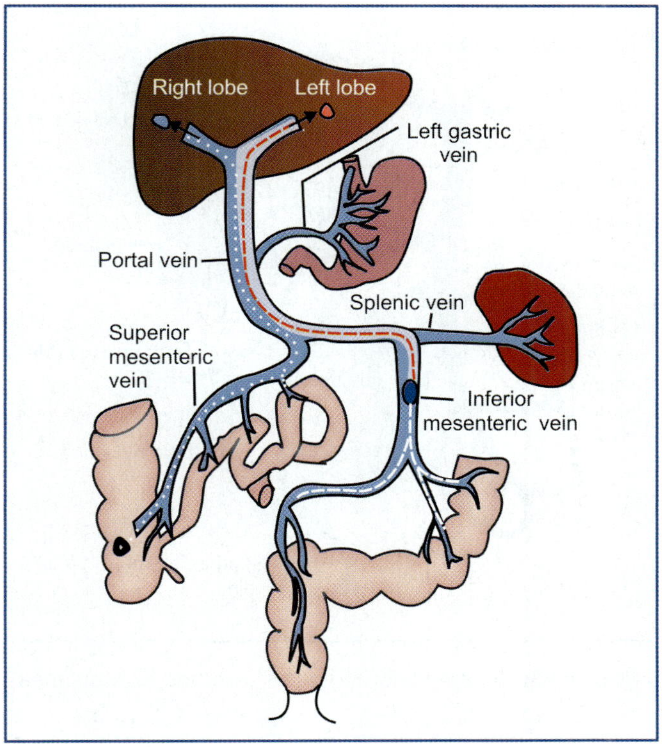

Fig. 143.2: Showing parallel streams of blood in portal vein. Infective focus in drainage area of superior mesenteric vein reaches right lobe and that of inferior mesenteric vein reaches left lobe

Tributaries (Fig. 143.3)

a. The direct tributaries of the portal vein are, superior mesenteric, splenic and right and left gastric veins.
b. The tributaries of the superior mesenteric vein are, ileocolic, right colic, middle colic, jejunal, ileal and right gastroepiploic veins.
c. The tributaries of the splenic vein are, short gastric, left gastroepiploic and inferior mesenteric veins.
d. The tributaries of the inferior mesenteric vein are superior rectal, sigmoid and left colic veins.

Paraumbilical, Cystic and Prepyloric Veins

a. The paraumbilical veins extend from the anterior abdominal wall along the ligamentum teres to the left branch of portal vein. They are connected to superficial veins of abdominal wall by potential anastomoses.
b. A few cystic veins open in the right branch of portal vein.
c. The prepyloric veins of Mayo are the anterior relation to the pylorus of the stomach. During surgery on

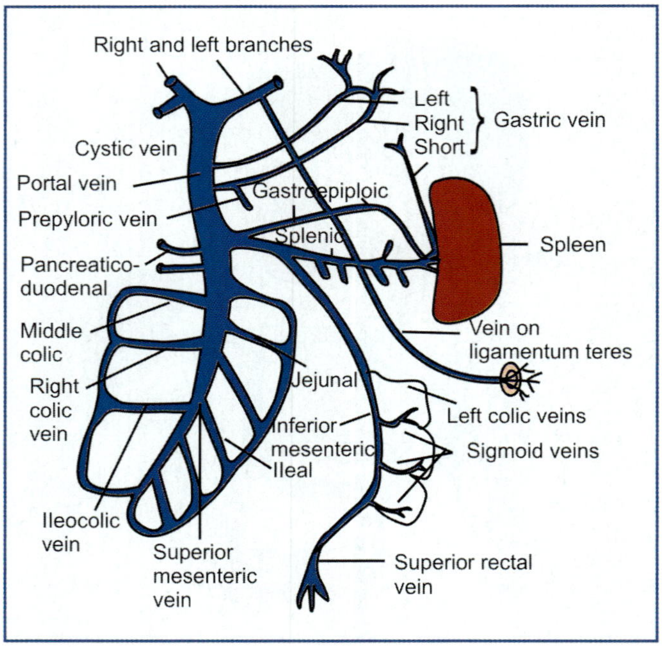

Fig. 143.3: Scheme showing portal vein and its tributaries

pylorus, these veins are helpful in identification of the pylorus. They ascend in front of the pylorus and drain into the right gastric vein.

Measurement of Portal Pressure

a. A direct method consists of the splenic puncture through which the pressure of the splenic pulp.
b. An indirect method of measuring the portal pressure is to record the hepatic vein pressure under radiographic control. The catheter passes in succession through the right median cubital, basilic, axillary, subclavian, and brachiocephalic veins and then through the SVC to the right atrium. It is further advanced to the IVC until it reaches the hepatic veins. When the tip of the catheter is wedged in the smaller tributaries of the hepatic vein, pressure is recorded.

Radiological Examination

To study the portal venous anatomy on a radiograph a contrast material is injected in the spleen (splenoportography)

Clinical Highlights

The obstruction of portal vein leads to portal hypertension. The causes of obstruction may be divided in intrahepatic and extrahepatic (Fig. 143.3). Among the intrahepatic causes, the most common is the cirrhosis of liver. Among the extrahepatic causes, portal vein thrombosis is one of the causes. The obstruction to blood flow leads to stasis and rise in portal pressure. The effects of portal hypertension are, splenomegaly (enlargement of spleen), ascites and those due to enlarged portosystemic collateral channels. The blood in portal circulation is diverted to the systemic circulation through portosystemic communications because of which the veins at such sites are dilated.

Sites of Portosystemic Anastomoses (Fig. 143.4)

a. At the lower end of esophagus, the left gastric vein (a portal vein tributary) and the esophageal veins (the hemiazygos vein—a systemic vein tributary) anastomose in the submucosa. This submucosal venous plexus is dilated and tortuous in portal hypertension giving rise to esophageal varices. The rupture of the varices leads to vomiting of blood (hematemesis).
b. Around the umbilicus, the paraumbilical veins (portal tributary) anastomose with the superficial tributaries of superior epigastric and inferior epigastric veins (systemic veins). Enlargement of the radiating veins in portal hypertension produces a characteristic pattern of dilated veins around the umbilicus (caput Medusae).

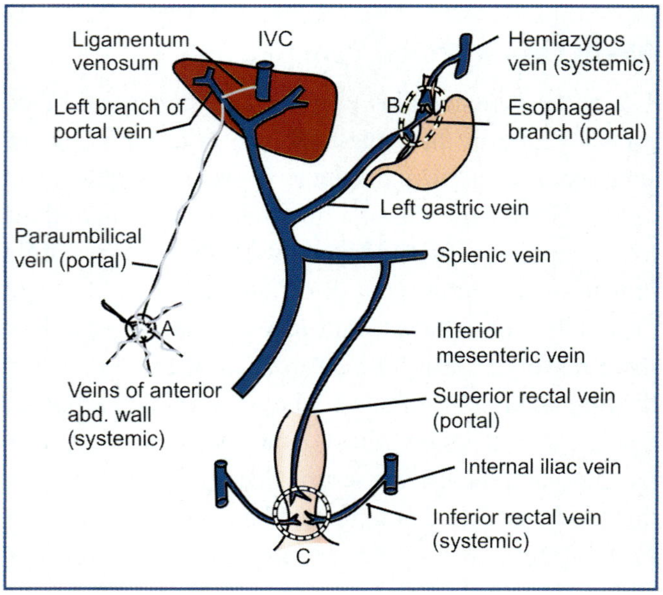

Fig. 143.4: Sites of portosystemic anastomosis (A—Umbilicus, B—lower end of esophagus, C—pectinate line of anal canal)

c. At the level of pectinate line in the anal canal, submucosal venous plexus contains potential anastomoses between the superior rectal vein (a portal vein tributary) with inferior rectal veins (systemic vein tributary) below the pectinate line. The enlargement of this venous plexus gives rise to internal piles, which may cause bleeding per rectum, on injury.
d. At bare area of liver, the hepatic portal radicles directly communicate with inferior phrenic veins.
e. Retroperitoneal areas of posterior abdominal wall are the areas in relation to retroperitoneal organs like ascending or descending colon. Here, the portal vein tributaries draining these organs may communicate with the systemic veins of posterior abdominal wall.

144 Abdominal Aorta

The abdominal aorta is the continuation of descending thoracic aorta at the aortic orifice of the diaphragm. Its vertebral extent is from the lower border of the twelfth thoracic vertebra to the fourth lumbar vertebra. It travels down on the anterior surfaces of upper four lumbar vertebrae. The aorta bifurcates into the right and left common iliac arteries a little to the left of the midline.

Surface Marking

The abdominal aorta can be indicated on the anterior abdominal wall by a 2 cm wide band drawn in the midline at the level of a point, which is 2.5 cm above the transpyloric plane. A point 1 cm below and to the left of umbilicus denotes the lower level of this band. The aortic pulsations can be felt or may be visible just below and slightly to the left of the umbilicus in thin individuals, when the abdominal muscles are relaxed.

Aortography

Abdominal aortography is the radiological procedure to visualize the aorta and its branches. The contrast is injected through the catheter passed in the femoral artery and extended via the external and common iliac arteries into the aorta. Ultrasound, CT and MRI are useful tools for visualizing the aorta.

Relations

a. The anterior relations from above downward are, the celiac trunk and its three branches, the origin of superior mesenteric artery, splenic vein, left renal vein, origin of inferior mesenteric artery, third part of duodenum and the root of the mesentery.
b. The posterior relations are, the vertebral column, the dorsal branches of aorta, namely, lumbar and median sacral arteries and the left third and fourth lumbar veins.
c. On the right side, it is related to the right crus of diaphragm and right celiac ganglion in the upper part. Below the level of second lumbar vertebra the right relation is inferior vena cava.
d. On the left side, there are left crus of diaphragm and left celiac ganglion in the upper part. At the level of second lumbar vertebra, the duodenojejunal junction is on the left side. Below this, the inferior mesenteric vessels are on the left side.

Branches

The branches are divided into two broad categories, visceral and parietal. The visceral branches supply the viscera and parietal branches mainly supply the body wall. The visceral branches are divisible into anterior and lateral groups. The parietal branches are divisible into posterior and lateral groups.

a. The anterior group consists of visceral branches (Fig. 134.5), celiac trunk, superior mesenteric artery and inferior mesenteric artery.
b. The lateral group of visceral branches are, middle suprarenal, renal and gonadal (ovarian or testicular) arteries.
c. The posterior group of parietal branches consists of lumbar arteries and a single median sacral artery.
d. The lateral group of parietal branches includes the right and left inferior phrenic arteries.

Celiac Trunk

The celiac trunk arises from abdominal aorta at the level of twelfth thoracic vertebra. It is a very short artery (1 cm long). It immediately divides into three branches, which diverge in three directions. Celiac plexus of nerves surrounds the celiac trunk and the suspensory ligament of Treitz splits to encircle it.

Surface Marking

The celiac trunk can be mapped out as a small circle drawn on the anterior abdominal wall 1.25 cm above the transpyloric plane in the midline.

Relations

It is surrounded by celiac plexus of nerves and is related anteriorly to the lesser omentum. On the right, it is related to right celiac ganglion and right crus of diaphragm. On the left side, it is related to left celiac ganglion and left crus of diaphragm. Inferiorly, it is related to tuber omentale of pancreas.

Celiac Arteriography

With the help of celiac arteriography the celiac artery and its branches can be visualized. The radiopaque dye is injected through a catheter that passes in succession through the femoral, external iliac, common iliac arteries and the aorta.

Branches of Celiac Trunk

a. The left gastric artery at first, runs upwards and to the left behind the parietal peritoneum to the cardiac end of the stomach. Then, it turns forwards and downwards raising the left gastropancreatic fold of peritoneum and enters the left end of the lesser omentum. Before entering the lesser omentum, it gives esophageal branches to the lower end of the esophagus. Inside the lesser omentum, it anastomoses with the right gastric artery along the lesser curvature of the stomach.
b. The common hepatic artery passes at first, to the right behind the parietal peritoneum and then turns forwards raising a right gastropancreatic fold of peritoneum. It passes forwards above the first part of duodenum to enter the free margin of the lesser omentum. Here, it gives origin to right gastric and gastroduodenal arteries. Beyond this point, it is called the hepatic artery proper, which ascends in the free margin of lesser omentum along with the common bile duct and portal vein. The hepatic artery proper divides very close to the porta hepatis into right and left hepatic branches. The cystic artery usually arises from the right branch of the hepatic artery. The right and left hepatic branches enter the porta hepatis.

Branches of Common Hepatic Artery

i. The right gastric artery passes to the left and enters the lesser omentum to anastomose.
ii. The gastroduodenal artery descends posterior to the first part of duodenum and divides into right gastroepiploic and superior pancreaticoduodenal arteries at its lower margin. The ulcer on the posterior wall of the first part of duodenum may perforate and erode the gastroduodenal artery causing massive bleeding in the peritoneal cavity. Hence, this artery is called the "artery of duodenal hemorrhage". It may give rise to supraduodenal artery of Wilkie and it frequently supplies retroduodenal branches to the first part of duodenum. The right gastroepiploic artery runs to the left to enter the greater omentum where it anastomoses with the left gastroepiploic artery. The superior pancreaticoduodenal arteries are two in number, anterior and posterior. They course along the junction of pancreatic head and second part of duodenum to anastomose with similar branches of inferior pancreaticoduodenal artery. The superior pancreaticoduodenal arteries give twigs to the head of pancreas and supply the duodenum till the major duodenal papilla.

c. The splenic artery is the largest branch of the celiac trunk. It is tortuous so as to allow for the expansion of the stomach because the artery is one of the constituents of the stomach bed. It runs retroperitoneally towards the left along the superior margin of the pancreas. After reaching the front of left kidney it enters the lienorenal ligament along with the tail of pancreas. It supplies several pancreatic branches (named and un-named) that arise along the superior margin of the gland. A few short gastric arteries and the left gastroepiploic artery arise near the hilum of the spleen and reach the stomach via the gastrosplenic ligament. The terminal splenic branches enter the splenic substance.

Superior Mesenteric Artery (SMA)

The superior mesenteric artery arises from the front of the abdominal aorta about 0.5 cm below the celiac trunk at the level of the disc between L1 and L2 vertebrae behind the body of pancreas. From its origin until its entry into the root of the mesentery, the artery lies on the posterior abdominal wall. Since the artery angles acutely in the first part of its course it forms a nutcracker with the aorta (Fig. 134.5). The structures enclosed inside the vascular nutcracker are, left renal vein, uncinate process of pancreas and third part of duodenum. The unusual venous relation at its origin, is the splenic vein embedded in the substance of the posterior surface of pancreas in front and the left renal vein behind.

Course

From behind the pancreas the artery emerges on the anterior aspect by passing between the uncinate process and body of the pancreas. It crosses in front of the third part of the duodenum to enter the root of the mesentery, in which it travels downwards and to the right to reach the ileocecal junction.

Surface Marking

The upper point is in the midline just above the transpyloric plane. The lower point lies at the intersection of right lateral and transtubercular planes. The line joining the two points should have a slight convexity to the left.

Branches

a. The inferior pancreaticoduodenal artery may arise from the superior mesenteric artery or its first jejunal branch. Its anterior and posterior branches make anastomoses with the corresponding branches of superior pancreaticoduodenal artery. This anastomosis is the only communication among the branches celiac and superior mesenteric arteries (arteries of the foregut and midgut).
b. The jejunal and ileal branches are several in numbers and arise from the left side of the superior mesenteric artery. These arteries pass through the mesentery to reach the gut.
c. The ileocolic artery is actually the continuation of the superior mesenteric artery. It divides in ascending and descending branches. The ascending branch anastomoses with descending branch of right colic artery. The descending branch supplies terminal ileum by its ileal branch, cecum by anterior and posterior cecal branches, appendix by appendicular branch and the lower part of ascending colon by colic branch.
d. The right colic artery arises from the right side and travels on the posterior abdominal wall behind the peritoneum. On reaching the ascending colon, it divides into ascending and descending branches, which anastomose with branches of ileocolic and middle colic arteries to form marginal artery.
e. The middle colic artery arises from the right side of superior mesenteric artery. It enters the transverse mesocolon and divides in right and left branches that anastomose with branches of right colic and left colic arteries to complete the marginal artery. The anastomosis between left colic and middle colic at the level of marginal artery may be deficient. This break in the marginal artery is usually compensated by presence of an artery called an arc of Riolan between the trunk of middle colic artery and ascending branch of left colic artery. In case the arc of Riolan is not developed, the blood supply of left colic flexure is in danger.

Intestinal Angina

Stenosis of superior mesenteric artery may produce colicky abdominal pain referred to the umbilicus (intestinal angina).

Superior Mesenteric Arteriography

The artery and its branches can be visualized by injecting a radiopaque dye into it. For this purpose, the artery is approached via the femoral artery, external iliac artery, common iliac artery and the abdominal aorta.

Inferior Mesenteric Artery (IMA)

This artery arises from the aorta at the level of L3 vertebra, posterior to the third part of duodenum. It courses down on the front of aorta and then on the posterior abdominal wall on the left side of the aorta. It continues as the superior rectal artery.

Surface Marking

The upper end of the artery is in the midline 4 cm below the transpyloric plane. The lower end lies 4 cm below the umbilicus and 4 cm to the left of the midline.

Branches (Fig. 137.8)

a. Left colic artery runs upwards and to the left behind the peritoneum and divides into ascending and descending branches. The descending branches communicate with sigmoid arteries and ascending branches meet the left branches of middle colic artery and thus form the marginal artery.
b. Sigmoid arteries enter the left limb of sigmoid mesocolon and their branches take part in completing the marginal artery. It has been observed that there is a constant anastomosis between the lowest sigmoid artery and a branch of superior rectal artery.
c. Superior rectal artery is the continuation of inferior mesenteric artery in the true pelvis. It descends in the right limb of the sigmoid mesocolon. At the level of third piece of sacrum, it divides into two branches. These branches course down on either side of rectum and give twigs that pierce the rectal wall to supply the mucous membrane of the rectum and that of anal canal up to the level of pectinate line, where they anastomose with branches of inferior rectal arteries.

Inferior Mesenteric Arteriography

It is possible to visualize the artery by injecting a radio-opaque dye in it. The approach is similar to that for the superior mesenteric artery.

Lateral Group of Visceral Branches of Aorta

a. The middle suprarenal arteries arise at level of origin of the superior mesenteric artery.
b. The renal arteries arise from the lateral sides and at right angles to the aorta below the superior mesenteric artery. The right artery, which is longer than the left, passes behind the inferior vena cava, head of pancreas and second part of duodenum to reach the hilum of right kidney. The left renal artery passes behind the body of pancreas, the left renal and splenic veins. Each renal artery gives off the inferior suprarenal artery.
c. The gonadal arteries consist of testicular arteries in male and ovarian arteries in female. The gonadal arteries originate a little below the renal arteries from the anterolateral aspect of the aorta.

The slender testicular arteries have a long intra-abdominal course. Each artery passes in inferolateral direction lying on the psoas major muscle to enter the deep inguinal ring and become the content of the spermatic cord in which it reaches the testis. The ovarian arteries are shorter in length than the testicular arteries. They enter the true pelvis by crossing the external iliac vessels at the pelvic brim. Each artery enters the infundibulopelvic ligament to reach the broad ligament of uterus, from where it enters the ovary through the mesovarium.

Lateral Group of Parietal Branches

The inferior phrenic arteries are the first branches of abdominal aorta. They supply the diaphragm and give origin to the superior suprarenal arteries.

Posterior Group of Parietal Branches

a. Four pairs of lumbar arteries arise from the back of the aorta. The lumbar arteries travel posterolaterally in contact with the upper four lumbar vertebral bodies and pass under the tendinous arches of the psoas major muscle. At the lateral border of the quadratus lumborum muscle the arteries enter the anterior abdominal wall, where they make anastomotic connections with the lower intercostal, sucostal, iliolumbar, inferior epigastric and deep circumflex iliac arteries.
b. Median sacral artery is a small branch from the dorsal aspect of aorta just above its bifurcation. It descends in the midline on the anterior surfaces of L4 and L5 vertebrae, sacrum and coccyx, ending in the coccygeal body. It may give a small lumbar artery called arteria lumbalis ima, which supplies branches to the rectum.

Clinical Highlights

a. Leriche syndrome is due to chronic atherosclerosis of the distal abdominal aorta below the origin of the renal arteries. The disease gradually occludes the abdominal aorta near its bifurcation and encroaches on the iliac arteries also. Claudication (pain on exercise) characteristically involves lower back, buttocks, thighs and calves. This may cause impotence in males, if the internal iliac arteries are occluded. The clinical findings include bilateral absence of femoral pulses and the detection of audible bruit on the abdomen below the umbilicus.

b. The acute occlusion in the distal abdominal aorta occurs as a result of occlusive embolus usually arising from the heart. This gives rise to acute pain in the lower limbs accompanied by coolness and pallor. Gangrene of the lower limb is the dreaded complication of this condition.

c. The aneurysm of abdominal aorta due to atherosclerosis, is common. It presents as a pulsatile, palpable nontender mass just below the umbilicus.

Common Iliac Arteries

The right and left common iliac arteries are the terminal branches of the abdominal aorta at the level of the L4 vertebra. The common iliac arteries divide into external and internal arteries at the level of the disc between sacrum and the L5 vertebra in front of the sacroiliac joints. The right common iliac artery is slightly longer than the left. To mark the artery on the surface, first take a point of aortic bifurcation 1 cm below and to the left of umbilicus. Join this point to the midinguinal point by a broad line. The upper one-third of this line represents the common iliac artery. The right common iliac artery is about 5 cm long. It is crossed anteriorly at its bifurcation by the right ureter. The venous relations of the common iliac artery are unusual. Three veins form its posterior relation below and at the level of L5 vertebra. They are the terminal parts of right and left common iliac veins and their union to form IVC. The left common iliac artery is about 4 cm long. It is crossed anteriorly by the left ureter at the bifurcation. The left common iliac vein is posterior to the artery in the lower part and medial to it in the upper part. The common iliac arteries give a few peritoneal and ureteric branches besides the terminal branches.

Terminal Branches of Common Iliac Arteries

a. The external iliac artery is larger and is the major artery supplying the lower limb. It descends along the medial margin of psoas major muscle to the midinguinal point, where it continues as the femoral artery. Its surface marking is as follows. The lower two-thirds of a broad line joining the point of aortic bifurcation to the midinguinal point represents the external iliac artery. Its branches are, the deep circumflex iliac artery and the inferior epigastric artery.

b. The internal iliac arteries enter the true pelvis. The description of its branches in the male and female, is given in Chapter 157.

145 Inferior Vena Cava

This largest vein drains the blood from the body below the level of diaphragm. It extends from the right of the L5 vertebra to the level of T8 vertebra, where it pierces the central tendon of diaphragm. It opens into the right atrium immediately thereafter.

Formation

The IVC is formed by the union of the right and left common iliac veins on the front of the body of the L5 vertebra about two cm to the right of the midline. The IVC has no valves.

Length

The IVC is 20 to 23 cm long (almost double the length of the abdominal aorta).

Surface Marking

The IVC is represented by a band 2.5 cm wide drawn to the right of the median plane. The left margin of the band is 1 cm from the median plane and the right margin is 3.5 cm from the median plane. The lower limit of the band corresponds to a line just below the transtubercular plane and its upper limit is at the sternal end of the right sixth costal cartilage.

Relations of Abdominal Part

a. The anterior relations, starting from its commencement to its opening in the diaphragm are, the right common iliac artery, root of mesentery, third part of duodenum, head of pancreas, bile duct and portal vein, epiploic foramen and caval groove on the posterior surface of the liver.
b. The posterior relations are the bodies of lumbar vertebrae, right psoas major muscle, right crus of diaphragm and the antero-medial surface of the right suprarenal gland. Besides these, the arteries that pass posterior to the IVC are, right lumbar arteries, right renal artery, right middle suprarenal artery and the right inferior phrenic artery.
c. To the left of IVC, runs the abdominal aorta and to its right are the second part of duodenum and medial margin of right kidney.

Tributaries of IVC

a. Four pairs of lumbar veins drain blood from the abdominal wall and the vertebral venous plexus. In front of the roots of the transverse processes of the lumbar vertebrae, the lumbar veins join each other by a vertical channel called the ascending lumbar vein, which joins the azygos vein. There is another vertical channel called lumbar azygos vein, which lies parallel and medial to the ascending lumbar vein. The first and second lumbar veins open in either the ascending lumbar vein or the azygos lumbar vein. The third and fourth lumbar veins directly open in the IVC.
b. Inferior phrenic veins open directly in the IVC.
c. Right gonadal vein (testicular or ovarian) is a direct tributary of the IVC (but the left is not).
d. Renal veins are the direct tributaries. The right vein is about 2.5 cm long and the left is much longer (7.5 cm). The left renal vein crosses in front of the aorta. The left renal vein receives the left suprarenal and left gonadal veins.
e. Right suprarenal vein opens directly in IVC (but the left does not).
f. Hepatic veins are usually three in upper set (right, middle and left) and a variable number in the lower set. They are extremely short so that as soon as they emerge from the posterior surface of liver in the groove

for IVC they enter it. Hence, they cannot be seen as, separate veins. They are identified by their openings in the lumen of IVC.

Collateral Circulation

If there is obstruction to the IVC, the blood from below the level of obstruction is carried to the right atrium through SVC. The blood bypasses the IVC if the potential collateral channels are opened up. Such collateral anastomotic channels develop in the following sites:

a. In the anterior abdominal wall the tributaries of the inferior epigastric veins (tributaries of external iliac veins) are in communication with the lateral thoracic veins (tributaries of axillary veins) by thoraco-epigastric veins. So, the blood from femoral vein goes to the external vein and from there is carried by the inferior epigastric vein to the thoraco-epigastric vein and thence to the axillary vein for onward passage to SVC. There are dilated and tortuous veins in the lateral part of anterior abdominal wall in obstruction of IVC.
b. The veins of vertebral system become dilated. The lumbar veins communicate in the anterior abdominal wall with lower intercostal, subcostal, inferior epigastric and iliolumbar veins. The posterior parts of lumbar veins receive intervertebral veins, which make communications with vertebral venous plexus. Similarly the lateral sacral veins carry blood from pelvic organs to the vertebral venous plexus. In obstruction of IVC the lumbar veins and the lateral sacral veins carry the blood in reverse direction to the vertebral venous plexus, the cranial venous sinuses and ultimately via the internal jugular vein to the SVC. This venous route is responsible for cancer deposits from the primary in pelvic organs to the vertebral column and cranial bones.
c. The azygos system of veins forms an important alternate venous pathway. The ascending lumbar, lumbar azygos and subcostal veins become dilated to carry additional load of blood from the anterior and posterior abdominal walls to the azygos vein, which empties into the SVC.

146 Clinicoanatomical Problems and Solutions

CASE 1

A 65-year-old man with a history of chronic bronchitis noticed a gradually increasing swelling in the left inguinal region. After physical examination the surgeon noted the following:

a. A lemon sized swelling above the pubic tubercle.
b. The swelling increased in size on coughing.
c. After manually reducing the swelling, the surgeon occluded the deep ring with the thumb and then asked the patient to cough. The swelling appeared medial to the thumb.

Questions

a. Which findings in the physical examination are confirmatory of inguinal hernia?
b. Give the type of inguinal hernia from finding "c".
c. Give the surface marking of deep inguinal ring.
d. Name the boundaries of Hesselbach's triangle.
e. Write a note on the conjoint tendon.
f. Name the artery in lateral relation to the neck of above type of hernia. Give its two named branches in this region.
g. Give the boundaries and contents of inguinal canal.

Solutions

a. The swelling is above the pubic tubercle and it increased on coughing.
b. Direct inguinal hernia.
c. It is marked by a point located 1.25 cm above the midinguinal point.
d. Hesselbach's triangle is bounded inferiorly by inguinal ligament, medially by lateral margin of rectus abdominis muscle and laterally by inferior epigastric artery.
e. Refer to Anterior Abdominal Wall in Chapter 127.
f. Inferior epigastric artery (branch of external iliac artery). Its two named branches here are, pubic artery and cremasteric artery in male or artery of the round ligament in female.
g. Refer to Inguinal Canal in Chapter 129.

CASE 2

A 60-year-old man (with a history of chronic duodenal ulcer) was admitted to the hospital in an unconscious state. His pulse was weak and blood pressure was very low. Ultrasound scan revealed fluid in the peritoneal cavity. This case was diagnosed as perforation of the first part of duodenum.

Questions

a. Which artery is eroded in the perforation of peptic ulcer on the posterior wall of the first part of duodenum? What is it a branch of?
b. What is the length of first part of duodenum?
c. Enumerate the special features of the first part of duodenum.
d. Give the relations of the second and third parts of the duodenum.
e. Describe the internal features of the second part of the duodenum.
f. Mention the development of the duodenum.
g. What is the effect of annular pancreas on duodenum?

Solutions

a. Gastroduodenal artery is eroded in perforation of the first part, being posterior relation of this part. It is known as artery of duodenal hemorrhage. It is a branch of common hepatic artery.

b. The length of the first part is 5 cm.
c. For special features of the first part of duodenum refer to Chapter 134.
d. For relations, refer to Chapter 134.
e. Generally there are circular folds of mucous membrane. There are two apertures lying on two raised papillae. The larger papilla located at a distance of 8 to 10 cm from the pylorus is known as major duodenal papilla. It is present at the proximal end of a longitudinal fold on the posteromedial wall. On its summit, open the hepatopancreatic ampulla pouring pancreatic juice and bile in this part. The minor duodenal papilla is located about 2 cm proximal to the opening of hepatopancreatic ampulla. On its summit, opens the accessory pancreatic duct.
f. The mucosa of the first part of the duodenum develops entirely from the endoderm of the foregut. The mucosa of the second part has dual development. The part above the major duodenal papilla develops from foregut and below that from midgut. The third and fourth parts develop from the midgut. The muscles in the wall and the supporting connective tissue develop from splanchnopleuric mesoderm. The duodenum loses its primitive mesentery (except for the proximal 2.5 cm of the first part) very early in embryonic life.
g. The annular pancreas surrounds the second part of the duodenum like a ring. This is a developmental anomaly. The pancreatic ring may compress the second part, causing duodenal obstruction in newborn.

CASE 3

A 70-year-old man with complaints of progressive jaundice, frequent bowel movements with pale greasy stools, back pain and weight loss was diagnosed as having carcinoma of the head of pancreas after ultrasound examination and other appropriate investigations.

Questions

a. What is the anatomical and physiological basis of jaundice in cancer of pancreatic head? Mention the type of jaundice.
b. Which cells secrete bile?
c. Draw a diagram of the extrahepatic biliary apparatus.
d. Name the boundaries and contents of Calot's triangle.
e. Draw a diagram to show the arterial supply of common bile duct.
f. Describe the development of the common bile and the main pancreatic ducts.
g. Give the anterior relations and development of the uncinate process.

Solutions

a. The common bile duct is embedded in the posterior surface of the head of the pancreas before joining the pancreatic duct. Therefore, in cancer of pancreatic head the CBD is blocked by cancer infiltration. The bile with contained bilirubin accumulates in the biliary tree leading to stasis in the biliary canaliculi. The bile escapes either through the lymph vessels of liver or through ruptured bile canaliculi into blood circulation. The type of jaundice in this case is obstructive or surgical jaundice.
b. Hepatocytes secrete bile.
c. Refer to Figure 141.1
d. The Calot's (cystohepatic) triangle has following boundaries, superiorly by inferior surface of right lobe of liver close to porta hepatis (some descriptions include cystic artery as the upper margin), inferiorly by cystic duct and to medially by common hepatic duct. The contents of the triangle are, cystic artery, cystic lymph node of Lund and right hepatic artery (cystic artery cannot be a content if it forms the upper boundary).
e. Refer to Figure 141.3.
f. The common bile duct develops from the proximal part of hepatic bud, which takes origin from endoderm of foregut. The duodenal side of the main pancreatic duct develops from the duct of ventral pancreatic bud and the remaining from the duct of dorsal pancreatic bud.
g. Superior mesenteric vessels. The uncinate process develops from ventral bud.

CASE 4

A young boy, about 17 years old was brought to the hospital with complaints of acute pain around the umbilicus, fever and vomiting. On examination, the surgeon found the area of maximum tenderness at the McBurney's point. The psoas test was positive.

Questions

a. Name the clinical condition.
b. Give the surface marking of McBurney's point. What is the importance of this point?
c. Name the different positions of the affected organ mentioning the most common position.
d. Comment on the arterial supply of the affected organ.
e. Which organ is known as abdominal tonsil and why?
f. What is the anatomical basis of psoas test?

Solutions

a. Acute appendicitis
b. McBurney's point is located at the junction of lateral one-third and medial two-thirds of a line joining anterior superior iliac spine and pubic tubercle on the right side. It indicates the base of the appendix and is used for placing incision for appendicectomy.
c. For different positions of appendix refer to Figure 137.7. The most common position of appendix is retrocecal.
d. The appendix receives arterial supply from a single appendicular artery, which is a branch of ileocolic artery. The appendicular artery travels in the mesoappendix from its base to the apex, where the mesoappendix is very short. As a result, the artery comes in direct contact with appendix at the tip. In acute appendicitis, the artery is at risk of thrombosis in this location. As a result, tip undergoes necrosis and gangrene and finally may perforate.
e. The vermiform appendix is known as the abdominal tonsil because its submucosa contains the lymphatic aggregations.
f. The retrocaecal appendix is in direct contact with the psoas major muscle. In inflammation of appendix, the muscle goes in spasm. So, when the right thigh is extended there is pain due to stretch on the psoas major, which is the flexor of the thigh at the hip joint. A positive psoas test suggests inflammation of retrocecal appendix.

CASE 5

An alcoholic man aged 65 years complained of repeated episodes of vomiting of blood and pain in the right upper part of abdomen. On examination of anterior abdominal wall, there were dilated veins radiating from the umbilicus. The liver and spleen were enlarged.

Questions

a. Name the clinical condition and the vessel affected in this.
b. What is the normal pressure in this vessel? Is it increased or decreased in this condition?
c. Give the formation, course, termination and tributaries of the vessel.
d. Remnants of which blood vessels are attached to the intrahepatic part of this vessel?
e. Give the reason for vomiting of blood in this case mentioning the source.
f. What is the term used for dilated radiating veins around the umbilicus?
g. How much a normal spleen must enlarge to become palpable?

Solutions

a. Cirrhosis of liver is the diagnosis and the blood vessels affected in cirrhosis are the intrahepatic branches of portal vein.
b. The normal portal pressure is higher than systemic venous pressure. It is about 5 to 15 mm Hg. It is increased in cirrhosis of liver.
c. Refer to Chapter 143 on Portal Vein.
d. The left branch of portal vein is attached to the ligamentum teres and ligamentum venosum inside the liver. The ligamentum teres is the remnant of left umbilical vein of fetal circulation, which brings oxygenated blood from the placenta. The ligamentum venosum is the remnant of ductus venosus, which short-circuits the oxygenated blood from the left branch of portal vein to the inferior vena cava.
e. Vomiting of blood is due to rupture of esophageal varices, which are the dilated veins in the submucosa of lower end of esophagus. This is one of the sites of portosystemic anastomosis, in which tributaries of left gastric vein and those of esophageal tributaries of hemiazygos vein take part.
f. Caput medusae
g. The spleen must enlarge double its normal size to become palpable under the left costal margin.

CASE 6

An overweight 40-year-old woman (mother of four children) was brought to the casualty with complaint of spasmodic colicky pain in the right upper quadrant of abdomen, nausea, vomiting and fever. The pain radiated to the back (coinciding with inferior angle of scapula). She was very much uncomfortable, when asked to take deep inspiration. While palpating right upper quadrant at the tip of 9th costal cartilage, the pain was unbearable.

Questions

a. Identify the organ that is inflamed mentioning the common reason for this.
b. Give the location of the organ mentioning the right and left boundaries of this location.
c. Explain the radiation of pain to the inferior angle of right scapula.
d. Name the different parts of the organ.
e. Name its inferior relations from before backwards.
f. What is the function of this organ?
g. Describe Hartman's pouch and Phrygian cap.

Solutions

a. Gallbladder is inflamed. The most common cause for cholecystitis is gallstones.
b. The gallbladder is located in the fossa on the inferior surface of the liver. The fossa for gallbladder lies between the right lobe on right and the quadrate lobe on the left.
c. The sympathetic nerve supply of gallbladder is from T7 to T9 segments of spinal cord. In cholecystitis the pain is radiated to inferior angle of scapula where the skin is supplied by seventh intercostal nerve.
d. Fundus, body and neck.
e. Transverse colon, superior duodenal flexure and first part of duodenum.
f. The gallbladder stores and concentrates the bile.
g. Hartman's pouch or infundibulum is a projection from the right side of the neck in the downward direction. Impaction of gallstone in this pouch may cause adhesion with first part of duodenum or with bile duct and injury. Phrygian cap is a congenitally present peculiar shape of the gallbladder. The fundus folds on itself to form a cap like structure because of a constriction.

CASE 7

An elderly woman gave a history of passing bloodstained stools for three months. After the proctoscopic examination the case was diagnosed as that of internal hemorrhoids.

Questions

a. Name the venous plexus, which is enlarged in the internal hemorrhoids.
b. Draw a diagram to show the three common positions of the internal piles.
c. Describe the internal features of the anal canal.
d. Tabulate the differences in the blood supply of anal canal above and below the pectinate line.
e. Name the parts of the external anal sphincter and give its nerve supply.

Solutions

a. Internal rectal venous plexus.
b. Refer to Figure 139.7.
c. The anal canal is subdivided into three parts by pectinate line and Hilton's line into upper 15 mm, middle 15 mm or pecten and lower 8 mm. The upper 15mm is lined by columnar epithelium, which is raised in to 6 to 10 longitudinal folds of Morgagni. Each column contains radicles of superior rectal vessels. The venous radicles in left lateral (3 o' clock), right anterior 11 o' clock) and right posterior (7 o' clock) become enlarged in portal hypertension causing primary internal piles. The anal valves are the crescentic mucous folds connecting the lower ends of the anal columns. The position of the valves corresponds to the wavy pectinate line. If the anal valve is torn it results in a painful condition called the anal fissure. The anal sinuses are the recesses above the valves and between the columns. The sinuses are deeper in the posterior wall of anal canal. The floor of the sinuses receives the ducts of anal glands.

The intermediate area (pecten) is lined by non-keratinized stratified squamous epithelium.

The lower area is also known as anal verge and is lined by true skin.

Pectinate line divides the anal canal into two areas, which are different in development, arterial supply, venous drainage, lymphatic drainage and nerve supply. Hilton's line is somewhat white in color. It corresponds to intersphincteric groove in the wall of the anal canal.

d. Refer to Chapter 139.

e. The external anal sphincter is subdivided into three parts, deep, superficial and subcutaneous. The inferior rectal nerve supplies the external sphincter.

CASE 8

A 6-week-old first-born male child was brought to the hospital because the mother complained that the boy was vomiting after every feed. Palpation of the abdomen, showed a button like mass in the epigastrium. The diagnosis of congenital hypertrophic pyloric stenosis was confirmed by ultrasound examination. Ramstedt's operation was performed.

Questions

a. What is the reason for narrowing of the pyloric orifice in this condition?
b. Give the surface marking of the pyloric orifice.
c. Which blood vessel helps in the identification of the pylorus during surgery?
d. Where does this blood vessel open?
e. Enumerate the layers of the pylorus (from without inwards) that are cut during Ramstedt's operation.
f. Describe the nerve supply of stomach and add a note on its clinical anatomy.

Solutions

a. The circular muscle layer at the pylorus is hypertrophied.
b. The midpoint of the pyloric orifice (which is 2 cm wide) lies at a point drawn 1.2 cm to the right of the midline on the transpyloric plane.
c. Prepyloric vein of Mayo passes in front of the pylorus lying in a groove demarcating pyloric canal and pylorus
d. The prepyloric vein opens into the right gastric vein.
e. Visceral peritoneum, longitudinal muscle layer and circular muscle layer.
f. Refer to Chapter 133 on Stomach.

CASE 9

A 62-year-old man came for consultation to the gastroenterologist because of the complaints of blood stained stools and altered bowel habits for the last two months. His other complaints were pain radiating down the back of both thighs and weakness of thigh muscles. On per rectum examination, a growth was palpable on the posterior rectal wall.

Questions

a. Give the extent of the rectum.
b. Mention the characteristic features of rectosigmoid junction.
c. What is ampulla of rectum?
d. Name the posterior relations of the rectum.
e. Which nerve is involved by the growth?
f. Describe with the help of diagram the lymphatic drainage of rectum.
g. Describe the peritoneal relations of the rectum in male and female.
h. Describe the development of rectum.

Solutions

a. The rectum extends from rectosigmoid junction (third sacral vertebra) to anorectal junction (just below the tip of coccyx).
b. The rectosigmoid junction is characterized externally by absence of the distinguishing features of large intestine and end of pelvic mesocolon. Internally, the junction presents an acute angulation, which lies at a distance of 15 to 17 cm from the anal orifice.
c. Ampulla is the part of cavity of the Rectum below the level of middle valve.
d. Refer to Chapter 138 on Rectum.
e. Sciatic nerve, a branch of sacral plexus (which is in posterior relation).
f. Refer to Chapter 138 on Rectum.
g. The peritoneum reflects from the junction of middle and lower third of rectum on to the urinary bladder in male, to form rectovesical pouch. In the female, the peritoneum reflects from the same level on to the posterior fornix of vagina to form rectouterine pouch of Douglas.
h. The rectal mucosa up to the level of middle valve develops from endoderm of preallantoic gut and below that from dorsal part of postallantoic gut (endodermal cloaca).

SINGLE BEST RESPONSE MCQs

1. **Which dermatome overlies the pubic symphysis?**
   A. T11 B. T12
   C. L1 D. L2
2. **Surgeon's guide to the base of vermiform appendix during surgery is:**
   A. Mesoappendix
   B. Anterior taenia coli of caecum
   C. Terminal ileum
   D. McBurney's point
3. **Which is the bilateral tributary of the IVC?**
   A. Hepatic B. Ovarian
   C. Suprarenal D. Renal
4. **The following part of pancreas develops from ventral pancreatic bud:**
   A. Accessory duct B. Entire main duct
   C. Upper part of head D. Lower part of head
5. **Which is not the posterior relation of the horizontal part of duodenum?**
   A. Inferior vena cava B. Abdominal aorta
   C. Right renal vessels D. Gonadal artery
6. **Lateral cutaneous branches of the following nerves enter the gluteal region:**
   A. T10 and T11
   B. Subcostal, ilioinguinal and iliohypogastric
   C. Subcostal and ilioinguinal
   D. Subcostal and iliohypogastric
7. **The following is true about splenic flexure:**
   A. Forms part of stomach bed
   B. Is derived from midgut
   C. Is located in transpyloric plane
   D. Is supplied by vagus nerve
8. **The anterior abdominal muscles actively contract in:**
   A. Normal expiration B. Forced expiration
   C. Forced inspiration D. Normal inspiration
9. **The following is true of the upper 15 mm of anal canal:**
   A. Lined with cuboidal epithelium
   B. Supplied with inferior rectal nerve
   C. Drained by superior rectal vein
   D. Develops from proctodeum
10. **The ureter lies along the following bony points, *except:***
    A. Tips of transverse processes of L2 to L5 vertebrae
    B. Ischial spine
    C. Sacroiliac joint
    D. Bodies of L2 to L5 vertebrae
11. **Which nerve is injured in a man who developed meralgia parasthetica after an operation on inguinal hernia?**
    A. Genitofemoral
    B. Lateral cutaneous nerve of thigh
    C. Iliohypogastric
    D. Ilioinguinal
12. **The vermiform appendix is characterized by:**
    A. Mesentery B. Sacculations
    C. Taenia coli D. Appendices epiploicae
13. **What is true about rectus abdominis muscle?**
    A. Tendinous insertion
    B. Fleshy origin
    C. Tendinous intersections on posterior aspect
    D. Flexor of vertebral column
14. **The part of the liver, where four layers of peritoneum are attached:**
    A. Porta hepatis
    B. Groove for IVC
    C. Fissure for ligamentum venosum
    D. Fissure for ligamentum teres
15. **Which vessel is not a content of the spermatic cord?**
    A. Testicular artery
    B. Testicular vein
    C. Artery to vas deferens
    D. Cremasteric artery
16. **The rectum begins in front of the following vertebra:**
    A. S2 B. S3
    C. S4 D. S5
17. **The anal canal develops from:**
    A. Preallantoic hindgut and proctodeum
    B. Allantois and urogenital sinus
    C. Postallantoic hindgut only
    D. Postallantoic hindgut and proctodeum

18. The part of the spleen that comes in contact with the lesser sac:
- **A.** Gastric area
- **B.** Renal area
- **C.** Hilum
- **D.** Intermediate margin

19. The transpyloric plane corresponds to the following, *except:*
- **A.** Upper part of the hilum of right kidney
- **B.** Origin of inferior mesenteric artery
- **C.** Lower end of spinal cord
- **D.** Fundus of gallbladder

20. Which forms the medial boundary of cystohepatic triangle?
- **A.** Porta hepatis
- **B.** Cystic duct
- **C.** Common hepatic duct
- **D.** Right branch of hepatic artery

Key for Single Best Response MCQs

1 C	2 B	3 D	4 D	5 C	7 A	8 B
9 C	10 D	11 B	12 A	13 D	14 C	15 B
16 B	17 D	18 C	19 B	20 C		

MULTIPLE RESPONSE MCQs (TRUE OR FALSE)

1. Morison's hepatorenal pouch is:
- **A.** Right anterior intraperitoneal space
- **B.** The most dependent space in supine position
- **C.** Right posterior intraperitoneal space
- **D.** Located posterior to inferior surface of liver

2. Metanephros:
- **A.** Is the permanent kidney
- **B.** Develops in pelvis
- **C.** Mesonephric duct forms its nephrons
- **D.** Nephrogenesis stops before birth

3. Traube's space:
- **A.** Is tympanic to percussion
- **B.** Overlies the fundus of stomach
- **C.** Bounded inferiorly by transverse colon
- **D.** Is obliterated in splenomegaly

4. The Meckel's diverticulum:
- **A.** Is a remnant of vitellointestinal duct
- **B.** Attached to jejunum 60 cm proximal to ileocaecal junction
- **C.** Also known as diverticulum ilei
- **D.** Occurs in 2 percent of population

5. Thoracolumbar fascia:
- **A.** Consists of three layers
- **B.** Quadratus lumborum is enclosed between anterior and middle layers
- **C.** Gives origin to quadratus lumborum muscle
- **D.** Medial attachment of anterior layer is to spines of lumbar vertebrae

6. The external oblique aponeurosis:
- **A.** Forms anterior wall of inguinal canal
- **B.** Prolongs as external spermatic fascia at deep ring
- **C.** Interfoveolar ligament is its extension
- **D.** Forms anterior wall of rectus sheath

7. Gastric canal:
- **A.** Located along greater curvature of stomach
- **B.** Produced due to absence of longitudinal folds
- **C.** Prone to ulceration
- **D.** Known as gastric magenstrasse

8. Portal vein:
- **A.** Is located in front of IVC
- **B.** Is formed behind the head of pancreas
- **C.** Inferior mesenteric vein is its indirect tributary
- **D.** Develops from "figure of 8" anastomosis

9. The rectus sheath:
- **A.** Inferior epigastric artery enters the sheath at arcuate line
- **B.** Arcuate line is a feature of its posterior wall
- **C.** Lower six intercostal nerves are its content
- **D.** Iliohypogastric nerve is its content

10. The embryonic midgut:
- **A.** Is connected to yolk sac
- **B.** Herniates into umbilical cord
- **C.** Caecum develops from its prearterial segment
- **D.** Undergoes 90° rotation in umbilical coelom

147 Lumbar Fascia

The **lumbar fascia** (thoracolumbar fascia) is the deep fascia of lumbar region on the back between the iliac crest and the last rib. It is divisible into three layers, the posterior, middle and anterior (Fig. 147.1).

Posterior Layer

a. Medially, it is attached to the tips of spines of the lumbar vertebrae and the supraspinous ligaments.
b. Above, it is continuous with the deep fascia on the posterior thoracic wall.
c. Below, it is continuous with the deep fascia over the sacral region.
d. Laterally, it fuses with the middle layer along the lateral margin of erector spinae.

Middle Layer

a. Medially, it is attached, to the tips of transverse processes of lumbar vertebrae.
b Above, it is attached to the lower border of the twelfth rib.
c. Below, it is attached to the posterior part of the iliac crest.
d. Laterally, it fuses with the posterior layer along the lateral margin of the erector spinae muscle.

Anterior Layer

a. Medially, it is attached to the middle of the anterior surface of transverse processes of lumbar vertebrae.
b. Above, it is attached to the lower border of twelfth rib.
c. Below, it is attached to the iliolumbar ligament and iliac crest.
d. Laterally, it fuses with the middle and posterior layers, lateral to quadratus lumborum muscle.

The special relations of anterior layer are as follows: It is located immediately behind the posterior surface of

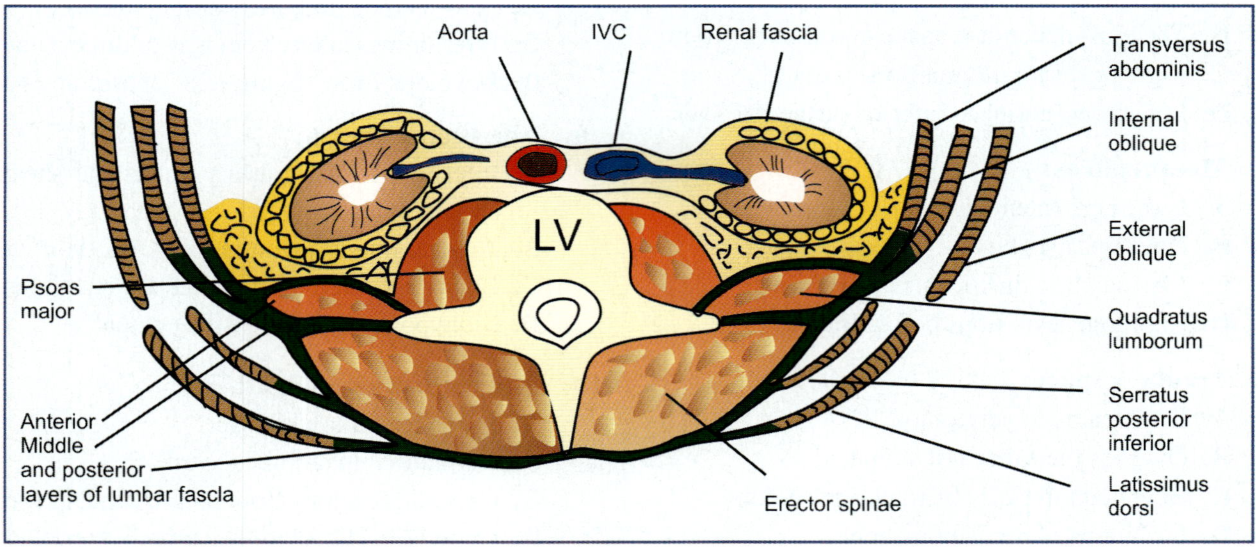

Fig. 147.1: Vertebral attachments of layers of lumbar fascia and muscles enclosed in them as well as muscles originating from them

the kidney. Its upper margin is thickened to form the lateral arcuate ligament, which extends from the front of the transverse process of first lumbar vertebra to the last rib. The quadratus lumborum muscle lies between the anterior and middle layers of lumbar fascia. The subcostal nerve and vessels, iliohypogastric and ilioinguinal nerves pass between the quadratus lumborum muscle and the anterior layer of lumbar fascia.

Muscles Attached to Lumbar Fascia

The posterior layer gives origin to the latissimus dorsi and serratus posterior inferior muscles. The lateral margin of the fused layers of the fascia gives origin to transversus abdominis and internal oblique muscles. The upper margin of the anterior layer (lateral arcuate ligament) gives origin to the diaphragm.

148 Muscles of Posterior Abdominal Wall

Quadratus Lumborum (Fig. 148.1)

The quadratus lumborum is the most lateral muscle of the posterior abdominal wall. It extends between the iliac crest and the twelfth rib. The muscle arises from the iliolumbar ligament, adjacent part of the iliac crest and second to fourth lumbar transverse processes. It is inserted into the anterior aspect of the medial part of the twelfth rib and into the upper four lumbar transverse processes posterior to its own slips of origin.

Nerve Supply

The muscle receives nerve supply from the direct branches of the ventral rami of upper lumbar nerves and subcostal nerve.

Relations

The relations of quadratus lumborum are important during surgery on kidney by lumbar route. The muscle is enclosed within the anterior and middle layers of thoracolumbar fascia. It is related anteriorly to the posterior surface of the kidney. The subcostal nerve and vessels and ilioinguinal and iliohypogastric nerves are in close relation to the anterior surface of the muscle.

Actions

The quadratus lumborum helps in inspiration by fixing the twelfth rib in lower position, when the diaphragm contracts. Acting singly, the muscle is a lateral flexor of lumbar vertebral column. Acting together, the muscles extend the lumbar vertebral column.

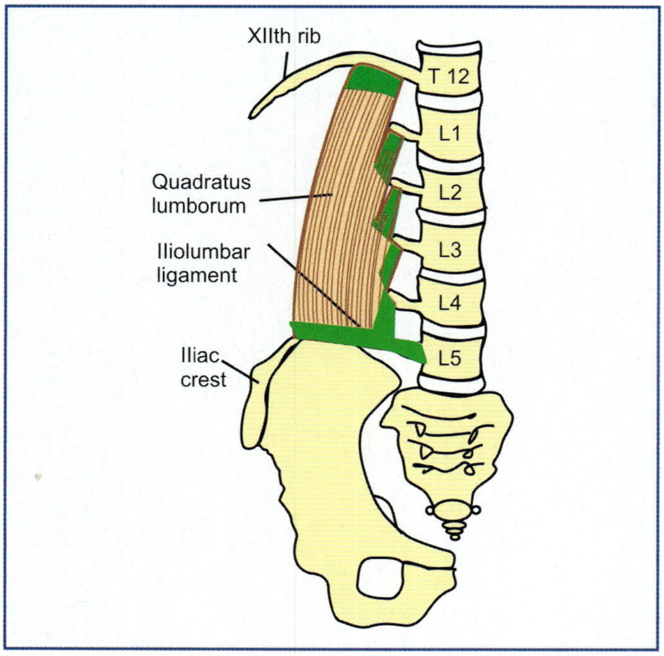

Fig. 148.1: Showing attachments of quadratus lumborum

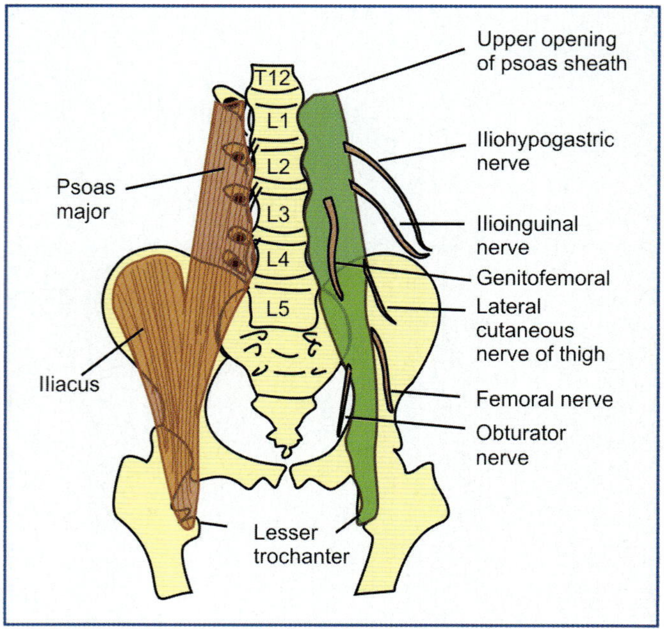

Fig. 148.2: Attachments of iliopsoas (Note: The psoas sheath on left side and the branches of lumbar plexus emerging from it)

Psoas Major (Fig. 148.2)

This muscle is located on posterior abdominal wall and in the femoral triangle.

Origin

It has a wide origin from the anterior surfaces of medial parts of transverse processes of all lumbar vertebrae, sides of bodies of all lumbar vertebrae and of twelfth thoracic vertebra, intervertebral discs between twelfth thoracic and fifth lumbar vertebrae and the tendinous arches between adjacent bodies of lumbar vertebrae.

Insertion

It is inserted by a tendon on the lesser trochanter of femur along with the iliacus.

(Psoas minor muscle, if present lies anterior to the psoas major and is confined to abdomen only. It has a common origin with psoas major from the twelfth thoracic and first lumbar vertebrae and is inserted into the iliopubic eminence.)

Nerve Supply

The psoas major is supplied by the ventral rami of upper four lumbar spinal nerves and minor is supplied by first lumbar ventral ramus.

Relations of Psoas Major in Abdomen

As the lumbar plexus is located in the substance of the psoas major, the branches of the plexus emerge from the muscle as shown in Figure 148.2. The iliohypogastric, ilioinguinal, lateral cutaneous nerve of thigh and the femoral nerve emerge from its lateral margin. The genitofemoral nerve emerges from its anterior surface and the obturator nerve and accessory obturator nerve (if present) emerge from its medial margin.

The psoas major muscle is enclosed in the psoas sheath, which is open only at its upper end. The upper margin of the psoas sheath is thickened to form medial arcuate ligament, which gives origin to muscle fibers of diaphragm.

Relations in Femoral Triangle

The psoas major lies in the floor of the femoral triangle, where it is related anteriorly to the femoral artery. Posteriorly, it is related to the capsule of hip joint with a large psoas bursa intervening between them (Fig. 189.2). The pectineus and femoral vein are related medially and the femoral nerve and iliacus are related laterally.

Actions

a. Main action along with iliacus is flexion of hip joint.
b. Since its insertion is lateral to the axis of rotation, which passes through the head of femur, it is medial rotator of the hip joint.
c. The muscles help in flexion of the trunk as in getting up from the supine position.
d. The action of the psoas in fracture of the neck of femur is noteworthy. It rotates the thigh laterally because the axis of rotation passes through the shaft of femur (medial to the insertion of psoas).

Testing Function of Psoas Major

In the sitting position, with lower limb at right angles to the trunk, the subject is asked to lift the limb (flexion at the hip is tested).

Clinical Highlights

a. The right psoas major muscle is related to the retrocaecal vermiform appendix. An inflamed appendix causes spasm of psoas major muscle. So, to reduce pain the patient keeps the right thigh in the flexed and medially rotated position. This anatomical relation is the basis of psoas test in appendicitis. In this test, on asking the patient to extend the thigh pain is experienced due to the stretch on the muscle.
b. Psoas abscess is accumulation of pus inside the psoas sheath. Since the sheath opens superiorly in the posterior mediastinum, pus from tuberculous thoracic vertebrae can enter it giving rise to abscess, which may track down along the sheath and appear as a swelling in the groin.

Iliacus Muscle (Fig. 148.2)

The iliacus is a triangular muscle that arises mainly from the floor of iliac fossa and also from the lateral part of the sacrum. The iliacus and psoas major muscles have a common insertion at lesser trochanter of femur. The abdominal part of the muscle is covered with fascia iliaca. This fascia merges medially with psoas sheath and is attached to the iliopectineal eminence. Inferiorly, it is attached to the inguinal ligament and is fused with the fascia transversalis. However, in the region of the femoral vessels the fascia iliaca forms the posterior wall of the femoral sheath. The caecum is related to the anterior surface of right iliacus while the descending colon is related to the left iliacus.

Actions

The iliacus flexes the trunk and the hip joint along with the psoas major muscle.

Nerve Supply

The femoral nerve supplies the muscle in the iliac fossa.

149 Lumbar Plexus

The lumbar plexus of nerves is formed on the posterior abdominal wall in the substance of psoas major muscle (Fig. 148.2). The lumbar plexus is formed from the upper three and the upper part of the fourth lumbar ventral rami. The lower part of the fourth and the fifth rami unite to form the lumbosacral trunk, which takes part in the sacral plexus. The ventral ramus of fourth lumbar nerve bifurcates to take part in the lumbar plexus and in formation of lumbosacral trunk. Hence, it is called the nervus furcalis. All the ventral rami receive gray rami communicantes (GRC) carrying postganglionic fibers from the sympathetic ganglia. The ventral rami of the first and the second lumbar nerves are connected to the sympathetic ganglia by white rami communicantes (WRC), which carry preganglionic fibers to the sympathetic chain from the spinal cord.

Formation

The ventral ramus of the first lumbar nerve receives a twig from ventral ramus of twelfth thoracic nerve and divides into upper larger division and lower smaller division. The upper division bifurcates to give rise to the iliohypogastric and ilioinguinal nerves. The lower division unites with a branch from the second lumbar ventral ramus to form the genitofemoral nerve. The second, third and fourth ventral rami divide into dorsal and ventral divisions. The dorsal divisions of second and third give off smaller branches, which unite to form the lateral cutaneous nerve of thigh. The remaining parts of the dorsal divisions of second and third and the entire dorsal division of fourth unite to form femoral nerve. All the three ventral divisions unite to form obturator nerve. Accessory obturator nerve, if present, receives fibers from the third and fourth ventral divisions. In addition to the aforementioned six branches, the lumbar plexus gives direct muscular branches to the quadratus lumborum, psoas major and minor muscles.

Iliohypogastric and Ilioinguinal Nerves

The iliohypogastric and ilioinguinal nerves (L1) come out of the lateral margin of psoas major muscle and then, descend laterally on the front of quadratus lumborum. They enter the neurovascular plane of the anterior abdominal wall at the lateral border of quadratus lumborum muscle. Their further course and distribution are described with the Anterior Abdominal Wall in Chapter 127.

Genitofemoral Nerve

The genitofemoral nerve (L1, L2) emerges from the anterior surface of the psoas major muscle. It pierces the psoas sheath and then ends by dividing in genital and femoral branches at a variable distance above the inguinal ligament. The genital branch enters the deep inguinal ring in the fascia transversalis and traverses the inguinal canal to come out through the superficial inguinal ring. It supplies the cremaster muscle and is sensory to the scrotal skin in male and skin of mons pubis and labium majus in female. The femoral branch descends posterior to the inguinal ligament and enters the femoral sheath lateral to the femoral artery. It pierces the anterior wall of the sheath and fascia lata to supply the skin of the upper part of femoral triangle.

Lateral Cutaneous Nerve of Thigh

The lateral cutaneous nerve of thigh is also known as the lateral femoral cutaneous nerve. It emerges from the lateral margin of psoas major muscle and descends on the iliacus muscle. In the iliac fossa, it is posterior to the lower part of descending colon on left side and caecum on the right side. It enters the thigh by passing behind or through the lateral end of inguinal ligament. At this site, the nerve is vulnerable to compression, which may give rise to a condition called meralgia parasthetica. The nerve is distributed to the skin of the anterolateral surface of the thigh.

Obturator Nerve

The obturator nerve (L2, L3, L4) takes origin from the ventral divisions of ventral rami of lumbar second to the fourth spinal nerves. It has abdominal and intrapelvic course before it reaches the obturator foramen, through which it enters the medial compartment of the thigh. The obturator nerve is the only nerve that emerges from the medial border of the psoas muscle. It enters the true pelvis behind the common iliac vessels and in front of the sacroiliac joint. In its intrapelvic course, the nerve travels forwards on the medial surface of the obturator internus along the lateral wall of the true pelvis. The obturator vessels accompany the obturator nerve lying below it. At the obturator foramen, the nerve terminates into anterior and posterior divisions. The relation of the obturator nerve to the ovarian fossa deserves special mention. The lateral surface of the ovary is in contact with the parietal peritoneum of ovarian fossa. The obturator nerve and vessels are retroperitoneal structures in this location. Inflammation of ovary may produce localized peritonitis in the ovarian fossa and consequent irritation of the obturator nerve. The patient may experience pain along the medial side of thigh and knee. The course and distribution of the obturator nerve in the thigh is described in Chapter 184.

Accessory Obturator Nerve

In some subjects, an accessory obturator nerve (L2, L3) is present. It descends along the medial margin of psoas major muscle and follows the external iliac vessels. It passes behind the inguinal ligament to enter the thigh and supplies the pectineus and the hip joint. It may communicate with anterior division of obturator nerve in the thigh.

Femoral Nerve

The main distribution of the femoral nerve (L2, L3, L4) is to the lower limb. But, its origin is on the posterior abdominal wall in the substance of psoas muscle from dorsal divisions of ventral rami of second to fourth lumbar nerves. The nerve emerges from the lateral border of psoas major a little distance above the inguinal ligament. At this position it is located between the iliacus laterally and psoas major medially. It supplies branches to iliacus muscle and enters the femoral triangle behind the inguinal ligament. For its course and distribution in thigh, refer to Chapter 180.

150 Suprarenal Gland

The suprarenal or the adrenal gland is located in close proximity to the superomedial part of each kidney, on the posterior abdominal wall. The suprarenal and kidney are enclosed in a common fascial sheath called the renal fascia. However, they occupy separate compartments inside the fascial sheath.

Parts

The suprarenal gland is composed of an outer cortex and an inner medulla, which are developmentally, structurally and functionally distinct from each other. Hence, the cortex and medulla are regarded as two separate endocrine glands.

Development

The cortex of the suprarenal gland is mesodermal and medulla is neuroectodermal. The cortex develops from the proliferation of coelomic epithelium on either side of the root of dorsal mesentery on the dorsal body wall of the embryo. The medulla develops from the cells of neural crest, which invade the coelomic epithelium. The fetal suprarenal gland is characterized by 2 types of cortex. The definitive cortex is limited to the subcapsular cortical cells. The fetal cortex comprises the main mass of the cortex. Within two weeks of birth, the involution of fetal cortex is completed. The subcapsular cells proliferate and differentiate to form three zones of the definitive cortex. Accessory suprarenal tissue may be found around the main gland, in greater omentum, or in broad ligament of uterus. In the female fetus, the hyperplasia of cortex leads to excess of androgens, due to which the external genitalia resemble that of male (female pseudohermaphroditism). In the male fetus, the cortical hyperplasia causes excessive development of external genitalia.

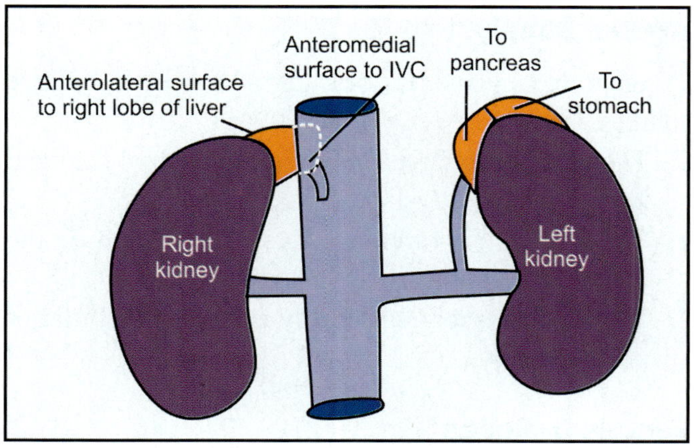

Fig. 150.1: Anterior relations of suprarenal glands (Note that short right suprarenal vein drains into IVC and long left vein into left renal vein)

Weight and Shape

Each gland weighs about 4 to 5 gm and measures 50 × 30 × 10 mm. The right and left suprarenal glands differ in shape. The right gland is an irregular tetrahedron and the left gland is of semilunar or crescentic shape.

Relations of Suprarenal (Fig. 150.1)

a. The right gland has three borders (anterior, medial and lateral) and three surfaces (anteromedial, anterolateral and posterior), a base and an apex. The anterior border bears a hilum nearer the apex. A very short and wide right suprarenal vein leaves the hilum to open in the inferior vena cava immediately after its exit. The anteromedial surface is related to the inferior vena cava and the anterolateral surface is related to the right lobe of liver. The upper part of this surface is in direct contact with bare area of liver while the lower part is related to visceral surface of right lobe. The posterior surface is divided in upper and lower portions

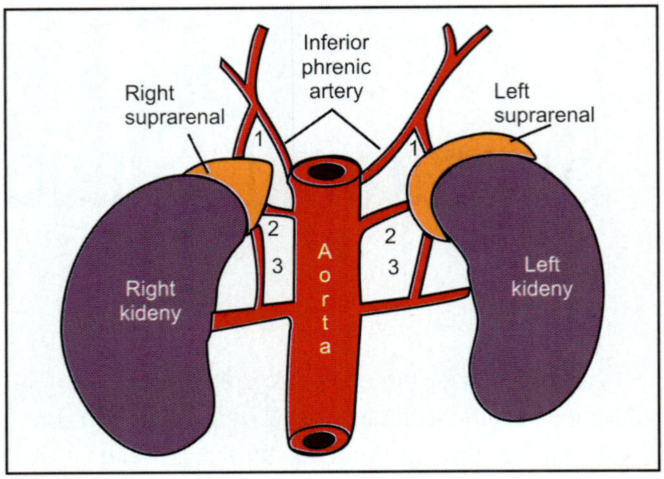

Fig. 150.2: Arterial supply of suprarenal gland (Note: The origin of suprarenal arteries: 1–superior, 2–middle 3– inferior)

for the diaphragm and the upper pole of right kidney respectively.

b. The left gland has anterior and posterior surfaces, lateral and medial borders and upper and lower poles. The anterior surface bears the hilum nearer the lower end. The hilum gives exit to the left suprarenal vein, which, is longer than but as wide as the right suprarenal vein. The upper part of the anterior surface is related to the posterior aspect of cardiac end of the stomach and the lower part to the body of pancreas with splenic vessels. The left suprarenal gland forms a part of the stomach bed. The posterior surface is in contact with the left crus of diaphragm medially and medial margin and adjacent upper pole of left kidney laterally.

Hormones of Suprarenal Cortex

The suprarenal cortex is divisible in three zones, which secrete three different hormones. The zona glomerulosa secretes mineralocorticoids or aldosterone responsible for maintenance of water and electrolyte balance. The zona fasciculata secretes glucocorticoids responsible for maintenance of carbohydrate balance and immune mechanism. The zona reticularis secretes androgens and other sex steroids. The cortex is essential to life. Its complete removal is fatal without replacement therapy.

Clinical Highlights

a. Deficiency of aldosterone leads to Addison's disease.

b. Adrenal hyperplasia with excessive aldosterone secretion results in Conn's syndrome, which is characterized by hypertension, edema due to sodium and water retention and hypokalemia.

c. Adrenal hyperplasia with excessive secretion of sex steroids leads to feminization of male and masculanization of female. Adrenal hyperplasia with excessive glucocorticoid secretion leads to Cushing's syndrome. The clinical features of this syndrome consist of, moon-shaped face, hirsutism, acne, hypertension, central distribution of fat, weakness and wasting of limbs and purple skin striae.

Hormones of Suprarenal Medulla

The medulla consists of chromaffin cells or pheochromocytes, which are the modified sympathetic ganglion cells. They synapse with the preganglionic sympathetic fibers and secrete epinephrine and norepinephrine in blood circulation. Under normal conditions very small quantity of the hormones is released but under stress situations the output is increased.

Clinical Highlights

Pheochromocytoma is the tumor of adrenal medulla, which causes excessive secretion of catecholamines in blood circulation. Typically, this produces paroxysms of palpitation, perspiration, pallor, headache and hypertension. The excretory product of catecholamines is vaniyll-mandelic acid (VMA). Elevation of VMA in urine confirms the diagnosis of pheochromocytoma.

Arterial Supply (Fig. 150.2)

The suprarenal gland receives arterial supply from three sources.

a. The inferior suprarenal artery is a branch of the renal artery.

b. The middle suprarenal artery is a branch of the abdominal aorta.

c. The superior suprarenal artery is a branch of inferior phrenic artery.

Venous Drainage (Fig. 150.1)

Only one vein emerges from the hilum of the suprarenal gland. The right suprarenal vein is extremely short. As soon as it emerges from the hilum on the anterior border, it opens in the IVC. This may pose difficulty during surgical removal of the right suprarenal gland. The left suprarenal vein is longer. It emerges from the hilum on the anterior surface and opens in the left renal vein. The surgical removal of left suprarenal gland is easier because the identification and clamping of the left suprarenal vein is easy.

Nerve Supply

The postganglionic sympathetic innervation to cortex and medulla is vasomotor in function. But, the medulla receives preganglionic sympathetic fibers from the greater and lesser splanchnic nerves via the suprarenal plexus, which is the extension coeliac plexus. The preganglionic fibers make synaptic contacts with each and every chromaffin cell.

151 Development of Urinary Organs

The urinary organs consist of kidneys, ureters, urinary bladder and urethra. Following is the account of the development and anomalies of kidney, ureter and urinary bladder. The development of urethra is described along with development of the external genitalia in Chapter 170.

Development of Kidney

The kidney develops from intermediate mesoderm of the embryo. In the fourth week of intrauterine life, bilateral nephrogenic cords (extending from the cervical to the sacral region) develop in the intermediate mesoderm, on the posterior abdominal wall. Three different kidney systems, the pronephros, mesonephros and the metanephros (permanent kidney) appear in succession in the nephrogenic cord (Fig. 151.1). Thus, kidney development is an example of ontogeny repeats phylogeny.

Pronephros

In the human embryo, the pronephros is rudimentary. It appears in the cervical part of the nephrogenic cord as 7 to 10 solid cell clusters, which regress completely by the end of fourth week. The pronephrenic duct develops but the tubules do not open into it.

Mesonephros

The mesonephric kidney comprises of mesonephric tubules and mesonephric duct (Wolffian duct). About 70 to 80 mesonephric tubules develop in the thoracolumbar part of the nephogenic cord. These tubules are more differentiated and are functional in the human embryo during 6-8 weeks. After the take over of the pronephric duct by the mesonephros, it is renamed as the mesonephric or the Wolffian duct. The right and left ducts open caudally in the urogenital sinus. After eight weeks, the mesonephric tubules begin to regress. However, a few mesonephric tubules are utilized in the formation of vasa efferentia in the male.

Common Derivatives of Wolffian Ducts in Male and Female

a. Ureteric bud arises from the caudal part of the Wolffian or mesonephric duct. Its cranial end forms the entire

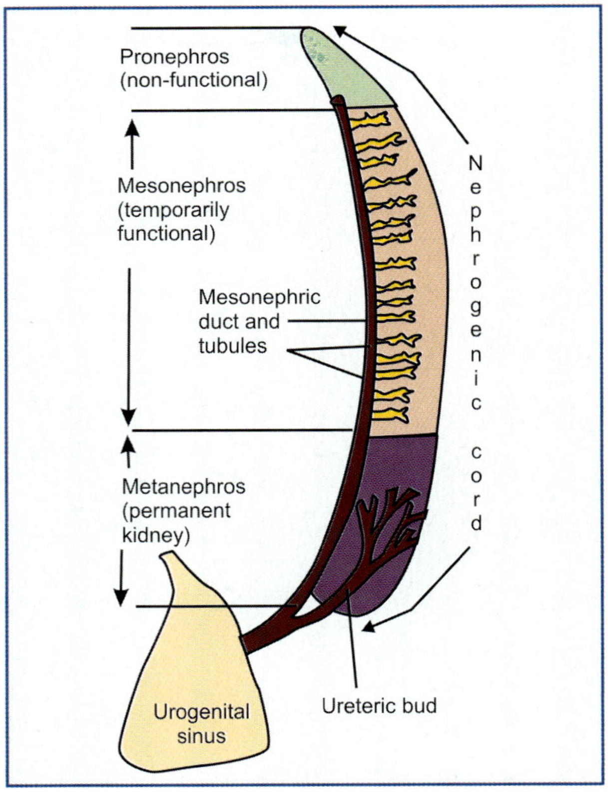

Fig. 151.1: Stages in development of permanent kidney (Note that metanephros and ureteric bud are developmental sources of this kidney)

collecting part of the metanephric kidney, which includes pelvis, calyces and all the collecting ducts. The rest of the bud becomes the ureter.

b. Caudal to the origin of the ureteric bud, the Wolffian duct of each side is absorbed in the urogenital sinus to form the trigone of the urinary bladder.

Metanephros or Permanent Kidney

The nephrogenic cord in the sacral region becomes condensed to form the metanephric blastema, which is invaded by the ureteric bud in the fifth week. Thus, the permanent kidney develops from two sources (Fig. 151.1). The nephrons develop from the metanephric blastema and the collecting part from the ureteric bud.

a. The collecting system develops from the ureteric bud, which undergoes dichotomous divisions in the metanephric blastema. This pattern of divisions continues till about 13 to 15 generations of branches are formed. The dilated upper end of the bud forms the pelvis of kidney. Its first division transforms in to the major calyces. The subsequent 2 to 4 generations are fused to form minor calyces. Its further divisions give rise to all the collecting ducts and collecting tubules. However, the contribution of branches of the ureteric bud to the formation of pelvis and calyces may be variable.

b. The process of development of nephrons is called nephrogenesis. The growing tip of each of the divisions of the ureteric bud becomes dilated to form ampulla. The metanephric tissue condenses around the ampulla (under its inductive influence) and gives rise to the nephron in a sequence. At first, a solid clump of metanephric cells is converted in a circular metanephric vesicle with a lumen. With growth, the vesicle becomes pear-shaped and later the S-shaped tube. One end of this tube is invaginated by the tuft of capillaries. The rest of the tube differentiates in PCT, loop of Henle and DCT. The crucial stage in nephrogenesis is to establish the luminal continuity between the developing nephron and the collecting tubule. The process of nephrogenesis is continued for some time in the postnatal life. The fetal kidney is lobulated.

Ascent and Rotation of Kidney

The kidney undergoes ascent and rotation during development. The metanephric kidney is a pelvic organ. Therefore, the kidney must ascend to gain its definitive position in the lumbar region. This is achieved by the differential growth of the body wall. With each new position on the body wall, a new artery, which is higher in location supplies the kidney. This is a physiological necessity because a direct branch from the aorta maintains a high-pressure head in the glomerular capillaries. To begin with, the hilum of the kidney faces anteriorly. As development progresses, the kidney undergoes 90° rotation in medial direction so that the hilum comes to face medially.

Function of Fetal Kidney

The fetal kidney becomes functional at the end of first trimester. Urine is passed in the amniotic cavity and mixes with the amniotic fluid, which is swallowed by the fetus. From the intestinal tract the fluid is absorbed in the blood and brought back to the kidneys. The fetal kidneys do not excrete the waste products like the adult kidney since the placenta is the excretory organ. However, the fetal kidneys are believed to play some role in the regulation of volume of the amniotic fluid. In cases of renal agenesis, volume of the amniotic fluid is small.

Congenital Anomalies

a. Agenesis of kidney can be unilateral or bilateral. The bilateral agenesis is incompatible with life. Unilateral kidney undergoes compensatory hypertrophy, so, a person can live a normal life.

b. Lobulated kidney means the retention of fetal lobulation in postnatal life. After birth, the growth of nephrons and connective tissue smoothens the kidney surface. So, the cause of the lobulated kidney is failure of postnatal growth in the kidney.

c. Pelvic kidney is an unascended kidney. It receives arterial supply from the common iliac or internal iliac artery. Pelvic kidney has a short ureter.
d. Crossed renal ectopia is a condition in which both kidneys are located on one side. The kidneys may be fused or separate.
e. Malrotated kidney is the one in which the hilum faces anteriorly or laterally.
f. Horseshoe kidney is caused by fusion of lower poles of the two kidneys by means of an isthmus. The inferior mesenteric artery arrests the ascent of the horseshoe kidney. This anomaly gives rise to urinary obstruction because the ureters cross in front of the isthmus.
g. The aberrant renal artery usually is due to failure of one of the lower arteries to regress as the kidney ascends. The aberrant artery entering the lower pole may cause compression of pelviureteric junction producing hydronephrosis. Sometimes, the aberrant artery is the sole supply of one vascular segment of the kidney.
h. In congenital hydronephrosis, there is dilatation of pelvis and calyces due to obstruction to the outflow of urine. The common reasons for congenital obstruction are the pinhole external meatus and valves and folds in the urethra.
i. Congenital polycystic kidney is an inherited disorder and almost always bilateral. There is failure in establishing luminal continuity between the nephrons and collecting tubules. The glomeruli continue to function and the filtrate accumulates in the tubules for lack of outlet. Thus, the tubules show cystic enlargement.

Development of Ureter

The ureter develops from the ureteric bud given off from the caudal end of the mesonephric duct. The congenital anomalies of the ureter are, its partial or complete duplication, congenital hydroureter due to obstruction to lower end of ureter and the postcaval ureter in which the right ureter lies behind the IVC instead of to its right.

Development of Urinary Bladder

The special feature of the transitional epithelium lining the urinary bladder is that it develops from 2 germ layers. The epithelium of the trigone is derived from mesoderm of the absorbed parts of mesonephric ducts and that of the rest of the bladder from the endoderm of the vesico-urethral canal of the urogenital sinus (Fig. 151.2). The urogenital sinus is continuous cranially with the allantois, which is a diverticulum projecting from the cranial end of the sinus into the umbilical cord. After birth, the allantois atrophies and turns into a fibrous band called urachus, which extends from the apex of the bladder to the umbilicus. The allantois is important because of the congenital anomalies related to it.

(Early in embryonic life the endodermal cloaca is divided in ventral urogenital sinus and dorsal hindgut by the formation of urorectal septum. The urogenital sinus is

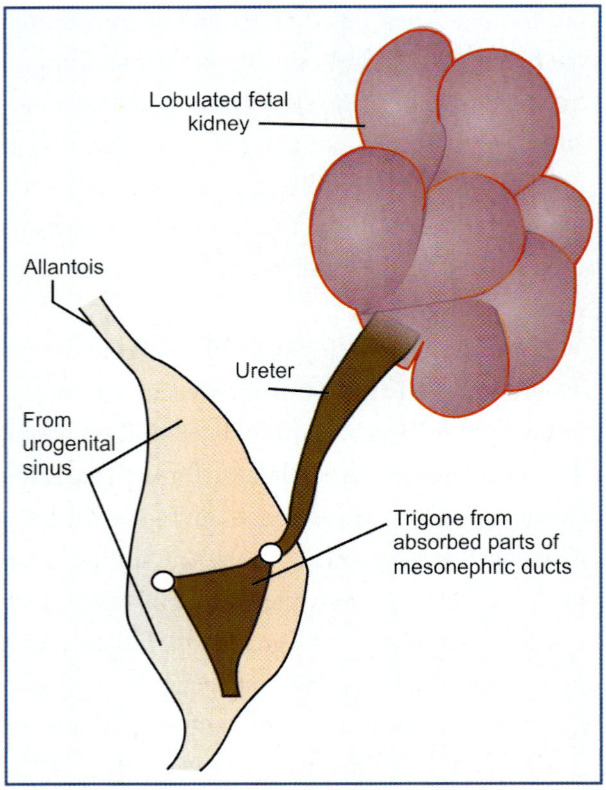

Fig. 151.2: Developmental sources of urinary bladder (Note: Endoderm and mesoderm contribute to development of bladder mucosa)

so named because it gives rise to parts of both urinary and genital tracts. The sinus is divisible in cranial part called vesicourethral canal [since it gives rise to urinary bladder and urethra] and the definitive sinus, which is further divided in upper pelvic part and lower phallic part.)

Congenital Anomalies of Urinary Bladder

a. Ectopia vesicae is the condition in which the infraumbilical abdominal wall and the anterior wall of bladder are deficient. As a result, the trigone of the bladder is exposed to the surface.
b. Congenital vesicovaginal or rectovesical fistula occurs due to incomplete septation of endodermal cloaca by defective urorectal septum.
c. Urachal cyst occurs due to partial patency of allantois.
d. Umbilical urinary fistula occurs due to complete patency of urachus.

152 Kidney

The kidneys function as the primary organs of excretion. They are reddish brown in color and present a smooth and glistening appearance in the living.

Measurements

Each kidney, in adult, measures about 11 to 12 cm in length, 6 cm in breadth and 3 cm in thickness. Its weight ranges from 130 to 170 gm.

Position

Each kidney is located on the posterior abdominal wall in the paravertebral gutter. It is retroperitoneal. The position of the kidney varies with respiration and the posture of the body. The upper extent of the right kidney approximately, corresponds to the twelfth rib and that of left kidney to the eleventh rib. The transpyloric plane passes through the lower part of the hilum of the left kidney and upper part of the hilum of the right kidney. This difference is on account of the fact that the massive liver pushes the right kidney slightly downwards.

Surfaces and Borders (Fig. 152.1)

Each kidney has two poles, two surfaces and two borders. The bulge of the vertebral column and the adjacent psoas major muscle affect the orientation of the kidney. The longitudinal axis of the kidney runs obliquely downward and laterally and hence the upper pole is situated 2.5 cm and the lower pole 7.5 cm away from the midline. The transverse axis of the kidney runs laterally and backwards, hence its medial border faces slightly anteriorly. The anterior surface faces anterolaterally and posterior surface posteromedially. The lateral border of the kidney is smoothly convex while the concave medial border shows the depression of hilum at its middle. The hilum gives passage to the renal vessels and the pelvis of the ureter. It is situated five cm away from the midline. The relations of the structures at the hilum in anteroposterior order are, renal vein, renal artery and renal pelvis. If the renal artery divides at the hilum, into its two main divisions then the order of the structures at the hilum from before backwards is, renal vein, anterior division of artery, renal pelvis and posterior division of artery.

Surface Marking (Fig. 152.1)

The kidneys can be marked on the anterior and posterior aspects of the trunk. The point to note while marking the width of the kidney is that on the surface of the body, the projected width is reduced compared to its actual width due to the obliquity of the transverse axis of the kidney. Hence, in the surface drawings of the kidney the width is taken as 4.5 cm.

a. In the anterior surface marking, the center of the hilum is marked on the transpyloric plane 5 cm from the midline and slightly medial to the tip of ninth costal

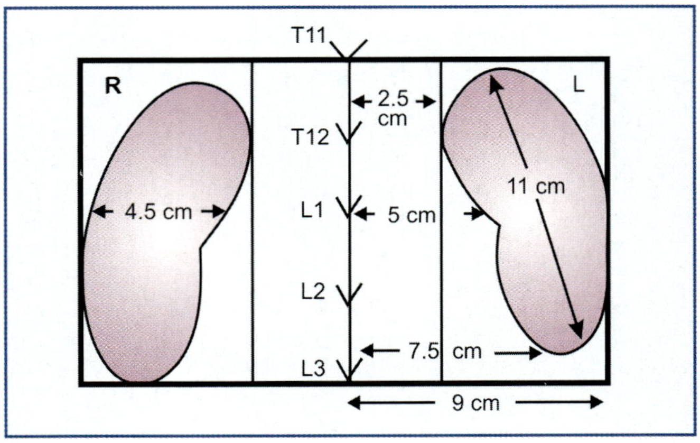

Fig. 152.1: Morris' parallelogram illustrating surface marking of kidney on the back

cartilage (left hilum, just above the transpyloric plane and right just below it). In relation to the hilum, an outline of the kidney (length of 11 cm and breadth of 4.5 cm) is drawn. The upper pole of the outline is drawn 2.5 cm away and the lower pole 7.5 cm from the midline.

b. On the posterior surface of the trunk, a quadrilateral or parallelogram is drawn (named after Morris) in which the outline of the kidney is mapped. Two points are marked at the level of eleventh thoracic spine situated 2.5 cm and 9 cm away from the midline. Two more points are marked at the level of third lumbar spine same distances away from the midline. On joining these points, we get a quadrilateral space. The medial margin of the kidney is represented by a line joining three points as follows, first point 2.5 cm away from midline (at T11 on left and T12 on right), second point (at L1) 5 cm away and third (at L3) 7.5 cm away from the midline. Join the upper and lower points at a distance of 4.5 cm, which is the width of the kidney, to mark the convex lateral border.

Renal Angle

It is an angle between the lower margin of twelfth rib and lateral margin of erector spinae muscle. At this angle, the kidney lies close to the body surface. The following points about the renal angle are clinically relevant.

i. Renal pain is usually felt at the renal angle as a dull ache.
ii. The perinephric abscess causes swelling and tenderness at the renal angle.
iii. The lower border of pleura runs horizontally, crossing the twelfth rib at the lateral margin of erector spinae muscle. Hence, the upper end of the skin incision for approaching the kidney by the lumbar route should begin below the renal angle. Any upward extension of the incision will injure the pleura.

Coverings (Fig. 152.2)

Each kidney has four coverings. From within outward, they are, true capsule (fibrous capsule), fatty capsule (perinephric fat), fascial capsule (false capsule, renal fascia or fascia of Gerota) and paranephric fat.

a. The true capsule is mainly composed of collagen fibers, a few elastic fibers and smooth muscle fibers. In a healthy kidney, the true capsule is easily stripped off and it gives the shining appearance to the kidney. The capsule becomes adherent in renal disease.
b. The fatty capsule is traversed by a number of fibrous strands connecting the true and false capsules.
c. The fascial capsule (fascia of Gerota) forms a common covering to the kidney and the suprarenal gland. Its anterior layer is called fascia of Toldt and posterior layer is called fascia of Zuckerkandl. On horizontal tracing (Fig. 147.1), laterally, these layers meet and fuse along the lateral border of kidney to become continuous with the transversalis fascia. Medially, the anterior layer passes in front of the renal vessels and becomes continuous with the anterior layer of the opposite side in front of the abdominal aorta and inferior vena cava while the posterior layer blends with the psoas fascia and is attached to the bodies of the lumbar vertebrae. On vertical tracing, the fascial layers fuse above the suprarenal gland and become continuous with the diaphragmatic fascia. Inferiorly, fascial layers continue downwards along the ureter and merge with the fascia iliaca. Thus, the fascial capsule is open inferiorly. In nephroptosis, the kidney descends to a very low level through the lower opening. The renal

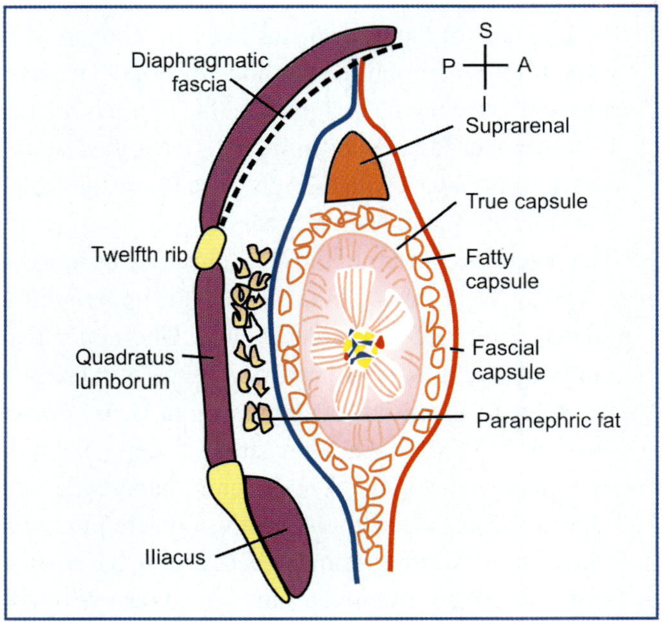

Fig. 152.2: Schematic diagram to depict the coverings of kidney (Note that the fascial capsule is open inferiorly)

Section four

vessels alone form the support of such a displaced kidney. This may cause kinking of ureter and urinary obstruction. The perinephric abscess collects in the space between the true and fascial capsules. It tends to descend along the periureteral sheath downwards and may reach pelvic cavity.

d. The paranephric fat, which is part of the retroperitoneal fat, lies outside the false capsule and is abundant on the posterior aspect.

Supports of Kidney

The kidney moves minimally with regular breathing. But, on deep inspiration it descends vertically by about 2 to 2.5 cm. The factors that maintain the kidney in position are the fatty capsule, fascial capsule and the renal vessels. If the fatty capsule is entirely absent, the weight of the kidney is borne by the renal pedicle and hence the kidney tends to fall down, which is known as nephroptosis (floating kidney).

Relations of Kidney

The relations of the anterior surface are different on the right and left sides but the posterior relations are similar.

a. The anterior relations on the right side, are as follows (Fig. 152.3). The superior pole and the adjacent part of medial border are in relation to the right suprarenal. A large area of the anterior surface is in contact with renal impression on the right lobe of liver. The area adjacent to the medial margin near the hilum is related to descending part of duodenum. Inferiorly, the anterior surface is in contact with the right colic flexure, laterally and coils of small intestine, medially.

b. The anterior relations of the left kidney are as follows (Fig. 152.3). A small medial area on the upper pole is related to the left suprarenal gland. The upper two thirds of lateral half of anterior surface is related to the spleen. A central rectangular area is in contact with body of pancreas and splenic vein. A small triangular area bounded by splenic, pancreatic and suprarenal areas is in contact with stomach. This area takes part in forming stomach bed. Below the splenic area, the narrow lateral margin is in contact with left colic flexure and beginning of descending colon. Below

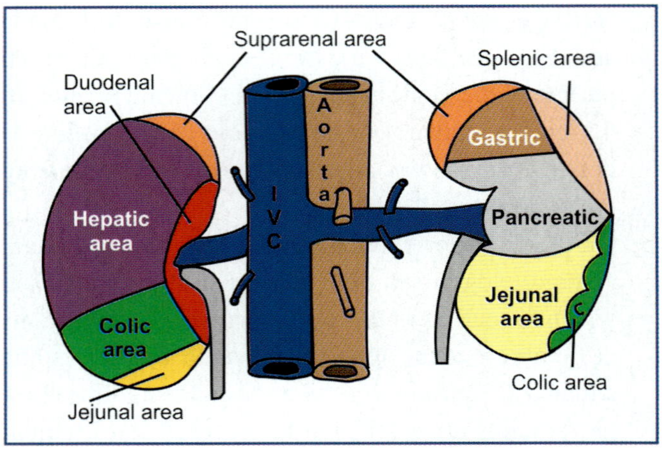

Fig. 152.3: Visceral relations of anterior surface of right and left kidneys

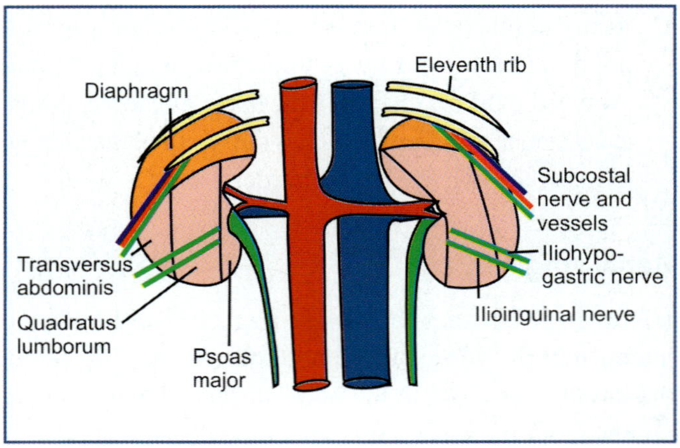

Fig. 152.4: Posterior relations of the kidneys

the pancreatic area, an extensive area is in contact with doudenojejunal flexure and beginning coils of small intestine.

c. The posterior relations of both the kidneys are similar (Fig. 152.4). The upper part is related to the diaphragm. The right kidney is related to twelfth ribs while left kidney is in relation to the eleventh and twelfth ribs. Below the twelfth rib, the posterior surface is related from medial to lateral, to the psoas major, quadratus lumborum and the transversus abdominis muscles. Between the quadratus lumborum and the posterior surface of kidney, the subcostal nerve and vessels, iliohypogastric and ilioinguinal nerves pass inferolaterally.

Gross Appearance of a Kidney Section (Fig. 152.5)

The kidney substance is composed of outer cortex and inner medulla. The sinus of the kidney is a large area lateral to the hilum and surrounded by the kidney substance. The walls of the sinus are lined with the continuation of the capsule in the interior. The sinus contains the branches of renal artery, accompanying veins, major and minor calyces, pelvis of kidney, nerve plexuses and fatty tissue. The cortex is pale and granular while the medulla is dark and striated in appearance. The cortex is composed of about a million or more nephrons per kidney. The medulla consists of about 6-12 pyramids, but this number is variable. The cortical tissue that extends in between the adjacent pyramids in the medulla is known as renal columns. The apex of each pyramid extends in the minor calyx as a small projection called the renal papilla. The pyramid is composed of collecting ducts and the apparatus for concentration of urine. The base of the pyramid is directed toward the cortex. The cortical area that caps the base of a pyramid is called the cortical arch. This unit of cortical arch and adjacent pyramid is called the renal lobe. The renal calyces are of two orders, greater or major and lesser or minor. Calyx is the Latin word for glass or cup. The minor calyces receive the papillae of the pyramids. One minor calyx may receive one papilla or more than one. Therefore, the number of the pyramids need not coincide with the number of minor calyces, which is very variable. There is a structural continuity between the papilla and the minor calyx. The major calyces are less in number, usually 2 to 3 and are formed by fusion of minor calyces. The major calyces unite to form the pelvis of kidney. The combined volume of the pelvis and calyces is nearly 8 ml. This fact has to be borne in mind while injecting radio-opaque material through the ureter to outline these spaces. Excess of the material may tear the sites of continuity between the minor calyces and renal papillae.

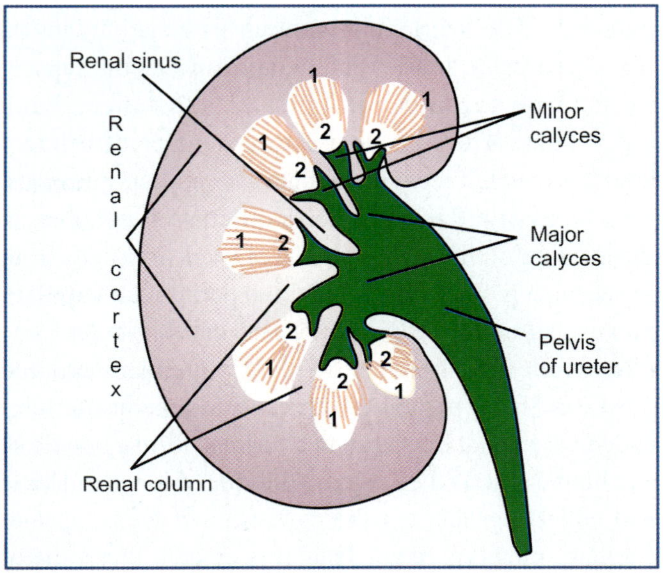

Fig. 152.5: Coronal section of kidney to depict its gross features 1–Pyramids, 2–Papillae (Note that collectively pyramids form the medulla and papillae are apical parts of pyramids)

Microstructure and Functional Correlation

The cortex consists of nephrons, which are the structural and functional units of the kidney. The nephrons consist of four parts, renal corpuscle, proximal convoluted tubule (PCT), loop of Henle and distal convoluted tubule (DCT). The renal corpuscles are concerned with filtration of blood and the other parts of the nephrons are concerned with selective resorption from the glomerular filtrate. The renal corpuscle consists of central glomerulus (lobulated tuft of capillaries) and Bowman's capsule, which is the blind expanded end of the nephron. The endothelium of the glomerular capillaries is fenestrated. The glomerulus invaginates in the Bowman's capsule, as a result of which the latter is divided in a parietal layer and a visceral (glomerular) layer enclosing a capsular space. The visceral layer closely invests the capillary endothelium. The cells of the visceral layer are called podocytes since they are attached to the basal lamina by numerous pedicles. The filtration barrier between capillary lumen and the capsular space is composed of, endothelial cells, fused basement membranes of the endothelial cells and podocytes and discontinuous footplates of the podocytes. The PCT begins at the lower end of the renal corpuscle and is lined by simple columnar or tall cuboidal cells. The apical aspects of the cells present striated or brush border, which is made of microvilli. The basal aspects of the cells show infoldings of the plasma membrane and plenty of mitochondria. All these structural features are indicative of the active functional status of the cells of

PCT. The PCT helps in absorption of water, sodium and potassium, glucose and amino acids from the glomerular filtrate back in the peritubular capillaries. The loop of Henle begins as the continuation of PCT and extends in the medulla. The simple squamous cells line the descending limb of the Henle's loop. There is passive ionic transfer across these cells. The ascending loop of Henle is lined by cuboidal cells, which help in transfer of the chloride and sodium from the tubules into the medulla. The countercurrent multiplier system in the ascending and descending limbs of the loop of Henle builds up high concentration of sodium and chloride in medullary interstitial spaces. The countercurrent exchange system between the vasa recta, which run parallel to the Henle's loops, help to conserve the high osmotic pressure in medulla. The distal convoluted tubules (DCT) are located in the cortex. Their lining epithelium is of low cuboidal type without microvilli. The water absorption from DCT is under the influence of antidiuretic hormone. Thus, the isotonic filtrate is passed on to the collecting tubules, which while passing through the high osmotic pressure in the interstitial spaces of medulla, let out more water in to the medulla so that finally the urine becomes hypertonic.

Juxtaglomerular (JG) Complex

The juxtaglomerular complex consists of three parts, macula densa of DCT, juxtaglomerular cells of afferent arteriole and the mesangial cells of glomerulus. Each glomerulus has a vascular pole consisting of an afferent arteriole and an efferent arteriole. At its beginning, each distal convoluted tubule is very close to the afferent arteriole. The lining cells of the adjacent walls of the DCT and the afferent arteriole show structural changes. The modified cells of the DCT in this location have secretory granules and are called macula densa. The adjacent smooth muscles of the afferent arteriole undergo epithelioid change, contain secretory granules and are called, the juxtaglomerular cells. The fluid pressure in the DCT activates the cells of macula densa to secrete some substances, which activate the JG cells to secrete renin. The renin has the property to convert angiotensinogen in the blood circulation to angiotensin I, which is changed to angiotensin II in pulmonary endothelial cells. The final effect is rise in blood pressure. The other function of JG cells is to produce erythropoietin. So, the JG complex plays a role in regulation of blood pressure and production of RBCs.

Arterial Supply

The renal arteries bring a large volume of blood to the kidneys. The renal arteries are the direct branches of abdominal aorta. In majority of cases, the renal arteries alone supply the blood to kidneys but in a few cases, accessory renal arteries in addition to the normal renal arteries are present. Each renal artery divides into an anterior and posterior division near the hilum. The primary branches of these divisions are segmental arteries, which are the end arteries and supply renal vascular segments. The anterior division passes in front of the renal pelvis and subdivides into four segmental arteries. The posterior division passes behind the pelvis and is continued as a segmental artery. However, the origin of segmental arteries may be variable. As the segmental arteries travel in the renal sinus they divide into lobar arteries, which further divide into interlobar arteries. These arteries pass through the renal columns in the medulla. At the corticomedullary junction, each interlobar artery divides into arcuate arteries, which arch over the bases of adjacent pyramids. The interlobular arteries arise at right angles from the arcuate arteries and radiate towards the capsule by passing through the cortical substance. Each interlobular artery gives rise to a number of afferent arterioles, which feed the glomerular capillary plexuses. Two types of efferent arterioles originate depending on the location of the nephrons. The efferent arterioles from the cortical glomeruli break up into peritubular capillary plexuses around the proximal and distal tubules. The efferent arterioles from juxtamedullary glomeruli proceed downward in the pyramid and break into straight arterioles called vasa recta. The straight arterioles form a bundle of smaller vessels as they pass by the side of loops of Henle and collecting ducts in the pyramid and break up into capillary plexuses there. Thus it is evident that a major part of renal blood circulates through the cortex while the medulla is dependent for its blood supply on the efferent arterioles of juxtamedullary glomeruli.

Venous Drainage

Interlobular veins drain the peritubular plexuses in the cortex, which drain in succession in arcuate, interlobular, interlobar, segmental and lastly in renal vein. The right and left renal veins open into the IVC.

Special Features of Renal Circulation

a. The renal arteries are large compared to the size of the kidneys and are the direct branches of aorta so as to maintain higher pressure in them.
b. The intrarenal branching of the renal artery, at all levels, is usually at right angles to ensure high pressure in the arterial tree.
c. The glomerular capillary plexus (filtration apparatus) is unique because it is the only capillary plexus in the body, which is fed by an arteriole and drained by an arteriole and moreover the efferent arteriole is narrower in diameter than the afferent. This specialization is necessary to maintain high hydrostatic pressure in the glomerular capillaries.
d. Efferent arterioles in kidney are unique because they begin in capillaries and end in capillaries.
e. Two types of circulation operate in the kidney (Fig. 152.6) due to different behavior of the efferent arterioles of cortical and juxtamedullary glomeruli. The larger circulation operates in the cortex and is concerned with filtration of blood. The smaller circulation operates in medulla and is responsible for the concentration of urine by a very complicated mechanism.
f. Percentage of toxic substances like urea is more in the renal artery than in the corresponding vein.
g. Stenotic or occluded renal artery may cause systemic hypertension because diminished arterial supply stimulates the production of renin, which is the precursor of angiotensin.

Vascular Segments (Fig. 152.7)

Based on the distribution of the five segmental arteries, each kidney is divided into five vascular segments, apical, upper anterior, middle anterior, lower and posterior segments. Apical segment occupies both anterior and posterior surfaces. The upper anterior segment is confined to the anterior surface only. The middle anterior segment is confined to the anterior surface only. The lower segment occupies the entire inferior pole and includes both anterior and posterior surfaces. The posterior segment occupies the posterior surface only (between the apical and lower segments). In summary, the apical and lower segments extend on both the surfaces of kidney. The segmental resection of kidney is possible if the disease is localized to one or more segments.

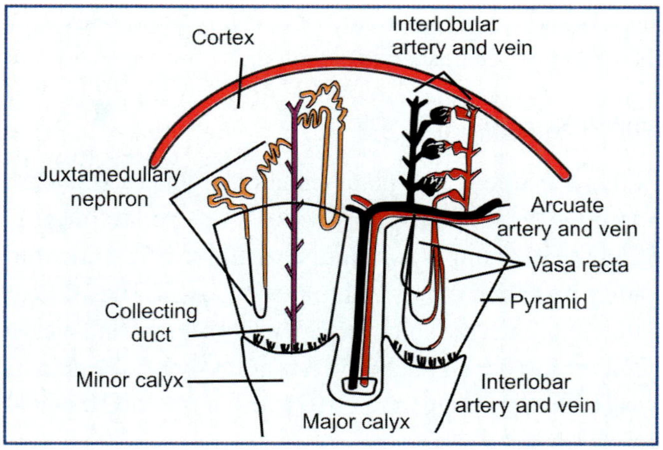

Fig. 152.6: Disposition of nephrons and blood vessels in cortex and medulla of kidney

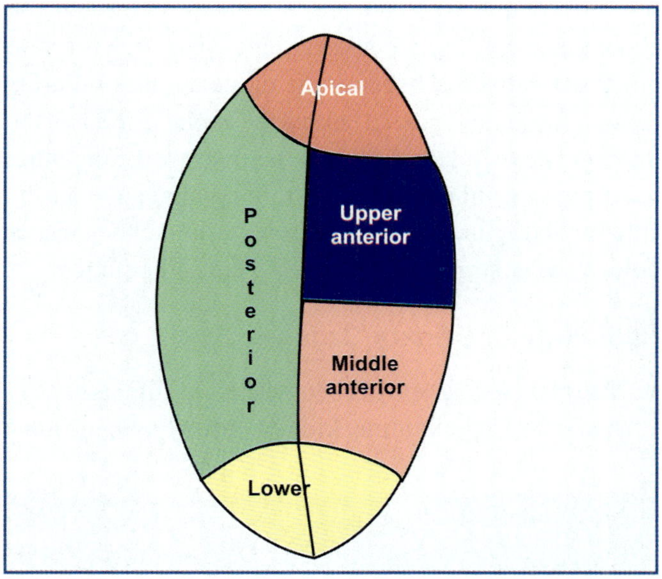

Fig. 152.7: Opened book view from the exterior showing vascular segments of right kidney (from lateral aspect)

Lymphatic Drainage

There are rich lymphatic plexuses in the substance of the kidney. The lymphatic vessels accompany the renal vessels and terminate in lateral aortic lymph nodes near the origin of renal arteries.

Nerve Supply

Both sympathetic and parasympathetic innervations are provided to the kidney through the renal plexus. Sympathetic supply is mainly vasomotor in function. Parasympathetic supply is through the vagus. The afferent pathways reach the spinal cord via least splanchnic nerve (T12) or lumbar splanchnic nerve (L1). Thus, the pain of renal or ureteric origin is referred to the lumbar and inguinal regions (loin to groin pain).

Palpation of Kidneys

It is not possible to palpate the normal kidney through the abdominal wall. The method of kidney palpation is called bimanual palpation because the clinician uses both the hands. One hand is placed behind the supine patient in the interval between lower rib and the iliac crest. The other hand presses simultaneously the lumbar region on the anterior abdominal wall. On deep inspiration, the inferior pole of the enlarged kidney is felt against the fingers.

Radiology of Urinary Organs

a. The plain radiograph of abdomen (KUB film) is usually inspected to examine kidney, ureter and urinary bladder. It is possible to detect the faint soft tissue shadow of kidney on plain radiograph.

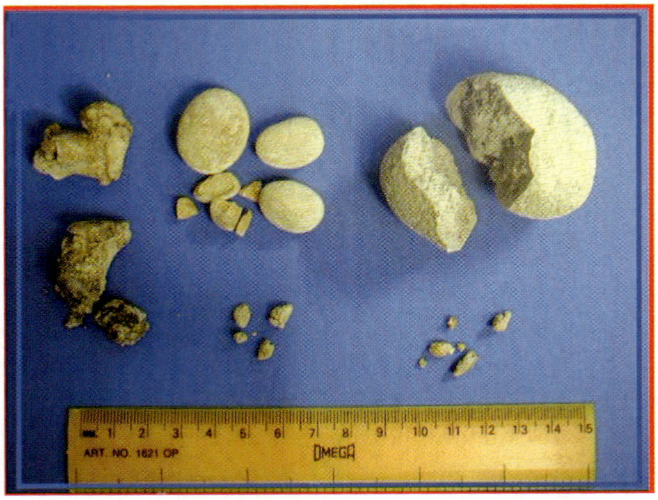

Fig. 152.8: Showing varieties of renal stones (staghorn, ureteric, bladder and passed stones (*Courtesy:* Personal collection of Dr. Fazil Maricker, Former Professor of Surgery, Medical College, Trivandrum)

b. The intravenous pyelography (IVP) consists of injecting the contrast material by the IV route. The patient is prepared for IVP as follows. To clear the bowel of gas, tablets of activated charcoal are given two days prior to the procedure and on the previous night, purgative is given to clear the bowel. Nothing is given orally for 6 to 8 hours before the procedure. The contrast agent (urograffin) is injected intravenously through median cubital or other superficial vein of the forearm. X-rays are taken at the interval of one, three, five, ten, fifteen and thirty minutes and postmicturition. The cupping of the minor calyces is distinctly visible in a normal kidney.

c. In retrograde pyelography, the contrast material is introduced in the ureter through a catheter. First a cystoscope is passed in urinary bladder through the urethra and then a catheter is passed through the cystoscope in the ureteric orifice in the urinary bladder. About 8 ml of dye is injected directly in the ureter and radiographs are taken.

d. Ultrasound, CT and MRI are useful techniques to study the morphology of the kidneys.

Clinical Highlights

a. The kidney is usually approached surgically through the lumbar region; the advantage being it is a retroperitoneal approach. For this approach, it is very essential to understand the posterior relations of kidney (Fig. 152.4) and the layers of lumbar fascia (Fig. 147.1).

b. Stone formation in kidney is a common cause of renal disease. Small stones pass out through urinary passages without causing symptoms. A very large stone occupying the renal calyces and pelvis is called staghorn stone. A larger stone if impacted in the ureter causes severe colicky pain. Stones are present in the urinary bladder also. Figure 152.8 shows different varieties of renal stones. Percutaneous removal of stones with the help of a nephroscope is possible. In another method, called extracorporeal shock wave lithotripsy (ESWL), an instrument called lithotriptor generates shock waves, which pass through body tissues and crush the stones to sand like particles, which are washed out through urinary passages.

c. The artificial kidney (hemodialysis) is used to maintain life in a patient with bilateral renal failure, for whom a suitable renal transplant is not available or possible. A subcutaneous arteriovenous fistula of Cimino between the radial artery and cephalic vein, at the wrist, is ideal for repeated vascular access. The patient's blood is drawn from the enlarged cephalic vein in the arterial line of the cannula to the kidney machine, where it comes in contact with a semipermeable membrane. This allows water, salts, and products of body's metabolism (urea) to diffuse freely but retains the blood cells and plasma proteins. The purified blood is returned to the cephalic vein through the venous line of the cannula.

153 Ureter

Each ureter is a thick muscular tube, which conveys urine from the renal pelvis to the urinary bladder. The ureter shows active peristaltic contractions, which are visible during surgical operation. The average length of the ureter is 25 cm and its diameter is 3 mm. It is retroperitoneal is position.

Extent

The ureter extends from the pelviureteric region to the urinary bladder. Normally, it is not possible to determine precisely the site of pelviureteric junction (where the renal pelvis ceases and the ureter begins). Usually, the pelviureteric region is extrahilar and lies adjacent to the lower part of medial border of the kidney. In subjects, where the entire renal pelvis is inside the renal sinus, the pelviureteric region is inside or at the hilum.

Parts

The ureter is divisible into two parts of equal lengths, abdominal and pelvic. The relations of abdominal part are different on the right and left sides while the relations of the pelvic parts are different in the male and female.

Constrictions (Fig. 153.1)

According to anatomical descriptions, the ureter shows narrowing, at pelviureteric region, at pelvic brim and in the wall of urinary bladder (intramural part). According to surgical descriptions, the ureter shows five constrictions, at pelviureteric junction, pelvic brim, where it is crossed by vas deferens in male (where it passes through a canal in the transverse ligament in the base of the broad ligament in female), intramural part and at the ureteric orifice. The renal stones tend to get impacted or pass slowly through these sites and produce ureteric colic. The pain of ureteric colic typically begins in loin and radiates to the groin. In the spasm of the intramural ureter, the pain radiates to external genitalia and anterior thigh.

Surface Marking

a. For the surface marking of ureter from the anterior aspect, join the tip of the ninth costal cartilage to the pubic tubercle.
b. For the surface marking of ureter from the posterior aspect, take a point about 4 cm lateral to the spine of L2 vertebra and join it to posterior superior iliac spine (indicated by the dimple).

Relations of Abdominal Part of Right Ureter

a. Anteriorly, the right ureter is related to the horizontal part of duodenum at the beginning. Below this, it is related to the right gonadal vessels followed by right

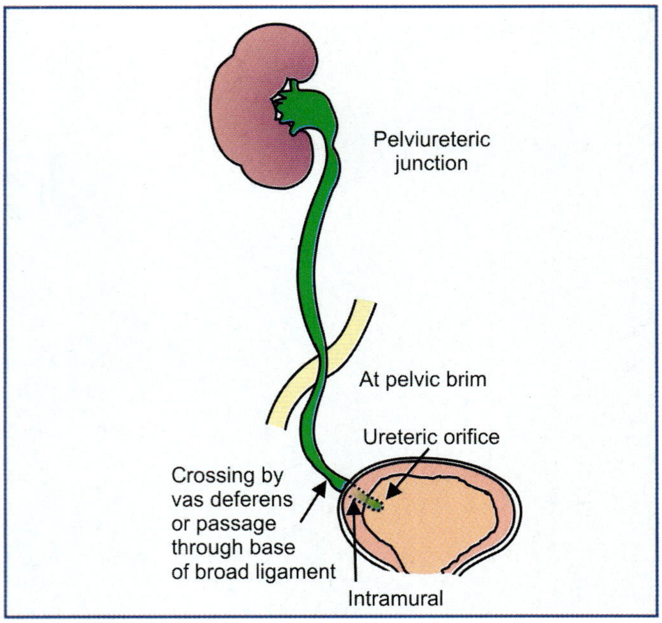

Fig. 153.1: Sites of constrictions of ureter

colic and iliocolic vessels. The root of the mesentery and coils of intestine are anterior to the lower part of the ureter.

b. On its left, it is in close relation to the inferior vena cava.
c. Posteriorly, the right ureter lies on the right psoas major muscle and the right genitofemoral nerve. At the pelvic brim, the ureter crosses in front of the bifurcation of right common iliac vessels.

Relations of Abdominal Part of Left Ureter

a. Anteriorly, the left ureter is mainly crossed by left gonadal, left colic and sigmoidal vessels. The sigmoid mesocolon lies anterior at its lower part.
b. Posteriorly, the ureter lies on the left psoas major muscle and left genitofemoral nerve. At the pelvic brim, the ureter crosses in front of the bifurcation of left common iliac vessels at the intersigmoid recess.

Pelvic Part of Ureter in Male

The pelvic part of ureter can be divided into two parts, namely, posterolateral (first part) and anteromedial (second part). The posterolateral part is in contact with lateral pelvic wall. It is related posteriorly, to the internal iliac vessels, lumbosacral trunk and sacroiliac joint, from before backwards. Anteriorly, it is covered with parietal peritoneum. Laterally, is related to the obliterated umbilical artery, obturator nerve and vessels, inferior vesical vessels and middle rectal vessels, from above downwards. The anteromedial or second part lies on the floor of the pelvic cavity. It is related superiorly, to the parietal peritoneum and inferiorly, to the levator ani muscle. Near its termination in the bladder, it is crossed by vas deferens anteriorly and is related to the upper end of the seminal vesicle.

Pelvic Part of Ureter in Female

The posterolateral or the first part is related posteriorly to the internal iliac vessels, lumbosacral trunk and sacroiliac joint. It is covered with parietal peritoneum anteriorly. It forms the posterior boundary of ovarian fossa and hence related to ovary and fimbriated end of uterine tube. In this position, the ureter is likely to be injured if clamped along with ovarian vessels in the infundibulopelvic ligament. Lateral to the ureter, are the obliterated umbilical artery, obturator nerve and vessels, uterine and vaginal arteries and middle rectal vessels from above downwards. The anteromedial or second part of the ureter lies in the extraperitoneal connective tissue along the lower margin of the broad ligament. Here, it pierces the transverse cervical ligament, in which it passes through the ureteric canal, which provides room for the peristaltic movements of the ureter. Uterine artery crosses the ureter in front from lateral to medial at a point nearly 2 to 2.5 cm from the cervix. The ureter is liable to be injured during surgery for removal of uterus as the ureter may be mistakenly clamped along with uterine vessels. Injury to the ureter may lead to extravasation of urine and peritonitis. Inferiorly, the ureter rests on the pelvic floor. Near its termination, the ureter is closely related to the lateral fornix of vagina and then lies on the anterior wall of the vagina.

Intravesical (Intramural) Part

The ureter has an oblique course in the wall of the urinary bladder. The ureteric openings are five cm apart in a distended bladder. The intramural part of the ureter is the narrowest. The oblique passage of the ureter prevents the reflux acting as a flap valve. The ureteric longitudinal muscle is continuous with trigonal muscle of bladder. When the ureteric stone is in the intramural ureter, the pain is felt in the tip of penis or clitoris.

Blood Supply

In view of its long course, several arteries supply the ureter. The arteries form longitudinal anastomoses on the wall of the ureter. The abdominal part of ureter receives twigs from renal artery, abdominal aorta and gonadal artery (from medially related arteries). As the ureter crosses the pelvic brim it receives twigs from common iliac and internal iliac arteries and inside the pelvis from the inferior vesical artery in male and uterine artery in female (from laterally related arteries). The veins correspond to the arteries.

Nerve Supply

Sympathetic innervation, to the upper part of ureter, is through the least splanchnic nerve from T12. Lumbar splanchnic nerve from L1 and L2 supplies the remaining part of abdominal and pelvic ureter through the abdominal autonomic plexuses. Parasympathetic supply is given from pelvic splanchnic nerve (S2 to S4), which reaches the ureter through the autonomic plexuses. Visceral afferents travel along the least splanchnic, lumbar splanchnic and pelvic splanchnic nerves. In distension of the renal pelvis, pain is referred to lumbar region. In distension of abdominal ureter, the pain is referred to inguinal and pubic regions (a typical loin to groin pain). In distension of pelvic ureter, the pain is referred to the perineum.

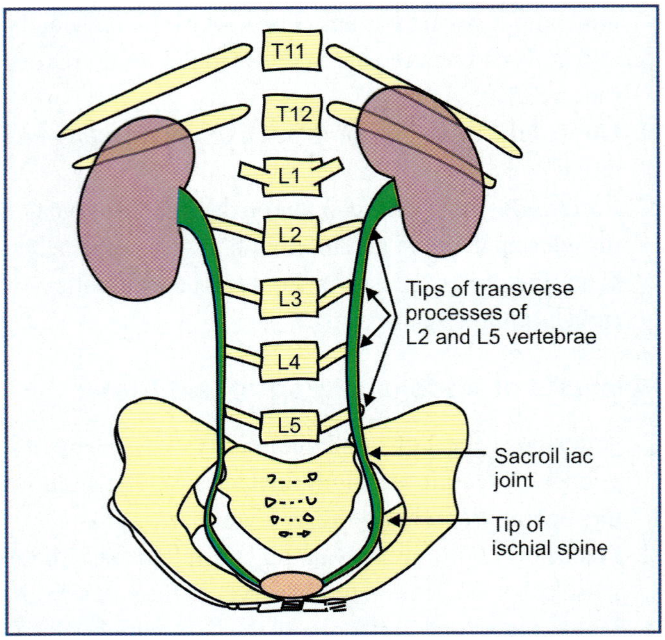

Fig. 153.2: Scheme to show skeletal relations of ureter

Skeletal Relations (Fig. 153.2)

Knowing the course of the ureter in relation to bony landmarks is clinically useful as this helps in identifying the course of the ureter in a plain X-ray of the abdomen and pelvis. The ureter starts at the tip of the transverse process of the second lumbar vertebra and then follows the line of the tips of the transverse processes of the remaining lumbar vertebrae. It crosses in front of the sacroiliac joint. It further courses slightly laterally along the anterior margin of the greater sciatic notch till it reaches the ischial spine. From here, it runs medially to enter the bladder about 1.5 to 2.5 cm from the midline. The positions of the ureteric constrictions can be located as follows. The first constriction at the pelviureteric junction lies at the tip of transverse process of the second lumbar vertebra. The second constriction at the pelvic brim overlies the sacroiliac joint. The third constriction lies medial to the tip of ischial spine. Thus, these bony landmarks help in locating a tiny stone in the ureter in the plain X-ray.

154 Urinary Bladder

The urinary bladder is a hollow muscular organ, which acts as a temporary reservoir of urine brought to it by the ureters. The stored urine is passed out through the urethra, when the bladder is distended enough to feel the desire to micturate.

Position

The position of the urinary bladder varies with age. At birth, the bladder is an abdominal organ, the internal urethral meatus being at the level of the upper border of symphysis pubis. The bladder starts descending at the age of 6 years and becomes a pelvic organ shortly after puberty, when the internal urethral meatus is just above the plane of the inferior margin of the symphysis pubis. In adult, the empty bladder is entirely in the pelvic cavity but a distended bladder rises in the abdominal cavity. The position of the empty bladder in the adult, is described as lying on the front part of pelvic floor, below the peritoneum and behind the pubic symphysis.

Shape and Capacity

The shape of the urinary bladder is described as tetrahedral when empty and globular or ovoid when distended. The capacity of the bladder varies from 120 to 250 ml. The maximum capacity is 500 ml, when tension builds up in the bladder wall and pain is experienced. The pain is referred to T11 to L2 and S2 to S4 dermatomes.

Surfaces, Borders and Angles (Fig. 154.1)

The urinary bladder has 4 triangular surfaces, 4 borders and 4 angles. The borders are, anterior, right and left lateral (inferolateral) and posterior. The base or fundus (or the posterior surface) is an inverted triangle with its narrow end pointed inferiorly and its broad end (posterior border) superiorly. The apex or anterior angle is the meeting point of superior and inferolateral surfaces. It gives attachment to the median umbilical ligament. The neck or inferior angle is the lowest and most fixed part of the bladder and is the meeting point of inferolateral surfaces and the narrow end of the posterior surface. The urethra begins at the neck. The right and left lateral angles are located at the meeting points of inferolateral, posterior and superior surfaces. This coincides with the lateral ends of the posterior border and the ureter opens at this angle on each side.

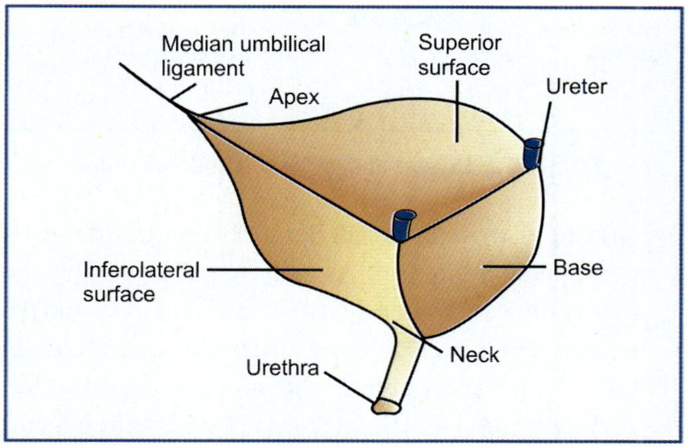

Fig. 154.1: Scheme to show tetrahedral shape of urinary bladder and its four surfaces

Relations in Male (Fig. 154.2)

a. The peritoneum covers the superior surface completely and is reflected from the upper part of the base on to the anterior surface of the rectum forming the rectovesical pouch of peritoneum. Anteriorly, the peritoneum is a reflected on the anterior abdominal wall. The superior surface is in relation to coils of small intestine and sigmoid colon. As the bladder rises

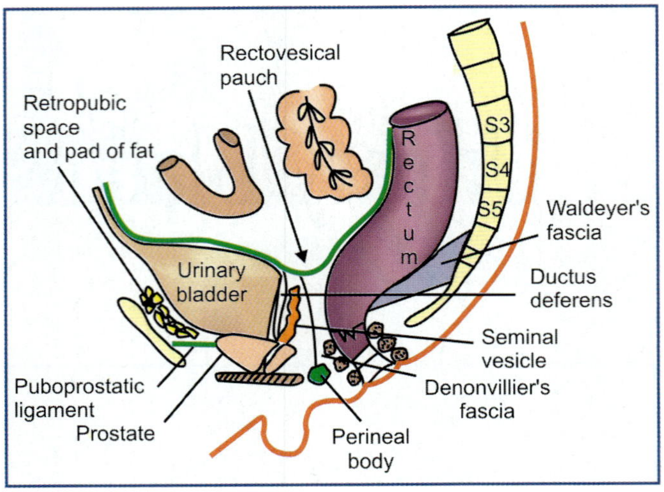

Fig. 154.2: Relations of urinary bladder in male

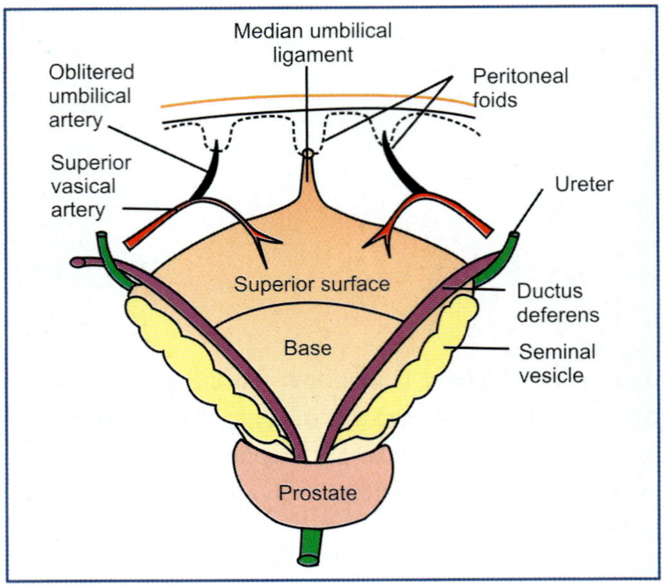

Fig. 154.3: Relations of the base of urinary bladder in male

with the distension, its superior surface and the covering peritoneum are raised. As a consequence of this, the anterior line of peritoneal reflection is lifted up and the peritoneum is peeled off the infraumbilical abdominal wall. In this way, more and more of inferolateral surfaces come in direct contact with the anterior abdominal wall. So, an extraperitoneal approach for suprapubic cystotomy (making an opening in the urinary bladder) is possible if the bladder is distended.

b. The inferolateral surfaces face downwards and laterally and the anterior border intervenes between them. The retropubic space or cave of Retzius with its pad of fat separates them from the pelvic surface of pubis and puboprostatic ligaments. On a slight posterior plane, these surfaces are in contact with fascia covering the levator ani and obturator internus.

c. The base or the posterior surface has important relations. On either side, it is intimately related to the seminal vesicle and ductus deferens. A triangular area of the base bounded above, by the line of peritoneal reflection and on each side, by vas deferens, is called the external trigone (Fig. 154.3). The external trigone is closely related to the rectum, the only structure intervening between them is rectovesical or Denonvillier's fascia.

Relations in Female (Fig. 154.4)

a. The superior surface of the bladder is not completely covered with peritoneum. Anteriorly, the peritoneum is reflected on the anterior abdominal wall as in the case of male. Posteriorly, the peritoneum is reflected from the superior surface on to the isthmus of uterus and forms a shallow uterovesical pouch of peritoneum. The peritoneum covered superior surface is related to coils of small intestine, sigmoid colon and body of uterus. A small nonperitoneal posterior part of superior surface is in contact with the cervix of uterus.

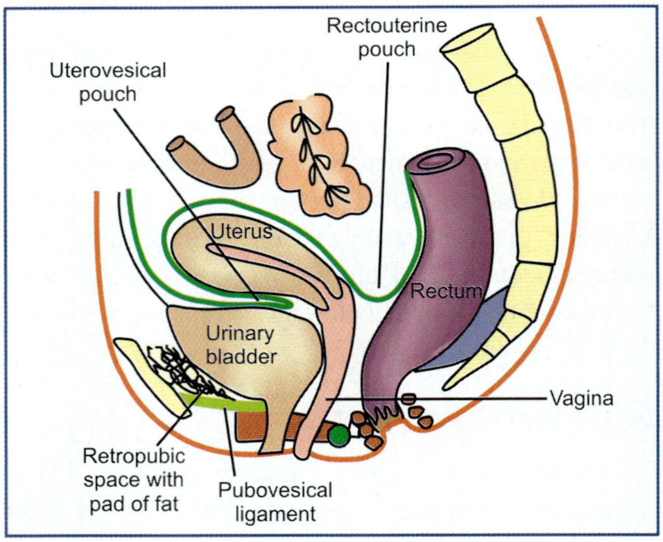

Fig. 154.4: Relations of urinary bladder in female (Note that superior surface of bladder is not fully covered with peritoneum)

b. The relations of the inferolateral surfaces are similar to those of male, except that in place of puboprostatic ligaments (in the floor of cave of Retzius) there are pubovesical ligaments in female.

c. The base or posterior surface is in direct contact with anterior wall of vagina.

Neck of the Bladder

The neck of the bladder alters very little with varying positions of the bladder or rectum. It is pierced by the internal urethral meatus. At the neck, the circular fibers of detrusor muscle show slight aggregation to form internal sphincter of the bladder. In male, the neck is in direct contact with the base of the prostate while in female it rests on the pelvic fascia.

Ligaments

The ligaments of the urinary bladder are divided into true and false. The true ligaments are the condensations of the pelvic fascia around the base and neck of the bladder or fibrous bands mixed with a few fibers of smooth muscles or the developmental remnants. The false ligaments are the peritoneal folds.

True Ligaments

a. The median umbilical ligament extends from the apex of the bladder to the umbilicus. It is the remnant of urachus.
b. The medial and lateral puboprostatic (male) or pubovesical (female) ligaments are composed of both smooth muscle fibers and condensation of pelvic fascia. The medial puboprostatic or pubovesical ligaments extend from the neck of bladder to the pubic symphysis while the lateral ligaments attach the neck to the anterior end of the tendinous arch of obturator fascia. The puboprostatic or pubovesical ligaments form the floor of cave of Retzius. These ligaments are of surgical importance because of their intimate relation to the vesical venous plexus. Hence, when they are divided, it is advisable to cut as laterally as possible and as close to the pubis as possible.
c. The lateral true ligaments are condensation of pelvic fascia and extend from the inferolateral surface to the tendinous arch.
d. The posterior true ligaments are condensations of the pelvic fascia. They attach the neck and the base of the bladder to the lateral pelvic wall along the internal iliac vein and contain the vesical venous plexus.

False Ligaments

a. The median umbilical fold is due to median umbilical ligament.
b. The medial umbilical folds are due obliterated umbilical arteries.
c. The lateral false ligaments are the reflections of peritoneum from the urinary bladder to the lateral pelvic wall.
d. The posterior false ligaments are the sacrogenital folds, which are the peritoneal folds from the sides of the bladder to the sacrum.

Interior

In the living, the mucous membrane of bladder is smooth and pale in color. It is very loosely attached to the submucosa hence is thrown up in folds, when the bladder is empty.

Internal Trigone (Fig. 154.5)

The internal trigone is a triangular area on the posterior surface of the interior, where the mucosa is pink in color and is firmly attached to the subjacent muscle layer (the submucosa being absent at the internal trigone). The internal trigone is shaped like an equilateral triangle. The interureteric ridge of Marcier, which is formed by fibers of the inner longitudinal muscle coat of the ureter, forms the upper margin of the trigone. The other two sides of the trigone are formed by uretero-urethral ridges, which are produced by the longitudinal muscle of ureter. The orifices of the ureters form the superolateral angles while the internal urethral orifice forms the inferior angle of the trigone. In the male, internal urethral orifice is guarded by an elevation of the trigone called uvula vesicae produced by the projection of the median lobe of the prostate. The hypertrophy of the median lobe blocks the internal urethral meatus causing retention of urine. The trigone differs from the rest of the bladder in being more vascular, more sensitive and being mesodermal in development. The calculi in the urinary bladder eroding

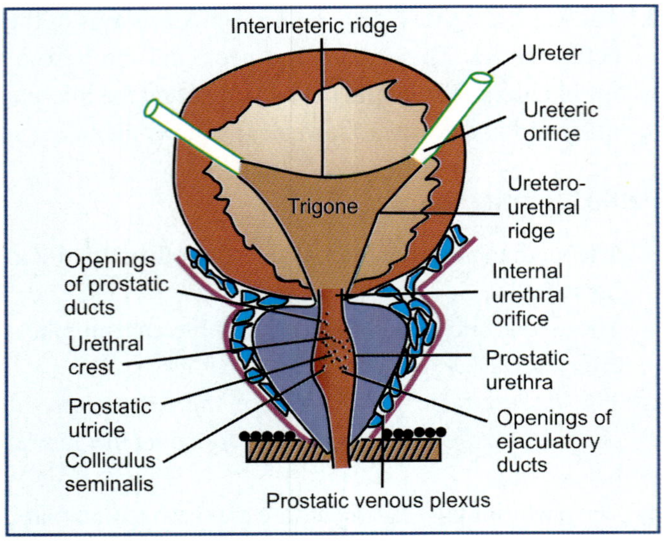

Fig. 154.5: Coronal section showing internal trigone of bladder and internal features of prostatic urethra

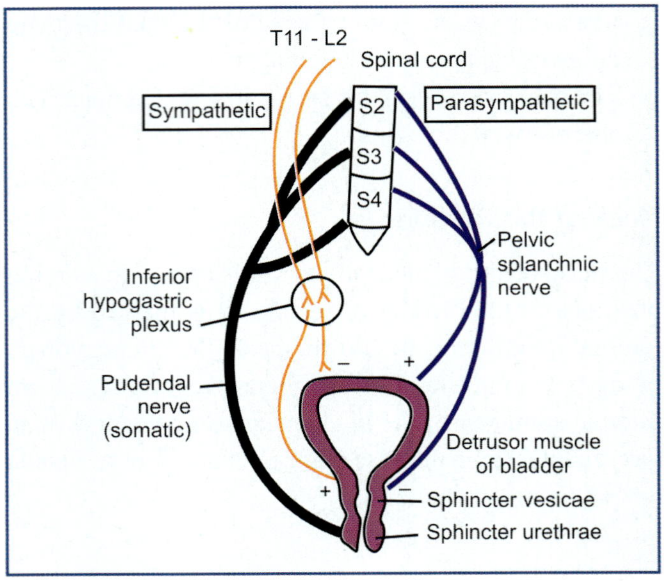

Fig. 154.6: Nerve supply of urinary bladder, sphincter vesicae and sphincter urethrae

the trigone and cancer involving the trigone are extremely painful. The pain from the trigone is referred to the perineum mainly to the tip of penis or clitoris.

Blood Supply

In the male, the urinary bladder receives branches mainly from the superior vesical and inferior vesical arteries. In addition, a few other sources of supply are obturator and inferior gluteal arteries. In the female, superior vesical arteries and the vaginal arteries (which replace the inferior vesical arteries in male) supply the bladder. Additional supply comes from uterine arteries. The venous drainage consists of a complicated plexus of veins lying on the inferolateral surfaces. These plexuses pass backwards along the posterior true ligaments to open in the internal iliac veins and are in communication with the internal vertebral venous plexus.

Lymphatic Drainage

The lymphatic vessels of the bladder leave it at various points but, all ultimately converge to the external iliac lymph nodes.

Nerve Supply (Fig. 154.6)

Both parasympathetic and sympathetic components of autonomic nerves supply the bladder through the vesical plexus of nerves.

a. The parasympathetic supply is via the pelvic splanchnic nerve or nervi erigentes (S2 to S4). These nerves terminate in the postganglionic neurons in the bladder wall. The postganglionic fibers are motor to the bladder. On stimulation, they cause contraction of the detrusor and relaxation of the internal sphincter. So, parasympathetic is described as "nerve of emptying or voiding."
b. The sympathetic fibers arise from lower thoracic and upper 2 lumbar segments of spinal cord. They reach the inferior hypogastric plexus, where synapse takes place and reach the bladder via the vesical plexus. It is regarded as mainly vasomotor. Its action on the detrusor is either inhibitory or it has no action on it but, it closes the internal sphincter. So, sympathetic efferent mainly acts on the muscle surrounding the bladder neck.
c. The afferent fibers from the bladder carry pain impulse from the mucosa and the sense of awareness of bladder filling. The pain impulse is carried by both parasympathetic and sympathetic nerves to the spinal cord via the posterior roots of the respective spinal nerves. The pain from the endodermal bladder is referred to the hypogastric region but that from the trigone, a mesodermal area is referred to the tip of the penis or clitoris. The pelvic splanchnic nerves carry the sensation

of awareness of bladder filling to the S2-S4 segments of the spinal cord. Therefore, the pelvic splanchnic nerves contain both the afferent and the efferent components of the micturition reflex, the center of the reflex arc being intermediolateral cells of S2-S4 spiral segments (spinal micturition center). The ventral horn cells of these segments control the voluntary component of the micturition through the nerve supply of the external urethral sphincter by the pudendal nerve (root value-S2, 3, 4). The spinal micturition center is governed by cortical micturition center in paracentral lobule. The pain fibers are carried in the anterior and lateral funiculi of spinal cord but the fibers subserving sensation of bladder fullness are carried in posterior funiculus.

Examination of Urinary Bladder

a. Cystoscopy is examination of the interior of the bladder with a help of a cystoscope passed through the urethra. It is possible to pass the catheter in the ureteric orifice through the cystoscope for retrograde pyelography or for collecting urine samples directly from the ureter. The pale interureteric ridge is a visible landmark, which helps in guiding the catheter in the ureteral orifice.
b. Cystogram is the radiograph of the urinary bladder after instilling contrast medium.
c. The ultrasound and CT scans are the best methods to examine the bladder.

Clinical Highlights

a. The urinary bladder may rupture in the fracture of the pubic bone causing intraperitoneal or extraperitoneal extravasation of urine.
b. The retention of urine may be due to enlarged prostate or stricture of urethra. In these conditions, the obstruction to urine outflow is slow and progressive. The bladder musculature hypertrophies and results in enlarged and trabeculated bladder. Gradual back-pressure builds up and affects the ureter and the entire collecting system of the kidney resulting in hydroureter and hydronephrosis.
c. Cystitis means the inflammation of urinary bladder. It gives rise to frequency and urgency of urination with suprapubic discomfort. The urine may be cloudy and offensive.
d. The transitional cell carcinoma of the bladder is usually due to chemical cause. The incidence of bladder cancer is more common in workers in aniline dye factories.
e. The suprapubic cystotomy provides an extraperitoneal surgical approach to bladder. For this procedure, first, the bladder is filled with distilled water so that its nonperitoneal superior surface comes in contact with anterior abdominal wall.
f. The spinal cord injuries affect the function of the urinary bladder giving rise to neurogenic bladder. The automatic reflex bladder is seen in spinal cord injury above the level of spinal micturition center. Due to injury at this level the cortical control or voluntary control is lost. As a result, the bladder fills and empties reflexly every one to four hours. The autonomous bladder is the condition produced due to destruction of S2 to S4 segments of spinal cord (located in the vertebral canal at the level of first lumbar vertebra). Here both voluntary and reflex control over micturition is lost. The bladder capacity is greatly increased because of loss of tone of detrusor. The bladder overfills and then overflows.

For development and anomalies of urinary bladder refer to Chapter 151.

155 Muscles of True Pelvis

The true pelvis or the lesser pelvis has the following boundaries. Its short anteroinferior wall is formed by pubic symphysis and pubic bones. The anterolateral wall is formed by part of hipbone below the level of arcuate line, pubic crest and the obturator internus muscle. The long and curved posterosuperior wall is composed of sacrum and coccyx and the posterolateral wall has greater and lesser sciatic foramina and the sacrotuberous and sacrospinous ligaments. Superiorly, the walls end in the margins of superior aperture of pelvis. Inferiorly, the walls end in the margins of inferior aperture of pelvis. The pubic symphysis, inferior pubic and ischial rami, ischial tuberosities, sacrotuberous ligaments and coccyx bound the diamond-shaped inferior aperture. The muscles of pelvic diaphragm and of urogenital diaphragm close the inferior aperture. The muscles of the true pelvis consist of obturator internus, levator ani, coccygeus and piriformis.

Obturator Internus

This muscle is located on the lateral wall of the pelvis. It takes origin from the inner surface of the obturator membrane and the margins of obtuartor foramen. A strong tendon emerges from the obturator internus muscle and leaves the pelvis through the lesser sciatic foramen to enter the gluteal region. The superior and inferior gemelli muscles are attached to the tendon of obturator internus on either side. These three structures form part of the bed for the sciatic nerve in the gluteal region and together they are inserted into the anterior part of medial aspect of greater trochanter of femur. The tendon turns through 90° and runs laterally behind the hip joint to reach its insertion.

Nerve Supply

The nerve to obturator internus (a branch of sacral plexus) supplies the muscle. It leaves the pelvis through the greater sciatic foramen and reenters it through the lesser sciatic foramen to supply the obturator internus and gemellus superior muscles.

Actions

The obturator internus muscle is the lateral rotator of the femur in the erect posture. It helps to maintain the head of femur in the acetabulum.

Obturator Fascia

The obturator fascia is a dense fascia covering the pelvic surface of the obturator internus muscle and is fused with the periosteum of the margins of the obturator foramen except at the obturator sulcus, where it leaves a gap for the obturator nerves and vessels to pass through the obturator foramen. There is a thickened tendinous arch (arcus tendinalis) in the obturator fascia extending between the body of pubis and the ischial spine. The tendinous arch gives origin to levator ani muscle. The part of the obturator internus below the level of the tendinous arch lies below the pelvic floor and forms the lateral wall of the ischiorectal fossa, which in located in the anal triangle of perineum.

Pelvic Diaphragm or Pelvic Floor (Fig. 155.1)

The pelvic diaphragm is the V-shaped floor of the true pelvis, which separates the pelvis from the perineum. The pelvic floor has evolved with assumption of erect posture by Man to support the pelvic viscera. The urethra and anorectal junction pass through it in the male. The vagina is the additional tube that passes through it in female. The right and left levator ani and coccygeus muscles enclosed in the superior and inferior layers of fasciae, form the pelvic diaphragm.

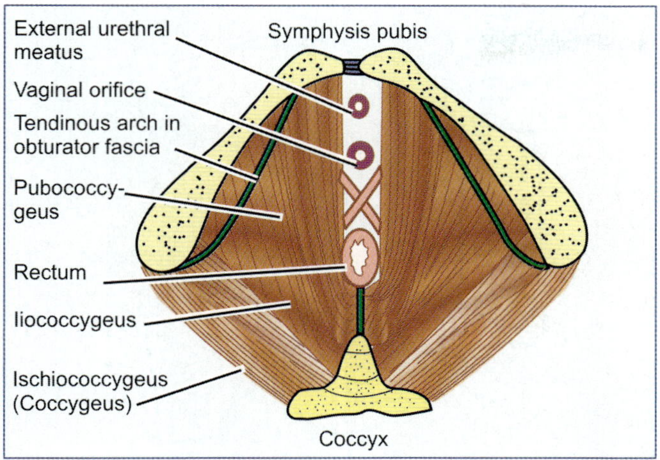

Fig. 155.1: Pelvic diaphragm in female

Levator Ani

This muscle has a broad origin from the inner side of the pelvis along a line extending from the body of pubis in front to the ischial spine behind. The muscle fibers sweep downwards and backwards to unite in the midline with fibers of the opposite side. The levator ani is broadly divided into pubococcygeus and iliococcygeus.

a. The pubococcygeus arises from the pelvic surface of the body of the pubis and anterior part of tendinous arch in obturator fascia. The fibers arising from the body of pubis (except those forming puborectalis sling) are inserted into perineal body while those arising from tendinous arch are inserted into the anococcygeal ligament and tip of the coccyx. According to the attachment of fibers, the pubococcygeus is subdivided in several components.
   i. Fibers that surround the prostate (levator prostatae) in male, are inserted in the perineal body (part of this muscle surrounding the urethra is peri-urithralis muscle). Fibers attached to the vaginal wall (pubovaginalis) in female, are inserted in the perineal body (part of this muscle surrounding the urethra is peri-urithralis muscle).
   ii. Fibers attached to rectum decussate and blend with the longitudinal rectal muscle to form conjoint longitudinal coat of anal canal.
   iii. The thick puborectal parts of the two sides join each other to form a sling at the anorectal junction.
   iv. Behind the rectum, majority of pubococcygeal fibers are attached to the tip of the coccyx and anococcygeal ligament.
b. The iliococcygeus arises from the posterior part of the tendinous arch in the obturator fascia and the ischial spine. It is inserted into the anococcygeal ligament and sides of the last two pieces of coccyx.

Coccygeus (Ischiococcygeus)

This muscle is posterior to the levaror ani. It arises from the pelvic surface and tip if ischial spine and is fused with the sacrospinous ligament. It is inserted into the coccyx and the fifth sacral vertebra. The sacrospinous ligament is regarded as degenerated tendon of this muscle.

Nerve Supply

Levator ani is supplied on its pelvic surface by the direct branches from the ventral ramus of fourth sacral nerve and on its lower surface by branches from either the perineal branch or the inferior rectal branch of the pudendal nerve. The coccygeus receives twigs from the third and fourth sacral nerves.

Fascia of Pelvic Diaphragm

The pelvic diaphragm is covered on inferior and superior aspects by the fascia. The inferior fascia of pelvic diaphragm is continuous with the obturator fascia laterally and after covering the medial wall of ischiorectal fossa blends with the fascia on sphincter ani externus. The superior fascia of pelvic diaphragm is attached anteriorly to the back of the body of pubis and to the superior ramus of pubis. It is continuous laterally with the obturator fascia and is continuous posteriorly with fascia on the piriformis and the anterior sacrococcygeal ligament.

Relations of Pelvic Diaphragm

The superior relations in the male, are the urinary bladder, prostate and rectum while those in the female, are the urinary bladder, uterus, vagina and rectum. The inferior relations are the ischiorectal fossae. Laterally, it has bony and fascial attachments. Medially, the pelvic floor gives passage to viscearal outlet, through which pass the urethra, anorectal junction in male and in addition, the vagina in female.

Actions

a. The most important function of the pelvic diaphragm is to support the pelvic viscera. Whenever there is rise in intra-abominal pressure (due to contraction of thoracic diaphragm and abdominal muscles) the muscles of pelvic floor contract to counter the downward pull on the pelvic viscera.
b. Puborectalis helps to create anorectal angle by pulling the anorectal junction upwards and forwards. This is an important factor in rectal continence. During defaecation, however, levator ani supports the viscera but the puborectalis relaxes along with the anal sphincters.
c. Pubovaginalis acts as a vaginal sphincter.
d. During the second stage of labor, the pelvic floor guides the fetal head into the anteroposterior diameter of the pelvic outlet. As the head passes under the pubic arch, the small urogenital hiatus in the anterior part of pelvic diaphragm becomes enormously enlarged. This may cause tear of the anterior fibers of the levator ani. The prompt repair of the perineal tears restores the normal function of the muscle.
e. Periurethralis muscle contracts for short spells thus helping the sphincter urethrae muscle.

Clinical Highlights

Pelvic diaphragm may be injured during difficult childbirth. This weakens the muscles of the pelvic diaphragm. The effects of weak pelvic floor are, uterine or vaginal prolapse, cystocele or herniation of bladder in the vagina, urinary stress incontinence (due to alteration in the position of bladder neck and urethra or urethrocele) and prolapse of rectum. Perineal exercises of Kegel are useful in increasing the tone of the muscles of perineum and levator ani.

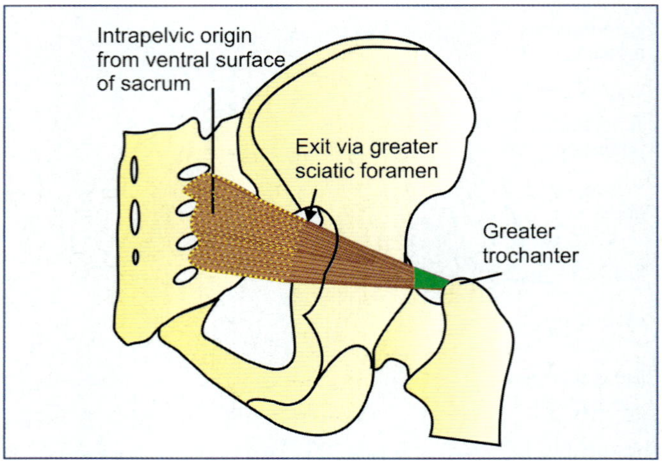

Fig. 155.2: Attachments of piriformis muscle

Piriformis (Figs 138.2 and 155.2)

The piriformis is located on the posterior wall of the pelvis. It is partly intrapelvic and partly extrapelvic.

It takes origin from the anterior surface of the sacrum by 3 digitations (inverted E-shaped origin) and passes inferolaterally to leave through the greater sciatic foramen, which it almost fills. It inserts by a rounded tendon on the upper border of greater trochanter of femur. Inside the pelvis, it is related anteriorly to the rectum, sacral plexus and branches of internal iliac artery. Its posterior surface is in contact with sacrum.

Nerve Supply

The piriformis receives direct branches from L5, S1 and S2 ventral rami inside the pelvis. (For its extrahepatic course and actions, refer to Chapter 185.)

156 Sacral and Coccygeal Plexuses

The sacral plexus is located in the pelvis in front of the sacrum. The nerves that take part in the sacral plexus are the lumbosacral trunk (L4, L5) and the ventral rami of the S1, S2, S3 spinal nerves and part of S4 spinal nerve.

Plan of Sacral Plexus

All the nerves mentioned above, converge towards the greater sciatic foramen and unite to form upper larger band and a lower smaller band. The upper band mainly consists of the nerves forming the two components of sciatic nerve. The ventral rami of L4, L5, S1 and S2 divide in ventral and dorsal divisions while that of S3 remains undivided. The lower band is more plexiform and receives contributions from ventral divisions of S2, S3 and from the undivided S4.

Branches of Communications

a. Each ventral ramus receives a gray ramus communicans from the sympathetic chain, through which each nerve receives postganglionic sympathetic fibers for distribution in their cutaneous territories.
b. The ventral rami of S2 to S4 sacral nerves carry preganglionic parasympathetic fibers form S2 to S4 segments of spinal cord. These parasympathetic fibers leave the ventral rami to form the pelvic splanchnic nerve or nervi erigentis, which terminates in the appropriate parasympathetic ganglia located close to the target organs.

Branches from Dorsal Divisions

a. Superior gluteal nerve (L4, L5, S1)
b. Inferior gluteal nerve (L5, S1, S2)
c. Perforating cutaneous nerve (S2, S3)
d. Perineal branch of the fourth sacral nerve
e. Direct branches to piriformis from S1, S2.

Branches from Ventral Divisions

a. Nerve to quadratus femoris and inferior gemellus (L4, L5, S1).
b. Nerve to obturator internus and superior gemellus (L5, S1, S2).
c. Direct branches from S4 to levator ani and coccygeus.
d. Pudendal nerve from S2, S3 and S4 ventral divisions.

Branches from Both Divisions

a. Posterior cutaneous nerve of thigh from ventral division of S2 and S3 and dorsal division of S2 and S3.
b. The common peroneal component of sciatic nerve from L4, L5, S1, S2 dorsal divisions and the tibial component from L4, L5, S1, S2 and S3 ventral divisions.

Except the intrapelvic muscular branches to piriformis, levator ani and coccygeus all the other branches of sacral plexus leave the pelvis through the greater sciatic foramen, where they are arranged in relation to piriformis muscle. Their extrapelvic course and distribution are described along with lower limb and perineum.

Clinical Highlights

a. Cancer of the uterus, cervix, or rectum may spread to the sacral plexus. Severe intractable pain in the lower limb is the most common symptom.
b. When the fetal head descends in the pelvis during the last trimester of pregnancy, the sacral plexus is likely to be compressed, which results in pain and discomfort.

Coccygeal Plexus

The nerves taking part in this plexus are as follows: A small branch from the fourth sacral, fifth sacral and the coccygeal ventral rami. These unite to form a common trunk on the surface of the coccygeus. Anococcygeal nerves are the fine filaments, which arise from it. They supply a few twigs to the coccygeus and levator ani. A few filaments pierce the sacrotuberous ligament to supply the skin from the coccyx to the anus.

157 Blood Vessels of Pelvis

The internal iliac arteries supply the pelvic walls, pelvic viscera, gluteal region, perineum and adductor compartment of thigh. They are the smaller of the two terminal branches of the common iliac arteries. In the fetus, the internal iliac arteries give origin to umbilical arteries through which blood reaches the placenta for purification. Because of this extra function, the internal iliac arteries are very large in fetal life. Each umbilical artery gives superior vesical branches to the urinary bladder. After birth, the entire umbilical artery does not undergo degeneration. Its patent segment forms the superior vesical artery while the rest of the umbilical artery (from the superior vesical artery until the umbilicus) is reduced to a fibrous ligament called lateral umbilical ligament.

Internal Iliac Artery (Figs 157.1 and 157.2)

Each internal iliac artery begins at the bifurcation of common iliac artery at the level of the disc between fifth lumbar vertebra and the sacrum, in front of the sacroiliac joint. It descends in posterior direction towards superior margin of the greater sciatic notch, where it divides into anterior and posterior trunks (divisions). The anterior trunk gives off both visceral and parietal branches while the posterior trunk gives only parietal branches.

Visceral Branches of Anterior Trunk

The visceral branches of the anterior trunk are three in male and four in female.

a. Superior vesical artery supplies the urinary bladder and often gives a branch to the ductus deferens in male.
b. Inferior vesical artery runs forward to the base of the bladder and supplies the structures related to the base in the male, including a long branch to the ductus deferens. In the female, the vaginal artery replaces the inferior vesical artery. It supplies the urinary bladder, vagina and urethra.
c. Middle rectal artery is a small branch, which may arise in common with inferior vesical artery. This artery

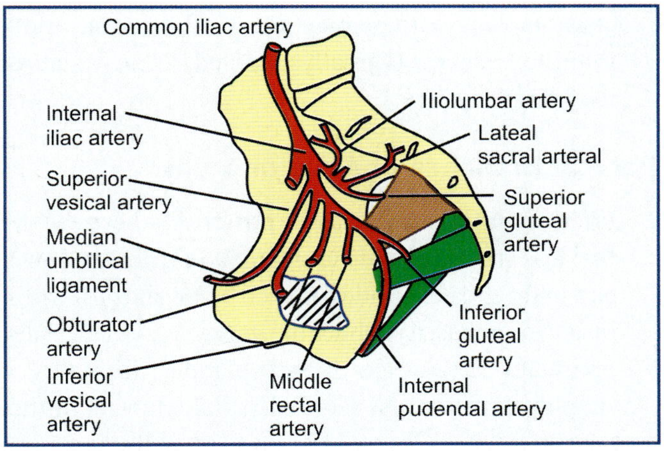

Fig. 157.1: Branches of internal iliac artery in male

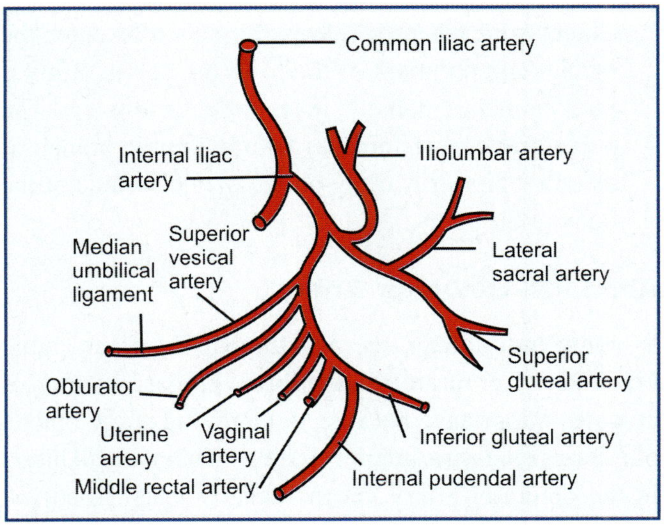

Fig. 157.2: Branches of internal iliac artery in female

supplies the rectum. It gives branches to the vagina in female and to the prostate and seminal vesicle in male.

d. Uterine artery describes a C-shaped course in the pelvis. At first, it passes medially along the floor in the root of the broad ligament. On reaching the lateral vaginal fornix (at a distance of 2 cm from the cervix), it crosses the ureter superiorly. This is a very important relationship described as "water under the bridge" by the surgeons. At this level, the artery gives off its descending branch to supply vagina. The uterine artery now turns forward and then upward in the broad ligament by the side of the uterus to which it supplies numerous branches. Reaching the medial end of uterine tube, the uterine artery turns laterally along the lower margin of uterine tube to end in the mesovarium by anastomosing with ovarian artery. The uterine artery is tortuous since it is greatly enlarged in gravid state of the uterus.

Parietal Branches of Anterior Trunk

a. Inferior gluteal artery passes posteriorly between the first and second sacral ventral rami to reach the lower part of the greater sciatic foramen below the piriformis. Inside the pelvis, it supplies the muscles of pelvic walls, perirectal fat and the urinary bladder. In males, it supplies prostate and seminal vesicle. For its further course, refer to Chapter 185 on Gluteal Region.

b. Obturator artery along with the nerve and vein of the same name (NAV from above downward) passes in anterior and inferior direction towards the obturator canal, from where it leaves the pelvis to enter the medial compartment of thigh. In the pelvis, it gives three branches, namely, iliac, vesical and pubic. The pubic branch anastomoses with the pubic branch of inferior epigastric artery on the pelvic surface of the body of the pubis.

Abnormal Obturator Artery

In some individuals, the anastomosis between pubic branches of obturator and inferior epigastric arteries assumes importance because in them, the pubic branch of inferior epigastric artery is large as it helps to fill blood in the obturator artery via this anastomosis. In such a situation, the anastomosis is called the abnormal obturator artery. This artery is closely related to femoral ring hence it is of surgical importance. Depending on its relation to femoral ring, the abnormal obturator artery has safe and unsafe positions (Fig. 178.3). Either it may be lateral to the ring (safe position) or it may pass medial to the ring on the lacunar ligament (unsafe position). In the latter case, it is prone to injury during surgical treatment of strangulated femoral hernia.

c. Internal pudendal artery leaves the pelvis through the lowest part of greater sciatic foramen. It is accompanied by the pudendal nerve and nerve to obturator internus. These three structures enter the gluteal region, hook round the ischial spine to enter the lesser sciatic foramen. The extrapelvic course of the artery is described in gluteal region and perineum.

Branches of Posterior Trunk

a. Superior gluteal artery is the largest branch and is the continuation of the posterior trunk. It passes between the lumbosacral trunk and first sacral ramus to reach the uppermost part of the greater sciatic foramen. It is accompanied by corresponding vein and superior gluteal nerve. Its further course is described with gluteal region.

b. Iliolumbar artery ascends anterior to the sacroiliac joint in close relation to lumbosacral trunk and obturator nerve. After reaching the medial border of psoas major muscle it divided into iliac and lumbar branches and may give rise to the fifth lumbar artery.

c. Lateral sacral arteries are two on each side. They enter the pelvic sacral foramina to supply the contents of sacral canal.

Veins of Pelvis

The following veins drain blood from pelvic viscera and pelvic walls. The internal iliac veins are the main venous channels. The superior rectal vein drains the rectum and upper part of anal canal into the portal vein. Besides this, these are ovarian veins in female and median sacral vein.

a. The internal iliac vein is the main vein of the pelvis and receives tributaries corresponding to the branches of the internal iliac artery. It is formed at the upper end of greater sciatic foramen by the confluence of all the veins accompanying the branches of internal iliac artery except the iliolumbar vein, which drains in the common iliac vein. The internal iliac vein joins the external iliac vein in front of the sacroiliac joint to form the common iliac vein.

b. The pelvic venous plexuses around the pelvic viscera give rise to the veins of the pelvis. These plexuses are thin-walled and intercommunicating.

   i. The vesical venous plexus in the male, lies in the retropubic space in relation to the inferolateral surfaces of the urinary bladder. It receives communication from the prostatic plexus and drains by inferior vesical veins into the internal iliac vein. Some part of it that travels along the posterior ligament of bladder drains in the internal vertebral venous plexus. This communication provides a route for spread of cancer from prostate into the vertebral column and skull bones.

   ii. The prostatic venous plexus lies within the fascial sheath of the prostate. It receives the deep dorsal vein of the penis and drains in vesical plexus.

   iii. In the female, the vesical plexus surrounds the neck of the bladder and the beginning of urethra. It receives the dorsal vein of clitoris and drains in the vaginal plexuses.

   iv. The uterine plexuses lie lateral to the uterus in the broad ligaments. They communicate with ovarian and vaginal plexuses and drain by two veins in the internal iliac veins. The vaginal plexuses (on the sides of vagina and in its mucosa) intercommunicate with uterine, rectal and vesical plexuses and drain by right and left vaginal veins in respective internal iliac veins.

   v. The rectal venous plexuses are of two types, internal and external. The internal plexuses are present in the submucosa of rectum and anal canal up to the pectinate line. The internal plexuses are important site of portocaval anastomosis and get enlarged in portal hypertension. The superior and inferior rectal veins drain these plexuses. The external rectal plexus lies outside the muscular layer and is drained by all the three rectal veins. The rectal plexuses are in free communications with vesical and other pelvic venous plexuses.

158 Abdominopelvic Part of Autonomic Nervous System

The efferent nerves of the autonomic nervous system supply the smooth muscles of the abdominal viscera, smooth muscles of the blood vessels and the glands inside the viscera. The afferent nerves carry sensation of pain and distension of viscera to the CNS. The viscera receive the nerves by means of the periarterial nerve plexuses, which arise in the central autonomic plexuses surrounding the major blood vessels situated on the posterior abdominal and lateral pelvic walls. The autonomic plexuses are composed of both afferent and efferent fibers belonging to sympathetic and parasympathetic systems. The plexuses also consist of collateral sympathetic ganglia and scattered postganglionic neurons.

Sympathetic Part

The following preganglionic visceral branches of the sympathetic chain take part in the central autonomic plexuses:

a. The greater, lesser and least splanchnic nerves arise from the thoracic sympathetic chain.
b. The lumbar splanchnic nerves arise from the lumbar chain.
c. The sacral splanchnic nerves arise from the sacral chain.

Parasympathetic Part

a. The right and left vagus nerves bring preganglionic fibers, which terminate on postganglionic neurons in the wall of the viscera via the plexuses.
b. The pelvic splanchnic nerves from sacral parasympathetic outflow carry preganglionic fibers, which terminate in the postganglionic neurons in the walls of the viscera via the plexuses.

Sympathetic Chains in Abdomen and Pelvis

The thoracic parts of the right and left sympathetic chains enter the posterior abdominal wall behind the respective medial arcuate ligaments to continue as the lumbar parts. Each lumbar sympathetic chain descends along the medial margin of psoas major muscle and usually possesses four ganglia. The lumbar part continues as the sacral part of the chain as it passes behind the common iliac vessels the crossing the pelvic brim. Each chain lies in front of the sacrum medial to anterior sacral foramina and behind the rectum. The sacral part of the chain also has four or five ganglia. At their lower ends, the right and left sympathetic chains converge in front of the first piece of coccyx to unite and form the ganglion impair.

Branches of Lumbar Part of Sympathetic Chain

a. Gray rami communicantes join each lumbar nerve for the pilomotor, sudomotor and vasomotor supply.
b. White rami communicantes from first and second lumbar ventral rami are given to the first and second lumbar ganglia.
c. The lumbar splanchnic nerves carry preganglionic fibers to the abdominal and pelvic plexuses.

Branches of Sacral Part of Sympathetic Chain

a. Gray rami communicantes join each sacral and coccygeal nerve for the pilomotor, sudomotor and vasomotor supply.
b. Sacral splanchnic nerves carry preganglionic sympathetic fibers to the inferior hypogastric plexuses.

Intra-abdominal Branches of Vagus Nerves

The gastric, coeliac, hepatic and renal branches of the vagus nerves join the autonomic plexuses in the abdomen.

Intrapelvic Branches of Sacral Parasympathetic Outflow

The pelvic splanchnic nerves or nervi erigentes carry the preganglionic parasympathetic fibers that arise in the intermediomedial column of spinal cord segments S2 to S4. They leave the cord through the second, third and fourth ventral roots of sacral nerves and unite outside the sacral canal to form the pelvic splanchnic nerve (nervi erigentes) on each side. The pelvic splanchnic nerves join the inferior hypogastric plexuses for supply of the digestive tract from the splenic flexure downwards upto the upper part of anal canal and for the supply of other pelvic viscera.

Celiac Plexus

The celiac plexus (solar plexus) is the largest autonomic plexus in the abdomen. It is a dense network surrounding the celiac artery and the root of superior mesenteric artery. Its main constituents are the right and left celiac ganglia and nerve fibers. The celiac ganglia are irregular masses made of postganglionic neurons situated on the crus of diaphragm on either side of the celiac trunk. They are grouped as collateral ganglia of sympathetic system. The lower part of each ganglion is detached to form aorticorenal ganglion. The greater splanchnic nerve (T5 to T9 sympathetic ganglia) ends in celiac ganglion for relay. The lesser splanchnic nerve (T10 to T11 ganglia of sympathetic chain) ends in the aorticorenal ganglion for relay.

Constituents

a. Postganglionic sympathetic fibers from the celiac ganglia.
b. Preganglionic parasympathetic fibers from the right and left vagi.
c. Afferent fibers from the abdominal viscera. The pain sensation is carried by sympathetic afferents to the spinal cord while the vagal afferents from abdominal organs are carried to medulla oblongata.
d. Phrenic nerves bring sensory fibers.

Secondary Plexuses from Celiac Plexus

The following secondary plexuses originate from the celiac plexus:

a. The phrenic plexus receives the branches of the phrenic nerve. On the right side at the junction of phrenic nerve and the plexus there is a small ganglion called phrenic ganglion, which distributes branches to IVC, suprarenal gland and hepatic plexus.
b. The hepatic plexus receives fibers from both vagi and from the right phrenic nerve. It accompanies the hepatic artery and its branches and portal vein and its tributaries.
c. The left gastric plexus accompanies the left gastric artery and receives the vagal gastric branches.
d. The splenic plexus is continued from the celiac plexus along the splenic artery. The parasympathetic fibers are distributed along the branches of splenic artery to the stomach and pancreas. The spleen receives sympathetic innervation only for its blood vessels and smooth muscle of capsule and trabeculae.
e. The suprarenal plexus receives a massive autonomic connection from the celiac plexus. The sympathetic fibers are preganglionic from the greater and lesser splanchnic nerves, which pass through the celiac ganglion uninterrupted and synapse on the chromaffin cells in the suprarenal medulla.
f. The renal plexus is quite dense, being composed of a few small ganglia and fibers from the celiac ganglion and plexus, parasympathetic fibers from vagus, aorticorenal ganglion, least splanchnic nerve, and first lumbar splanchnic nerve. The renal plexus enters the kidney along with branches of renal artery. It gives connections to ureteric and gonadal plexuses.
g. The testicular or ovarian plexuses receive fibers from renal and aortic plexuses and travel along the testicular or ovarian artery to the target organs. The efferent sympathetic fibers are from T10 and T11 segments of spinal cord. The afferent fibers reach the same segments of spinal cord. The connections with inferior hypogastric plexus bring pelvic parasympathetic fibers responsible for vasodilatation.
h. The superior mesenteric plexus is a downward continuation of the celiac plexus and accompanies the superior mesenteric artery into the mesentery. This

plexus has a superior mesenteric ganglion in it. It supplies the viscera along the branches of superior mesenteric artery.

i. The intermesenteric or abdominal aortic plexus is located on the sides and front of abdominal aorta between the origin of superior and inferior mesenteric arteries. It is formed from celiac plexus and from contribution of first and second lumbar splanchnic nerves.

j. The inferior mesenteric plexus is continuous above with the aortic plexus and receives additional branches from second and third lumbar splanchnic nerves. The preganglionic parasympathetic fibers reach the plexus indirectly (through branches of pelvic splanchnic nerves to the inferior hypogastric plexus travelling upto the superior hypogastric plexus) or by direct branches from the pelvic splanchnic nerves to the inferior mesenteric plexus. The plexus gives parasympathetic supply to the derivatives of hindgut by following the inferior mesenteric artery and its branches.

Superior Hypogastric Plexus

This plexus lies anterior to aortic bifurcation, the body of fifth lumbar vertebra and promontory of sacrum. It was earlier referred to as presacral nerve though it is never a single nerve and its main position is in front of the fifth lumbar vertebra rather than in front of sacrum. This plexus is composed of scattered neurons and small ganglia. It is mainly derived from the downward continuation of aortic plexus. It is joined by third and fourth lumbar splanchnic nerves and ascending fibers of pelvic splanchnic nerves. The afferent sympathetic fibers carry pain sensation from pelvic viscera to the dorsal root ganglia of lower thoracic and upper two lumbar spinal nerves. The superior hypogastric plexus supplies branches to ureteric, testicular, ovarian and common iliac plexuses. It divides in to right and left hypogastric nerves, which descend in the pelvis to become the inferior hypogastric plexus.

Inferior Hypogastric Plexus

This plexus is present along the lateral wall of pelvis on each side of midline pelvic viscera.

Constituents of Inferior Hypogastric Plexus

a. Pelvic splanchnic nerves carry preganglionic parasympathetic fibers.
b. Preganglionic and postganglionic sympathetic fibers from thoracic tenth to twelfth and first two lumbar segments of the spinal cord are brought in the hypogastric nerves.
c. Sacral splanchnic nerves are derived from sacral part of the sympathetic chain.
d. Small ganglia and scattered neurons.

The pelvic viscera are supplied through several secondary plexuses arising from the inferior hypogastric plexus. The secondary plexuses reach the viscera along the branches of internal iliac arteries.

Secondary Plexuses from Inferior Hypogastric Plexus

a. The middle rectal plexus surrounds the middle rectal branch of internal iliac artery and supplies the smooth muscle of the rectum and anal canal.
b. The vesical plexus goes along the vesical arteries or artery depending on the sex to supply bladder, and terminal parts of ureters. In males it also gives twigs to seminal vesicles.
c. The prostatic plexus supplies the prostate, seminal vesicles and ejaculatory ducts. It extends as cavernous nerves of penis for supply of cavernous tissue of bulb and crura of the penis.
d. The uterovaginal plexus follows the uterine and vaginal arteries and is located in the base of the broad ligaments. The plexus supplies the uterus, cervix, vagina, and the erectile tissue of the vestibule and the clitoris.

Clinical Highlights

Pain sensations from cervix of uterus and distended urinary bladder are carried in pelvic splanchnic nerves to S2- S4 segments of the spinal cord. Pain sensations from the majority of organs are carried by sympathetic afferents. Due to this dual path for pain, surgically removing superior hypogastric plexus (presacral neurectomy) does not fully abolish the pain sensation from the pelvic viscera in intractable pain of cancer in these viscera.

159 Lymph Nodes of Abdomen and Pelvis

The main lymph nodes of the abdomen are retroperitoneal and are located in relation to the abdominal aorta. These nodes are called lumbar nodes and are divisible in three groups, each having a specific area of drainage.

a. Preaortic group comprising of intercommunicating coeliac, superior mesenteric and inferior mesenteric nodes.
b. Right lateral aortic group.
c. Left lateral aortic group.

Preaortic Lymph Nodes

The preaortic lymph nodes are located in front of the abdominal aorta around the origin of its three-midline branches. They receive lymph from the alimentary canal below the diaphragm and the associated glands. The efferent vessels from the celiac group unite to form intestinal trunks, which empty in the cisterna chyli. The celiac lymph nodes receive lymph from the regional or intermediate nodes lying along the branches of coeliac trunk. Three main groups fall under this category, namely, gastric, hepatic and gastrosplenic. These are further subdivided in outlying nodes associated with specific viscera. The superior and inferior mesenteric nodes lie around the origin of the arteries of the same names. They receive lymph from regional nodes draining the digestive tract from duodenojejunal flexure to the pectinate line of anal canal. The regional lymph nodes comprise of 100 to 150 mesenteric nodes. Ileocolic, colonic and the pararectal nodes.

Lateral Aortic Lymph Nodes (Para-aortic)

These nodes receive lymph from the viscera and other structures supplied by the lateral and dorsal branches of aorta and from the nodes in relation to the iliac vessels in the pelvis. Their efferent vessels form right and left lumbar trunks, which open in cisterna chyli. These nodes receive the lymph vessels directly from the kidney, suprarenal gland, abdominal ureter, posterior abdominal wall, gonad, uterine tube and upper part of uterus. They also receive lymph from regional nodes, namely, common, external and internal iliac nodes. Thus, it is very clear that lateral aortic nodes receive lymph from both the lower limb and the pelvis.

Pelvic Lymph Nodes

a. The common iliac lymph nodes lie around the common iliac vessels and receive lymph from the external and internal iliac nodes and drain in lateral aortic group.
b. The external iliac nodes are more in number and collect lymph from the inguinal nodes, deeper layers of infraumbilical anterior abdominal wall, adductor region of thigh, membranous urethra, prostate, base of bladder, cervix of uterus and upper vagina. Their efferent vessels pass to the common iliac nodes.
c. The internal iliac nodes receive lymph from all the pelvic viscera, deeper parts of perineum, gluteal region and posterior part of the thigh. They receive lymph from sacral nodes found along the median sacral and lateral sacral vessels. The efferent vessels from the internal iliac nodes reach the common iliac nodes.
d. There are other groups called obturator and sacral nodes.

Cisterna Chyli

This is a thin-walled elongated lymphatic sac situated in front of the first two lumbar vertebral bodies. It lies on the right side of abdominal aorta and is normally overlapped by the right crus of diaphragm. In this situation it is very deeply placed on the posterior abdominal wall. It receives the intestinal trunks from the celiac lymph nodes and the right and left lumbar lymph trunks from the lateral aortic lymph nodes. The cisterna chyli continues superiorly as the thoracic duct.

160 Development of Reproductive Organs

Initially, when the reproductive organs make their appearance in the embryonic stage, they are similar in both sexes. This is referred to as indifferent stage. Later on, development proceeds on different paths.

Male Reproductive Organs

Following is the account of male reproductive organs, which include testes, epididymis, ductus deferens, seminal vesicles and the prostate (Fig. 160.1).

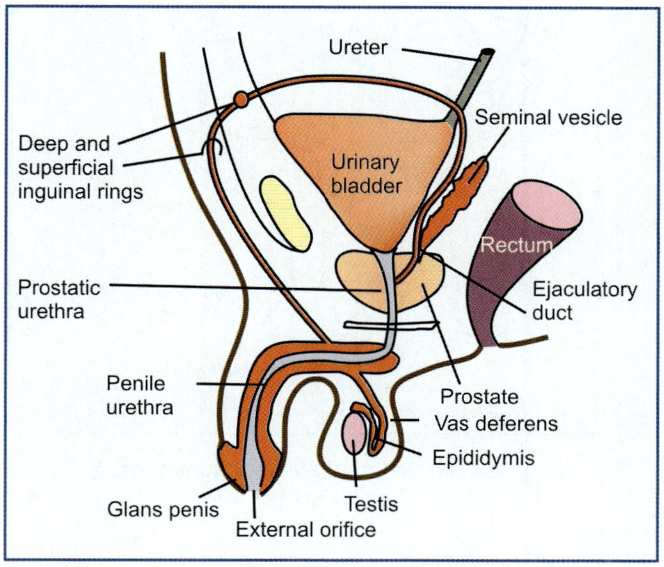

Fig. 160.1: Sagittal section depicting the location of various components of male reproductive organs

Development of Testis

The genital ridge is formed on each side by proliferation of coelomic epithelium on the dorsal body wall of the embryo during the fifth week (Fig. 160.2). The primordial germ cells migrate in the genital ridge in the sixth week from endoderm of the yolk sac. At this stage, the gonad is unidentifiable as testis or ovary. Under the influence of TDF (testis determining factor) gene on the short arm of Y chromosome the indifferent gonad differentiates into testis. The cells of coelomic epithelium form the rete testis and seminiferous tubules. The primordial germ cells, which are incorporated in the seminiferous tubules develop into spermatogonia.

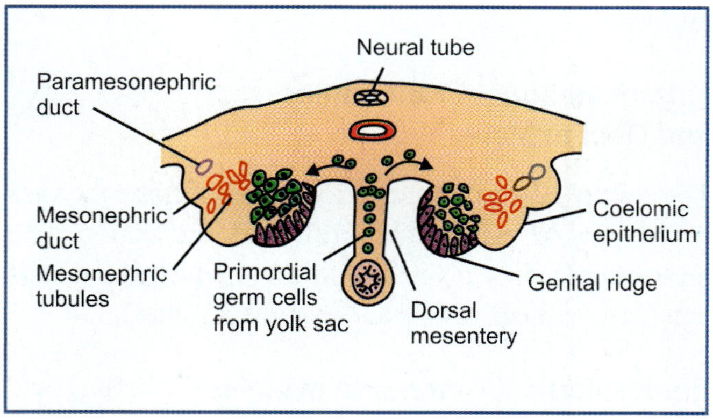

Fig. 160.2: Developmental sources of gonad

Differentiation of Genital Ducts

Early in embryonic life, two genital ducts develop during indifferent stage. They are called mesonephric (Wolffian duct) and paramesonephric (Müllerian's duct) as shown in Figure 160.3. The paramesonephric duct is formed by the invagination of the coelomic epithelium. It is located lateral to the mesonephric duct. The right and left paramesonephric ducts fuse at their caudal ends. Their fused end abuts on the posterior wall of the urogenital sinus to produce a bulge in the interior of latter. This bulge is called Müllerian's tubercle. Under the influence of the testosterone secreted by the Leydig cells of fetal testes, the mesonephros and the mesonephrenic ducts become

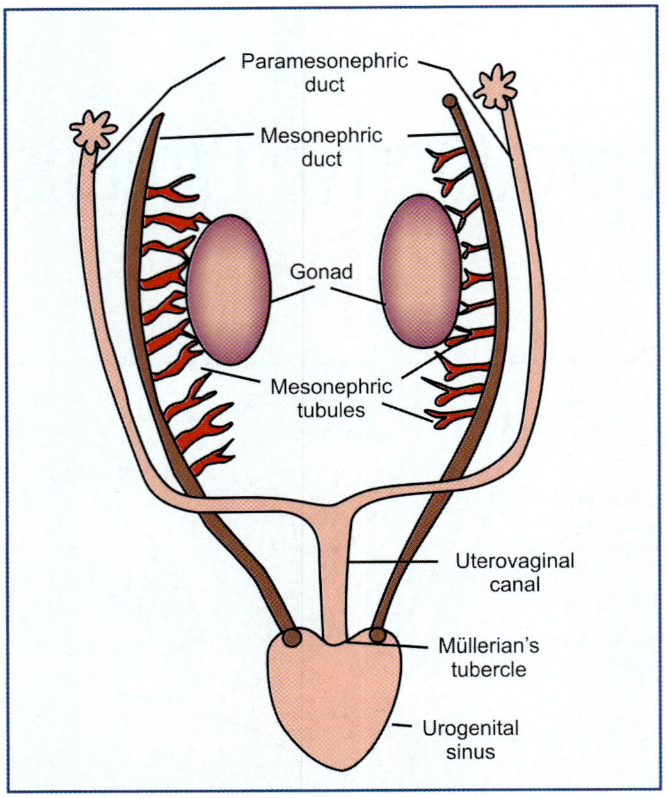

Fig. 160.3: Indifferent stage of gonad and genital ducts

functionally linked to the testes. Simultaneously, under the influence of Mullerian inhibiting substance secreted by Sertoli cells of fetal testes, the paramesonephric ducts regress.

Fate of Mesonephric Tubules and Duct in Male (Fig. 160.4)

The cranial 12-15 mesonephric tubules become the vasa efferentia or efferent ductules of the testis. The mesonephric duct gives rise to the epididymis, ductus deferens, seminal vesicle and ejaculatory duct.

Embryological Remnants in Male (Fig. 160.4)

a. A few cranial mesonephric tubules become the superior aberrant ductules and a few caudal mesonephrenic tubules become the inferior aberrant ductules and the paradidymis.
b. The cranial end of the mesonephrenic duct becomes the appendix epididymis. It is a small pedunculated structure on the head of the epididymis.

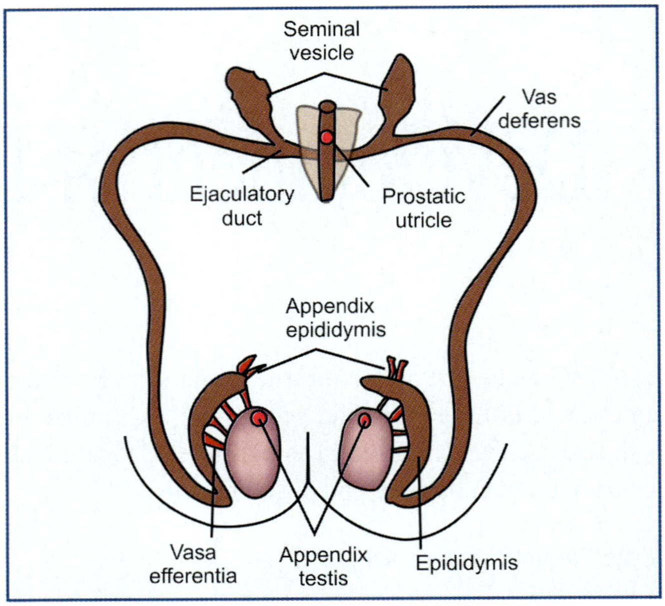

Fig. 160.4: Fate of mesonephric and paramesonephric ducts in male (Note that prostatic utricle and appendix testis are remants of paramesonephric ducts and appendix epididymis of mesonephric ducts)

c. The remnants of paramesonephric duct are, appendix testis and prostatic utricle inside the prostate gland.
d. The remnant of Müllerian's tubercle is colliculus seminalis inside the prostate gland.

Descent of Testis

The descent of testis from the posterior abdominal wall to the scrotum is a gradual process. The spermatogenesis needs lower temperature than that of the body. Hence, the testis descends to the scrotum with the help of gubernaculum testis and processus vaginalis. The gubernaculum testis (mesenchymal band) extends from the lower pole of the testis, traverses the inguinal canal to reach the bottom of the developing scrotum. It pulls the testis downwards. The processus vaginalis is a peritoneal pouch, which precedes the testis and lies in front of gubernaculum. The testis invaginates the processus vaginalis after reaching the scrotum and acquires a serous envelope (tunica vaginalis).

Fate of Gubernaculum Testis and Processus Vaginalis

The gubernaculum is reduced to the scrotal ligament, which connects the lower pole of testis to the scrotal wall.

The distal part of processus vaginalis forms the tunica vaginalis testis. The part of processus vaginalis between tunica vaginalis and peritoneal cavity is obliterated and reduced to a fibrous strand.

Chronology of Descent (Fig. 160.5)

The testis descends in the iliac fossa at third month of intrauterine life. It reaches the deep inguinal ring at seventh month, passes through the inguinal canal during the eighth month. It is in the scrotum at term or immediately after birth.

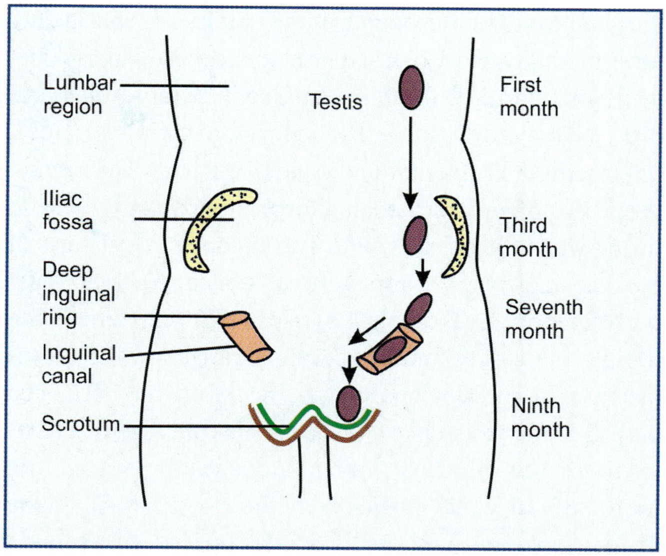

Fig. 160.5: Simplified scheme to depict chronology of descent of testis

Anomalies of Descent

a. Cryptorchidism or undescended testis may be unilateral or bilateral. The testis may be arrested anywhere in the path of its descent. An undescended testis in incapable spermatogenesis and is more liable to malignancy. Surgical correction is necessary early in childhood.
b. Ectopic testis is a normally descended testis but in abnormal position. The ectopic testis may be found in the anterior abdominal wall, thigh, femoral canal, perineum or at the root of the penis. The ectopic testis is functionally normal but it is more liable to injury.

Development of Prostate

It is described in Chapter 162.

Female Reproductive Organs

Following is an account of the development of ovaries, fallopian tubes, uterus and vagina. Some embryological remnants are also described.

Ovaries

In the indifferent stage, the gonads and duct systems are identical in both sexes. The female gonad is associated with the mesonephros, mesonephric ducts and paramesonephric ducts. The genital ridge and the primordial germ cells form the indifferent gonad like in the male. The proliferating coelomic epithelium forms sex cords, which invade the mesenchyme of the genital ridge and surround each primordial germ cell to give rise to the primordial ovarian follicles. The surface epithelium of the ovary is called germinal epithelium, which contributes the follicular cells. The primordial germ cells become oogonia, which begin maturation in intrauterine life itself. By the time of birth all oogonia in the fetal ovary have entered the metaphase of first miotic division and they remain arrested in that phase up to the time of ovulation.

Descent of Ovary

The ovary descends from the posterior abdominal wall to the true pelvis. The process of descent is similar in the two sexes. The gubernaculum ovarii and processus vaginalis are formed. The gubernaculum ovarii becomes attached to the paramesonephric duct (at the future site of junction of uterine tube and uterus) and then passes through the inguinal canal to the genital swelling, which will later on form the labium majus. Thus, it is clear that the attachment of gubernaculum to the paramesonephric duct prevents the descent of ovary outside the abdomen. The gubernaculum ovarii remains long and is changed in to ligament of ovary and round ligament of uterus. If the gubernaculum ovarii fails to contact the paramesonephric duct the ovary may be pulled out of the abdomen, giving rise to ectopic ovary. The processus vaginalis or canal of Nuck is very small. It normally obliterates completely.

Genital Ducts in Female

The paramesonephric or Müllerian's ducts (Figs 160.3 and 160.6) give rise to the uterus and uterine tubes. At the caudal end of mesonephros the paramesonephric duct turns medially and crosses ventral to the mesonephric duct to lie medial to it. At this stage, each paramesonephric duct is divisible into three parts, cranial vertical, intermediate horizontal and caudal vertical. The cranial vertical and the intermediate horizontal parts give rise to the uterine tube on each side. The caudal vertical parts of the two sides fuse to form uterovaginal canal. The cranial part of uterovaginal canal gives rise to the epithelium lining the uterine cavity and the cervical canal. As the uterus increases in size, small portions of medial ends of horizontal parts of paramesonephric ducts are absorbed in the uterus to form the fundus. The blind caudal end of the uterovaginal canal projects in the dorsal wall of the urogenital sinus, where it produces the Müllerian's eminence or Müllerian's sinus tubercle.

Congenital Anomalies of Uterus

a. Uterus didelphys is complete duplication of uterus, cervix and vagina due to failure of fusion of the caudal parts of paramesonephric ducts.
b. Uterus bicornis bicollis is characterized by double uterus and cervix but single vagina. This is due to incomplete fusion of the caudal parts of the paramesonephric ducts.
c. Septate uterus shows an incomplete septum in the uterine cavity.
d. Unicornuate uterus is due to unilateral suppression of paramesonephric duct.

Embryological Remnants (Fig. 160.6)

a. The epoophoron and paroophoron are the remains of the mesonephric tubules and are located in the broad ligament.
b. Gartner's duct is the remnant of mesonephric duct. It runs parallel to but below the uterine tube in mesosalpinx and then passes downward by the side of uterus to the level of internal os, where it passes in the tissues of the cervix. The duct sometimes forms a cyst called Gartner's cyst in the broad ligament.

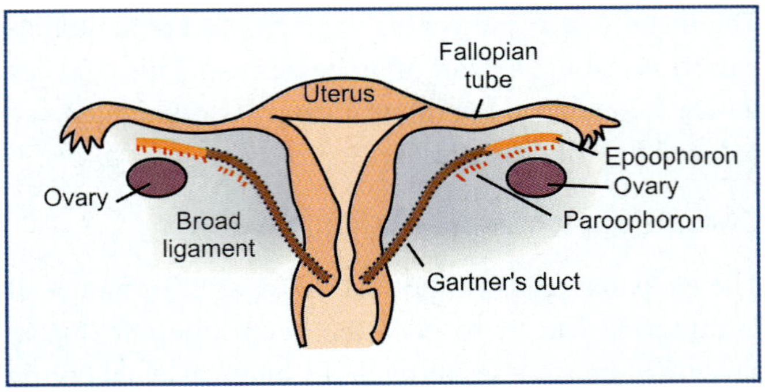

Fig. 160.6: Fate of paramesonephric and mesonephric ducts in female

Vagina

According to one theory, the vagina is of composite origin. Its upper one-fifth develops from the mesoderm of uterovaginal canal and the lower two-fifths from the endodermal vaginal plate, which develops from the proliferation of sinuvaginal bulbs of the urogenital sinus. According to another theory, the epithelium of the entire vagina develops from the sinuvaginal bulbs and hence is endodermal. The central part of Müllerian's eminence degenerates to form hymenal orifice and the peripheral part is retained as the hymen.

Congenital Anomalies of Vagina

a. Duplicate vagina is associated with duplication of uterus and cervix.
b. Imperforate hymen causes hematocolpos (accumulation of menstrual blood in vagina) after the onset of puberty. The imperforate hymen is the result of failure of the central part of Müllerian's eminence to disintegrate.
c. Congenital rectovaginal or vesicovaginal fistulae are common anomalies.

161 Testes and Duct System

The testes are responsible for the production of sperms and the secretion of testosterone. The sperms are transported by a series of ducts, which include epididymes, ductus deferens (vas deferens) and ejaculatory ducts to the prostatic urethra. The associated glands, which pour their secretions for providing nourishing liquid medium for sperms in the semen, are the seminal vesicles, prostate and bulbourethral glands. The testes, epididymes and the part of vasa deferentia are located outside the abdominal cavity and remaining part of the vasa deferentia, seminal vesicles, ejaculatory ducts and prostate are inside the pelvic cavity.

Gross Features of Testis

The testis and epididymis are suspended in one half the scrotum by the spermatic cord (Fig. 161.1). The left testis usually lies at a slightly lower level than the right because the left spermatic cord is longer than the right. The testis is oval-shaped structure of rubbery consistency and measures 5×3×2.5 cm in the adult.

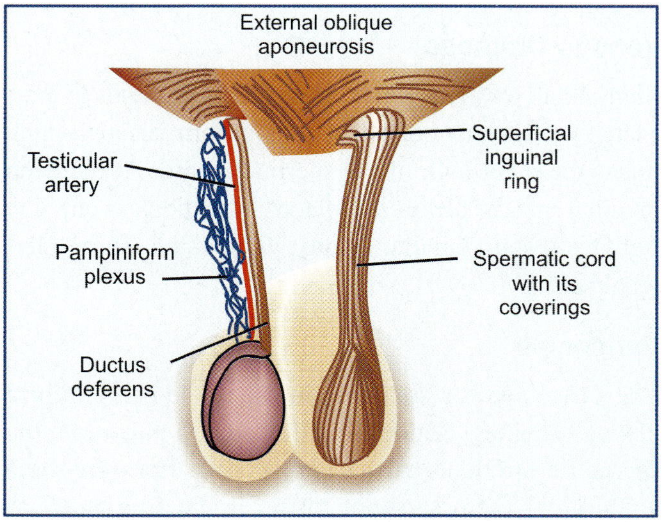

Fig. 161.1: Schematic diagram to show the extra-abdominal part of spermatic cord and its main contents (right side)

Each testis has superior and inferior poles, anterior and posterior borders and lateral and medial surfaces. The inferior pole of the testis is attached to the scrotal wall by scrotal ligament (Fig. 161.2), which is the remnant of the gubernaculum testis.

Epididymis

The epididymis is a very long and highly coiled tube attached to the posterior margin of testis. It consists of the head, body and tail. The head of epididymis is applied to the superior pole of the testis and the body lies against the posterolateral surface. Hence, the swelling of the epididymis is posterolateral to testis.

Tunica Vaginalis

The tunica vaginalis is a serous sac. Both the testis and epididymis are covered by the two layers of the tunica vaginalis on all sides, except along the posterior aspect of

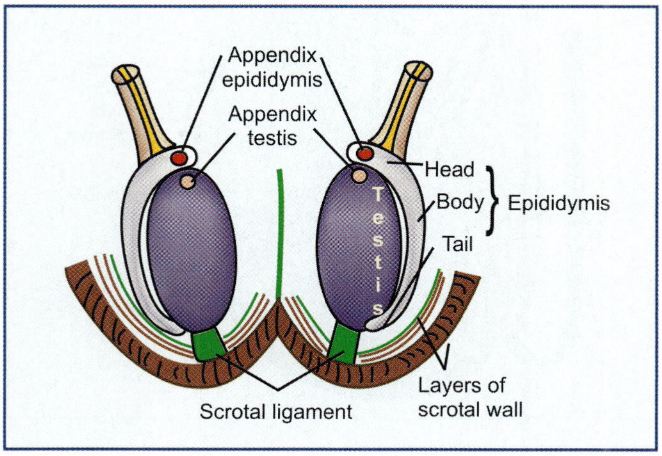

Fig. 161.2: Testis and epididymis inside scrotum

testis. The parietal layer of the tunica vaginalis lines the innermost layer of scrotal wall and the visceral layer covers the front and sides of the testis and epididymis. The two layers enclose a potential space. On the lateral aspect, the visceral layer dips in the space between the body of epididymis and the testis to form sinus of epididymis, which helps in side determination of an isolated testis.

Coverings of Testis

There are three coverings for the testis, which collectively form its capsule. The tunica vaginalis is a serous sac for both testis and epididymis. The tunica albuginea is a thick layer of fibrous tissue, which is thickest along the posterior margin of the testis. The tunica vasculosa lies deeper to tunica albuginea. In addition to the above three immediate coverings, there are others forming the wall of the scrotum, which also cover the testis and epididymis.

Testis and Epididymis on Section (Fig. 161.3)

The tunica albuginea projects from the posterior margin of the testis, into the interior of the testis, as a septum called mediastinum testis. This septum is traversed by blood and lymph vessels and by the intercommunicating network of channels called rete testis. The fibrous septa divide the testis in 200 to 300 lobules. Each lobule contains convoluted seminiferous tubules, which are the seats of sperm production. The seminiferous tubules join the rete testis and discharge their contents in the spaces of the rete from where the sperms are discharged in efferent ductules for onward transmission in to the duct of epididymis. The head of the epididymis consists of highly convoluted efferent ductules, which connect the duct of the epididymis and the testis. The highly coiled duct of epididymis is about 6 to 7 m long and forms the body and tail of epididymis, where it becomes continuous with the ductus deferens.

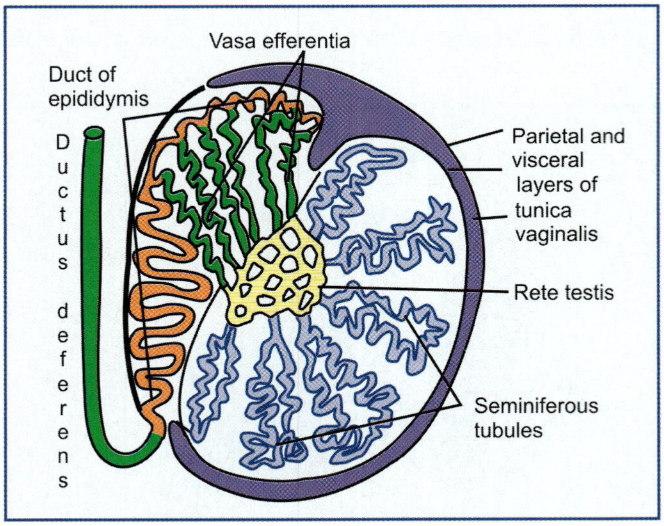

Fig. 161.3: Schematic vertical section of testis and epididymis to show their components

Microscopic Structure of Seminiferous Tubule

The germ cells (spermatogonia) rest on rest on a basement membrane of the seminiferous tubules. In addition there are spermatocytes and spermatids also. In between the germ cells there are supporting or Sertoli cells. The nuclei of these cells are of cartwheel shape hence the Sertoli cells lose the capacity for mitosis. These tall cells bear pits on their sides, where the germ cells come in close contact. The function of the Sertoli cells is to support and nourish the immature germ cells. They help in phagocytosis of residual bodies. They secrete estrogen and provide blood testis barrier.

Arterial Supply (Fig. 161.4)

The testicular artery is a branch of abdominal aorta. It enters the deep inguinal ring and travels in the spermatic cord to the testis. The other sources of arterial blood are, the artery to vas from the superior or inferior vesical artery and cremasteric artery from the inferior epigastric artery.

Venous Drainage

Many small testicular veins emerge from the testis to form a large venous network called pampiniform plexus, which forms the main bulk of the spermatic cord. At the deep inguinal ring the plexus is replaced by testicular vein. The right testicular vein drains into IVC and the left into left renal vein.

Varicocele

The varicocele is a condition in which the pampiniform plexus becomes tortuous and dilated. On palpation, the spermatic cord feels like a bag of worms. There are some anatomical factors responsible for the frequency of varicocele on the left side compared to the right. The left testicular vein is longer than the right. The left vein opens

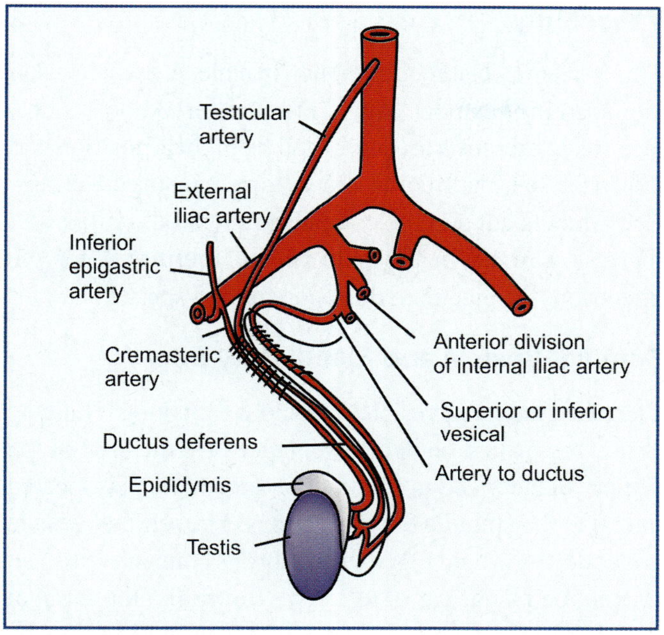

Fig. 161.4: Scheme depicting arterial supply of testis, epididymis and ductus deferens

in the left renal vein at right angle while the right vein opens in the inferior vena cava at an acute angle. The left testicular vein ascends posterior to the descending colon, which when loaded may compress the vein.

Tumors of the left kidney may grow along the left renal vein and may block the opening of left testicular vein causing varicocele.

The rise in scrotal temperature due to varicocele may sometimes interfere with spermatogenesis.

Lymphatic Drainage

The testis and epididymis are drained by lymphatics that open in preaortic and lateral aortic lymph nodes on the posterior abdominal wall. At times, enlargement of these lymph nodes may be the only sign of testicular cancer.

Nerve Supply

The testis and epididymis receive sympathetic efferent nerve supply through coeliac and testicular plexuses from T10 to T12 segments of spinal cord. The afferent fibres travel in sympathetic nerves in the same plexuses to the lesser and least splanchnic nerves, which carry them to the same segments of spinal cord. The testicular pain is referred to the middle and lower abdominal wall.

Testicular Thermoregulation

Scrotal temperature is 30° lower than the body temperature. The factors responsible for maintaining the temperature of scrotum are as follows. The scrotal sweat glands are numerous and the subcutaneous fat is absent in scrotal skin. The contraction of dartos muscle in cold conditions reduces the surface area of scrotal skin. The countercurrent heat exchange mechanism is said to exist between the testicular artery and veins in pampiniform plexus in the spermatic cord. The artery is entwined in venous plexus so that heat is absorbed from the artery in to the veins. In this way pre-cooled blood reaches the testis.

Clinical Highlights

a. The carcinoma of testis called seminoma arises from the germ cells. It spreads by lymphatics to the preaortic lymph nodes on the posterior abdominal wall.
b. The torsion of testis is the rotation of testis around the spermatic cord within the scrotum. It is associated with excessively large tunica vaginalis and commonly occurs in adolescent boys. The torsion may lead to occlusion of testicular artery and necrosis of testis.

Ductus Deferens or Vas Deferens

The ductus deferens is a thick-walled muscular tube, measuring 45 cm in length. The sperms are stored and transported to the prostatic urethra through it. The vas can be felt superomedial to the pubic tubercle and can be easily identified in the spermatic cord because it has the consistency of a plastic tube. The ductus is divisible into three parts.

Course (Fig. 160.1)

a. The first part of ductus deferens is in the scrotum and begins at the tail of epididymis. It is highly coiled. It ascends along the posteromedial aspect of testis to its superior pole.
b. The second part is the component of spermatic cord and extends from the superior pole of testis to the deep inguinal ring. It passes through the superficial inguinal ring, travels the inguinal canal and enters the abdominal cavity via deep inguinal ring.

c. The third part (pelvic part) begins at the deep inguinal ring after it separates from the spermatic cord. It turns medially by hooking around the inferior epigastric artery and then turns backward to cross the external iliac vessels and come to lie in the lateral wall of true pelvis after crossing the pelvic brim. On its way to the base of the urinary bladder, it crosses in succession, the superior vesical artery, obturator nerve and vessels, inferior vesical artery, and lastly the ureter. The vas, then, turns downwards and medially towards the base of bladder medial to the seminal vesicle, where it ends by joining the duct of seminal vesicle to form ejaculatory duct. The terminal dilated part of the vas deferens that lies behind the urinary bladder is called the ampulla.

Spermatic Cord

The spermatic cord is 7.5 cm long and extends from the upper end of the posterior border of testis to the deep inguinal ring. It is composed of tubular sheaths enclosing the ductus deferens and the associated blood vessels and nerves.

Coverings of Spermatic Cord

The coverings of the spermatic cord are derived from the muscles and fascia of the anterior abdominal wall. The outer covering is the external spermatic fascia, which is continuous with external oblique aponeurosis at the superficial ring. The intermediate covering is the cremaster muscle and fascia which is derived from internal oblique muscle. The inner covering is the internal spermatic fascia derived from the transversalis fascia at the deep ring.

Contents of Spermatic Cord (Fig. 161.5)

a. Vas deferens lies in the posterior part of the cord.
b. Pampiniform venous plexus gives the bulk to the cord
c. There are three arteries, namely, the testicular, deferential and cremasteric.
d. The lymphatics of the testis and epididymis
e. The autonomic nerves and the genital branch of genitofemoral nerve
f. Fibrous remnant of the embryonic processus vaginalis.

Vasectomy

This is a family planning operation in male. A small incision is placed in the upper part of the scrotum on both sides. The vasa deferentia are identified from their position and feel in the spermatic cords after cutting open the coverings. Each duct is cut and the cut ends are ligated. In this way there is a break in the path of the sperms. After the operation, the ejaculate does not contain sperms.

Seminal Vesicle and Ejaculatory Duct

The paired seminal vesicles are about 5 cm long lobulated structures, which lie in close contact with the base of the urinary bladder and in front of the rectum. Each is located lateral to the ampulla of vas deferens. The seminal vesicle is a coiled tube held together by fibrous connective tissue. Its uncoiled length is 10 to 15 cm. Inferiorly, the seminal vesicle narrows to form a duct, which joins with the ductus deferens to form ejaculatory duct. The function of the seminal vesicle is to produce secretion rich in fructose, which is added to the seminal fluid.

The ejaculatory ducts pierce the posterior surface of prostate and open in the prostatic part of urethra. Their function is to pour the seminal fluid in the prostatic urethra.

Arterial Supply

The artery to vas deferens or deferential artery, either a branch of superior vesical artery or the inferior vesical artery supplies the vas deferens. The seminal vesicle,

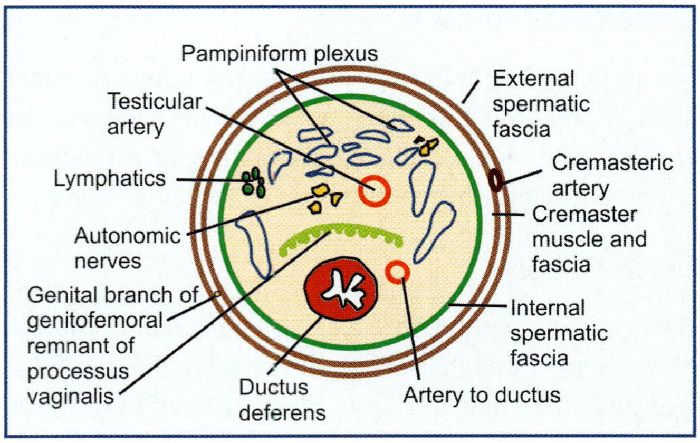

Fig. 161.5: Schematic transverse section of spermatic cord to show details of its contents

ejaculatory duct and ampulla of vas deferens receive branches from inferior vesical and middle rectal arteries.

Nerve Supply

The testicular plexus supplemented by hypogastric plexuses, supplies the sympathetic efferent fibres to the smooth muscle in the wall of the ductus, seminal vesicle and ejaculatory duct. The fibers originate in L1 segment of the spinal cord. On sympathetic stimulation, the contraction of the smooth muscle helps in pouring of the contents and secretions of the above structures in the urethra as seminal fluid.

162 Prostate

The prostate is an accessory sex gland in the male. It is located deep in the pelvic cavity. The prostate is composed of glandular and fibromuscular tissue. Hence, it is firm in consistency. The size and activity of prostate are under the influence of testosterone. The prostate becomes functionally active from the age of puberty. Its secretion is added to seminal fluid in the prostatic urethra. The prostatic secretion is rich in acid phosphatase.

Shape and Size of Prostate

The shape of the prostate resembles an inverted cone, with broad base upward and pointed apex downward. Its vertical diameter is 3 cm, anteroposterior diameter is 2 cm and the transverse diameter at the base is 4 cm (length is smaller than width).

Location (Fig. 162.1)

The prostate is located between the urinary bladder and urogenital diaphragm. It lies behind the lower margin of pubic symphysis and in front of rectal ampulla. It surrounds the initial three cm of the urethra.

Development

The prostate develops from both endoderm and mesoderm. It originates as endodermal buds from the caudal part of vesicourethral canal and from the cranial part of the pelvic part of definitive urogenital sinus. The buds that arise from the posterior wall of prostatic urethra are mesodermal because this wall of the urethra develops from the mesonephric ducts. The mesodermal buds form the glands of internal submucosal zone, which are prone to benign hypertrophy of prostate in later life. The endodermal buds form the glands of peripheral zone, which are more prone to malignancy in later life. The fibromuscular stroma develops from the surrounding splanchnopleuric mesoderm. The embryological remnants inside the substance of prostate, are the prostatic utricle derived from the caudal end of the fused paramesonephric ducts and the colliculus seminalis derived from the Mullerian tubercle.

Capsules

The prostate has two capsules called true and false between which prostatic venous plexus (Fig. 154.5) is located. True capsule is the condensation of connective tissue stroma of the prostate around it. It is adherent to the prostate. False capsule lies outside the true capsule and is the part of pelvic fascia. It is continuous with puboprostatic ligaments anteriorly, true ligaments of bladder posteriorly and rectovesical fascia.

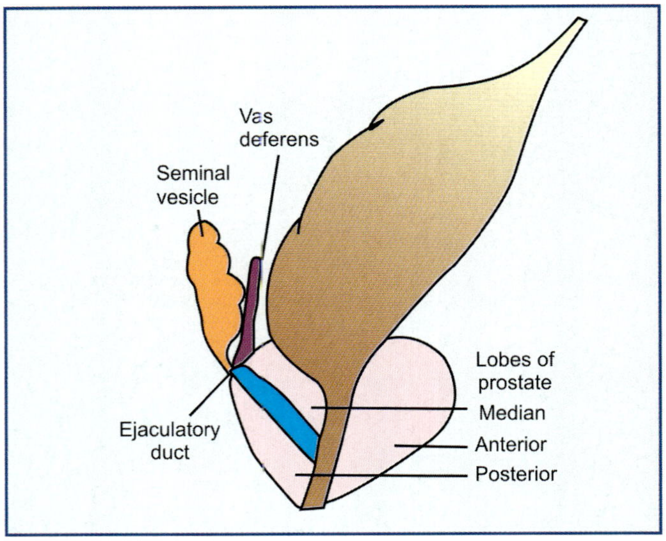

Fig. 162.1: Lateral view of prostate gland to show its lobes in relation to ejaculatory duct and prostatic urethra

Relations (Fig. 154.2)

The prostate has five surfaces, superior (base), posterior, right and left inferolateral and anterior.

a. The superior surface is also called vesical surface since it is in contact with neck of the bladder. This surface is pierced by urethra nearer the anterior aspect.
b. The posterior surface is separated from the ampulla of rectum by rectovesical fascia of Denonvillier. The right and left ejaculatory ducts pierce this surface to enter the prostate and open into the prostatic urethra.
c. The anterior surface lies about 2 cm behind the pubic symphysis. It is related to the retropubic space, which contains retropubic pad of fat and vesical venous plexus. This surface is connected to the pubic bones by puboprostatic ligaments, which form the floor of the retropubic space.
d. The right and left inferolateral surfaces are supported by anterior parts of levator ani muscles. The medial fibres of this muscle constitute levator prostatae.

Internal Features

The prostatic urethra passes through the gland. The right and left ejaculatory ducts enter the prostate to open into the prostatic urethra. Numerous ducts of prostatic glands open in the prostatic urethra. Prostatic utricle, which is the remnant of caudal end of paramesonephric duct, lies inside the prostate.

Surgical Lobes (Figs 162.1 and 162.2)

The prostate is incompletely divided into five lobes.

a. Anterior lobe or isthmus lies in front of urethra. This lobe is the connecting bridge between the anterior ends of the two lateral lobes. It is devoid of glandular tissue hence, adenoma never occurs in this lobe.
b. Posterior lobe is situated behind the urethra and below the ejaculatory duct. It connects the posterior ends of the two lateral lobes. It contains glandular tissue and is the site of primary carcinoma. This lobe is palpable per rectum.
c. Median lobe lies between the urethra and the ejaculatory duct. It is a wedge shaped lobe in contact with trigone of bladder. The bulge produced by it on the lower end of trigone is called the uvula of bladder. It contains more glandular tissue than other lobes and is more susceptible to benign hypertrophy of prostate (BHP). The median lobe is not palpable per rectum because it lies anterior to the posterior lobe and the ejaculatory ducts.
d. Right lateral lobe on the right side of urethra and the left lateral lobe on its left side contain numerous glands, which may give rise to adenoma.

Prostatic Urethra

The prostatic urethra is the proximal 3 cm of male urethra lying inside the prostate gland. It pierces the base of the prostate and leaves it at the apex. It lies nearer the anterior surface. It is the most dilatable and widest part of male urethra.

Features of Prostatic Urethra (Fig. 154.5)

The posterior wall of prostatic urethra shows following features:

a. Urethral crest is a midline longitudinal ridge.
b. Seminal colliculus is an elevation at the middle of urethral crest. It has three openings on it a median for prostatic utricle and lateral for ejaculatory duct of each side.
c. Prostatic sinus is a groove on each side of the crest. About 15 to 20 prostatic ducts open in the prostatic sinus and pour the secretion of prostate in the urethra.

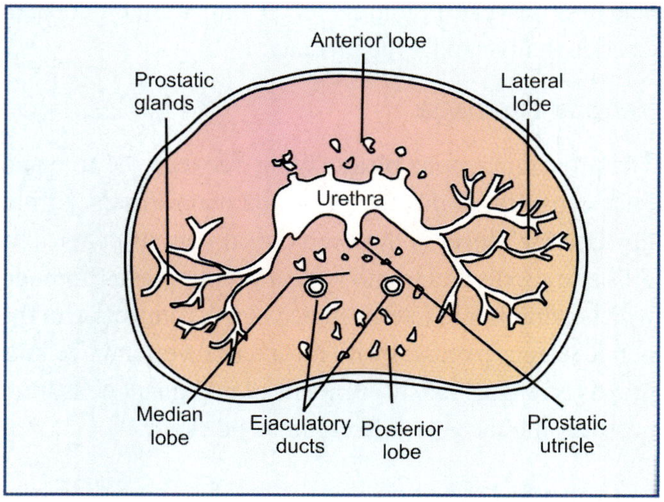

Fig. 162.2: Cross-section through prostate to depict internal structures

Structure of Prostate

The fibromuscular stroma consists of smooth muscle and fibrous tissue. The smooth muscle of the stroma is continuous above with the smooth muscle of bladder wall. A peculiar feature is the presence of striated muscle subjacent to the true capsule. This band of striated muscle is in continuity with the striated muscle of sphincter urethrae surrounding the membranous urethra in the deep perineal pouch. The intraprostatic striated muscle is connected to the true capsule and stroma by collagen tissue. The function of the smooth muscle is to compress the follicles to facilitate their drainage in prostatic urethra. The function, of the striated muscle is, probably, to expand the prostatic urethra to accommodate seminal fluid (3-5 ml) prior to ejaculation. The glandular tissue is arranged in three concentric layers or zones. The peripheral zone consists of long branching glands, whose ducts curve to reach the posterior wall of the prostatic sinuses below the level of colliculus seminalis. The glands in this zone develop from endoderm and are prone to carcinoma. The internal zone consists of submucosal glands, whose ducts open on the floor of prostatic sinuses at the level of colliculus seminalis. The glands in this zone develop from mesoderm and are prone to benign hypertrophy of prostate (BHP). The innermost zone consists of simple mucosal glands surrounding the upper part of the prostatic urethra.

Arterial Supply

The inferior vesical, middle rectal and internal pudendal arteries richly supply the prostate.

Venous Drainage

The prostatic venous plexus lying between the true and false capsules, drains the gland. Its main tributary from the anterior aspect is the deep dorsal vein of penis. The prostatic plexus drains into vesical venous plexus, through which it drains into internal iliac vein. A connection of the pelvic venous plexuses with the internal vertebral venous plexus is responsible for deposits of malignant cells from prostate into the vertebral column and skull.

Lymphatic Drainage

The lymph from prostate is drained into internal iliac, external iliac and sacral group of lymph nodes.

Nerve Supply

The parasympathetic supply is from the pelvic splanchnic nerves via the inferior hypogastric plexus. The sympathetic nerves originating in L1 segment of spinal cord and reaching the gland through the hypogastric plexuses, supply the smooth muscle of the prostate. The sympathetic supply of the prostate, the seminal vesicles and vas deferens is responsible for ejaculation. The striated muscle inside the prostate is supplied by pudendal nerve.

Age Changes

a. In the newborn and childhood, the prostate has fibromuscular stroma and the rudiments of duct system.
b. At the age of puberty, there is a spurt in the growth of prostate under the influence of testosterone. The prostatic follicles develop and proliferate and begin secretion of acid phosphatase and prostate specific antigen (PSA) in addition, to other constituents like prostaglandins.
c. During the third decade, glandular epithelium of the follicles grows by irregular multiplication of epithelial infoldings in the lumen of follicles.
d. After third decade, amyloid concretions start forming in the follicles.
e. After 45 to 50 years, the prostate may show gradual benign hypertrophy or progressive atrophy.

Clinical Highlights

a. The prostate is easily palpable per rectum. Hence, prostatic pathology can be easily detected by rectal examination.
b. The benign hypertrophy of prostate affects the median lobe, which projects in the urinary bladder and obstructs the urinary outflow. As the patient strains to urinate, the median lobe blocks the internal urethral opening more. This may give rise to chronic obstruction to bladder outflow leading to effects of backpressure on the bladder, ureter and renal pelvis and calyces.
c. The carcinoma of prostate is the most common malignant tumour in men over 65 years. It may spread locally involving bladder neck, seminal vesicle, ureters and rectum. The spread by lymphatic route is common.

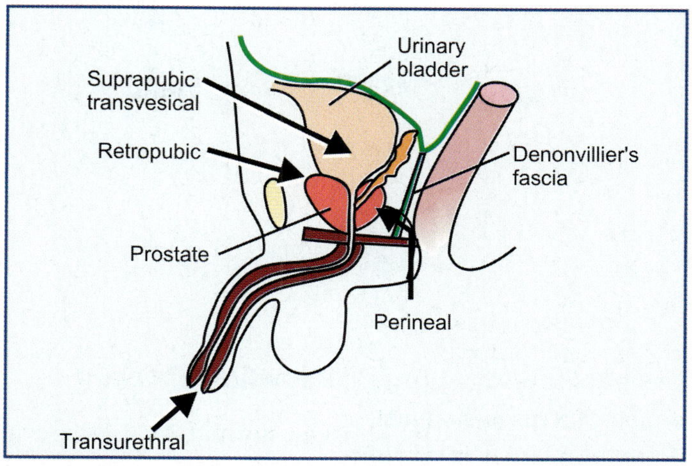

Fig. 162.3: Schematic representation of anatomical basis of surgical approaches to prostate

The external and internal iliac nodes besides the sacral nodes are enlarged. The spread by venous route occurs to the pelvic bones, lower lumbar vertebrae, femoral head, ribs and skull.

d. Surgical removal of the prostate is called prostatectomy. There are four approaches to the prostate (Fig. 162.3). The retropubic approach is through the retropubic space or cave of Retzius. It is an extraperitoneal approach. The suprapubic transvesical approach is through the urinary bladder, which is opened and prostate enucleated by a finger in the urethra. Perineal approach is an almost outdated technique, where the prostate is approached through the rectovesical fascia. The transurethral approach is the most accepted approach, nowadays. It is known as transurethral resection of prostate (TURP).

163 Ovary

The female reproductive organs consist of the ovaries (female gonads), the fallopian tubes, uterus and vagina. The ovaries, tubes and uterus form the internal organs of reproduction since they are located inside the true pelvis. The process of oogenesis, which begins during the intrauterine life, is completed during each ovarian cycle throughout the reproductive life of the female. The lateral end of fallopian tube picks up the secondary oocyte liberated by the ovary, at ovulation, in the peritoneal cavity. The normal site of fertilization is the ampulla of fallopian tube. The zygote, which is the product of fertilization, is transported to the uterus for implantation and for further growth and development of the embryo and fetus. If the secondary oocyte is not fertilized, it is transported to the uterus for discharging through the menstrual flow.

Position of Ovary

The ovaries are located in the true pelvis on the lateral pelvic wall in the ovarian fossa in the nulliparous woman. The location of the ovary is not constant in women who have borne children. The ovaries rise in the abdominal cavity along with expanding pregnant uterus. After parturition, when the uterus returns to pelvic cavity the ovaries do so but not in the same position. Frequently, the ovaries lie in rectouterine pouch.

External Appearance

Each ovary is almond shaped. In the living, the ovaries are grayish pink and present smooth appearance before regular ovulation begins. After the onset of puberty, the surface of ovary is rough because of the scarring, which results from repeated ovulation and degeneration of successive corpora lutea.

Palpation of Ovary

The normal ovaries are not palpable on vaginal or abdominal examination. Enlarged ovaries or the ovaries prolapsed in rectouterine pouch are palpable by vaginal examination. The inspection of ovaries is possible by peritoneoscope inserted through the anterior abdominal wall. Ultrasound examination is useful in detecting pathologies of ovary.

Functional Importance

Normally, the ovaries liberate one secondary oocyte per ovarian cycle at ovulation (Fig. 163.1) in the peritoneal cavity. The maturation of ovarian follicles, ovulation and development of corpus luteum are sequential events, which constitute the ovarian cycle. The maturation of Graafian

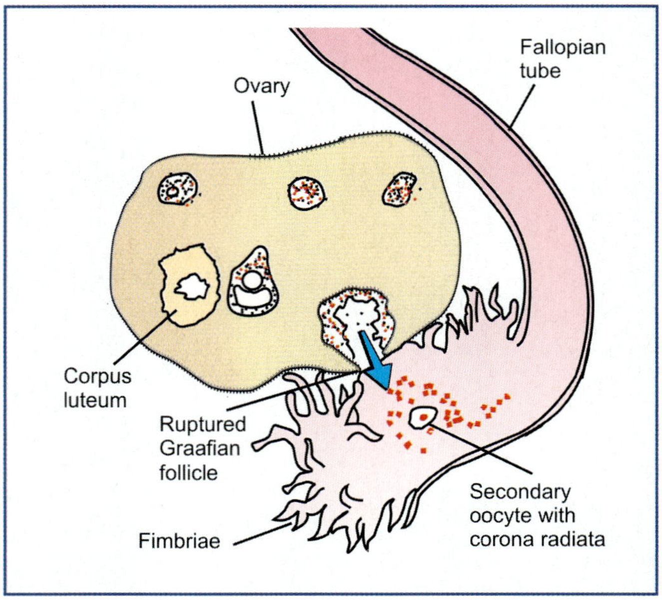

Fig. 163.1: Scheme to show relationship of fimbriated end of tube to ovary at the time of ovulation

follicle is under the influence of FSH of anterior pituitary. The granulosa calls of Graafian follicle secrete estrogen, which acts on the endometrium. After ovulation, the ruptured Graafian follicle becomes the corpus luteum, which is under the influence of leutinising hormone of pituitary and produces progesterone and estrogen. The progesterone acts on the endometrium and prepares it for implantation. Thus the ovary releases the secondary oocyte and prepares the endometrium through the actions of its hormones for implantation of blastocyst, each month.

Parts of Ovary

The long axis of ovary is nearly vertical. The ovary has lateral and medial surfaces, upper and lower poles and anterior and posterior borders. The boundaries and relations of the ovarian fossa are also the relations of the ovary. The ovarian fossa (Fig. 163.2) is a shallow recess of the peritoneal cavity situated on the lateral wall of pelvis. The lateral surface of the ovary rests on the floor of the ovarian fossa, which is formed by the parietal peritoneum, obturator nerve and vessels, obturator fascia, obturator internus muscle from within outwards. The relationship with the obturator nerve explains why ovarian pathology gives rise to pain radiating down to the knee. The external iliac vessels form the superior or anterior boundary of the fossa while the internal iliac vessels and the ureter form its posterior boundary. The medial surface of the ovary is in contact with ovarian fimbria of the uterine tube.

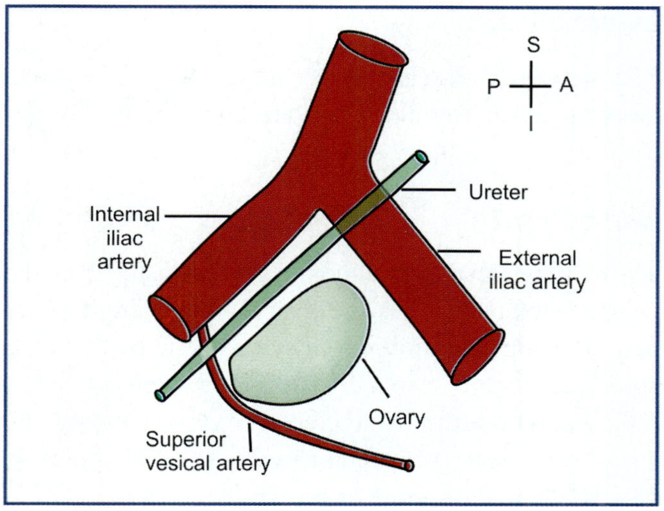

Fig. 163.2: Boundaries of left ovarian fossa (Note that lateral boundary (obturator nerve and vessels) is not shown in the figure)

Peritoneal Relation

The ovary is covered with germinal epithelium, which is the modified mesothelium. At the anterior or mesovarian border, the germinal epithelium of ovary is continuous with mesothelium of the peritoneum of mesovarium.

Ligaments of Ovary

a. The mesovarium suspends the ovary from the back of broad ligament. It is a double fold of peritoneum attaching the posterior layer of broad ligament to the anterior border of ovary. It carries ovarian blood vessels.
b. The infundibulopelvic ligament or suspensory ligament of ovary extends from the upper pole of ovary and adjoining infundibulum to the lateral wall of pelvis. It is a part of broad ligament lateral to the attachment of mesovarium. The ovarian vessels and accompanying nerve plexuses reach broad ligament via suspensory ligament of ovary. The ovarian vein is in the form of pampiniform plexus in this ligament. Occasionally, this plexus becomes varicose giving rise to varicocele (a condition usually more common in male). Ovarian torsion is due to very long mesovarium or suspensory ligament. The torsion compresses the ovarian blood vessels producing ischaemia and abdominal pain.
c. The ligament of ovary, a derivative of gubernaculum, attaches the lower pole of ovary to the tubouterine junction.

Arterial Supply

Each ovarian artery arises from the abdominal aorta just below the renal artery. It crosses the pelvic brim to enter the infundibulopelvic ligament and to reach the ovary via the mesovarium.

Venous Drainage

The right ovarian vein drains into inferior vena cava and the left drains into left renal vein.

Lymphatic Drainage

The lymphatic vessels of ovary travel along the ovarian blood vessels and terminate in lateral aortic group of lymph nodes.

Nerve Supply

The ovarian plexus of autonomic nerves arising from the coeliac plexus supplies the ovary. The afferent fibres carrying pain sensation run in sympathetic pathways to spinal segments T10 to T12. The ovarian pain is referred to lower abdominal and pubic region. Cutting the suspensory ligament, which carries the ovarian plexus, may alleviate intractable ovarian pain.

Clinical Highlights

a. Ovarian tumors are common disorders of ovary. They are of three types. The functional tumors arise from the cells of Graafian follicle or from the cells of corpus luteum. The teratoma of the ovary arises from undifferentiated cells persisting from embryonic life. The teratoma occurs in young age and contains a mixture of hair, bone, and nail inside it. The malignant growths of ovary may arise from germ cells, follicular cells and connective tissue. The secondary deposits from other places into the ovary are common. This normally occurs by retrograde lymphatic spread or transcoelomic spread from breast or abdominal organs. Bilateral secondary deposits are called Krukenberg's tumors.
b. Ovarian dysgenesis is found in Turner's syndrome (45×0). In this condition, the ovary is devoid of germ cells. The patients show characteristic phenotype. They show short stature, webbed neck, cubitus valgus and amenorrhea.
c. The surgical removal of ovary is called oophorectomy.

164 Fallopian Tube

Each fallopian tube (uterine tube) extends from the tubouterine junction laterally, in the free margin of the broad ligament. Its lateral end is fimbriated and bears 5 to 6 fimbriae. This end is very close to the ovary. The fallopian tube communicates the uterine cavity with the peritoneal cavity.

Length and Shape

The length of the fallopian tube is 10 cm. The shape of the tube is like that of a trumpet (salpinx).

Functions

a. The fallopian tube transports the secondary oocyte liberated from the ovary to the uterine cavity in normal menstrual cycle.
b. It plays a coordinating role in the meeting of the sperms and the secondary oocyte, for fertilization to take place in the ampulla of the tube.
c. It nourishes the zygote and the subsequent stage, morula. It transports the morula to the uterine cavity.

Parts (Fig. 164.1)

The tube is divided into four parts, from medial to lateral side, they are interstitial, isthmus, ampulla and infundibulum.

a. The interstitial or intramural part passes through the myometrium to open in the uterine cavity. This segment is the shortest (1.25 cm) and narrowest.
b. The isthmus lies immediately outside the uterus. Its length is 2.5 cm.
c. The ampulla is lateral to the isthmus and is the longest (5 cm) and widest part of the tube. It is the site of fertilization.
d. The infundibulum (1.25 cm) is the most lateral part of the tube, which opens into the peritoneal cavity. The infundibulum is funnel-shaped and provided with finger like projections called fimbriae. The tubal ostium is guarded by these motile and prehensile fimbriae. Of the 5 to 6 fimbriae, one is longer than the rest and is called ovarian fimbria since it is attached to the medial surface of the ovary.

Peritoneal Relations

The fallopian tube is located in the upper part of broad ligament. It is covered with peritoneum completely except a small area inferiorly, which is left bare by the reflection of the peritoneum to form two layers of mesosalpinx.

Relation to Ovary

The infundibulum of fallopian tube reaches the lower end of the ovary and then follows its anterior border to reach its upper pole. It arches over the upper pole and turns down to end in relation to the posterior free margin and

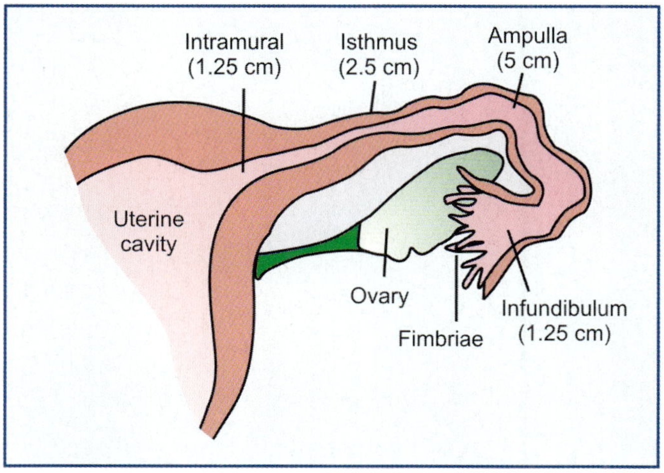

Fig. 164.1: Showing the parts of fallopian tube and length of each part

medial surface. Thus, the lateral end of the fallopian tube is related to all parts of the ovary except its lateral surface.

Blood Supply and Lymphatic Drainage

The medial two-thirds of the tube is supplied by uterine artery while the lateral one third is supplied by ovarian artery. The blood drains through corresponding veins. The lymph vessels travel along ovarian vessels to terminate in lateral aortic lymph nodes.

Nerve Supply

The fallopian tube is supplied through the ovarian and inferior hypogastric plexuses. Therefore its parasympathetic supply is from vagus as well as pelvic splanchnic nerves. The sympathetic innervation is through spinal segments T10 to L2.

Radiological Examination

a. Hysterosalpingography is a radiological method to investigate the female genital passages. The radiopaque dye is injected through the cannula into the uterine cavity, under direct vision. About 15 ml of medium is injected to outline the uterus and tubes. If the tubes are patent, there will be spillage of dye in the peritoneal cavity.
b. The tubes are inspected by means of the ultrasound.

Clinical Highlights

a. Tubectomy is the operation of female sterilization as it prevents the meeting of sperm and secondary oocyte. In mini-laparotomy, a small suprapubic incision is given to approach the fallopian tube. Then, each tube is brought out of the incision, ligated at two points and the segment of the tube between the ligatures is cut.
b. In laparoscopic sterilization a small subumbilical incision is placed under local anesthesia. An operating laparoscope is introduced to visualize the pelvic viscera. The fallopian tubes are identified and clipped at both ends.
c. The inflammation of the tube is called salpingitis, which is the commonest cause of tubal block leading to sterility.
d. The tubal block can be detected by a test called tubal insufflation. In this test, carbon dioxide is introduced in the fallopian tube via the vaginal route. On auscultation of lower abdomen, a bubbling sound is heard if the tube is patent.
e. Tubal implantation is a common type of ectopic pregnancy. In this condition, the morula fails to move to the uterine cavity so the blastocyst is formed in the tube and is implanted in the tube. The natural course of tubal pregnancy is rupture of the fallopian tube with internal bleeding in peritoneal cavity. This is a surgical emergency and needs immediate resection of the affected tube.

165 Uterus

The uterus is a hollow muscular organ situated between the urinary bladder in front and the rectum behind, in the pelvic cavity. Its wall has three layers, the perimetrium, myometrium and endometrium, from without inward. The endometrium (mucosa) shows cyclical changes in response to ovarian hormones, from the age of puberty to the menopause. The implantation of blastocyst takes place in the uterine decidua (endometrium after implantation is called decidua). All the layers of uterus increase in size considerably during pregnancy because the uterus houses not only the foetus but also the placenta and the amniotic sac.

Shape and Size

In the adult, the uterus is pear-shaped (piriform) and measures 7.5 × 5 × 2.5 cm. The fundus and body together are 5 cm long and the cervix is 2.5 cm long.

Parts (Fig. 165.1)

The uterus consists of fundus, body and cervix. The fundus is the rounded upper part above the level of the entrance of uterine tubes. The uterus gives attachment to two ligaments at the uterotubal (also described as tubo-uteral) junction or the lateral angle of uterus. The ligament of ovary is attached posteroinferior and round ligament of uterus anteroinferior to this junction. The body of uterus is between the fundus and the isthmus. The isthmus is the constricted part measuring about 0.5 cm between the body and the cervix. The cervix is cylindrical in shape. It extends from the isthmus and ends at external os, which opens in the vagina by perforating its anterior wall. Thus, cervix is divisible into supravaginal and vaginal parts.

Uterine Cavity

The uterine cavity is divisible into the cavity of the body and that of cervix. The shape of the cavity of the body is inverted isosceles triangle while that of the cervix is spindle shaped. The cavity of cervix (cervical canal) communicates with that of body at internal os and with that of vagina at external os. Therefore, the cervical canal extends between internal and external os. The uterine cavity, as measured by an instrument called uterine sound is 6 cm long from the external os to the wall of fundus. The ratio of length of cervix and of uterus varies with age. From birth till the age of puberty, the ratio is 2:1 while after puberty it becomes 1:2.

Normal Position (Fig. 165.2)

When the urinary bladder is empty, the position of uterus is described as anteverted and anteflexed. The body of the uterus is tilted forward on the superior surface of bladder, which provides support to the uterus. The term anteversion is defined as the angulation between the long axis of the cervix and the long axis of the vagina. The angle of version is 90°. Due to this angulation, the uterus is bent forward. When the bladder is fully distended, the uterus lies in line with the vagina. Then the position of uterus becomes retroverted. So, retroverted position can

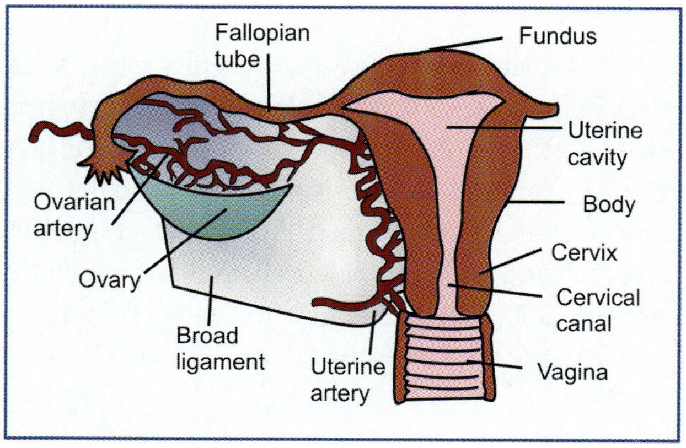

Fig. 165.1: Uterus, fallopian tube and ovary seen from posterior aspect

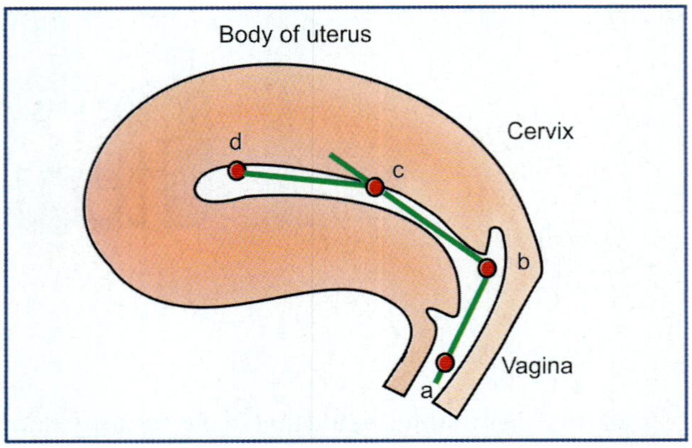

Fig. 165.2: Normal position of uterus angle of anteversion < abc = 90°, angle of anteflexion < bcd = 125~170°

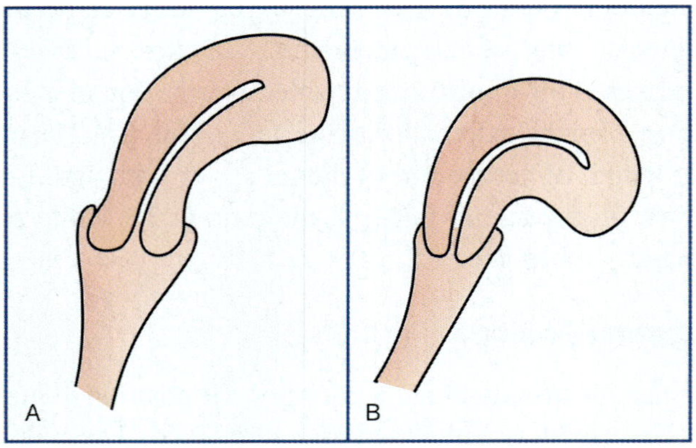

Fig. 165.3: Abnormal positions of uterus (A) Retroversion, (B) Retroversion and retroflexion

be normal in fully distended state of the bladder. The term anteflexion is defined as the angulation between the long axis of the body of uterus and long axis of the cervix. The angle of flexion is 120 to 170°. Due to this angulation the uterus is bent downward.

Abnormal Positions (Fig. 165.3)

In some women, the uterus is permanently retroverted so that the body of uterus bends backwards in the rectouterine pouch. Retroversion predisposes to prolapse of uterus because the bladder cannot provide support to the uterus, which is straight. Sometimes, the axis of uterine body passes upwards or backwards as a result of which there is no angulation between the uterus and cervix. In such cases, the uterus bends back on the cervix causing narrowing of the cervical canal. This is known as retroflexion, which may cause painful menstruation and reduce the chances of conception.

Peritoneal Relations (Fig. 132.1)

The uterus is intraperitoneal. The uterus is held from the lateral wall of pelvis by a flat sheet of peritoneum on either side, called broad ligament.

a. The peritoneum covers the anterior surface of the body of uterus upto the level of isthmus and gets reflected on the superior surface of bladder. This reflection gives rise to a shallow peritoneal pouch called uterovesical pouch. The anterior or vesical surface of uterus is thus related to urinary bladder.
b. The peritoneum covers the entire posterior surface of the body and cervix of the uterus and then goes down to cover the posterior fornix of vagina. From this level, it is reflected on the anterior surface of rectum. This reflection forms a deep peritoneal pouch called rectouerine pouch of Douglas. The bottom of this pouch is 5.5 cm above the anal orifice. This is the lowest part of female peritoneal cavity. This pouch can be approached surgically through the posterior fornix of vagina for aspiration of accumulated fluid. The rectouterine pouch normally contains sigmoid colon and coils of intestine, which make contact with the posterior or intestinal surface of uterus.

Cervix

The cervix is the most fixed part of the uterus. The cervix is divisible into the supravaginal cervix and vaginal cervix.

a. The anterior wall of the supravaginal cervix is not covered with peritoneum. It is directly related to the base of the urinary bladder. Laterally, at a distance of 2 cm this part of the cervix is related to the uterine artery crossing in front of the ureter. This relation is of surgical importance because during clamping the uterine artery in the operation of hysterectomy, the ureter is in danger of injury. The posterior wall of the supravaginal cervix is covered with peritoneum of rectouterine pouch, which separates it from the rectum.
b. The vaginal part of the cervix lies in the interior of the upper part of the vagina and is encircled by vaginal fornices. Its rounded lower end bears an aperture called the external os. At the lower end of cervical canal, the simple columnar epithelium changes to the stratified squamous nonkeratinized type covering the lips of the external os and the outer surface of the vaginal cervix. The shape of the external os is circular

in nulliparous women but the shape changes to a transverse slit in parous women. A shorter, thicker and more projecting anterior lip and a longer and thinner posterior lip, bound the external os.

Cervical Canal (Fig. 165.1)

It is a cavity of the cervix extending from the internal to the external os. Its lining epithelium is simple columnar. It does not show periodic changes during menstrual cycle. The cervical glands are branched tubular in type and secrete mucus with high content of fructose. The mucus collects as a plug in the cervical canal. The palmate folds arise from the longitudinal mucosal ridge of the anterior and posterior wall and interdigitate. The palmar folds resemble the branches of a tree (arbor vitae uteri) and they close the cervical canal.

Functional Isthmus

The upper third of cervix including the internal os is called the functional isthmus. It behaves more like the body of uterus in having same epithelium like the uterus and in its response to ovarian hormones. From second month of pregnancy, it is taken up in the body of the uterus to form the lower uterine segment. An incision is placed in the lower segment in the operation of lower segment caesarian section (LSCS).

Examination of Cervix

Direct inspection by per speculum examination, exposes the interior of the vagina including the vaginal cervix. The digital palpation helps in assessing the shape and consistency of the cervix.

Ligaments Attached to Cervix (Fig. 165.4)

The cervix being the most fixed part of the uterus, gives attachments to the ligaments. There are three ligaments, which form a three-spoked triradiate ligament, consisting of, Mackenrodt's ligament laterally, uterosacral ligament posteriorly and pubovesical ligament anteriorly.

Blood Supply of Uterus (Fig. 165.1)

The uterus receives blood from a pair of uterine arteries supplemented by a pair of ovarian arteries. Each uterine artery is a branch of anterior division of internal iliac artery. The uterine arteries are highly tortuous in nonpregnant state. As the uterine artery ascends by the lateral margin of uterus, it gives a series of arcuate arteries, which run transversely on the anterior and posterior surfaces of the body of uterus. The branches of the two sides anastomose in the midline. The radial branches of the arcuate arteries enter the inner longitudinal layer of the myometrium (stratum vasculare). The muscle bundles in this layer are arranged in the pattern of figure of eight and hence on their contraction the blood vessels are clamped. This is the reason why these muscle fibres are known as living ligatures of the uterus. This action is important in controlling uterine bleeding during parturition and menstruation. The uterine veins drain into the internal iliac veins.

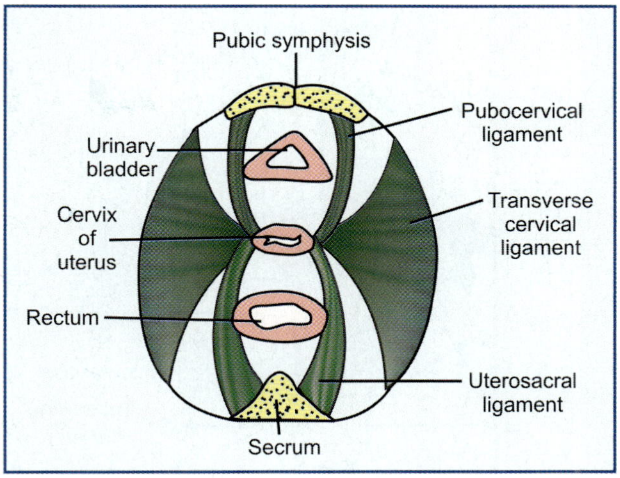

Fig. 165.4: Schematic illustration of ligaments attached to cervix uteri

Lymphatic Drainage (Fig. 165.5)

a. The lymph vessels from the fundus pass along the ovarian vessels to drain into the lateral aortic and preaortic lymph nodes. A few vessels from the lateral angle of uterus (uterotubal junction) reach the superficial inguinal nodes along the round ligament of uterus.
b. The lymph vessels from the body travel via the broad ligament to the external iliac lymph nodes.
c. The cervix drains laterally into the external iliac and obturator lymph nodes. A few vessels terminate in paracervical nodes, which are located at the crossing of ureter and uterine artery. The enlarged paracervical

Section four

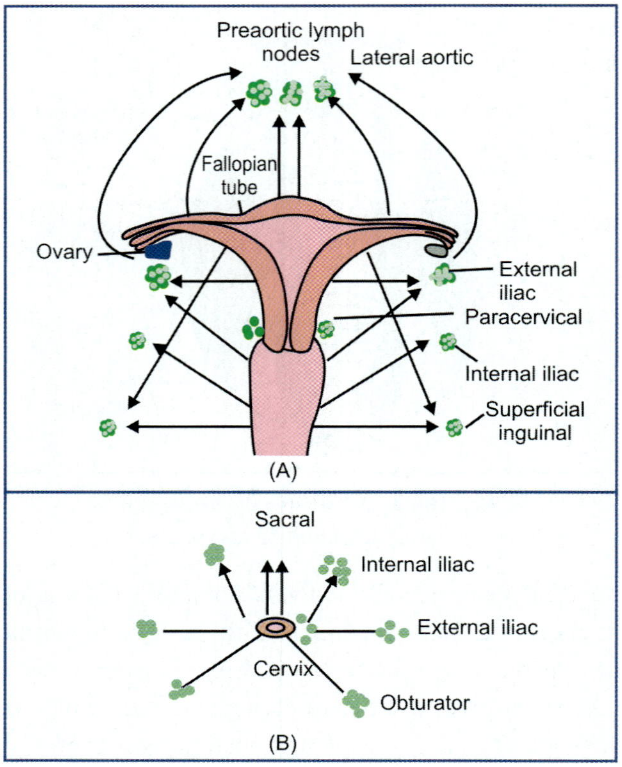

Fig. 165.5: Lymphatic drainage of (A) uterus, ovary, fallopian tube and vagina and (B) cervix

node (due to cervical cancer) may block the ureter. Some lymph vessels travel in posterior direction to drain in sacral lymph nodes. A few lymph vessels pass along the uterine vessels to terminate in internal iliac nodes.

Nerve Supply

The autonomic nerve supply to the uterus is derived from uterovaginal plexuses, which lie in the broad ligaments. The efferent sympathetic fibres arise from T12 to L1 segment of spinal cord. The efferent parasympathetic fibres arise from S2 to S4 segments of spinal cord. The pain sensation from cervix and uterus during childbirth passes through parasympathetic pathways (pelvic splanchnic nerves) to the S2-S4 sacral segments of spinal cord. The caudal analgesia is a method to give nerve block to achieve painless labor.

Ligaments of Uterus

The ligaments are divided into peritoneal and non-peritoneal. The broad ligament is the peritoneal and round

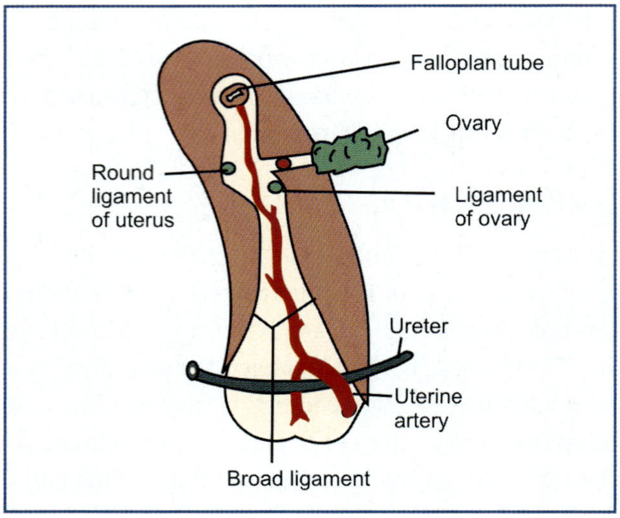

Fig. 165.6: Sagittal section of broad ligament near its attachment to uterus showing its contents

ligament is the nonperitoneal one (These may be regarded as false ligaments of uterus).

a. The broad ligament of uterus is a large peritoneal fold enclosing the parametrium (connective tissue of the pelvis fascia) and extending from the body of uterus to the lateral pelvic wall. It has two margins, free anterior margin and fixed posterior margin or base (Fig. 165.6). It has anteroinferior and posterosuperior layers forming corresponding surfaces. The broad ligament consists of four parts. The mesovarium is the part of the posterior layer attached to the anterior margin of ovary. The suspensory ligament of ovary is the part lateral to the ovary. The mesosalpinx is that part which lies between the uterine tube and the ovary. The mesometrium is the remaining part.

   A large number of structures are located inside the different parts of the broad ligament. The mesolsalpinx contains the uterine tube, round ligament of uterus, ligament of ovary, paroophoron and epoophoron. The mesovarium transmits the ovarian blood vessels and nerve plexuses. The contents of the infundibulopelvic ligament are the ovarian vessels, lymph vessels and nerve plexuses. The contents of the mesometrium are the uterine vessels, uterovaginal nerve plexuses, lymphatic vessels and the duct of Gartner.

b. The round ligament of the uterus is the remnant of gubernaculum ovarii and extends from uterotubal junction to the labium majus. It is about 10-12 cm long and passes through the broad ligament diagonally down and laterally to the pelvic floor. On its way to the deep inguinal ring, it crosses the pelvic brim and hooks round the inferior epigastric artery. It passes through the inguinal canal. After coming out of the superficial ring, it splits in fibrous strands, which attach to the skin of labium majus. It is accompanied by lymphatics, which drain into the superficial inguinal lymph nodes.

Supports of Uterus

The following factors that maintain the uterus in the anteverted and anteflexed position in the pelvic cavity.

a. Pelvic diaphragm is the most important support since it cradles the uterus from below. It is constantly subjected to strain due to rise in intra-abdominal pressure during the acts of coughing, sneezing and straining at stools. The vaginal delivery puts an extra strain on the pelvic diaphragm.
b. The true ligaments of the uterus are the condensation of the pelvic fascia. These ligaments pass from the cervix in three different directions and fix it to the pelvic walls. These ligaments form a hammock of condensed pelvic fascia and support the uterus against vertical descent. In the operation of hysterectomy, it is not possible to free the cervix and vagina unless these ligaments are cut. Mackenrodt's ligament or transverse cervical ligament or cardinal ligament connects the lateral aspect of vagina and cervix to the lateral pelvic wall. It passes through the base of the broad ligament. The uterine artery may pass through a special tunnel in the ligament or it may pass superior to it. The uterosacral ligament extends from the posterior aspect of cervix backward, lateral to rectum, to gain attachment to the sacrum. The pubocervical ligament extends from the anterior aspect to the back of pubic symphysis.
c. The urogenital diaphragm and the perineal body provide additional support to the uterus by supporting the vagina.

Radiological Examination

Ultrasound examination of the pelvis reveals the anatomy of uterus and ovaries and other pelvic organs. The hysterosalpingography is another method of visualizing the genital tract.

Clinical Highlights

a. If the supports of the uterus become weak due to any cause the uterus descends in the vagina. This is called prolapse of the uterus. The loss of tone of the muscles of pelvic diaphragm, perineal tears and repeated childbirths are the main causes of the prolapse. There are different degrees of uterine prolapse. In the first degree prolapse, the cervix descends in the vagina. In the second degree, the cervix descends to the level of vulva. In the third degree, the cervix protrudes outside the vaginal orifice. In procidentia, the whole uterus protrudes outside the vaginal orifice.
b. To diagnose the disorders of endometrium, a procedure called dilatation and curettage (D and C) is very common in gynaecology. At first, the size of the uterine cavity is measured with the help of an instrument called the uterine sound. The cervix is then gradually dilated and the endometrium is scraped with a curette. This is useful in detecting endometrial cancer and in assessing the hormonal status of the ovaries after histological examination of the curettings.
c. The myoma or fibroid is a tumour of myometrium. It is more common in younger age group. If single, myomectomy alone is possible but if multiple, hysterectomy is required.
d. Placental pathologies affect the uterus. The vesicular mole is the cystic degeneration of the chorionic villi. Choriocarcinoma is the malignancy of the vesicular mole.
e. Among the intrauterine contraceptive devices (IUCD), copper-T is commonly used. The principle underlying occluding the uterine cavity is to prevent implantation of the blastocyst.
f. The surgical removal of uterus is called hysterectomy and can be performed by vaginal or abdominal route.
g. Hysterotomy is the operative removal of products of conception from the uterus before 28 weeks of gestation by cutting through the anterior wall of uterus. It is usually done for medical termination of pregnancy (MTP).
h. In some women, it is not possible to have normal vaginal delivery. The baby is born through an operation

called the lower segment cesarian section (LSCS). The abdomen is opened either through a vertical infraumbilical midline incision or through a low transverse incision (modified Pfannenstiel). The peritoneum of the uterovesical pouch and the lower segment of uterus are incised transversely.

166 Vagina

The vagina is a fibromuscular tube connecting the cervical canal to the exterior, at the vestibule. It is lined by stratified squamous nonkeratinized epithelium. It functions as an excretory passage for menstrual flow, which consists of blood and pieces of endometrium. It is a female organ of sexual intercourse. It serves as a birth canal. The upper half of vagina lies in the pelvic cavity and the lower half in the perineum. The vagina passes through two diaphragms, namely, the pelvic and urogenital.

Length

The length of its posterior wall is 9 cm as against that of anterior wall, which is 7 to 7.5 cm.

Vaginal Fornices

The anterior and posterior walls of vagina are in apposition except at the upper end of vagina where the cervix projects in it. Here, the vagina is wide and forms anterior, posterior, right and left lateral fornices around the projecting cervix. The posterior fornix is the deepest and through it, rectouerine pouch can be approached surgically.

Relations

a. The upper part of the anterior wall is related to the base of the urinary bladder and terminal parts of ureters. The lower part of the anterior wall is intimately related to the urethra.
b. The upper third of the posterior wall, is covered with peritoneum of rectouterine pouch and related to the contents of the pouch. In the middle third, the posterior wall is related to the ampulla of rectum and in the lower third, it is related to perineal body.
c. The lateral wall on each side is related (from above downwards) to the crossing of ureter and uterine artery, transverse cervical ligament, medial fibers of levator ani (sphincter vaginae), urogenital diaphragm, bulb of the vestibule and greater vestibular gland.

Blood Supply

The vagina receives blood from multiple branches of internal iliac artery (vaginal, uterine, middle rectal arteries) and inferior rectal branch of internal pudendal artery. The veins drain into the internal iliac veins.

Nerve Supply

The upper part of vagina receives autonomic nerve supply. Hence, it is pain insensitive. The lower part receives twigs from the inferior rectal and labial nerves (branches of pudendal nerve). It is pain sensitive.

Lymphatic Drainage (Fig.165.5)

The upper third of vagina drains into external and internal iliac lymph nodes. The middle third drains into internal iliac nodes. The lower third drains into superficial inguinal nodes.

Clinical Highlights

a. Digital examination of vagina (per vaginum examination) is routinely done in obstetrics and gynecology practice. It provides an easy route for palpation of pelvic organs.
   i. The form and size of the body of the uterus can be examined by bimanual palpation with two fingers in the vagina and the other hand on anterior abdominal wall above the pubic symphysis.
   ii. The urinary ladder and urethra are felt through the anterior wall.
   iii. Through the posterior wall, the rectal ampulla can be palpated. In the pouch of Douglas, loops of intestine and sigmoid colon can be felt.

   iv. Through the lateral fornices the ureter and pulsations of uterine artery can be felt.
   v. The size of the pelvis is often assessed digital examination (internal pelvimetry).

b. The cystocele is the prolapse of the anterior wall of vagina. During rise in the intra-abdominal pressure the anterior vaginal wall is pushed down by the urinary bladder. The rectocele is the prolapse of posterior vaginal wall by the pressure of rectum. These conditions are usually due to severe injury to perineal body during repeated childbirths.

c. For aspiration of pus or blood from the pouch of Douglas, a needle is introduced through the posterior wall of posterior fornix (colpotomy).

d. The cells of the vaginal mucosa are rich in glycogen during the reproductive life (from puberty to menopause). The glycogen production is under the control of estorgen. The vaginal cytology is a laboratory investigation done to assess the hormonal status during ovarian cycle and during early pregnancy.

167 Perineum

The perineum is the lowest region of the trunk in the erect position. It lies below the level of pelvic diaphragm. The perineum is traversed by the anal canal and urethra in male and by the anal canal, urethra and vagina in female. The male external genital organs are suspended from the perineum while the female external genitalia form the surface features of the perineum.

Bony Boundaries (Fig. 167.1)

Anteriorly, the perineum is bounded by the inferior margin of pubic symphysis and posteriorly, by the coccyx. The lateral boundary on each side, is formed by the ischiopubic ramus, ischial tuberosity and sacrotuberous ligament from before backward.

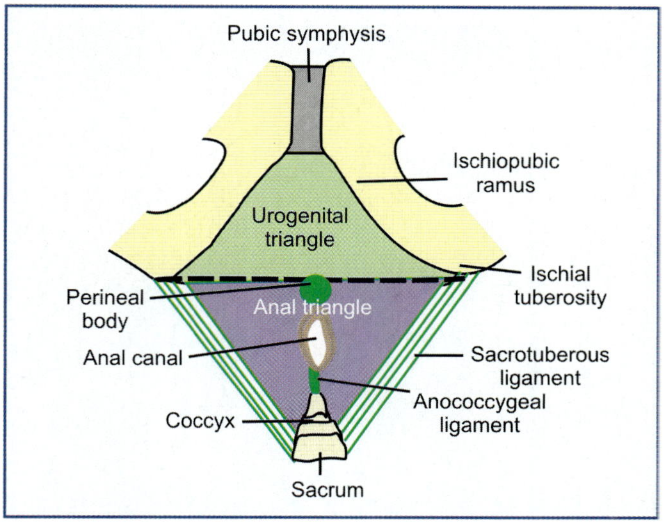

Fig. 167.1: Boundaries and subdivisions of perineum

Subdivisions

The perineum is divided into the anterior urogenital triangle and a posterior anal triangle by an imaginary line in the coronal plane, passing through the anterior ends of the ischial tuberosities.

Contents of Anal Triangle

The anal triangle contains the anal canal in the midline and the ischiorectal fossa on either side of anal canal. The anal canal is described in Chapter 135.

Contents of Urogenital Triangle

The urogenital triangle contains the superficial and deep perineal pouches, which differ in the two sexes. The details of the contents are described in Chapter 169.

Superficial Fascia

The superficial fascia in the perineum is subdivided into superficial fatty (Camper) and deep membranous (Colles) layers. The attachments of the membranous layer are clinically important. Laterally, it is attached to the ischial tuberosities and to the lateral margins of ischiopubic rami. Anteriorly, it crosses the front of the bodies of pubic bones up to the pubic tubercles, and then it becomes continuous above with the membranous layer of superficial fascia of the anterior abdominal wall (Scarpa). In the male, this layer forms the fascial sheath and fundiform ligament of penis and continues as dartos muscle of scrotum. Posteriorly, the membranous layer fuses with the posterior margin of the perineal membrane or inferior layer of the urogenital diaphragm.

Fascial Boundaries of Urogenital Triangle

The urogenital triangle consists of two perineal pouches bounded by three fascial layers. In the erect position of the body these three layers are placed one above the other.

The lowermost layer is the membranous layer of superficial fascia of the perineum. Superior to the membranous layer is the perineal membrane or inferior layer of urogenital diaphragm. Above the perineal membrane lies the superior fascia of urogenital diaphragm. These three layers of fasciae fuse posteriorly with each other. The superficial perineal space (pouch) is enclosed by the membranous layer of superficial fascia and the perineal membrane. This space is open arteriorly, where it is continuous with the anterior abdominal wall. In the male, the rupture of the bulbar urethra in the superficial pouch may cause extravasation of urine into the anterior abdominal wall due to fascial continuity. The deep perineal space (pouch) is enclosed by the perineal membrane and the superior fascia of urogenital diaphragm. This is a completely closed space. Thus, the perineal pouches lie one above the other in the narrow space bounded by the ischiopubic rami and pubic arch, in the erect position of body.

168 Ischiorectal Fossa

The ischiorectal fossa is renamed as the ischioanal space in the most recent edition of Nomina Anatomica. This is because it is located between the ischial tuberosity and the anal canal (not the rectum). However, in the following account the old name is retained. The fossa is a fat- filled space on either side of the anal canal. The right and left fossae allow distension of anal canal during defaecation. The ischiorectal fossa is wedge-shaped having a base, apex, anterior, posterior, lateral and medial walls.

Boundaries (Fig. 168.1)

a. The vertical lateral wall is partly muscular and partly bony. The obturator internus muscle and the fascia covering it form the upper larger part and the medial surface of the ischial tuberosity forms the lower smaller part of this wall.
b. The sloping medial wall is formed by the perineal surface of the levator ani above and sphincter ani externus below.
c. The linear apex is the meeting of the fascia lining the perineal aspect of levator ani and the fascia covering the obturator internus muscle. Herniation of pelvic viscera in the ischiorectal fossa may occur if there is a gap at the apex of the fossa due to separation of levator ani from obturator fascia. The gap is called hiatus of Schwalbe.
d. The perineal skin forms the base or floor of the fossa.
e. Posteriorly, the fossa is bounded by the sacrotuberous ligament and lower margin of gluteus maximus muscle.
f. Anteriorly, it is bounded by posterior margin of perineal pouches. Above the level of deep perineal pouch, the fossa projects as anterior recess upto the level of pubic bone.

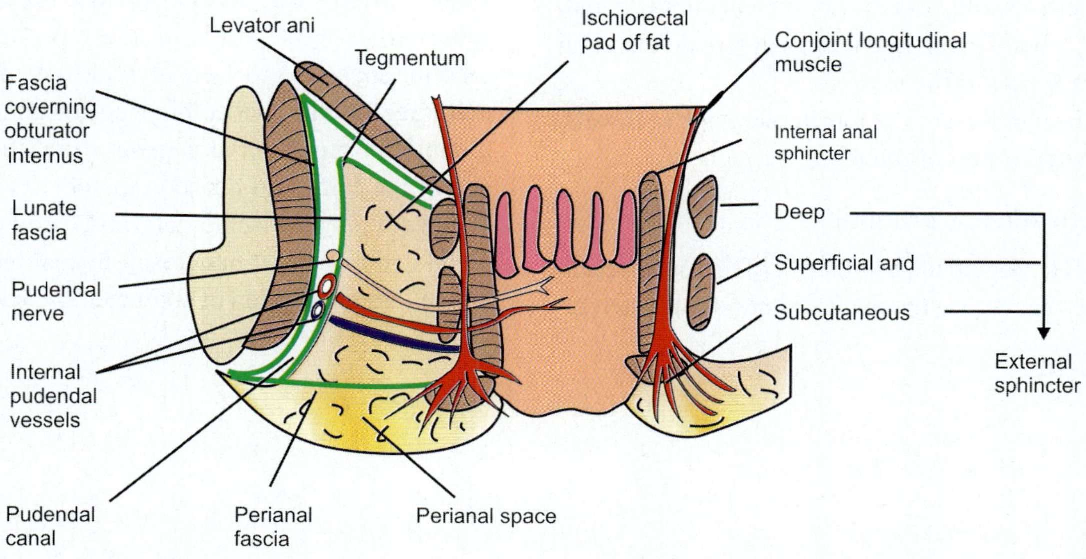

Fig. 168.1: Boundaries and contents of ischiorectal fossa

Fascial Relations

The ischiorectal fossa is a fascial space. Its lateral wall is lined by obturator fascia and the medial wall is lined by inferior fascia of pelvic diaphragm. The subcutaneous pad of fat raises the deep fascia inside the fossa to form a dome-shaped lunate fascia. The summit of lunate fascia is called the tegmentum. Medially and laterally, the lunate fascia comes very close to the fasciae of the respective walls. The perianal fascia is the most lateral septum from the lower end of the conjoint longitudinal tendon in the wall of anal canal. The perianal fascia is attached to the skin. Therefore, the lunate and perianal fasciae divide the fossa in three compartments, namely, suprategmental space, ischioanal space proper and perianal space. The last named space contains loculated fat. The pudendal or Alcock's canal in the lateral wall is the fascial canal bounded by the lunate and obturator fasciae.

Contents

a. The fossa is filled with a pad of fat, which is the fibrofatty tissue of the superficial fascia. Tension of the gluteus maximus muscles during standing compresses the fat around the anal canal contributing to anal continence.
b. The inferior rectal nerve and vessels (branches of pudendal nerve and internal pudendal vessels in the pudendal canal) cross the fossa from lateral to medial side.
c. The posterior scrotal nerves and vessels in male and posterior labial vessels and nerves in female travel in the anterior part of the fossa.
d. The perineal branch of the fourth sacral nerve travels in the posterior part of the fossa.

Pudendal or Alcock's Canal

This is a fascial canal in the lateral wall of the ischiorectal fossa. It gives passage to the pudendal nerve and internal pudendal vessels. The canal extends from the lesser sciatic foramen to the anterior wall of the fossa. Regarding formation of the canal, there are two views as follows. The obturator internus fascia splits to enclose the canal or the obturator internus fascia and lunate fascia enclose the canal. The pudendal nerve divides in the canal into its terminal branches namely, dorsal nerve of penis or clitoris and perineal nerve. In the posterior part of the canal the pudendal nerve is below the internal pudendal vessels. In the anterior part of the canal, the relation of the neurovascular bundle is dorsal nerve, internal pudental vessels and perineal nerve, from above downwards.

Clinical Highlights

a. Ischiorectal or ischioanal abscess is quite common because the fat in the fossa is poorly vascularized and may be infected from anal canal or from boils in the perianal skin. The ischiorectal abscess is very painful because of the compression of the sensory nerves passing through the fossa. The abscess may burst on the skin forming a sinus. It may open on the skin and in the anal canal-forming fistula. The abscess on one side may spread to the other side behind the anal canal forming a horseshoe-shaped abscess.
b. The pudendal nerve block by perineal route is given in the pudendal canal. In this procedure, the anesthetic solution is injected in the canal about 2.5 cm from the surface along the medial surface of the ischial tuberosity. This may cause temporary urinary incontinence due to loss of function of sphincter urethrae. But, the anal continence is retained because the inferior rectal nerve is given off at the posterior end of the canal and hence is spared.
c. While draining the ischiorectal abscess, if the inferior rectal nerve is cut, it may result in anal incontinence due to loss of function of sphincter ani externus.

169 Urogenital Triangles

The urogenital triangle consists of superficial and deep perineal pouches, which differ in the male and female.

Superficial Perineal Pouch in Male

The boundaries of the superficial pouch are as follows. The membranous layer of the superficial fascia of perineum (Colles fascia) forms the inferior boundary and the inferior fascia of the urogenital diaphragm or the perineal membrane forms its superior boundary. The lateral limits are the conjoint ischiopubic rami. Posteriorly, the pouch is closed by the fusion of the superior and inferior walls. Anteriorly, the pouch is open, where it is continuous via the scrotum and penis with the anterior abdominal wall. The bulbar part of the urethra passes through the bulb of penis in the superficial perineal pouch. If this part of the urethra ruptures (for example in straddle injuries), the urine leaks in superficial pouch distending the pouch as well as the external genitalia (Fig. 169.1). The urine may ascend in the anterior abdominal wall in the space between the membranous layer of superficial fascia (fascia Scarpa) and the aponeurosis of external oblique muscle. The extravasation of urine in these regions produces a circumscribed swelling of the perineum, scrotum and infraumbilical anterior abdominal wall. The urine cannot enter the thigh because of the fusion of membranous layer of superficial fascia of thigh and fascia lata at the Holden's line (Fig. 177.1).

Contents

The superficial pouch in male, contains the structures forming the root of penis, muscles, nerves and vessels.

a. The root of penis consists of three structures, the bulb of penis and two crura (Fig. 169.2). The bulb is attached to the inferior surface of perineal membrane and is traversed by the bulbar part of penile urethra. The bulb extends in the body of penis as corpus spongiosum. The crus is attached to the medial surface of conjoint ischiopubic ramus and adjoining perineal membrane and continues in the body of penis as corpus cavernosus, on each side. The eversion of the

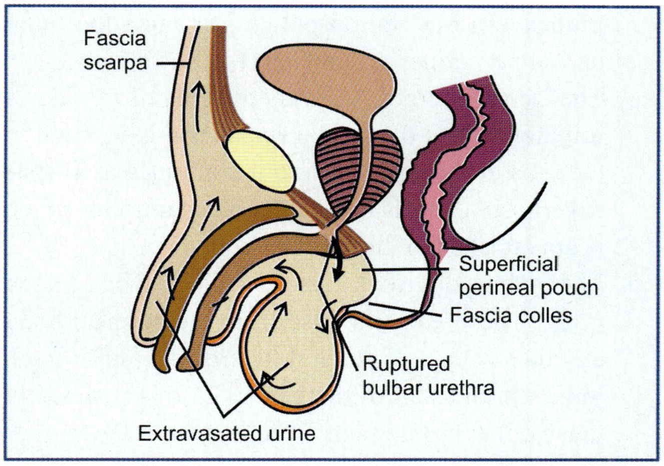

Fig. 169.1: Rupture of bulbar urethra (Note: The direction of spread of urine via superficial perineal pouch into anterior abdominal wall)

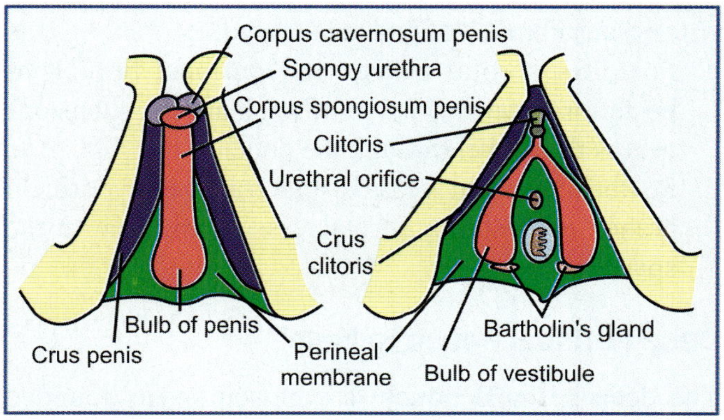

Fig. 169.2: Superficial perineal pouch in male and female showing root of penis and clitoris respectively, attached to inferior surface of perineal membrane

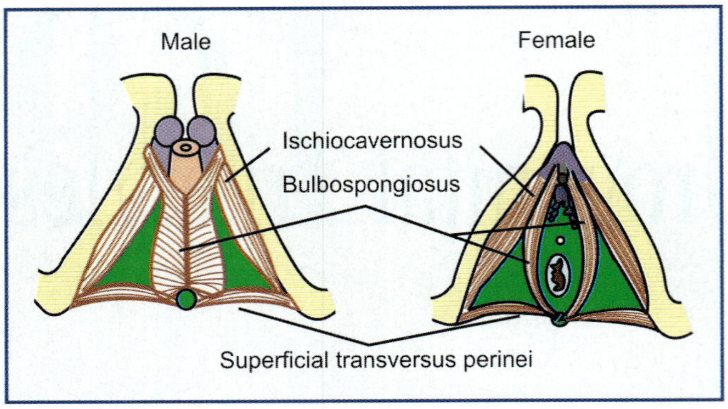

Fig. 169.3: Muscles of superficial perineal pouch in male and female

ischiopubic rami in male is due to attachments of crus and ischiocavernosus muscle.

b. There are three muscles on each side, namely, ischiocavernosus, bulbospongiosus and superficial transversus perinei as shown in Figure 169.3.
   i. The ischiocavernosus covers the crus of its side. It originates from the ischial ramus and is inserted in the crus at the point, where it continues as corpus cavernosus. This is the only perineal muscle, which is not attached to the perineal body.
   ii. The bulbospongiosus muscles cover the bulb of the penis. These muscles arise from the perineal body and fuse with each other at the median raphe. Each inserts in the skin of the penis. So, this is the only muscle that has no bony attachments.
   iii. The superficial transversus perinei muscle arises on each side from ischial tuberosity and inserts in the perineal body.
   The muscles of the superficial pouch are supplied by perineal branch of pudendal nerve.
c. Posterior scrotal nerves and perineal branch of posterior cutaneous nerve of thigh are the cutaneous nerves that travel through the pouch.
d. Posterior scrotal vessels and transverse perineal branch of posterior scrotal vessels are seen in the space.

Deep Perineal Pouch in Male

The deep perineal pouch is a closed space bounded superiorly by the superior fascia of urogenital diaphragm and inferiorly by the inferior fascia of the urogenital diaphragm or perineal membrane. The conjoint ischiopubic rami limit the space laterally on each side. The fusion of the two fascial layers limits it posteriorly. The posterior margin is intimately fused with the perineal body. Anteriorly, the space is closed due to fusion of the superior and inferior fascial layers. The thickened anterior border of the perineal membrane forms transverse perineal ligament. There is gap between this ligament and the arcuate pubic ligament at the inferior margin of pubis.

Contents of Deep Pouch (Fig. 169.4)

a. Membranous part of urethra.
b. Bulbourethral glands (Cowper's glands) on either side of the urethra.
c. Two striated muscles, sphincter urethrae surrounding the urethra and deep transversus perinei.
d. Dorsal nerve of penis courses forwards near the ischiopubic ramus on each side.
e. Internal pudendal artery, artery to the bulb, deep and dorsal artery of penis course along the ischiopubic ramus.

Muscles of Deep Pouch

a. The sphincter urethrae muscle arises from the medial surface of inferior pubic ramus. The fibres of the two sides unite in front and behind the urethra. The posterior fibres attach to the perineal body. The perineal branch of pudendal nerve supplies the sphincter urethrae. It is the voluntary sphincter of urethra.
b. The deep transversus perinei muscles are situated on each side but behind the sphincter urethrae. Each arises from the medial surface of ischial ramus and is inserted in the perineal body. Perineal branches of pudendal nerve supply the muscle.

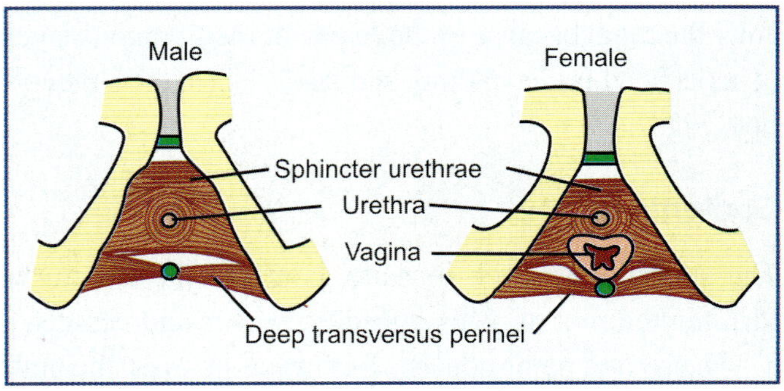

Fig. 169.4: Muscles of deep perineal pouches in male and female

Urogenital Diaphragm (Figs 169.5A and B)

The urogenital diaphragm is a muscular sheet (consisting of the two muscles of the deep perineal pouch) enclosed between the superior and inferior fasciae of urogenital diaphragm. Along the narrow anterior margin of the diaphragm, the two fasciae fuse to form the transverse perineal ligament. At the midpoint of its posterior margin, the diaphragm gives attachment to the perineal body. This diaphragm lies below the anterior part of the pelvic diaphragm and it reinforces the pelvic diaphragm at the urogenital hiatus. The diaphragm is pierced by membranous urethra in male and urethra and vagina in female. It supports the prostate and neck of urinary bladder in male and the neck of urinary bladder and vagina in female. It provides voluntary control of urethra in both sexes. There are differing views regarding the true nature of the urogenital diaphragm. According to one view, it is poorly defined in female. According to another view, its presence is questioned in both sexes.

Perineal Membrane (Fig. 169.6A)

The perineal membrane is the key structure in the urogenital triangle. It lies between the deep and superficial pouches. In the anatomical position, the deep pouch is the superior relation while the superficial pouch forms the inferior relation of the membrane. The membrane is triangular in shape. Its base is directed posteriorly and gives attachment to the perineal body near its midpoint. All the three fascial layers fuse along the base of the perineal membrane. Its lateral margins are attached to the medial surfaces of ischiopubic rami. Its apex is directed forward and is thickened to form transverse perineal ligament. Through the gap between this ligament and arcuate pubic ligament, the deep dorsal vein of penis enters the pelvis. The structures that pierce the perineal membrane in male are, the urethra in the midline, ducts of the bulbourethral glands by side of the urethra on each side and the artery to the bulb of the penis. At the base of the membrane two posterior scrotal nerves and vessels pierce on each side. The anterior part of the membrane is pierced by dorsal nerve and deep and dorsal arteries of penis.

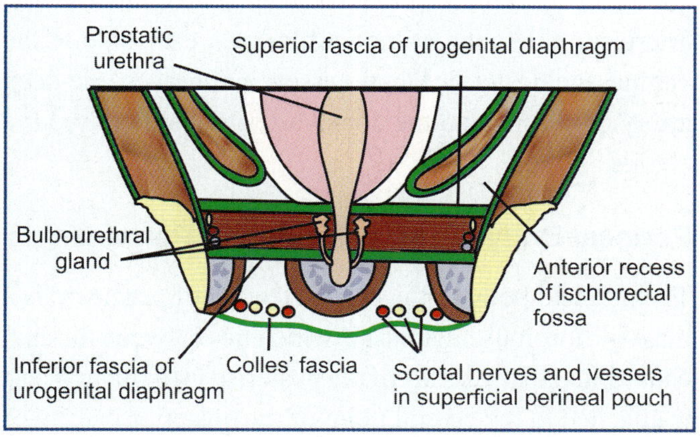

Fig. 169.5A: Coronal section through urogenital diaphragm in male

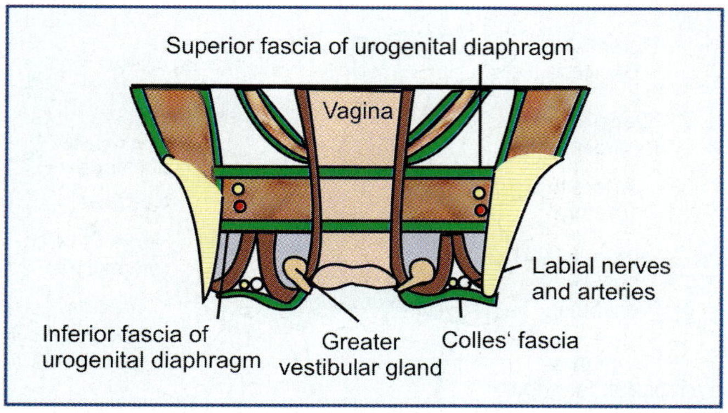

Fig. 169.5B: Coronal section through urogenital diaphragm in female

Perineal Body or Central Tendon of Perineum

This is a mass of fibromuscular tissue lying between the bulb of penis in front and the anal canal behind. It provides

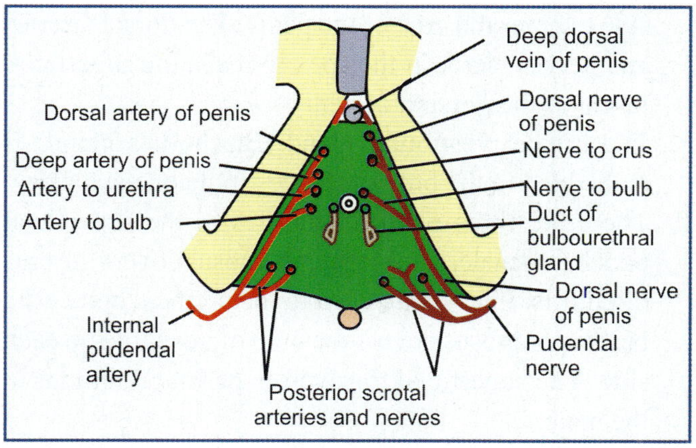

Fig. 169.6A: To show structures piercing perineal membrane from above (in male) Note that deep dorsal vein does not pierce the membrane. (Nerves are shown on right side and arteries on left side)

Section four

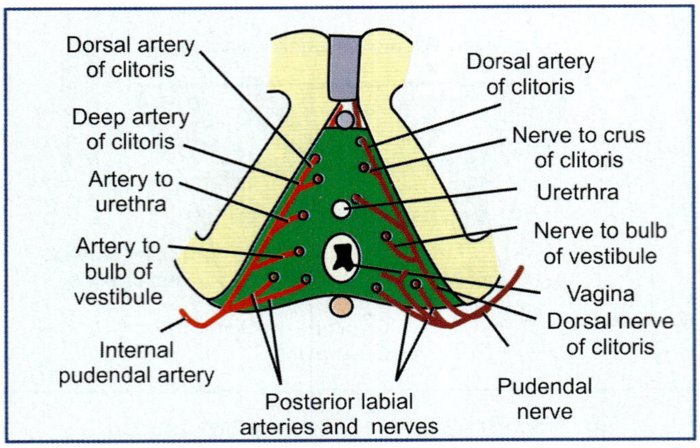

Fig. 169.6B: To show structures piercing perineal membrane from above in female

attachment to a large number of muscles. The importance of perineal body in male is to support the prostate gland and anal canal.

Superficial Perineal Pouch in Female

The boundaries of the superficial pouch are the same as in male.

Contents (Figs 169.2 and 169.3)

a. The urethra and vagina pass through the space.
b. The crura of the clitoris are attached on each side to the ischiopubic ramus. The bulb of vestibule is seen on each side of vagina but attached to the lower aspect of the perineal membrane. The deep artery of the penis pierces at the central part of the lateral margin on each side to enter the crus of the penis. The dorsal arteries and nerves pierce at the apex to reach the superficial fascia of the dorsum of penis.
c. The greater vestibular gland (Bartholin's gland) is embedded in the bulb of the vestibule on each side.
d. There are three pairs of muscles in the superficial pouch in female. The ischiocavernosus covers the crus of clitoris. It is not attached to the perineal body. The bulbospongiosus covers the bulb of vestibule on each side. The superficial transverses perinei is similar to the male.
e. Three blood vessels pass through the space, two posterior labial and the transverse perineal vessels.
f. Three sensory pass through the space to reach the labium majus of its side, two posterior labial nerves and the perineal branch of the posterior cutaneous nerve of thigh.

Greater Vestibular Gland (Bartholin's Gland)

This gland is embedded in the erectile tissue of the bulb of the vestibule and is covered by the bulbospongiosus muscle. Its 25 mm long duct opens in the vagina below the hymen. It is a compound racemose gland, which secretes lubricating mucus. The gland becomes infected in gonorrhoea (bartholinitis). The bulbourethral glands in male are the homologue of Bartholin's glands in female.

Deep Perineal Pouch in Female

The boundaries of the deep perineal pouch in the female are the same as in the male.

Contents (Fig. 169.4)

The urethra and the vagina pass through the deep space. The sphincter urethrae and the deep transverses perinei are the striated muscles, whose attachments and nerve supply are similar to corresponding muscles of male. The dorsal nerve of the clitoris enters the space from the ischiorectal fossa. The internal pudendal artery and its terminal branches, the artery to bulb, dorsal and deep artery of clitoris pass through the space.

Perineal Membrane (Fig. 169.6B)

In the female, the perineal membrane is very thin because it is pierced by the vagina apart from other structures like, urethra in the midline (urethra being in front of the vagina), arteries to the bulbs of the vestibule on each side of the vagina, the posterior labial vessels and nerves, the deep artery of clitoris and the dorsal arteries and nerve of the clitoris.

Perineal Body (Central Tendon of Perineum)

The perineal body or the central tendon of perineum is a mass of fibromuscular tissue, which lies between the anal canal and the lower part of the posterior wall of vagina. It is attached to the central point of the posterior margin of urogenital diaphragm. It gives attachment to the following muscles:

a. Right and left superficial transversus perinei
b. Right and left bulbospongiosus
c. Right and left deep transversus perinei
d. Sphincter urethrae
e. Sphincter ani externus
f. Right and left pubovaginalis part of levator ani.

Clinical Highlights

a. The perineal body is very important structure in the female during childbirth. It is stretched during the second stage of labour and is liable to tears, when the fetal head passes through the vaginal orifice. The tears of the perineal body may be accompanied by tear of the posterior wall of the vagina and of the anal sphincters. Rectal incontinence may result if the perineal tears are not repaired immediately. Weakened perineal body may predispose to prolapse of uterus.
b. Episiotomy is a simple surgical procedure performed in third stage of labour to prevent irregular and uncontrolled tears in the perineum during vaginal childbirth. A planned incision in the posterolateral direction in the perianal skin includes perineal muscles that are inserted in perineal body and the posterior wall of vagina. This facilitates the easy passage of head through the vaginal orifice.

170 External Genitalia

Development (Fig. 170.1)

The external genitalia pass through an indifferent stage before the sex can be distinguished at the third month of fetal life. The external genitalia first appear as five swellings around the urogenital membrane.

a. The genital tubercle appears at the cranial end of the urogenital membrane. Soon, glans is recognizable at the tip of the elongated genital tubercle.
b. The urethral or genital folds appear on each side of the membrane.
c. The genital swellings or labioscrotal swellings appear at the base of the genital tubercle.

Development of Male External Genitalia

a. The scrotum develops from the fusion of genital swellings.
b. The penis develops from the genital tubercle and genital or urethral folds. Its development is intimately related to the development of penile urethra (Fig. 170.2). With the elongation of the genital tubercle, the urogenital membrane and the genital folds also elongate. The elongated genital tubercle forms the primitive phallus, which shows the cranial and caudal surfaces. The phallic part of urogenital sinus extends on the superior surface of the urogenital membrane. The endoderm of the sinus proliferates to form urethral plate. After the breakdown of the membrane around five to six weeks, the endoderm of the urethral plate and the surface ectoderm become continuous with each other at the edges of the disrupted membrane. With the canalization of urethral plate, the fusion of genital folds occurs and during this process, the endoderm fuses with endoderm, mesoderm with mesoderm and ectoderm with ectoderm. The site of fusion of genital folds is indicated by the penile raphe. In this way, the penile urethra is formed from the endoderm. However, the urethra in the glans develops from the ingrowth of surface ectoderm. Thus, the external urethral orifice is carried to the tip of the penis.

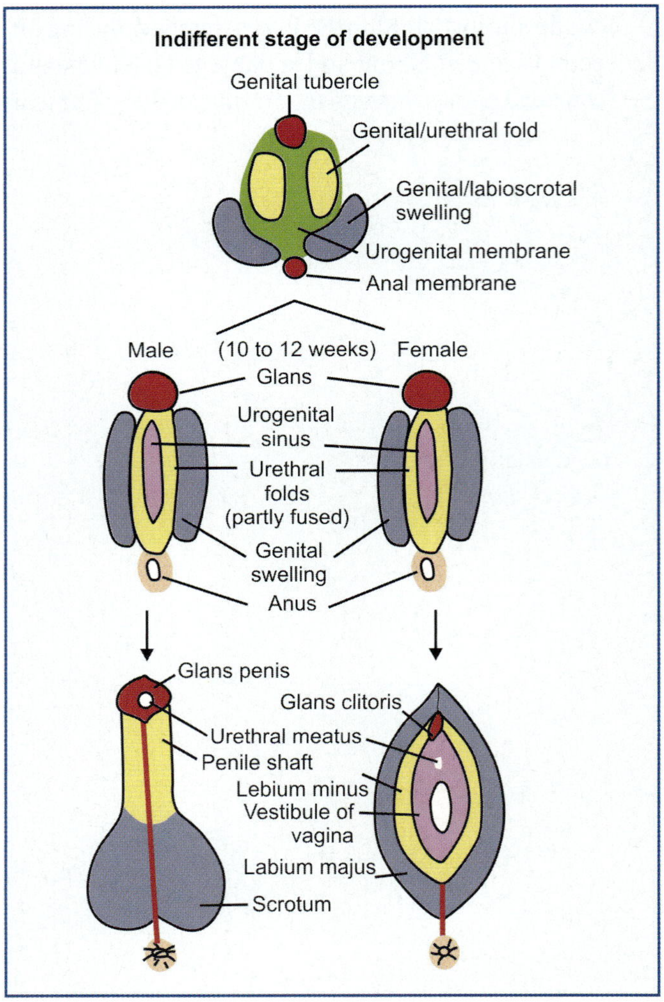

Fig. 170.1: Scheme to show development of external genitalia

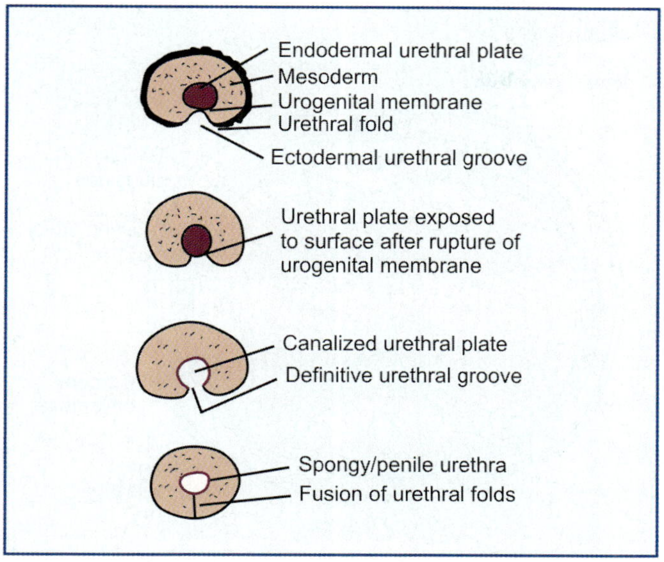

Fig. 170.2: Transverse section through phallus to depict development of penile urethra

Congenital Anomalies (Fig. 170.3)

a. Cleft scrotum is a condition in which there is complete failure of fusion of genital swellings and folds. The external genitalia resemble that of female.
b. Hypospadias is the condition in which the urethral orifice lies on the undersurface of the penis. This defect is due to partial failure of the fusion of the genital or urethral folds. The location of the urethral meatus varies and accordingly hypospadias is of different types. In this defect, the tip of penis is curved inwards (ventrally), which is known as chordee.
c. Epispadias means the urethral orifice opens on the dorsal surface of penis. This defect is associated with ectopia vesicae.

Development of Female External Genitalia

a. The genital tubercle, which exceeds that of male in length initially, becomes the clitoris.
b. The genital folds remain separate to form the labia minora.
c. The genital swellings remain separate to form the labia majora.
d. The pelvic and phallic parts of urogenital sinus are compressed and pulled down in female to form the vestibule of vagina, which receives the openings of urethra and vagina.

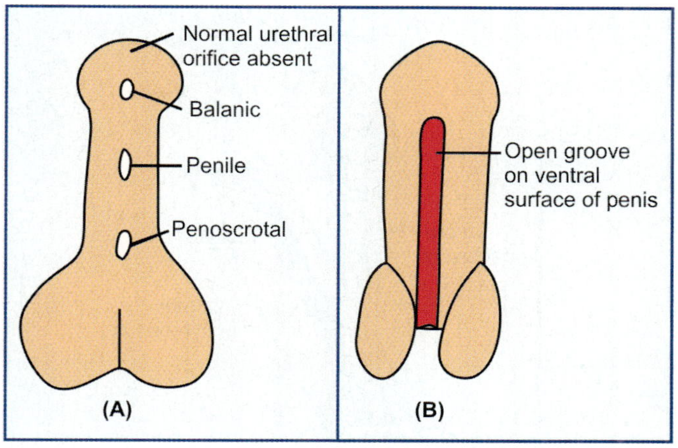

Fig. 170.3: Anomalies of male external genitalia (A) Types of hypospadias, (B) Cleft scrotum

Gross Anatomy of Male External Genitalia

The external genital organs of male consist of the penis and scrotum. The penis is the male copulatory organ. It gives passage to the urine and semen. The scrotum houses both testes and epididymes.

The penis consists of two parts, namely the root or fixed part, which lies in the superficial perineal space and the free part called body, which is enveloped in the skin. So, the penis is suspended from the perineal membrane and the conjoint ischiopubic rami (Fig. 170.4).

a. The root of the penis is formed by three masses of erectile tissues. The midline bulb of penis carries the bulbar urethra (the initial segment of penile urethra) and is pierced by both right and left arteries to the bulb. On each side of the bulb, there is crus, which is pierced by the deep artery.
b. The body of penis is elongated and ends in glans penis. It consists of three elongated masses of erectile tissue, which are the continuation of the root of penis. The crura continue as the corpora cavernosa while the bulb continues as corpus spongiosum, which lies in a groove on the ventral surface of fused corpora cavernosa. The distal end of the corpus spongiosum is expanded to form the glans penis. The corpus spongiosum carries the penile or spongy urethra inside it. The external urethral meatus lies at the tip of the glans. The tapered ends of the corpora cavernosa are attached to the hollowed proximal surface of the glans. The slightly everted margin of glans is called the

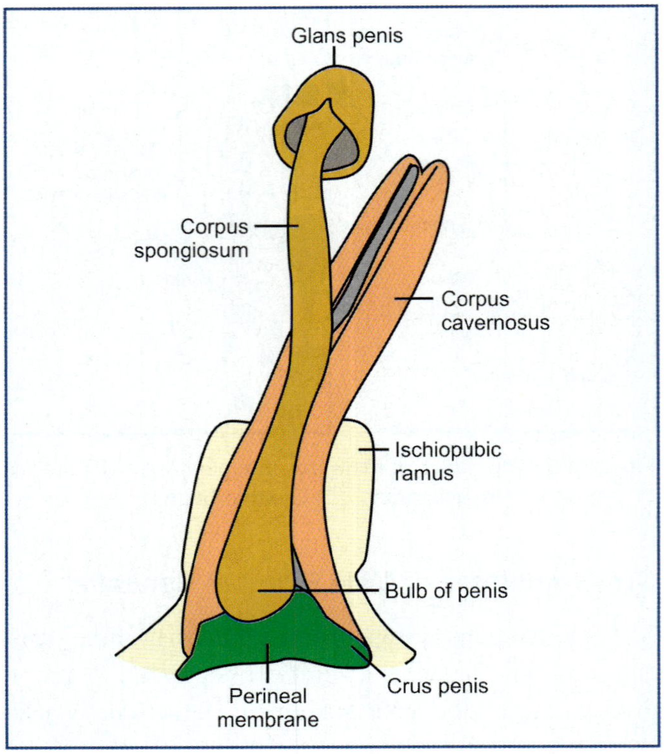

Fig. 170.4: Showing continuity of structures forming the root of penis into its body

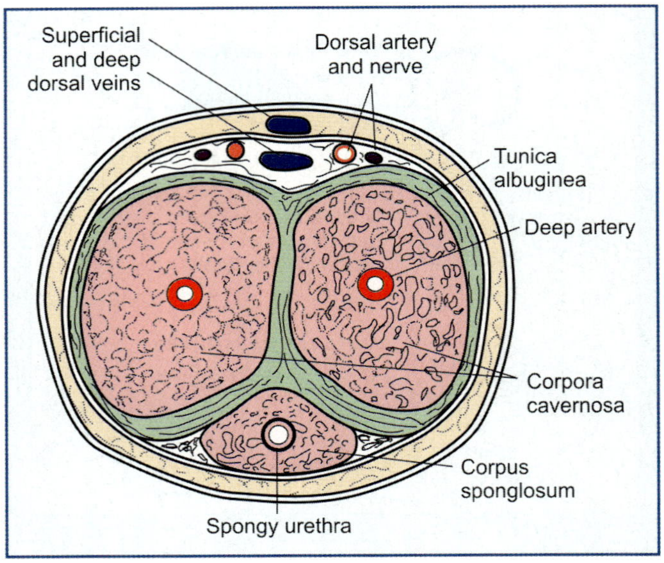

Fig. 170.5: Cross-section of the body of penis to depict its contents

corona glandis and the narrowing of body proximal to corona glandis is called the neck of penis. The dorsal surface of the erect penis becomes the ventral surface in flaccid state. The ventral surface or the urethral surface of penis bears the penile raphe and faces dorsally in flaccid state. The erect penis is regarded as anatomical position of the penis.

Cross-section of Penis (Fig. 170.5)

a. The skin covering the body of penis is loose, thin and hairless. At the neck of the penis, the skin is reflected upon itself to form prepuce or foreskin, which covers the glans. The prepuce is attached to the ventral surface of glans by a fold of skin called frenulum of the prepuce. Phimosis is the condition where the prepuce is too tight to retract over the glans penis. Accumulation of secretions (smegma) under the prepuce predisposes to infection and malignancy. It can also cause narrowing of external urethral meatus. Circumcision is the operation in which redundant part of prepuce is removed.

b. The superficial fascia of penis contains no fat. The superficial dorsal vein lies in the midline.

c. The fascia of penis or Buck's fascia forms a common covering for the three erectile masses but it does not cover the glans. It is continuous with fascia of Scarpa of the anterior abdominal wall and dartos muscle of the scrotum. The suspensory ligament connects the pubic symphysis to the fascia of penis. Five structures lie deep to this fascia on the dorsal aspect of penis, single deep dorsal vein in the midline, flanked on either side by dorsal arteries and still laterally by dorsal nerves.

d. Fibrous layer or tunica albuginea is a fibrous covering for each mass of erectile tissue.

Arterial Supply

Penis is a highly vascular organ. The corpora cavernosa receive deep artery of penis on each side while the corpus spongiosum receives a pair of artery to the bulb. In addition, the dorsal arteries lie along the dorsal surface and supply the superficial parts of the penis. Erection of penis is a vascular phenomenon. There is vasodilation in the cavernous tissue as a result of parasympathetic stimulation (pelvic splanchnic nerves). The engorged corpora cavernosa and corpus spongiosum compress the veins thereby retarding the outflow of blood. Both arterial and venous factors are responsible for increasing and maintaining the internal pressure.

Venous Drainage

The veins of the penis do not correspond to the arteries. There are two veins, superficial dorsal vein and deep dorsal vein of penis.

a. The superficial dorsal vein drains the prepuce and the skin of the penis. It runs backwards in the superficial fascia of the dorsum and either ends in right or left superficial external pudendal vein or divides in two and each ends in the superficial external pudendal vein of its side.
b. The deep dorsal vein drains blood from the glans penis and corpora cavernosa. It courses back in the midline between the right and left dorsal arteries of the penis lying deep to the fibrous sheath of the penis. At the root of the penis, it enters the space between the transverse perineal ligament and the arcuate pubic ligament to reach the pelvis. It divides in right and left branches, which empty in to prostatic venous plexus. The deep dorsal communicates with internal pudendal veins before dividing in right and left branches.

Lymphatic Drainage

The skin of the penis including the prepuce is drained in superficial inguinal lymph nodes. The glans penis is drained in deep inguinal nodes (gland of Cloquet). The deeper tissues are drained in internal iliac nodes.

Nerve Supply

The somatic and autonomic nerves supply the penis. The somatic innervation is by the dorsal nerves of penis to the skin of the body, prepuce and glans. The pelvic splanchnic nerves supply parasympathetic innervation through cavernous nerves, which arise from prostatic nerve plexuses. The cavernous nerves supply vasodilator fibres to blood vessels in erectile masses. The sympathetic fibres from the L1 segment of spinal cord reach through the inferior hypogastric plexus. Their role is opposite to that of the parasympathetic.

Scrotum

The scrotum is a pendulous sac of skin, hung from the medial part of inguinal region of the lower abdominal wall and located between the thighs behind the flaccid penis. It houses testes and epididymes along with the lower parts of spermatic cords. A midline raphe is the indication of its internal division in two halves. The left half is at a slightly lower level compared to the right due to the greater length of the left spermatic cord.

Layers of Scrotal Wall (Fig. 127.3)

The layers of the scrotal wall are the skin, dartos muscle, external spermatic fascia, cremaster muscle, cremaster fascia and the internal spermatic fascia.

Characteristics of Scrotal Skin

The scrotal skin is thin, pigmented and rugose. It bears thinly scattered hairs and the dermis contains sebaceous and numerous sweat glands. Subcutaneous fat is absent. The dartos muscle is a thin layer of subcutaneous smooth muscle of scrotum. It extends in the scrotal septum, which divides the scrotum in two halves. The septum contains all the layers of scrotal wall except the skin. The sympathetic nerves reach the dartos via genitofemoral nerve. The dartos contracts reflexly on exposure to cold. This makes the scrotal skin wrinkled and it is brought very close to the testes, thus helping in preservation of heat. In warm climate, the dartos relaxes and the scrotal skin becomes smooth and elongated, thus helping in dissipation of heat. The scrotal temperature is lower by about three degrees than that of the body temperature.

Blood Supply

The external pudendal branches of femoral artery, posterior scrotal branches from inferior rectal artery and the cremasteric branch from inferior epigastric artery supply the scrotal skin. The veins follow the arteries.

Lymphatic Drainage

The lymph drains from the scrotum to the superficial inguinal lymph nodes. Scrotal swellings due to carcinoma of scrotal skin or due to seminoma can be differentiated from the examination of the appropriate lymph nodes.

Nerve Supply

The anterior one-third of the scrotal skin receives supply from the ilioinguinal nerve and genital branch of genitofemoral nerve (L1). The posterior two-thirds is supplied by posterior scrotal and perineal branch of posterior cutaneous nerve of thigh (S3). It is important to note that two discontinuous dermatomes (L1 and S3) come in apposition at the junction of anterior third and posterior two-thirds of scrotum. The spinal anaesthesia at S3 level may not be sufficient to anesthetize the entire scrotum.

Clinical Highlights

a. The commonest cause of scrotal swelling is a hydrocele in which there is collection of fluid in tunica vaginalis of testis. Elephantiasis is the commonest cause of huge swelling of the scrotum. To drain the fluid a needle in passed through successive layers (skin, dartos, external spermatic fascia, cremaster fascia, internal spermatic fascia and parietal layer of tunica vaginalis). This procedure is called tapping the hydrocele. The eversion of the sac is another method of treating the hydrocele. The other causes of scrotal swelling, are, inguinal hernia, varicocele, diseases of the testis and epididymis.
b. Empty scrotum occurs, when the testis fails to descend in to the scrotum.

Female External Genitalia (Fig. 170.6)

The external genitalia in the female consist of the following structures: The mons pubis is a fat filled, hair bearing skin superficial to the pubic bones. The vulva or the pudendal cleft begins at its lower margin. The vulva is the cleft between the two labia majora, which are fat filled and hair bearing folds of skin. The right and left labia majora join to form posterior commissure in front of the anus. The inner surfaces of the labia majora are hairless. The round ligaments terminate at their upper ends. The labia minora are a pair of smooth mucous folds. The anterior ends of labia minora split to form two folds. The posterior folds fuse and attach to the inferior surface of clitoris as the frenulum of clitoris. The pair of anterior folds unites to form prepuce over the tip of the clitoris. The vestibule is the area between labia minora and contains openings

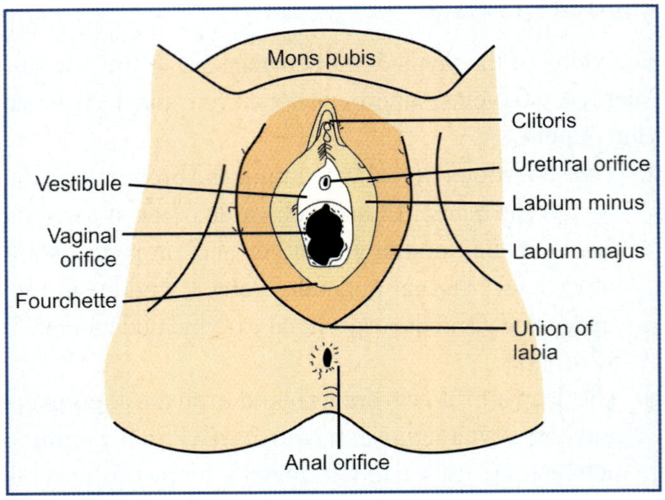

Fig. 170.6: Female external genitalia

of urethra, vagina and ducts of greater vestibular glands. The clitoris resembles the penis but is not traversed by urethra. It lies in the anterior part of vulva. The sensitive tip of the clitoris is called the glans. Vaginal orifice lies in the posterior part of vestibule. It is partly closed in virgin by hymen. The urethral orifice lies anterior to the vaginal orifice. It lies two cm posterior to the clitoris. Its margins are palpable.

Homologous Structures of Male and Female External Genitalia

a. The dorsal part of penis is equivalent to clitoris (genital tubercle).
b. The ventral part of penis is equivalent to labia minora (urethral or genital folds).
c. The scrotum is equivalent to labia majora (genital swellings).
d. The lower prostatic, membranous and penile parts of urethra (except the urethra in the glans) are equivalent to vestibule of vagina (pelvic and phallic parts of urogenital sinus).
e. The corpus spongiosum is equivalent to bulb of vestibule.
f. The bulbourethral glands are equivalent to greater vestibular glands.

Pudendal Nerve and Vessels of Perineum

171

Pudendal Nerve

The pudendal nerve (Fig. 171.1) takes origin from the sacral plexus inside the pelvic cavity. Its root value is S2, S3, S4. It supplies the urogenital and anal triangles of the perineum and the external genitalia.

Course of Pudendal Nerve

This is divisible in three parts, namely, intrapelvic, gluteal, and perineal.

a. Intrapelvic part of pudendal nerve extends from its origin till it reaches the lower margin of the greater sciatic foramen, below the piriformis muscle. The nerve leaves via this foramen to enter the gluteal region in company with internal pudendal vessels and nerve to obturator internus muscle.
b. Gluteal part of pudendal nerve is very short as it immediately leaves through the lesser sciatic foramen to enter the lateral wall of ischiorectal fossa. In the gluteal region, it is in contact with the apex of the sacrospinous ligament close to its attachment to the ischial spine. The nerve lies medial to internal pudendal artery, as it crosses the dorsal surface of ischial spine and nerve to obturator internus.
c. Perineal part of the pudendal nerve begins at the posterior end of the pudendal or Alcock's canal, which lies on the lateral wall of the ischiorectal fossa. In the posterior part of the canal, the pudendal nerve lies superior to the internal pudendal artery. It gives off the inferior rectal nerve here. In the anterior part of the canal, the pudendal nerve divides in to its terminal branches, perineal nerve and dorsal nerve of penis or clitoris. The dorsal nerve, internal pudendal artery and the perineal nerve lie from above downward in the anterior part of the canal.

Branches of Pudendal Nerve

a. Inferior rectal or hemorrhoidal nerve crosses the ischiorectal fossa from lateral to medial side. Since it is a mixed nerve, it supplies the sphincter ani externus and provides sensory branches to lower one third of anal canal, perianal skin and lower two cm of vaginal mucosa.
b. The perineal nerve is the larger terminal branch of the pudendal nerve. In the anterior part of the pudendal canal it divides in to the posterior scrotal or labial and muscular branches. The posterior scrotal or labial branches enter and course through the superficial perineal pouch to supply the posterior two thirds of the scrotal or labial skin. The muscular branches supply all the five muscles of the urogenital triangle

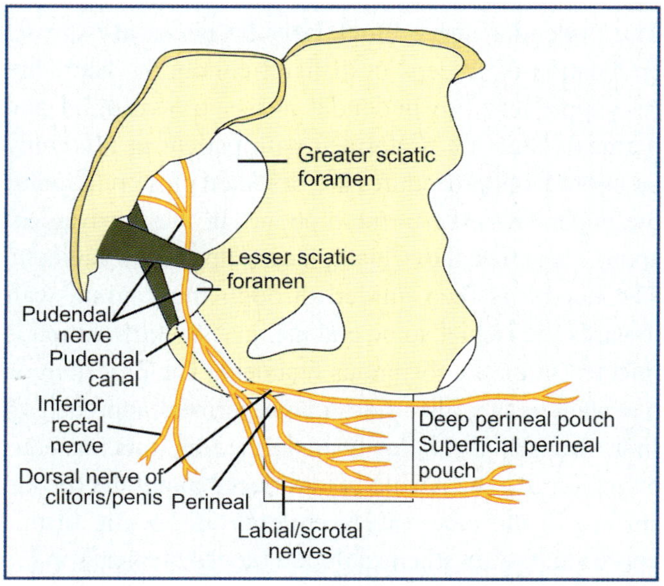

Fig. 171.1: Schematic diagram depicting course and branches of pudenal nerve

(superficial transverse, bulbospongiosus, ischiocavernosus, deep transverse and sphincter urethrae). The branch to bulbospongiosus supplies the urethra and corpus spongiosum also. The perineal nerve sends twigs to anterior part of levator ani muscle. These twigs enter the muscle from below.

c. The dorsal nerve of clitoris is much smaller than that of penis. The nerve enters the deep perineal pouch from its posterior margin. It travels forwards on the superior surface of the perineal membrane in contact with the medial surface of ischiopubic ramus. Near the anterior end of the deep space the nerve pierces the perineal membrane and enters the gap between the transverse perineal ligament and the arcuate pubic ligament. The nerve and accompanying artery enter the dorsal surface of the penis or clitoris. The dorsal nerve of penis lies deep to penile fascia. It is located lateral to the dorsal artery of its side. The dorsal nerves of penis supply the penile skin, glans penis and prepuce.

To sum up the functions of the pudendal nerve, through nerve supply of sphincter urethrae it controls micturition, through its supply of external anal sphincter it controls defecation and through its sensory supply of penis or clitoris it performs sexual functions as well.

Pudendal Nerve Block

The pudendal nerve block may be necessary during application of forceps in difficult childbirth. There are two approaches to pudendal nerve, transvaginal and perineal. Both are performed with patient in lithotomy position. Both procedures are based on close relation of the pudendal nerve to the hipbone. In the transvaginal approach, at first, the ischial spine is palpated per vaginum. The needle is then guided through the vaginal wall towards the ischial spine and the anaesthetic solution is injected in the sacrospinous ligament. The procedure is repeated on the other side. In the perineal approach, at first, the ischial tuberosity is defined by subcutaneous palpation and the needle is introduced along the medial surface of the tuberosity at a depth of 2.5 cm. In this approach, the anesthetic solution blocks the nerve in the pudendal canal. The procedure is repeated on the opposite side.

Internal Pudendal Artery

The internal pudendal artery (Fig. 171.2) is larger in male compared to the female. However, the course and distribution is similar in the two sexes. It takes origin from the anterior division of internal iliac artery inside the pelvic cavity. It descends in lateral direction towards the inferior margin of greater sciatic foramen, where it leaves the pelvis in company with pudendal nerve and nerve to obturator internus. The three structures enter the gluteal region for a short course. The artery turns around the dorsal aspect of the ischial spine to enter the ischiorectal fossa via lesser sciatic foramen. Then, the internal pudendal artery traverses the pudendal canal by lying below the pudendal nerve at first and then between the latter's two terminal branches. It enters the deep perineal pouch and runs along the ischiopubic ramus forwards to terminate behind the inferior pubic ligament by dividing in dorsal artery of penis or clitoris and deep artery of penis or clitoris.

Branches

a. Muscular branches are given in the pelvis and gluteal region.
b. Inferior rectal artery supplies the lower part of anal canal and perianal skin.

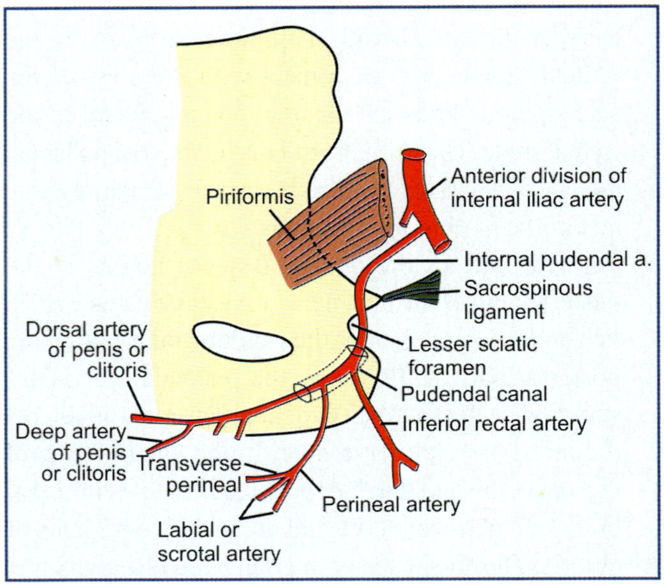

Fig. 171.2: Origin, course and branches of internal pudendal artery

c. Perineal artery gives rise to posterior scrotal or labial arteries and transverse perineal branch in the superficial perineal pouch.
d. Artery to the bulb of penis, on each side, enters the bulb of penis, from where the two arteries travel in the corpus spongiosum. The artery to bulb of vestibule in female supplies the bulb of the vestibule on each side and also lower vagina.
e. Urethral artery in male supplies the urethra.
f. Deep artery of penis or clitoris enters the corpus cavernosum of its side.
g. Dorsal artery of the penis or clitoris reaches the anterior end of the deep perineal pouch and by piercing the perineal membrane enters the suspensory ligament to reach the dorsum of penis or the clitoris. On the dorsum of penis or clitoris, the artery lies between the deep dorsal vein medially and dorsal nerve laterally.

Internal Pudendal Vein

This vein accompanies the internal pudendal artery. Inside the pelvis it makes connections with prostatic venous plexus in male or vesical venous plexus in female and terminates in internal iliac vein. The deep dorsal vein of penis or clitoris ends directly in the prostatic or vesical plexuses respectively. The superficial dorsal vein of penis or clitoris ends in external pudendal vein of its own side or of other side.

172 Urethra

The urethra is very long in male compared to female. It performs dual function of transmission of urine and semen in the male. There is marked difference in the development of urethra in two sexes.

Development of Male Urethra

The male urethra develops from multiple sources, which are derived from endoderm, mesoderm and ectoderm. Contribution of mesoderm and ectoderm much less compared to the endoderm.

a. The prostatic urethra develops from two sources above the level of colliculus seminalis but form one source below this level. Except the posterior wall, which is derived from mesoderm of the absorbed part of mesonephric ducts, the rest of upper urethra is from endoderm of vesicourethral canal. The prostatic urethra below the level of colliculus seminalis develops from the endoderm of pelvic part of the definitive urogenital sinus.
b. The membranous urethra develops from the pelvic part of definitive urogenital sinus.
c. The penile urethra (except the part inside the glans) develops from canalization of the urethral plate derived from the endoderm of phallic part of the urogenital sinus (Fig. 170.2).
d. The part of urethra inside the glans develops from surface ectoderm.

Development of Female Urethra

The female urethra is developmentally equivalent to the prostatic urethra upto the level of colliculus seminalis. Therefore, it is derived from endoderm of vesicourethral canal and mesoderm of the absorbed parts of mesonephric ducts.

Male Urethra (Fig. 172.1)

The male urethra is a long fibromuscular tube functioning as a conduit for both urine and seminal fluid. It begins in the neck of the urinary bladder and passes in succession through the pelvic diaphragm, prostate, perineal pouches and the penis to reach the external urethral meatus at the tip of the glans. The male urethra presents a double curve when the penis is in the flaccid state. The length of the male urethra is 18 to 20 cm.

Parts

The male urethra is divisible into four parts, preprostatic, prostatic, membranous and spongy or penile. The shape of urethral lumen varies in its different parts.

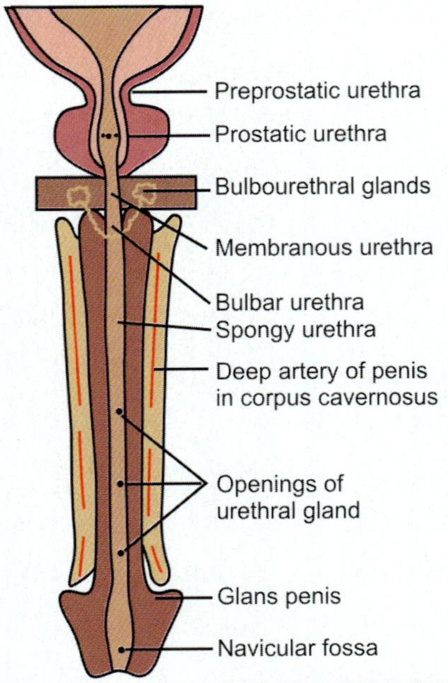

Fig. 172.1: Schematic diagram depicting different parts of male urethra

a. The preprostatic part extends from the bladder neck to the base of the prostate. It is just over 1 cm in length. The smooth muscle of its wall (part of sphincter vesicae) is richly innervated with sympathetic fibers. It contracts to prevent retrograde ejaculation of semen.
b. The prostatic part is the widest and most dilatable part of urethra. It is 2.5 cm long and its lumen is crescentic in shape. The features on its posterior wall are shown in Figure 154.5. A midline ridge like projection of mucosa is called the urethral crest. The linear depression on either side of the crest on either side of the crest is the prostatic sinus in which large number of prostatic ducts open. The widest part of urethral crest bears a rounded swelling called colliculus seminalis (verumontanum). At the summit of this eminence lies a blindly ending prostatic utricle. The ejaculatory ducts open on either side of the prostatic utricle, which is a remnant of the fused paramesonephric ducts in male.
c. The membranous urethra begins at the apex of prostate and passes through the anterior part of levator ani to enter the deep perineal pouch, where it is surrounded by sphincter urethrae muscle. This is the short (1.5 cm), narrow and least dilatable part of male urethra. The mucous membrane of the membranous urethra is thrown in folds hence on cross-section its lumen is stellate. The bulbourethral gland lies on either side of it. The membranous urethra pierces the perineal membrane about 2.5 cm posterior to the lower margin of pubic symphysis and enters the bulb of penis. The rigid perineal membrane fixes the urethra firmly to the bony pelvis. This makes the membranous urethra more vulnerable to injury.
d. The penile part is the longest part of the male urethra being 15 cm in length. It traverses the bulb of penis in superficial perineal pouch, corpus spongiosum in penile body and glans penis. The part in the bulb is called bulbar part or intrabulbar fossa, as it is a dilated part. The floor and sides of its walls are greater in dimensions than its anterior wall hence its shape on cross section is described as trapezoid. It is this part, which receives the ducts of the bulbourethral glands. The part in the corpus spongiosum is called the spongy urethra. It is uniform in diameter and its shape on cross-section is a transverse slit. The part in the glans penis is dilated and called navicular or terminal fossa. It opens to the exterior by external urethral meatus, which is the narrowest part of the urethra. The shape of the navicular fossa is a vertical slit. Thus it is very important to know, especially during passage of instruments in the urethra that the penile urethra has two dilatations. Urethral glands (glands of Littre) open in the entire length of spongy urethra in small out-pouchings of the mucosa called lacunae. The lacuna in the roof of the navicular fossa, which is called lacuna magna, is quite deep. The urethral glands are prone to gonococcal infection, which may cause scarring and strictures in the urethra.

Mucosa of Urethra

a. The prostatic urethra is lined by transitional epithelium above the level of colliculus seminalis, below which it is lined by patchy stratified columnar or pseudostratified columnar epithelium.
b. The membranous urethra is lined by patchy stratified columnar or pseudostratified columnar epithelium.
c. The spongy urethra is lined by stratified columnar epithelium.
d. The navicular fossa is lined by stratified squamous epithelium.

Urethral Sphincters

a. The internal sphincter (vesical sphincter) controls the bladder neck and preprostatic part of urethra. It is composed of nonstriated muscle, collagen and elastic fibres. Its nerve supply is mainly sympathetic. On sympathetic stimulation the smooth muscle in the male genital tracts and the internal sphincter contract simultaneously. This causes closure of the internal sphincter during ejaculation so that seminal fluid does not enter the urinary bladder. The significant role of internal sphincter in genital function is established. Postoperative urinary incontinence does not follow surgical excision of bladder neck or prostate. This observation is suggestive of the insignificant role of the internal urethral sphincter in continence of urine.
b. The sphincter urethrae muscle around the membranous urethra in the deep perineal pouch forms

the external sphincter. It is composed of striated muscle and is supplied by pudendal nerve. It is a voluntary sphincter after early infancy.

Arterial Supply

The inferior vesical, middle rectal and penile branches of internal pudendal arteries supply the male urethra.

Venous Drainage

The proximal part of urethra blood drains directly in prostatic venous plexuses. The remaining part of urethra drains in the prostatic plexuses indirectly through the deep dorsal vein of penis.

Lymph Drainage

Lymph vessels drain in internal and external lymph nodes. The distal part drains in superficial inguinal nodes.

Clinical Highlights

a. Straddle injuries damage the bulbar urethra. In such injuries, the urine leaks in the superficial perineal pouch and may extravasate in the anterior abdominal wall after filling the superficial perineal pouch, scrotum and penis.
b. In rupture of the membranous urethra, there is accumulation of urine in deep perineal pouch.
c. In the fracture of pelvic bones, the junctional area between prostatic and membranous urethra is ruptured. In such cases, extravasation of urine occurs in extraperitoneal tissue of pelvis.
d. Injury to the preprostatic urethra may cause damage to the vesical sphincter and its sympathetic nerve supply. This results in retrograde ejaculation and consequent sterility.
e. While passing a catheter in the male urethra (catheterization), following anatomical facts must be borne in mind. The external urethral meatus is the narrowest part of urethra hence maximum resistance is encountered to the passage of instrument at this site. The lacuna magna in the roof of navicular fossa, which is large enough to receive the tip of catheter, may be perforated. To avoid this, the catheter is kept as close to the floor of navicular fossa as possible. The double curve of the urethra is made in a single continuous curve by elevating the penis during passage of the catheter.
The membranous urethra is thin walled, narrow and most fixed. Any force applied during the passage of catheter through this part results in rupture of urethra.

Female Urethra

The female urethra is about 4 cm long. It extends from the bladder neck to the external urethral meatus in the vestibule of vagina. The urinary tract infections are more common in female due to shortness of the urethra. The urethra is intimately related to the anterior wall of vagina. Its initial part lies behind the pubic symphysis and is fixed to the pubic rami by pubourethral ligaments. The paraurethral glands of Skene (homologous to prostate) and urethral glands open in the urethra. The female urethra is lined by transitional epithelium in the uppermost part followed by pseudostratified or stratified epithelium. Nearer the external urethral meatus, the epithelium is stratified squamous in type. The wall of the female urethra is composed of outer circularly arranged sphincter urethrae muscle and the inner longitudinally arranged smooth muscle.

Sphincters of Female Urethra

a. The internal sphincter like in the male is composed of elastic and collagen fibers and a negligible amount of smooth muscle. It has been suggested that the passive elastic resistance offered by the elastic fibers is the major factor in the mechanism of internal sphincter in female
b. The periurethral part of levator ani muscle plays a role in female continence. This muscle provides additional occlusive force during raised intra-abdominal pressure.
c. The sphincter urethrae muscle (voluntary sphincter) surrounds the female urethra in the deep perineal pouch.

Clinical Highlights

Urinary stress incontinence is an extremely common symptom, particularly in women, who have borne children.

During childbirth, injury to perineal body (periurethral part of pubococcygeus and sphincter urethrae) is common. This may result in increase in the angle between neck of bladder and urethra leading to herniation of urethral mucosa in vagina (urethrocele). In this condition, a very small quantity of urine dribbles every time the intra-abdominal pressure rises during laughing, coughing or lifting heavy weight. Alternate contraction and relaxation of perineal muscles (Kegel's exercises) strengthen the sphincter urethrae and pubococcygeus muscles. Sometimes, surgical repair is necessary to relieve the symptoms.

173 Clinicoanatomical Problems and Solutions

CASE 1

A 15-year-old boy, who was riding a bicycle, hit the bar forcibly in an accident. He did not pass urine after the fall. After a gap of ten hours the boy observed a swelling of the scrotum, penis and lower part of the anterior abdominal wall.

Questions

a. Name the structure that is ruptured and enumerate the parts of this structure in male.
b. Which part is located in the superficial perineal pouch?
c. Which glands open in this part?
d. Which is the shortest and least dilatable part of male urethra?
e. Draw a diagram to show the path of urine in rupture of male urethra in superficial perineal pouch.
f. Does the urine enter the thigh from the anterior abdominal wall? Give reason for the answer.
g. Describe the voluntary sphincter of urethra.
h. Name the anomaly in which the external meatus opens on the ventral surface of penis.

Solutions

a. Urethra is ruptured. The parts of the male urethra are, preprostatic, prostatic, membranous and spongy.
b. Bulbar urethra in the bulb of penis.
c. Bulbourethral glands
d. Membranous urethra
e. Refer to Figure 169.1
f. The urine does not enter the thigh because of the fusion of membranous part of superficial fascia of thigh and the fascia lata along Holden's line in upper thigh.
g. The voluntary sphincter of urethra or sphincter urethrae is present in the deep perineal pouch. It surrounds the membranous urethra in male and urethra in female. It takes origin from the ischiopubic rami on either side and surrounds the urethra in male and urethra and vagina in female. It is partially fused with perineal body. It is supplied by perineal branch of pudendal nerve.
h. Hypospadias (chordee).

CASE 2

A postmenopausal woman came to the hospital with complaint of the sensation of something coming down the vagina, dribbling of urine while bending down and frequency of micturition. Per vaginum examination revealed the descent of cervix in the vagina (uterovaginal prolapse) and a prominent cystocele (bulging of the anterior wall of vagina during straining).

Questions

a. What is the normal position of the uterus?
b. Describe the ligamentous supports of the uterus with the help of a diagram.
c. Describe broad ligament of uterus.
d. What is embryological importance of round ligament?
e. What is arterial supply of uterus and vagina?
f. Which part of levator ani surrounds the vagina and the urethra?
g. Which organ pushes down the anterior wall of vagina in cystocele?

Solutions

a. Anteversion and anteflexion
b. The true ligaments of the uterus that retain it in position are, uterosacral, transverse cervical and pubovesical ligaments (Fig. 165.4). These ligaments

are the condensations of pelvic fascia and extend from the cervix in three different directions thus ensuring that cervix is the most fixed part.

c. The broad ligament of the uterus is a peritoneal fold that passes from the uterus to the sidewall of pelvis on each side. This peritoneal fold faces antero-inferiorly and posterosuperiorly because of the anteverted position of the uterus. It has free upper margin, which contains fallopian tube. The ligament of ovary lies in it posterior to the tube and round ligament of uterus is contained anterior to the tube. The other contents are, vestigial remnants- paroophoron, epoophoron and Gartner's duct. These embryonic vestiges may undergo cystic changes and enlarge to form cysts of broad ligament. The broad ligament also contains, connective tissue called parametrium supporting uterine and ovarian blood vessels, nerves and lymphatics.
d. Round ligament of uterus is the remnant of gubernaculum ovarii.
e. The uterine artery, a branch of anterior division of internal iliac artery and the ovarian artery, a branch of abdominal aorta supply the uterus. The vagina receives blood from multiple branches of internal iliac (a direct vaginal branch, uterine artery and middle rectal artery) and also from artery to bulb of vestibule (from internal pudendal branch of internal iliac artery).
f. The pubovaginalis surrounds the vagina and pubourethralis surrounds the urethra. Both are parts of pubococcygeus subdivision of levator ani.
g. In cystocele, the anterior wall of vagina is pushed down by urinary bladder.

CASE 3

A 45-year-old man was admitted to the hospital with complaints of dull and intermittent pain in both flanks and passage of blood clots in urine. On examination, there was fullness in both flanks and kidneys were enlarged, which was confirmed on ultrasound examination. On intravenous pyelography, the diagnosis of bilateral polycystic kidney was made.

Questions

a. Name the developmental sources of permanent kidney.
b. Give the embryological explanation of multiple cyst formation in polycystic kidney.
c. What is the embryological explanation of pelvic kidney?
d. What is horseshoe kidney?
e. Name the blood vessel, which prevents the ascent of the horseshoe kidney.

Solutions

a. The nephrons (secretory part of kidney) develop from metanephric blastema and the collecting part of the kidney develops from ureteric diverticulum of mesonephrenic duct.
b. A simple embryological explanation of the cyst formation is as follows. There is failure of the process of luminal continuity between the developing nephrons and the collecting tubules, during nephro-genesis. So, the urine that is secreted by the nephrons accumulates in them for want of outlet. Thus, the nephrons undergo cystic enlargement.
c. A kidney located in pelvis (instead of lumbar region) is known as pelvic kidney. It may be unilateral or bilateral. This occurs due to arrest of the process of ascent of embryonic kidney. The permanent kidney develops in sacral region, where the metanephric blastema is invaded by the ureteric bud. Differential growth of the abdominal wall is responsible for the ascent of the low placed embryonic kidney. Occasionally, the peritoneal folds carrying the umbilical arteries arrest the ascent of the kidneys.
d. Horseshoe kidney is the one that resembles a horseshoe in shape. In this case the lower poles of the two kidneys are connected by an isthmus, which usually lies anterior to aorta and IVC.
e. The inferior mesenteric artery (lowest midline ventral branch of abdominal aorta) prevents the ascent of horseshoe kidney.

CASE 4

A 26-year-old woman with acute pain in the lower abdomen was rushed to the hospital in a state of shock. A history of two missed periods suggested early pregnancy. The abdominal wall showed tenderness and guarding. Ultrasound revealed empty and enlarged uterus and fluid in the pouch of Douglas.

Questions

a. Name the structure that is ruptured in the above case giving the cause of the rupture.
b. What is the normal site of fertilization?
c. Give the normal length and name the parts of the fallopian tube.
d. What is the normal site of implantation?
e. What is the reason of tenderness and muscle guarding in the abdominal wall?
f. What is the development of fallopian tube?
g. Tubectomy prevents which physiological process?

Solutions

a. Fallopian tube is ruptured due to tubal pregnancy.
b. Normal site of fertilization is ampulla of fallopian tube.
c. Normal length of fallopian tube is 10 cm. Its parts from ovarian end are, infundibulum, ampulla, isthmus and intramural.
d. Normal site of implantation is posterior wall of uterus near the fundus.
e. Due to tubal rupture there is haemorrhage in the peritoneal cavity including in the pouch of Douglas. There is irritation of parietal peritoneum, which results in tenderness and muscle guarding.
f. Fallopian tube develops from the cranial unfused part of paramesonephric duct.
g. Tubectomy prevents fertilization.

CASE 5

A 75-year-old man had a one-year history of difficulty and frequency in micturition. Per rectum examination confirmed the enlargement of prostate. Investigations ruled our cancer of prostate.

Questions

a. What is the probable diagnosis?
b. Describe the age changes in prostate.
c. What is uvula vesicae?
d. Give the posterior relations of the prostate.
e. Name the embryological remnants inside the prostate.
f. Describe the capsules of the prostate.
g. Draw a diagram to show the surgical approaches to the prostate.

Solutions

a. Benign hypertrophy of prostate (BPH).
b. In childhood, the prostate is small and is composed of fibromuscular stroma and rudiments of ducts. At puberty, there is sudden increase in size under the influence of testosterone. There is proliferation of prostatic follicles, which begin to secrete acid phosphatase, prostate specific antigen and prostaglandins. During third decade of life, there is irregular epithelial infoldings in the lumen of follicles. During fourth decade, formation of amyloid concretions in the follicles begins. After 50 years, the prostate may show gradual benign hypertrophy or progressive atrophy.
c. The bulge produced by the median lobe of prostate on the apex of trigone of urinary bladder is called uvula vesicae.
d. Posteriorly, the prostate is related to Denonvillier's fascia, which separates it from the ampulla of rectum. The ejaculatory ducts pierce the posterior surface of the prostate.
e. The embryological remnants inside the prostate are found in relation to the prostatic urethra. An elevation in the middle part of the urethral crest on the posterior wall of prostatic urethra is known as colliculus seminalis (verumontanum). This is a remnant of Mullerian tubercle. The prostatic utricle (uterus masculinus) opens on this elevation in the midline. The prostatic utricle is a remnant of fused part of paramesonephric ducts.
f. The prostate gland is covered with inner true capsule and outer false capsule. True capsule is the condensation of the prostatic stroma and the false capsule is part of pelvic fascia. The prostatic venous plexus is located between the two capsules.
g. Refer to Figure 162.3 for surgical approaches to prostate.

CASE 6

A 30-year-old man was brought to the casualty with a bleeding stab wound in left loin. There was marked swelling in the left renal angle. Plain X-ray of abdomen revealed fracture of left 11th and 12th ribs. Urine specimen showed frank blood.

Questions

a. Name the organ that is injured giving its side.
b. Give the bony, muscular and neural relations of the posterior surface of this organ.
c. Name the coverings of this organ from inner to outer side. Describe the fascial capsule in detail.
d. Draw a diagram to show the Morris' parallelogram.
e. Write note on renal angle.
f. Name the vascular segments of this organ.

Solutions

a. Left kidney
b. Posterior surface of left kidney is related to 11th and 12th ribs. The muscles in relation are, diaphragm above and transversus abdominis, quadratus lumborum and psoas major muscles from lateral to medial side below the area related to diaphragm. The subcostal, iliohypogastric and ilioinguinal nerves are related to this surface.
c. Coverings of kidney from inner to outer side are, true capsule, perinephric fat, fascial capsule and paranephric fat. The fascial capsule (fascia of Gerota) provides a common covering for the kidney and the suprarenal gland. It anterior layer is called fascia of Toldt and posterior layer is called fascia of Zuckerkandl. On horizontal tracing, the anterior and posterior layers fuse along the lateral margin of kidney. Medially, the anterior layer passes in front of the renal vessels to become continuous with the corresponding layer of the opposite side in front of the aorta and IVC. The posterior layer blends with psoas fascia and is attached to the bodies of lumbar vertebrae. On vertical tracing, superiorly the two layers fuse above the suprarenal gland, where they are continuous with diaphragmatic fascia. Anterior and posterior layers are joined to each other by a septum, which separates kidney and suprarenal gland. Inferiorly, fascial capsule is open since its two layers continue downward along the ureter to merge with fascia iliaca. In nephroptosis, (dropped kidney) kidney is displaced downwards from its normal position due to the opening in the fascial capsule. The renal vessels alone form the support to the kidney. This may give rise to kinking of ureter and consequent urinary obstruction. Another importance of the lower opening of the fascial capsule is that perinephric abscess may track down along the ureter into the pelvic cavity.
d. Refer to Figure 152.1.
e. It is the angle between the lower margin of twelfth rib and lateral margin of erector spinae muscle. At this angle, the kidney lies close to the surface. The renal pain is felt at the renal angle as dull ache. The lower margin of pleura crosses the renal angle. Therefore, upper end of skin incision for approaching kidney by lumbar route must begin below the renal angle.
f. The vascular segments of the kidney are, apical, anterior, middle, lower, and posterior.

CASE 7

A 2-month-old male child was brought to the hospital because the mother noticed that the left scrotum of the boy was empty. On examination it was noticed that the right testis was in the scrotum. A swelling of 1.5 cm diameter was noted in the left inguinal region.

Questions

a. Mention two common conditions resulting in empty scrotum in newborn.
b. Differentiate between these two conditions.
c. Of the above two conditions which one is seen in this case?
d. Describe the process of descent of testis including its chronology.
e. Give the fate of the structures responsible for descent of testis.
f. Differentiate between the lymphatic drainage of testis and scrotum.

Solutions

a. Undescended testis (cryptorchidism) and ectopic testis are the common causes of empty scrotum in newborn.
b. If the descent of testis is arrested inside the abdominal cavity, in the lumbar region or in the inguinal canal or at the superficial inguinal ring, it is known as

undescended testis. The effects of undescended testis are, nonformation of seminiferous tubules, small size of testis and infertility. Moreover, such testis is more prone to malignancy. Ectopic testis is the one that has descended normally but is placed in abnormal position. In this condition, the testis descends normally until it comes put of the superficial ring. After this, due to abnormal attachment of the gubernaculum the testis may be found in the superficial fascia of anterior abdominal wall, perineum, root of penis or in the femoral triangle. The ectopic testis is functionally normal but it is more liable to injury.

c. This case is that of cryptorchidism or undescended testis.
d. Refer to Chapter 160.
e. The processus vaginalis, which is a peritoneal pouch preceding the testis forma the tunica vaginalis testis at its distal end. The remaining part of processus vaginalis is obliterated and reduced to a fibrous remnant in the spermatic cord. The gubernaculum testis is shortened and becomes the scrotal ligament, which attaches the lower pole of the testis to the scrotal wall.
f. The lymphatics of the testis drain into the lateral aortic nodes or preaortic nodes and those of scrotum into the superficial inguinal nodes.

CASE 8

A 32-year-old man presented with the complaint of dragging feeling in the left side of scrotum. On examination of scrotum, the surgeon could feel the normal testis. Palpation of the spermatic cord gave a "bag of worms" feeling to the examining fingers.

Questions

a. Name the blood vessels, which when dilated give the feeling of bag of worms on palpation.
b. What is this condition called and on which side it is more common?
c. What is the extent and length of the spermatic cord?
d. Give the extent and length of the vas deferens.
e. Give the constituents of spermatic cord.
f. Name the coverings of the spermatic cord giving their derivation.
g. At what point does the pampiniform plexus become the testicular vein?
h. Where does the left testicular vein drain?
i. Give anatomical reasons for proneness of varicocele on left side.

Solutions

a. The dilated pampiniform plexus gives a" bag of worms" feeling.
b. This condition is called varicocele and it is more common on left side.
c. The spermatic cord extends from the superior pole of the testis to the deep inguinal ring. Its length is about 7.5 cm.
d. The vas deferens extends from the tail of epididymis to the ejaculatory duct. Its length is 45 cm.
e. For constituents of the spermatic cord refer Chapter 161 and Figure 161.2.
f. The spermatic cord has three concentric coverings. The external spermatic fascia is derived from external oblique aponeurosis. The cremaster muscle and fascia are derived from internal oblique muscle and internal spermatic fascia is derived from fascia transversalis.
g. The pampiniform plexus becomes the testicular vein at the deep inguinal ring.
h. The left testicular vein drains into left renal vein.
i. The longer left testicular vein opens in to left renal vein at right angles. The left vein ascends posterior to the descending colon, which when loaded with fecal matter presses on the vein.

SINGLE BEST RESPONSE MCQs

1. The embryonic source of primordial germ cells is:

A. Mesoderm of genital ridge
B. Mesoderm of mesonephros
C. Endoderm of yolk sac
D. Endoderm of allantois

2. The lymph vessels of the testis drain into following nodes:

A. Superficial inguinal B. Deep inguinal
C. Internal iliac D. Preaortic

3. **The infundibulopelvic ligament contains:**
   A. Uterine vessels
   B. Ligament of ovary
   C. Ovarian vessels
   D. Infundibulum of tube
4. **Which discontinuous dermatomes meet on the scrotum?**
   A. L1 and S4 B. L1 and S3
   C. L5 and S1 D. L4 and S3
5. **The longest part of fallopian tube is:**
   A. Intramural B. Isthmus
   C. Ampulla D. Infundibulum
6. **What is true about the suprarenal medulla?**
   A. Develops from neural crest
   B. Essential for life
   C. Cells arranged in zones
   D. Receives postganglionic sympathetic nerves
7. **The external trigone of urinary bladder is related posteriorly to:**
   A. Prostate B. Seminal vesicle
   C. Urethra D. Rectum
8. **The inferior vena cava begins at the level of:**
   A. Sacral promontory B. L5
   C. L4 D. L1
9. **Membranous layer of superficial fascia of perineum is called:**
   A. Fascia lunata B. Colles fascia
   C. Scarpa's fascia D. Camper's fascia
10. **The cervix of uterus drains into following lymph nodes:**
    A. Preaortic B. Superficial inguinal
    C. Deep inguinal D. Sacral
11. **The term chordee is used for the anomaly of:**
    A. Seminal vesicle B. Penis
    C. Scrotum D. Ductus deferens
12. **Which joint is not of secondary cartilaginous type?**
    A. Lumbosacral B. Pubic symphysis
    C. Sacrococcygeal D. Sacroiliac
13. **Length of the uterine cavity is:**
    A. Two cm B. Six cm
    C. Twelve cm D. Fifteen cm
14. **Which of the following pairs is correctly associated?**
    A. Bulbourethral gland—deep perineal pouch
    B. Sphincter urethrae—superficial perineal pouch
    C. Greater vestibular glands—deep perineal pouch
    D. Bulbs of the vestibule—deep perineal pouch
15. **What is not true about trigone of urinary bladder?**
    A. Endodermal development
    B. Lacks submucosa
    C. Highly sensitive
    D. Transitional epithelium
16. **What is untrue about pelvic splanchnic nerve?**
    A. Represents sacral parasympathetic
    B. Arises from S2, S3 and S4 segments of spinal cord
    C. Is inhibitory to detrusor
    D. Also known as nervi erigentes
17. **A girl with short stature, webbed neck, ovarian dysgenesis will show following karyotype:**
    A. 47, XXX B. 47, XXY
    C. 46, XX D. 45, XO
18. **Pelvic splanchnic nerves carry the following fibers:**
    A. Preganglionic sympathetic
    B. Postganglionic sympathetic
    C. Preganglionic parasympathetic
    D. Postganglionic parasympathetic
19. **The ureter is related to the following bony parts, *except:***
    A. Anterior superior iliac spine
    B. Ischial spine
    C. Sacroiliac joint
    D. Tips of lumbar transverse processes
20. **Which of the following is known as coccygeus?**
    A. Puborectalis B. Ischiococcygeus
    C. Pubococcygeus D. Iliococcygeus

Key to MCQs

1 C	2 D	3 C	4 B	5 C	6 A	7 D
8 B	9 B	10 D	11 B	12 D	13 B	14 A
15 A	16 C	17 D	18 C	19 A	20 B	

MULTIPLE RESPONSE MCQs (TRUE OR FALSE)

1. **About levator ani:**
   A. Partly bony and partly tendinous origin
   B. Bony insertion in coccyx
   C. Funnel-shaped muscle
   D. Forms lateral wall of ischiorectal fossa

2. **Embryonic midgut:**
   A. Is connected to yolk sac
   B. Contains coeliac artery in its mesentery
   C. Supplied by vagus
   D. Undergoes 270° rotation

3. **The anterior relation of right kidney:**
   A. Visceral surface of right lobe of liver
   B. Gallbladder
   C. Second part of duodenum
   D. Splenic flexure of colon

4. **Regarding cervix of uterus:**
   A. Longer than body of uterus in infancy
   B. Cervical canal is closed by arbor vitae
   C. Vaginal part of cervix is lined by columnar epithelium
   D. Cervix is the most mobile part of uterus

5. **The rectum:**
   A. Is related posteriorly to upper three pieces of sacrum
   B. Is entirely intraperitoneal
   C. Develops from proctodeum
   D. Contains valves of Houston

6. **Pudendal nerve:**
   A. Traverses through both greater and lesser sciatic foramina
   B. Supplies sphincter ani externus
   C. Supplies sphincter ani internus
   D. Supplies sphincter urethrae

7. **Paramesonephric duct:**
   A. Is mesodermal in origin
   B. Crosses the mesonephric duct from medial to lateral side
   C. Is vestigial in male
   D. Unfused part develops into uterine tube

8. **Remnants of mesonephric tubules:**
   A. Paroophoron
   B. Epoophoron
   C. Appendix testis
   D. Appendix epididymis

9. **Prostate gland:**
   A. Contains uterus masculinus
   B. Secretion rich in acid phosphatase
   C. Median lobe is palpable per rectum
   D. Width is greater than length

10. **Epididymis:**
   A. Is related to posterolateral surface of testis
   B. Duct of epididymis is 6 meters long
   C. Head consists of coiled vasa efferentia
   D. Is a store of sperms

Annexure: Radiographs of Abdomen and Pelvis

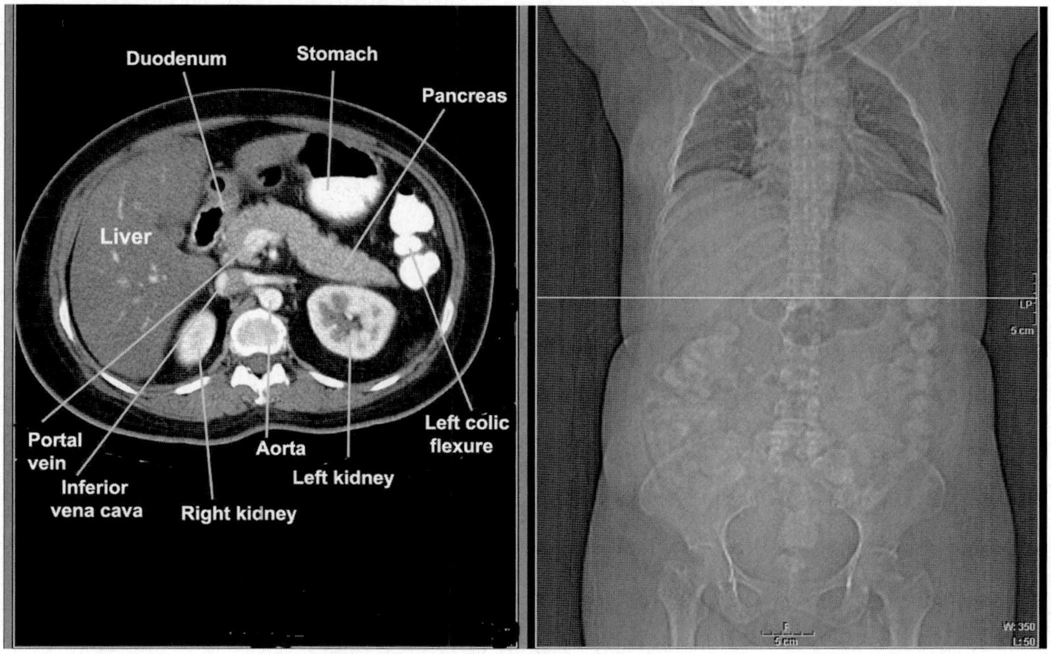

ABD-R1. Cross-section of abdomen at L1 level obtained by CT scan with contrast

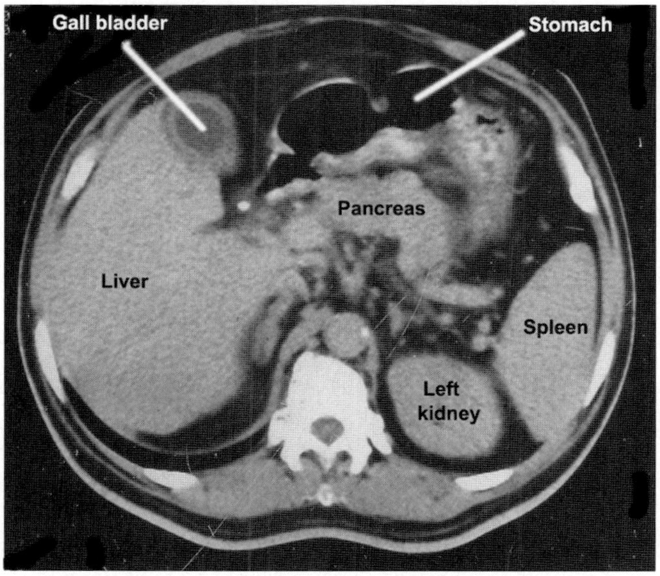

ABD-R2. CT scan of abdomen at the level of pancreas

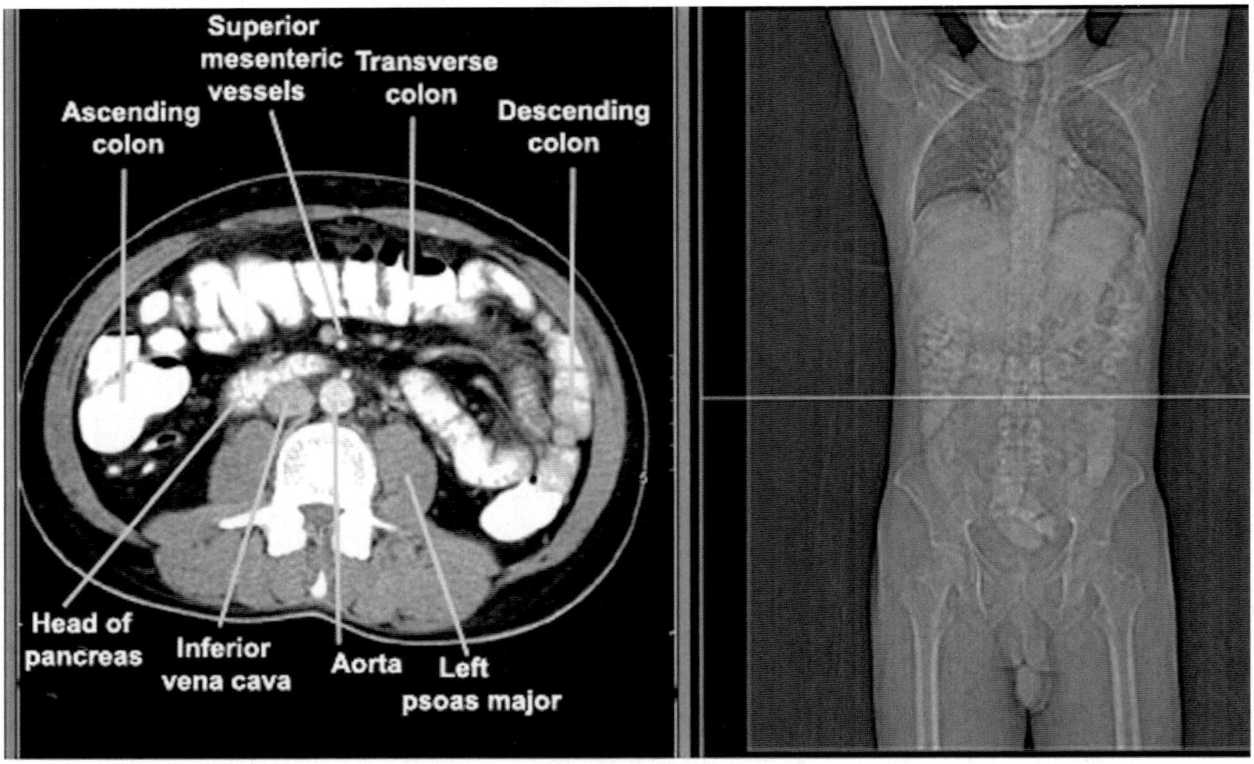

ABD-R3. Cross-section of abdomen at L3 level obtained by CT scan with contrast

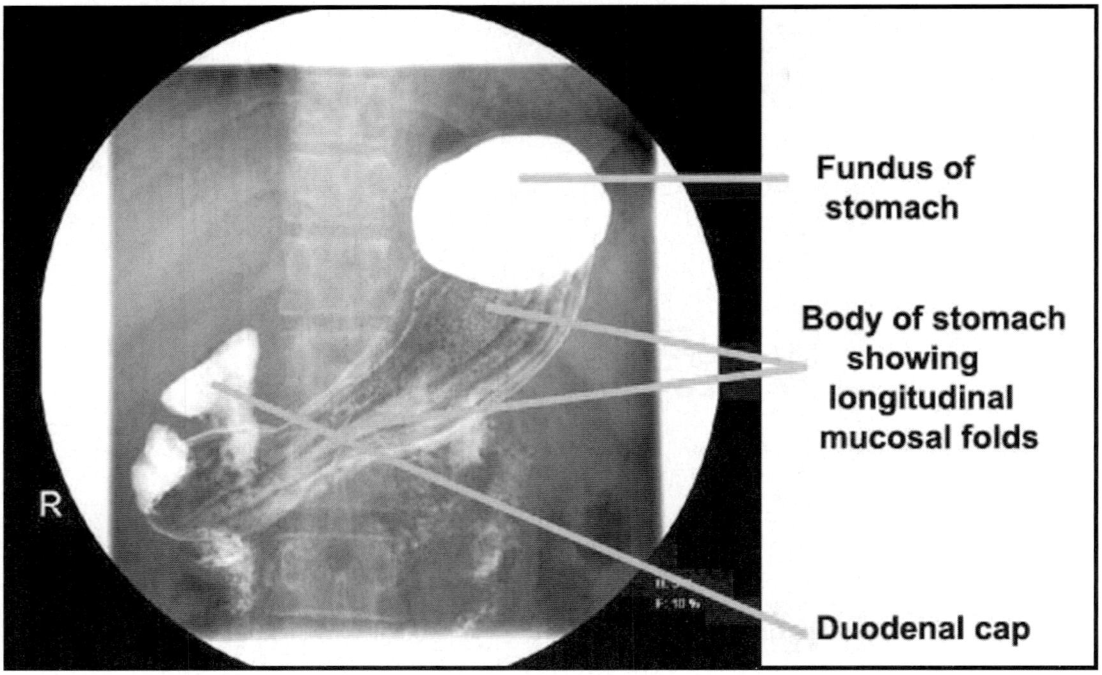

ABD-R4. Barium meal radiograph. (Note: Stomach is of transverse type, hence the fundus is filled with contrast medium and gas bubble outlines the folds in the body of stomach)

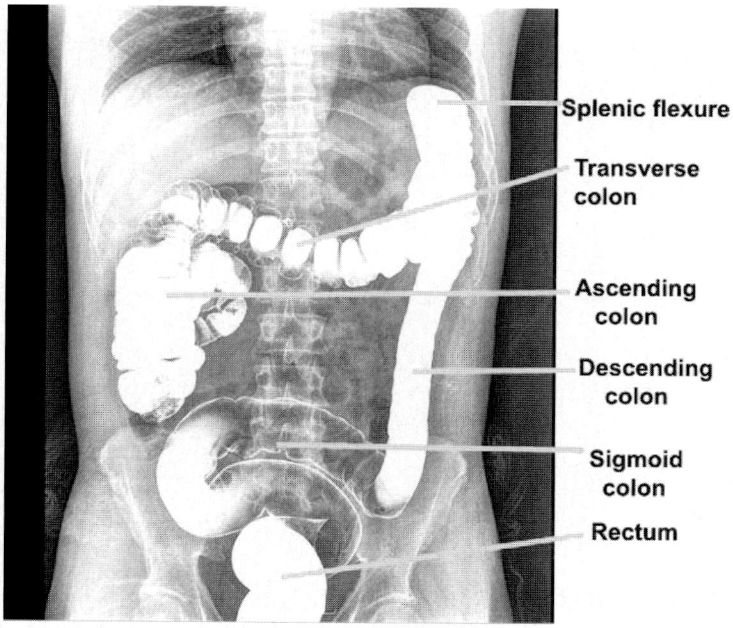

ABD-R5. Contrast radiograph of large intestine using barium enema

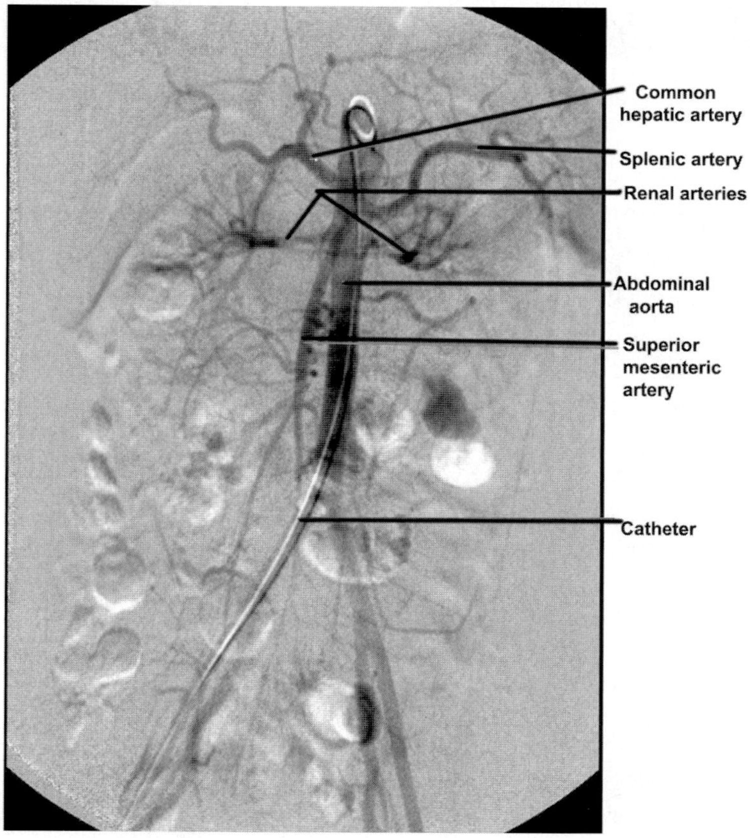

ABD-R6. Digital substraction angiogram of abdominal aorta showing few of its branches (Note: Path of catheter via femoral, external iliac and common iliac arteries to reach aorta)

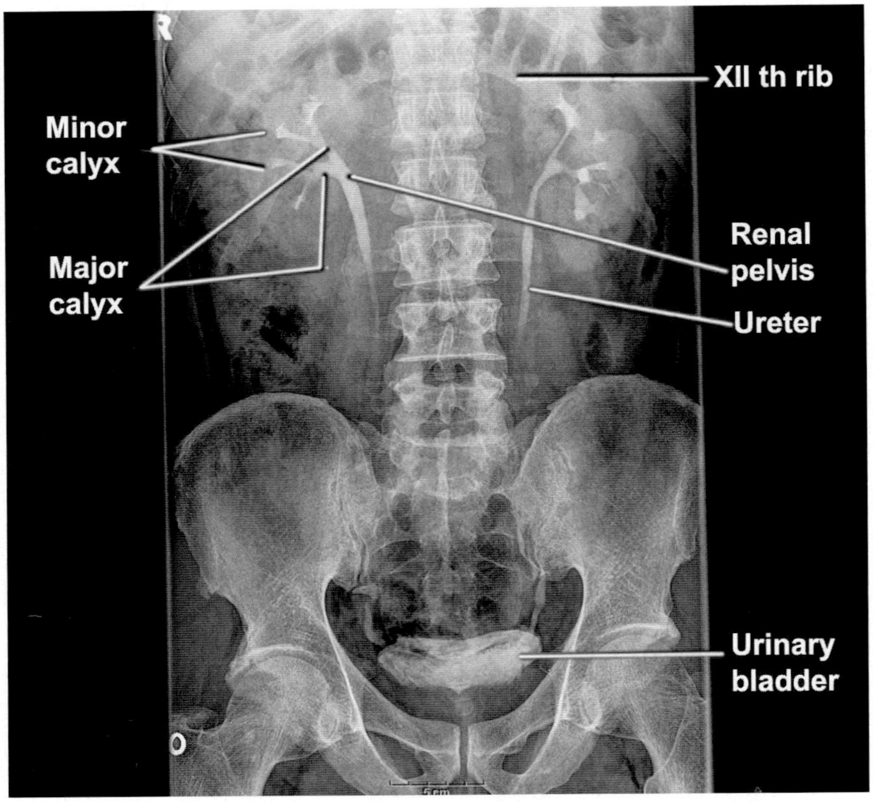

ABD-R7. Intravenous urogram (IVU) or pyelogram (IVP) to visualize renal calyces and renal pelvis, ureter and bladder

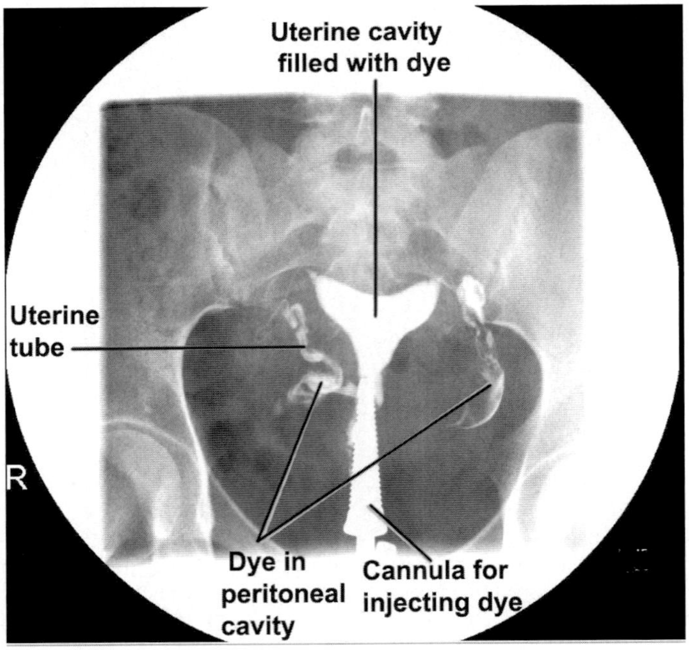

ABD-R8. Hysterosalpingogram to visualize uterine cavity and uterine tubes

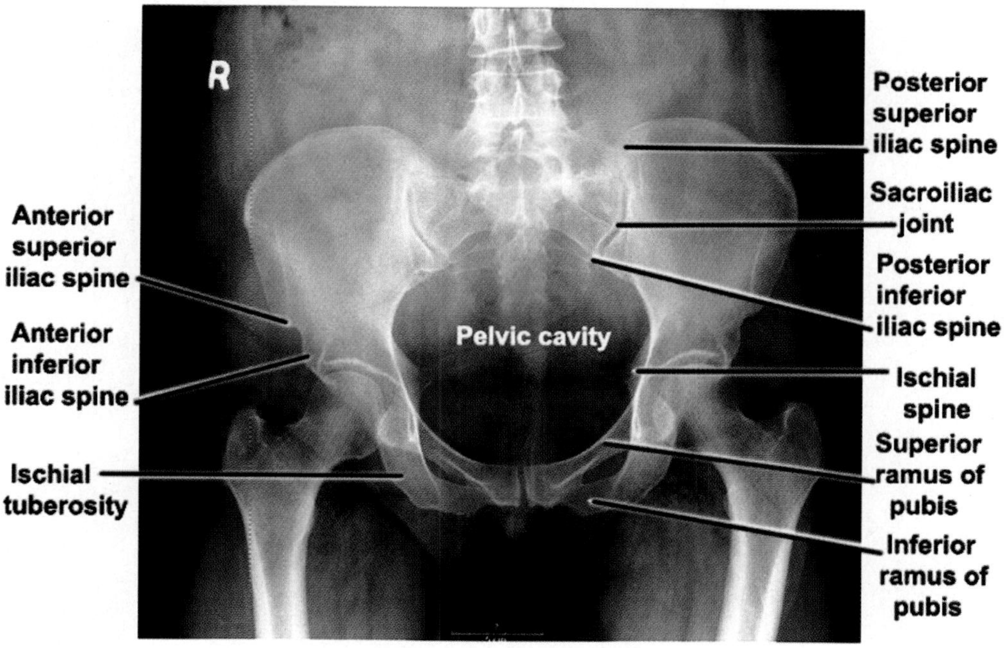

ABD-R9. Anteroposterior radiograph of female pelvis (Note: The wide subpubic angle)

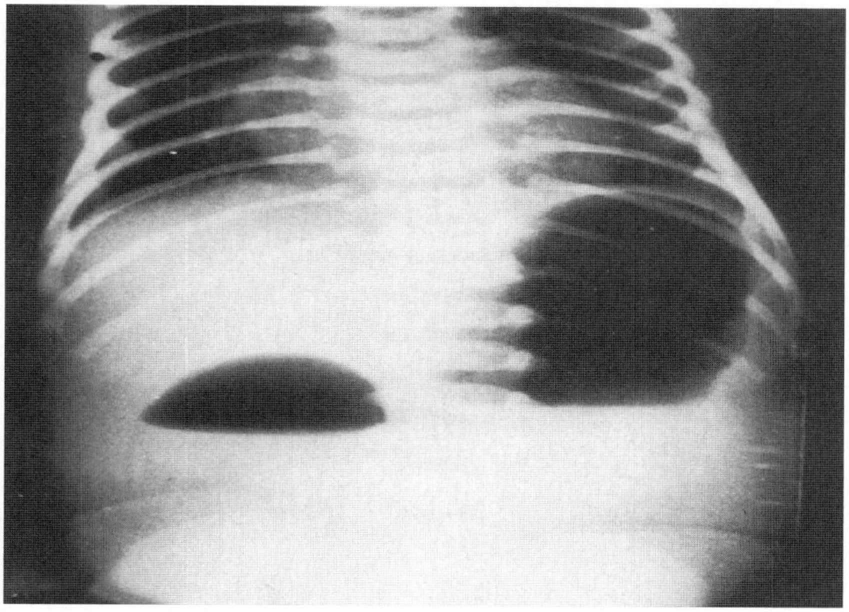

ABD-R10. Anteroposterior radiograph of upper abdomen of a child to show double bubble sign (typical of duodenal obstruction due to congenital anomaly called annular pancreas) (*Courtesy:* Department of Pediatrics Surgery, DR SMCSI Medical College, Karakonam)

SECTION FIVE

Lower Extremity

174 Introduction

INTRODUCTION

The basic function of the lower limbs is to support the body during standing and in locomotion. The lower limbs are connected to the bony pelvis at hip joints, through which the body weight is transmitted to the lower limbs or the propulsive forces from the lower limbs are transmitted to the axial skeleton. The lower limb consists of the gluteal region, thigh, popliteal fossa, leg, ankle and the foot. The gluteal region is separated from the thigh by the gluteal sulcus, which is a skin crease inferior to the gluteal fold produced by the inferior margin of gluteus maximus (Fig.174.1).

Surface Landmarks

a. The iliac crest, which is palpable in its entire extent, forms the superior limit of the gluteal region. The highest point of the iliac crest is at the level of the spine of L4 vertebra and the plane passing through it is known as the supracristal plane (Fig.174.1).
b. The anterior superior iliac spine is easily palpable in thin individuals.
c. The tubercle of the iliac crest lies five cm behind the anterior superior iliac spine. The plane passing through it, is known as trans-tubercular plane and it corresponds to the spine of L5 vertebra.
d. The posterior superior iliac spine is difficult to palpate but a skin dimple indicates its position. The dimple is located four cm lateral to the spine of second sacral vertebra. This landmark is clinically useful. One can palpate the sacroiliac joint at this site. The iliac crest can be easily approached here for bone marrow aspiration or for taking pieces of bone for grafting.
e. The pubic symphysis is felt in the inferior aspect of abdominal wall in the median plane. The pubic crest, which is the superior margin of the pubis and its lateral end, called pubic tubercle, are palpable parts of the pubic bone.
f. The ischial tuberosity is easily palpable in sitting position. The weight of the body is supported by the ischial tuberosities in this position.
g. The greater trochanter of femur can be felt a hand's breadth below the midpoint of the iliac crest.
h. The condyles of femur are subcutaneous, hence, easily palpable, when the knee is flexed or extended.
i. The adductor tubercle is felt above and behind the medial epicondyle of femur and is continuous with the lower end of medial supracondylar line. The lower epiphyseal line passes through the adductor tubercle (Fig 190.1).

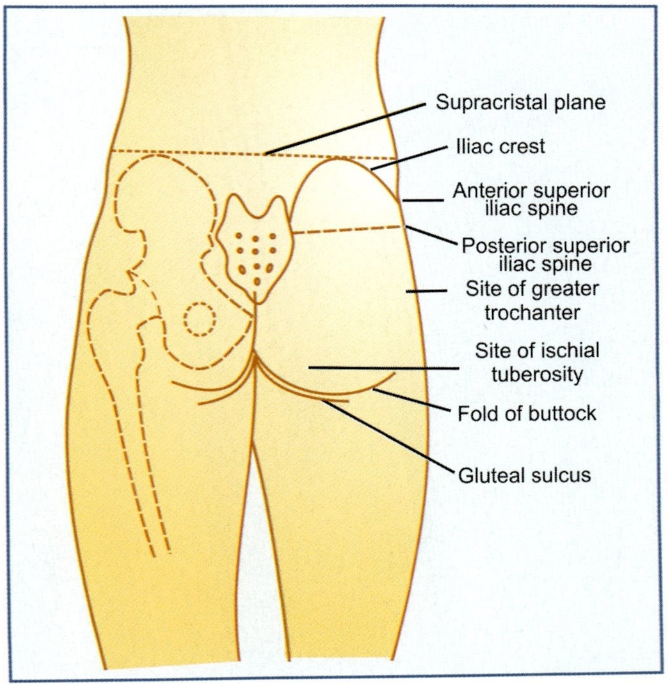

Fig. 174.1: Surface landmarks of gluteal region

j. The patella or kneecap moves during flexion and extension of knee joint. Its lateral and medial margins can be felt, when the knee is flexed.
k. The tibial tuberosity is felt five cm below the apex of patella. The tibial condyles form visible and palpable landmarks at the medial and lateral sides of ligamentum patellae. The medial surface of tibia lies between the anterior and medial borders and is subcutaneous. It is easily accessible and hence, used for taking pieces for bone grafting.
l. The anterior border of tibia (shin) is sharp and palpable throughout.
m. The medial malleolus at the lower end of tibia is subcutaneous and the great saphenous vein runs along its anterior margin.
n. The head of fibula is subcutaneous at the posterolateral aspect of the knee and is palpable at the level of the superior margin of tibial tuberosity. The neck of the fibula is palpable distal to the head. The lower end of shaft of fibula is subcutaneous.
o. The lateral malleolus is subcutaneous and its tip extends further distally than that of medial malleolus.
p. The posterior, lateral and medial surfaces of calcaneus can be palpated. The sustentaculum tali can usually be felt as a small prominence about a fingerbreadth below the tip of medial malleolus.
q. The peroneal trochlea is felt as a small tubercle on the lateral aspect of the calcaneus, two cm distal to the tip of lateral malleolus. The tendon of peroneus brevis passes above and the tendon of peroneus longus passes below the peroneal trochlea.
r. The head of talus is palpable anteromedial to the lateral malleolus if the foot is inverted and anterior to the medial malleolus if the foot is everted.
s. The head of the first metatarsal is a prominent landmark on the medial aspect of foot. The tuberosity of the fifth metatarsal bone is palpable at the midpoint of the lateral border of foot. The shafts of metatarsals and phalanges are palpable on the dorsum of the foot.

175 Cutaneous Nerves and Dermatomes of Lower Limb

The cutaneous nerves of the lower limb are derived from five sources, subcostal nerve (T12), branches of lumbar plexus, branches of sacral plexus, and the dorsal rami of lumbar and sacral nerves.

Gluteal Region (Fig. 175.1)

The gluteal region is the only part of the lower limb that receives sensory supply from dorsal as well as ventral rami. The region may be divided into four unequal areas, which receive cutaneous nerves from different sources.

a. The superolateral area receives twigs from the lateral cutaneous branch of subcostal nerve (T12) and of iliohypogastric nerve (L1). These branches pass anterior and posterior to the iliac tubercle to reach the level of greater trochanter.
b. The inferolateral area receives branches from lateral cutaneous nerve of thigh (L2, L3), which is a branch of lumbar plexus.
c. The superomedial area receives branches from the dorsal rami of L1, L2, L3 nerves and of S1, S2, S3 nerves.
d. The inferomedial area receives twigs from the gluteal branches of posterior cutaneous nerve of thigh (S1, S2, S3) and a few twigs from perforating cutaneous nerve (S2, S3), both branches of sacral plexus. The last named cutaneous nerve perforates the sacrotuberous ligament as well as the gluteus maximus muscle.

Thigh

a. The skin of the back of thigh receives branches from the posterior cutaneous nerve of thigh and the lateral cutaneous nerve of thigh. The medial anterior femoral cutaneous nerve of thigh may also supply.
b. As many as six nerves supply the skin of the front of thigh. Direct sensory branches of the lumbar plexus are, ilioinguinal nerve, femoral branch of genito-femoral nerve and lateral cutaneous nerve of thigh. The femoral nerve supplies through its medial femoral and intermediate femoral cutaneous branches and the saphenous nerve. The obturator nerve also supplies skin of the medial side through its contribution to the subsartorial plexus.

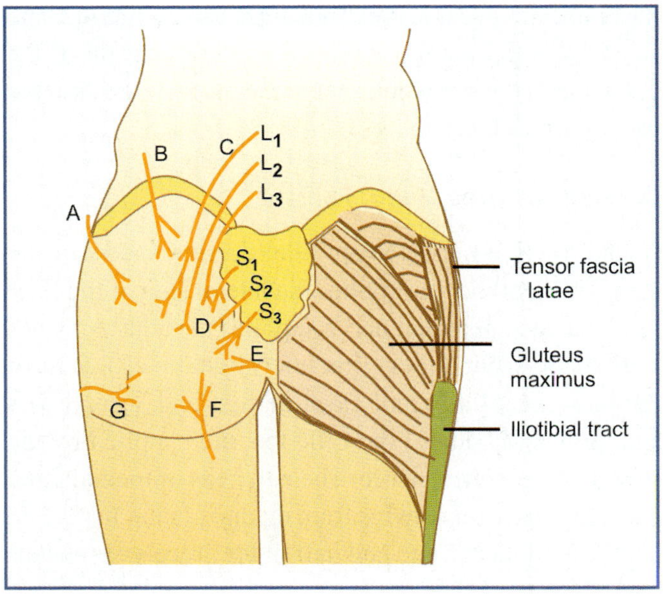

Fig. 175.1: Cutaneous nerves of gluteal region shown on left side. A-Lateral cutaneous branch of subcostal nerve. B-Lateral cutaneous branch of iliohypogastric nerve. C-Dorsal rami of lumbar nerves. D-Dorsal rami of sacral nerves. E-Perforating cutaneous nerve. F-Gluteal branch of posterior cutaneous nerve of thigh G-Branch from lateral cutaneous nerve of thigh

Popliteal Fossa

The skin of the popliteal fossa receives branches mainly from the posterior cutaneous nerve of thigh with a contribution from posterior branch of medial femoral cutaneous nerve.

Back of Leg

The back of the leg receives branches from sural nerve, a branch of tibial nerve in popliteal fossa and sural communicating nerve, a branch of common peroneal nerve in popliteal fossa. A few twigs are supplied from posterior cutaneous nerve of thigh and branch of medial femoral cutaneous nerve of thigh.

Front of Leg (Fig. 175.2)

The front of the leg is supplied mainly by three nerves. The saphenous nerve supplies medially and lateral cutaneous nerve of leg laterally, in the upper part of leg. However, in the lower part, saphenous nerve supplies medially and superficial peroneal nerve laterally.

Dorsum of Foot (Fig. 175.2)

Three nerves basically supply the dorsum of foot. The superficial peroneal nerve supplies the larger intermediate area. The sural nerve supplies the lateral margin of the dorsum and the saphenous nerve the medial side upto the base of great toe.

Dorsum of Toes (Fig. 175.2)

A total of five nerves supply the dorsal aspects of the toes. The sural nerve supplies the lateral side of the little toe. The deep peroneal nerve supplies the adjacent sides of first and second toes (first inter-digital cleft). Rest of the toes except adjacent sides of first and second toes and the lateral side of the little toe, are supplied by the superficial peroneal nerve. The nail beds of medial three and half toes receive twigs from medial plantar nerve and nail beds of lateral one and half of toes receive branches from the lateral plantar nerve.

Sole of Foot (Fig. 175.3)

The medial calcanean nerve, which is a branch of tibial nerve supplies the skin covering the heel. The cutaneous branches of medial plantar and lateral plantar nerves supply the rest of the sole including the plantar aspects of the toes.

Dermatomes of Lower Limb (Fig.1.5)

The ventral rami of lumbar and sacral nerves pleat together to form lumbar and sacral plexuses through which the cutaneous supply of the lower limb is derived. However, the gluteal region receives sensory nerves through the dorsal rami also. In the case of the limbs, dermatome is the area of skin supplied by one ventral ramus through its

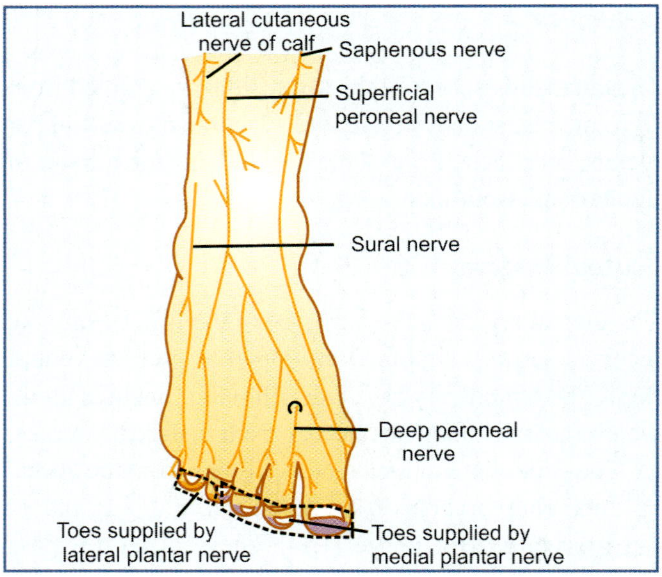

Fig. 175.2: Cutaneous nerves of front of leg, dorsum of foot and dorsum of toes

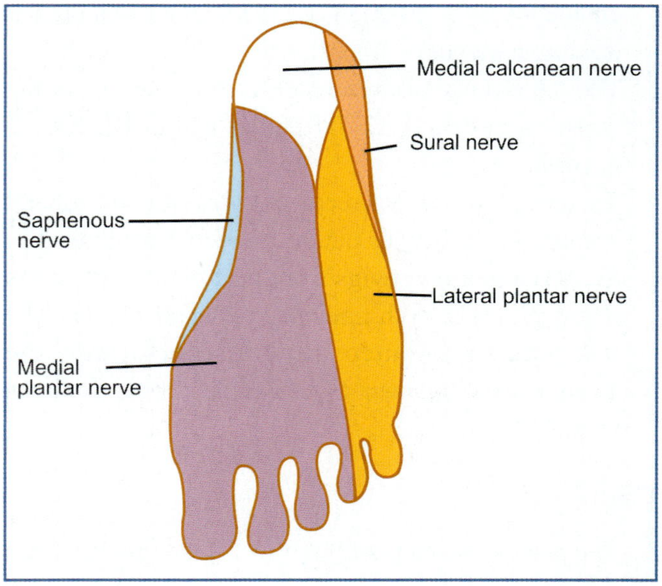

Fig. 175.3: Sensory nerve supply of sole

various cutaneous branches. Therefore, S1 dermatome receives S1 fibres from the cutaneous branches of several peripheral nerves carrying S1 fibres. Only if the sensory rootlets of first sacral nerve are damaged will there be complete anesthesia in S1 dermatome. In injury to the peripheral nerve, the nerve fibres belonging to more than one segment of the spinal cord will be involved and hence the sensory effects will not coincide with the entire cutaneous area of that nerve neither with any dermatome. The embryonic development of the lower limb helps to understand its dermatomal map. The lower limb bud originates against L1 to S3 segments of the spinal cord. When the limb bud elongates, it drags down the dermatomes along with the spinal nerves. Due to the medial rotation of the lower limb bud, its borders and surfaces are exactly opposite to that of upper limb. The preaxial digit of the lower limb comes to occupy medial side while the postaxial digit on the lateral side of the foot. The dorsal or extensor surface except the gluteal region comes to lie anteriorly while the ventral or flexor surface faces posteriorly. The preaxial border starts near the midpoint of thigh and descends to the knee. It then curves medially to descend to the medial malleolus and reach the great toe along the medial margin of the foot. In broad terms, the lumbar dermatomes lie in succession from L1 to L5 on the front of the limb. The L4 and L5 lie side by side in the front of leg. However, L5 dermatome occupies the middle of the dorsum of foot and middle three toes while the L4 dermatome occupies the medial side of the foot including the great toe. The S1 dermatome begins on the lateral aspect of dorsum as well as of the sole of the foot and includes the little toe. While eliciting Babinski sign, the clinician scratches the skin in the S1 dermatome. The S1 dermatome ascends on the back of the leg to be followed by the S2 dermatome up to the gluteal fold and S3 dermatome above it in the gluteal region including the saddle area of the perineum.

176 Venous and Lymphatic Drainage of Lower Limb

It is essential to know the anatomy of the veins of the lower limb to understand the pathogenesis, diagnosis and surgical treatment of the varicosity of the veins of lower limb. Varicosity is a condition in which veins become tortuous and dilated.

The veins of the lower limb are divided into three groups for descriptive purposes.

a. Superficial or subcutaneous veins in the superficial fascia.
b. Deep veins accompanying the arteries located deep to the deep fascia.
c. Perforating veins connecting the above two by passing through the deep fascia.

Superficial Veins (Fig. 176.1)

The superficial veins consist of dorsal venous arch on the dorsum of foot, great or long saphenous vein and small or short saphenous vein.

Dorsal Venous Arch

The dorsal venous arch lies on the distal parts of the metatarsal bones. It receives the dorsal digital and dorsal metatarsal veins and communicates with proximally, located dorsal venous network. Along the sides of foot, there are medial and lateral marginal veins which drain both the dorsal and plantar aspects of the respective sides in to the dorsal venous arch. The medial end of the arch along with medial marginal vein continues as the great saphenous vein. Similarly, the lateral end of the arch along with lateral marginal vein continues as the small saphenous vein.

Great (Long) Saphenous Vein

The word saphenous, which is Greek in origin, means easily seen. Since the saphenous vein lies in the superficial fascia it is easily seen. The great saphenous vein is the longest vein in the body. It is thick-walled and contains numerous valves, which allow the blood to flow towards heart. The valves divide the long column of blood in short segments so as to reduce the pressure on the distal part of the vein during prolonged standing.

Formation

The formation of great saphenous vein is described in two ways.

a. The medial end of dorsal venous arch and medial marginal vein of the foot continue as great saphenous vein.
b. The union of dorsal digital vein of the medial side of big toe and the medial end of dorsal venous arch form the great saphenous vein.

Course and Relations (Fig. 176.1A)

a. At the ankle, the great saphenous vein enters the leg at a very constant point. It ascends in the interval between the anterior aspect of the medial malleolus and the tendon of tibialis anterior muscle. Then, it lies in contact for a short distance with the distal third of medial subcutaneous surface of the tibia. In this part of its course it is accompanied by saphenous nerve. Further, it ascends along the medial border of tibia to reach the posterior aspect of the medial side of the knee.

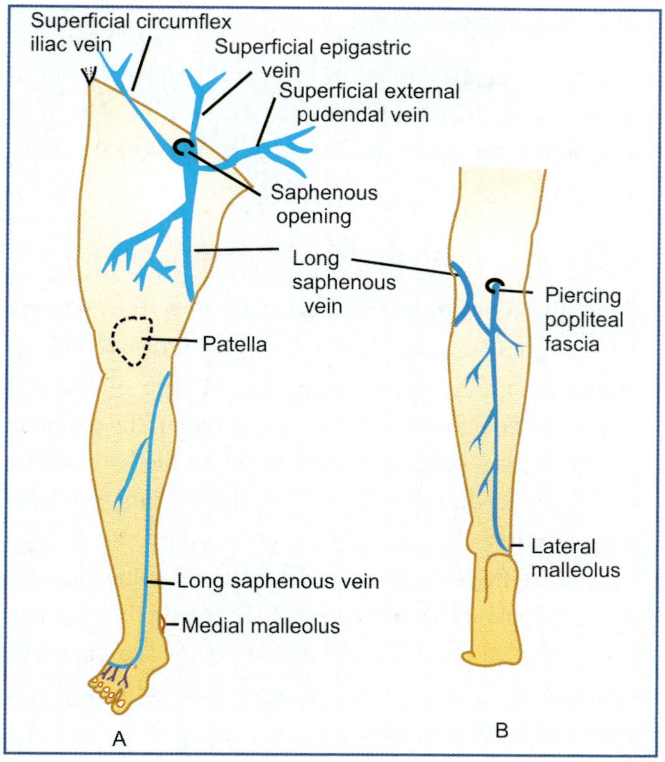

Fig. 176.1: Superficial veins of lower limb
A-Long saphenous vein, B-Short saphenous vein

b. At the back of the knee, it lies about a handbreadth behind the medial border of patella.
c. In the thigh, the vein ascends along the medial aspect of the front of thigh until it reaches the saphenous opening in the fascia lata. A few branches of medial cutaneous nerve of thigh are closely related to it here. The great saphenous vein pierces the cribriform fascia at the saphenous opening along with the three superficial branches of the femoral artery (superficial circumflex iliac, superficial epigastric and superficial external pudendal arteries) and lymph vessels. It terminates in the femoral vein after piercing the anterior wall of the femoral sheath. A valve guarding the saphenofemoral junction lies at a point about 3.5 to 4 cm inferolateral to the pubic tubercle.

Tributaries

a. At the ankle, it receives blood from the sole and the dorsum of foot.
b. In the leg, it receives anterior vein of the leg and posterior arch vein, which is formed on the medial malleolus and ascends on the medial aspect of the calf to join the great saphenous vein. The posterior arch vein is connected to the posterior tibial venae comitantes (deep veins) by three ankle perforators. Some surgeons refer the posterior arch vein as vein of Leonardo da Vinci.
c. In the thigh, the great saphenous vein receives the anterolateral vein of thigh and posteromedial vein of thigh. Before it passes through the saphenous opening it receives three tributaries, namely, superficial epigastric, superficial external pudendal and superficial circumflex iliac veins (Fig. 176.1A).
After passing through the saphenous opening but before piercing the femoral sheath it receives deep external pudendal vein (last tributary).

Perforating Veins or Perforators

There are about five perforating veins, which connect the great saphenous vein to the deep veins of leg and thigh. These veins are called perforators because they perforate the deep fascia. Their unique feature is that they contain unidirectional valves, which allow the blood to flow only from the superficial veins to the deep veins. In this way, the perforating veins minimize the load of the superficial veins. The incompetence of the valves of the perforators is one of the causes of dilatation of superficial veins of lower limb.

Position of Perforating Veins (Fig. 176. 2)

a. Between the medial malleolus and midcalf there are three ankle perforators of Cockett connecting the posterior arch vein to the venae comitantes of posterior tibial artery. Therefore, these perforators indirectly connect the great saphenous vein to the deep veins of leg
b. At the upper end of the calf, there is tibial tubercle perforator or Boyd's perforator that connects the venae comitantes of the posterior tibial artery to the great saphenous vein
c. In the intermediate third of thigh, one vein called Hunterian perforator or perforator of Dodd connects the great saphenous vein to the femoral vein in the subsartorial canal. This perforator passes through the fascial roof of the canal.

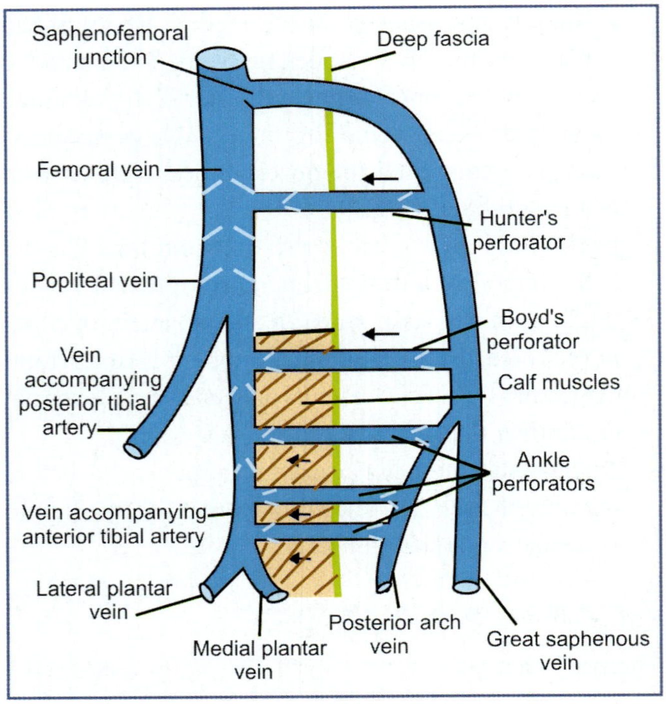

Fig. 176.2: Schematic representation of perforating veins connecting great saphenous vein to deep veins

Surface Marking of Great Saphenous Vein

Though one can see the long saphenous vein in thin people in its course in the foot and leg it is necessary to know its surface marking in the entire extent because this vein is used for venous cut downs and for coronary artery bypass graft.

a. At the ankle the vein passes upwards about 2.5 cm anterior to the medial malleolus.
b. In the leg it ascends crossing the medial surface and the medial border of tibia to reach the posteromdial aspect of the knee.
c. At the knee it lies about a hand's-breadth posterior to the medial margin of patella.
d. In the thigh, it ascends along the medial aspect of the front of thigh to enter the saphenous opening. The termination of the vein is indicated by the center of the saphenous opening, which is roughly four cm below and lateral to the pubic tubercle. One should know the surface marking of termination of the vein while performing various tests to assess saphenofemoral valve competency.

Small Saphenous Vein

It begins as the continuation of lateral marginal vein of foot or is formed by the union of dorsal digital vein of lateral side of the little toe and lateral end of dorsal venous arch.

Course and Relations (Fig. 176.1B)

At first, the short saphenous vein ascends posterior to the lateral malleolus and then on the lateral side of the tendocalcaneus. It passes along the middle of the calf and pierces the deep fascia in the lower part of the popliteal fossa to open in the popliteal vein above the level of the back of the knee joint. However, the termination may show variations. It may join the great saphenous vein in the proximal thigh, or it may bifurcate, one branch joining the great saphenous vein and the other joining the popliteal vein. In the leg, the short saphenous vein is accompanied by sural nerve. Like the great saphenous vein, this vein too has numerous valves.

Tributaries

At the ankle it receives veins from the sole and dorsum of foot. It receives several cutaneous tributaries of the leg and communications from the great saphenous vein. Perforating vein may connect it to the deep veins of the calf.

Deep Veins of Lower Limb

The deep veins accompany the arteries. The contractions of the muscles (soleus and gastrocnemius) supporting the deep veins, propel the venous blood upward. Valves are more in deep veins compared to the superficial veins. The deep veins receive blood from superficial veins through perforators. The major deep veins of lower limb include the deep veins of the sole (medial and lateral plantar veins), venae comitantes accompanying the dorsalis pedis, posterior tibial and anterior tibial arteries, the popliteal vein and the femoral vein.

Factors Facilitating Venous Return

In the standing position the venous blood has to flow against gravity. The following factors help the venous return.

a. The deep veins of the leg lie in the tight fascial compartment along with the arteries. When the muscles of the calf contract there is rise in the pressure inside the compartment, which compresses the deep veins. The valves open up and blood is propelled in upward direction. The soleus contains venous sinuses filled with blood and on contraction it squeezes the blood out in the deep veins. For this reason the soleus is regarded as the peripheral heart and the calf muscles collectively work as a venous pump. During relaxed state of the muscles, the blood is sucked from the superficial to the deep veins through the perforators.
b. The pulsations of accompanying arteries help in propelling the blood in the veins.
c. The valves in superficial and deep sets of veins allow the blood to flow in upward direction only.
d. The negative pressure in the thoracic cavity sucks the blood in the venous system towards heart in standing or recumbent position.

Clinical Highlights

a. The great saphenous vein is often chosen for a venous cut down in an emergency, when the superficial veins elsewhere are collapsed and invisible. A small skin incision is placed just in front of the medial malleolus (taking care not to injure the accompanying saphenous nerve) to expose the great saphenous vein. The vein can be cannulated here for giving intravenous fluids.
b. Being a muscular vein the great saphenous vein is ideally suited for coronary arterial graft. A segment of the patient's vein from the thigh is removed for this purpose. While suturing in place of the blocked coronary artery, the venous graft is reversed so that its valves do not obstruct the arterial flow.
c. Deep vein thrombosis (DVT) or phlebothrombosis in deep veins of calf is the most feared complication after surgical operation. During postoperative period, there is minimum activity of the legs, which favors venous stasis and thrombosis. The emboli from the thrombus enter venous circulation to reach the right side of heart and may cause life-threatening pulmonary embolism.
d. In varicosity of lower limb, the superficial veins are dilated and tortuous. This is a common affliction of lower limb, especially in people, whose jobs require prolonged standing (bus conductors or traffic police or nurses). Incompetence of valves may be another cause of varicosity. If the valves in perforating veins are incompetent, it will cause reversal of blood flow from the deep to the superficial veins leading to dilatation of the latter. If the saphenofemoral valve is incompetent there may be flow of blood from the femoral in to the saphenous vein.
e. Complications of varicose veins include thrombophlebitis or inflammation of superficial veins causing pain, local swelling, redness and tenderness in affected area. Venous ulcers are common in the skin near the medial malleolus. The reason for this is as follows. The venous stasis affects the oxygen supply of the skin, which initially becomes dry and discolored and later sloughs producing ulcer.
f. Trendelenburg test is performed to find out whether the saphenofemoral valve is incompetent or the valves in the perforators are incompetent. The patient is asked to lie down in supine position and then to raise the leg to empty the superficial veins. The saphenofemoral junction is closed by thumb and the patient is asked to stand up. Immediate filling of the great saphenous vein from above after release of the pressure indicates the incompetency of saphenofemoral valve. This is positive Trendelenburg test. Slow filling from below without releasing the pressure indicates the incompetent valves in the perforating vein or veins. This is also a positive test. The positive tests are indications for operation.

Lymphatic Drainage of Lower Limb

The lymph nodes and lymph vessels of the lower limb are divided in superficial and deep groups.

Superficial Group of Lymph Nodes (Fig. 176.3)

The superficial inguinal lymph nodes are located in the superficial fascia of the inguinal region and are normally palpable. They are arranged in two groups resembling the letter T. The horizontally disposed nodes lie parallel to and just below the inguinal ligament. The vertically disposed nodes lie along the great saphenous vein before it pierces the deep fascia. The superficial lymph vessels (running along the superficial veins) drain into these nodes.

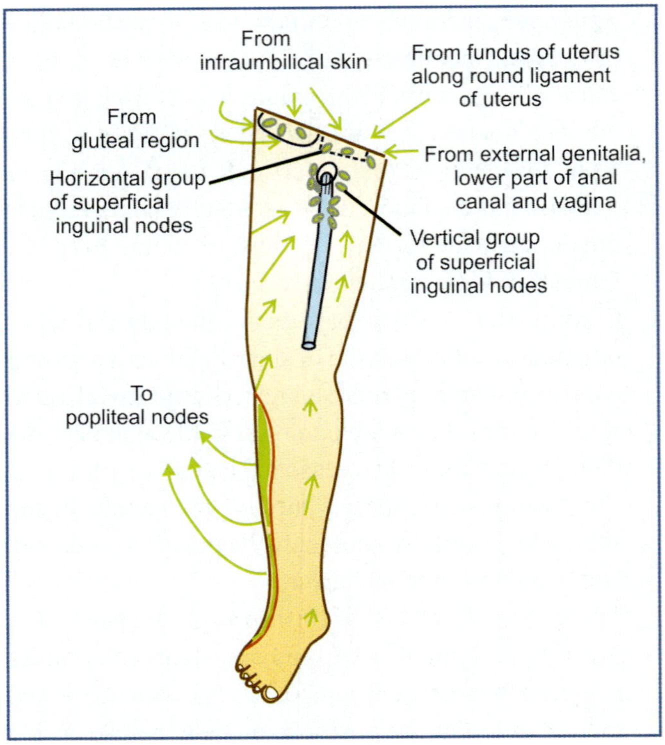

Fig. 176.3: Scheme to show superficial lymph vessels and nodes of lower limb

Areas of Drainage

The medial nodes of the horizontal group receive lymph from the external genitalia in both sexes except the glans penis or clitoris, lower end of vagina in female, terminal part of male urethra, lower part of anal canal, medial-half of the anterior abdominal wall below the umbilicus and part of fundus of uterus along the tubouterine junction in female. The lateral nodes of the horizontal group receive lymph directly from the gluteal region and adjoining part of the trunk, lateral half of the anterior abdominal wall below the umbilicus, the entire lower limb except the following areas namely, the lateral part of foot, the heel and lateral part of the back of leg.

Deep Group of Lymph Nodes (Fig. 176.4)

This group includes the deep inguinal nodes and the popliteal nodes. The deep nodes lie deep to the deep fascia.

a. The deep inguinal nodes lie along the medial side of femoral vein in femoral triangle. One node, which is inside the femoral canal, is called the node of Cloquet and it receives lymph from the glans penis or clitoris. The other nodes of this group receive lymph from the deeper tissues of the thigh, the popliteal lymph nodes and from the superficial lymph nodes. The efferent vessels from the deep group drain into the external iliac nodes.
b. The popliteal lymph nodes (Fig. 190.7) lie embedded in the fat in the popliteal fossa. They are about three to six in number and are disposed in three sets. The most posterior or superficial node lies at the sapheno-popliteal junction. The most anterior or deepest node lies between the knee joint and the popliteal artery. The nodes in the intermediate set lie on either side of the popliteal vessels. The popliteal nodes are unique because they are the only deep nodes that receive both superficial and deep lymph vessels. The posterior or superficial node receives superficial vessels from lateral side of foot, the heel and the lateral half of the back of the leg because these lymph vessels travel with small saphenous vein, which opens in popliteal vein. The intermediate set receives deep lymph vessels accompanying the deep blood vessels (anterior and posterior tibial) from the entire leg and foot. The most anterior node

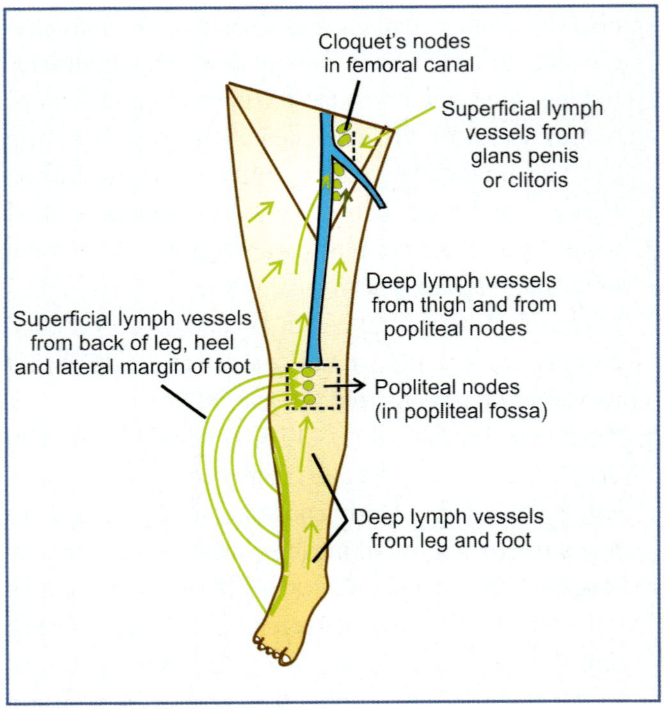

Fig. 176.4: Scheme to show areas of drainage of deep lymph nodes of lower limb

Section five

receives the lymph from the knee joint. The efferent vessels from the popliteal nodes reach the deep inguinal nodes.

Clinical Highlights

a. The lymphatic vessels of the lower limb may be blocked by microfilarial parasites (*Wuchereria bancrofti*). This usually manifests as massive edema of the lower limb (elephantiasis).
b. In inflammatory lesions of the lower limb the inguinal lymph nodes in vertical chain are enlarged and painful.
c. The malignant melanoma usually affects the medial toes. The melanoma originates from the melanocytes of the skin. Since this cancer spreads by lymphatics there is enlargement of inguinal nodes. Therefore, in the treatment of malignant melanoma the affected toe is amputated along with complete removal of the inguinal lymph nodes.
d. The lesion of prepuce, penis, labia majora, scrotum, lower part of vagina, utero-tubal junction (part of fundus of uterus), lower part of anal canal and terminal urethra in male will cause enlargement of horizontal chain of super-ficial inguinal lymph nodes. A boil or abscess in the gluteal region will cause inflammation and swelling of lateral nodes of horizontal group.
f. Enlargement of popliteal lymph nodes may occur in lesions of heel, lateral side of the foot and back of leg.

177 Thigh

The thigh extends from the hip to the knee. The proximal extent of the thigh is the inguinal region or groin anteriorly, perineum medially and the gluteal fold posteriorly. The distal extent of the thigh anteriorly is the front of the knee and posteriorly it is the popliteal fossa. The thigh is divided in three osteofascial compartments by intermuscular septa, which pass from the deep fascia of the thigh to the linea aspera of femur. The compartments are the anterior or extensor, posterior or flexor and medial or adductor (Fig. 177.2).

Superficial Fascia

In the upper part of the front of thigh, the superficial fascia consists of two layers, a superficial fatty layer and deep membranous layer. These two layers are continuous in front of the inguinal ligament with the corresponding layers of anterior abdominal wall. The membranous layer is fused with the deep fascia of thigh along a horizontal line starting from the pubic tubercle and passing for about eight cm laterally. This line is referred to as Holden's line (Fig. 177.1). This line of fascial fusion seals the space between the membranous layer of superficial fascia and the external oblique aponeuroses in the infraumbilical abdominal wall. This explains why the extravasated urine (in rupture of urethra in perineum) deep to the membranous layer of superficial fascia in the anterior abdominal wall does not descend in to the thigh below this line.

Deep Fascia of Thigh

The deep fascia of the thigh (the fascia lata) encircles the thigh like a stocking. It has a wide attachment above and below, it is attached to all the bony prominences at the knee.

a. Superiorly, on the anterior aspect it is attached to the inguinal ligament. The downward pull of the fascia lata on the inguinal ligament is responsible for the upper concavity of the inguinal ligament. On the lateral aspect, it is attached to the iliac crest. On the medial side, it is attached to the body and inferior ramus of pubis and the ramus and tuberosity of ischium. On the posterior aspect, it is attached to the sacrotuberous ligament, sacrum and coccyx. In the gluteal region, it splits to enclose the gluteus maximus muscle.
b. Inferiorly, on the anterior aspect it is attached to the patella, condyles of femur and tibia and head of fibula. The patella is held to the tibial condyles by lateral and medial patellar retinacula (thickened bands of deep fascia) through which lateral and medial vasti are inserted in respective margins of the patella. On the posterior aspect, the deep fascia continues as the popliteal fascia.

Special Features of Deep Fascia

a. The saphenous opening is the deficiency in deep fascia. It is covered by cribriform fascia, which is pierced by multiple structures giving it a sieve like appearance.

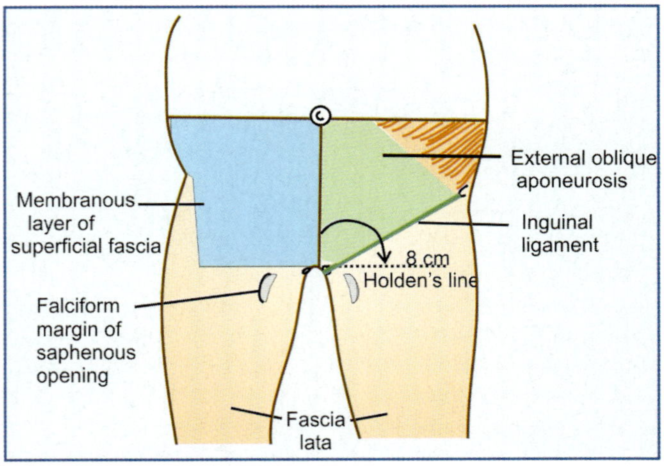

Fig. 177.1: Scheme to show Holden's line (line of fusion of membranous layer of superficial fascia with fascia lata)

b. Iliotibial tract is the thickened part of deep fascia laterally, extending like a band from the iliac crest to the lateral tibial condyle. It splits superiorly to enclose the tensor fasciae latae.
c. The intermuscular septa arising from the deep fascia course internally towards the linea aspera of the femur (Fig. 177.2). The lateral, medial and posterior intermuscular septa divide the thigh in to three osteo-fascial compartments. The anterior compartment consists of extensor muscles supplied by branches of femoral nerve. The posterior compartment consists of hamstring or flexor muscles supplied by branches of sciatic nerve. The medial compartment consists of adductor muscles supplied by branches of obturator nerve.

Saphenous Opening

This is an oval aperture (Fig. 177.1) in the deep fascia of the thigh. It is about 3 cm long and 1.5 cm wide. The center of the opening lies about 3 to 4 cm inferolateral to the pubic tubercle. It has a sharp falciform margin, which bounds it on superior, lateral and inferior aspects. The medial margin, however, is smooth and sloping and merges with fascia covering the anterior surface of pectineus. It should be borne in mind that the falciform margin, which is at a superficial plane forms the anterior relation of the femoral sheath while the medial margin, which is at a deeper plane passes posterior to the sheath. The two margins of the opening are connected by the cribriform fascia, which is so called because of its sieve-like appearance. The long saphenous vein, lymph vessels and the superficial external pudendal, superficial epigastric and superficial circumflex iliac arteries (branches of the femoral artery) pierce the cribriform fascia.

Iliotibial Tract (Fig. 175.1)

It is a thickened part of deep fascia on the lateral aspect of thigh. It is attached to the anterior part of iliac crest and to the front of the lateral condyle of tibia on a circumscribed area. Superiorly, it splits to enclose the tensor fasciae latae muscle. In the thigh, it provides insertion to the tensor fasciae latae and the gluteus maximus muscles. It is interesting to note that the muscles inserted into it are supplied through different nerves (gluteus maximus by inferior gluteal nerve and tensor fasciae latae by superior gluteal nerve). Through the iliotibial tract, the insertion of these two muscles is extended to the tibia. The function of iliotibial tract is to stabilize the knee joint in extended position.

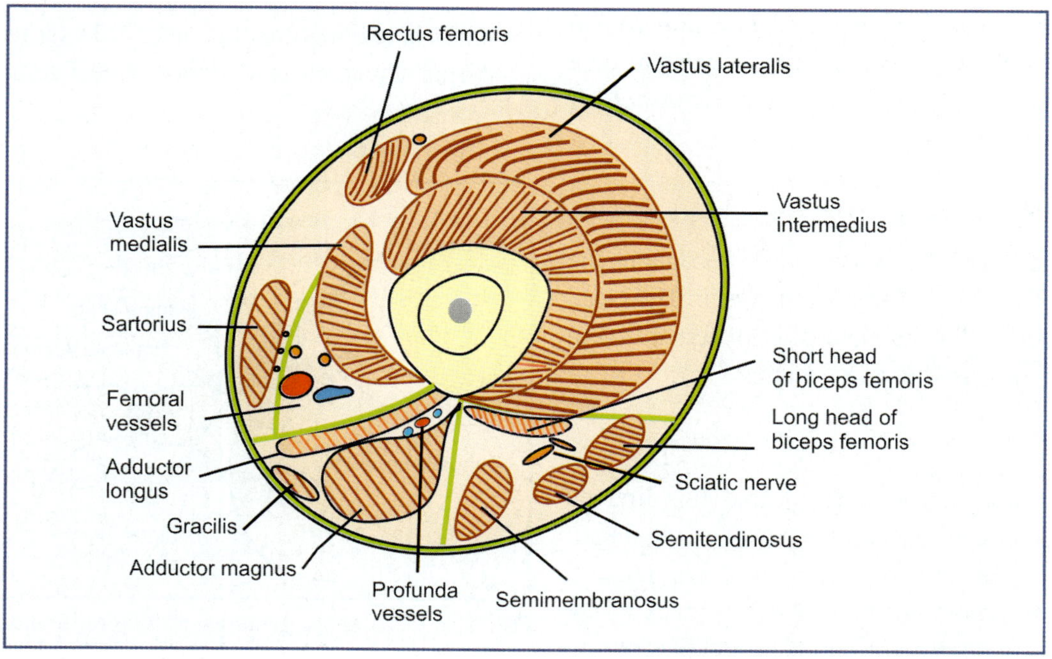

Fig. 177.2: Cross-section at the level of mid-thigh to depict osteofascial compartments (Note: Structures attached to linea aspera (vastus medialis, medial intermuscular septum, adductor longus, adductor magnus, posterior intermuscular septum, short-head of biceps femoris, lateral intermuscular septum and vastus lateralis)

178 Femoral Sheath

The femoral sheath is a funnel-shaped fascial envelope around the femoral vessels as they descend behind the medial half of inguinal ligament in the thigh.

Formation

The fascia transversalis forms the anterior wall of the sheath and the fascia iliaca forms the posterior wall. The lateral wall of the sheath is straight while its medial wall is sloping. The femoral sheath closes inferiorly because its anterior and posterior walls fuse with the tunica adventitia of femoral vessels.

Compartments (Fig. 178.1)

The femoral sheath is divided in three compartments by two antero-posterior septa. The medial compartment is called the femoral canal. The intermediate compartment contains the femoral vein and the lateral compartment contains the femoral artery and femoral branch of genitofemoral nerve.

Femoral Canal

The femoral canal is about two cm long. It contains the lymph node of Cloquet and fibro-fatty tissue. The canal provides dead space for the expansion of femoral vein during times of increased venous return.

Femoral Ring

It is the upper opening of the femoral canal. It is directed towards the abdomen. It can admit the tip of a little finger. It is wider in females due to wider pelvis. The femoral ring is closed by femoral septum, which is made of the extraperitoneal fatty tissue. The boundaries of the femoral ring are of surgical importance. The lateral margin is formed by femoral vein, anterior margin by inguinal ligament, posterior margin by pectineus muscle and the medial margin by the base of lacunar ligament. If the abnormal obturator artery is present, it lies on the base of the lacunar ligament (medial boundary of femoral ring).

Clinical Highlights

a. The femoral ring is the weak area in the lower part of the abdominal wall. The protrusion of abdominal contents covered by parietal peritoneum through the femoral ring, into the femoral canal, is called the femoral hernia. It is more common in females due to the greater width of the femoral ring. The femoral hernia presents as a globular swelling in the groin. Its distinguishing features are its relations to the pubic tubercle and inguinal ligament. It lies inferolateral to the pubic tubercle and inferior to the inguinal ligament.

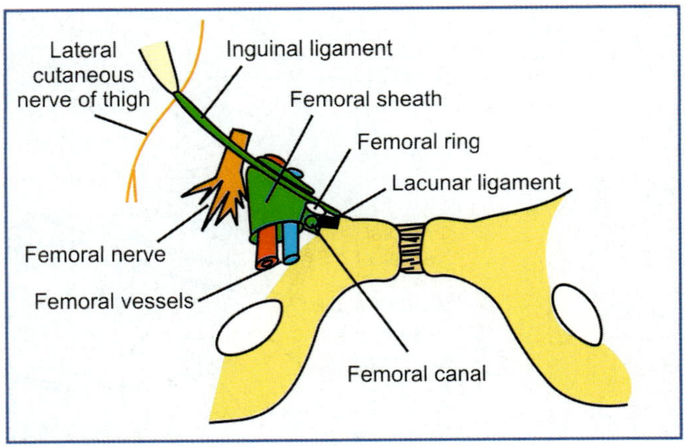

Fig. 178.1: To show contents of femoral sheath. Note that femoral nerve is outside the sheath and Cloquet's lymph node is inside the femoral canal

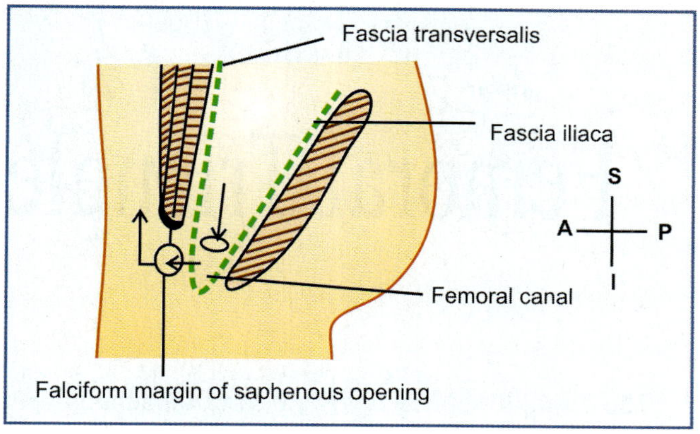

Fig. 178.2: Simplified diagram showing path of femoral hernia as indicated by arrows. The path of hernia is downwards, anteriorly and upwards

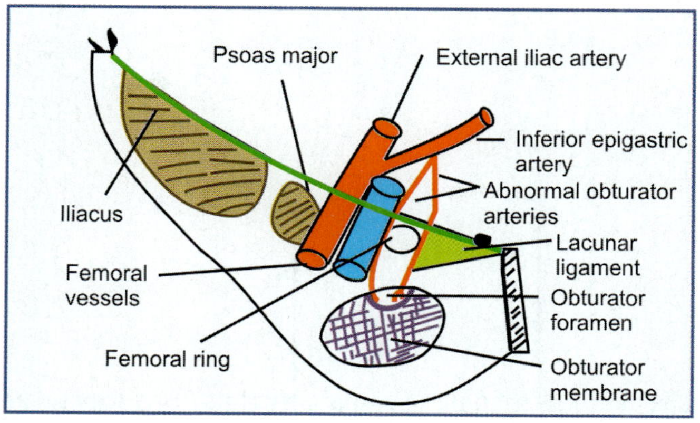

Fig. 178.3: Abnormal obturator arteries (enlarged pubic branches of inferior epigastric artery). Note that it is dangerous, when the artery is in medial relation to femoral ring

b. The path of the femoral hernia is at first downward, then anterior and then upward (Fig. 178.2). First, it enters the femoral canal and then passes through its anterior wall into the saphenous opening, where it turns upwards around the sharp falciform margin (Fig. 177.1). It is useful for the surgeon to know the path of the hernia in order to reverse the path while manually reducing the hernia.
c. The femoral hernia is prone to strangulation because of the compression of the neck of the hernial sac at the narrow femoral ring. The strangulation endangers the blood supply of the herniated intestinal loop. The relief of the strangulated loop is obtained by cutting the lacunar ligament in order to enlarge the femoral ring. The surgeon must be familiar with the anatomical relations of the abnormal obturator artery to the femoral ring while incising the lacunar ligament. If the abnormal obturator artery (Fig. 178.3) is in lateral relation to the ring it is its safe position. If it is in medial relation to the ring (in contact with lacunar ligament) it is prone to inadvertent injury and bleeding while cutting the lacunar ligament.

179 Femoral Triangle

The femoral triangle (Scarpa's triangle) is a triangular space in the upper third of the thigh below the inguinal ligament and medial to the sartorius muscle.

Boundaries (Fig. 179.1)

The inguinal ligament forms the base of the triangle. The medial border of the adductor logus muscle bounds the triangle medially and the medial border of sartorius laterally. The apex of the triangle is the meeting of the adductor longus and sartorius muscles. At the apex, the femoral triangle is continuous with subsartorial canal. The gutter- shaped floor has four muscles (medial to lateral), adductor longus, pectineus, psoas major and iliacus. The fascia lata forms the roof, which presents some features like saphenous opening and cribriform fascia.

Contents

The main contents of the femoral triangle are, from lateral medial, femoral nerve and its branches, femoral artery and its branches and femoral vein with its tributaries. The lateral cutaneous nerve of thigh enters the lateral angle of the triangle, usually after piercing the inguinal ligament.

a. The femoral nerve breaks up into a bunch of three sensory and six muscular branches. The sensory branches are, intermediate and medial femoral cutaneous nerves and the saphenous nerve. The muscular branches supply the sartorius, pectineus and four heads of quadriceps femoris.
b. The femoral artery enters the base of the triangle at midinguinal point. Its upper part, along with femoral vein is enclosed in femoral sheath. The femoral artery gives three superficial branches, deep external pudendal and profunda femoris artery. Two branches of the profunda femoris artery (lateral and medial circumflex femoral) originate in the femoral triangle.
c. The femoral vein receives the long saphenous vein besides smaller tributaries.
d. The deep inguinal lymph nodes, the lateral cutaneous nerve of thigh and the femoral branch of genitofemoral nerve are the other contents.

Exit of Contents from the Triangle (Fig. 179.2)

a. The femoral vessels leave through the apex to enter the subsartorial canal.
b. The profunda femoris vessels leave through the floor, via a gap between pectineus and adductor longus muscles.
c. The medial circumflex femoral vessels pass through the gap between psoas major and pectineus muscles.
d. The lateral circumflex femoral vessels pass behind the sartorius.
e. The superficial branches of the femoral artery pierce the cribriform fascia.
f. The saphenous nerve and nerve to vastus medialis leave through the apex. The other muscular branches

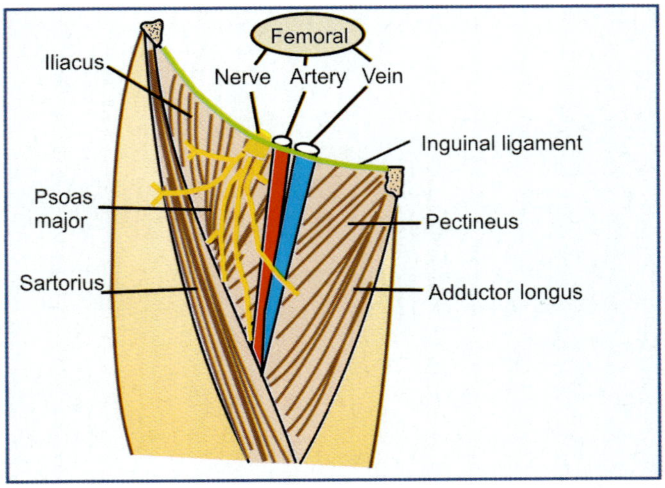

Fig. 179.1: Boundaries of femoral triangle

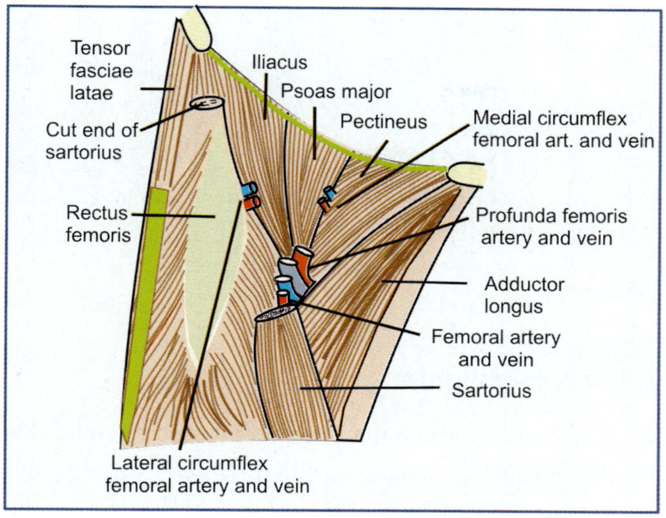

Fig. 179.2: Sites of exit of vessels through femoral triangle (Note that a stab wound at the apex of the triangle is likely to injure four blood vessels)

enter the respective muscles in the triangle itself while the other cutaneous nerves pierce the deep fascia of the triangle.

Relations at Apex of the Triangle (Fig. 179.2)

At the apex of the triangle, four vessels and two nerves are crowded. The femoral vessels passing through the apex are separated by the adductor longus from the profunda vessels. These four vessels are of fairly large size and are arranged from anterior to posterior in the following order, femoral artery, femoral vein, profunda vein, and profunda artery. The saphenous nerve and nerve to vastus medialis also pass through the apex. All these structures are involved in a stab or bullet injury at the apex of the femoral triangle.

Clinical Highlights

A number of anatomical structures in the base of femoral triangle may give rise to swelling in the groin. Therefore, while examining a case of lump in the groin a clinician thinks of following anatomical structures:

a. The subcutaneous fatty tissue may form a lipoma.
b. The femoral and inguinal hernia present as swellings. The pubic tubercle helps in distinguishing the swelling of femoral hernia from that of inguinal hernia. The neck of the femoral hernia lies inferolateral to the pubic tubercle while that of inguinal hernia is superior to the pubic tubercle. This relationship corresponds to the positions of superficial ring and saphenous opening in relation to the pubic tubercle.
c. The dilatation or aneurysm of femoral artery forms a pulsatile swelling.
d. An injury to the femoral vein (for example, during venipuncture) may result in hematoma.
e. The great saphenous vein may dilate at its termination.
f. The femoral nerve may give rise to neuroma.
g. The psoas abscess arising high up from the tuberculosis of thoracic vertebrae, presents as a swelling in the groin.
h. The inguinal lymph nodes enlarge due to inflammatory lesions or malignancy in the areas of their drainage.
i. The ectopic testis may present as lump in the groin.

180 Femoral Nerve

The femoral nerve is a branch of lumbar plexus, which is housed inside the substance of the psoas major muscle located on the posterior abdominal wall. The dorsal branches of the ventral rami of second, third and fourth lumbar spinal nerves join to form the femoral nerve (root value—L2, L3, L4).

Course (Fig. 180.1)

The femoral nerve emerges from the lateral margin of psoas major muscle and descends to reach the iliac fossa, where it lies between the iliacus and psoas major muscles. It enters the femoral triangle behind the inguinal ligament lying outside the femoral sheath. Here, it is in lateral relation to the femoral artery, which is inside the femoral sheath. In the femoral triangle, the femoral nerve lies in the groove between psoas and iliacus. The femoral nerve divides into anterior and posterior divisions just below the inguinal ligament. Hence, it has a very short trunk in the femoral triangle.

Branches of Femoral Nerve

a. In iliac fossa—to iliacus muscle
b. In femoral triangle

Muscular branches

- From trunk—to pectineus
- From anterior division—to sartorius
- From posterior division—to rectus femoris, three vasti and articularis genu

Articular branches

- From branch to rectus femoris—to hip and knee joints
- From branches to vasti—to knee joint

Cutaneous branches

- From anterior division—medial and intermediate femoral cutaneous nerve of thigh
- From posterior division—saphenous nerve

Clinical Highlights

a. The femoral nerve may be compressed or injured at the base of the triangle, where it lies in the groove between the iliacus and psoas muscles due to accumulation of pus or blood in the psoas sheath or neuropathy.
b. Injury to nerve results in atrophy of extensor muscles of thigh with inability to extend the leg at the knee joint and loss of knee jerk.
c. The femoral nerve block can be easily achieved in the femoral triangle by injecting the anesthetic solution at a point one-finger breadth lateral to the point of femoral pulse, which is just below the midinguinal point.

Saphenous Nerve

It is a branch of the posterior division of femoral nerve. It is the longest cutaneous nerve.

Course (Fig. 180.1)

The saphenous nerve leaves the femoral triangle along with femoral vessels through the apex of triangle to enter the subsartorial canal. During its course through the canal it crosses in front of the femoral artery to come on medial side. It leaves the subsartorial canal along with saphenous branch of descending genicular artery by piercing the fibrous roof at the lower end of the canal. In its further course, it descends vertically along the medial side of knee lying behind the sartorius. The saphenous nerve pierces the deep fascia between the tendons of sartorius and gracilis to become superficial. In the leg, it descends with the great saphenous vein along the medial side and passes in front of the medial malleolus to enter the dorsum of the foot, where it reaches upto the base of great toe.

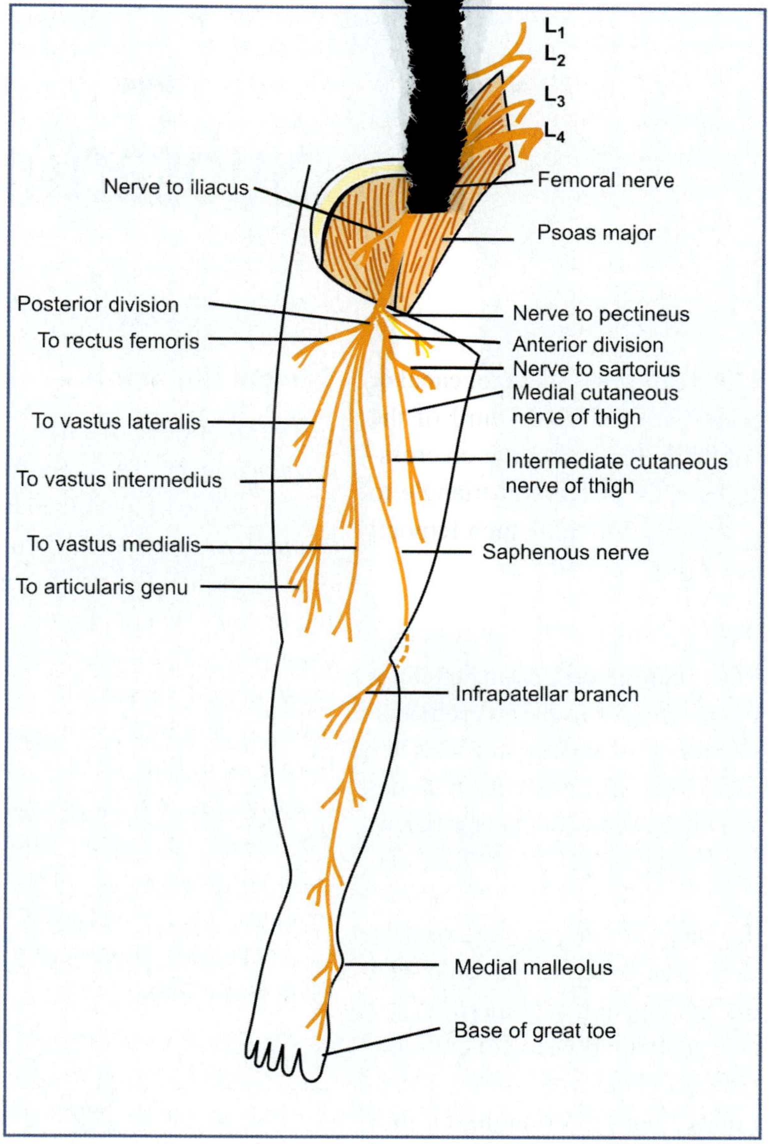

Fig. 180.1: Schematic diagram showing course and branches of femoral nerve (Note that saphenous nerve extends upto the base of great toe)

Branches

a. In the thigh, the saphenous nerve gives a twig to the subsartorial plexus. Its infrapatellar branch contributes to the patellar plexus along with medial, intermediate and lateral femoral cutaneous nerves of thigh.

b. In the leg, it supplies the skin of medial side of front of leg and the medial side of ankle.

c. In the foot, it supplies the skin of the medial side of the dorsum of foot upto the base of great toe.

Clinical Highlights

Being superficial in location, the saphenous nerve is often used for nerve grafting.

181 Subsartorial Canal

The subsartorial canal is also called the adduct[illegible] or Hunter's canal. It is located in the middle-th[illegible]e medial side of the front of thigh. It is triangula[illegible] section. It extends from the apex of femoral [illegible] the opening in adductor magnus through whi[illegible] vessels enter the popliteal fossa.

Boundaries (Fig. 181.1)

The vastus medialis is the anterolateral boundary. The fibrous roof covered with sartorius forms the anteromedial boundary. Between the fibrous roof and the sartorius lies the subsartorial plexus of nerves. The posterior wall has the adductor longus above and the adductor magnus below.

Contents

The main contents of the canal are the femoral vessels, saphenous nerve and the nerve to vastus medialis. (A vascular branch of the anterior division of obturator nerve and genicular branch of the posterior division of obturator nerve enter the canal briefly). The four main contents enter through the apex of the femoral triangle but they leave by different routes. The femoral vessels leave through the posterior wall at the tendinous opening in the adductor magnus. The saphenous nerve leaves by piercing the roof. The nerve to vastus medialis leaves by entering the anterolateral wall, which means the vastus medialis muscle.

Subsartorial Plexus

The subsartorial plexus of nerves is not a content of the canal as it lies between the fibrous roof and the sartorius. This plexus receives contributions from saphenous nerve, medial cutaneous femoral nerve and anterior division of obturator nerve. The plexus supplies the skin of the medial side of thigh.

Clinical Highlights

In the treatment of aneurysm of popliteal artery, the surgeons ligate the femoral artery in subsartorial canal. The principle of this procedure depends on the existence of anastomotic channels around the knee, through which blood reaches the popliteal artery despite ligation of femoral artery. For approaching the femoral artery in the canal, the surgeon must be well-versed with the surgeon must be well-versed with the relations of the artery in the canal. A skin incision is placed along the line of anterior border of middle third of sartorius. The superficial and deep fasciae are divided and the sartorius is retracted. The fibrous roof of the canal is incised to enter the canal. John Hunter was the first to describe the exposure and ligation of the femoral artery in subsartorial canal in treating the aneurysm of popliteal artery. That is why the canal is named after him.

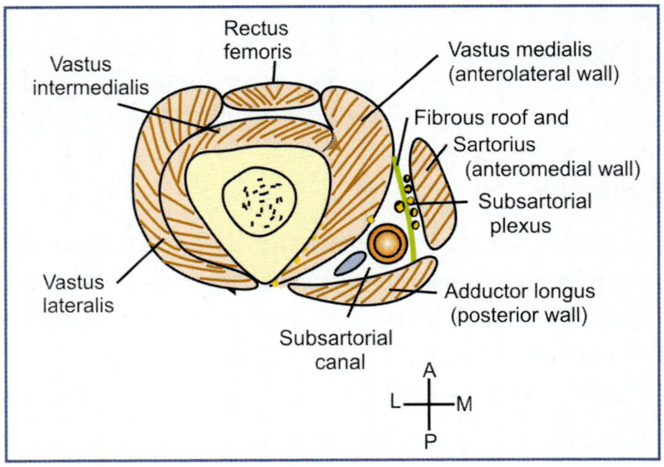

Fig. 181.1: Boundaries and contents of subsartorial canal (left side). Note, femoral vessels, saphenous nerve and nerve to vastus medialis inside the canal

182 Femoral Vessels

FEMORAL ARTERY

The femoral artery is the chief artery of the lower limb. It begins as the continuation of the external iliac artery at the midinguinal point. The femoral artery enters the thigh by passing behind the inguinal ligament. After coursing through the femoral triangle and subsartorial canal, it leaves the thigh through adductor hiatus or tendinous opening in the adductor magnus muscle and enters the popliteal fossa to continue as popliteal artery.

Surface Marking

To draw the femoral artery on the surface, the thigh is kept in a position of slight flexion, abduction and lateral rotation. The upper two-thirds of a line drawn from the midinguinal point to the adductor tubercle represents the femoral artery in the thigh. The upper one-third of this line represents the femoral artery in femoral triangle while the middle third represents the femoral artery in the subsartorial canal.

Femoral Pulse (Fig. 182.1)

The clinicians feel the femoral artery in the femoral triangle just below the midinguinal point (a point half way between the anterior superior iliac spine and pubic symphysis) by palpating against the head of femur (Fig. 182.2). Bilateral weak femoral pulse compared to the radial pulse is indicative of coarctation (narrowing) of arch of aorta. The femoral pulse may be reduced or obliterated by atheroscelorotic changes or by blockage of common iliac or external iliac artery or arteries by an embolus.

Relations of Femoral Artery in Femoral Triangle

Anterior relations from superficial to deep, are the skin, superficial fascia with inguinal lymph nodes, fascia lata and anterior wall of femoral sheath. The posterior relations are the posterior wall of the femoral sheath, nerve to pectineus and tendon of psoas major muscle. This tendon separates the artery from the capsule of hip joint. At this site, the artery can be compressed against the head of the femur through the skin. The femoral nerve and its branches form the lateral relation. The femoral vein lies medial to the artery (Fig. 179.1) except at the apex, where it lies posterior to the artery (Fig. 179.2).

Relations in Subsartorial Canal

The saphenous nerve crosses the femoral artery anteriorly to reach its medial side. The femoral vein, which is posterior to the artery in the upper part of the canal, becomes its lateral relation distally. The artery is related posteriorly to the adductor longus and magnus muscles (Fig. 182.2).

Branches in Femoral Triangle (Fig. 182.3)

Three superficial and three deep branches originate in femoral triangle.

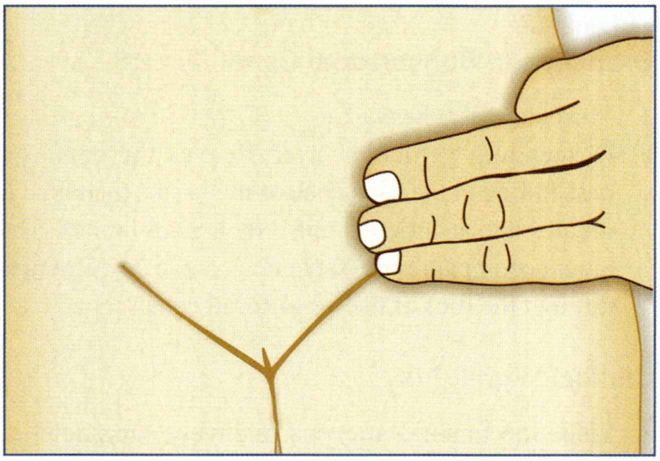

Fig. 182.1: Site of palpation of femoral pulse

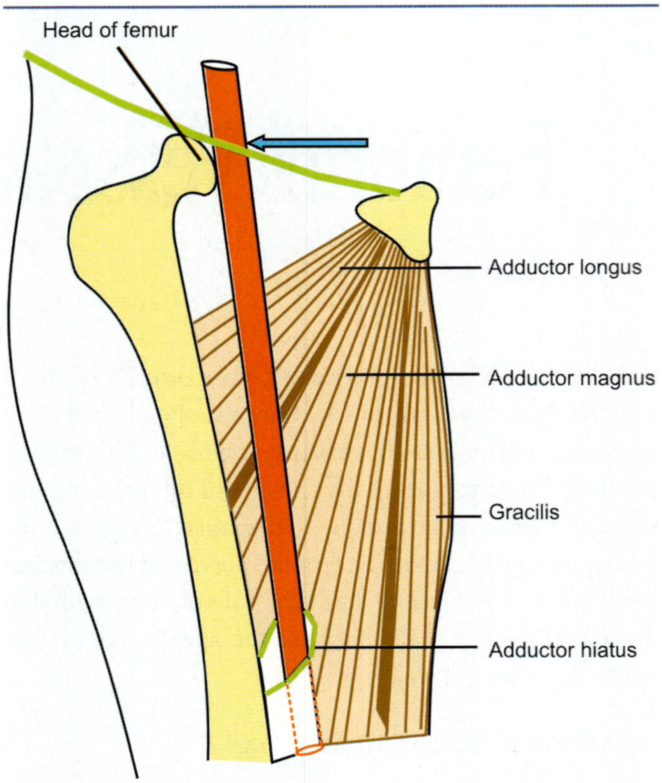

Fig. 182.2: Showing relation of femoral artery to head of femur. Arrow indicates site of compression of femoral artery against head of femur

a. The superficial branches are superficial epigastric, superficial external pudendal and superficial circumflex iliac arteries.
b. The deep branches are deep external pudendal, profunda femoris and the muscular branches.

Branches in Subsartorial Canal (Fig. 182.3)

a. Muscular branches
b. Descending genicular artery leaves the canal by descending in the substance of the vastus medialis. It divides into an articular and a saphenous branch. The latter accompanies the saphenous nerve as it emerges through the roof of the subsartorial canal.

Clinical Highlights

a Since the femoral artery is relatively superficial in position in the thigh; it is easy to approach the artery for various procedures. To inject radiopaque dye in the arteries of abdomen (aortic angiography, celiac artery angiography, superior and inferior mesenteric angiography, etc.) the catheter is introduced through the femoral artery. It is also a favored vessel for coronary angiography or for coronary angioplasty (retrograde catheterization), in which after entering the femoral artery the catheter passes in succession the external iliac artery, common iliac artery, abdominal aorta, descending thoracic aorta, arch of aorta and the ascending aorta to reach the coronary arteries. The complication that may occur after the procedure of femoral puncture is thrombus formation in the artery at this site. Therefore, after this procedure, routinely the dorsalis pedis pulse of the patient is tested.
b. The femoral angiography is done for visualizing the artery and its branches in suspected cases of femoral artery occlusion.

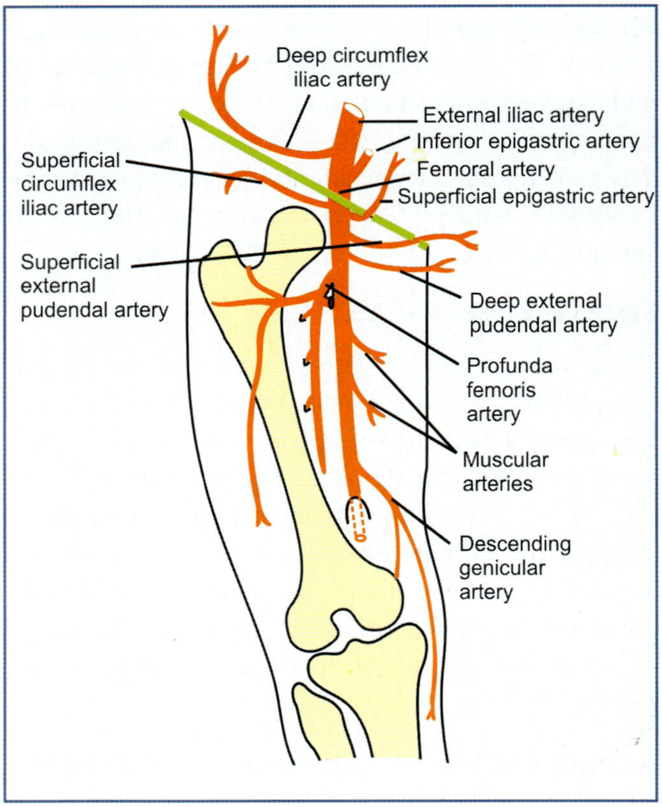

Fig. 182.3: Schematic depiction of branches of femoral artery

c. Sudden occlusion or block in the femoral artery usually occurs due to emboli from the heart (myocardial infarction or thrombi in the left atrium in mitral stenosis) or due to traumatic injury to the artery as in the fracture of femur or due to diabetes. It presents as five "P"s—pain, pallor, paraesthesia (altered sensations), paralysis and pulselessness. The serious complication of acute occlusion is gangrene of the lower limb. Gangrene means death of tissues with putrefaction.
d. In gradual narrowing of the femoral artery as a result of atherosclerosis, circulation to lower limb is maintained through collateral channels. If the narrowing is in the proximal part of femoral artery (proximal to origin of profunda femoris) cruciate and trochanteric anastomoses maintain the blood circulation. Narrowing in the distal part opens up anastomosis between the perforating branches of profunda femoris artery and the branches of the popliteal artery.

Femoral Vein

The extent and course of the femoral vein correspond to that of the femoral artery. The femoral vein begins at the tendinous opening in the adductor magnus as the continuation of popliteal vein. It ascends in the subsartorial canal and then enters the femoral triangle. After traversing the intermediate compartment of the femoral sheath the vein continues upward as the external iliac vein just medial to the midinguinal point.

Relations

The vein has different relation to the femoral artery at different levels. At the tendinous opening in the adductor magnus, the vein is lateral to the artery. During its course through the subsartorial canal the vein, gradually crosses posterior to the artery so that at the apex of the femoral triangle it becomes posterior. In the base of the femoral triangle, the vein lies medial to the artery. The femoral vein contains four to five valves, the most constant being the saphenofemoral valve (competency of this valve is determined by Trendelenburg test).

Tributaries

The great saphenous vein is its longest tributary. The other important veins that open in it are the profunda femoris vein, lateral and medial circumflex femoral veins and the direct muscular tributaries.

Clinical Highlights

The femoral vein is the preferred site for intravenous lines in infants and children. It is also used for passing a catheter in the right side of the heart for blood samples or for pressure recordings or to approach the pulmonary arteries. To reach the right ventricle, a long slender catheter is passed in succession through the femoral, external iliac and common iliac veins, IVC, right atrium, tricuspid orifice and right ventricle. Femoral vein puncture may give rise to hematoma due to injury to the wall of the vein and oozing of blood.

183 Muscles in Anterior Compartment of Thigh

The psoas major and iliacus muscles are described with along with posterior abdominal wall. The pectineus muscle is described with medial compartment of thigh.

Tensor Fasciae Latae

This muscle is located at the junction of thigh and gluteal region at the lateral side of thigh (Fig. 175.1). It shares its insertion with gluteus maximus muscle and shares its nerve supply and actions with gluteus medius and minimus muscles. The muscle is enclosed in the upper part of iliotibial tract.

Attachments

The tensor fasciae latae takes origin from the anterior part of the iliac crest and the lateral surface of the anterior superior iliac spine. Its insertion is into the iliotibial tract through which it gains attachment to the lateral tibial condyle.

Nerve Supply

The superior gluteal nerve supplies the muscle.

Actions

The tensor fasciae latae assists the gluteus medius and minimus in abduction and medial rotation of the hip. It stabilizes the knee joint in standing position and helps in extension of the knee joint through the iliotibial tract.

Sartorius

The word sartorius is derived from the Latin word sartor meaning tailor. Hence, sartorius is called the tailor's muscle. Tailors adopt while sitting, a position of lower limbs, in which both hip and knee joints are flexed. It is a long strap-like muscle composed of parallel muscle fibers.

Attachments

The sartorius takes origin from anterior superior iliac spine and is inserted into the upper part of the subcutaneous medial surface of the shaft of tibia. The tendinous insertion of sartorius is separated on the posterior aspect by bursa anserina from the insertions of gracilis and semitendinosus.

Relations

The sartorius courses obliquely in latero-medial direction from its origin to insertion. It forms the lateral boundary of the femoral triangle and covers the fibrous roof of the subsartorial canal. On its way to insertion, it passes close to the medial boundary of the popliteal fossa.

Nerve Supply

The femoral nerve, supplies the muscle.

Actions

It is the only muscle that flexes both hip and knee joints. It may help in lateral rotation of thigh.

Quadriceps Femoris

It is a very bulky muscle, which almost fills the anterior compartment of thigh. It has four parts having separate names (rectus femoris, vastus lateralis, vastus medialis and vastus intermedius). Each part has a separate origin but a common insertion.

Origin

a. Rectus femoris has two heads of origin. The straight head arises from the anterior inferior iliac spine and the reflected head from the ilium above the acetabulum. The two heads unite to form the bipennate muscle, which passes vertically downwards to join the other parts of quadriceps femoris. The rectus femoris crosses the hip and knee joints.

b. Vastus lateralis, which is the largest part, takes origin from the root of greater trochanter, lateral lip of gluteal tuberosity and lateral lip of linea aspera. Because of its bulk, the vastus lateralis is preferred for the intramuscular injection.

c. Vastus medialis takes origin from intertrochanteric and spiral lines, medial lip of linea aspera and medial supracondylar line.

d. Vastus intermedius arises from the lateral and anterior surfaces of the femoral shaft. Its lowest fibers called articularis genu, arise from the front of the lower part of shaft of femur.

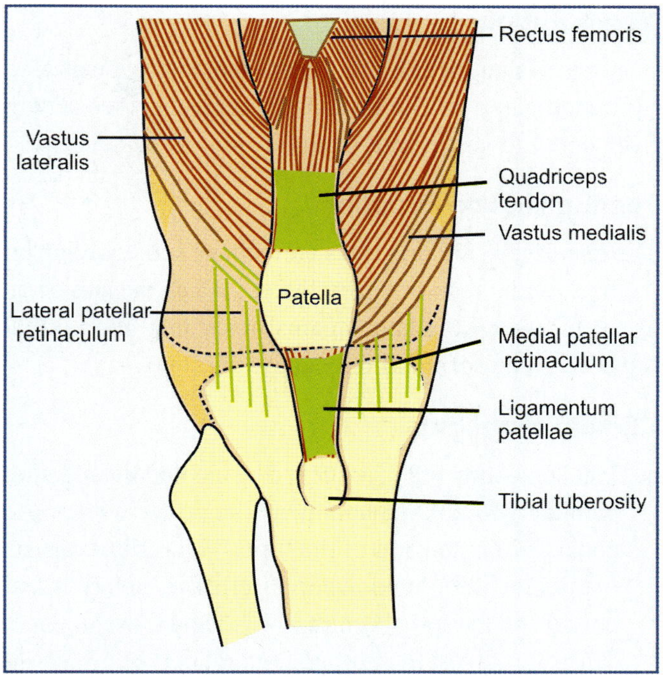

Fig. 183.1: Schematic representation of insertion of quadriceps femoris

Insertion (Fig. 183.1)

a. The tendons of the above four parts unite to form a single tendon, which is attached to the margins of patella. The insertion is prolonged over the front of patella as the strong ligamentum patellae to the tuberosity of tibia. The rectus femoris and vastus intermedius are inserted in the upper margin of patella. The lower horizontal fleshy fibers of vastus medialis insert into the medial margin of patella. Moreover, the attachment of vastus medialis extends longer than that of vastus lateralis to the lateral margin of patella. This part of vastus medialis is known as vastus medialis oblique as against its remaining part, which is known as vastus medialis longus. The medial and lateral patellar retinacula are the expansions from the sides of patella to the respective condyles of tibia. The patella, which is a sesamoid bone in the tendon of quadriceps femoris, increases the power of the muscle by holding the tendon of quadriceps away from the distal end of femur. This brings the tendon in line with the tibial tuberosity, thereby increasing its leverage. The combination of quadriceps tendon, patella and ligamentum patellae is known as patello-femoral complex.

b. Articularis genu is inserted in to the synovial membrane of the suprapatellar bursa of knee joint.

Actions

a. The quadriceps muscle is a powerful extensor of the knee joint. It straightens the lower limb (extends) during the act of standing from sitting position. The tone of the quadriceps muscle is very important to the stability of the knee joint.

b. The tendinous expansions of medial and lateral vasti form the patellar retinacula, which blend with the joint capsule to reinforce it.

c. Among the four parts, rectus femoris alone acts on the hip joint. It is the flexor of this joint.

d. The function of articularis genu is to retract the synovial membrane superiorly during extension of the joint so as to prevent it getting caught between femur and patella.

Nerve Supply

All parts of quadriceps femoris are separately innervated by femoral nerve. The articularis genu receives a twig from nerve to vastus intermedius.

Testing Muscle Function

The quadriceps femoris is tested with the subject lying on the back with the knee partly flexed. When the subject is asked to extend the knee against resistance the normal muscle can be seen and felt easily.

Clinical Highlights

a. Patellar tendon reflex is elicited by tapping ligamentum patellae with a knee hammer. The positive response consists of extension of the limb. The reflex consists of afferent limb (femoral nerve), efferent limb (femoral nerve) and the spinal centre (L2, L3 and L4 segments). The reflex is lost in injury to femoral nerve or injury to spinal reflex center.
b. The disuse atrophy of quadriceps femoris results due to immobilization of knee joint due to any cause (arthritis or plaster cast). Reduction in size of the quadriceps femoris due to atrophy is found out by measuring the circumference of each thigh. For preventing the disuse atrophy active exercises (physiotherapy) must be started as early as possible in patients in whom lower limbs are not moved.
c. Normally, between the obliquity of the line of quadriceps muscle and the straight line of patellar ligament there is valgus angle opening on lateral side. The supplement of the valgus angle is called the quadriceps angle or Q angle (normal value is around 10 to 12°). Wider pelvis in female increases the obliquity of femur and the Q angle. In fact, it is the Q angle that is responsible for the natural tendency of patella to dislocate laterally. To counteract this tendency the vastus medialis oblique muscle pulls the patella medially in addition to the bony factor (Chapter 204). If the value of Q angle is greater than 15° there is lateral pull on patella, which rubs against the lateral condyle of femur resulting in patellar pain initially and later lateral dislocation of patella.

Medial Compartment of Thigh

184

The medial compartment of thigh contains six muscles, obturator nerve, obturator vessels and the profunda femoris vessels. The muscles are arranged in three strata (Fig. 184.1). The superficial stratum contains the pectineus, adductor longus and gracilis. The intermediate stratum contains the obturator externus and adductor brevis and the deep stratum contains the large adductor magnus muscle. The adductor muscles collectively are called rider's muscles.

Pectineus

The pectineus is a composite muscle that belongs to medial and anterior compartments of thigh. It is located in the medial part of the floor of femoral triangle. It takes origin from the pecten pubis of the superior ramus of pubis and is inserted into the posterior aspect of femur on a line extending from the lesser trochanter to the linea aspera.

Relations

The anterior surface of the pectineus is directed towards the femoral triangle. The posterior wall of femoral sheath and the femoral vessels contained in it forms its immediate anterior relation. The posterior surface of pectineus is related to the capsule of the hip joint, obturator externus and the adductor brevis from above downward. The anterior division of obturator nerve descends between the posterior surface of the pectineus and the obturator externus and adductor brevis muscles. The adductor longus lies on the medial side of pectineus and the profunda femoris vessels enter the gap between the two. The psoas major lies on the lateral side of pectineus and the medial circumflex femoral vessels enter the gap between the two.

Nerve Supply

The pectineus receives double nerve supply. It receives a branch from the femoral nerve from its anterior aspect and from a branch of anterior division of obturator nerve (or by accessory obturator nerve when present) from its posterior aspect.

Actions

It is a flexor of the hip joint. It aids in adduction also.

Adductor Longus

It is a triangular muscle. It arises from the front of the body of pubis (just below the pubic tubercle) by a narrow

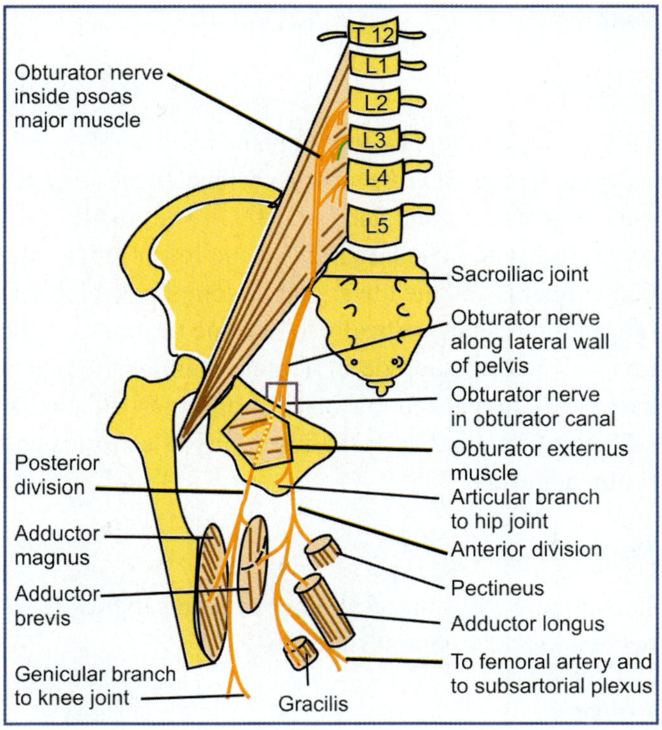

Fig. 184.1: Schematic depiction of course and distribution of obturator nerve

tendon and widens at its aponeurotic insertion on the linea aspera. If the tendinous origin of the adductor longus is ossified, it forms a sesamoid bone (rider's bone).

Relations (Fig. 179.1)

The medial margin of adductor longus forms the medial margin of the femoral triangle. It also forms the medial-most part of the floor of femoral triangle, where it lies edge to edge with pectineus on lateral side. Medially it is closely related to gracilis muscle.

Its anterior relations are as follows. Near its origin it is crossed by spermatic cord in male. In the femoral triangle and subsartorial canal it is related to femoral vessels (Fig. 182.2). Its posterior relations are, profunda vessels, anterior branch of obturator nerve and adductor brevis muscle.

Nerve Supply

Anterior division of obturator nerve supplies the muscle.

Actions

It is the adductor and medial rotator of thigh at the hip joint.

Gracilis

This muscle derives its name from the Latin word gracilis meaning slender. It is the most superficial of the adductor muscles and is thin and flat (Fig. 182.2). The gracilis takes origin from the medial margin of the lower half of the body of pubis and the lower part of conjoint ischiopubic ramus. It descends vertically to become tendinous at the level of medial condyle of femur. It is inserted by a narrow, flattened tendon in the upper part of medial surface of tibia between the insertions of sartorius and semitendinosus.

Nerve Supply

The anterior division of obturator nerve supplies it. Its nerve and artery enter it superiorly.

Actions

It is an adductor and medial rotator of thigh at the hip joint and accessory flexor of leg at the knee joint.

Clinical Highlights

Being easily accessible and functionally a weak muscle, the gracilis is suitable for muscle graft to replace the damaged muscle in some part of the body, where muscle function cannot be compromised.

Obturator Externus

Though this muscle lies in the adductor compartment and is innervated by obturator nerve it does not function like other five muscles in this compartment.

Attachments

The obturator externus takes origin from the external surface of obturator membrane and the bony margins of the obturator foramen. Its tendon passes through the gluteal region behind the neck of the femur (with which it is in intimate contact) for insertion in the trochanteric fossa. From the site of origin the muscle takes a posterior, upward and lateral direction to reach its insertion. A communicating bursa intervenes between the tendon and the capsule of hip joint.

Nerve Supply

The posterior division of obturator nerve, which passes through its substance, supplies it.

Actions

The obturator externus is a lateral rotator of thigh. The tendon of obturator externus spirals round the back of neck of the femur. This enables it to act like a ligament steadying the head of femur in acetabulum.

Adductor Brevis

It is triangular in shape and takes origin from the external aspect of body and inferior ramus of pubis. It expands in an aponeurosis at its insertion along a line extending from the base of the lesser trochanter to upper part of linea aspera just behind the attachment of upper part of adductor longus.

Relations

The adductor brevis lies between the pectineus and adductor longus in front and the adductor magnus behind.

It is sandwiched between the anterior and posterior divisions of obturator nerve (Fig. 184.1). Its vascular relations to branches of profunda femoris are as follows. The medial circumflex femoral artery runs along its upper margin between it and obturator externus. The relations of the first, second and third perforating arteries are shown in Figure 184.2.

Nerve Supply

It is usually supplied by anterior division of obturator nerve but may receive a branch from the posterior division as well.

Actions

It is the adductor of thigh.

Adductor Magnus

This is a large muscle, which is composed of two functionally different parts, adductor and hamstring, which have different origin, insertion and nerve supply.

Attachments

a. The adductor part of the muscle takes origin from the ischiopubic ramus. The short, horizontal fibers from the pubic ramus insert in the gluteal tuberosity. This part of the muscle is called adductor minimus. The middle oblique fibers from the ischial ramus insert by a broad aponeurosis in the linea aspera and the proximal medial supracondylar line. This long insertion of the muscle is interrupted by five osseo-aponeurotic openings, bridged by tendinous arches attached to the bone. The upper four openings are small and transmit the four perforating arteries. The lowest opening is large and called adductor or tendinous hiatus (Fig. 182.2). It transmits the femoral vessels in to the popliteal fossa. The opening lies on the medial supracondylar line of femur at the junction of middle and lower thirds of thigh.
b. The ischial part is composed of posterior vertical fibers, which take origin from the inferolateral quadrant of the ischial tuberosity (Fig. 186.1). This part descends to end in the lower-third of thigh as a rounded tendon, which can be palpated proximal to its attachment to the adductor tubercle.

Relations

Anterior relations are, pectineus, adductor brevis and adductor longus muscles from above downwards. The other anterior relations are, posterior division of obturator nerve, profunda vessels (between the lower margins of the adductor brevis and adductor longus muscles) and femoral vessels in the lower part of subsartorial canal. The posterior relations of adductor magnus are, the sciatic nerve and the hamstring muscles.

Nerve Supply

The adductor part receives nerve supply from the posterior division of obturator nerve and the ischial part from the tibial component of the sciatic nerve.

Actions

The adductor part adducts and medially rotates the thigh. The ischial part acts with the hamstring muscles to extend the hip joint and flex the knee joint.

Obturator Nerve (Fig.184.1)

The obturator nerve is a branch of the lumbar plexus, which is located in the substance of the psoas major muscle on the posterior abdominal wall. It is formed by the union of the ventral divisions of the ventral rami of L1, L2 and L3 spinal nerves. It emerges from the medial margin of the psoas major muscle and crosses the pelvic brim anterior to the sacroiliac joint (Fig. 184.1) to enter the pelvic cavity. The obturator nerve courses forwards along the lateral pelvic wall along the upper margin of obturator internus muscle. In female it is related to lateral surface of the ovary. The obturator artery, which is a branch of anterior division of internal iliac artery, accompanies the nerve. The obturator nerve terminates in anterior and posterior divisions in the obturator canal. The terminal branches leave the pelvic cavity through the obturator foramen to enter the medial compartment of thigh along with obturator artery.

Course in Medial Compartment of Thigh

a. The anterior division of the obturator nerve descends at first, in front of the obturator externus muscle and then in front of adductor brevis. It passes behind the pectineus and adductor longus muscles. It gives following branches:

i. Articular branch supplies the hip joint.
ii. Muscular branches supply the pectineus, adductor longus, adductor brevis and gracilis.
iii. Vascular filament enters the subsartorial canal to supply the femoral artery.
iv. Cutaneous branch communicates with the branches of medial femoral cutaneous and saphenous nerves to form subsartorial plexus, which supplies the skin of medial side of the thigh.

b. The posterior division of obturator nerve passes through the substance of obturator externus and descends on the anterior surface of adductor magnus lying behind the adductor brevis. Distal to the lower limit of the adductor longus, the posterior division continues in the popliteal fossa as the slender genicular branch, which reaches the fossa by one of the two routes. It enters the subsartorial canal and then reaches the popliteal fossa along with femoral vessels through the tendinous opening or it may enter the popliteal fossa directly by passing through the substance of the adductor magnus muscle. The posterior division gives following branches:
i. Muscular branches supply the obturator externus, adductor brevis (if it does not receive supply from anterior division) and the adductor part of adductor magnus.
ii. Genicular branch supplies the articular capsule of the knee joint and after piercing the oblique popliteal ligament supplies the interior of the knee joint.

Clinical Highlights

a. Bilateral obturator neurectomy (cutting the nerve) is done to treat severe adductor spasm. Since the thighs are held in adducted position in adductor spasm, the lower limbs cross each other like the scissors. This is seen in some neurological cases.
b. The pain due to disease of hip joint may be referred to knee joint and to medial side of the thigh. This is because the common nerve supply of the joints through its articular branches and to medial side of thigh through its contribution to subsartorial plexus.

Blood Vessels in Medial Compartment

Three blood vessels enter the medial side of thigh. The obturator artery enters through the obturator canal. The profunda femoris artery enters through the gap between the pectineus and adductor longus muscles. The medial circumflex branch of the profunda enters through the gap between the pectineus and the psoas major muscle.

Obturator Artery

The obturator artery is a branch of anterior division of internal iliac artery. It accompanies the obturator nerve in the pelvis and like the nerve divides into anterior and posterior branches in the obturator canal. These branches along with branches of the medial circumflex femoral artery form an arterial arcade between the obturator membrane and the obturator externus muscle. This arterial arcade supplies the muscles in the medial compartment. It also sends an articular branch called acetabular branch to the hip joint through the acetabular notch, which reaches the head of femur via the ligament of the head of femur.

Profunda Femoris Artery (Deep Femoral Artery)

This is the main artery providing blood to all the muscles of thigh. Its origin is in the femoral triangle but its main course is in the medial compartment. Its branches, however, enter all the compartments and take part in the chain of arterial anastomoses in the back of thigh.

Origin (Figs 182.2 and 184.2)

The profunda femoris artery arises from the lateral aspect of the femoral artery in the femoral triangle about 3.5 to 4 cm below the inguinal ligament. However, the point of origin may be variable, being either much higher or lower.

Course and Branches in Femoral Triangle

From its origin the artery gradually turns medially to pass posterior to the femoral vessels. In this course it lies on the anterior aspect of pectineus muscle. It leaves the femoral triangle through the gap between the pectineus and adductor longus muscles to enter the adductor compartment. The branches of profunda artery in the femoral triangle are, medial circumflex femoral artery, lateral circumflex femoral artery and muscular arteries.

Course and Branches in Medial Compartment

At the level of the apex of femoral triangle, it is separated from the femoral vessels by adductor longus. The gunshot or stab injury at this level may injure all the four blood vessels. In its further descent it lies at first between the adductor longus in front and adductor brevis behind. Beyond the lower limit of adductor brevis it lies between the adductor longus in front and adductor magnus behind. At midthigh level it enters the substance of the adductor magnus to continue as the fourth perforating artery. The profunda vein lies anterior to the artery. The first to third perforating arteries arise in relation to the adductor brevis muscle, first at the level of its upper border, the second in front of it and the third at its lower border.

Medial Circumflex Femoral Artery

This artery usually arises from the posteromedial aspect of the profunda femoris artery in the femoral triangle. It takes a circuitous route as it passes through three regions, femoral triangle, medial compartment of thigh and gluteal region. It leaves the femoral triangle by passing between the psoas major and pectineus muscles (Fig. 179.2). It travels in posterior direction between the obturator externus and adductor brevis and then enters the gluteal region, where it passes between the quadratus femoris and upper margin of adductor magnus (Fig. 184.3). The medial circumflex femoral artery gives off following three branches.

a. Transverse branch takes part in cruciate anastomosis by anastomosing with the first perforating artery, inferior gluteal artery and the transverse branch of lateral circumflex femoral artery.
b. Ascending branch passes up in the gluteal region on the tendon of the obturator externus and takes part in trochanteric anastomosis along with superior gluteal and lateral femoral circumflex arteries. The ascending branch forms a vascular ring around the femoral neck by anastomosing with ascending branch of the lateral femoral circumflex artery. The retinacular branches from this vascular ring provide blood to the head and neck of the femur. The medial circumflex femoral artery is in fact the chief arterial source to the head of the femur.
c. Acetabular artery enters the acetabulum along with a similar branch from obturator artery to supply the femoral head.

Lateral Circumflex Femoral Artery

This is a lateral branch arising near the root of profunda femoris artery. It leaves the femoral triangle by passing deep to the sartorius and passes deep to rectus femoris, where it divides in three branches.

a. Ascending branch runs along the intertrochanteric line lateral to the hip joint and anastomoses with the superior gluteal artery, a branch of internal iliac artery and deep circumflex iliac branch of external iliac artery at spinous anastomosis. Through these connections the branches of internal and external iliac arteries communicate with branches of profunda artery. It also forms an anstomotic ring around the femoral neck with ascending branches of medial circumflex femoral artery.
b. Descending branch runs down along the anterior border of vastus lateralis. It supplies the vastus lateralis and its one long branch descends in the substance of vastus lateralis to anastomose with lateral superior genicular branch of popliteal artery.
c. Transverse branch passes laterally anterior to the vastus intermedius and pierces the vastus lateralis to come to the posterior aspect to take part in cruciate anastomosis.

Perforating Arteries (Fig. 184.2)

The upper three perforating arteries pierce the insertion of adductor magnus to reach the flexor compartment. They lie very close to the femur. They pass through the flexor compartment to supply the muscles there and connect with each other by anastomotic branches. They pierce the origin of short head of biceps femoris and the lateral intermuscular septum to terminate in the vastus lateralis in the extensor compartment. The first perforator takes part in cruciate anastomosis. The second perforator gives a nutrient branch to the femur. The terminal part of the profunda artery is called the fourth perforating artery. It anastomoses with the superior muscular branches of the popliteal artery and ends like other perforating arteries.

Anastomoses of Profunda Femoris

a. Spinous anastomosis at anterior superior iliac spine
b. Trochanteric anastomosis in the gluteal region

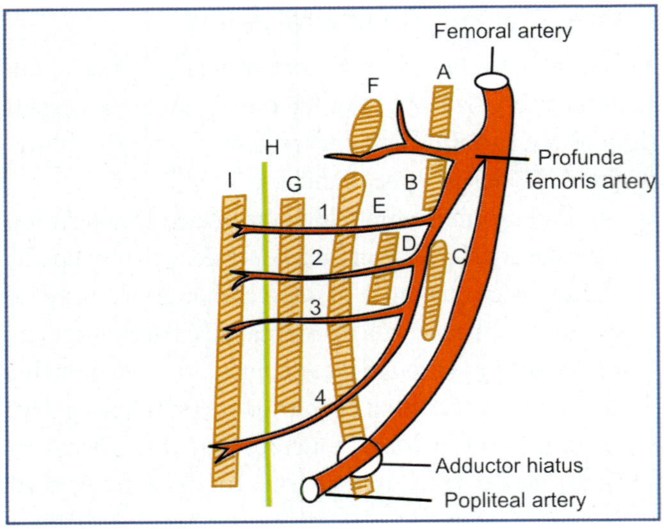

Fig. 184.2: Schematic diagram of profunda femoris artery and its perforating branches numbered 1 to 4. A-Psoas major, B-Pectineus, C-Adductor longus, D-Adductor brevis, E-Adductor magnus, F-Quadratus femoris, G-Short-head of biceps femoris, H-Lateral intermuscular septum, I-Vastus lateralis

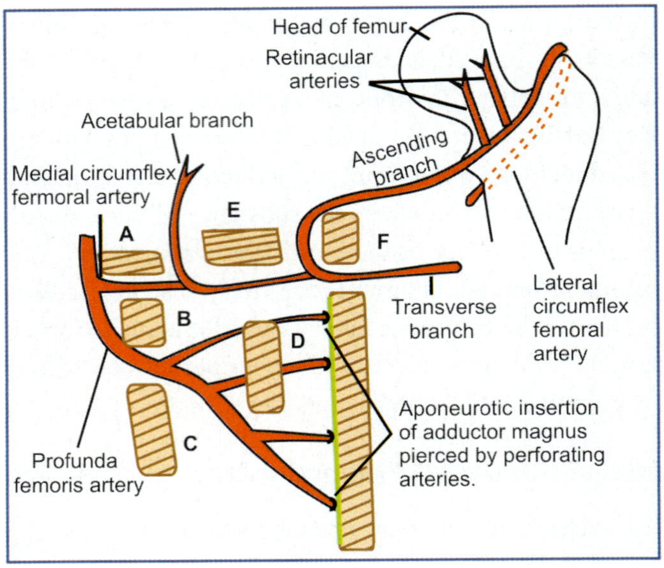

Fig. 184.3: Schematic diagram to show distribution of medial circumflex femoral artery (posterior view). A-Psoas major, B-Pectineus, C-Adductor longus, D-Adductor brevis, E-Obturator externus, F-Quadratus femoris

c. Cruciate anastomosis in the upper part of thigh at the level of lesser trochanter
d. Vertical anastomotic chains between branches of perforating arteries in the middle of thigh
e. In the lower part of thigh the branches of popliteal artery anastomose with fourth perforating and lateral circumflex femoral arteries (branches of profunda femoris).

Clinical Highlights

a. The deeply located profunda femoris artery is of great importance to the orthopedic surgeon. As this artery is in close proximity to the femoral shaft, it is prone to injury in fracture of femoral shaft. It may also be injured in blunt injury to the thigh without fracture of the femur. The artery is also liable to injury in surgical procedures like fixing metallic screws in the femur.
b. Rupture of the profunda femoris artery causes severe bleeding inside the thigh muscles, which may result in thigh compartment syndrome.
c. The preferred site of femoral artery ligation is proximal to the origin of profunda femoris. This ensures the arterial supply to lower limb via the anastomoses between branches of profunda and branches of internal and external iliac arteries.
d. In blockage of femoral artery beyond the origin of profunda femoris, the arterial supply of lower limb is maintained via the anastomoses of branches of profunda femoris with those of popliteal artery.

185 Gluteal Region

The gluteal region or buttock is a prominent bulge produced by the subcutaneous fat and a bulky gluteus maximus muscle.

Boundaries and Communications

The gluteal region is bounded superiorly by the iliac crest and superomedially by the sacrum. Inferiorly, the gluteal sulcus separates it from the thigh. Medially, there is natal cleft. A line joining the anterior superior iliac spine to the front of the greater trochanter of femur limits the region laterally.

Through greater sciatic foramen it communicates with pelvic cavity. Through lesser sciatic foramen it communicates with the ischiorectal fossa of the anal triangle of perineum. Inferiorly, the gluteal region continues in the posterior compartment of thigh.

Superficial Fascia

The superficial fascia of the gluteal region is thick and filled with fat. A number of cutaneous nerves are present in the superficial fascia (Fig. 175.1).

Deep Fascia

The deep fascia splits to enclose the gluteus maximus muscle, above which it continues as a single sheet covering the outer surface of gluteus medius muscle (gluteal aponeurosis). On the lateral aspect the deep fascia is thickened to form iliotibial tract. The tensor fasciae latae muscle is enclosed in the two layers of iliotibial tract. Thus, in the gluteal region the deep fascia splits twice to enclose two muscles, both of which insert in iliotibial tract lower down in the thigh.

Gluteus Maximus

The gluteus maximus (Fig. 175.1) is the largest and the most superficial muscle of the gluteal region. It has a coarse texture due to the presence of a large number of fibrous septa in its substance.

Origin

The gluteus maximus takes origin from outer surface of ilium behind the posterior gluteal line, posterior surface of adjacent sacrum and coccyx and the sacrotuberous ligament. The muscle slopes downwards and laterally over the greater trochanter of femur.

Insertion

Three fourth of the muscle is inserted by tendinous fibres in the posterior aspect of iliotobial tract and the deeper one fourth is inserted in the gluteal tuberosity of femur.

Nerve Supply

The inferior gluteal nerve supplies the muscle.

Actions

a. The gluteus maximus is a powerful extensor of thigh on the trunk or of trunk on the thigh at the hip joint in such activities as running, climbing steps and rising from sitting position (for these actions it acts from the origin).
b. It is a lateral rotator of thigh.
c. Acting from its insertion it can straighten the trunk after stooping by rotating the pelvis backward on the head of femur (this action is along with hamstring muscles).

d. It maintains the upright position of trunk by preventing the pelvis from rotating forward on the head of femur (thus retaining the center of gravity behind the hip joint).
e. The muscle stabilizes the knee joint through iliotibial tract

Testing Muscle Function

The subject lying in prone position is asked to raise the thigh against resistance. Inability to do so indicates weakness of the muscle.

Structures Under Cover of Gluteus Maximus

a. The bony structures include ischial spine, ischial tuberosity, greater trochanter in addition to greater and lesser sciatic foramina.
b. The sacrotuberous ligament extends from the ischial tuberosity to the lower lateral part of sacrum and coccyx and both posterior iliac spines. It is regarded as the continuation of biceps femoris muscle. The perforating cutaneous nerve from the sacral plexus pierces this ligament (Fig. 185.1) to enter the gluteal region. The triangular sacrospinous ligament extends from the tip of ischial spine to the lower lateral part of sacrum and coccyx. It lies deep to sacrotuberous ligament and is regarded as the aponeurotic posterior part of coccygeus muscle. The pudendal nerve passes over the apex of the ligament to enter the lesser sciatic foramen.
c. A large trochanteric bursa separates the gluteus maximus from the greater trochanter. The gluteofemoral bursa is present between the tendon of gluteus maximus and origin of vastus lateralis. Ischial bursa lies between the gluteus maximus and the lower medial part of ischial tuberosity. This bursa may become inflamed due to excessive friction producing ischial bursitis (Weaver's bottom).
d. The muscles under cover of gluteus maximus are, the gluteus medius and deep to it the gluteus minimus, piriformis, tendon of obturator internus with fleshy bellies of gemelli muscles, quadratus femoris (the tendon of obturator externus deep to it) and the origin of hamstring muscles from the ischial tuberosity.
e. The following seven branches of the sacral plexus (inside the pelvic cavity) enter the gluteal region via greater sciatic foramen, the sciatic nerve, posterior cutaneous nerve of thigh, superior and inferior gluteal nerves, nerve to obturator internus, nerve to quadratus femoris and pudendal nerve.
f. The following arteries are seen in the gluteal region. The branches of internal iliac artery are, superior and inferior gluteal arteries, which accompany the corresponding nerves. The internal pudendal artery is flanked by nerve to obturator internus laterally and pudendal nerve medially during its brief sojourn in the gluteal region. The medial circumflex femoral artery, which is the branch of profunda femoris artery, enters from the thigh.

Gluteus Medius and Minimus

These two muscles have common nerve supply and actions. The gluteus medius takes origin from the outer surface of ilium between the anterior and posterior gluteal lines. It is inserted in the lateral aspect of greater trochanter along an oblique ridge. The gluteus minimus is entirely

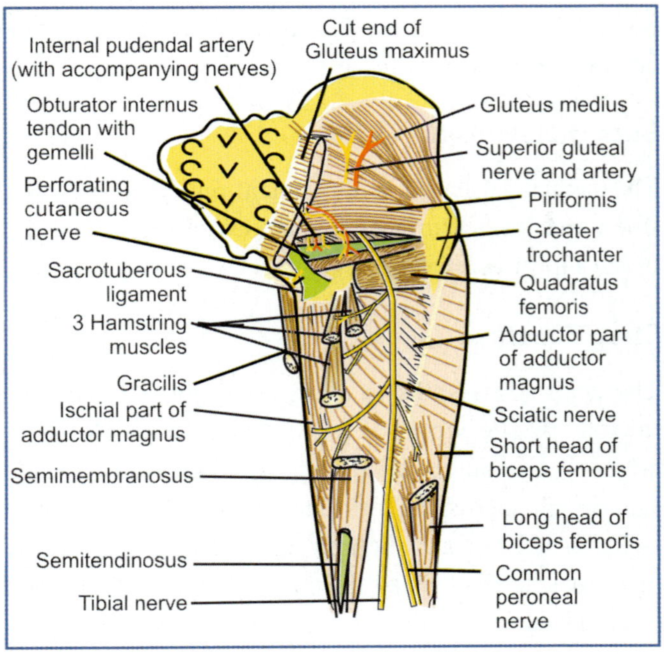

Fig. 185.1: Structures under cover of gluteus maximus and in the posterior compartment of thigh

under cover of gluteus medius. It arises from the outer surface of ilium between anterior and inferior gluteal lines and is inserted in the greater trochanter on the anterolateral ridge. The reflected head of rectus femoris and the capsule of hip joint are located deep to gluteus minimus.

Nerve Supply

Both gluteus medius and minimus muscles are supplied by superior gluteal nerve.

Actions

a. The gluteus medius and minimus muscles abduct the thigh at the hip joint, when the limb is free to move.
b. Their anterior fibres bring about medial rotation and flexion of thigh.
c. Their important function is to support the pelvis in walking. When a person stands on one foot and the foot of the opposite side is raised from the ground to take a step, the contraction of the glutei medius and minimus muscles of the supported side raises the contralateral pelvis a little (Fig. 185.2). In this way the contraction of the muscles on one side prevents the pelvis of the opposite side from sinking down, when the foot on that side is off the ground. These actions on the right and left sides of pelvis occur alternately during walking and depend on the integrity of three factors, namely, the normal glutei medius and minimus, normal hip joint and intact femoral neck with normal angulation with the shaft (125°).

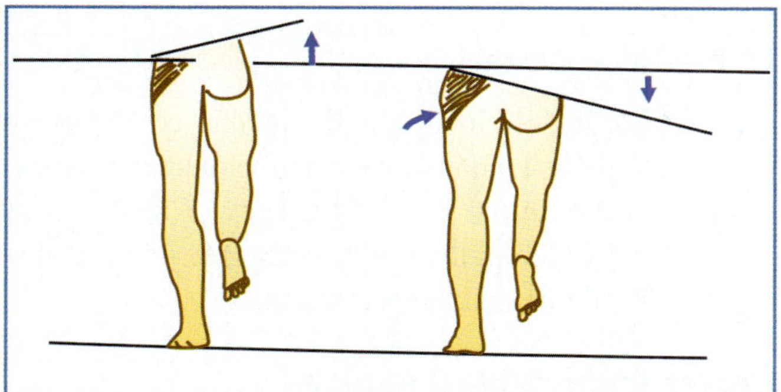

Normal action of left gluteus medius and minimus in locomotion | PositiveTrendelenburg sign in paralysis of same muscles

Fig.185.2: To show the action of normal and paralyzed glueteus medius and minimus muscles

Testing Muscle Function

The subject lies prone with knee flexed at 90°. The subject is asked to push the foot outward against resistance. Inability to do so means weakness of gluteus medius and minimus muscles.

Clinical Highlights

a. In paralysis of gluteus maximus muscle (for example, due to poliomyelitis or due to injury to inferior gluteal nerve) the gait of the person has a typical backward lurch during every step forward. This is explained by the fact that due to non-action of the muscle the center of gravity is retained by tilting the hip backward.
b. In paralysis of glutei medius and minimus the pelvis of the unsupported (normal side) side sinks, when the patient tries to stand on the limb of affected side. This is known as positive Trendelenburg's sign (Fig. 185.2). In an attempt to raise the opposite foot the centre of gravity is shifted lateral to the hip joint of supported side by flexing the trunk to that side. This produces a characteristic dipping or lurching gait (also known as abductor lurch). In bilateral paralysis of these muscles or bilateral congenital dislocation of hip joints the gait is described as waddling in which the trunk is flexed from side-to-side with each step.

Short Lateral Rotators of Thigh

There are four muscles, which fall in this category, piriformis, obturator internus with gemelli, obturator externus and quadratus femoris. These short muscles are collectively called the short lateral rotators thigh at the hip joint. However, their main function is to act as liga-ments, which retain the head of femur in the acetabulum.

Piriformis (Fig. 155.2)

This muscle is located partly in the pelvis and partly in the gluteal region. Its origin is inverted E-shaped from the anterior or pelvic surface of the sacrum.

Course and Relations

In its intra-pelvic course the piriformis turns laterally towards the greater sciatic foramen, through which it enters the gluteal region. Inside the pelvis its important anterior relations are, rectum, sacral plexus and branches of internal iliac artery. The piriformis almost fills the greater sciatic foramen. It is regarded as the key muscle of the gluteal region because the nerves and blood vessels entering the gluteal region are arranged in relation to it at the greater sciatic foramen. The superior gluteal nerve and vessels are related to the upper margin of the piriformis. The inferior gluteal nerve and vessels, sciatic nerve, posterior cutaneous nerve of thigh, nerve to quadratus femoris, nerve to obturator internus, pudendal nerve, nerve to obturator internus and internal pudendal vessels are related to its lower margin. When the sciatic nerve divides inside the pelvis, its common peroneal component passes through or above the piriformis but the tibial component passes below the piriformis (Fig. 187.1).

Insertion

The muscle is inserted on the superior border of the greater trochanter of femur.

Nerve Supply

The intrapelvic part of the piriformis receives direct branches from the ventral rami of the fifth lumbar and upper two sacral nerves.

Clinical Highlights

In piriformis syndrome the sciatic nerve is compressed due to spasm or hypertrophy of the piriformis muscle at the greater sciatic foramen.

Obturator Internus and Gemelli

The obturator internus muscle is partly intrapelvic and partly gluteal in course. Its intrapelvic part is described with muscles of the pelvis.

Origin

It takes origin from the inner surface of obturator membrane and the surrounding bony margin.

Course and Relations

The tendon of the obturator internus muscle enters the gluteal region through the lesser sciatic foramen. The tendon provides the site of insertion for the superior gemellus, which takes origin from the posterior aspect of ischial spine and for the inferior gemellus, which takes origin from the uppermost part of ischial tuberosity. The tendon of obturator internus passes horizontally across the capsule of the hip joint. The tendon and the gemelli together form the anterior relation of the sciatic nerve.

Insertion

The obturator internus and two gemelli insert on the trochanteric fossa of femur.

Nerve Supply

The nerve to obturator internus, a branch of sacral plexus supplies the obturator internus muscle and superior gemellus. The nerve to quadratus femoris supplies the inferior gemellus.

Quadratus Femoris

This is a small qudrilateral muscle lying between the inferior gemellus and superior margin of adductor magnus. It takes origin from the lateral border of ischial tuberosity and passes behind the neck of femur and capsule of hip joint, the tendon of obturator externus intervening. It is inserted in the quadrate tubercle located on the upper part of intertrochanteric crest of femur.

Nerve Supply

The quadratus femoris is innervated by nerve to quadratus femoris, a branch of sacral plexus. This muscle is a lateral rotator of hip joint.

Obturator Externus

This muscle is described with the medial compartment of thigh. Only its tendon appears in the gluteal region in close contact with the back of the neck of femur on its way to its insertion in the trochanteric fossa. The tendon lies anterior to the quadratus femoris.

Nerves in the Gluteal Region

a. The superior gluteal nerve (L4, L5, S1) arises from sacral plexus in pelvis and enters the gluteal region along the uppermost part of greater sciatic foramen above the piriformis and in company with superior gluteal vessels. Lying in the interval between gluteus medius and minimus, it divides into superior and inferior branches. The superior branch supplies the gluteus medius and the inferior branch supplies the gluteus medius, gluteus minimus and tensor fasciae latae. Since the superior gluteal nerve lies in the superomedial quadrant of the gluteal region, an inadvertent intramuscular injection here may injure it.

b. The inferior gluteal nerve (L5, S1, S2) arises from the sacral plexus and enters the gluteal region through the greater sciatic foramen below the piriformis and along with inferior gluteal vessels. It divides in branches, which enter the deep surface of the gluteus maximus muscle.

c. The nerve to quadratus femoris (L4, L5, S1) is a branch of sacral plexus. It enters the gluteal region through the greater sciatic foramen by passing below the piriformis. It descends initially behind the dorsal surface of ischium and in front of sciatic nerve, and then, in front of the superior gemellus and tendon of obturator internus muscle. It supplies two muscles, namely, gemellus inferior and quadratus femoris. It may also give an articular twig to hip joint.

d. The nerve to obturator internus (L5, S1, S2) is a branch of sacral plexus. It enters the gluteal region through the greater sciatic foramen along with pudendal nerve and internal pudendal vessels. It supplies a branch to the superior gemellus. It crosses the dorsal surface of the base of ischial spine and re-enters the lesser sciatic foramen to supply branches to the pelvic surface of obturator internus muscle.

e. The pudendal nerve (S2, S3, S4) is a branch of the sacral plexus. It enters the gluteal region with the internal pudendal vessels through the greater sciatic foramen below piriformis. It has a very short course in the gluteal region. It crosses the sacrospinous ligament to enter the lesser sciatic foramen. The internal pudendal artery, which is a branch of the internal iliac artery, accompanies the nerve. It crosses the dorsal aspect of the ischial spine near the tip and then enters the lesser sciatic foramen. The artery with the accompanying veins is sandwiched between nerve to obturator internus laterally and pudendal nerve medially in the gluteal region. Both the pudendal nerve and the internal pudendal artery are described in detail in chapter on perineum.

f. The posterior cutaneous nerve of thigh (S1, S2, S3) is also known as posterior femoral cutaneous nerve. It arises from the sacral plexus and contains fibres from the dorsal divisions of S1 and S2 ventral rami and from ventral divisions of S2 and S3 ventral rami. It enters the gluteal region by passing below the piriformis. Its course is divided in four parts, gluteal, posterior thigh, popliteal fossa and leg. In the gluteal region it lies on the superficial aspect (posterior) of the sciatic nerve immediately deep to the gluteus maximus. In the thigh it descends lying superficial to the long head of biceps femoris and deep to the deep fascia of thigh. It enters the popliteal fossa and pierces the deep fascia here and descends in the superficial fascia to the level of middle of the calf along with short saphenous vein. Its branches are as follows. Gluteal branches are two to three in number and wind round the lower margin of gluteus maximus to supply the skin of the lower and lateral part of gluteal region. Perineal branch travels medially below the ischial tuberosity. It pierces the fascia lata and fascia of Colles to enter the superficial perineal pouch. It travels in this pouch to reach the skin of the posterior aspect of scrotum or labia majora. Cutaneous twigs are distributed to the skin of the back of thigh, popliteal fossa and the upper half of back of leg.

g. Perforating cutaneous nerve (S2, S3) is a branch of sacral plexus. Unlike the other nerves, it enters the gluteal region by perforating the sacrotuberous ligament. It winds round the lower margin of gluteus maximus to supply the skin of postero-inferior area of gluteal region (Fig. 175.1).

h. The sciatic nerve, which is the thickest nerve in the body, enters the gluteal region via the greater sciatic foramen. Its course in the gluteal region and thigh is dealt with in Chapter 187.

Vessels of the Gluteal Region (Fig. 185.3)

The branches of internal iliac artery enter the gluteal region. Some branches of these arteries anastomose with the branches of femoral artery. Through these anasto-

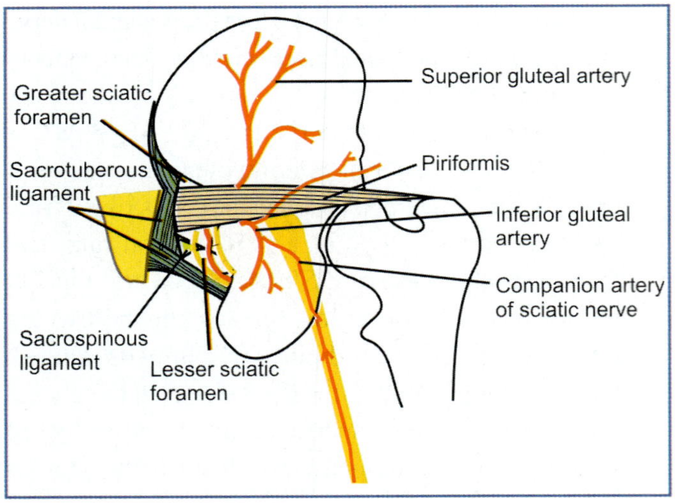

Fig. 185.3: Schematic depiction of greater and lesser sciatic foramina. Note the relation of nerve to obturator internus and internal pudendal artery to ischial spine and of pudendal nerve to sacrospinous ligament

moses collateral circulation can be established if either of the main artery is blocked.

a. The superior gluteal artery is a branch of the posterior division of internal iliac artery. It enters the gluteal region along with the corresponding nerve above the piriformis. It divides in superficial and deep branches. The superficial branch supplies the gluteus medius and maximus. The deep branch divides in upper and lower branches. The upper or ascending branch anastomoses with superficial and deep circumflex iliac and ascending branch of lateral circumflex and iliolumbar arteries near the anterior superior iliac spine. This anastomosis communicates the branches of internal and external iliac and the femoral arteries. The lower or descending branch takes part in trochanteric anastomosis.
b. The inferior gluteal artery is a branch of anterior division of internal iliac artery. Along with inferior gluteal nerve it enters the gluteal region below the piriformis. It gives muscular branches mainly to gluteus maximus muscle. Its most important branch is, an accompanying artery to sciatic nerve, which sinks in the substance of sciatic nerve. It also gives anastomotic branches that take part in trochanteric and cruciate anastomosis.

Trochanteric Anastomosis

It is located in the trochanteric fossa of femur and following four arteries take part into its formation.

a. Descending branch of the superior gluteal artery
b. A branch from inferior gluteal artery
c. Ascending branch of lateral circumflex femoral artery
d. Ascending branch of medial circumflex femoral artery.

The trochanteric anastomosis provides the chief source of blood supply to the head of femur.

Cruciate Anastomosis

The cruciate anastomosis is located in the interval between the upper margin of adductor magnus and lower margin of quadratus femoris. The following arteries take part in this anastomosis.

a. Transverse branch of medial circumflex femoral artery
b. Transverse branch of lateral circumflex femoral artery
c. Descending branch of inferior gluteal artery
d. Ascending branch of first perforating artery.

Since this anastomosis is the link between the internal iliac artery and profunda femoris artery, it provides collateral circulation to fill the femoral artery if it is blocked proximal to the origin of profunda femoris artery.

186 Posterior Compartment of Thigh

The posterior or flexor compartment of thigh contains a group of muscles called hamstrings. The tendons of these muscles are found in the region of ham (poples) in the lower part of the back of the thigh (popliteal region). This is according to the Cunningham's manual of practical anatomy. The dictionary meaning of ham is back of thigh and buttock.

Characteristics of Hamstring Muscles

To be called a hamstring the muscle must have following four features.

a. Origin from ischial tuberosity (Fig. 186.1)
b. Insertion in either tibia or fibula
c. Nerve supply by tibial part of sciatic nerve
d. Action as extensor of hip joint and flexor of knee joint.

Contents of Posterior Compartment

The posterior compartment of thigh (Fig. 185.1) contains four hamstring muscles (long head of biceps femoris, semitendinosus, semimembranosus and ischial part of adductor magnus), short head of biceps femoris and two nerves, which descend from the gluteal region (sciatic and posterior cutaneous nerve of thigh). There in no major artery in the back of thigh, however, the hamstrings and short head of biceps are supplied by perforating branches of profunda femoris artery.

Biceps Femoris (Fig. 186.2)

This muscle has two heads. The long head is a true hamstring muscle while the short head is not.

Origin

The long head takes origin from the muscular impression on the superomedial area of the ischial tuberosity along with semitendinosus and the short head takes origin from the lateral lip of linea aspera of femur.

Insertion

The two heads unite in the thigh and form a tendon, which can be palpated in the superolateral boundary of popliteal fossa. The tendon splits round the fibular collateral ligament and is inserted in the head of fibula.

Nerve Supply

The long head is supplied by tibial part of sciatic nerve at the level of ischial tuberosity while the short head is supplied by the common peroneal part of the sciatic nerve in the thigh.

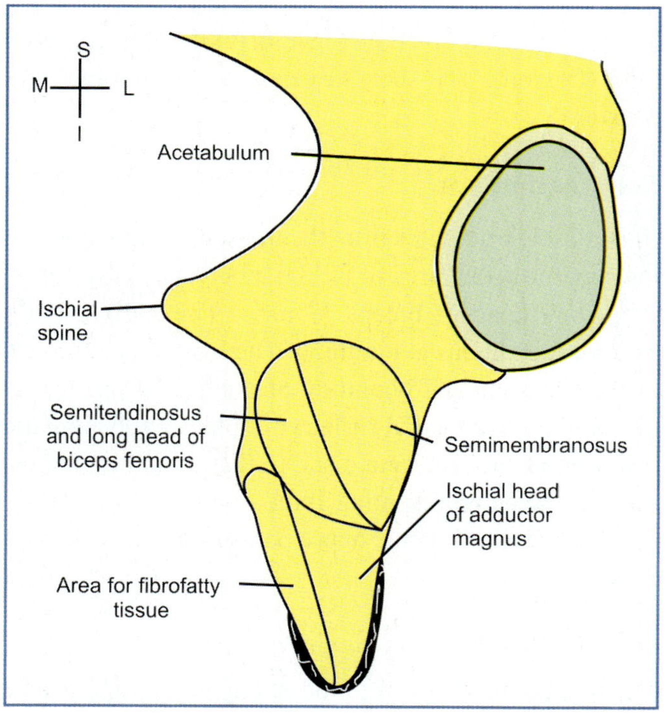

Fig. 186.1: Posteroinferior aspect of ischial tuberosity to depict origin of hamstring muscles (right side)

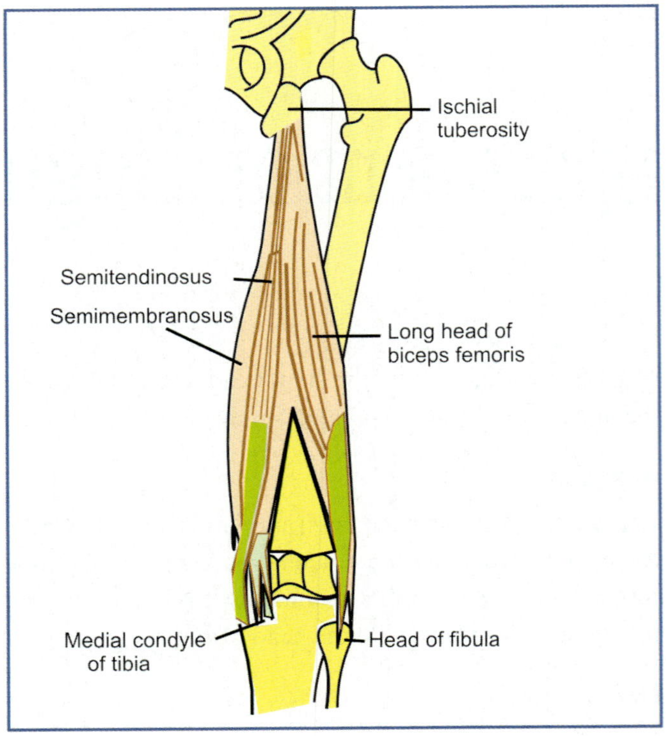

Fig. 186.2: Showing attachments of long head of biceps femoris, semitendinosus and semimembranosus

Actions

The long head acts on both hip joint (extension) and knee joint (flexion). The short head acts only on knee joint (flexion).

Semitendinosus

This muscle originates from the muscular impression on the supero-medial area of ischial tuberosity, in common with long head of biceps femoris. The muscle belly becomes tendinous at midthigh. The long tendon travels in the superomedial boundary of popliteal fossa and is inserted into the medial surface of tibial shaft behind the insertion of sartorius and distal to that of gracilis. Thus, three muscles representing three compartments of the thigh are inserted on the upper part of medial surface of tibia.

Nerve Supply

The tibial or medial part of the sciatic nerve supplies the muscle.

Semimembranosus

This muscle originates from the supero-lateral area of ischial tuberosity by a broad flat tendon. Its lower tendon forms the superomedial boundary of the popliteal fossa and is inserted mainly in the tuberculum tendinis at the back of the medial condyle of tibia. A number of slips extend from this insertion, oblique popliteal ligament of knee joint, fascia covering the popliteus muscle and a slip to the deep fascia of leg (Fig. 186.3).

Nerve Supply

The tibial or medial part of the sciatic nerve supplies the muscle.

Adductor Magnus

The ischial part of adductor magnus is described along with adductor group of muscles.

Actions of Hamstrings

The hamstring muscles extend the thigh at the hip and flex the leg at knee joint. With knee semiflexed, the biceps femoris acts as lateral rotator of knee and the semitendinosus and semimembranosus act as medial rotators of knee.

Testing Muscle Function

While testing the hamstring muscles the subject lies prone with knee extended. The subject is asked to flex the knee against resistance in this position.

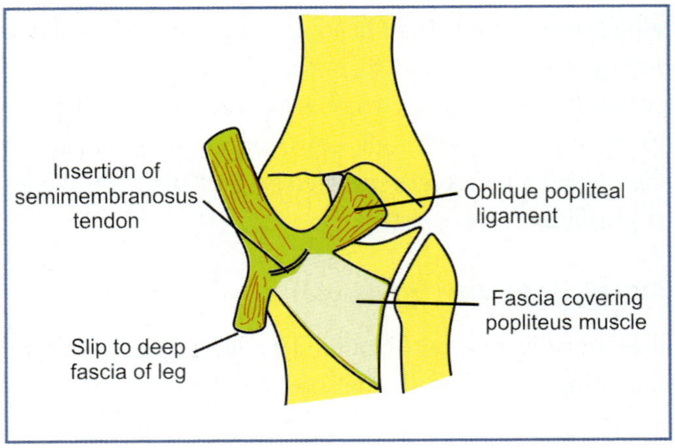

Fig. 186.3: To show insertion of semimembranosus on back of medial condyle of tibia and its extensions

Clinical Highlights

The professional runners are prone to a painful condition known as pulled hamstring. The attachment of hamstrings to the ischial tuberosity is torn in this condition. The extension of hip and flexion of knee is essential for running. So, the runners are liable to overstrain these muscles.

187 Sciatic Nerve

The sciatic nerve is the thickest nerve in the body. It is about 1.5 to 2 cm wide. The sciatic nerve extends from the pelvis to the upper angle of popliteal fossa (at the level of the junction of lower and middle thirds of thigh), where it divides in to terminal branches, which are known as tibial and common peroneal (common fibular) nerves. The sciatic nerve supplies the muscles of the posterior compartment of thigh and through its terminal branches, it supplies all the muscles of the leg and foot. It has a wide sensory supply, which includes the entire leg and foot except the area supplied by the saphenous nerve.

Root Value and Components

The sciatic nerve is the largest branch of the sacral plexus (root value- L4, L5, S1, S2, S3), which is located in the pelvis in front of the piriformis muscle. Its medial tibial component consists of ventral divisions of L4, L5, S1, S2, and S3 ventral rami and the lateral common peroneal component consists of the dorsal divisions of L4, L5, S1 and S2 ventral rami of spinal nerves. The two components are enclosed in a common connective tissue covering.

Exit from Pelvis

Normally the sciatic nerve enters the gluteal region through the greater sciatic foramen below the piriformis (Fig. 185.1). Intra-pelvic division of the sciatic nerve is a variation that is encountered in a few people. In such cases, to come out of the pelvis the common peroneal component either pierces the piriformis or passes above it and the tibial component passes below the piriformis (Fig. 187.1). Sometimes, there is high division of the sciatic nerve in the gluteal region or the thigh.

Relations in Gluteal Region

From the lower margin of the piriformis, the sciatic nerve descends to enter the posterior compartment of thigh. It passes downwards through the inferomedial quadrant of the gluteal region. From above downwards its anterior

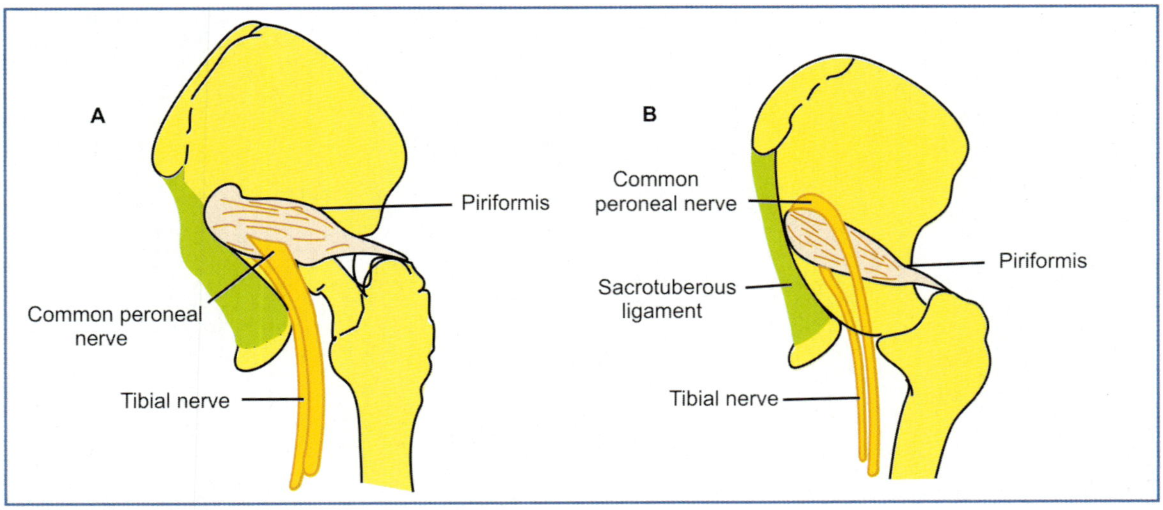

Fig. 187.1: Different modes of exit of branches of sciatic nerve in its intrapelvic division in 'A', common peroneal nerve pierces piriformis and in 'B' it emerges above the muscle

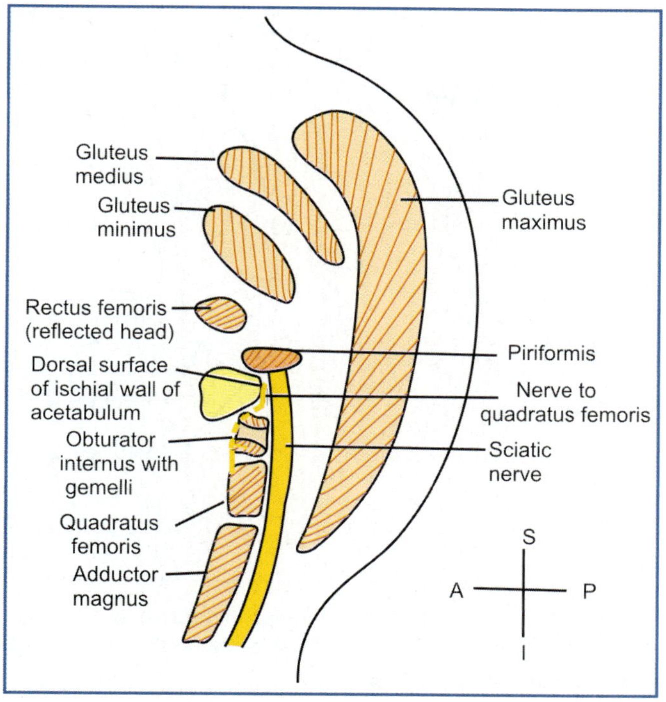

Fig. 187.2: Highly schematic depiction of anterior relations of sciatic nerve in gluteal region

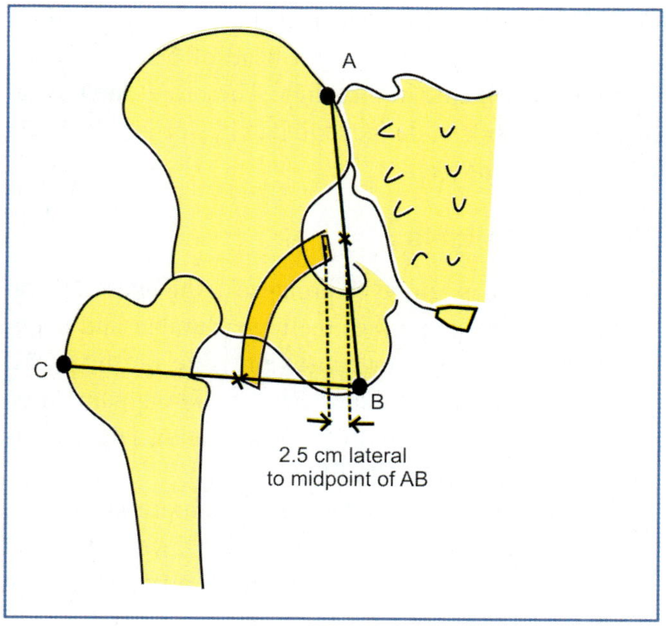

Fig. 187.3: Surface marking of sciatic nerve in gluteal region. A–Posterior, superior iliac spine, B–Ischial tuberosity, C–Greater trochanter

relations (Fig. 187.2) are, the dorsal surface of body of ischium close to acetabulum separated by nerve to quadratus femoris, superior gemellus, tendon of obturator internus, inferior gemellus, quadratus femoris and upper part of adductor magnus. The sciatic nerve is covered posteriorly by the gluteus maximus. The posterior cutaneous nerve of thigh forms its superficial or medial relation.

Relations in Posterior Compartment of Thigh

In the back of the thigh, the sciatic nerve descends vertically lying between the adductor magnus anteriorly and long head of biceps femoris posteriorly. The long head of the biceps crosses the sciatic nerve from medial to lateral side as it runs from ischial tuberosity to the head of fibula. It gives a branch to the short head of biceps femoris from its lateral side (common peroneal component). It usually terminates in the back of thigh at the upper angle of popliteal fossa by dividing into tibial and common peroneal nerves.

Surface Marking (Fig. 187.3)

To represent the gluteal course of the sciatic nerve two points are marked. The upper point is located about 2 to 2.5 cm lateral to the midpoint of a line joining the posterior superior iliac spine and the ischial tuberosity. The lower point lies midway between the greater trochanter and ischial tuberosity. A thick curved line (with outward convexity) joining these two points represents the nerve. To represent the sciatic nerve in the thigh, a straight line is drawn from the lower point to the apex of popliteal fossa.

Arterial Supply (Fig. 185.3)

The sciatic nerve receives a special artery called companion artery of sciatic nerve (arteria nervi ischiadici), a branch of inferior gluteal artery. This artery enters the substance of the sciatic nerve. Its surgical importance is that, when the sciatic nerve is cut, in above knee amputation, the companion artery should be secured and ligated to avoid profuse bleeding. Its embryological importance is that, it is one example of the remnant arteries representing the axis artery of lower limb.

Branches (Fig. 185.1)

The sciatic nerve gives articular branch to the hip joint in the gluteal region. Its muscular branches arise in the upper thigh from its medial side (tibial part) for long head of biceps femoris, semitendinosus, semimembranosus and ischial part of adductor magnus. Its common peroneal part provides a branch to short head of biceps femoris from the lateral side in the thigh. Therefore, the medial side is called side of danger and lateral side is called safe side of sciatic nerve.

Clinical Highlights

a. The sciatica is caused by prolapse of the intervertebral disc, which compresses the lower lumbar and upper sacral nerve roots or causes pressure on the sacral plexus. The patient experiences radiating pain down the posterior aspect of thigh, posterior and lateral sides of leg and lateral part of foot.
b. Sleeping foot is due to temporary compression of the sciatic nerve against femur, at the lower border of gluteus maximus, when a person sits on the hard edge of a chair for a long time.
c. The motor effect of injury to sciatic nerve (for example in posterior dislocation of hip joint) is paralysis of the muscles of posterior compartment of thigh and of the leg and foot. There is sensory loss below the knee with sparing of the skin supplied by saphenous nerve.
d. Injury to the tibial component of the sciatic nerve causes paralysis of all the muscles of posterior compartment of leg and of sole of the foot leading to inability to stand on the toes (due to loss of plantar flexion of foot) and loss of Achillis tendon reflex. There will be sensory loss on the sole of the foot. Trophic ulcers tend to develop in the sole of foot due to loss of sensation.
e. Injury to the common peroneal component of sciatic nerve results in paralysis of the muscles of anterior and lateral compartments of leg. This results in inability to stand on heel (foot drop due to involvement of deep peroneal nerve) and inability to evert foot (due to involvement of superficial peroneal nerve). There is loss of sensation on the anterolateral side of leg and dorsum of foot except for the area supplied by saphenous nerve (medial side of lower part of leg and medial border of foot as far as the root of great toe).

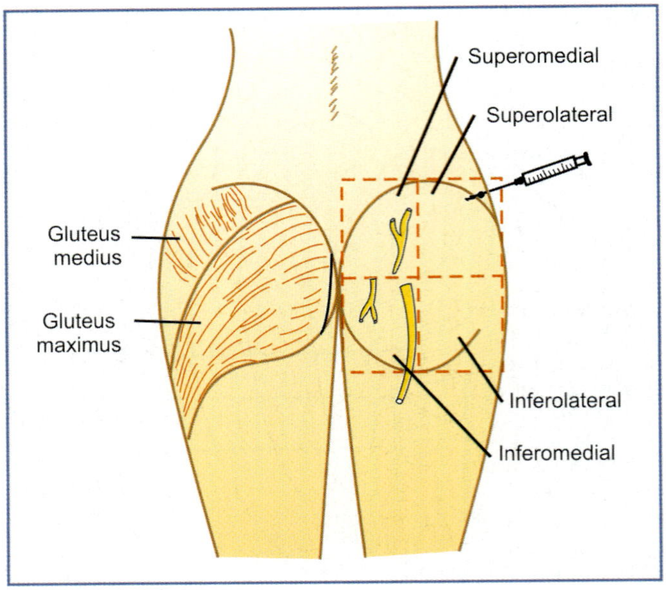

Fig. 187.4: Safe quadrant and site for intramuscular injection in gluteal region. Note that the muscle pierced by the needle is shown on the opposite side

f. Intragluteal injections (Fig. 187.4) are commonly used in clinical practice. The gluteal muscles provide a large surface area for absorption of drugs. Injecting in the superomedial quadrant will endanger the superior gluteal nerve and vessels. Injecting in inferomedial quadrant will endanger the sciatic nerve and inferior gluteal nerve and vessels. Sometimes, only the lateral part of the sciatic nerve may be injured causing effects of common peroneal nerve injury like foot drop. Therefore, superolateral quadrant is a safe site for intramuscular injection. Here, the needle will pierce in succession the skin, superficial fascia, deep fascia and gluteus medius. The point of injection should be just inferior and posterior to the anterior superior iliac spine.

188 Popliteal Fossa

The popliteal fossa is a diamond-shaped hollow situated behind the knee joint. It is an important region because it gives passage to the main vessels and nerves from the thigh to the leg.

Boundaries (Fig. 188.1)

The tendons of hamstring muscles form the superoleteral and superomedial boundaries. The fleshy origins of the flexor muscles of the leg form the inferolateral and inferomedial boundaries.

a. The tendon of biceps femoris forms the superolateral boundary.
b. The tendons of semitendinosus and semimembranosus muscles form the superomedial boundary.
c. The lateral head of gastrocnemius and plantaris muscles form the inferolateral boundary.
d. The medial head of gastrocnemius forms the inferomedial boundary.

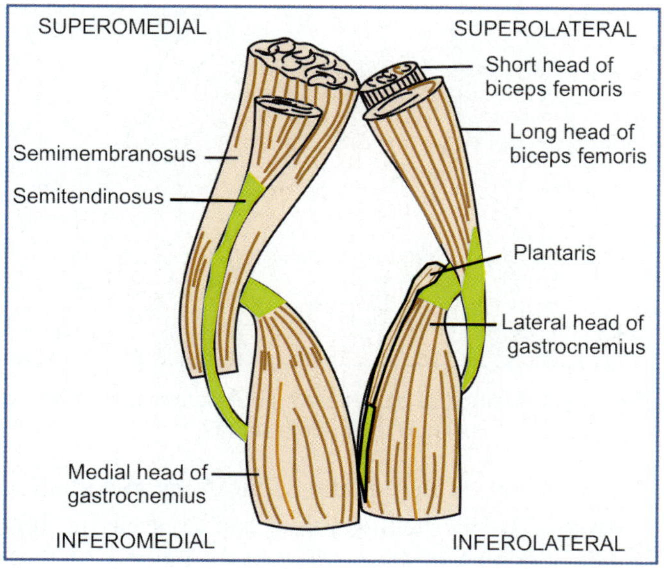

Fig. 188.1: Boundaries of popliteal fossa

e. The floor or anterior wall (Fig. 188.2) is divisible in three parts. Its bony upper part is formed by the popliteal surface of femur. The intermediate part is the capsule of the knee joint (oblique popliteal ligament). The lower part is the thick fascia, which is derived from semimembranosus insertion and which covers the popliteus muscle.
f. The roof or the posterior wall is the deep fascia called the popliteal fascia. The small saphenous vein, superficial lymphatics, and posterior cutaneous nerve of thigh pierce the roof.

Contents

The popliteal artery and its branches and the popliteal vein and its tributaries along with the two terminal

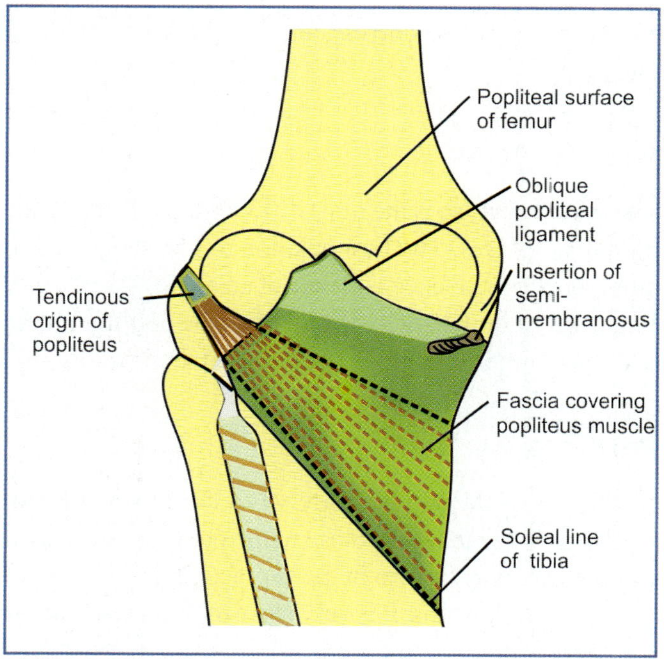

Fig. 188.2: Schematic diagram showing floor of popliteal fossa

branches of the sciatic nerve (tibial and common peroneal) are the main contents of the fossa. Two other nerves that enter the fossa are, the posterior cutaneous nerve of thigh and the descending genicular branch of the posterior division of the obtuartor nerve. The popliteal lymph nodes are present in close vicinity of the popliteal vessels. All the contents are packed in popliteal fat.

Popliteal Artery (Fig. 188.3)

The popliteal artery is the continuation of femoral artery at the level of tendinous opening in the adductor magnus. It is the deepest structure in the fossa and runs very close to the floor of the fossa. The artery runs obliquely across the fossa with a lateral inclination to reach the distal border of the popliteus muscle, where it terminates at the wide interosseous space into anterior and posterior tibial arteries. This artery is used for measuring blood pressure in lower limb for example, in cases of coarctation of aorta.

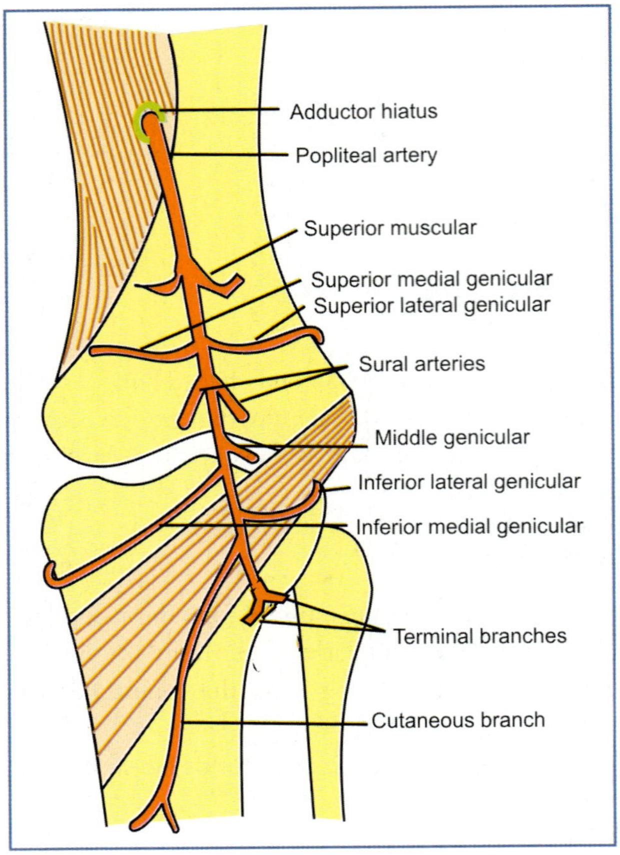

Fig. 188.3: Showing branches of popliteal artery

Surface Marking

The popliteal artery is marked on the popliteal fossa by joining the following three points. The upper point is 2.5 cm medial to the midline at the junction of middle and lower thirds of thigh. The second point is at the level of knee joint in the midline. The lower point in the midline on the back of leg corresponds to the level of tibial tuberosity.

Popliteal Pulse

The popliteal pulse is the most difficult to feel among the peripheral pulses. The best position to feel the popliteal pulse is, when the knee is flexed at an angle of 120°. The fingertips of both hands are placed in the popliteal fossa with the thumbs resting on patient's patella (Fig. 188.4).

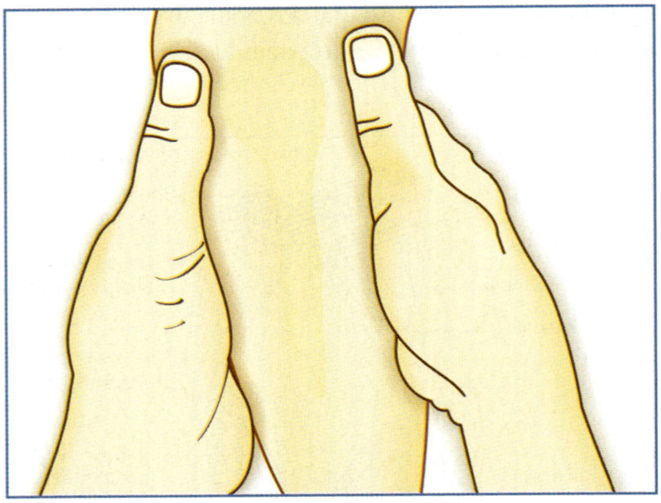

Fig. 188.4: Method of palpation of popliteal pulse in a flexed knee using both hands

Relations

a. Anteriorly the popliteal artery is related to the floor of fossa. Since it is very close to the popliteal surface of femur, it may be torn in the supracondylar fracture of femur. Below this, it is very close to the capsule of the knee joint and hence, endangered in posterior dislocation of knee joint.
b. Posteriorly, at the middle of the fossa the artery is crossed by the popliteal vein and tibial nerve from lateral to medial side, as a result of which the relations of the neurovascular structures differ at three levels

of the fossa (Fig. 188.5). At the upper end the mediolateral arrangement is—artery, vein and nerve. In the central part (at the site of crossing), the anteroposterior arrangement is—artery, vein and nerve. At the lower end of the fossa the mediolateral arrangement is—nerve, vein and artery.

c. One popliteal lymph node lies between the popliteal artery and the capsule of the knee joint and a few lymph nodes surround the popliteal vessels.

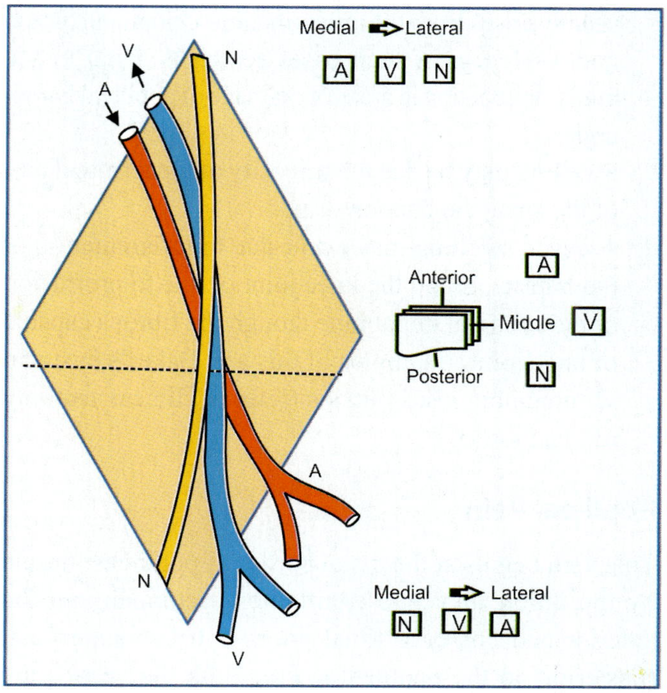

Fig.188.5: Highly schematic depiction of neurovascular relations in popliteal fossa. A–Popliteal artery, V–Popliteal vein, N–Tibial nerve

Branches (Fig. 188.3)

a. The superior muscular branches supply the muscles in the thigh (hamstrings).
b. The sural arteries supply the soleus, gastrocnemius and plantaris muscles.
c. The lateral and medial superior genicular, lateral and medial inferior genicular and middle genicular arteries supply the knee joint.

Genicular Anastomosis

The arterial anstomosis around the knee joint is called the genicular anastomosis. It maintains adequate blood flow during flexion of knee joint, when the popliteal artery is compressed. The following branches of popliteal, anterior and posterior tibial, femoral and profunda femoris arteries take part in the anastomosis.

a. The superior medial genicular artery anastomoses with descending genicular branch of femoral artery and inferior medial genicular artery.
b. The inferior medial genicular artery anastomoses with superior medial genicular and saphenous branch of descending genicular artery.
c. The superior lateral genicular artery anastomoses with descending branch of lateral circumflex iliac artery and inferior lateral genicular artery.
d. The inferior lateral genicular artery passes deep to the fibular collateral ligament to anastomose with superior lateral genicular artery, anterior and posterior tibial recurrent branches of anterior tibial artery and circumflex fibular branch of posterior tibial artery.

Clinical Highlights

The swellings in the popliteal fossa originate not only from structures in the fossa but also from structures associated with the knee joint (which is anatomically very close). Therefore, it is customary to examine knee joint in a case of popliteal swelling or to examine the popliteal fossa in the case of affliction of knee joint.

a. The popliteal aneurysm due to dilatation of popliteal artery presents as a pulsatile midline swelling in the popliteal fossa. This may cause edema of leg due to compression of popliteal vein. Stasis of blood in the aneurysm may favor formation of thrombosis and emboli, which may enter the distal arteries causing pain and ulceration in toes. The operative treatment of popliteal aneurysm consists of exposing and clamping the popliteal artery. Another method of treatment is to use saphenous vein graft to replace the dilated part of the popliteal artery. Yet another time-honored method pioneered by John Hunter, is to ligate the femoral artery in the subsartorial canal. This method is based on the knowledge that arteries taking part in genicular anastomosis enlarge to provide arterial supply to the leg.
b. Popliteal abscess is a painful swelling that presents as a red and edematous swelling in the popliteal fossa. It

usually arises from the inflammation of popliteal lymph nodes. Hence, in such cases search is made to see injury or infection in areas of drainage of popliteal lymph nodes.

c. Swelling may be due to varicosity of the terminal part of the small saphenous vein.
d. A cystic swelling may occur due to inflammation of the bursae around the knee joint or due to protrusion of the synovial membrane though the fibrous capsule of knee joint. Examples of this are, Baker's cyst and semimembranosus bursitis (refer to clinical anatomy of knee joint).

Popliteal Vein

This vein begins at the distal border of popliteus muscle by the union of venae comitantes accompanying the anterior and posterior tibial arteries. It lies superficial (posterior) to the popliteal artery. Both the vessels are enclosed in the same fibrous sheath. The vein has triple relation to the artery as follows. The vein lies medially in the lower part; it crosses superficially (posteriorly) in the middle part (between the two heads of gastrocnemius) and lies laterally at the upper part. The popliteal vein continues as the femoral vein at the adductor opening. The tributaries of the popliteal vein are the veins accompanying the branches of the popliteal artery and the small saphenous vein.

Tibial Nerve in Popliteal Fossa

The tibial nerve is the larger of the two terminal branches of sciatic nerve. It courses through the popliteal fossa and the posterior compartment of the leg. It enters the popliteal fossa through the upper angle. It bears triple relation to the popliteal vessels. In the upper part it lies lateral to the vessels. In the middle of the fossa it crosses the vessels superficially (posteriorly) and in the distal part it lies medial to the vessels. At the distal margin of popliteus muscle it continues in the posterior compartment of leg as the tibial nerve in company with posterior tibial vessels.

Branches (Fig. 188.6)

a. The articular branches are superior medial, inferior medial and middle articular (genicular) nerves. The middle genicular artery, middle genicular nerve and genicular branch of posterior division of obturator nerve pierce the oblique popliteal ligament (middle part of the floor of the fossa) to enter the knee joint.
b. Only one cutaneous nerve arises in the popliteal fossa. It is called sural nerve. It descends between the heads of gastrocnemius and after leaving the fossa pierces the deep fascia of leg to become superficial. It supplies the posterior part of leg and lateral border of foot including the lateral margin of little toe. Being superficial in location it is frequently used for nerve grafting.
c. Muscular branches are five in number, out of which four arise from the lateral aspect of the tibial nerve and one from the medial aspect. The muscles supplied by branches from lateral side are, lateral head of gastrocnemius, plantaris, soleus and popliteus. A branch arising from the medial side of the nerve supplies the medial head of gastrocnemius. The nerve to popliteus has peculiar course. It passes down lying on the posterior surface of the muscle and winds round its distal margin to supply the muscle from its anterior or deep aspect. Apart from popliteus, this nerve also supplies the superior tibiofibular joint, interosseous

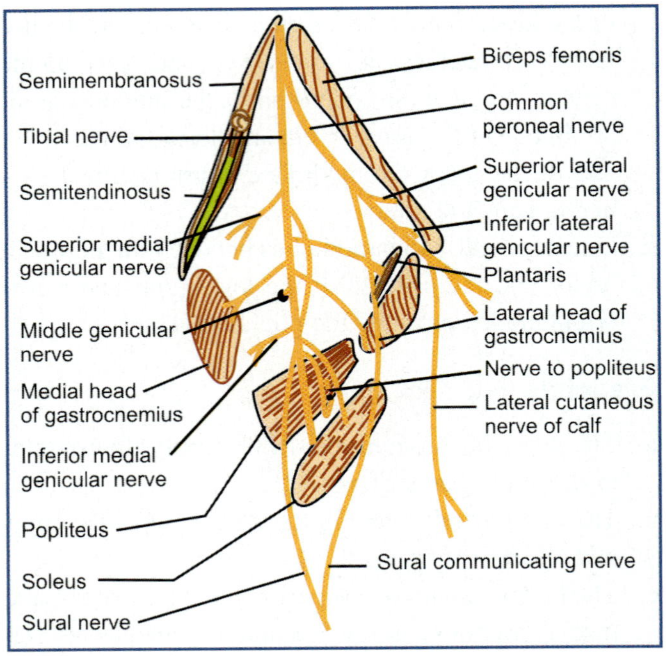

Fig. 188.6: Schematic diagram showing distribution of tibial and common peroneal nerves

membrane, inferior tibiofibular joint, medullary branch to tibia and a branch to the tibialis posterior muscle.

Surface Marking

The nerve can be represented by a straight vertical line starting from the upper angle of popliteal fossa to a point in the midline at the level of tibial tuberosity.

Clinical Highlights

The tibial nerve is rarely injured in popliteal fossa because of its relatively protected position in the fossa. However, if injured, all the muscles of calf and intrinsic muscles of foot are paralyzed. This will give rise to talipes calcaneovalgus deformity of foot (foot is everted and dorsiflexed). The patient will walk on the heel. The sensory loss mainly affects the sole.

Common Peroneal Nerve

The common peroneal nerve (dorsal branches of L4, L5, S1, S2) is the smaller terminal division of the sciatic nerve. It enters the popliteal fossa through the upper angle and lies medial to the biceps femoris tendon. It follows this tendon to the back of the head of the fibula. It then curves forward lying in close contact with the lateral side of the neck of fibula, where it divides in its terminal branches, deep to the peroneus longus muscle.

Branches in Popliteal Fossa (Fig. 188.6)

The common peroneal nerve has no muscular branches but, gives two articular and two cutaneous branches in the popliteal fossa. The articular branches are the superior lateral and inferior lateral, which accompany the corresponding arteries and supply the knee joint. The lateral cutaneous nerve of leg and sural (peroneal) communicating nerve are the cutaneous branches for the leg and foot.

Branches at the Neck of Fibula

The recurrent genicular nerve arises just before its termination (Fig. 191.2). This branch passes through the tibialis anterior muscle along with anterior tibial recurrent artery, supplies a twig to the muscle and reaches the knee joint. The terminal branches of the common peroneal nerve are called the superficial and deep peroneal nerves. The superficial peroneal nerve enters the peroneal compartment of leg while the deep peroneal nerve enters the anterior compartment of leg.

Surface Marking

The nerve can be indicated on the surface by a line starting from the upper angle of the popliteal fossa along the tendon of biceps femoris to the back of the head of fibula.

Clinical Highlights

a. The common peroneal nerve being relatively superficial, is unprotected, compared to the tibial nerve. Hence, it is a commonly injured nerve in the lower limb. It may be compressed in the substance of the peroneus longus muscle. It may be injured in fracture of the neck of fibula or due to direct pressure of a tightly applied plaster cast. It is affected in Hensen's disease along with other peripheral nerves and becomes tender and thickened.
b. The common peroneal nerve is palpated by rolling it against the neck of fibula.
c. Injury to common peroneal nerve leads to paralysis of dorsiflexors of the ankle joint and evertors of the foot supplied through its deep peroneal and superficial peroneal branches respectively. This results in foot drop deformity in which the foot is inverted and plantarflexed. This combination is called talipes equinovarus. The patient walks on the toes.

Popliteal Lymph Nodes (Fig. 190.7)

These nodes belong to the deep group of lymph nodes of lower limb. They are usually five to six in number. They are embedded in the fat of popliteal fossa. One node is present at the sapheno-popliteal junction. This node receives superficial lymph vessels draining the lateral side of the foot including the little toe, lateral side of heel and lateral side of the back of leg. One node is present between the popliteal artery and the capsule of knee joint. It receives lymph from the joint. The other nodes are grouped around the popliteal vessels. They receive lymph vessels draining all the deep structures below the knee.

The efferent vessels from the popliteal nodes travel with the popliteal vessels and so pass through the adductor hiatus. Then, they accompany the femoral vessels to reach the deep inguinal nodes.

Clinical Highlights

a. Popliteal lymph nodes are enlarged in injury to deeper tissues of the foot. Palpation of popliteal lymph nodes is as follows. The deep fascia of the popliteal fossa is relaxed by passively flexing the knee. The examiner holds the knee with hands and explores the fossa for enlarged lymph nodes with the fingers of both hands.
b. Popliteal abscess may form in cases of inflammation in foot, leg or knee joint. The abscess may remain unnoticed due to the strong popliteal fascia. It may press on the nerves and vessels of the popliteal fossa. The abscess is drained from the lateral aspect anterior to the biceps femoris tendon.

189 Hip Joint or Coxal Joint

The hip joint is an example of multiaxial ball and socket type of synovial joint. Its primary functions are to support the body weight in standing and to transmit the forces during movements of trunk upon the femur during walking and running. The range of movements in all directions is possible due to the presence of long and narrow neck of the femur, which makes an angle with the shaft.

Articular Surfaces

The bones taking part in the hip joint are the head of femur and the acetabulum of the hip bone.

Acetabulum

The acetabulum (in Latin cup) is a cup-shaped cavity formed by the union of ilium, ischium and pubis. The rim of the acetabulum presents a notch in its lower part. This notch gives attachment to the transverse acetabular ligament and its margins give attachment to the ligament of head of femur. The fibrocartilaginous labrum acetabulare deepens the acetabulum. The labrum, which is attached to the rim of acetabulum forms a tight fit around the head of femur. The horseshoe shaped articular surface (lunate surface) of acetabulum is covered with articular cartilage. It is thickest and widest superiorly, where the maximum body weight is transmitted to the femur. The nonarticular part of acetabulum is known as acetabular fossa. It is filled with Haversian pad of fat, which is intracapsular but extrasynovial.

Head of Femur

The spherical femoral head is covered by hyaline articular cartilage, except for a rough pit where the ligament of the head of femur is attached. The articular cartilage is thickest in the center and thins out toward the periphery.

Ligaments (Fig. 189.1)

The fibrous capsule covers the joint. The capsule is strengthened in three places to form the iliofemoral, pubofemoral and ischiofemoral ligaments. The transverse acetabular ligament converts the acetabular notch into the acetabular foramen through which, pass acetabular branch of obturator artery, acetabular branch of medial circumflex femoral artery and articular branch of anterior division of obturator nerve. The ligament of the head of femur carries the articular vessels and nerves to the head of the femur as this ligament extends from the acetabular notch to the fovea on the head of femur.

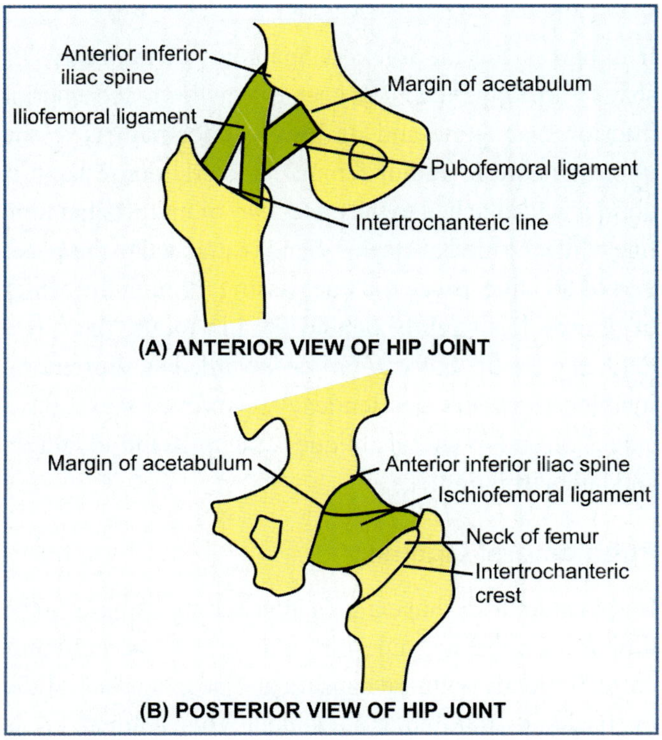

Fig. 189.1: Ligaments of hip joint

Fibrous Capsule

The capsule is very strong and hugs the joint tightly. It is attached medially to the margins of the acetabulum and laterally to the femur. Anteriorly, it is attached to the intertrochanteric line so that entire anterior surface of neck is intracapsular. Posteriorly, it is attached to the posterior surface of the neck a short distance medial to the intertrochanteric crest. Thus, the posterior surface of the neck is partly intracapsular.

Special Parts of Capsule

a. Zona orbicularis is the inner part of the capsule consisting of circularly arranged fibers, which forms a tight collar for the neck of the femur.
b. Retinacula are the longitudinal fibers on the anterior surface of the neck. These fibers originate from the capsular attachment to intertrochanteric line and proceed toward the femoral head in close contact with the anterior surface of the neck and produce grooves on it. Their main function is to support the retinacular arteries running toward the head.

Iliofemoral Ligament (Ligament of Bigelow)

It is one of the the thickest ligaments in the body. Its shape is like inverted Y. Its apex is attached to the anterior inferior iliac spine and its lower attachment is to the intertrochanteric line of femur. Its lateral dense band is oblique and attached to the upper part of intertrochanteric line while the medial vertical band is attached to the lower part of this line. Since the line passing through the center of gravity lies slightly behind the hip joints, there is a tendency for the body to fall backward. The iliofemoral ligament prevents this tendency. It prevents excessive extension and its lateral oblique band limits the adduction and lateral rotation.

Pubofemoral Ligament

It is triangular in shape and is attached by its base to the iliopubic eminence, superior pubic ramus and obturator crest. It blends with the capsule and deep surface of the medial band of iliofemoral ligament. This ligament limits abduction and lateral rotation movements.

Ischiofemoral Ligament

This ligament reinforces the back of the capsule. It is attached to the ischium below the lower margin of acetabulum. From this attachment the fibers spiral superolaterally to merge in the fibrous capsule. The ischiofemoral ligament limits the medial rotation of thigh.

Synovial Membrane (Fig. 189.2)

The synovial membrane lines the inner surface of the fibrous capsule. It covers the intracapsular part of the neck as far as the articular margin of the head of femur. It also covers the acetabular labrum, ligament of the head of femur and Haversian pad of fat inside acetabular fossa. The synovial fold surrounding the ligament of the head of femur carries the blood vessels and nerves entering the joint through the acetabular foramen. The synovial membrane lining the intracapsular part of the neck is raised in folds by the retinacular fibers. Occasionally, the synovial membrane may protrude through as opening in the anterior part of capsule between iliofemoral and ischiofemoral ligaments to become continuous with psoas bursa.

Relations of Joint (Fig. 189.3)

a. Anteriorly, the joint is related to the muscles in the floor of the femoral triangle, femoral nerve and femoral vessels. The pectineus separates the femoral

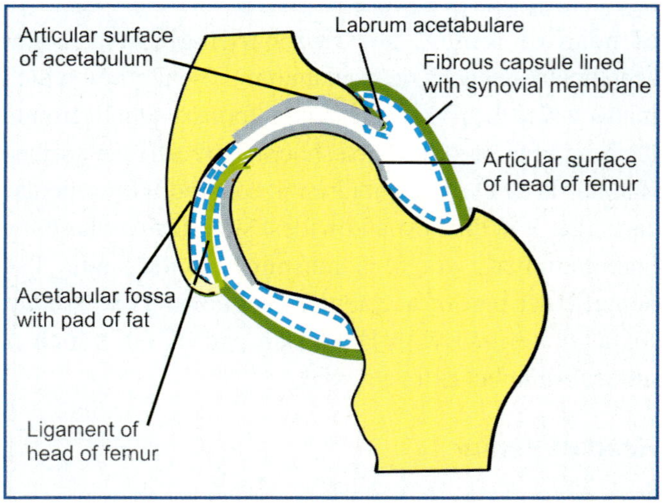

Fig. 189.2: Coronal section of hip joint (Note that synovial membrane covers labrum acetabulare, ligament of head of femur, acetabular pad of fat and intracapsular part of neck of femur)

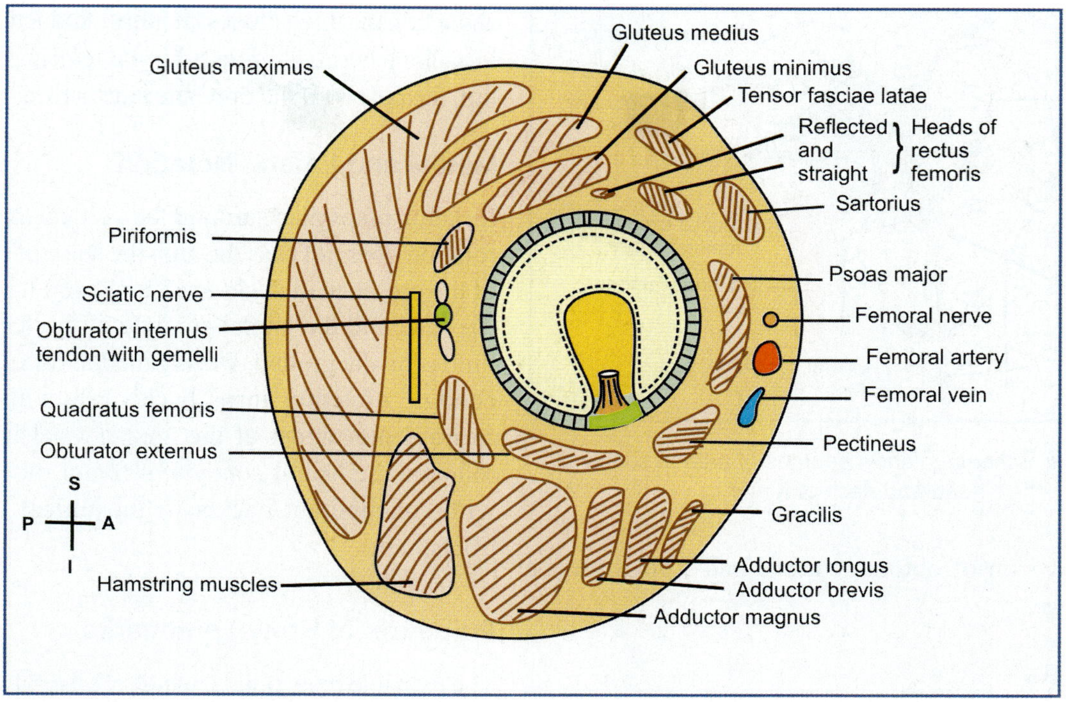

Fig. 189.3: Schematic diagram showing relations of hip joint

vein from the joint and the iliopsoas separates the femoral artery and nerve from the joint. The femoral artery can be palpated through the tendon of psoas against the inferolateral part of the head of femur. The sartorius, lateral cutaneous nerve of thigh and the rectus femoris are the other anterior relations.

b. Superiorly, the joint is related to the reflected head of rectus femoris medially and the gluteus minimus laterally. Above these, the gluteus medius and tensor fasciae late are related.
c. Inferior relations are the obturator externus and lateral fibers of pectineus muscles.
d. The posterior relations are very important. The short lateral rotator muscles in the gluteal region cover the posterior aspect of the capsule. From above downward they are, piriformis, obturator internus with two gemelli and quadratus femoris muscles. The obturator internus and the two gemelli separate the sciatic nerve from the joint. The obturator externus tendon lies in close contact with the posterior surface of the neck and separates the joint from the quadratus femoris. Superficial to these intimate relations, the gluteus maximus is related. In posterior dislocation of the joint the sciatic nerve is in danger of injury.

Arterial Supply (Fig. 189.4)

a. The area of femoral head around the fovea is supplied by acetabular branch of obturator artery and acetabular branch of medial circumflex femoral artery. The acetabular branches reach the head via ligament of the head of femur. This source is of little significance.
b. The rest of the head and the neck receive blood from arterial circle around the capsular attachment, in which the medial circumflex femoral artery is the chief source. The retinacular arteries arise from this vascular ring, pierce the capsule and run along the neck of femur to supply it and the head. The arterial supply of the head and neck is solely dependent on the retinacular arteries. In the rupture of these arteries (due to intracapsular fracture of the femoral neck) avascular necrosis of the head of femur sets in for want of adequate nutrition.
c. The nutrient artery of the femur gives a few branches to the head and neck of femur.

Nerve Supply

The joint receives articular twigs from femoral nerve via a branch to rectus femoris, nerve to quadratus femoris,

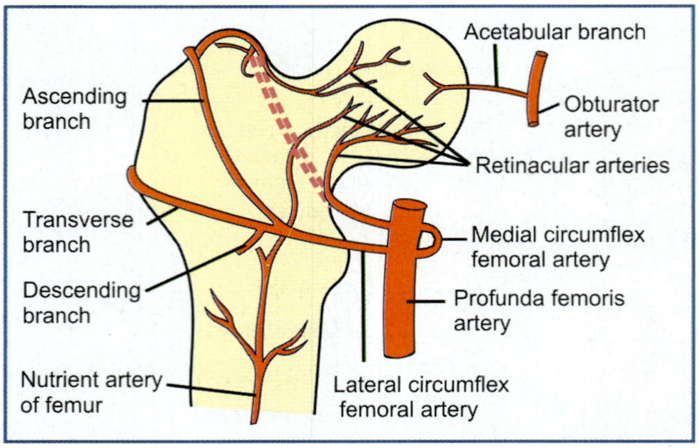

Fig. 189.4: Scheme to show sources of arterial supply of head and neck of femur

anterior division of obturator nerve and from superior gluteal nerve.

Movements

Being a multiaxial ball and socket type of joint, the movements around three axes are possible in the hip joint.

Flexion and Extension

These movements occur around transverse axis. The range of flexion is greater and it is limited when the anterior surface of thigh touches the anterior abdominal wall. The extension is limited when the thigh and trunk are in the same vertical line.

Adduction and Abduction

These movements occur around anteroposterior axis. Adduction is limited by contact with the opposite thigh. In abduction the thigh moves laterally. Abduction is important in walking because through this movement of the supported hip, the pelvis on the opposite side is lifted up.

Medial and Lateral Rotation

Rotation takes place around the vertical axis. The axis of rotation does not pass through the shaft of femur because of the presence of neck- shaft angle but it passes through the head and the lateral condyle of the femur, when the limb is on the ground. During medial rotation, the medial condyle of femur turns backwards with concomitant forward movement of the greater trochanter. In lateral rotation, the lateral condyle of femur moves backwards with concomitant backward movement of the greater trochanter.

Palpation of Bony Landmarks

The palpable bony points, which are useful in examination of the hip joint, are the anterior superior iliac spine, greater trochanter and the ischial tuberosity. The greater trochanter is located a hand's-breadth below the tubercle of iliac crest. Upward displacement of greater trochanter indicates shortening of the limb due to fracture dislocations in hip region. The orthopedic surgeons have devised various methods to find out the position of the greater trochanter with the help of bony landmarks. The simple methods are given below:

a. Nelaton's line is drawn with the patient lying on the normal side, from the anterior superior iliac spine to the most prominent part of ischial tuberosity. Normally, the tip of greater trochanter is at or just below this line.

Muscles Responsible for Each Movement

Movement	*Main muscles*	*Accessory muscles*
Flexion	Iliopsoas	Pectineus, sartorius, rectus femoris
Extension	Gluteus maximus	Hamstring muscles
Adduction	Adductors longus, brevis and magnus	Pectineus and gracilis
Abduction	Gluteus medius and minimus	Tensor fasciae latae
Medial rotation	Gluteus medius and minimus	Tensor fasciae latae and adductor muscles
Lateral rotation	Obturator externus and internus, gemelli,	Piriformis, gluteus maximus, sartorius quadratus femoris
Circumduction	Sequential contraction of all muscles responsible for above movements	

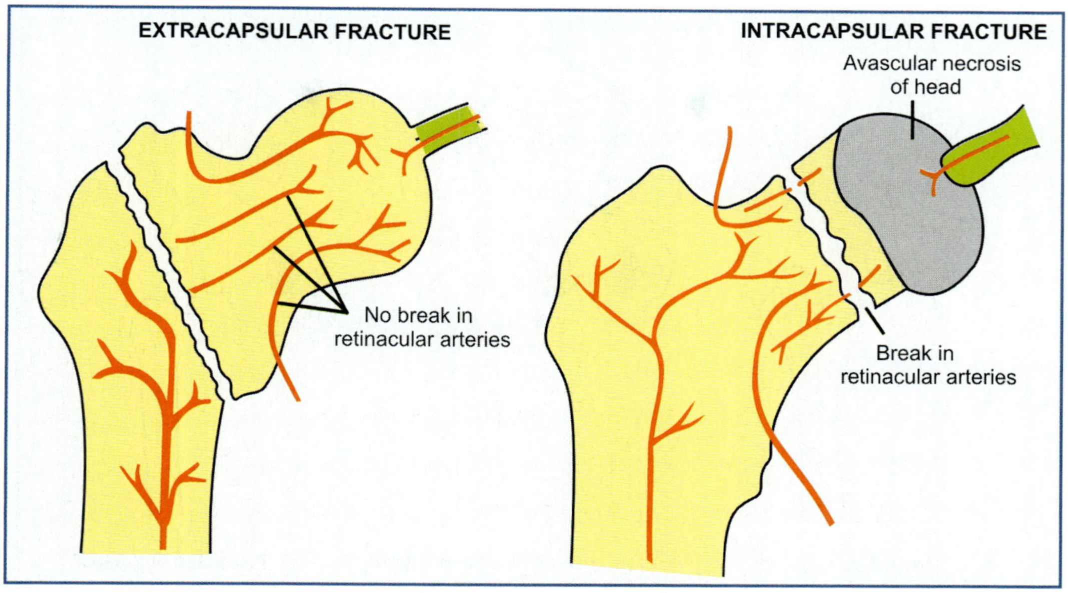

Fig. 189.5: Arterial supply of head of femur in extracapsular and intracapsular fracture of neck of femur

b. Schoemaker's line is a straight line that extends from the tip of greater trochanter to the anterior superior iliac spine and upward over the anterior abdominal wall to reach the umbilicus. If the greater trochanter is elevated the line passes below the umbilicus.

Radiological Anatomy

In the radiograph of a normal adult hipbone and upper end of femur, it is possible to identify the smooth curve of the femoral articular surface and the articular surface of acetabulum with the joint space in between. The neck and the greater trochanter of the femur are identifiable. The ischial tuberosity, ischiopubic ramus and the superior ramus of the pubis can be seen. By joining the medial margin of the femoral neck and the inferior margin of superior ramus of the pubis, a smoothly curved Shenton's line is visible. Fracture of neck or dislocation of hip joint distorts this line.

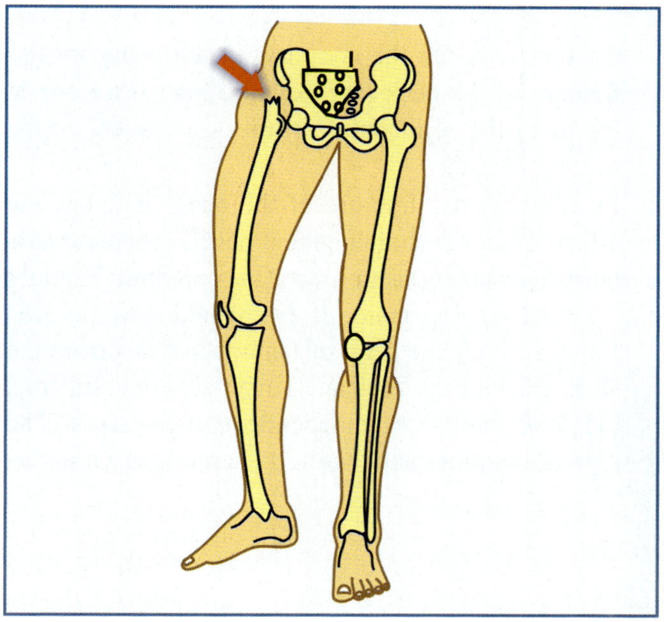

Fig. 189.6: Fracture of neck of right femur resulting in upward and posterior displacement of greater trochanter (indicated by arrow)

Clinical Highlights

a. The fracture of the neck of femur (Fig. 189.5) is very common in elderly due to osteoporotic changes in the neck. Postmenopausal women, who develop osteoporosis, are more prone to this fracture on trivial trauma. This fracture is of two types, intracapsular (subcapital, transcervical and basal) and extracapsular. In the intracapsular fracture, the retinacular arteries are injured leading to delay in healing or nonunion of fracture. Its serious complication is avascular necrosis of head of the femur with resultant loss function of

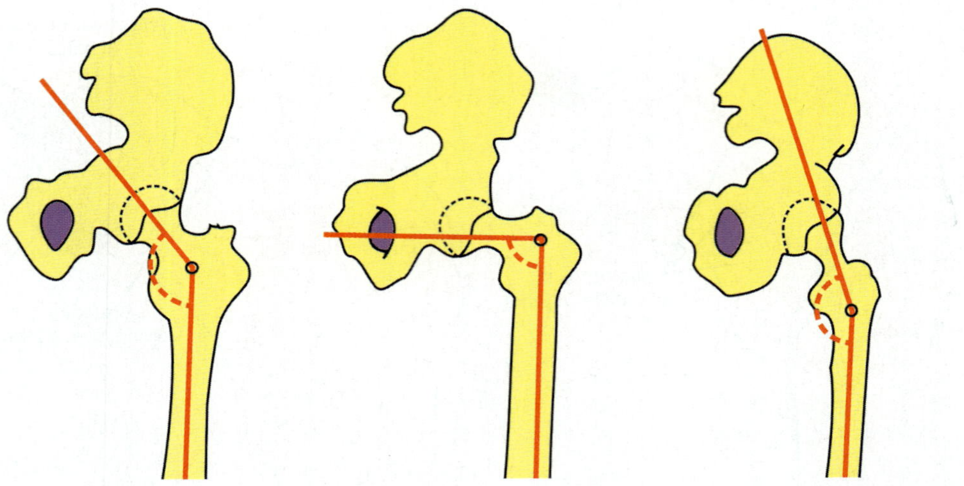

Fig. 189.7: Clinical importance of neck-shaft angle
(Angle between long axis of neck and long axis of shaft of femur)

the hip joint. On the contrary, in the extracapsular fracture of the neck (for example inter-trochanteric fracture) the retinacular arteries are saved, hence healing is faster.

b. In intracapsular fracture of the neck of femur the affected limb is shortened and held in characteristic laterally rotated position with toes pointing laterally (Fig. 189.6). The anatomical explanation of this is as follows. Since the head of femur separates from the shaft (carrying the trochanter) in intracapsular fracture, the shaft can rotate independent of the head. The gluteus maximus and the short lateral rotator muscles rotate the femur laterally. The psoas major becomes a lateral rotator after fracture due to shift in the axis of action. The muscles attaching the hipbone and femur pull the femur upward.

c. The neck-shaft angle is also known as angle of inclination (Fig. 189.7). The normal neck-shaft angle is 125° in adult and 160° in children. When there is increase in the angle it is called coxa valga. It is found in congenital dislocation of hip. Coxa valga limits the adduction movement of the hip joint. If the angle is reduced it is called coxa vara. It is seen in fracture of neck of femur and it limits the abduction at the hip.

190 Knee Joint

The knee joint is the largest and the most complicated synovial joint in the body. It is classified as a modified hinge joint with a mobile transverse axis. In addition to flexion and extension it allows a small degree of rotation. In fact, the knee joint is composed of three articulations, right and left condylar joints between the tibial and femoral condyles and a saddle joint between the patella and the patellar surface of the femur. It is a major weight- bearing joint and its stability depends on its ligaments and quadriceps mechanism (extensor apparatus).

Articular Surfaces

The articular surfaces are, the proximal articular surface on the lower end of femur, distal articular surface on the upper end of tibia and patellar articular surface. These articulating surfaces (covered with articular cartilage) are not congruent with each other.

Proximal or Femoral Articular Surface

The proximal articular surface covers the posterior, inferior and anterior surfaces of the medial and lateral condyles of femur. The articular surfaces of the two condyles are continuous with each other anteriorly but are separated by intercondylar notch posteriorly. The proximal articular surface is divided into three parts.

a. The patellar articular surface or trochlear surface is present on the anterior aspect and is subdivided in larger lateral and smaller medial areas by a vertical groove. The larger lateral articular surface is elevated (compared to the medial). A small semilunar area of the articular surface on the medial condyle adjoining the anterior margin of intercondylar fossa comes in contact with the medial articular facet of patella in full flexion.
b. The tibial articular surface on medial condyle is longer in antero-posterior axis and is obliquely set compared to the articular surface on lateral condyle.
c. The tibial articular surface on lateral condyle is straight, less curved and smaller by about two cm than the corresponding surface on the medial condyle.

Distal or Tibial Articular Surfaces

The distal articular surfaces are present on the upper surfaces of the two condyles of tibia as the lateral and medial condylar surfaces separated by a rough non-articular area. They are slightly concave centrally but flat peripherally, where they come in contact with the menisci. The articular surface on medial tibial condyle is oval and its anteroposterior diameter is greater than the transverse diameter. The articular surface on the lateral tibial condyle is circular and its posterior part extends on the posterior aspect of the lateral condyle, where the tendon of popliteus glides.

Patellar Articular Surface

The posterior surface of patella bears a large articular area, which is divided by a vertical groove in larger lateral and smaller medial areas. Near the medial margin of the patella, there is a narrow semilunar strip for contact with medial condyle of femur in full flexion. The rest of the lateral and medial areas are divided in three facets on each side. These facets come in contact with femur one by one as the knee passes from the position of full extension to that of flexion.

Fibrous Capsule

The unique feature of the capsule of knee joint is that it is deficient in the anterior part of the joint. The strong quadriceps tendon, patella and ligamentum patellae take the place of the deficient capsule. These three structures together form the extensor mechanism or apparatus of the knee joint.

Upper Attachment of Capsule (Fig. 190.1A)

a. Anteriorly, the capsule is attached to the expansions of vastus lateralis and medialis muscles called the lateral and medial patellar retinacula, which are attached to the lateral and medial margins of patella and to the margins of ligamentum patellae. The patella and the ligamentum patellae are present in place of the capsule anteriorly.
b. Posteriorly, the capsule is attached to the medial and posterior aspects of medial condyle of femur just beyond the articular surface. The line of attachment can be traced laterally, along the posterior margin of intercondylar notch to the posterior surface of lateral condyle, and then to its lateral surface along the upper margin of the popliteal groove, so that the origin of the popliteus becomes intracapsular.

Lower Attachment of Capsule (Fig. 190.1B)

a. Anteriorly, the capsule blends with the patellar retinacula through which it is attached to the anterior margins of tibial condyles and to the sides of the tibial tuberosity.
b. Posteriorly, the capsular attachment begins at the medial margin of medial condyle just beyond the articular surface. Then it can be traced along the posterior margin of medial condyle, intercondylar area, posterior margin of lateral condyle and the lateral margin of lateral condyle. There is a gap in the capsular attachment behind the lateral condyle for the exit of the tendon of popliteus.

Ligaments

There are five important ligaments, ligamentum patellae, oblique popliteal ligament, arcuate popliteal ligament, tibial collateral ligament and fibular collateral ligament.

a. The ligamentum patellae or patellar ligament is the continuation of the central part of the tendon of quadriceps femoris. It extends from the apex of the patella to the tibial tuberosity. It gives attachment to lateral and medial patellar retinacula. Posteriorly, it is related to a large infrapatellar pad of fat above and deep infrapatellar bursa below. In clinical practice this ligament is used for eliciting patellar reflex or knee jerk by tapping it with a knee hammer.
b. The oblique popliteal ligament is a broad band, which strengthens the capsule posteriorly and is an expansion from the tendon of insertion of semimembranosus (Fig. 186.2). It extends from the posterior aspect of the medial condyle of tibia to the lateral part of intercondylar line and lateral condyle of femur. The popliteal artery is in contact with this ligament. The middle genicular artery, middle genicular nerve and genicular branch of the posterior division of obturator nerve pierce the ligament to enter the joint.
c. The arcuate popliteal ligament is Y-shaped. Its stem is attached to the styloid process of head of fibula. Its posterior limb is attached to posterior end of the intercondylar area of tibia and the anterior limb extends to the lateral condyle of femur deep to fibular collateral ligament.

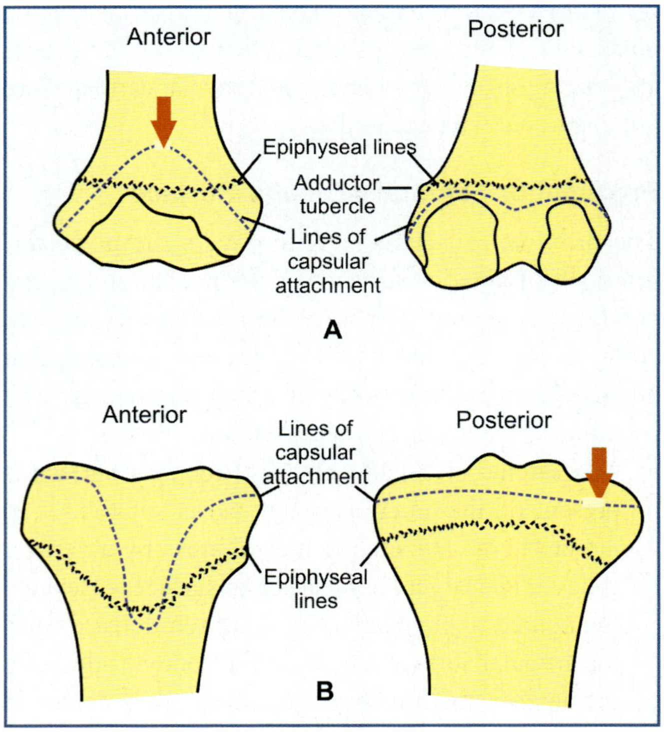

Fig. 190.1: Attachment of the capsule of knee joint to femur in (A) and to tibia in (B). Arrows indicate gaps in the capsule

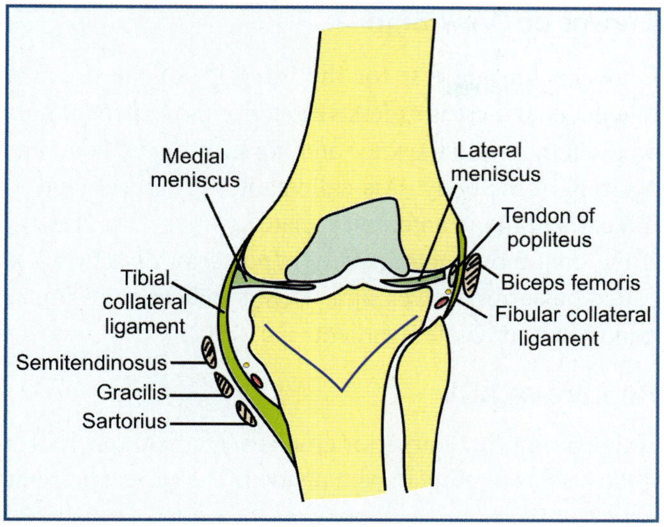

Fig. 190.2: Showing attachments and relations of collateral ligaments of knee joint (Note: Inferior genicular nerve and artery deep to collateral ligaments)

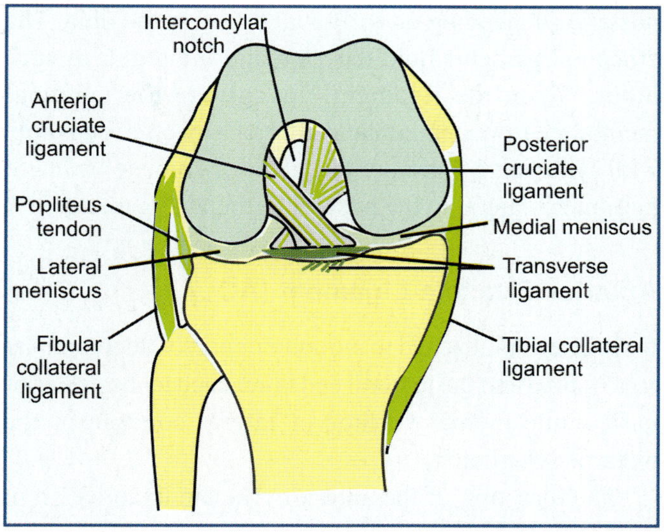

Fig. 190.3: Intra-articular structures of knee joint as seen from anterior aspect in a flexed knee

d. The tibial collateral ligament or TCL (Fig. 190.2) is the thickening of the medial part of the capsule and forms a very strong flat band, about eight to nine cm long. Its upper attachment is to the medial epicondyle of femur. It is divided in superficial and deep layers inferiorly. The deep layer is fused with the capsule and is attached to the articular margin of medial condyle of tibia. The superficial layer is attached to the medial surface of tibia between the medial border of tibia and the insertions of sartorius, gracilis and semitendinosus. Morphologically, this ligament is the lower part of the adductor magnus muscle. Superficially, it is related to the tendons of sartorius, gracilis and semitendinosus and on deeper side it is related to the inferior medial genicular artery and nerve. The medial meniscus is fused with the deep aspect of TCL.
e. The fibular collateral ligament or FCL (Fig. 190.2) is a rounded, cord-like and short. It extends from the lateral epicondyle of femur to the lateral surface of the head of fibula. The tendon of biceps femoris, which is split by the ligament, overlaps it. Morphologically, the fibular collateral ligament is the upper part of peroneus longus muscle. The deep relations of the ligament are the tendon of popliteus, which separates it from the lateral meniscus and the inferior lateral genicular nerve and vessels.

Functions of Collateral Ligaments

Both the collateral ligaments are taut in extension of knee. The fibular collateral ligament prevents adduction (medial rotation) of tibia on the femur while the tibial collateral ligament prevents the abduction (lateral rotation) of tibia on the femur.

Testing Integrity of Collateral Ligaments

The patient is seated on a high stool with legs hanging down but not touching the ground. The lower end of femur is grasped firmly with one hand. The tibia is moved in lateral or medial direction. Abnormal degree of lateral movement suggests rupture of TCL while excessive medial movement means rupture of FCL.

Intra-articular Structures (Fig. 190.3)

The structures inside the knee joint are the cruciate ligaments, semilunar cartilages or menisci, infrapatellar pad of fat, synovial membrane and the tendon of popliteus. The interior of the knee joint can be inspected with the help of arthroscope in the living.

Cruciate Ligaments

There are two cruciate ligaments inside the knee joint. The anterior and posterior cruciate ligaments cross each other like the letter X. They are named anterior and posterior depending on their attachment to the tibia. The cruciate ligaments bind the tibia and the femur to each other. Since the ligaments invaginate the synovial membrane from behind their anterior aspects are covered with synovial membrane. The anterior cruciate ligament lies antero-lateral to the posterior cruciate ligament.

Anterior Cruciate Ligament (ACL)

Its tibial end is attached to the anterior part of intercondylar area of tibia and the femoral end is attached to the posterior part of the medial surface of lateral condyle in the intercondylar notch.

The direction of the anterior cruciate ligament from its tibial to femoral ends is superior, posterior and lateral. This ligament prevents posterior dislocation of femur on tibia and anterior dislocation of tibia on femur. It becomes taut in extension along with all the other ligaments

Posterior Cruciate Ligament (PCL)

It tibial end is attached to the posterior part of the intercondylar area of tibia and the femoral end is attached to anterior part of the lateral surface of the medial condyle in the intercondylar notch.

The direction of the posterior cruciate ligament from its tibial to femoral ends is superior, anterior and medial. This ligament prevents anterior dislocation of femur on tibia and posterior dislocation of tibia on femur. It becomes taut during flexion along with anterior cruciate ligament.

Drawer or Draw Sign

Drawer sign is a test for the integrity of the cruciate ligaments. If there is excessive anterior movement of tibia on the femur with the knee and hip kept flexed in supine position of the body, it is called anterior drawer sign. It indicates injury to anterior cruciate ligament (Fig. 190.4). If the tibia moves excessively in posterior direction it is called posterior drawer sign. This is indicative of injury to posterior cruciate ligament (Fig. 190.5).

Rupture of ACL

Isolated rupture of anterior cruciate ligament may occur if the knee is forcibly hyperextended. The patient presents with acute pain and swelling of the knee joint. The anterior drawer sign is positive. Rupture of cruciate ligaments gives rise to bleeding inside the knee joint (hermarthrosis).

Menisci or Semilunar Cartilages

The menisci are two in number, medial and lateral. They are fibrocartilaginous discs situated on the articular surfaces of tibial condyles. The menisci divide the joint cavity in two chambers in each half, meniscofemoral above and meniscotibial below. They are wedge- shaped plates with thick peripheral and thin inner margins. Each meniscus has two horns, anterior and posterior and two surfaces, superior and inferior. The peripheral margin of the menisci is attached to the fibrous capsule and tibial condyles by the coronary ligaments. The transverse ligament connects the anterior horns of the two menisci to each other.

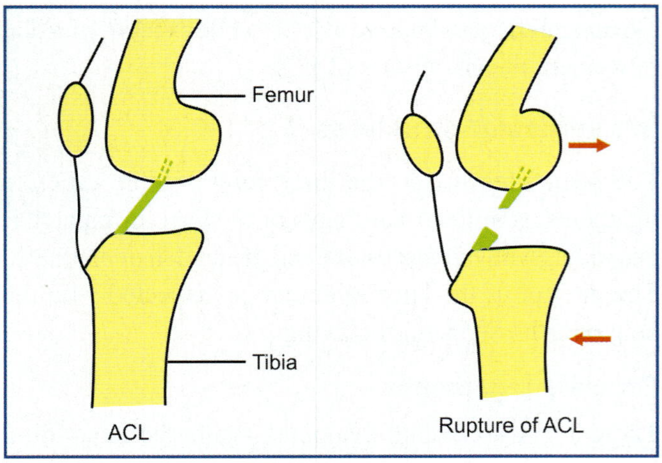

Fig. 190.4: Positive anterior drawer sign in rupture of anterior cruciate ligament

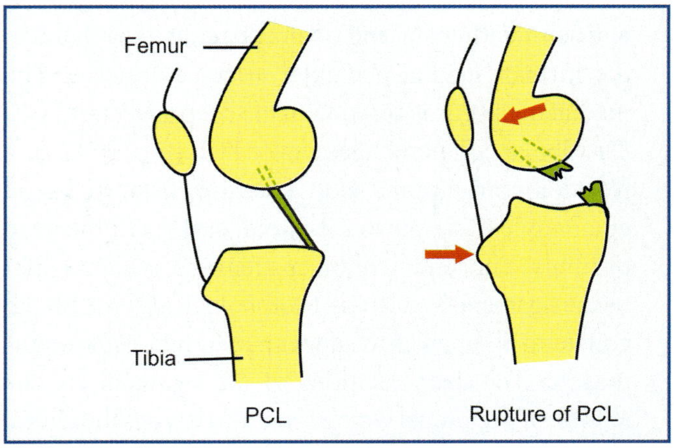

Fig. 190.5: Positive posterior drawer sign in rupture of posterior cruciate ligament

Medial Meniscus

It is a C- shaped cartilage. The two ends of the C represent the two horns of the meniscus, which are attached to the intercondylar area of tibia. Its periphery is fused with the fibrous capsule in the region of tibial collateral ligament. This close proximity of the meniscus and the ligament makes the medial meniscus less mobile and more prone to tears.

Lateral Meniscus

It is circular in shape. The points of attachments of the anterior and posterior horns of the lateral meniscus to the intercondylar area are very close to each other (within the points of attachments of the two horns of medial meniscus). The intracapsular tendon of popliteus intervenes between the lateral meniscus and the fibrous capsule. The peripheral attachment of the lateral meniscus to the capsule is lax hence, the lateral meniscus is more mobile compared to medial. Since a few fibers of popliteus are attached to the posterior horn of lateral meniscus the muscle pulls the meniscus back if the femur is rotated laterally. In this way, the popliteus protects the lateral meniscus from injuries. The posterior horn of lateral meniscus sends two slips, one in front and one behind the posterior cruciate ligament to gain attachment to the medial condyle of femur. These slips are referred to as anterior meniscofemoral ligament of Humphrey and posterior meniscofemoral ligament of Wrisberg.

Nutrition of Menisci

The peripheral thick part of the menisci is vascular and is supplied by the capsular blood vessels. The inner thin part is avascular and is nourished by synovial fluid.

Functions of Menisci

The menisci make the tibial articular surface more concave and congruent with the femoral condylar surface. They act as shock absorber and help in evenly spreading the synovial fluid on the articular surfaces. They divide the joint cavity in two chambers for independent movements. The flexion and extension takes place in meniscofemoral compartment while the rotation occurs in the meniscotibial compartment.

Synovial Membrane (Figs 190.6 and 190.7)

The knee joint has the most extensive synovial membrane. It lines the inner surface of the capsule and covers the nonarticular parts of tibial and femoral condyles inside the joint. The synovial membrane is attached to the margins of patella. Above the patella the synovial membrane extends upward deep to the tendon of quadriceps femoris for a short distance to form the suprapatellar bursa. The articularis genu attached to the synovial membrane of this bursa holds it in position. From the margins of patella the synovial membrane covers the inner aspects of lateral and medial patellar retinacula. Below the patella it extends deep to ligamentum patellae from which it is separated by infrapatellar pad of fat.

Anteriorly, the synovial membrane extends from the deep surface of the ligamentum patellae in the posterior direction covering the deep surface of the infrapatellar pad of fat. This layer of synovial membrane forms the right and left alar folds and in the midline, an infrapatellar fold. The infrapatellar and alar folds with the infrapatellar pad of fat make soft packing between the three bones in the anterior part of the joint cavity. The infrapatellar fold is attached to the most anterior point of the intercondylar notch of the femur. Posteriorly, the synovial membrane lines the posterior part of fibrous capsule and the posterior

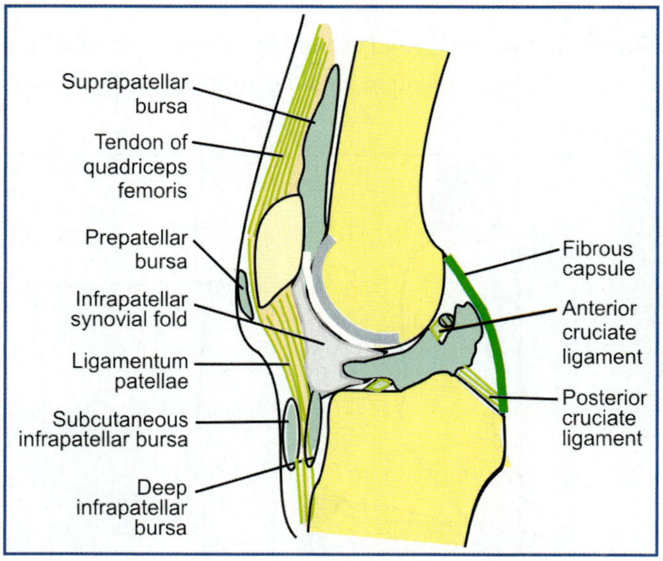

Fig. 190.6: Parasagittal section through knee joint to depict synovial membrane (Note: The anterior bursae in the vicinity of patella)

Section five

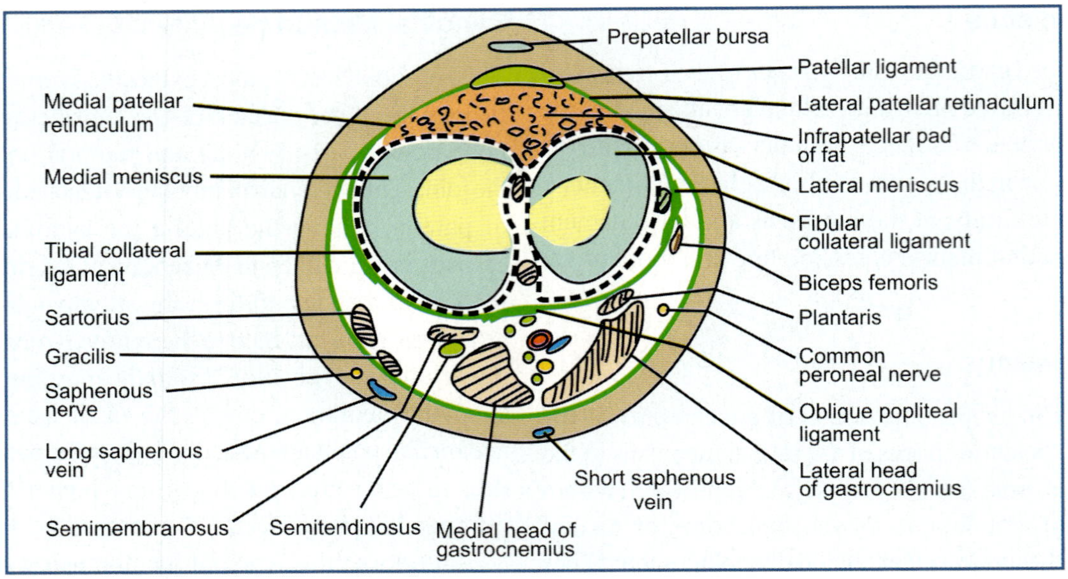

Fig. 190.7: Transverse section of right knee joint to show its relations (Note: Popliteal vessels, tibial nerve and popliteal lymph nodes in popliteal fossa posterior to the joint)

edges of the menisci. It extends anteriorly as a fold inside the intercondylar notch to cover the anterior and lateral aspects of the cruciate ligaments. This fold of synovial membrane is attached to the margins of intercondylar area of tibia and forms a partial partition between the two halves of the joint.

Bursae in Relation to Knee Joint

Several bursae are found around the knee joint, of which four are in communication with the joint cavity. The bursae are divided in three groups according to their relation to the knee as follows.

Anterior Group (Fig. 190.6)

a. Subcutaneous prepatellar bursa is present between the lower part of patella and the skin. When inflamed it gives rise to a painful swelling called prepatellar bursitis or housemaid's knee (Fig. 190.8A).
b. Subcutaneous infrapatellar bursa occupies the space between the ligamentum patellae and the skin.

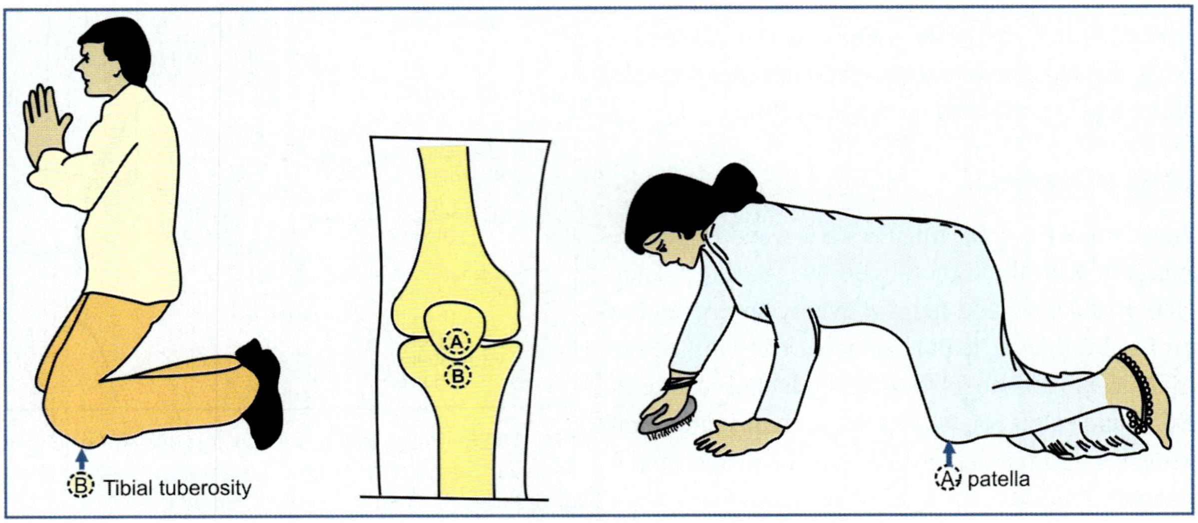

Fig.190.8: Anatomical basis of housemaid's knee (prepatellar bursitis) and clergyman's knee (inflammation of subcutaneous infrapatellar bursa) due to frequent adoption of specific postures

Inflammation of this bursa gives rise to clergyman's knee (Fig. 190.8B).

c. Deep infrapatellar bursa lies between the ligamentum patellae and tibial tuberosity.
d. Suprapatellar bursa is the extension of joint cavity superiorly behind the tendon of quadriceps femoris. Effusion in the knee joint distends this bursa, which is described as water on the knee. On physical examination the patella appears to float over the femur.

Lateral Group

a. Bursa between the lateral head of gastrocnemius and the joint capsule.
b. Bursa between the tendon of biceps femoris and fibular collateral ligament
c. Bursa between the tendon of popliteus and the fibular collateral ligament
d. Popliteus bursa between the lateral condyle of tibia and the tendon of popliteus communicates with the joint cavity.

Medial Group

a. A bursa between the medial head of gastrocnemius and the capsule is known Brodie's bursa. It communicates with the joint cavity.
b. A bursa between the tibial collateral ligament and the tendons of sartorius, gracilis and semitendinosus is called bursa anserine. The term pes anserinus (foot of the goose) is derived from the foot of the goose appearance of insertion of these three tendons on medial surface of tibia. This bursa is in communication with joint cavity.
c. Bursa between the superficial and deep parts of tibial collateral ligament.
d. Bursa between the insertion of semimembranosus and medial condyle of tibia may communicate with the knee joint. Semimembranosus bursitis is a chronic inflammation of the bursa, which may present as a cystic swelling in the medial part of the popliteal fossa. Baker's cyst is a fluctuant swelling in the popliteal fossa either due to inflammation of this bursa or due to projection of synovial membrane from a diseased joint.

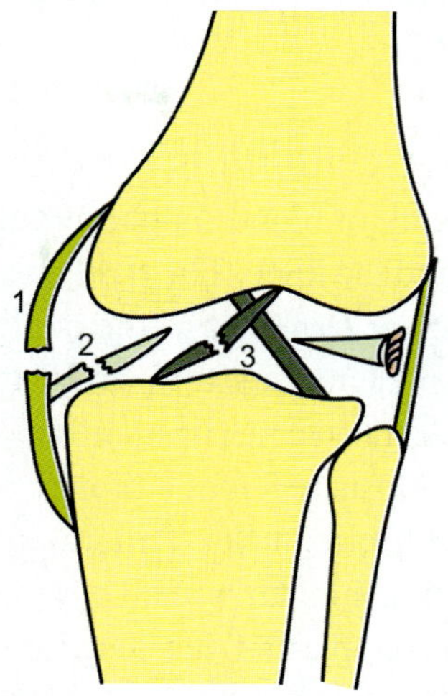

Fig. 190.9: Schematic representation of unhappy triad of knee joint

Relations of Knee Joint (Fig. 190.7)

Anteriorly the joint is related to the tendon of quadriceps femoris, patella and ligamentum patella. The medial patellar retinaculum lies anteromedially and the lateral patellar retinaculum anterolaterally. The tendon of semimembranosus and superficial to it sartorius and gracilis tendons, form the posteromedial relation. The tendon of biceps femoris and the common peroneal nerve outside the joint and tendon of popliteus inside the joint form the posterolateral relation. The popliteal artery and the associated lymph nodes with popliteal vein and tibial nerve are the posterior relations. Medial and lateral heads of gastrocnemius overlap the vessels and tibial nerve.

Nerve Supply

The articular branches of femoral, obturator, common peroneal and tibial nerves supply the knee joint. The femoral nerve supplies through its three branches to vasti. The posterior division of the obturator nerve supplies through its descending articular branch. The tibial nerve gives three genicular branches, superior medial, middle and inferior genicular in the popliteal fossa. The common peroneal nerve gives two genicular branches, superior lateral and inferior lateral in the popliteal fossa. The common peroneal nerve also gives recurrent genicular branch, which arises at its bifurcation (Fig. 191.2) deep to the peroneus longus muscle.

Arterial Supply

The knee joint receives plenty of blood supply through a complex anastomosis around the knee. The right and left superior and inferior genicular branches of the popliteal artery anastomose amongst each other to form bilateral vertical and upper and lower transverse anastomoses. The superior part of this anastomosis receives a branch from descending branch of lateral circumflex femoral artery laterally and the descending genicular branch of femoral artery medially. The inferior part of the anastomosis receives the circumflex fibular branch of posterior tibial artery and the anterior and posterior tibial recurrent branches from the anterior tibial artery. The middle genicular branch of popliteal artery does not take part in the anstomosis since it enters the knee joint by piercing the oblique popliteal ligament.

Movements

The knee joint permits flexion, extension, lateral rotation and medial rotation. The flexion- extension occurs on a mobile transverse axis, which shifts forward during extension and backward during flexion. In this movement the femoral condyles move on the tibia and the menisci in the meniscofemoral compartment. The rotation occurs around a vertical axis in the meniscotibial compartment. There are two types of rotation in the knee joint. The conjunct rotation (about 20-30°) is part of locking-unlocking mechanism. The adjunct rotation (about 50-70°) occurs in the semiflexed knee. Active muscle contraction is necessary for adjunct rotation.

Extension

The anteroposterior diameter of lateral condyle of femur is less than that of that of medial condyle. Therefore, the lateral femoral condylar surface comes in contact with the articular surface of tibial condyle earlier than that of the medial condyle in the process of extension. A small part of medial condylar articular surface of femur remains without making contact with the tibial articular surface. To achieve full congruity between the articular surfaces of the medial condyles of the two bones, the femur rotates medially on the tibia or the tibia rotates laterally on the femur. The femur can rotate on the tibia when the foot is on the ground while the tibia can rotate on the femur if the foot is off the ground. The 20 to 30° of rotation at the final stage of extension is part and parcel of the movement of extension, hence, called conjunct rotation. It is also described as screw home movement or locking mechanism. In this position the joint is maximally congruent and the ligaments are taut. A person is able to stand for hours together without strain to the quadriceps femoris when the knee joint is locked and the center of gravity lies in front of the transverse axis of the joint. The muscle responsible for extension is quadriceps femoris assisted by tensor fasciae latae.

Flexion

From a fully extended knee the flexion begins by the unlocking movement, which consists of lateral rotation of femur or medial rotation of tibia (depending on whether the foot is on or off the ground). This rotation is also integral at the beginning of flexion, hence, it is conjunct rotation though it requires contraction of popliteus muscle (key of knee joint). Hamstring group of muscles assisted by gastrocnemius, plantaris and popliteus brings about the flexion.

Rotation in Semiflexed Knee

In the semiflexed knee about 50 to 70° of adjunct rotation is possible with the help of active contraction of muscles. Popliteus, semitendinosus and semimembranosus are the medial rotators while the popliteus and biceps femoris are the lateral rotators.

Radiological Anatomy

In the anteroposterior view of the radiograph of knee, the adductor tubercle may be seen above the medial condyle of femur. The tibial and femoral condyles can be visualized with the shadow of patella overlying the femur. The intercondylar tubercles of tibia can be seen projecting in the joint space. The shadow of the infrapatellar fat pad may be visible. Fabella (a sesamoid bone in lateral head of gastrocnemius at its origin) is visible on lateral projection. The patella is also best visible in the lateral view. Arthrography is a special investigation in which air

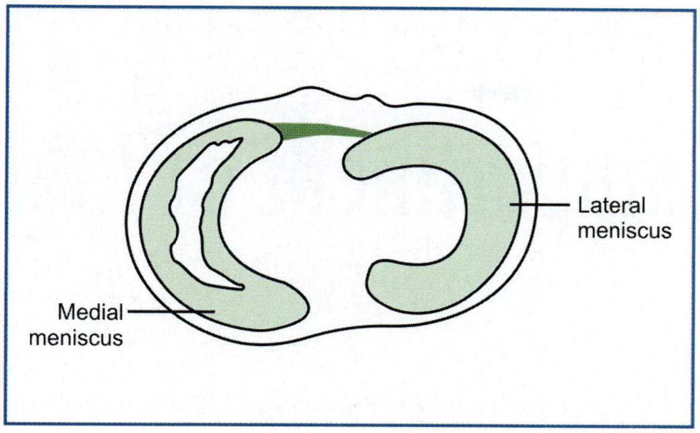

Fig. 190.10: Bucket handle tear of medial meniscus of right knee joint

or opaque fluids are injected in the joint cavity before taking radiographs. The menisci can be examined by this technique.

Clinical Highlights

a. The internal derangement of the knee joint causes serious interference with the joint function. The collateral ligaments, cruciate ligaments and the menisci are the structures that are injured. The injury to any of these structures is associated with traumatic synovitis. A combination of injury to the tibial collateral ligament, medial meniscus and anterior cruciate ligament is called 'unhappy triad' of knee joint (Fig. 190.9).

b. The medial meniscus injuries are more common than that of lateral meniscus because it is firmly fused with the tibial collateral ligament. A sudden blow on the lateral side of a flexed weight-bearing knee can cause rupture of the tibial collateral ligament with a concomitant tear in the medial meniscus. The bucket handle rupture (Fig. 190.10) of the medial meniscus is common in football players. On rupture of the meniscus the patient feels sudden pain in the knee. The knee gets locked in the flexed position and swollen due to synovitis. The chances of the knee getting struck on the medial side are far less in sports hence the injury to lateral collateral ligament is much less. Moreover, the injury to this ligament does not result in the tear of lateral meniscus because the lateral meniscus is more mobile and the tendon of popliteus protects it.

c. Runner's knee or patello-femoral pain syndrome is a very common condition in athletes. Symptoms of runner's knee include pain near the patella. Pain is also felt after sitting for a long stretch with the knees bent. This condition happens when the patella is not able to track smoothly on condyles of femur. Conditions that increase the Q angle like, wide pelvis, genu valgum, patella alta (high patella) and weak vastus medialis increase the chance of having runner's knee.

191 Anterior Compartment of Leg

The leg is the part of the lower limb between the knee and ankle. It is divided in three osteofascial compartments by bones and fasciae and intermuscular septae (Fig. 191.1).

Deep Fascia of Leg

The deep fascia of the leg is continuous above, with the fascia lata. It is strengthened in the region of knee by expansions from the tendons of sartorius, gracilis and semitendinosus medially and biceps femoris laterally. The deep fascia is attached to the condyles of tibia, head of fibula, tibial tuberosity and patella. The patella is attached to the tibial condyles by the medial and lateral patellar retinacula, which are thickened bands of deep fascia reinforced by tendons of vastus madialis and lateralis respectively. At the anterior and medial borders of tibia, the deep fascia becomes continuous with the periosteum covering the subcutaneous medial surface of the tibia. Two intermuscular septa pass from the deep aspect of the deep fascia towards the fibula. The anterior intermuscular septum, which intervenes between the lateral and anterior compartments, is attached to the anterior border of fibula. The posterior intermuscular septum, which intervenes between the lateral and posterior compartments, is attached to the posterior border of fibula. At the ankle, the deep fascia is modified to form flexor, extensor and peroneal retinacula, which help in strapping down the tendons at the ankle.

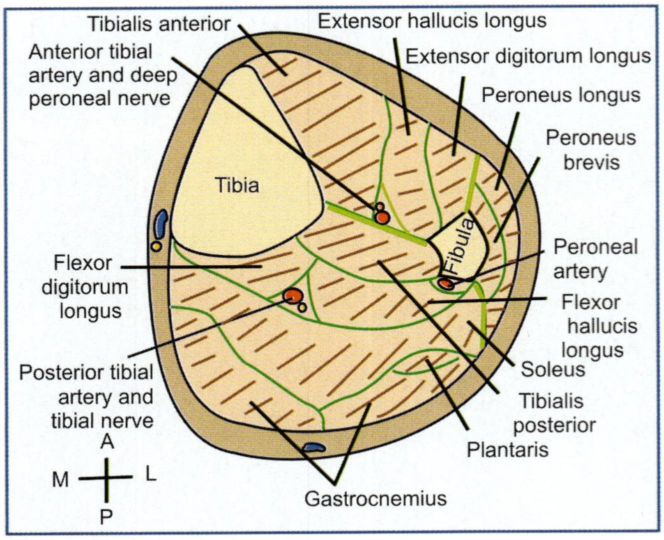

Fig.191.1: Cross-section through middle of leg to show boundaries and contents of osteofascial compartments (Note that anterior and posterior intermuscular septa and interosseous membrane are attached to respective borders of fibula)

Boundaries of Anterior Compartment (Fig. 191.1)

The anterior compartment is limited laterally by the anterior intermuscular septum and medially by the lateral surface of the tibia. The interosseous membrane and the narrow anteromedial surface of fibula limit it posteriorly and the investing layer of deep fascia of leg bound it anteriorly.

Contents (Fig. 191.2)

The anterior compartment contains four muscles (tibialis anterior, extensor digitorum longus, extensor hallucis longus and peroneus tertius), anterior tibial vessels and deep peroneal nerve. The perforating branch of peroneal artery enters the compartment from the posterior compartment of leg by piercing the interosseous membrane (this branch is described with peroneal artery in posterior compartment of leg).

Tibialis Anterior (TA)

This muscle takes origin from the upper two thirds of the lateral surface of tibia and adjacent interosseous membrane and is inserted on the medial surface of medial cuneiform and the base of first metatarsal bone. The anterior tibial recurrent artery (a branch of anterior tibial artery) and recurrent genicular nerve (a branch of common peroneal nerve at its bifurcation) pass through the substance of the tibialis anterior.

Nerve Supply

The muscle receives twigs from the deep peroneal nerve and recurrent genicular nerve.

Actions

The tibialis anterior is the dorsiflexior of foot at the ankle joint and invertor of the foot at the midtarsal and subtalar joints. It assists in maintenance of medial longitudinal arch of the foot.

Testing Function of TA

The subject is asked to dorsiflex the foot against the resistance of examiner's hand placed across the dorsum of the foot.

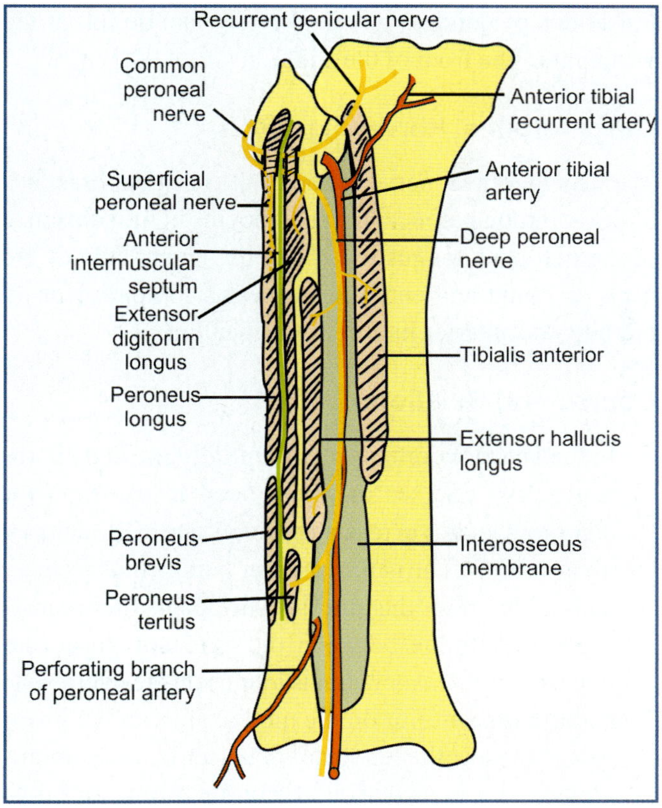

Fig. 191.2: Scheme showing structures in the anterior compartment of leg. (Figure also shows peroneus longus and brevis belonging to lateral compartment)

Extensor Hallucis Longus (EHL)

This muscle takes origin from the medial part of the anteromedial surface of the middle two fourths of fibula and adjacent interosseous membrane. The tendon of the muscle emerges between the extensor digitorum longus and tibialis anterior in the lower part of leg. It is inserted in the base of terminal phalanx of the great toe.

Nerve Supply

It is supplied by the deep peroneal nerve.

Actions

The extensor hallucis longus produces the dorsiflexion of foot at the ankle and dorsiflexion of the great toe. It is an important support of medial longitudinal arch.

Testing Function of EHL

The subject attempts to dorsiflex the great toe against resistance.

Extensor Digitorum Longus (EDL)

This muscle takes origin from the upper three fourths of the anteromedial surface of the fibula, adjacent interosseous membrane and anterior intermuscular septum. The extensor digitorum longus divides in to four tendons on the dorsum of foot. The tendons of second to fourth toes fuse with the tendons of extensor digitorum brevis and together they form the dorsal digital expansion. At the proximal interphalangeal joint each dorsal digital expansion divides into three slips. The median slip is attached to the base of middle phalanx and the collateral slips unite before inserting in the base of terminal phalanx.

Nerve Supply

It is supplied by the deep peroneal nerve.

Actions

The extensor digitorum longus produces the dorsiflexion of ankle joint and the dorsiflexion of lateral four toes.

Testing Function of EDL

The subject is asked to dorsiflex the toes against resistance.

Peroneus Tertius

It takes origin from the lower part of anteromedial surface of fibula (in continuation with the extensor digitorum longus) and is inserted into the dorsal surface of the base of fifth metatarsal bone.

Nerve Supply

It is supplied by the deep peroneal nerve.

Actions

It produces dorsiflexion at ankle joint and is a weak evertor of foot.

Anterior Tibial Artery (Fig. 191.2)

The anterior tibial artery is the smaller terminal branch of the popliteal artery in the back of the leg at the distal margin of the popliteus. It enters the anterior compartment by passing through the gap above the superior margin of the interosseous membrane. The artery lies very close to the medial aspect of the fibular neck in the uppermost part of the compartment. Then, it descends in contact with the anterior surface of the interosseous membrane and is flanked by venae comitantes. The anterior tibial artery continues as the dorsalis pedis artery in front of the ankle. The artery is deeply placed in the upper two-thirds of the leg, but, is superficial in the lower third.

Relations

a. Posteriorly, the proximal two-thirds of the artery is in direct contact with the interosseous membrane. Its lower third is in contact with the lateral surface of tibia and front of ankle joint.
b. Anteriorly, the three muscles namely, TA, EHL and EDL cover its proximal two-thirds. In the lower part of the leg the tendon of extensor hallucis longus crosses the artery in front. Below this level, it is superficial and covered by fasciae and extensor retinaculum.
c. Medially, it is related to the tibialis anterior muscle and lower down, to the tendon of extensor hallucis longus.
d. Laterally, it is related to the neck of fibula followed by extensor digitorum longus in the upper third and the extensor hallucis longus in the middle third. At the ankle, the extensor digitorum longus lies laterally.

Branches

a. The posterior tibial recurrent artery arises before the anterior tibial artery enters the anterior compartment. It takes part in genicular anastomosis.
b. The anterior tibial recurrent artery passes through the tibialis anterior muscle and takes part in genicular anastomosis.
c. The anterior medial malleolar artery takes part in medial malleolar network
d. The anterior lateral malleolar artery takes part in lateral malleolar network.
e. Besides the named branches, there are numerous muscular branches.

Surface Marking

The artery can be represented by a line, which begins about 2.5 cm inferior to the medial side of the head of fibula and ends at the midpoint between the malleoli.

Anterior Tibial Pulse

Pulsations of the anterior tibial artery can be felt at the midpoint of the front of the ankle.

Deep Peroneal Nerve (Fig. 191.2)

The deep peroneal nerve is one of the terminal branches of the common peroneal nerve. It begins in the substance of the peroneus longus muscle at the lateral side of the neck of fibula and enters the anterior compartment by piercing the anterior intermuscular septum.

Course and Relations

a. In the anterior compartment, initially the deep peroneal nerve courses medially deep to the extensor digitorum longus to reach the lateral side of the anterior tibial vessels. The neurovascular bundle thus formed, travels down on the anterior surface of the interosseous membrane between the extensor digitorum longus and extensor hallucis longus on the lateral side and tibialis anterior on the medial side. In the lower part of the leg, the tendon of extensor hallucis longus crosses the neurovascular bundle from lateral to medial side. The deep peroneal nerve is called the nervus hesitans due to its relations to the anterior tibial aretery. The nerve though initially lateral in position, gradually comes in front of the artery but at the lower level, again, goes back in lateral position (as if the nerve hesitates to cross the artery). It gives branches to the four muscles of the compartment and supplies articular branch to the ankle joint.

b. In front of the ankle, the deep peroneal nerve passes deep to the extensor retinaculum on way to the dosrum of foot. It is located midway between the two malleoli, between the tendons of extensor hallucis longus (medially) and extensor digitorum longus (laterally).

c. On the dorsum of the foot, the peroneal nerve terminates immediately into lateral and medial branches (Fig. 194.1). The medial terminal branch courses distally to reach the first interdigital cleft. During its course, it gives articular branches to the adjacent intertarsal joints, muscular branch to first dorsal interosseous muscle and dorsal digital nerves to the skin of first interdigital cleft (adjacent sides of first and second toes). The lateral terminal branch passes distally deep to the extensor digitorum brevis and enlarges into a pseudoganglion, which gives a muscular branch to the extensor digitorum brevis and three tiny interosseous branches to the tarsal and metatarsophalangeal joints of the middle three toes. The first interosseous branch also supplies the second dorsal interosseous muscle.

Clinical Highlights

a. Anterior compartment syndrome may develop as a result of unaccustomed strenuous exercise, which leads to marked swelling of the muscles of the compartment. This may impede venous return leading to more accumulation of fluid inside the compartment, which has unyielding walls. Other common cause of fluid accumulation is bleeding due to fracture of the tibia. The increased pressure in the closed space tends to compress the contents. Arterial insufficiency may lead to the gangrene of the leg or foot. The compression of deep peroneal nerve may cause severe pain in the leg and weakness of the muscles of the compartment. To relieve the compression, the deep fascia of the leg is surgically incised (fasciotomy) along the whole length of the compartment.

b. Shin splints is a condition that results from overexertion or traumatic injury to the tibialis anterior. Some people, who are not used to exercise, after a long walk, experience pain in the front of leg. Sudden exercise may cause micro-trauma to tibialis anterior or tears in the periosteum of tibia.

c. Injury to deep peroneal nerve leads to paralysis of dorsiflexors resulting in foot drop. The patient walks on the tips of the toes, on the affected side. There is loss of sensation on the skin along the adjacent sides of the first and second toes.

192 Peroneal Compartment of Leg

The peroneal or the lateral compartment of the leg is smallest in size. It is bounded by the anterior intermuscular septum anteriorly and posterior intermuscular septum posteriorly. The lateral surface of the fibula forms its medial boundary and the deep fascia of leg is on its lateral side (Fig. 191.1). This compartment contains the peroneus longus and brevis muscles. The termination of common peroneal nerve into deep peroneal and superficial peroneal nerves, occurs in the upper part of the compartment. The recurrent genicular branch of common peroneal nerve takes origin here (Fig. 191.2).

Muscles of Peroneal Compartment (Fig. 192.1)

a. The peroneus longus takes origin from the head and upper two thirds of the lateral surface of fibula. The common peroneal nerve passes through the gap between its two attachments to fibula. The muscle becomes tendinous in the lower part of the leg. Its long tendon changes direction around the lateral malleolus, where it is strapped by the superior peroneal retinaculum. On the lateral side of the calcaneus, it is strapped by the inferior peroneal retinaculum. It courses forwards in the foot below the peroneal trochlea of calcaneus to reach the lateral margin of foot, where it changes direction to enter the groove on the plantar surface of the cuboid. Further, it crosses the sole from lateral to medial side to reach its insertion on medial cuneiform and base of first metatarsal bone (Fig. 200.3).

Special Features of Peroneus Longus

i. The peroneus longus has a very long tendon, which changes direction at two places in its course, first at the lateral malleolus and second at the cuboid bone

ii. The tendon crosses across the sole from lateral to medial side deeply grooving the cuboid bone.

iii. The common peroneal, deep peroneal and superficial peroneal nerves lie deep to it at the neck of fibula. The superficial peroneal nerve passes through the substance of peroneus longus for a short distance.

b. Peroneus brevis takes origin from the lower two-thirds of the lateral surface of fibula. It lies deep to peroneus longus. The tendon of peroneus brevis is in direct contact with the lateral malleolus and that of peroneus longus lies superficial to it. Like the peroneus longus its tendon passes under the peroneal retinacula. The peroneus brevis courses forwards above the peroneal

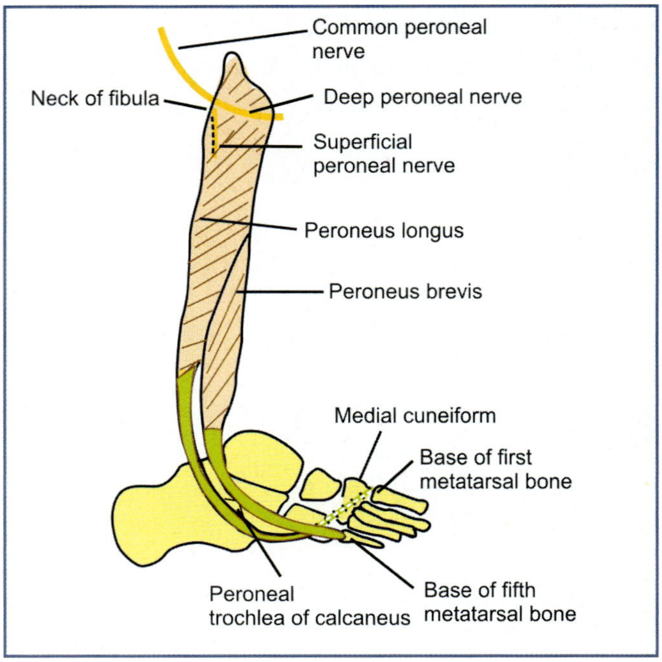

Fig. 192.1: Scheme to depict muscles of lateral compartment of leg

trochlea to insert in to the lateral aspect of the tuberosity of the base of the fifth metatarsal bone.

Synovial Sheath of Peroneal Tendons

The tendons of peroneus longus and brevis are very close to each other as they pass deep to the peroneal retinacula. They are covered with a common synovial sheath from the lateral malleolus to peroneal trochlea. Beyond this, there is a separate synovial sheath for each tendon upto its insertion (Fig. 194.2). The reason for two synovial sheaths at this level is that deep to inferior peroneal retinaculum separate osteofascial spaces are formed due to the presence of a septum from the inferior peroneal retinaculum to the peroneal trochlea.

Nerve Supply

The peroneus longus and brevis muscles are innervated by superficial peroneal nerve.

Actions

The peroneus longus and brevis muscles produce eversion of foot at subtalar and midtarsal joints. They assist in extreme plantar flexion of foot at ankle joint. The tendon of peroneus longus acts as a pulley that supports the arches of foot from above.

Testing Muscle Function

A subject in the supine position is asked to evert the foot against resistance, when the foot is raised from the bed. Isolated weakness of peroneal muscles thus found, may be the earliest sign of peroneal muscular atrophy.

Superficial Peroneal Nerve

The superficial peroneal nerve is the nerve of lateral compartment of leg. It is one of the terminal branches of the common peroneal nerve deep to the peroneus longus muscle (Fig. 191.2). From this level it travels down in the intermuscular plane between the two peroneal muscles, which it supplies. At the junction of upper two-thirds and lower one-third of the leg, it pierces the deep fascia to enter the superficial fascia of the leg and supplies the skin of the lower part of leg. The superficial peroneal nerve divides into medial and lateral branches in the lower part of leg. Both the terminal branches cross in front of the extensor retinaculum to enter the dorsum of the foot. Its course and distribution on the dorsum are shown in Figure 175.2. The medial terminal branch divides in two dorsal digital nerves, which supply the medial side of great toe and adjacent sides of second and third toes. The smaller lateral branch divides in two dorsal digital branches for the adjacent sides of third and fourth and fourth and fifth toes. In addition, the terminal branches supply the skin of the larger intermediate area of the dorsum.

Clinical Highlights

Lesion of the superficial peroneal nerve causes weakness of eversion of the foot and sensory loss on the lateral aspect of leg extending on the intermediate area of dorsum of foot and the toes except the first interdigital cleft and lateral side of fifth toe.

193 Posterior Compartment of Leg

The posterior compartment of the leg is the largest osteofascial compartment. Superiorly, it is continuous with the popliteal fossa. Inferiorly, it is continuous with the sole of foot behind the flexor retinaculum.

Boundaries and Subdivisions (Fig.191.1)

This compartment is bounded anteriorly by the posterior surfaces of tibia and fibula and the interosseous membrane. Its posterior limit is the deep fascia of the leg. Its lateral boundary is the posterior intermuscular septum and medial boundary is the attachment of the deep fascia to the medial border of tibia.

The compartment is subdivided into two parts (superficial and deep) by a transverse septum, which is attached to the soleal line above, medial border of tibia medially, posterior border of fibula laterally and is continuous with the flexor retinaculum below. The superficial subdivision of the compartment contains gastrocnemius, soleus and plantaris muscles, which are the superficial muscles of calf. The deep subdivision contains flexor digitorum longus, flexor hallucis longus, and tibialis posterior and popliteus muscles including the tibial nerve and posterior tibial artery and peroneal artery. The tibialis posterior is the deepest muscle lying on the interosseous membrane. Between it and the long flexors of the toes there is s fascial layer spanning between the tibia and fibula.

Gastrocnemius

This muscle arises by two heads from the lower end of femur. The lateral head arises from the lateral aspect of lateral condyle of femur by a tendon. Occasionally, a sesamoid bone, called fabella develops in the tendon of lateral head. The medial head arises from the upper and posterior part of medial condyle behind the adductor tubercle and part of the popliteal surface of femur just above the medial condyle. The tendinous origin of medial head is separated from the capsule of knee joint by a bursa. The plantaris, gastrocnemius and soleus insert in the middle one-third of posterior surface of calcaneus by tendocalcaneus.

Nerve Supply

The medial and lateral heads receive separate branches of the tibial nerve in popliteal fossa.

Tennis Leg

It is a painful calf injury in which there is a tear of medial belly of gastrocnemius at its musculotendinous junction, due to overstretching.

Plantaris

It is a fusiform muscle with small belly and long tendon, lying under cover of the lateral head of gastrocnemius. It arises from the lower third of lateral supracondylar ridge of femur. It is inserted in the calcaneus through the tendocalcaneus. Plantaris is a vestigeal muscle and plantar aponeurosis is said to be its degenerated part. A branch from tibial nerve in popliteal fossa, innervates it. The plantaris tendon is used for tendon grafting in the repair of ruptured long tendons in the hand (palmaris longus tendon serves similar purpose).

Soleus

It is a very powerful muscle situated deep to the gastrocnemius. It is multipennate flat muscle.

Attachments

It has a broad, horseshoe shaped origin from the upper one third of the posterior surface of fibula, soleal line and middle third of the medial border of tibia and the tendinous arch posterior to the neurovascular structures of the compartment. The massive muscle belly gives rise to a tendon, which fuses with the tendon of gastrocnemius to form tendocalcaneus by which it is inserted into the calcaneus.

Nerve Supply

The branches of the tibial nerve in the popliteal fossa supply the muscle.

Tendocalcaneus (Achillis Tendon)

The tendocalcaneus is the thickest and strongest tendon in the body (length 15 cm). It begins in the middle of calf, although its anterior aspect receives muscle fibres of soleus almost to its lower end. About four cm above the calcaneus, it becomes flattened and is inserted into the posterior surface of calcaneus. This tendon is very important in conserving the energy and releasing it in the next stage in gait cycle. Unlike the other long tendons at the ankle, the tendocalcaneus is not enveloped in the synovial sheath. The tendon is related to two bursae. The calcaneal bursa, between the calcaneus and the tendon is prone to inflammation in long distance runners. There is a bursa between the tendon and the skin (adventitious bursa).

Actions of Superficial Calf Muscles

a. The gastrocnemius and soleus muscles cause plantarflexion of foot at the ankle joint. In flexed position of knee, the gastrocnemius cannot act on the ankle, so soleus alone is the plantarflexor.
b. Both muscles provide the main propulsive force in walking and running, though gastrocnemius is more active in these movements. The gastrocnemius is an example of white muscle composed mainly of the fast fatigue-susceptible type of muscle fibres.
c. Gastrocnemius is a flexor of knee.
d. Soleus is a postural muscle. It is a red muscle consisting mainly of slow fatigue- resistant muscle fibres.
e. Gastrocnemius and soleus together make the calf muscle pump for facilitating venous return from the lower limb. The soleus is regarded as the peripheral heart because it houses large venous sinuses, which are connected to superficial veins by perforating veins, which veins pass through soleus. Thus contraction of soleus helps in sucking the blood in to the perforating veins and propelling it towards the deep veins of the posterior compartment.

Testing Function of Muscles

a. On asking the subject to plantarflex against resistance with knee in extended position, one can feel the contraction of the gastrocnemius.
b. For soleus, the subject is asked to plantarflex against resistance with knee in flexed position.

Clinical Highlights

a. The sprain and rupture of tendoaclcaneus (Fig. 193.1) are common injuries. The rupture causes sudden pain in the calf. Due to retraction of the muscle bellies of gastrocnemius proximally, a gap can be felt in the tendon. There is loss of plantarflexion of the foot. The ruptured tendon can be sutured and strengthened using fascia lata.
b. The ankle jerk or Achillis tendon reflex is elicited as follows. On tapping the tendon with knee hammer, there is reflex contraction of gastrocnemius with resultant plantarflexion of the foot. The nerve responsible for this is the tibial nerve and the spinal center is S1 segment. In paralysis of gastrocnemius the patient will not be able to stand on the toes and there will be loss of ankle jerk.

Posterior Tibial Artery

The posterior tibial artery is a terminal branch of the popliteal artery at the lower margin of popliteus muscle.

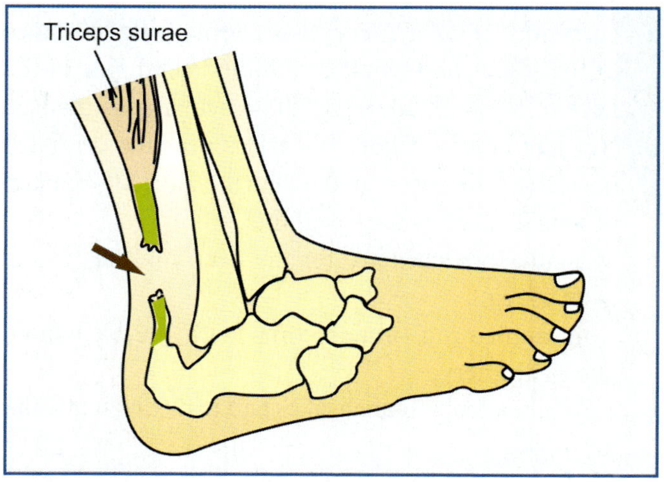

Fig. 193.1: Rupture of tendocalcaneus resulting in dorsiflexed foot

The venae comitantes and the tibial nerve are closely associated with the artery. The neurovascular structures enter the posterior compartment by passing under the tendinous arch.

Course and Relations (Fig. 193.2)

The artery passes vertically downwards in the posterior compartment and divides into lateral and medial plantar arteries deep to the flexor retinaculum. Anteriorly, the artery rests on the posterior surfaces of tibialis posterior and flexor digitorum longus muscles, posterior aspect of tibia and the capsule of the ankle joint. Posteriorly, it is separated by the transverse septum from the superficial calf muscles. Distally, it is covered by skin and fasciae and hence lies very close to the surface. Its terminal part is deep to the flexor retinaculum and abductor hallucis. The tibial nerve is at first medial to the artery but gradually changes to posterior position and in the lower part it lies posterolateral to the artery.

Surface Marking

It corresponds to a line from the midline on the back of the leg at the level of the neck of fibula to a point midway between the tendocalcaneus and medial malleolus.

Posterior Tibial Pulse (Fig. 193.3)

The posterior tibial pulse can be felt behind and below the medial malleolus between the tendons of flexor hallucis longus and flexor digitorum longus.

Branches

a. Circumflex fibular artery passes through the substance of the soleus and winds round the lateral side of the neck of fibula. It takes part in genicular anastomosis.
b. Nutrient artery of the tibia arises near the origin of posterior tibial artery and enters the nutrient foramen of tibia just below the soleal line.
c. Muscular branches are for the deep muscles of the back of leg.
d. Communicating branch joins with the branch of peroneal artery.
e. Medial malleolar branch takes part in medial malleolar network.
f. Medial calcanean branches pierce the flexor retinaculum and supply the skin of the heel.

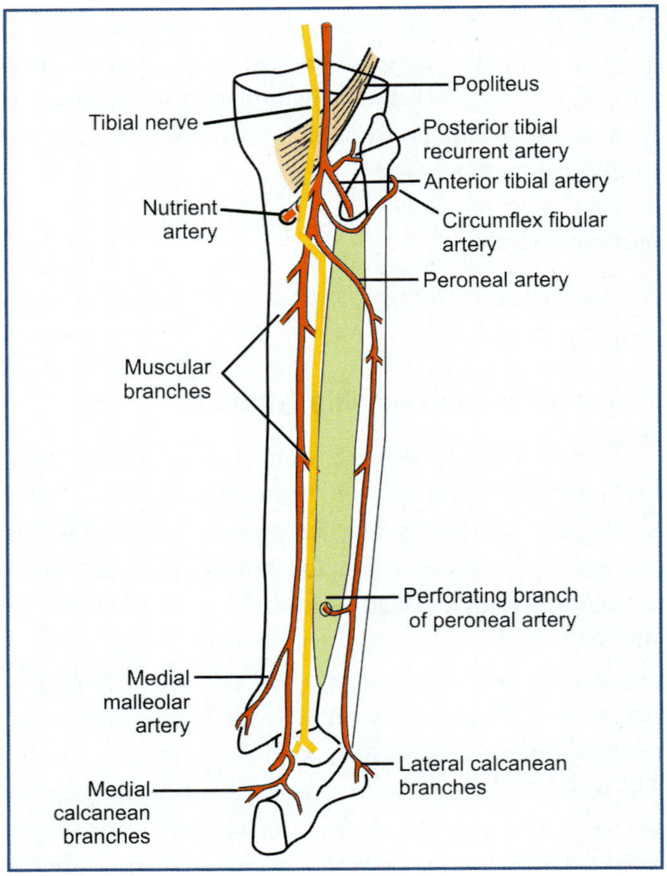

Fig. 193.2: Schematic depiction of the branches of arteries in posterior compartment of leg (Note: The tibialis posterior muscle lying anterior to posterior tibial artery)

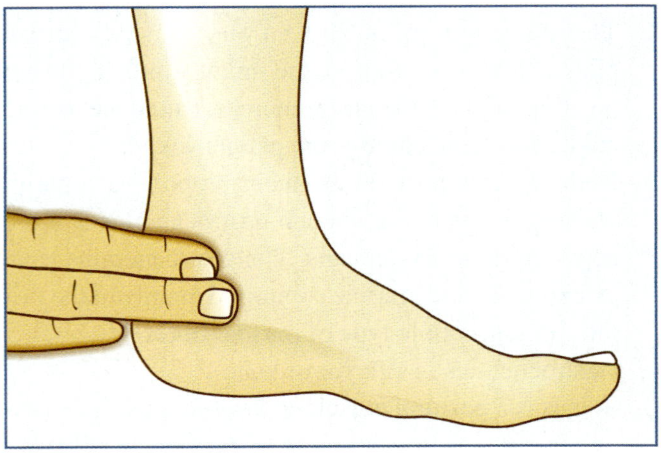

Fig. 193.3: Palpation of posterior tibial pulse

g. The peroneal artery (Fig. 193.2) is a large branch that arises very close to the beginning of the posterior tibial artery. It travels the entire length of the compartment lying in close contact with the medial crest of the fibula in a fibrous tunnel between the tibialis posterior and flexor hallucis longus muscles (Fig. 191.1). It terminates on the lateral aspect as the lateral calcanean branches, which take part in the lateral malleolar network. The branches of the peroneal artery are, muscular to the proneal muscles, nutrient to the fibula, the communicating branch to join with communicating branch of posterior tibial artery and the perforating branch, which passes through the lower part of interosseous membrane to enter the anterior compartment of leg. The perforating artery after reaching anterior aspect of the leg anastomoses with the lateral malleolar branch of anterior tibial artery and with the lateral tarsal artery (a branch of dorsalis pedis) to form lateral malleolar network. The perforating branch is sometimes enlarged in which case it may replace the dorsalis pedis artery.

Clinical Highlights

Arterial insufficiency in the leg is characterized by intermittent claudication, (pain in the calf muscles is felt on walking, but disappears after rest). On walking, when the demand for more blood is not met, the muscle ischemia causes pain. The causes of narrowing of the arteries are atherosclerosis, diabetes and hypertension. In young men, a condition called thromboangiitis obliterans (TAO) develops in blood vessels of leg due to chronic smoking. The serious complication of the arterial insufficiency is the gangrene of the toes or foot or the leg.

Posterior Tibial Veins

The veins accompanying the posterior tibial artery (venae comitantes) are the posterior tibial veins. These veins begin deep to the flexor retinaculum by the union of veins accompanying the lateral and medial plantar arteries. The tributaries of the posterior tibial veins are the veins from the muscles, especially the venous plexus in the soleus and peroneal veins. The perforating veins connecting these veins to the great saphenous vein are provided with unidirectional valves so that blood flows from the superficial to the deep veins. The venae comitantes of the posterior and anterior tibial arteries unite at the lower margin of popliteus muscle to form popliteal vein.

Clinical Highlights

The deep veins of the leg are clinically very important because they are prone to thrombosis, if the lower limb is immobilized for any reason (plaster cast on leg or postoperative period). If the thrombus is detached it may enter venous circulation and reach the pulmonary arteries via right side of heart causing fatal pulmonary embolism.

Tibial Nerve

The tibial nerve in the popliteal fossa continues as the tibial nerve of posterior compartment of leg, at the distal border of popliteus muscle. It enters the posterior compartment along with posterior tibial vessels deep to the tendinous arch of origin of the soleus.

Course and Relations

Its relations are similar to those of the posterior tibial artery. The tibial nerve lies applied to the anterior surface of the deep transverse septum throughout its course. The nerve lies medial to the posterior tibial vessels deep to the tendinous arch of soleus muscle. Below this level, the nerve crosses the vessels posteriorly from medial to lateral direction. At the ankle, the nerve is lateral to the artery. It divides deep to the flexor retinaculum into lateral and medial plantar nerves.

Branches

a. The muscular branches are given to tibialis posterior, flexor digitorum longus and flexor hallucis longus. The soleus may also receive a branch in the leg.
b. The articular branches supply the ankle joint.
c. The medial calcanean branches pierce the flexor retinaculum to supply the skin over the heel.

Clinical Highlights

Being deep in location, injury to tibial nerve is less common in both popliteal fossa and the posterior compartment of leg. However, in case of injury all the muscles of the posterior compartment of leg and all the intrinsic muscles of the foot are paralyzed. The foot is held in calcaneovalgus position due to unresisted action of dorsiflexors and evertors. There is sensory loss on the sole and trophic ulcers may develop as a consequence.

Popliteus

The popliteus is the muscle of the leg, which lies in the lower part of the floor of popliteal fossa. This muscle is important in unlocking a locked knee joint. Therefore, it is referred to as the key to the knee joint.

Attachments

The popliteus takes origin from the anterior end of the popliteal groove on the lateral condyle of femur. Its origin is tendinous and is located inside the capsule of knee joint. At origin it is attached to the back of lateral meniscus. The intracapsular tendon of popliteus intervenes between the lateral meniscus and fibular collateral ligament. The long tendon enclosed in synovial sheath pierces the posterior part of fibrous capsule, below the arcuate popliteal ligament. The tendon expands in a triangular fleshy belly, which is inserted on the posterior surface of tibia above the soleal line.

Relations (Fig. 188.2)

The posterior surface of the popliteus is covered with a strong fascia, which is an extension from the insertion of semimembranosus. This surface is related to the popliteal vessels and tibial nerve. Its anterior surface is in contact with the tibia. The following four events occur at its distal margin, division of popliteal artery, formation of popliteal vein, entry of the tibial nerve into the posterior compartment of leg and nerve to popliteus winds round this margin to reach the anterior surface of the muscle.

Nerve Supply

The nerve to popliteus is a branch of the tibial nerve in the popliteal fossa. This nerve travels to the lower margin of the muscle, where it winds round to reach its anterior surface. The branches of the nerve enter the anterior aspect of the popliteus. The nerve to popliteus also supplies a few twig to tibialis posterior, proximal and distal tibiofibular joints and interosseous membrane.

Actions

a. The popliteus rotates the tibia medially on the femur, when the foot is off the ground and it rotates the femur on the tibia laterally, when the foot is on the ground. This movement is known as unlocking as it occurs at the beginning of flexion of a fully extended or locked knee joint.
b. It is the flexor of knee joint and the lateral rotator of the semiflexed knee.
c. It protects the lateral meniscus from injury.

Flexor Digitorum Longus (FDL)

This muscle arises from the posterior surface of tibia below the soleal line and medial to the tibial origin of tibialis posterior and from the fascia covering the tibialis posterior. Its tendon crosses superficial to the tendon of tibialis posterior in the lower part of leg. At the ankle, it passes behind the flexor retinaculum and then enters the sole. In the sole, the tendon turns laterally and crosses superficial to the tendon of flexor hallucis longus. The flexor digitorum longus receives some fibres from the flexor hallucis longus tendon during the crossing (the connection being called William Turner's slip). This connection serves the purpose of strengthening the flexor digitorum longus muscle. The FDL tendon, also receives the insertion of flexor digitorum accessorius on its lateral side. This connection serves to straighten the pull of action of flexor digitorum longus on the toes. The common tendon splits in four digital tendons for four lateral toes. Each digital tendon gives origin to the lumbrical muscle of the foot. Finally, the digital tendon enters the fibrous flexor sheath, pierces the tendon of flexor digitorum brevis and is inserted into the plantar surface of the base of terminal phalanx of lateral four toes.

Nerve Supply

The tibial nerve supplies the FDL muscle in the posterior compartment of the leg.

Actions

The flexor digitorum longus causes the plantarflexion of lateral four toes at metatarsophalangeal and interphalangeal joints. It assists the plantarflexion at ankle joint and provides support to the arches of foot.

Flexor Hallucis Longus (FHL)

This muscle is much larger than the flexor digitorum longus. It arises from the posterior surface of fibula (Fig. 194.4) below the origin of soleus and from the fascia covering the tibialis posterior. It also takes origin from the lower part of interosseous membrane below the distal attachment of tibialis posterior. Its tendon passes obliquely downward and medially. It lies in a groove on the lower end of tibia, and then, passes deep to the flexor retinaculum. After entering the sole, it grooves the posterior surface of the talus and then, the sustentaculum tali of the calcaneus.

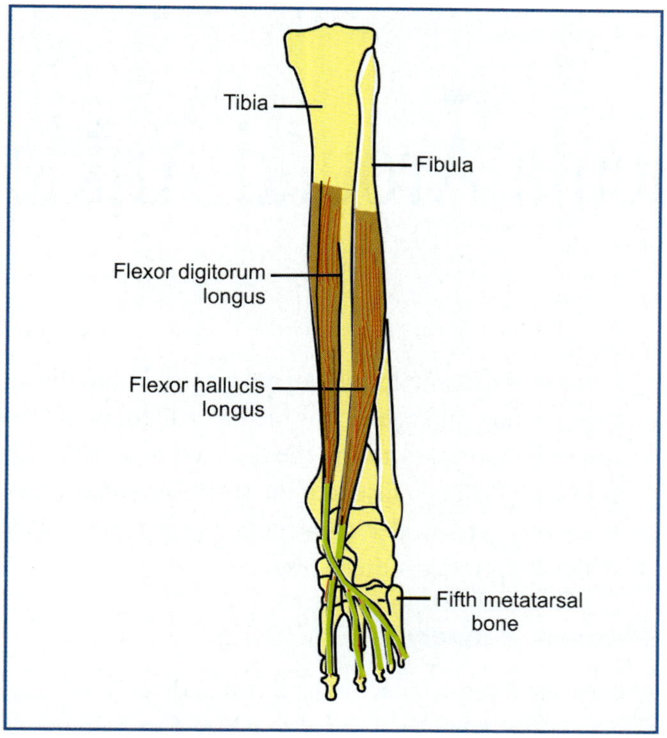

Fig.193.4: Attachments of long flexor muscles of leg (Note that tendons of flexor digitorum longus and flexor hallucis longus cross in second layer of sole to reach their insertion)

It crosses the tendon of flexor digitorum longus in the second layer of sole and in doing so, gives a fibrous slip (William Turner's slip) to it. Finally, it is inserted into the base of the distal phalanx of the great toe. To sum up, the FHL tendon grooves the following bones in succession, the posterior aspect of lower end of tibia, posterior surface of talus and inferior surface of sustentaculum tali.

Nerve Supply

The tibial nerve supplies the FHL muscle in the leg.

Actions

The FHL causes the plantarflexion of the great toe and of the ankle joint. Additional action is to provide support to the medial longitudinal arch of foot.

Tibialis Posterior

This muscle is the most anterior or deeply placed muscle in the posterior compartment. Though it lies between the two long flexor muscles, it is overlapped by both, but especially by the flexor hallucis longus.

Attachments

The tibialis posterior takes origin from the upper two-thirds of the posterior aspect of the interosseous membrane and adjacent parts of the posterior surfaces of both bones of the leg.

In the distal part of the leg, its tendon passes deep to the tendon of flexor digitorum longus. Then, it passes in a groove behind the medial malleolus enclosed in a synovial sheath and goes deep to the flexor retinaculum to reach the sole. In the sole, it lies inferior to the plantar calcaneo-navicular ligament (spring ligament).

The main insertion of the tendon is on the tuberosity of the navicular bone. The remaining part of the tendon sends slips of attachments to sustentaculum tali and the plantar surface of all the tarsal bones except the talus and to the bases of second to fourth metatarsal bones.

Nerve Supply

The tibial nerve supplies the tibialis posterior in the posterior compartment. It may also receive a twig from nerve to popliteus.

Actions

Tibialis posterior is the chief invertor of the foot at the calcaneocuboid, subtalar and midtarsal joints. It is a weak plantarflexor of the foot at the ankle. It gives the main support to the medial longitudinal arch.

Synovial Sheaths of Flexor Tendons

The sheath for tibialis posterior starts 4 cm above the medial malleolus and ends just proximal to its insertion in navicular bone. The sheath for the flexor hallucis longus extends from the malleolar level proximally and reaches the base of first metatarsal bone distally. The sheath for the flexor digitorum longus begins just above the medial malleolus and reaches the level of navicular. Inflammation of the synovial sheaths around the tendons gives rise to tenosynovitis.

194 Retinacula Around Ankle

The deep fascia of the leg shows thickened bands called retinacula around the ankle to strap down tendons, which cross the joint to enter the sole or dorsum of foot. These retinacula are named according to the compartments of the tendons, which pass deep to them. The tendons belonging to muscles of anterior or extensor compartment, pass deep to extensor retinaculum. The tendons belonging to posterior or flexor compartment pass deep to flexor retinaculum and those belonging to lateral or peroneal compartment pass deep to peroneal retinaculum.

Extensor Retinacula (Fig. 194.1)

There are two thickened bands in front of the ankle called superior and inferior extensor retinacula. The function of these bands is to hold the extensor tendons strapped to the ankle joint. In the absence of the retinacula, the tendons will jump forward during dorsiflexion.

a. The superior extensor retinaculum is attached laterally to the lower part of subcutaneous anterior surface of fibula and medially to the anterior border of tibia above the medial malleolus. It superficial relations from medial to lateral side, are the saphenous nerve and great saphenous vein and the medial and lateral terminal branches of the superficial peroneal nerve. Its deep relations (from medial to lateral) are the tibialis anterior, extensor hallucis longus, anterior tibial vessels, deep peroneal nerve, extensor digitorum longus and peroneus tertius. The extensor tendons, as they pass deep to the superior extensor retinaculum acquire synovial sheaths. The function of the synovial sheath is to permit frictionless movements of the tendons. Inflammation of the tendon synovial sheath is called tenosynovitis.
b. Y-shaped inferior extensor retinaculum is present on the dorsum of foot. Laterally, it is attached to the upper surface of the anterior part of calcaneus. Medially, its upper band is attached to the medial malleolus and the lower band passes to the medial side of the foot to fuse with the deep fascia of the sole. The same structures that pass under the superior retinaculum pass under the inferior retinaculum.

Peroneal Retinacula (Fig. 194.2)

The peroneal retinacula are the thickened bands of deep fascia on the lateral side of the ankle. The tendons of peroneus longus and brevis muscles pass deep to them. The small saphenous vein and sural nerve pass superficial to the superior peroneal retinaculum. The superior

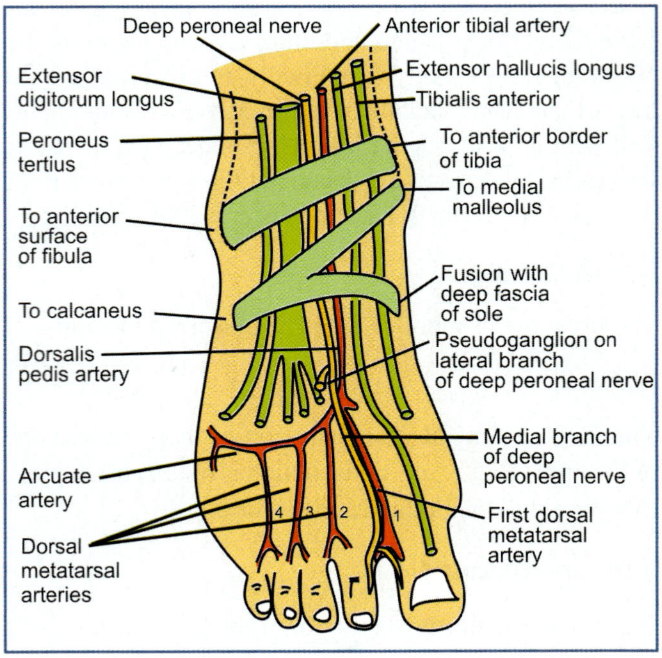

Fig. 194.1: Scheme to show attachments and deep relations of extensor retinacula of foot (Note: Dorsal metatarsal branches of dorsalis pedis and arcuate arteries as well as branches of deep peroneal nerve on dorsum of foot)

peroneal retinaculum is attached to the back of lateral malleolus above and to the lateral surface of calcaneus below. The inferior peroneal retinaculum is attached to the lateral surface of calcaneus posteriorly and to the stem of the inferior extensor retinaculum anteriorly. Some of the fibers of the retinaculum are attached to the periosteum of peroneal trochlea as it crosses the trochlea. This gives rise to two osteofascial canals for the tendons of peroneal muscles. This explains why the originally common synovial sheath of the peroneal tendons becomes double distally.

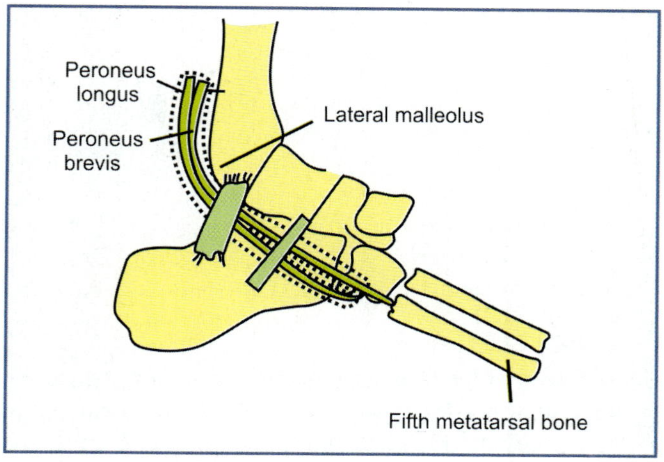

Fig.194.2: Attachments and deep relations of peroneal retinacula

Flexor Retinaculum (Fig. 194.3)

It is a thick band of deep fascia on the medial aspect of ankle. From its upper attachment, it is directed inferiorly, posteriorly and laterally. Its attachments are as follows. Medially or above, it is attached to the medial malleolus and laterally or below, to the medial process of the tubercle of calcaneus. Its distal border gives origin to the abductor hallucis muscle. The medial calcanean nerve (a branch of tibial nerve) and the medial calcanean artery (a branch of posterior tibial artery) pierce the retinaculum. Its deep relations from above downwards (or medio-laterally) are, tibialis posterior tendon, the flexor digitorum longus tendon, posterior tibial artery, tibial nerve and flexor hallucis longus tendon.

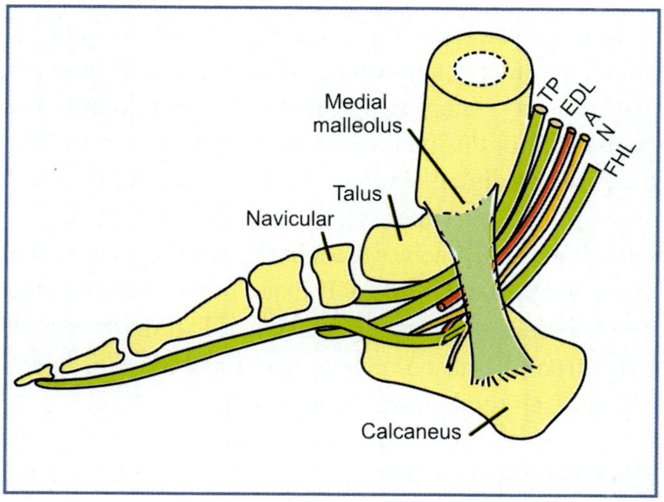

Fig.194.3: Attachments and deep relations of flexor retinaculum of foot (Note: The anteroposterior order of structures passing deep to retinaculum. TP–Tibialis posterior, FDL–Flexor digitorum longus, A–Posterior tibial artery, N–Tibial nerve, FHL–Flexor hallucis longus)

Clinical Highlights

In tarsal tunnel syndrome the tibial nerve is compressed in the osseofibrous tunnel behind the medial malleolus deep to flexor retinaculum. The symptoms are, burning and tingling and pain in the sole of the foot. Surgical division of the flexor retinaculum relieves the severe and persistent pain.

195 Dorsum of Foot

The dorsum of the foot contains the following structures, dorsal venous arch, extensor tendons, extensor digitorum brevis, nerves and the dorsalis pedis artery.

Sensory Nerve Supply (Fig. 175.2)

The saphenous nerve supplies the dorsum along the medial margin upto the base of big toe. The sural nerve supplies along the lateral side of the dorsum. The superficial peroneal nerve supplies the larger intermediate area. The medial side of the great toe and all the other toes (except the first interdigital cleft and the lateral side of fifth toe) are supplied by superficial peroneal nerve. The first interdigital cleft receives branches from the deep peroneal nerve and the lateral side of fifth toe from the sural nerve. The nail beds of the medial three and half digits receive twigs from the medial plantar nerve and those of lateral one and half digits from the lateral plantar nerve.

Dorsal Venous Arch

The dorsal venous arch drains the dorsum of the foot and toes via the dorsal metatarsal veins. The small saphenous vein on the lateral side and the great saphenous vein on the medial side begin on the dorsum.

Tendons on Dorsum of Foot (Fig. 194.1)

The tendons of the four muscles of the anterior compartment pass on the dorsum to reach their insertion. If the foot is dorsiflexed, the large tendon of tibialis anterior is visible and can be palpated on the medial side of the foot. The tendon of extensor hallucis longus can be felt just lateral to tibialis anterior tendon, when the great toe is dorsiflexed. The four tendons of extensor digitorum longus are visible in the distal part of dorsum on dorsiflexion of lateral four toes. In addition to tendons of these four muscles, there are four tendons of extensor digitorum brevis. This muscle can be identified in the living as a small elevation formed by contraction of its fleshy belly in front of the lateral malleolus, on dorsiflexion of medial four toes.

Extensor Digitorum Brevis (Fig.195.1)

This is the only muscle on the dorsum of the foot. It originates from the anterior part of the dorsal surface of calcaneus and from the stem of the inferior extensor retinaculum. It slants distally and medially across the dorsum of foot and ends in four tendons. The medial part of the muscle with its tendon forms an independent muscle called extensor hallucis brevis, which crosses the dorsalis pedis artery superficially. This tendon is inserted into the base of the proximal phalanx of big toe. The other three tendons join the tendons of extensor digitorum longus of the second to fourth toes. They extend the metatarso-phalangeal and interphanlangeal joints of middle three toes. In the big toe, the extensor hallucis brevis acts only on proximal phalanx.

Nerve Supply

The extensor digitorum brevis is supplied by lateral terminal branch of deep peroneal nerve through a pseudoganglion (Fig. 194.1).

Dorsalis Pedis Artery (Dorsal Artery of Foot)

The dorsalis pedis artery is the direct continuation of anterior tibial artery midway between the malleoli. It courses downwards and medially on the dorsum of the foot to reach the proximal end of the first intermetatarsal space (Fig. 194.1), where it turns downwards between the two heads of the first dorsal interosseous muscle. It

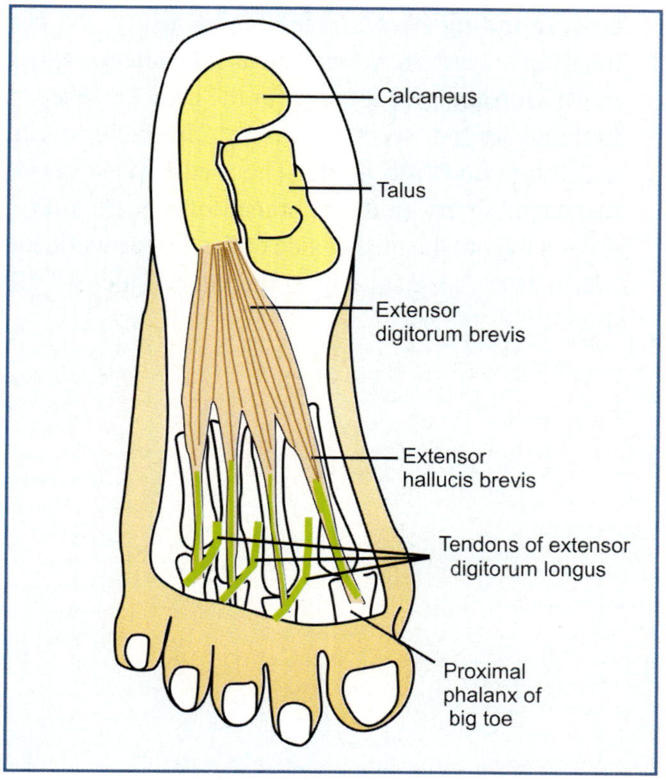

Fig. 195.1: Schematic diagram to show origin and insertion of extensor digitorum brevis

enters the sole and ends by completing the plantar arch medially.

Dorsalis Pedis Pulse (Fig. 195.2)

The palpation of dorsalis pedis artery is very easy because of the superficial location of the artery. It can be felt just lateral to the extensor hallucis longus tendon against the tarsal bones. A diminished or absent dorsalis pedis pulse indicates arterial insufficiency of the lower limb caused by block in any one of the proximal arteries of the lower limb (cause may be thrombosis, embolism or arteriosclerosis in femoral, popliteal or anterior tibial arteries).

Surface Marking

A line starting from the midpoint between the malleoli to the proximal end of first intermetatarsal space represents the dorsalis pedis artery.

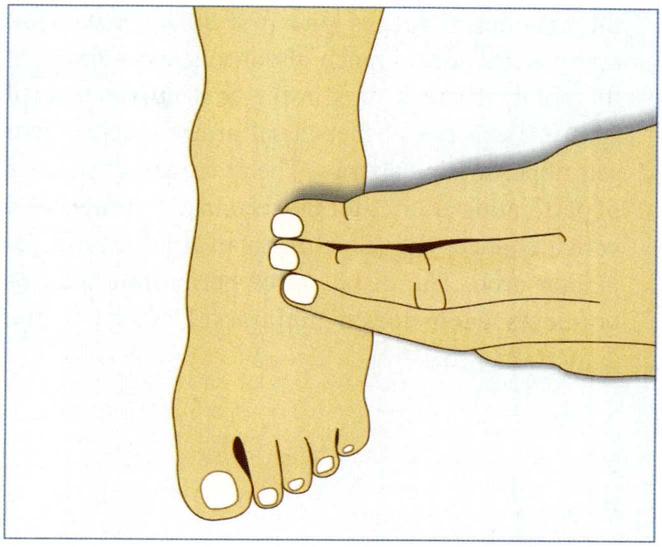

Fig. 195.2: Palpation of dorsalis pedis pulse

Relations

On the deep (inferior) aspect the artery lies successively on the capsule of ankle joint, talus, navicular and intermediate cuneiform bones. On the superficial or superior aspect the skin, fasciae, and inferior extensor retinaculum and extensor hallucis brevis cover it distally. Medial to it, is the tendon of extensor hallucis longus and laterally it is related to the medial tendon of extensor digitorum longus and medial terminal branch of deep peroneal nerve.

Branches

There are three named branches of dorsalis pedis on the dorsum, arcuate artery, lateral and medial tarsal arteries and the first dorsal metatarsal artery.

Arcuate Artery (Fig. 194.1)

The arcuate artery (a branch of dorsalis pedis) passes laterally across the bases of metatarsal bones deep to the extensor tendons. It terminates by taking part in the lateral malleolar network. The artery has the shape of the arch with forward convexity.

Branches

a. From the convexity of the arcuate artery three dorsal metatarsal arteries originate for the second to fourth intermetatarsal spaces (the first dorsal metatarsal artery is the direct branch of dorsalis pedis artery, at the point, where it dips in the first intermetatarsal space). Each dorsal metatarsal artery receives two sets of perforating arteries. The proximal set consists of perforating arteries for the second to fourth spaces, which connect the dorsal metatarsal arteries to the plantar arch. The distal set of perforating arteries connects each dorsal metatarsal artery to the corresponding plantar metatarsal artery. At the interdigital cleft each dorsal metatarsal artery divides in two dorsal digital arteries for the adjacent sides of first and second, second and third, third and fourth, and fourth and fifth digits. The medial-most dorsal metatarsal artery (a direct branch of arcuate artery) gives a twig to the medial side of the big toe while the fourth artery gives a twig to the lateral side of little toe.

196 Sole of Foot

The sole of the foot bears the weight of the body and is subjected to the maximum wear and tear. Hence, it is covered by thick skin with keratinized layer of epidermis. The subcutaneous fat is divided in small loculi by fibrous septa, which anchor the skin to the deep fascia. The fibrofatty tissue is particularly well-developed at three sites, which come in contact with the ground, namely, the heel, the heads of the metatarsals and the pulp of terminal digits.

Sensory Supply (Fig. 175.3)

The medial calcanean branches of tibial nerve supply the skin over the heel. The cutaneous branches of medial plantar nerve supply the skin of the medial half of the sole and the plantar digital branches supply the plantar aspect of the great, second, third and medial half of fourth toes. The cutaneous branches of lateral plantar nerve supply the lateral half of sole and the plantar digital branches supply the plantar aspect of lateral half of fourth toe and the entire fifth toe.

Arterial Supply of Heel

The heel receives blood from two sources, the medial aspect from the medial calcanean branches of the posterior tibial artery and the lateral aspect from the lateral calcanean branch of peroneal artery. If the posterior tibial artery is blocked above the origin of its medial calcanean branch or if the medial calcanean artery is injured, it may cause necrosis of the skin covering the heel.

Deep Fascia of Sole

The deep fascia of sole is described as plantar fascia. The central part of the plantar fascia is much thicker than its lateral and medial parts.

Plantar Aponeurosis (Fig. 196.1)

Plantar aponeurosis is the thick central part of deep fascia. It is triangular in shape. It is regarded as the degenerated tendon of plantaris muscle.

Attachments

The apex of plantar aponeurosis is directed posteriorly and is attached to the medial process of the calcaneal tubercle. Its base splits in five slips (one for each toe) proximal to the metatarsal heads. Each slip divides in a superficial and a deep stratum. The superficial stratum is connected to the superficial transverse metatarsal ligament. The deep stratum of each slip divides in two slips, which pass on either side of flexor tendons and are attached to deep transverse metatarsal ligaments, plantar

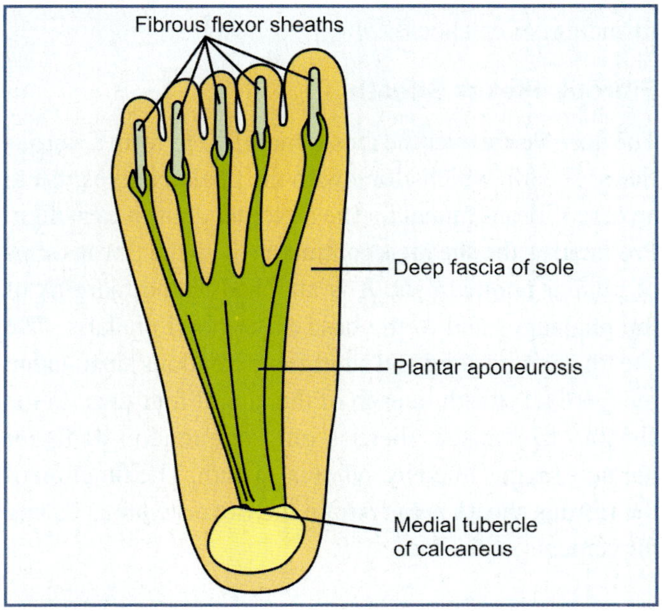

Fig. 196.1: Scheme to show plantar aponeurosis and its division into five slips, distally

ligaments of metatarsophalangeal joints and fibrous flexor sheath at the base of each proximal phalanx.

The plantar aponeurosis is continuous laterally with the plantar fascia covering the abductor digiti minimi and medially with the plantar fascia covering the abductor hallucis. A lateral intermuscular septum projects from the lateral margin of plantar aponeurosis. It is attached to the fibrous sheath of peroneus longus tendon and the fifth metatarsal bone. A medial intermuscular septum projects from the medial margin of the plantar aponeurosis. It is attached to a large number of ligaments, tarsal bones and fascia over the muscles and tendons. These two septa divide the sole in three compartments.

Function

The aponeurosis gives protection to the plantar nerves and blood vessels. It also provides support to the arches of foot.

Clinical Highlights

The chronic inflammation of the posterior bony attachment of the plantar aponeurosis is called plantar fascitis. This gives rise to pain in the heel. This condition is common in people, who have to stand for long periods of time. The plantar fascia may tear at its apex. This condition is more common in policemen hence called policeman's heel. Ossification at the apex of the aponeurosis leads to formation of calcaneal spur.

Fibrous Flexor Sheath

The deep fascia over the toes is modified to form a fibrous flexor sheath, which along with the phalanx gives rise to an osseofibrous tunnel for the flexor tendons in each digit. Proximally, the sheath is continuous with the fibrous slips of plantar aponeurosis. It is attached to the margins of the phalanges and to the base of terminal phalanx. The sheath contains long and short flexor tendons surrounded by synovial sheath in each of the lateral four toes. In the sheath of great toe, there is only one tendon of flexor hallucis longus lined by synovial sheath. The function of the fibrous sheath is to restrain the flexor tendons during movements of the toes.

Muscles of Sole

The intrinsic muscles of the sole and the tendons passing through the sole are arranged in four layers from superficial to the deep aspect of the sole. There are total eighteen intrinsic muscles of the sole and tendons of four extrinsic muscles. These tendons pass through the sole for reaching their sites of insertion. The nerves and vessels travel through two neurovasculr planes. The first neurovascular plane lies between the first and second layers of muscles while the second neurovascular plane lies between the third and fourth layers.

Muscles in First Layer

There are three muscles in the first layer, abductor hallucis, flexor digitorum brevis and abductor digiti minimi (Fig. 196.2).

a. The abductor hallucis muscle takes origin from the medial tubercle of calcaneus and the flexor retinaculum. The plantar nerves and vessels enter the sole deep to this muscle. The muscle runs forwards along the medial margin of the foot. Along with slip from medial part of flexor hallucis brevis and an extension from medial part of extensor hallucis longus tendon, it is inserted mainly in to the plantar surface and partly in to the medial surface of the base of the proximal phalanx of great toe. The plantar position of insertion is responsible for weak abduction. This may cause permanent adducted great toe, which passes transversely under the lateral toes (hallux valgus). This will eventually give rise to bunion due to pressure of shoe on the head of first metatarsal bone. The actions of the muscle on the great toe are, to move it away from second toe (abduction) and flexion. The trunk of the medial plantar nerve supplies a branch to abductor hallucis.
b. The flexor digitorum brevis lies immediately deep or superior to the plantar aponeurosis. It arises by a narrow tendon from the medial tubercle of calcaneus and from plantar aponeurosis. Distally, it divides in four tendons for the lateral four toes. Each tendon of flexor digitorum brevis enters the fibrous flexor sheath along with the tendon of flexor digitorum longus. At the base of proximal phalanx the tendon of flexor digitorum longus perforates the tendon of flexor digitorum brevis, which divides again and is inserted in both sides of the plantar surface of the middle phalanx (Fig. 196.2). The mode of insertion of the flexor digitorum brevis is similar to that of flexor digitorum

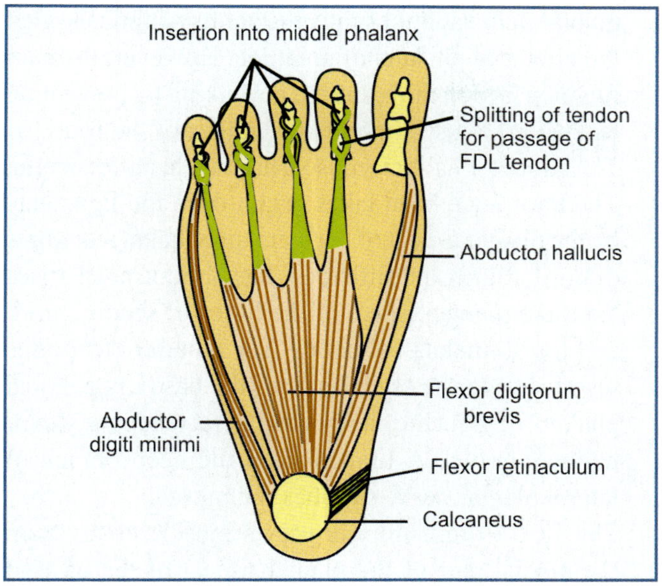

Fig. 196.2: Muscles in the first layer of sole (Note that mode of insertion of flexor digitorum brevis tendons is similar to that of flexor digitorum superficialis of hand)

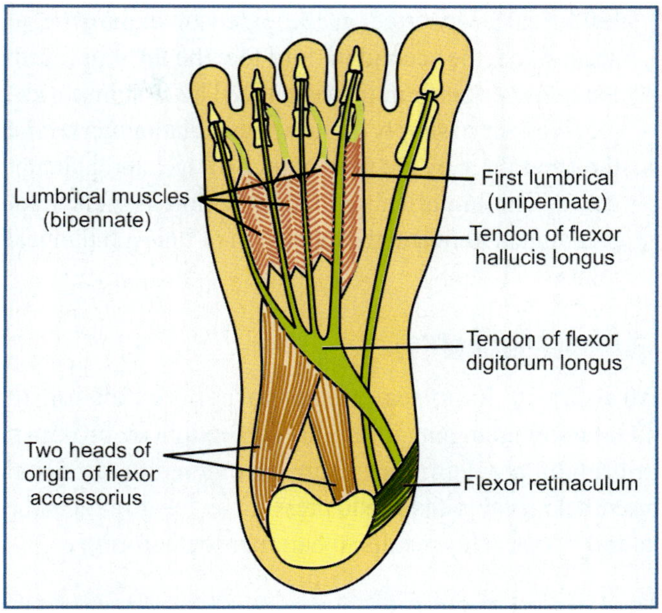

Fig. 196.3: Muscles and tendons in the second layer of sole

superficialis of the hand. The flexor digitorum brevis receives nerve supply from the trunk of the medial plantar nerve.

c. The abductor digiti minimi muscle lies along the lateral margin of the foot. It arises from the lateral and medial tubercles of calcaneus and from the deep aspect of plantar aponeurosis. It ends in a tendon, which is inserted in the lateral side of the proximal phalanx of little toe. A branch from the lateral plantar nerve supplies it.

Muscles and Tendons in Second Layer

The second layer contains the tendons of flexor hallucis longus and of flexor digitorum longus. It also contains the lumbricals and flexor digitorum accessorius muscles (Fig. 196.3).

a. The flexor digitorum accessorius or quadratus plantae is the intrinsic muscle of the second layer of sole. It takes origin by two heads. The fleshy medial head arises from medial surface of calcaneus. The tendinous lateral head arises from the lateral tubercle of calcaneus. The two heads unite and are inserted in the lateral side of the tendons of the flexor digitorum longus. A branch from the trunk of lateral plantar nerve supplies this muscle. This muscle straightens the oblique pull of action of the flexor digitorum longus on the lateral four toes. It assists in the plantarflexion of the same toes.

b. The long flexor tendons that pass through the second layer are the tendons of the flexor hallucis longus and flexor digitorum longus. There is a crossing of these tendons in the second layer. The flexor tendon of the great toe gives a few fibres through the William Turner's slip to the flexor digitorum longus tendons to strengthen the long flexors of the digits. The tendons of the flexor digitorum longus give origin to the lumbrical muscles. The common tendon of the muscle receives insertion of the flexor accessorius.

c. There are four lumbrical muscles, which are numbered from medial to lateral side. Each lumbrical muscle takes origin from the tendon of flexor digitorum longus. Except the first lumbrical the rest are bipennate muscles. The first lumbrical takes origin from the medial side of the tendon for second toe hence it is unipennate. Each muscle ends in a tiny tendon, which curves round the medial side of the corresponding metatarsophalangeal joint and is inserted in the extensor expansion and through it in the base of middle and terminal phalanges of lateral four toes. The first lumbrical is inserted in the extensor expansion of second toe, the second in third toe, the third in fourth toe and the fourth in the fifth toe. The first lumbrical receives nerve supply by the medial plantar nerve and the other three by the deep branch of the lateral plantar nerve. The lumbricals produce flexion at metatarso-phalangeal joint and the extension of inter-phalangeal joints.

Clinical Highlights

Paralysis of lumbricals leads to hyperextension of metatarsophalangeal joints, hyperflexion of proximal interphalangeal joints. There is extension of distal interphalangeal joints due to pressure on the ground in the lateral 4 toes. This results in hammer toe deformity.

Muscles in Third Layer

The third layer consists of three muscles namely, flexor hallucis brevis, adductor hallucis, and flexor digiti minimi brevis muscles (Fig. 196.4).

a. The flexor hallucis brevis muscle has double origin from the medial part of the plantar surface of cuboid bone and from the lateral cuneiform bone. Distally, the common muscle belly divides in medial and lateral parts, which end into two tendons, which are inserted in the respective side of the base of proximal phalanx of great toe. A well-developed sesamoid bone occurs in each tendon near its insertion. A branch of medial plantar nerve supplies the muscle. Its action is to flex the proximal phalanx of great toe. However, its main function is to stabilize the toe in walking by preventing extension. It also supports the arches of the foot.
b. The adductor hallucis muscle has two heads of origin. The transverse head takes origin from the ligaments on the plantar aspect of the metatarsophalangeal joints of third, fourth and fifth toes. The oblique head arises from the plantar aspect of the bases of second, third and fourth metatarsal bones. The common tendon is inserted in to the lateral part of the base of proximal phalanx of great toe along with lateral tendon of flexor hallucis brevis. A branch from the deep branch of lateral plantar nerve supplies the muscle.
c. The flexor digiti minimi brevis muscle arises from the medial part of the plantar aspect of the base of fifth metatarsal bone and from the sheath around the peroneus longus tendon. It is inserted in the lateral side of the base of the proximal phalanx of little toe. The superficial branch of the lateral plantar nerve supplies the muscle.

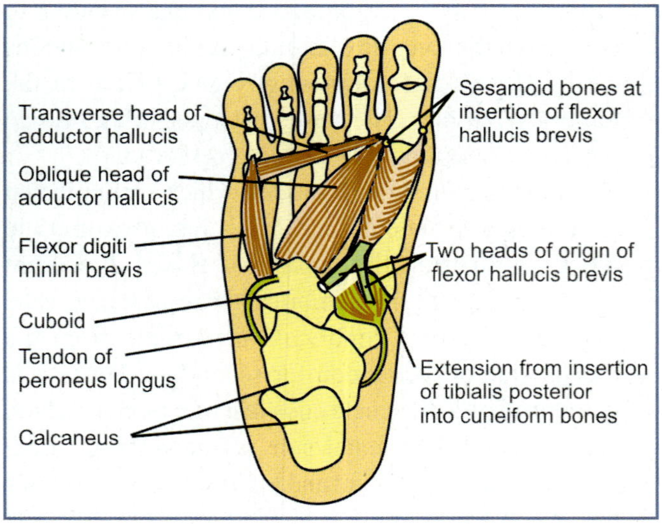

Fig. 196.4: Muscles in the third layer of sole

Muscles and Tendons in Fourth Layer

The fourth layer contains the tendons of the peroneus longus and tibialis posterior muscles in addition to the four dorsal interossei and three plantar interossei.

Interossei Muscles of Foot

The interossei muscles are located between the metatarsal bones. The interossei are numbered from medial to lateral side.

Plantar Interossei (Fig. 196.5)

There are three plantar interossei, which are unipennate. The first plantar interosseous muscle arises from the plantar aspect of the shaft of the third metatarsal bone. The second arises from the fourth metatarsal and the third from the fifth metatarsal bone. Each plantar interosseous muscle is inserted in the medial side of the base of the proximal phalanx of its own digit and partly in the extensor expansion.

Dorsal Interossei (Fig. 196.6)

There are four dorsal interossei, which are the bipennate muscles. They arise from the shafts of the adjacent

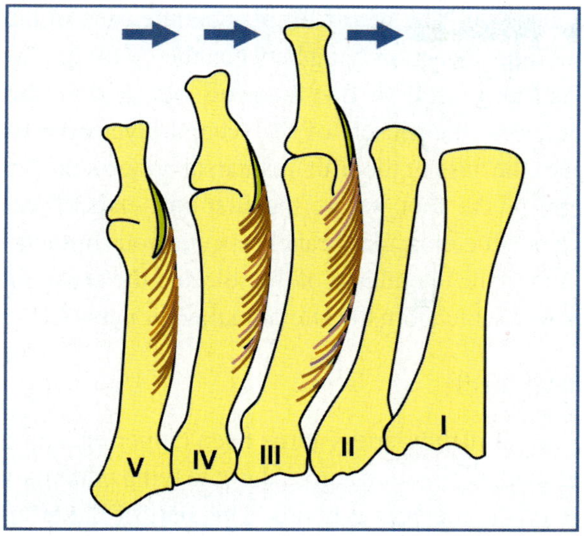

Fig. 196.5: Plantar interossei muscles. The axis of action of interossei passes through second toe

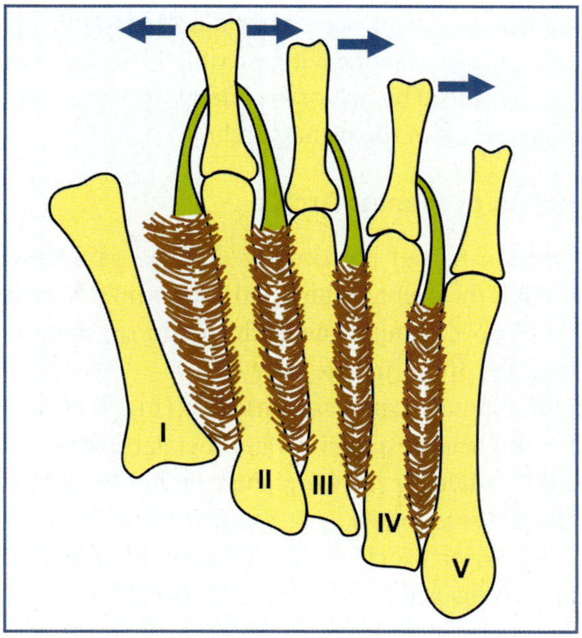

Fig. 196.6: Scheme to show dorsal interossei of foot
The axis of action of interossei passes through second toe

metatarsal bones. Each dorsal interosseous muscle ends in a tendon, which is inserted in the base of the proximal phalanx and the extensor expansion as follows. The first muscle is inserted in the medial side of second toe. The second muscle is inserted in the lateral side of second toe. The third muscle is inserted in the lateral side of third toe and the fourth muscle is attached to the lateral side of the fourth toe.

Nerve Supply of Interossei

The lateral plantar nerve supplies both plantar and dorsal interossei. The interossei of the fourth space (third plantar and fourth dorsal) are supplied through its superficial branch and all others by the deep branch of the lateral plantar nerve. In addition, the dorsal interossei of first and second spaces receive twigs from the deep peroneal nerve.

Actions

The action of the interossei takes place around an axis passing through the second toe. The plantar interossei adduct the toes towards the second toe. The dorsal interossei abduct the toes away from the second toe. In the case of the second toe either the lateral or medial movement is abduction. Besides this, the interossei and the lumbricals cause the dorsiflexion of the interphalangeal joints and the plantarflexion of the metatarsophalangeal joints.

Tendons in the Deep layer of Sole

The peroneus longus tendon crosses the sole from lateral to medial side to reach its insertion in the medial cuneiform and the base of first metatarsal bone. From its main insertion in the tuberosity of navicular bone, the tibialis posterior sends slips for attachment to all the tarsal bones except the talus and to the middle three metatarsal bones.

Collective Action of Intrinsic Muscles of Sole

The intrinsic muscles of the sole support the foot during standing and walking.

Arteries of Sole (Fig. 196.7)

Branches of medial plantar artery, branches of lateral plantar artery and branches of plantar arch supply the structures in the sole.

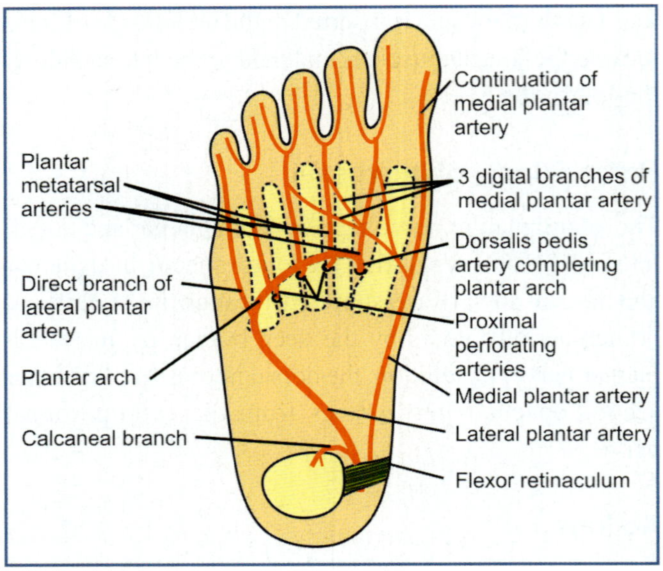

Fig. 196.7: Schematic diagram to show branches of plantar arteries and plantar arch

Medial Plantar Artery

This is the smaller terminal branch of the posterior tibial artery. It begins deep to the flexor retinaculum and enters the sole under cover of the abductor hallucis along the medial plantar nerve. It runs forward lying in the interval between the abductor hallucis and flexor digitorum brevis. The medial plantar nerve is on its lateral side. It branches include the cutaneous branches to the skin of the medial side of sole, muscular branches and three digital branches, which are often small or absent and end by joining the first, second and third plantar metatarsal arteries. The terminal part of medial plantar artery anastomoses with the branch of first plantar metatarsal artery to the medial side of big toe.

Lateral Plantar Artery

This is the larger terminal branch of the posterior tibial artery deep to the flexor retinaculum. The lateral plantar artery can be divided in two parts, first part being the lateral plantar artery proper and the second part, which takes part in the plantar arch.

Course and Relations

The lateral plantar artery enters the sole under cover of the abductor hallucis muscle in company with the lateral plantar nerve. The neurovascular bundle runs in lateral and oblique direction lying between the flexor digitorum brevis (the muscle of first layer of sole) and the flexor accessorius (the muscle of the second layer of sole). It reaches the base of the fifth metatarsal bone on the lateral margin of the foot, where the first part ends. The first part gives the muscular branches, cutaneous branches to the skin of the lateral half of the sole and the anastomotic branches, which join the lateral malleolar network.

Plantar Arch

The lateral plantar artery turns deep (superior) and runs in the medial direction across the sole lying plantar to the bases of the metatarsal bones. This part of the artery is called the plantar arch. It ends by joining the termination of dorsalis pedis artery in the first intermetatarsal space. The plantar arch thus, extends from the fifth metatarsal base to the proximal end of the first intermetatarsal space located between the muscles of the third and fourth layers. The arch presents a concavity proximally and convexity distally. The deep branch of the lateral plantar nerve lies in the concavity of the plantar arch.

Branches of Plantar Arch

a. Three proximal perforating arteries pass upward through the second, third and fourth intermetatarsal spaces to communicate with the dorsal metatarsal branches of the arcuate artery.
b. Four plantar metatarsal arteries (Fig. 196.7) run forward in corresponding inter-metatarsal spaces and end by dividing in two plantar digital branches for adjacent sides of the toes. The first plantar metatarsal artery arises exactly at the anastomotic junction of the dorsalis pedis and the lateral plantar artery and it sends a proper plantar digital branch to the medial side of big toe. The lateral side of the little toe receives a proper plantar digital branch directly from the lateral end of the plantar arch. The plantar metatarsal arteries are called the common plantar digital arteries after uniting with the digital branches of medial plantar artery. The distal part of each plantar metatarsal artery gives rise to a distal perforating artery, which joins the distal part of the dorsal metatarsal artery. The common arteries divide in two proper plantar digital arteries for the adjacent sides of the two toes.

Clinical Highlights

It is difficult to control the bleeding from the plantar arch by direct ligature due to its deep location. The immediate treatment consists of compression of the femoral artery. The compression of anterior tibial alone or posterior tibial alone or of both the tibial arteries may not be effective due to presence of anastomoses around the ankle, in which the peroneal artery also takes part.

Veins of Sole

The veins in the sole accompany the arterial trunks and their branches. The venae comitantes accompanying the lateral and medial plantar arteries unite deep to the flexor retinaculum to form the venae comitantes accompanying the posterior tibial artery.

Nerves of Sole

The sole of the foot contains the lateral and medial plantar nerves, which are the terminal branches of the tibial nerve (deep to the flexor retinaculum). They enter the sole with the corresponding branches of the posterior tibial artery under cover of the abductor hallucis. The medial plantar nerve is comparable to the distribution of median nerve in the hand and the lateral plantar nerve to that of ulnar nerve in the hand.

Medial Plantar Nerve (Fig. 196.8)

This is the larger terminal branch of the tibial nerve. At first it passes deep to the abdductor hallucis and then appears between it and the flexor digitorum brevis. It gives the medial proper digital nerve for the big toe and then divides at the bases of the metatarsal bones in three common plantar digital nerves.

Branches

The medial plantar nerve gives cutaneous branches to the skin of medial half of sole. Its muscular branches arise at different levels. The branches to abductor hallucis and flexor digitorum brevis arise from the trunk of the nerve. The branch to flexor hallucis brevis originates from the medial proper digital nerve to the big toe. The branch for the first lumbrical arises from the first common plantar

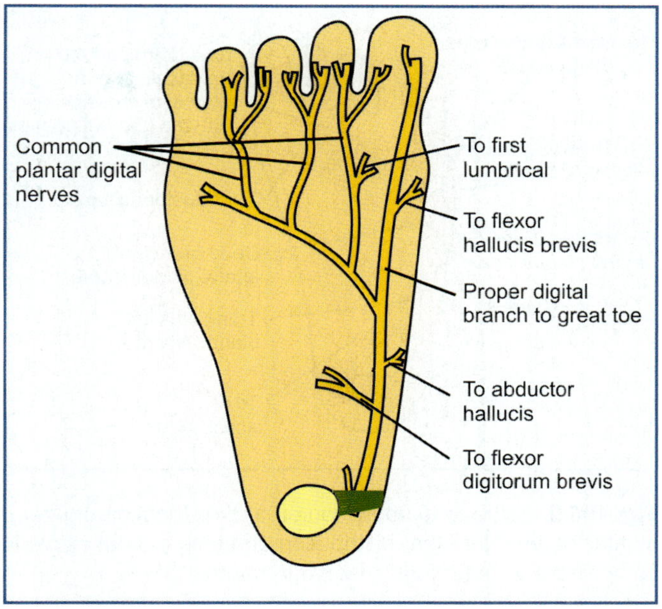

Fig. 196.8: Scheme to show course and distribution of medial plantar nerve (Note that distribution of medial plantar nerve is comparable to that of median nerve in hand)

digital nerve. The articular branches supply the joints of the foot. The proper digital branches supply the skin of the plantar aspect of the toes and also the nail bed on the dorsal aspect of the toes. The three common plantar digital nerves supply the adjacent sides of the first and second toes, second and third toes, and third and fourth toes. The distribution of common digital branches of medial plantar nerve is similar to that of median nerve in the hand.

Clinical Highlights

Morton's metatarsalgia is a condition in which a neurofibroma occurs on the digital nerve supplying the adjacent sides of third and fourth toes. There is usually a communication between the most lateral digital branch of medial plantar nerve and the medial branch of lateral plantar nerve. The neurofibroma may arise in this communication. The pressure of the tight fitting shoe may be the cause of this condition, which results in severe pain in the third and fourth toes.

Lateral Plantar Nerve (Fig. 196.9)

This nerve is one of the terminal branches of the tibial nerve deep to the flexor retinaculum. It enters the sole

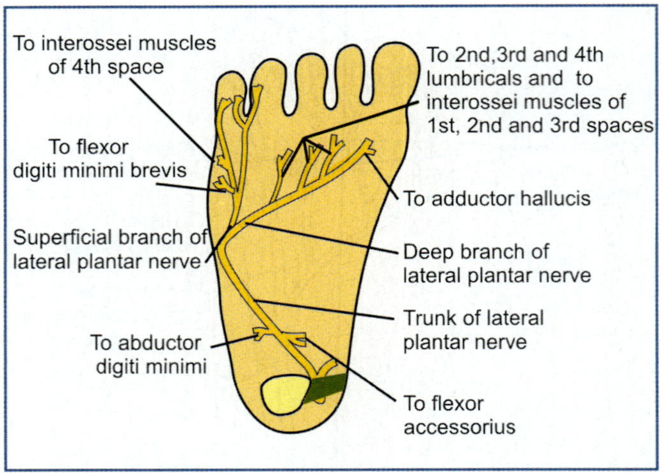

Fig. 196.9: Scheme to show course and distribution of lateral plantar nerve (Note that distribution of lateral plantar nerve is comparable to that of ulnar nerve in hand)

under cover of abductor hallucis. The nerve then passes forward and laterally across the sole in oblique direction to reach the tuberosity of the fifth metatarsal, where it divides in superficial and deep branches. During its oblique course it lies between the flexor accessorius muscle of the second layer and the flexor digitorum brevis muscle of the first layer. At its termination the nerve lies between the flexor digitorum brevis and the abductor digiti minimi.

Branches of Trunk

The trunk of the lateral plantar nerve supplies the flexor digitorum accessorius and the abductor digiti minimi. It gives sensory branches to the skin of lateral part of the sole.

Superficial Branch

The superficial branch runs distally along the lateral border of sole and divides in two common plantar digital nerves. The lateral common plantar digital nerve supplies three muscles, namely, flexor digiti minimi brevis, fourth dorsal interosseous and third plantar interosseous muscles (both in the fourth intermetatarsal space). The remaining common plantar digital nerve becomes the proper plantar digital nerve for the lateral side of the little toe. The medial common plantar digital nerve often connects with the third common plantar digital branch of the medial plantar nerve. It divides in to proper plantar digital nerves for the adjacent sides of the fourth and fifth toes. In summary, the superficial branch of the lateral plantar nerve supplies three muscles and the skin of the lateral one and half toes.

Deep Branch

The deep branch of the lateral plantar nerve turns medially from the base of fifth metatarsal bone and travels across the sole between the muscles of the third and fourth layers to terminate in the adductor hallucis. It carries only motor fibres and supplies the lateral three lumbricals, first, second and third dorsal interossei, first and second plantar interossei and adductor hallucis.

In summary, the lateral plantar nerve is comparable to ulnar nerve in the hand.

Clinical Highlights

The hammertoe deformity in the lateral four toes is produced due to paralysis of lumbricals. There is hyperextension at the metatarsophalangeal joint, hyperflexion of proximal interphalangeal joint and extension at the distal interphalangeal joint.

197 Tibiofibular Joints

There are three joints between the tibia and the fibula. The proximal (superior) tibiofibular joint is of synovial type. The middle tibiofibular joint is of the fibrous type. The distal (inferior) tibiofibular joint belongs to syndesmosis type of fibrous joint.

Proximal Tibiofibular Joint

It is plane type of synovial joint between the facet on the posterolateral aspect of lateral condyle of tibia and the medial aspect of the head of the fibula. The joint capsule is thick anteriorly and posteriorly. The fibular collateral ligament and the tendon of biceps femoris are related to the superolateral aspect of the joint. The tendon of the popliteus enclosed in the synovial sheath passes across the posteromedial aspect of the joint. In 10 percent of people the synovial sheath of the popliteus may communicate with the synovial cavity of the joint. A slight amount of gliding movement is permitted in the joint. The nerve to popliteus and the recurrent genicular nerve (a branch of common peroneal nerve just before its termination) innervate the joint.

Interosseous Membrane of Leg

This is a fibrous membrane that stretches between the interosseous borders of tibia and fibula thus, intervening between the anterior and the posterior compartments of the leg. The direction of fibers in the membrane is downward and laterally from the tibia to fibula. At the lower end, the interosseous membrane is in continuity with the interosseous ligament of distal tibiofibular joint. The anterior tibial artery enters the anterior compartment of leg through a large oval opening above the superior margin of the membrane. The perforating branch of peroneal artery pierces the membrane near its lower margin and enters the anterior compartment. The nerve to popliteus supplies the membrane. The relations of the membrane are as follows:

a. The anterior surface is related to the anterior tibial vessels and deep peroneal nerve. The muscles that have a partial origin from the anterior surface are, the tibialis anterior, extensor hallucis longus, and extensor digitorum longus and peroneus tertius.
b. The posterior surface of the membrane gives partial origin to the tibialis posterior and the flexor hallucis longus.

Distal Tibiofibular Joint

The interosseous ligament is the connecting bond between the medial convex surface of the distal end of fibula and the rough fibular notch of the lateral surface of tibia. The anterior tibiofibular ligament lies in front of the joint between the adjacent margins of tibia and fibula. The stronger posterior tibiofibular ligament strengthens the joint on the posterior aspect. The inferior margin of this ligament forms a separate ligament called inferior transverse tibiofibular ligament, which is yellow in color due rich content of elastic fibers. The inferior transverse ligament extends beyond the lower limits of tibia and fibula as it stretches from the proximal end of lateral malleolar fossa to the posterior border of tibial articular surface. It forms the posterior lip of the socket of ankle joint and makes contact with the posterolateral part of the body of talus. The inferior tibiofibular syndesmosis receives twigs from the nerve to popliteus, deep peroneal nerve and saphenous nerve.

198 Ankle Joint

The ankle joint is a strong weight-bearing joint of the lower limb. The ankle joint belongs to the uniaxial hinge variety of synovial joint.

Articulating Bones

The bones, which take part in this articulation are, the lower end of tibia, lower end of fibula and the talus (Fig. 198.1).

Articular Surfaces

a. Proximally, the articular facets of the lower end of tibia, fibula and inferior transverse tibiofibular ligament form the tibiofibular socket. The tibial articular surface covers the lower end of tibia and lateral surface of medial malleolus. The fibular articular surface is a triangular facet on the medial aspect of lateral malleolus.

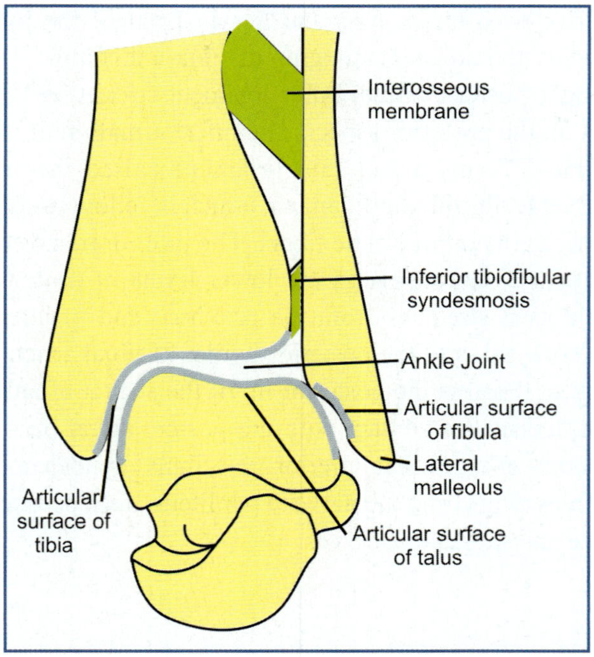

Fig. 198.1: To show bones taking part in ankle joint

b. Distally, the articular facets are present on the superior, lateral and medial surfaces of the talus. These facets form a continuous articular area. The comma-shaped facet on the medial aspect of the talus articulates with the facet on the medial malleolus. The triangular facet on the lateral aspect of talus articulates with the facet on lateral malleolus. The trochlea on the superior aspect of talus is wider in front than behind. During dorsiflexion of the ankle, the grip of the malleoli on the talus is strongest because this movement forces the anterior wider part of trochlea posteriorly between the malleoli. The ankle joint is relatively unstable during plantarflexion because the narrower posterior part of the trochlea does not fill the tibiofibular socket.

Fibrous Capsule

The capsule is attached superiorly to the margins of articular surfaces of the tibia and the malleoli. It is attached inferiorly to the margins of articular surfaces of talus.

Ligaments

a. The medial ligament of the ankle joint is very strong. It is triangular in shape hence it is also known as the deltoid ligament (Fig. 198.2). The ligament is attached to the medial malleolus above. Its lower attachment extends from the medial margin of plantar calcaneonavicular ligament, navicular tuberosity, neck of talus, sustentaculum tali and medial aspect of body of talus, from before backwards.
b. The lateral ligament of the ankle joint is thick and divided in three discrete parts, namely, anterior talofibular, posterior talofibular and calcaneofibular (Fig. 198.3). The anterior talofibular ligament extends from the anterior border of lateral malleolus to the lateral aspect of the neck of talus. The posterior

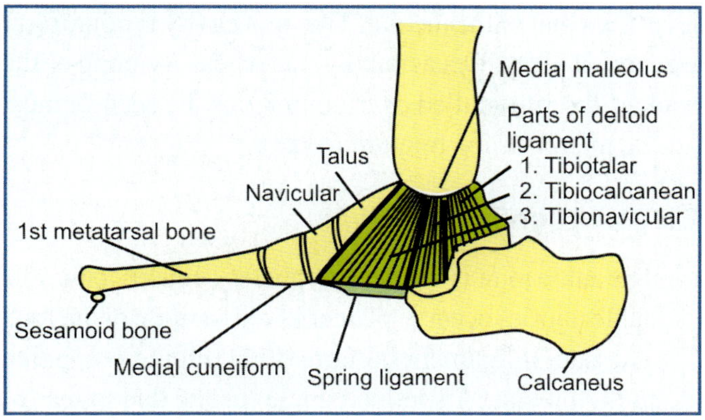

Fig. 198.2: Showing attachments of deltoid ligament of ankle joint

talofibular ligament runs from the distal part of malleolar fossa of lower end of fibula to the posterior tubercle of talus. The calcaneofibular ligament is cord like and extends from the distal end of lateral malleolus to the lateral surface of calcaneus.

Synovial Membrane

The synovial membrane lines the fibrous capsule except the anterior and posterior aspects of the capsule, where fatty pads intervene between the capsule and the synovial membrane. It is attached to the margins of the articulating surfaces. There is an extension of synovial membrane between the tibia and fibula just below the interosseous ligament of the distal tibiofibular joint.

Relations (Fig. 198.4)

a. The anterior relations of the ankle joint are the structures that pass deep to the extensor retinaculum (tibialis anterior, extensor hallucis longus, anterior tibial artery, deep peroneal nerve, extensor digitorum longus and peroneus tertius).
b. The posteromedial relations are the structures that pass deep to flexor retinaculum (tibialis posterior, flexor digitorum longus, posterior tibial artery, tibial nerve and flexor hallucis longus).
c. The posterolateral relations are the tendons of peroneus longus and brevis lying deep to the peroneal retinacula.
d. The direct posterior relation is tendocalcaneus separated from the joint by fibrofatty tissue.

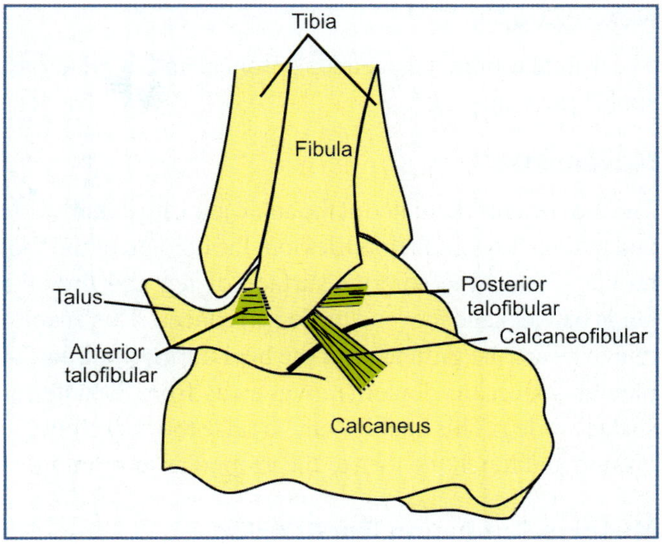

Fig. 198.3: Scheme to show three parts of lateral ligament of ankle joint

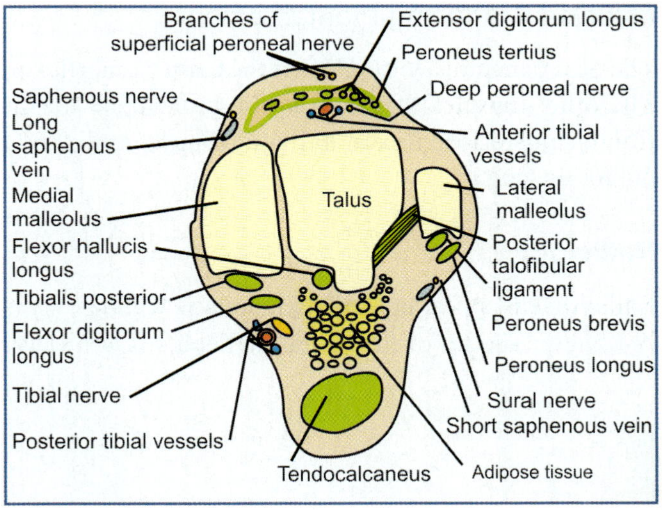

Fig. 198.4: Horizontal section through ankle joint at the level of inferior extensor retinaculum depicting the structures surrounding it

Arterial Supply

The joint receives arterial supply through the rich arterial anastomoses around the ankle, which consists of vascular networks around the malleoli. A large number of arteries take part in the formation of the medial and lateral malleolar networks.

Nerve Supply

The articular branches of deep peroneal and tibial nerves supply the joint.

Movements

The movements permitted at the ankle joint are dorsiflexion and plantarflexion. In dorsiflexion, the dorsum of the foot moves toward the anterior surface of leg and thus the angle between the foot and the leg is reduced. This enables one to strike the ground with the heel during walking. In plantarflexion, the dorsum moves away from the anterior surface of leg. This enables one to raise the heel from the ground and touch the toes to the ground as in running.

Muscles Producing Dorsiflexion

The tibialis anterior, extensor digitorum longus, extensor hallucis longus and peroneus tertius are the dorsiflexors.

Muscles Producing Plantarflexion

The gastrocnemius with soleus is the main plantarflexor. The other muscles that help in the movement are the tibialis posterior, flexor hallucis longus and flexor digitorum longus.

Radiology

Radiological appearance of ankle joint is well-shown in A-P view. The tip of the lateral malleolus is at a lower level than that of the medial. The joint cavity is of uniform size on all sides. Occasionally, an accessory bone at the back of the talus called os trigonum may be seen. It must not be mistaken for fracture of talus.

Clinical Highlights

a. The ankle joint is the most frequently injured joint. The ankle injuries occur in plantarflexed position of the foot. The lateral ligament in more often injured compared to the medial. A sprained ankle results due to tear of anterior talofibular and calcaneofibular ligaments, when the foot is twisted in lateral direction (inversion injury). In forcible eversion of foot the deltoid ligament may be torn. At times, the deltoid ligament pulls the medial malleolus thereby causing avulsion fracture of the malleolus.
b. Pott's fracture (fracture- dislocation of the ankle) occurs when the foot is caught in the rabbit hole in the ground and the foot is forcibly everted. In this condition, at first, there is an oblique fracture of the shaft and lateral malleolus of fibula. The strong eversion pull on the deltoid ligament causes transverse fracture of the medial malleolus. If the tibia is carried anteriorly, the posterior margin of the distal end of tibia is also broken by the talus producing trimalleolar fracture (because here the distal end of tibia is regarded as a third malleolus).

199 Joints of Foot

There are numerous joints between the tarsal, metatarsal and phalangeal bones of the foot (Fig. 199.1). They include inter-phalangeal, metatarsophalangeal, tarso-metatarsal, inter-metatarsal and intertarsal joints.

Intertarsal Joints

The intertarsal joints are divided into two subtypes.

a. The major intertarsal joints include the subtalar or posterior talocalcanean joint and the midtarsal or transverse tarsal joint, which is composed of two articulations, the talocalcaneonavicular joint and calcaneocuboid joint.
b. The small intertarsal joints include the cuneonavicular joint, cuboideonavicular joint, cuneocuboid joint and intercuneiform joints. The articular surfaces of all the small joints are flat, and all have dorsal and plantar ligaments. These joints give certain amount of resilience to the tarsus but the amount of movement in each is very small.

Subtalar Joint

This is the posterior talocalcanean joint belonging to the plane variety of synovial joint. The upper articular surface is the concave posterior facet on the inferior surface of talus and the lower one is the convex posterior facet on the superior surface of calcaneus. The joint is surrounded by fibrous capsule.

Ligaments

a. The lateral and medial talocalcanean ligaments strengthen the joint on each side.
b. The interosseous talocalcanean ligament is a bilaminar band, which occupies the sinus tarsi (tarsal canal). It descends obliquely from the sulcus tali to sulcus calcanei. The ligament separates the talocalcaneo-navicular and posterior talocalcanlean joints.
c. The cervical ligament is lateral to the sinus tarsi and extends from the upper surface of calcaneus to the inferolateral tubercle of the neck of talus.

Talocalcaneonavicular Joint

This is a compound articulation consisting of anterior talocalcanean and talonavicular articulations. It belongs to the ball and socket type of synovial joint. The articular

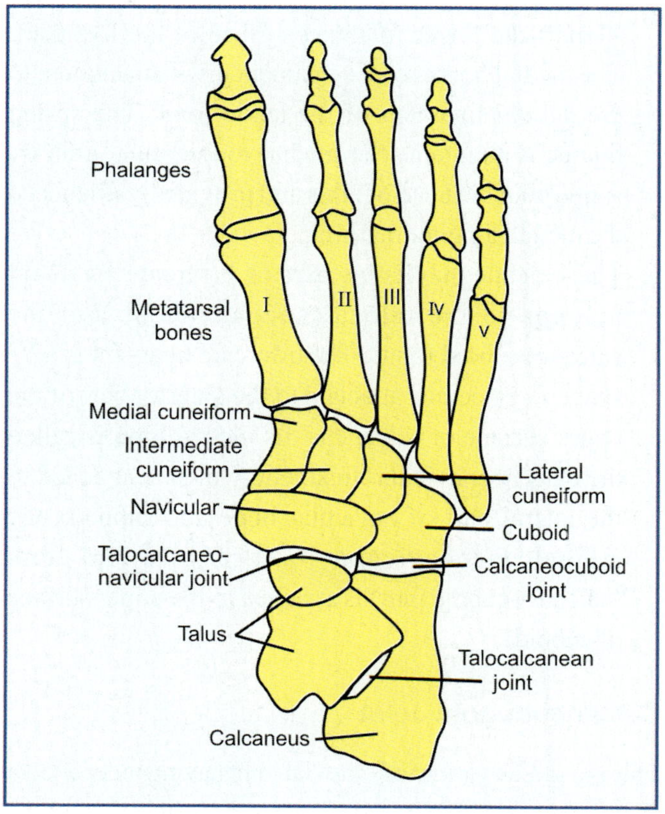

Fig.199.1: Showing bones and major joints of the foot

surface of the rounded head of the talus fits into the socket formed by the posterior surface of navicular, middle and anterior talar facets on the calcaneus and the superior surface of the spring ligament.

Ligaments

A fibrous capsule surrounds the articulating bones. The synovial cavity is separate from the other joints. The plantar calcaneonavicular ligament and the calcaneonavicular part of bifurcate ligament connect the calcaneus to the navicular bone (there being no direct articulation between them).

a. The spring (plantar calcaneonavicular) ligament (Fig. 198.2) is a fibrocartilaginous band, which extends from the anterior margin of sustentaculum tali to the plantar aspect of navicular bone. It takes part in forming the socket for the head of talus. The upper surface of the ligament has a fibrocartilaginous facet, which supports the infero-medial part of the head of talus. The tendons of the tibialis posterior and of flexor hallucis longus support the lower (plantar) surface of the ligament. The medial border of the ligament gives attachment to the deltoid ligament of the ankle joint. The spring ligament maintains the medial longitudinal arch by supporting the head of talus and provides resilience to the medial longitudinal arch.
b. The calcaneonavicular part of bifurcate ligament belongs to the talocalcaneonavicular and the calcaneocuboid joints. The bifurcate ligament is a Y-shaped. Its stem is attached to the anterior part of the upper surface of calcaneus. Its medial limb is called the calcaneonavicular ligament, which is attached to the lateral part of navicular bone and supports the talocalcaneonavicular joint. The lateral limb (calcaneocuboid part) is attached to the upper surface of cuboid.

Calcaneocuboid Joint

This is a saddle variety of synovial joint having independent synovial cavity. The bones taking part in this joint are the anterior surface of calcaneus and the posterior surface of cuboid. The joint lies along the lateral side of foot.

Important Ligaments

a. The long plantar ligament is the longest ligament, which extends from the plantar surface of calcaneus to the to the plantar surface of cuboid and beyond it to the bases of the three metatarsal bones (second to fourth). It converts the groove on the plantar surface of cuboid in a tunnel for the tendon of peroneus longus.
b. The short plantar ligament is called the plantar calcaneocuboid ligament. It lies superior to the long plantar ligament. It stretches from the anterior tubercle of the calcaneus to the adjoining part of cuboid.
c. The calcaneocuboid part of bifurcate ligament extends from the stem of the bifurcate ligament to the dorsal aspect of cuboid.

Movements

The inversion and eversion of the foot take place at the subtalar and midtarsal joints.

Inversion and Eversion

The inversion and eversion are the movements of the foot, which take place at the subtalar and midtarsal joints. These movements occur along an oblique axis and are basically rotation movements of the foot on the talus.

Definition

The inversion is defined as a movement in which the medial border of the foot is raised so that the sole faces medially. Eversion is defined as a movement in which the lateral border of the foot is raised so that the sole faces laterally. There is difference in the rotation movements when the foot is off the ground and on the ground.

Movements When the Foot is off the Ground

The degree of inversion is greater when the foot is off the ground. Inversion is a combination of adduction of forefoot, lateral rotation or supination of forefoot and plantarflexion at ankle. Similarly the degree of eversion is also greater when the foot is off the ground. Eversion is a combination of abduction of the forefoot, medial rotation or pronation of forefoot and dorsiflexion at the ankle.

Movements When the Foot is on the Ground

When the foot is on the ground it is bearing the weight of the body. Therefore, inversion and eversion are more restricted. They consist of only one movement and that is lateral rotation or supination of the forefoot in inversion and medial rotation or pronation of the forefoot in eversion. Pronation raises the heads of lateral metatarsals and supination raises the heads of medial one or two metatarsals. This type of rotation allows us to stand upright on a sloping ground.

Functional Importance

The movements of inversion and eversion are necessary while walking on uneven and sloping ground. They enable the body to move sideways over the foot while the foot is fixed. It is not possible to reproduce the movements of inversion and eversion in an artificial limb. Therefore, an amputee wearing an artificial limb finds difficulty in walking on uneven ground.

Muscles Producing Inversion and Eversion

Tibialis anterior and tibialis posterior are the main invertors of the foot. Both the muscles pass medial to the axis of rotation. The peroneus longus, brevis and tertius are the evertors of the foot. These muscles pass lateral to the axis of rotation.

200 Arches of Foot

The human foot is aptly described as an architectural marvel. Its construction is the best example of the structural adaptation to function. The foot has two major functions. It supports the body weight during standing and progression and it acts as a lever to propel the body forwards during walking, running and jumping. To fulfill the first function the foot must be pliable to withstand the stresses and to fulfill its second function it must be transformable in a lever. A segmented arched lever converts the foot in to a spring hence is ideally suited for its functions. The bones of the foot are arranged to form transverse and longitudinal arches (Fig. 199.1). The arches of the foot are present from birth. Due to the presence of subcutaneous fat, the arching is not apparent during infancy and childhood. Gradually the plantar surface acquires the concave appearance and the characteristic footprint.

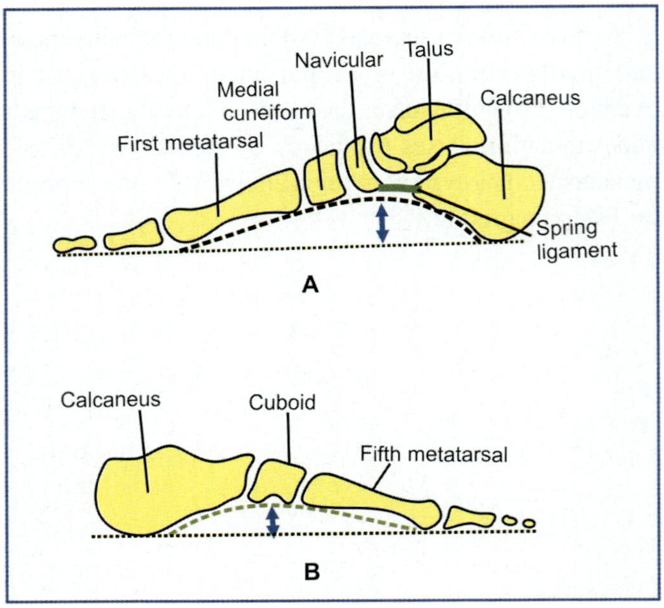

Fig. 200.1: Showing height of arches of foot from ground: (A-Medial view of medial longitudinal arch, B-Lateral view of lateral longitudinal arch)

Types of Arches

There are two longitudinal arches per foot, medial and lateral. There is only half a transverse arch per foot. Only when the two feet are held close to each other the transverse arch becomes complete.

General Principles of Construction

The longitudinal arches have anterior and posterior pillars, summit and joints. The supports of the arches are more or less similar to the mechanical supports of the overhead bridges.

Medial Longitudinal Arch (Figs 199.1and 200.1)

The bones of the medial longitudinal arch from behind forward are, calcaneus, talus, navicular, cuneiforms and medial three metatarsal bones including the two sesamoid bones under the head of the first metatarsal bone. The short and sturdy calcaneus forms the posterior pillar of the medial longitudinal arch. The head of the talus lies at the summit of the arch. Therefore, the talus is the keystone of this arch. The heads of the medial three metatarsal bones and the sesamoid bones contribute to the formation of the anterior pillar. The medial longitudinal arch is taller than the lateral. It is more dynamic and pliant due to the presence of joints in this arch (talocalcaneonavicular and subtalar joints).

Supporting Factors of Medial Arch (Fig. 200.2)

a. The summit of the arch (head of the talus) transfers the body weight to the other bones of the foot. Therefore, support to the talus is very important. The

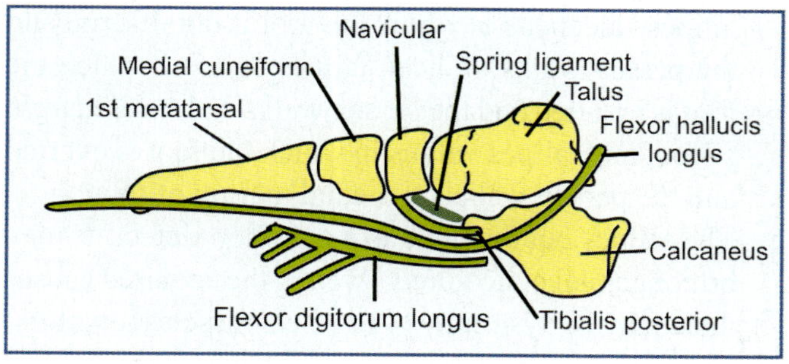

Fig. 200.2: Schematic diagram to show main supports of medial longitudinal arch

head of the talus is held in a socket provided by the navicular, sustentaculum tali and the spring ligament. The combination of the spring ligament and the underlying tibialis posterior tendon forms a dynamic support to the head of talus. In addition the flexor hallucis longus and flexor digitorum longus assist.

b. The anterior and posterior pillars of the medial arch are held together by the plantar aponeurosis, abductor hallucis and flexor hallucis brevis. These structures act as tie beams of the arch.

c. The combined action of the tendon of tibialis anterior and deltoid ligament of the ankle joint is to exert a sling action from above. The slips of insertion of the tibialis posterior in all the tarsal bones (except the talus) provide the support from below.

Lateral Longitudinal Arch (Figs 199.1 and 200.1)

The bones forming the lateral longitudinal arch from behind forwards are calcaneus, cuboid and lateral two metatarsals. This arch being very short it almost touches the ground. The heads of lateral two metatarsal bones form the anterior pillar while the posterior pillar is the calcaneus. The calcaneocuboid joint is the important joint in this arch. The lateral arch being lower and less mobile than the medial is adapted to transmit weight and thrusts.

Supporting Factors of Lateral Arch

The long plantar and short plantar (plantar calcaneocuboid) ligaments are the main ligamentous supports of this arch. The plantar aponeurosis and the intrinsic muscles of little toe function as tie beam of this arch. The tendons of peroneus brevis and tertius, which are inserted in the base of the fifth metatarsal bone act as slings from above. The tendon of peroneus longus, which grooves the cuboid and courses transversely across the sole, provides the support to the cuboid bone (and the calcaneocuboid joint) from above, through its pulley like action (Fig. 200.3).

Transverse Arch

Each foot is composed of a series of transverse arches. The bony components of the transverse arch are the bases of the metatarsals and the cuboid and the three cuneiform bones. The factors that maintain the transverse arch are the interosseous ligaments and the dorsal interossei muscles. The tendon of peroneus longus and the adductor hallucis muscle play a major role in support to this arch.

Functions of Arches

The medial longitudinal arch functions as a propulsive force during locomotion being more elastic and dynamic. The lateral longitudinal arch functions as a static organ of support and weight transmission. Besides this the arches act as shock absorbers. The concavity of the arches provides protection to the deeply located nerves and vessels of the sole.

Clinical Highlights

a. The pes planus or flat foot is due to collapse of medial longitudinal arch. The support to the head of the talus is lost hence it is pushed downward between the calcaneus and navicular bones. During long periods

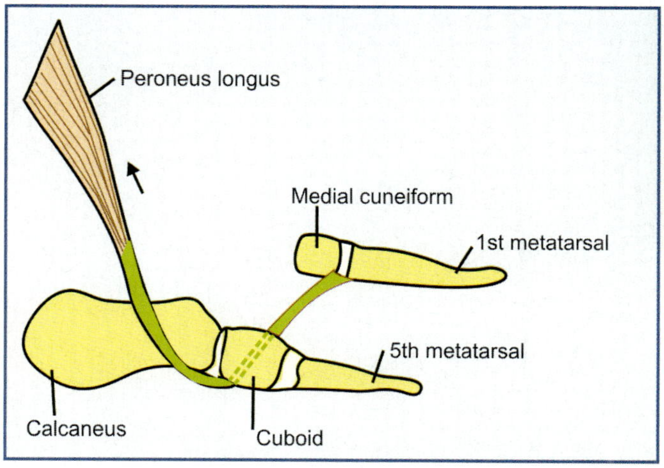

Fig. 200.3: Schematic depiction of the support provided by peroneus longus tendon to lateral longitudinal arch

of standing, the plantar aponeurosis and other plantar ligaments including the spring ligament are overstretched, which may gradually result in flattening of the medial arch with lateral deviation of foot. The person with flat foot usually has clumsy gait and susceptibility to trauma. Pressure on nerves and vessels of the sole results in neurovascular symptoms (for example pain and swelling in the foot).

b. The pes cavus is a highly arches foot. It is associated with claw foot in which there is dorsiflexion of metatarso-phalangeal joints and plantar flexion of interphalangeal joints.

c. Rocker bottom feet are the ones in which plantar concavity is replaced by convexity. This is found in babies born with trisomy 18 (Edward syndrome).

d. The talipes is a Latin word meaning clubfoot. The types of talipes are, talipes equinus (horse like) in which the foot is plantarflexed and the person walks on toes, talipes calcaneus in which the foot is dorsiflexed and the person walks on heel, talipes varus in which the foot is inverted and the person walks on lateral margin of foot and talipes valgus in which the foot is everted and the person walks on medial margin of foot.

e. The talipes equinovarus is a common defect. It may be congenital or acquired. Among the acquired causes there may be dystrophy of peroneal muscles (evertors) or damage to common peroneal nerve (combined paralysis of peroneal and extensor muscles). The foot is held in plantarflexion and inversion.

f. In hallux valgus the great toe is deviated laterally at the metatarsophalangeal joint. Constant wearing of pointed shoes with high heel is said to be the cause of this deformity. Due to lateral deviation of great toe underneath the other toes there is prominence of head of first metatarsal bone. The head tends to rub on the shoe, giving rise to a protective adventitious bursa (bunion) on its medial side.

201 Clinicoanatomical Problems and Solutions

CASE 1

A patient with 4 gm hemoglobin was given intramuscular injections of iron in the gluteal region. After a few weeks, the patient complained of numbness in the intermediate part of dorsum of foot and dorsum of all toes except lateral side of little toe and first interdigital cleft. On examination, it was noted that the patient was not able to dorsiflex and evert the right foot.

Question

a. Name the nerve that is injured.
b. Name the two components of this nerve giving the root value of each.
c. Based on the symptoms and signs, which component is injured?
d. Give the origin and termination of the nerve.
e. Give its surface marking.
f. What is the peculiarity of its arterial supply?
g. Intramuscular injection in which quadrant of gluteal region will cause injury to this nerve?
h. Name the structures that are its anterior relations in the gluteal region.
i. Name the muscle that crosses it in the thigh from medial to lateral side.

Solutions

a. Sciatic nerve
b. Tibial (root value- L4, 5, S1, 2, 3) and common peroneal (root value- L4, 5, S1, 2) components.
c. Common peroneal nerve
d. The sciatic nerve originates from sacral plexus in the pelvis. It enters the gluteal region via the greater sciatic foramen below the piriformis. It passes through the posterior compartment of thigh and terminates into tibial and common peroneal nerves at the apex of popliteal fossa.
e. Draw a line joining the posterior superior iliac spine and ischial tuberosity. Take the first point about 2.5 cm lateral to the midpoint of the above line. Second point is the midpoint of a line joining the ischial tuberosity and greater trochanter. Trace the line joining the above two points to the apex of popliteal fossa.
f. The companion artery of the sciatic nerve (a branch of inferior gluteal artery) enters the substance of the nerve. It bleeds profusely, when the nerve is cut in amputation of limb. To avoid this, the artery is dissected out and ligated. It is an example of axis artery of the lower limb.
g. Inferomedial quadrant
h. From above downwards, dorsal surface of ischium with nerve to quadratus femoris, obturator internus with gemelli, quadratus femoris, adductor magnus.
i. Long head of biceps femoris.

CASE 2

A 50-year-old policeman with a history of chronic dull ache in both legs, came to the hospital, when he noticed dilated and tortuous veins on the medial side of his both legs. The skin on the medial malleolus was found to be discolored, dry and scaly.

Questions

a. Name the clinical condition mentioning the vein involved.

b. What is the relation of the vein to medial malleolus?
c. Name closely related cutaneous nerves along its course.
d. Name the veins that connect it to deep veins of lower limb.
e. What is the direction of flow of blood in them?
f. Name the perforating veins according to the position.
g. Write briefly on saphenous opening.
h. Name the terminal tributaries of this vein before it pierces cribriform fascia.
i. Write a note on saphenous vein graft.
j. What is the reason for dry scaly skin at medial malleolus?

Solutions

a. Varicose veins (varicosity) of lower limb due to dilatation of long saphenous vein
b. Ascends 2.5 cm in front of medial malleolus
c. In the leg- saphenous nerve and in the thigh- medial femoral cutaneous nerve
d. Perforating veins
e. From superficial to deep veins
f. Adductor canal perforator or Hunter's perforator in thigh, Boyd's perforator near knee, three ankle perforators in leg
g. Saphenous opening is 3 cm long and 1.5 cm long. It is a deficiency in fascia lata. Its center lies 3.5- 4 cm below and lateral to the pubic tubercle. It is covered with a thin cribriform fascia. Except on its medial side it is bounded by a sharp falciform margin. The long saphenous vein passes through the cribriform fascia and saphenous opening. The surface marking of this opening is important to the surgeon while testing for patency of saphenofemoral valve. Since, the saphenous opening lies in front of femoral sheath the femoral hernia enters it from the femoral canal and then the hernia turns upwards around the falciform margin.
h. Terminal tributaries of long saphenous vein are, superficial epigastric vein, superficial circumflex iliac vein and superficial external pudendal vein.
i. Saphenous vein, being a muscular vein is ideal for coronary artery graft. The blocked segment of the artery is replaced by a segment of patient's own saphenous vein in the thigh. While suturing the venous graft, the venous segment is reversed so that its valves do not impede the arterial blood flow.
j. Due to venous stasis in varicose veins at medial malleolus, the oxygen supply of the skin is lowered.

CASE 3

A 78-year-old woman was not able to move her right lower limb after a minor fall. On examination, it was noted that the toes of her right foot were pointing laterally. The right limb was found to be shorter, on measuring the length. X-ray showed subcapital intra-capsular fracture of femoral neck and general osteoporosis.

Questions

a. How is the length of the lower limb measured?
b. What is the reason for shortening of right lower limb in this patient?
c. Which anatomical factors are responsible for the characteristic position of the right foot?
d. Draw a diagram to show the arterial supply of head and neck of femur.
e. What is the serious complication of this type of fracture. Give reason for the same.
f. Write notes on Nelaton's line and Shenton's line.

Solutions

a. From anterior superior iliac spine to medial malleolus.
b. Contraction of hamstrings and adductor muscles pulls the shaft of femur upwards.
c. The thigh is laterally rotated by contraction of gluteus maximus and short lateral rotators of thigh. In fracture of neck of femur, the psoas major muscle becomes lateral rotator due to shift in its axis.
d. Refer to Figure 189.4.
e. Avascular necrosis of femur occurs due to rupture of the retinacular arteries that pass along the neck of femur.
f. Joining the anterior superior iliac spine to ischial tuberosity draws Nelaton's line, which is used in assessing the position of the greater trochanter. Normally the line passes through the highest point of greater trochanter. If the trochanter is above this line it suggestive of fracture of neck of femur. Shenton's line is visible in a radiograph of hip joint. It is a smooth curve formed by lower margin of neck of femur and the lower margin of superior ramus of pubis. This line is distorted in fracture of neck of femur or dislocation of hip joint.

CASE 4

A football player, on receiving a blow on the lateral side of the right knee, felt a sharp pain on the medial aspect and was not able to extend the leg. His right knee was swollen especially above the patella. Drawer signs were negative. Radiological examination did not show any fracture.

Questions

a. Which intra-articular structure is torn in this patient?
b. Name the type of tear that usually occurs in it in the sports injury.
c. Give the shape, attachments and nutrition of this structure.
d. Illustrate the 'unhappy triad' of knee joint with the help of simple diagram.
e. What is suprapatellar bursa? Which muscle is inserted in it?
f. What is housemaid's knee?
g. Write short note on the muscle that originates inside the capsule of knee joint.

Solutions

a. Medial meniscus
b. Bucket handle tear
c. The medial meniscus is C-shaped. It related to the superior surface of the medial condyle of tibia. Its anterior horn is attached to the front of inter-condylar area of tibia and the posterior horn to the posterior part of inter-condylar area between the attachment of posterior horn of lateral meniscus and posterior cruciate ligament.
d. Refer to Figure 190.9.
e. Suprapatellar bursa is an extension of the synovial cavity above the patella and behind the quadriceps tendon in the thigh. Articularis genu is inserted in to it.
f. The popliteus muscle has intracapsular and extrasynovial tendinous origin from the anterior part of the groove on the lateral condyle of femur. A few fibres are attached to the meniscus also. The tendon of popliteus intervenes between the lateral meniscus and fibular collateral ligament. The tendon pierces the posterior part of the capsule and expands into a triangular fleshy part, which is inserted in the posterior surface of tibia above the soleal line. The popliteus is covered with fascia, which is an extension from semimembranosus insertion. The fascia and the muscle form the lower part of the floor of the popliteal fossa. The muscle receives nerve supply from tibial nerve in popliteal fossa. This nerve is unique in that it travels on the posterior surface of the popliteus, wind round its inferior margin to reach its anterior surface to supply the muscle. This nerve also supplies motor branch to tibialis posterior, tibiofibular joints and interosseous membrane. The action of the popliteus is to unlock the locked knee joint (key muscle of knee joint).

CASE 5

A few days following the removal of plaster cast for fracture of the upper end of left fibula, the patient complained of loss of sensation on the lateral and anterior aspect of leg and on the intermediate area of the dorsum of foot including toes except the lateral side of little toe and first interdigital cleft. On examination, the patient was unable to dorsiflex and evert the left foot.

Questions

a. Name the nerve that is injured in this patient.
b. Give the site where this nerve is palpated.
c. Name the deformity in which the foot cannot be dorsiflexed.
d. Inability to dorsiflex the foot is due to loss of function of which nerve?
e. Describe the course and distribution of this nerve.
f. Describe the muscles that are the chief evertors of foot.

Solutions

a. Common peroneal nerve
b. Lateral side of neck of fibula
c. Foot drop
d. Deep peroneal nerve
e. For course and distribution of deep peroneal nerve refer to anterior compartment of leg.
f. Peroneus longus and brevis are the chief evertors of foot. For description of these muscles refer to lateral compartment of leg.

CASE 6

A candidate for recruitment in the army was rejected because he was found to have pes planus (flat foot) in the medical check up.

Questions

a. Define pes planus and explain anatomical factors that are responsible for it.
b. Draw a diagram to show the bones forming the medial longitudinal arch of foot.
c. Which bone is the keystone of this arch?
d. Describe the main ligament that supports the head of the talus.
e. Name few effects of flat foot.
f. Define inversion and eversion.
g. Name the joints where these movements take place.
h. Describe plantar aponeurosis and how does it differ from palmar aponeurosis?

Solutions

a. Pes planus means flat foot. In this condition, there is collapse of medial longitudinal arch. There are two reasons for it. Due to loss of support to the head of the talus, it is pushed downwards between navicular and calcaneus. The ligaments supporting the arch (spring, long and short plantar, plantar aponeuroses) are overstretched due to strain.
b. Refer to Figure 199.1.
c. Talus
d. Spring ligament or plantar calcaneonavicular ligament supports the head of the talus from below. It is a thick band that extends from anterior margin of sustentaculum tali to the plantar surface of navicular bone. Its upper surface presents fibrocartilaginous facet for the head of talus. Its lower surface is in contact with tendons of tibialis posterior and flexor hallucis longus. Its medial margin gives attachment to deltoid ligament of ankle joint. The spring ligament not only supports the keystone of the medial arch but also provides resilience to it needed for propulsion.
e. The flat foot leads to loss of elasticity in the foot, which makes it liable to trauma and arthritic changes. Loss of concavity of the plantar aspect of foot leads to compression of nerves and vessels in the sole.
f. Inversion is the movement in which the medial margin of foot is raised and the sole faces medially. Eversion is the movement in which lateral margin of foot is raised and the sole faces laterally.
g. Subtalar joint and midtarsal joints (calcaneocuboid and talocalcaneonavicular).
h. Refer to Chapter 196.

CASE 7

A 50-year-old woman came to the hospital, when she noticed a lemon sized swelling in the upper thigh. O/E The swelling was inferior and lateral to the pubic tubercle and it was seen to push into the saphenous opening.

Questions

a. Which hernia gives rise to swelling below and lateral to pubic tubercle?
b. Name the passage through which the hernia entered the thigh.
c. Give the name and the boundaries of the upper opening of the passage.
d. Describe the direction of the hernia and the importance of this knowledge to the surgeon.
e. In case of strangulation of this hernia how is the upper opening of the passage enlarged?
f. Describe abnormal obturator artery.

Solutions

a. Femoral hernia
b. Femoral canal
c. Femoral ring, Its boundaries are, in front-inguinal ligament, medially-lacunar ligament, laterally-femoral vein in the middle compartment of femoral sheath, posteriorly-pectineus and fascia.
d. The femoral hernia, at first comes downwards in the femoral canal then, it goes anteriorly in to the saphenous opening and finally turns upwards against the falciform margin of the saphenous opening. In manual reduction of the hernia, the surgeon reverses the order by pushing the hernia, downwards, posteriorly and upwards.
e. In case of strangulation of femoral hernia its medial boundary (lacunar ligament) is cut.
f. For abnormal obturator artery refer to Figure 178.3 and Chapter 157.

CASE 8

A policeman sustained a bullet shot injury in his left buttock in a street encounter. After convalescence, he developed a characteristic limp during walking. There was sagging of right hip while taking a step on left foot. On examination, Trendelenburg sign was positive.

Questions

a. Identify the nerve of the gluteal region that is injured.
b. Give its origin, course and branches.
c. Explain positive Trendelenburg sign.
d. Name the characteristic gait in unilateral injury and in bilateral injury to the nerve.
e. Describe the attachments and actions of the muscles supplied by this nerve.

Solutions

a. Superior gluteal nerve (L4, 5 ,S1)
b. Surperior gluteal nerve is a branch sacral plexus inside the pelvic cavity. It enters the gluteal region above the piriformis through the greater sciatic foramen. It is accompanied by superior gluteal artery, which is a branch of posterior division of internal iliac artery. It runs between the glutei medius and minimus muscles and supplies them and the tensor fasciae latae.
c. When left foot is raised from the ground, the right hip sags due to the failure of gluteus medius and minimus of left side to contract and support the pelvis on the opposite side.
d. Unilateral injury to superior gluteal nerve results in lurching or dipping gait and bilateral injury results in waddling gait.
e. Refer to Chapter 185.

SINGLE BEST RESPONSE MCQs

1. Which of the following is not attached to fibula?
A. Tibialis anterior
B. Extensor hallucis longus
C. Extensor digitorum longus
D. Peroneus tertius

2. The number of ossification centers in the lower limb (on one side) in full term newborn:
A. Six B. Five
C. Two D. One

3. Profunda femoris artery leaves the femoral triangle through:
A. Apex
B. Behind sartorius
C. Between psoas major and pectineus
D. Between pectineus and adductor longus

4. In clergyman's knee which bursa is affected?
A. Prepatellar
B. Suprapatellar
C. Subcutaneous infrapatellar
D. Semimembranous

5. Which is not a branch of common peroneal nerve?
A. Lateral inferior genicular
B. Recurrent genicular
C. Sural
D. Sural communicating

6. Femoral branch of genito-femoral nerve is located in:
A. Femoral canal
B. Inguinal canal
C. Middle compartment of femoral sheath
D. Lateral compartment of femoral sheath

7. Which vein pierces the cribriform fascia?
A. Superficial epigastric
B. Superficial external pudendal
C. Deep external pudendal
D. Great saphenous

8. The relation of neck of the femoral hernia to pubic tubercle:
A. Above and lateral B. Above and medial
C. Below and lateral D. Below and medial

9. Dorsalis pedis pulse is present in the block of the following artery:
A. Anterior tibial B. Popliteal
C. Posterior tibial D. Femoral

10. The structure that comes out of the lesser sciatic foramen:
A. Tendon of obturator internus
B. Pudendal nerve
C. Internal pudendal artery
D. Nerve to obturator internus

11. **Which of the following muscles of thigh has no attachment to femur?**
A. Quadratus femoris B. Rectus femoris
C. Vastus intermedius D. Pectineus

12. **Rider's bone is found in the tendinous origin of:**
A. Adductor longus
B. Adductor brevis
C. Lateral head of gastrocnemius
D. Medial head of gastrocnemius

13. **Which is the main joint of the medial longitudinal arch?**
A. Calcanocuboid B. Subtalar
C. Talocalcaneonavicular D. Ankle

14. **Pes anserinus is the term used for insertion of the following muscles, *except:***
A. Semitendinosus
B. Semimembranosus
C. Sartorius
D. Gracilis

15. **Which pair of muscles does not share the nerve supply?**
A. Soleus and popliteus
B. Gluteus medius and tensor fasciae latae
C. Quadratus femoris and superior gemellus
D. Obturator externus and adductor brevis

16. **Paralysis of which muscle predisposes to lateral dislocation of patella?**
A. Vastus medialis
B. Vastus lateralis
C. Vastus intermedius
D. Rectus femoris

17. **Which dermatome is located over the little toe?**
A. L4 B. L5
C. S1 D. S2

18. **In talipes equinus the patient walks on:**
A. Heel
B. Toes
C. Lateral margin of foot
D. Medial margin of foot

19. **What is true about the lateral meniscus?**
A. Attached to popliteus tendon
B. Restricted mobility
C. Bucket handle tear common
D. Semicircular shape

20. **Which nerve is tested if the physician pinches the skin between big toe and second toe?**
A. Superficial peroneal B. Deep peroneal
C. Sural D. Saphenous

Key to MCQs

1 A	2 B	3 D	4 C	5 C	6 D	7 D
8 C	9 C	10 A	11 B	12 A	13 C	14 B
15 C	16 A	17 C	18 B	19 A	20 B	

MULTIPLE TRUE OR FALSE (WRITE T OR F AGAINST EACH STATEMENT)

1. **The popliteal lymph nodes:**
A. Receive superficial lymph vessels from great toe
B. Receive lymph from knee joint
C. Are organized in three groups
D. Drain into vertical chain of superficial inguinal nodes

2. **The femoral ring:**
A. Is the upper opening of femoral sheath
B. Is covered by lymph node
C. Its lateral boundary is femoral artery
D. Its medial boundary is lacunar ligament

3. **Patella:**
A. Is the largest sesamoid bone
B. Lacks periosteum
C. Acts as a pulley as well as lever
D. Has natural tendency to dislocate laterally

4. **Sciatic nerve:**
A. Supplies all the muscles below the knee
B. Supplies the entire skin below the knee
C. Is inferior to piriformis
D. Supplies the skin of the back of the thigh

5. **The hamstring muscles:**
   A. Act both on hip and knee joints
   B. Are supplied by tibial part of sciatic nerve
   C. Short head of biceps femoris is a hamstring muscle
   D. Ischial part of adductor magnus is a hamstring muscle

6. **Contribution to patellar plexus of nerves from:**
   A. Nerve to sartorius
   B. Posterior division of obturator
   C. Anterior division of obturator
   D. Saphenous

7. **Medial rotator of hip joint:**
   A. Gluteus maximus
   B. Gluteus medius
   C. Gluteus minimus
   D. Reflected head of rectus femoris

8. **Popliteal artery:**
   A. Is the most anterior content of the popliteal fossa
   B. Gives five genicular branches
   C. Divides at distal margin of popliteus
   D. Gives sural branches to supply the skin

9. **Locations of readily palpable arterial pulsation in lower limb:**
   A. Just below the midpoint of inguinal ligament
   B. In the popliteal fossa
   C. In front of medial malleolus
   D. Medial to tendon of tibialis anterior on dorsum of foot

10. **Obturator nerve:**
   A. Emerges from lateral margin of psoas major
   B. Is branch of sacral plexus
   C. Supplies obturator externus
   D. Is sectioned to relieve adductor spasm

Annexure: Radiographs of Lower Extremity

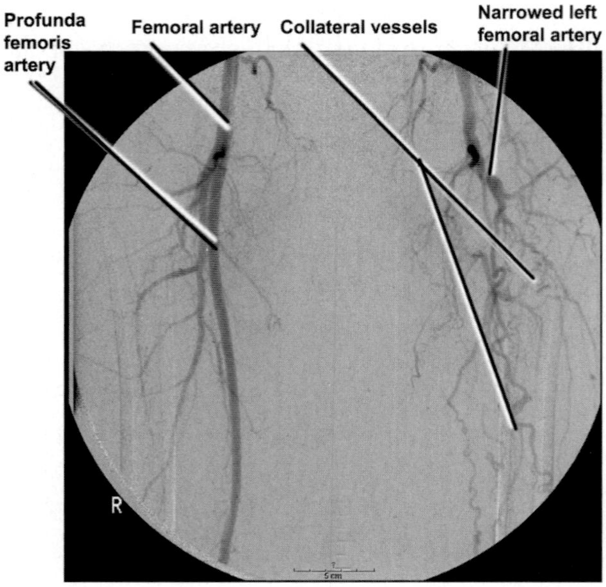

LL-R1. Femoral angiogram showing normal right femoral artery and constricted left femoral

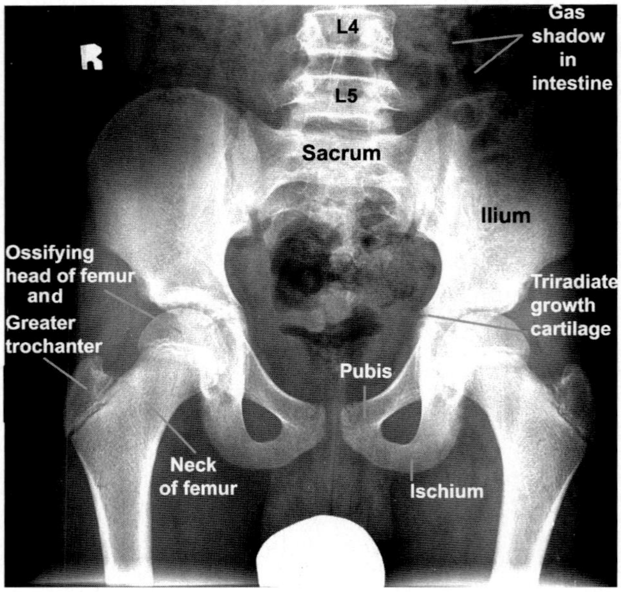

LL-R2. Anteroposterior radiograph of hip bones and femurs of a boy aged about 12 years (Note that neck of femur is ossified from the diaphysis)

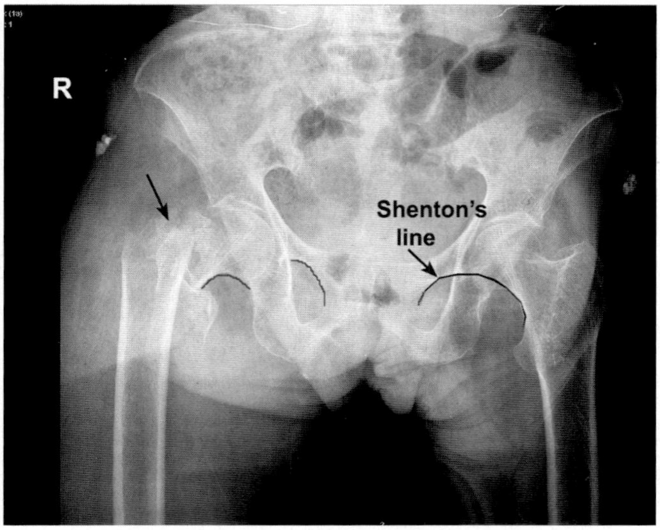

LL-R3. Radiograph of hip joints showing fractured neck of femur and distorted Shenton's line on right side

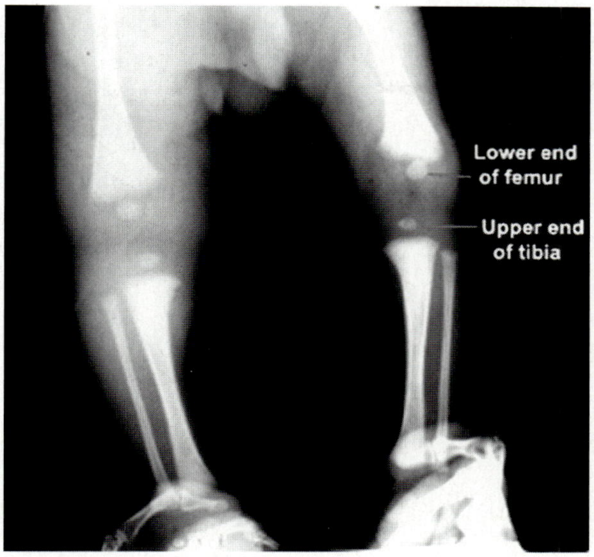

LL-R4. Radiograph of lower limbs of full-term neonates showing two of the secondary centers of ossifying, which appear before birth

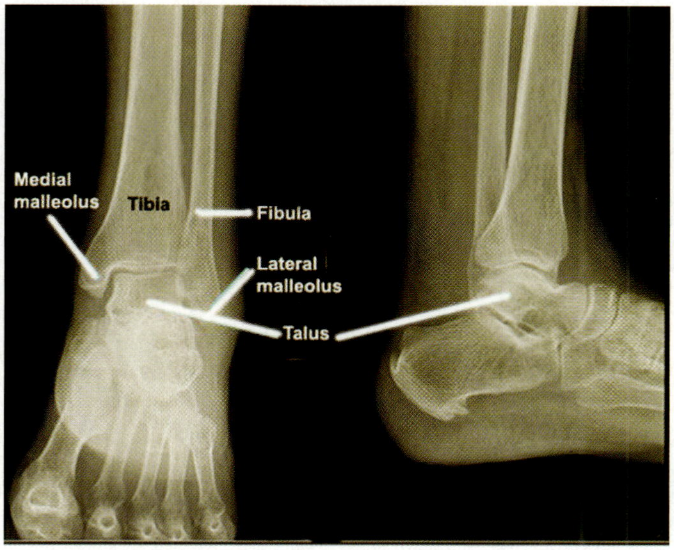

LL-R5. Showing bones taking part in ankle joint

SECTION SIX

Overview of Osteology

Introduction

Osteology is the study of bones. The bones take part in the joints. The bones and joints together form the skeletal system of the body. The human skeleton has 206 bones, which includes 64 in upper limbs, 62 in lower limbs, 22 in cranium, 6 ear ossicles, 1hyoid, 24 ribs, 1 sternum and 26 vertebrae.

GENERAL STRUCTURE OF BONE

Though extremely hard, the bone is a living tissue. It is constantly changing in response to stresses to which it is subjected. It is a special type of highly vascularized connective tissue, consisting of cells and mineralized matrix.

Functions of Skeleton

Skeleton gives framework to the body. It provides levers for the muscles and thereby helps in movements. The skull gives protection to brain, vertebral column to spinal cord, thoracic cage to the thoracic and upper abdominal viscera and pelvis protects reproductive organs and other pelvic viscera. The bones store 97% of total calcium of body and phosphorus. The ends of long bones, bodies of vertebrae, sternum and ribs and iliac crests contain red bone marrow throughout life and are responsible for production of blood cells.

Clinical Uses of Bones

a. Bone marrow aspiration is a commonly used method for carrying out histological study of bone marrow cells to diagnose diseases. The preferred sites are, posterior superior iliac spine, iliac crest, manubrium sterni and upper part of medial surface of tibia (only in children under 2 years).
b. Intraosseous infusion is used in children below 5years to directly inject fluids in the bone marrow in cases where the peripheral veins have collapsed. The preferred site is on the medial subcutaneous surface of tibia 1-2 cm below and slightly medial to the tibial tuberosity.
c. Bone grafting is done certain cases. For this purpose the iliac crest, ribs and subcutaneous surface of tibia are preferred.

Types of Bones

a. According to position, the bones are either axial (skull bones, vertebrae, ribs and sternum) or appendicular (upper limb and lower limb bones).
b. According to the shape, the bones are long, short, flat, irregular, pneumatic and sesamoid, etc.

Ossification of Bones

The bones develop by intramembranous or endochondral ossification. Some bones of cranium develop by both membranous and endochondral ossification.

The primary center of ossification usually appears before birth. However, in carpal bones and tarsal bones except talus, calcaneus and cuboid they appear after birth. By and large, the secondary center or centers appear after birth with the exception of lower end of femur, upper end of tibia and head of humerus (in 20% individuals).

Long Bones

The part of long bone that develops from primary center is called diaphysis and that from secondary center is called epiphysis. If there are more than one secondary centers there will be more than one epiphyses. The epiphyses are of three types. The traction epiphysis is nonarticular and gives muscular attachments (greater trochanter of femur). The pressure epiphysis is articular and transmits weight (head of femur). Atavistic epiphysis is phylogenetically a separate bone, which in Man has become part of another bone to derive nutrition (coracoid process of scapula, posterior tubercle of talus or os trigonum). A typical long bone presents epiphysis at both ends. There is usually, a law of union of epiphysis. The law states that the epiphysis that appears first unites last. The fibula is the only long bone that breaks this law.

Epiphyseal Cartilage (Growth Cartilage) and Growing End

Epiphyseal cartilage is a plate of hyaline cartilage that is located between diaphysis and epiphysis of a growing bone. As long as the bone grows in length, the epiphyseal cartilage persists. At the growing end of a long bone the secondary center appears first but fuses last with the diaphysis. The direction of the nutrient foramen is opposite to that of the growing end. The dictum " towards the elbow I go and away from the knee I flee" tells the directions of the nutrient foramina of the limb bones. From this it is apparent that the upper end of humerus and lower ends of forearm bones are the growing ends in upper limbs while lower end of the femur and upper ends of the leg bones are the growing ends in the lower limbs.

Metaphysis

The end of the diaphysis facing the epiphyseal cartilage is known as metaphysis. It is the most actively growing area of the bone and is highly vascular, being supplied by nutrient artery, periosteal arteries and juxta-epiphyseal arteries. The microorganism may settle in the hairpin like capillary loops formed by branches of nutrient arteries here. Hence, in the long bone, metaphysis is prone to infections (osteomyelitis).

Sesamoid Bones

These bones develop in tendons as seed hence the name sesamoid (seed). Sesamoid bones act as pulleys for muscular contraction. The unique features of the sesamoid bones are, they develop in tendons, ossify after birth, are devoid of periosteum and lack Haversian system. The examples of sesamoid bones are, patella in quadriceps femoris, pisiform in flexor carpi ulnaris, fabella in lateral head of gastrocnemius, two bones in the two heads of flexor hallucis brevis, in tendon of peroneus longus and rider's bone in adductor longus origin.

Classification of Joints

The joints are known as arthroses. Broadly, the joints are grouped in two types, movable (diarthroses or synovial) and immovable (synarthroses). The movable joints have cavity within them. In immovable joints, the bones are united by solid bond of special connective tissue. There are two types of synarthroses, fibrous (in which the connecting bond is connective tissue) and cartilaginous (in which the connecting bond is a plate of cartilage).

Types of Fibrous Joints

The three types of fibrous joints are, suture, syndesmosis and gomphosis.

a. The suture is the most common type. A large number of flat cranial bones unite by sutural ligaments. The types of sutures are, serrate, denticulate, plane, squamous and schindylesis (or wedge and groove). The only example of the last type is the joint between vomer and rostrum of sphenoid.
b. In syndesmosis two bones are united by interosseous membrane or ligament, for example, inferior tibiofibular joint, middle radioulnar joint and middle tibiofibular joint.
c. Gomphosis is a peg and socket type of fibrous joint seen between the teeth and alveolar sockets.

Types of Cartilaginous Joints

a. In synchondroses or primary cartilaginous joints the articulating bones are joined by hyaline cartilage. The primary function of these joints is growth. Once the growth is achieved the synchondroses become the synostoses (ossified). Hence, synchondroses are temporary joints. The best examples of this variety are, joint between diaphysis and epiphysis of long bones and the joint between basisphenoid and basiocciput at the base of the skull. The first costosternal or chondrosternal joint is traditionally included in this category based on the assumption that first costal cartilage undergoes calcification and ossification after the completion of growth.

b. The examples of unclassified arthroses are the costochondral joints, in which the union between the cartilage and the bone is by continuity of the perichondrium and periosteum. Nowadays, first chondrosternal joint is regarded as unclassified variety of synarthroses since the first costal cartilage is united to the manubrium by a thin lamina of fibrocartilage. It must be understood that in both costochondral and sternochondral joints the union is between cartilage and bone.
c. In symphyses or secondary cartilaginous joints the articulating bones are united by fibrocartilaginous plate. These joints are midline in location in the body and are permanent. The examples are, joints between vertebral bodies, symphysis pubis, manubriosternal joint, lumbosacral joint and sacrococcygeal joint.

Types of Synovial Joints

a. Plane joints are between the flat surfaces of articulating bones (examples being, intercarpal joints, intertarsal joints, facet joints of vertebrae and sacroiliac joints).
b. Hinge joint allows movements around transverse axis (examples being, elbow joint, ankle joint and interphalangeal joints).
c. Pivot joint allows rotation movements along a vertical axis (examples being, superior radioulnar joint and median atlantoaxial joint).
d. Bicondylar or condylar joints allow conjunct and adjunct rotations (examples being, temporomandibular joint and knee joint).
e. Ellipsoidal joints are biaxial joints (examples being, wrist joint and the metacarpophalangeal joints).
f. Saddle or sellar joint is biaxial and the articulating surfaces are reciprocally concavo-convex. The first carpometacarpal joint (trapeziometacarpal joint) belongs to this type.
g. Ball and socket type of joints are freely mobile as they are multiaxial (examples being, hip joint, shoulder joint, talocalcaneonavicular joint and incudostapedial joint).

203 Bones of Upper Limb

CLAVICLE OR COLLAR BONE

The clavicle is an unusual bone. It is an S-shaped subcutaneous long bone that lies horizontally in the body. It is the first long bone to ossify having two primary centres, which appear during 5th to 6th weeks of intra-uterine life. It is the only long bone to ossify in membrane. However, its two ends grow by endochondral ossification.

Cleidocranial dysostosis is the autosomal recessive disorder in which the clavicles may be absent or show defective ossification along with defects in cranial bones that ossify in membrane. Persons without clavicles can bring the two shoulders close together in front of the chest. Bilateral dislocation of sternoclavicular joints causes instability of clavicle (floating clavicle).

Relations of Posterior Surface of Medial 2/3rds of Clavicle

a. At the medial end related to three veins (terminal parts of internal jugular and subclavian veins and the beginning of brachiocephalic vein)
b. Divisions of the trunks of the brachial plexus
c. Third part of subclavian vessels
d. Suprascapular vessels along the upper part of its posterior surface.

Growing End

The sternal end is the growing end. An epiphysis appears in this end at 18 to 20 years of life and unites with the shaft at 25 years. It is the last of all epiphyses of the body to unite with the shaft of its bone.

Blood Supply

The nutrient artery of the clavicle arises from clavicular branch of acromiothoracic artery.

Fracture of Clavicle

The clavicle is commonly fractured at the junction of medial two- thirds and lateral one-third. This part is weak because it is located between two differently-shaped and differently curved parts of clavicle. The medial two-thirds of clavicle is cylindrical in shape and convex forwards while the lateral one-third is fattened and concave forwards. When the clavicle fractures medial to the attachment of the coracoclavicular ligament, its two fragments are displaced in different directions, corresponding to the muscle pull. The medial fragment is displaced upwards due to sternomastoid while the lateral fragment is drawn downwards by the weight of the upper limb. The contraction of pectoralis major pulls the lateral fragment medially. This leads to overriding of the two fragments and shortening of the clavicle. In fracture of the clavicle the subclavian artery and the pleura (lying posterior to the artery) may be injured causing serious bleeding into the pleural cavity. The tearing of the communicating vein between the cephalic vein and the external jugular vein, which passes anterior to the clavicle, may cause bleeding. The divisions of the trunks of the brachial plexus are in danger in the fracture due to their close proximity.

Scapula

This is a flat triangular bone, which is located on the posterior thoracic wall. It articulates with the humerus at the shoulder joint and with the clavicle at the acromio-clavicular joint. It provides attachments to a large number of muscles. The scapula is suspended from the cranium by trapezius and held close to the posterior thoracic wall by the serratus anterior.

Features

The scapula has three borders (superior, medial or vertebral and lateral), three angles (lateral or glenoid, superior and inferior) and three processes (coracoid, acromion and spinous). It has two surfaces, costal facing anteriorly and dorsal facing posteriorly. It is the only bone in the body having three types of epiphyses. The upper part of the glenoid cavity is a pressure epiphysis, acromion is a traction epiphysis and coracoid process is an atavistic epiphysis.

Palpable Parts

Tip of coracoid process is felt through the lateral side of infraclavicular fossa. The acromion and the crest of the spine are subcutaneous. The inferior angle is palpable at the level of seventh thoracic vertebra and seventh rib. It is used to count the ribs and vertebrae. The medial border is palpable below the spine. The meeting of the crest of the spine with the medial margin is at the level of third thoracic spine.

Vascular Relations

a. The superior border presents suprascapular notch, which is converted into suprascapular foramen by superior transverse ligament. The suprascapular artery passes above the ligament to enter the supraspinous fossa (suprascapular nerve passes through the foramen).
b. The lateral border is related to circumflex scapular artery and thoracodorsal artery. The circumflex scapular (a branch of subscapular) turns round the lateral border between two sets of fibers of teres minor muscle. The thoracodorsal artery, the continuation of subscapular artery below the origin of circumflex scapular, follows the lateral margin of scapula to its inferior angle.
c. The medial border is related to the deep branch of the transverse cervical artery or the dorsal scapular artery.
d. The branches of the above mentioned arteries form anastomosis around the scapula on its dorsal and costal aspects. Enlargements of the scapular anastomoses may occur in arterial obstruction between the first part of subclavian artery and the third part of axillary artery. This may give rise to pulsating scapula.

Triangle of Auscultation

The lower part of the medial border of scapula laterally, lateral margin of trapezius medially and latissimus dorsi below, are the boundaries of the triangle.

Winged Scapula

Winged scapula is the deformity in which the vertebral border and inferior angle of scapula protrude posteriorly due to paralysis of serratus anterior muscle.

Humerus

It is the bone of arm and is the longest bone of upper limb. The humerus is intimately related to three nerves.

a. The upper end of the humerus presents head, greater tuberosity, lesser tuberosity, bicipital sulcus and three necks.
   i. The anatomical neck surrounds the margin of head and gives attachment to the capsule of shoulder joint except at its inferomedial part.
   ii. The surgical neck is the part of the upper end, where the upper end joins the shaft of humerus. Being thin, the surgical neck is vulnerable to fracture in which case axillary nerve and posterior circumflex humeral vessels are liable to be injured.
   iii. The morphological neck corresponds to the epiphyseal line between the upper end and the shaft of the humerus. In the adult, its position is about half cm above the surgical neck.
b. The shaft of the humerus is clothed with muscles. Its posterior aspect presents a spiral groove, which houses the radial nerve and profunda brachi artery. In fracture of the shaft, the radial nerve is in danger of injury.
c. The lower end presents medial epicondyle, trochlea, capitulum and lateral epicondyle. The posterior surface of medial epicondyle is closely related to ulnar nerve, which can be palpated against it. The medial epicondyle is called funny bone because a hit on the epicondyle by a hard object gives rise to painful and tingling sensations along the medial side of forearm and hand. In the fracture of the medial epicondyle, the ulnar nerve is likely to be injured. The anterior aspect of medial epicondyle presents area for common flexor origin for five muscles. Similarly, the anterior surface of lateral epicondyle presents area for common

extensor origin for four muscles below which it gives origin to supinator. The posterior surface of lateral epicondyle gives origin to anconeus. Both epicondyles give attachments to respective collateral ligaments of elbow joint.

Three Bony Points Behind the Elbow

The tip of the olecranon process of ulna and the tips of the medial and lateral epicondyles of humerus form a triangle in the flexed position of the elbow. However, these bony points are in a transverse line in the extended elbow. This knowledge is helpful in differentiating the supracondylar fracture of humerus from the posterior dislocation of the elbow joint. In supracondylar fracture, the distal fragment of humerus along with the olecranon moves posteriorly without any change in the positions of the three bony points. On the contrary, in the posterior dislocation of the elbow joint, the olecranon moves posteriorly away from the humerus changing the normal relations with the epicondyles.

Growing End

The upper end of humerus is its growing end (the nutrient foramen is directed towards the elbow). The nutrient artery is a branch of profunda brachii artery.

Supracondylar Fracture

This is the fracture at the distal end of humerus just above the epicondyles. It occurs most often in children as a result of a fall on the outstretched hand. The distal fragment of humerus moves backwards and upwards. The proximal fragment moves forwards causing compression of the brachial artery and the median nerve, which are the anterior relations of the humeral shaft.

Radius

The radius is the lateral bone of the forearm. It is the weight bearing bone hence fractures of radius amongst the forearm bones are more common. It has a broader distal end and disc-like head and a neck proximally. The head moves in the annular ligament during movements of pronation and supination. It is felt in a depression just below the lateral epicondyle of humerus. The movements of the head in supination and pronation in this location can be appreciated in the flexed position of the elbow. The interosseous borders of radius and ulna are connected by the interosseous membrane, through which weight is transmitted from the radius to ulna. The distal end has Lister's tubercle on the dorsal aspect. The tendon of EPL grooves the medial aspect of the tubercle as it changes direction around this tubercle. The styloid process of radius extends for a longer distance than ulnar styloid process. The radial styloid process lies in the floor of anatomical snuff-box.. The radial artery is palpated against the shaft of the distal end of radius lateral to the tendon of flexor carpi radialis.

Section Six

Growing End

The lower end of the radius is the growing end.

Colles' Fracture

This is the fracture of the lower end of radius. It commonly occurs in elderly women due to a fall on outstretched hand. The wrist and hand show a dinner fork deformity, which occurs due to the displacement of the lower fragment of radius in the posterior and upward direction. As a result, the radial styloid process moves upwards so that it is at the same level or at a higher level than that of ulnar styloid process.

Smith's Fracture or Reversed Colles' Fracture

In this fracture the displacement of the lower fragment is opposite to that of Colles' fracture. The distal fragment is displaced anteriorly and downwards.

Ulna

The ulna is the medial bone of the forearm. Its proximal end looks like a hook and bears the olecranon and coracoid processes. The upper articular surface (trochlear notch) articulates with the trochlea of humerus. The olecranon process and the posterior border of ulna are subcutaneous. The tip of olecranon process provides insertion to triceps brachii muscle. The violent contraction of this muscle may fracture the olecranon process. The lower tapering end of ulna shows head and styloid process. The ulnar styloid process is palpable is supinated position of forearm about one cm proximal to the plane of radial styloid process. The ulnar head is excluded from wrist joint by articular disc of the inferior radioulnar joint.

Growing End

Lower end of ulna is its growing end.

Carpal Bones

There are eight carpal bones arranged in two rows. The proximal row consists of (from lateral to medial) scaphoid, lunate, triquetral, pisiform and the distal row consists of trapezium, trapezoid, capitate and hamate. Carpal bones are small irregular bones. The pisiform is the sesamoid bone in the tendon of flexor carpi ulnaris.

Ossifiaction

The ossification of carpus is important. It helps in determining the bone age. Each carpal bone ossifies from one primary center, which appears after birth. Capitate is the first bone to show ossification followed by hamate. Pisiform is the last to ossify.

Time of Appearance of Ossification Centers

- Capitate—second month
- Hamate—end of third month
- Triquetral—third year
- Lunate—fourth year
- Scaphoid, trapezium and trapezoid—fourth to fifth year
- Pisiform—tenth to twelfth year.

Fracture of Scaphoid

Of all the carpal bones, the scaphoid is the most commonly fractured. The reason for this is that the distal half of scaphoid belongs to the distal row and proximal half belongs to proximal row of carpal bones. The waist or narrow part between the two-halves of the bone lies in intercarpal line, which is subjected to maximum stresses. Hence, waist is the common site of fracture. The artery supplying the scaphoid enters through its distal half. Hence, if the waist is fractured blood supply to the proximal half is engendered and it undergoes avascular necrosis resulting in the non-union of fracture. Scaphoid can be palpated in the floor of anatomical snuff-box. In fracture of scaphoid pain and tenderness are felt in the snuff-box.

Dislocation of Lunate

The lunate is commonly dislocated in the anterior direction, which may cause compression of the median nerve in the carpal tunnel.

Metacarpal Bones

The five metacarpal bones numbered from lateral to medial are the miniature long bones. The first metacarpal is shortest and strongest. It is the modified first phalanx of thumb. It is not in line with the other four metacarpals. It gives great mobility to the thumb by its articulation with the trapezium. It's mode of ossification is like the phalanx.

Bennet's Fracture

It is the fracture of the base of first metacarpal involving the first carpometacarpal joint. This is often caused by direct blow with closed fist, as in boxing.

204 Bones of Lower Limb

HIP BONE OR INNOMINATE BONE

The hipbone is an irregular bone made up of three components, the ilium, pubis and ischium, which are united to each other at the acetabulum. The articulations of the hipbone are, pubic symphysis between the pubic bones, the sacroiliac joint between the sacrum and ilium and the hip joint between the acetabulum and the head of femur. The right and left hipbones, the sacrum and coccyx together, form the bony pelvis. Because of its location, the hipbone belongs to lower limb, pelvis and perineum. Therefore, the attachments and relations of the hipbone can be best appreciated only after familiarity with the anatomy of the lower limb, pelvis and perineum.

Anatomical Position

To hold the hipbone in anatomical position, one has to see that the pubic tubercle and anterior superior iliac spine lie in the same coronal plane. In this position, the pelvic surface of the body of pubis faces postero-superiorly and the medial surface of the body of pubis lies in the midline.

Ilium

The ilium consists of upper end, (iliac crest), lower end, anterior, posterior and medial margins, iliac fossa, sacro-pelvic surface and gluteal surface.

Iliac Crest

It is the subcutaneous curved upper end of ilium extending from the anterior superior iliac spine (ASIS) to the posterior superior iliac spine (PSIS). It consists of outer lip, intermediate area and inner lip in its ventral two-thirds. The tubercle of the iliac crest lies about 5 cm behind the anterior end of the crest on its outer lip. The supracristal plane is the line passing through the highest points of iliac crests and it corresponds to the spine of L4 vertebra or passes between the third and fourth lumbar vertebra. This plane is used to determine the site of lumbar puncture. The transtubercular plane passes through the upper margin of L5 vertebra.

Structures Attached to Ventral Segment

Outer lip gives attachment to tensor fasciae latae from ASIS to iliac tubercle to external oblique abdominis in its anterior two-thirds and to latissimus dorsi in its posterior one-third (part of the crest between the two muscles forms the base of lumbar triangle).

a. Intermediate area gives attachment to internal oblique abdominis.
b. Inner lip gives attachment to transversus abdominis in anterior two-thirds and quadratus lumborum in posterior one-third.
c. Important vascular relation of the inner lip of iliac crest is the deep circumflex iliac artery.

Structures Attached to Dorsal Segment

Outer surface gives attachment to gluteus maximum and inner surface to erector spinae.

Anterior Border of Ilium

The anterior superior iliac spine gives attachments to-sartorius and inguinal ligament and anterior inferior iliac spine to straight head of rectus femoris and iliofemoral ligament.

Posterior Border of Ilium

The posterior superior iliac spine is not visible externally but lies subjacent to the skin dimple called dimple of Venus (well-marked in female) in the upper part of the gluteal region. It corresponds to the spine of second sacral vertebra (level with lower end of subarachnoid space). This site is often used to draw bone marrow from the iliac crest for studying the cells of bone marrow.

Greater Sciatic Notch

The greater sciatic notch with the help of sacrotuberous and sacrospinous ligaments forms the greater sciatic foramen, which gives passage to the piriformis muscle and 2 structures above it and 8 structures below it.

- Structures above the piriformis are, superior gluteal nerve and vessels
- Structures below the piriformis are, inferior gluteal nerve and vessels, posterior cutaneous nerve of thigh, sciatic nerve, nerve to quadratus femoris, internal pudendal vessels, pudendal nerve and nerve to obturator internus.

Medial Border of Ilium

The posterior one-third is rough; middle third is sharp and the anterior third forms arcuate line, which is continuous with pecten pubis at ilio-pubic eminence. The linea terminalis (lateral boundary of pelvic inlet) is composed of arcuate line, pecten pubis and pubic crest. Some structures cross it to enter the lesser pelvis (internal iliac vessels, ureter, ovarian vessels in female and vas deferens in male). The round ligament of uterus also crosses the linea terminalis to leave the lesser pelvis.

Surfaces of Ilium

a. Iliac fossa gives origin to iliacus muscle.
b. Sacro-pelvic surface has sacral part dorsally and pelvic part ventrally. The sacral part presents an auricular surface covered with articular cartilage and non-articular area (iliac tuberosity). Auricular surface articulates with sacrum at sacroiliac joint. The iliac tuberosity gives attachment to iliolumbar ligament, dorsal sacroiliac and interosseous sacroiliac ligaments. The smooth pelvic surface presents pre-auricular sulcus, which is well marked in female. This sulcus gives attachment to ventral sacroiliac ligament.
c. Gluteal surface is divided into four areas by posterior, anterior and inferior gluteal lines.
   - Gluteus maximus—to the area behind posterior gluteal line.
   - Gluteus medius—to area between posterior and anterior lines.
   - Gluteus minimus—to area between anterior and inferior lines.
   - Reflected head of rectus femoris—below inferior gluteal line.

Ischium

This part of hip bone consists of body and a ramus. The upper end of the body is united with ilium and pubis in acetabulum. The dorsal part of this area is in direct contact with sciatic nerve. The lower end forms the ischial tuberosity. The posterior margin of the body presents the ischial spine.

Relations and Attachments of Ischial Spine

a. Ligaments—sacrospinous ligament is attached to the apex.
b. Muscles—coccygeus and most posterior fibers of levator ani muscle take origin from the pelvic surface.
c. Internal pudendal vessels and nerve to obturator internus cross the dorsal surface.
d. Ureter—related to pelvic surface.
e. In pudendal nerve block by vaginal approach the ischial spine is the landmark as the pudendal nerve crosses the dorsal aspect of the sacrospinous ligament near the apex of the ischial spine.

Lesser Sciatic Notch

The structures that pass through the lesser sciatic foramen are, tendon of obturator internus, nerve to obturator internus, internal pudendal vessels and pudendal nerve.

Relations of Ischial Tuberosity

The lower part of the smooth pelvic aspect of the ischial tuberosity is related to the lateral wall of the ischiorectal fossa (pudendal or Alcock's canal). In pudendal nerve block by perineal approach the needle is inserted along the medial side of ischial tuberosity for the depth of about 4 cm to reach the pudendal canal.

Attachments of Ischial Tuberosity

a. The sacrotuberous ligament is attached to medial margin.
b. The quadratus femoris muscle is attached to lateral margin.
c. Its gluteal surface is divided by a transverse ridge into upper quadrangular and lower triangular areas. The upper area is unequally divided by an oblique line into a superolateral area for semimembranosus and the superomedial area (placed at lower level compared to the superolateral area) for the semitendinosus and long head of biceps femoris. A vertical line divides the lower area in a larger lateral area (for origin of ischial part of adductor magnus) and smaller medial area, which is covered with fibrofatty tissue since this area comes in contact with the ground in sitting position. The ischial bursa intervenes between the tuberosity and the gluteus maximus. The inflammation of this bursa is called weaver's bottom.

Pubis

The pubis is the anterior part of the hip bone and consists of the body and superior and inferior rami. The two pubic bones articulate at the pubic symphysis.

Pubic Crest

The upper palpable margin of the body of pubis is called pubic crest. The rounded lateral end of the pubic crest is called pubic tubercle, which is a very important bony landmark. The pubic tubercle is partly covered in male by spermatic cord. The hernia that is superomedial to this tubercle is inguinal and the one that is inferolateral to it is femoral.

Posterior or pelvic surface forms the anterior wall of retropubic space (cave of Retzius), which separates it from urinary bladder (hence fracture of the body of pubis may injure urinary bladder). The posterior surface gives origin to pubococcygeus part of levator ani.

Superior Ramus

Its superior border (pecten pubis or pectineal line) is sharp. It extends from pubic tubercle to the iliopubic eminence and provides attachments to conjoint tendon, lacunar ligament and the pectineus muscle. The anterior border is called obturator crest, which extends from the pubic tubercle to the acetabular notch. The inferior border is sharp and takes part in the formation of obtuartor foramen. The inferior margin of the superior ramus and the medial (lower) margin of femoral neck together form a smoothly curved line (Shenton's line) in normal radiographs.

Inferior Ramus

It extends from the body of pubis to the ischial ramus, medial to the obturator foramen. The two rami unite to form conjoint ischiopubic ramus.

Conjoint Ischiopubic Ramus

The lower border of the conjoint ramus is everted in males. It provides attachment to fascia lata of thigh and membranous layer of superficial fascia of perineum (Colle's fascia). The inner surface is smooth. It forms the lateral limit of the urogenital triangle of the perineum. This surface is divided in three areas by attachment of two fascial layers, namely, superior fascia of urogenital diaphragm and inferior fascia of urogenital diaphragm (perineal membrane). The uppermost area gives origin to intrapelvic muscle, namely, obturator internus. The intermediate area gives attachment to muscles of deep perineal pouch (sphincter urethrae and deep transversus perinei). The lower area gives attachment to some contents of superficial perineal pouch (crus of clitoris or penis in front, ischiocavernosus muscle around the crus and superficial transversus perinei muscle behind). Fusion of the ischial and pubic rami occurs by the age of 6 to 8 years.

Femur

The femur is the longest and strongest bone in the body. Its length is one-fourth of the height of the individual (approximately 45 cm in a six feet person). The shaft of the femur is convex forwards because the line of gravity of the body passes behind the hip joint and in front of the knee joint. The weakness caused by the forward convexity of the shaft is compensated by linea aspera (a thickened ridge) on the posterior aspect of middle third of the shaft.

At the lower end, the lips of linea aspera continue as lateral and medial supracondylar lines. The lateral supracondylar line ends in lateral epicondyle. The medial supracondylar line is interrupted, where the femoral vessels cross it (at the lowest osseoaponeurotic opening). It reappears below this point and ends in adductor tubercle.

Vascular Relations

a. The inferomedial part of the head of femur is separated by psoas major tendon from the femoral artery at the midinguinal point. The artery can be compressed against the head of femur to stop bleeding if the distal arteries of the lower limb are injured.
b. The lowest osseo-aponeurotic opening or adductor hiatus lies at the medial supracondylar line about the junction of middle and lower thirds of the femur. At this opening the femoral vessels become the popliteal vessels.
c. Popliteal surface of femur is in direct contact with the popliteal artery.
d. Linea aspera is in close relation to profunda femoris vessels.
e. The perforating arteries (branches of profunda femoris) cross the linea aspera at the osseo-aponeurotic openings in the insertion of adductor magnus.
f. Retinacular arteries produce grooves on the anterior surface of the neck of femur.

Upper End

The upper end presents head, neck, greater trochanter and lesser trochanter. The tip of the greater trochanter is palpable about a hand's breadth below the midpoint of iliac crest.

Neck

The neck is very long and narrow and connects the head to the shaft. It is obliquely set on the femoral shaft. The neck-shaft angle or angle of inclination is 125° in adult. In coax vara the angle of inclination is decreased while in coax valga it is increased. The neck represents the metaphysis of the developing bone as it is ossified from the primary center. The anterior surface of the neck is fully intracapsular but the posterior surface is partly intracapsular. The anterior surface is marked with longitudinal grooves produced by the retinacular arteries arising from the vascular ring around the capsular attachment. There are numerous vascular foramina on this surface. The neck is strengthened by calcar femorale, which is a plate of compact bone extending from the linea aspera to the neck. In old age, maximum osteoporosis occurs in the neck hence it is liable for fractures with slightest trauma.

Fracture of Femoral Neck

This fracture is very common in postmenopausal women because of the osteoporotic changes in the bones. The fracture may be intracapsular or extracapsular. In intracapsular fracture the proximal fragment often loses part of its blood supply hence the union of this fracture is difficult. The injured limb lies in the position of lateral rotation and the lower limb is shortened. The shaft of femur carrying the trochanters is laterally rotated (by lateral rotators of thigh and psoas major) and is elevated due to the upward pull of hamstring and adductor muscles) on the injured side. The complication of this fracture is avascular necrosis of head of femur. In extracapsular fracture of the neck the blood supply to the proximal fragment is retained hence the fracture heals faster.

Shenton's Line

This is visible only on X-ray. It is a smoothly curved line (concavity facing downwards) formed by medial margin of the neck and the lower margin of the superior ramus of pubis. Fracture of the neck may distort the line.

Fractures of Shaft of Femur

When the shaft of femur breaks in two fragments it is difficult to keep the fragments together due to pull of the muscles attached to the femur. The flexors are inserted in lesser trochanter, the abductors in greater trochanter and the adductors into the linea aspera. The gastrocnemius muscles are attached to the lower end of femur.

a. In the fracture in the proximal third of the shaft (subtrochanteric), the small proximal fragment is drawn in flexed position by iliopsoas muscle and abducted by gluteus medius and minimus muscles.

b. In the fracture of middle third of the shaft (midshaft) the adductor muscles pull the distal fragment upward and medially.
c. In the fracture of the distal third of the shaft (the supracondylar) gastrocnemius muscles flex the distal fragment backward thereby injuring the popliteal artery.

Popliteal Surface of Femur

The popliteal surface is present at the lower part of the posterior aspect of shaft, between the lateral and medial supracondylar lines. It forms the upper part of the floor of popliteal fossa. The popliteal artery is in contact with this surface.

Lower End of Femur

The lower end of the femur bears two large condyles separated by an intercondylar fossa. The ossification center for the lower end appears just before birth at the ninth month of intrauterine life. This is of medicolegal importance. The presence of this center is a proof of the viability of the newborn that is born dead. The medial condyle presents adductor tubercle, which is a palpable landmark. The lower epiphyseal line passes through the adductor tubercle. Any injury to the epiphyseal plate (during childhood) will shorten the limb.

Growing End

The lower end is the growing end of femur. The direction of nutrient foramen is towards the upper end. The nutrient artery is usually derived from the second perforating branch of profunda femoris artery.

Length of Femur

The length of femur is measured from the tip of greater trochanter to the lateral condyle.

Patella (Kneecap)

The patella is the largest sesamoid bone and develops in the tendon of quadriceps femoris. The insertion of quadriceps femoris in it is extended to the tibial tuberosity via ligamentum patellae. Normally, the patella lies in front of the knee joint. Sometimes it may be placed quite high (patella alta) and sometimes, it may be placed low (patella baja). The patella functions as both lever and pulley. As a lever the patella magnifies the force exerted by quadriceps during extension of knee. As a pulley the patella alters the direction of the pull of quadriceps for better efficiency. It keeps the quadriceps away from the bones of knee joint so as to protect it during extension movement. However, in flexion movement, the patella straddles the knee joint as in this position it is in contact with both condyles of femur.

Ossification

Patella ossifies from several centers that develop in quadriceps tendon during 3 to 6 years. Fusion is complete at puberty.

Arterial Supply

The transverse anastomosis (between the inferior genicular arteries) that lies deep to ligamentum patellae supplies blood to the patella.

Clinical Highlights

a. The patella has a natural tendency to dislocate laterally. The explanation for this is as follows. The quadriceps femoris is obliquely placed in line with femur but the ligamentum patellae is in line with tibial tuberosity. As a result of this inclination, whenever quadriceps femoris contracts it pulls the patella upwards and laterally (rectus femoris is attached to anterior inferior iliac spine, which is laterally placed compared to patella). This tendency is counteracted by bony and muscular factors. The forward projection of lateral condyle of femur prevents lateral movement of patella. Similarly, the medial pull of vastus medialis oblique on the patella is stronger than the lateral pull by the vastus lateralis. The recurrent dislocation of patella on extension of knee, may occur if the factors, which keep its position are diseased, for example, weakness of quadriceps muscle, traumatic rupture of medial patellar retinaculum and congenitally underdeveloped lateral condyle of femur.
b. The patella may be fractured by direct trauma or by sudden and forceful contraction of quadriceps femoris.
c. Bipartite patella is a bilateral condition in which a separate process of the bone develops from separate center of ossification at the superolateral angle. This may be mistaken for fracture.

Tibia

The tibia is the medial bone of the leg. It is a robust bone as it is the main weight-bearing bone of the leg. The upper end of tibia bears lateral and medial condyles and on the anterior aspect there is tibial tuberosity, to which ligamentum patellae is attached. The ossification center for tibial tuberosity is usually present at birth.

Intercondylar Area

An intercondylar non-articular area is present between the articular surfaces of the two condyles. This area provides attachments to following structures from before backward, anterior horn of medial meniscus, anterior cruciate ligament, anterior horn of lateral meniscus, posterior horn of lateral meniscus, posterior horn of medial meniscus and posterior cruciate ligament.

The shaft of tibia has three surfaces and three borders. The anterior border or shin is entirely subcutaneous and extends from tibial tuberosity to the medial margin of medial malleolus. The medial surface is entirely subcutaneous. At its upper end the medial surface receives insertion of three muscles representing the three compartments of thigh (sartorius, gracilis and semitendinosus). The pattern created by linear insertions of these tendons resembles the foot of a goose, which in Greek is *Pes anserinus*. Therefore, these three muscles are called anserine muscles and the bursa in between these tendons is known as anserine bursa. Long saphenous vein (accompanied by saphenous nerve) crosses the lower third of this surface. The long saphenous vein is often cannulated on this surface, in front of the medial malleolus. The medial surface and anterior border are used for taking pieces of bone for bone grafting. The upper part of medial surface is the favored site for marrow puncture and intraosseous infusion in very small children.

The lower end of the tibia is smaller than the upper end. It projects medially as medial malleous, which is subcutaneous. The apex of the medial malleolus gives attachment to deltoid ligament of ankle joint. The anterior aspect of the lower end is crossed by structures in the anterior compartment of leg. From medial to lateral side, they are, tibialis anterior, extensor hallucis longus, anterior tibial artery, deep peroneal nerve, extensor digitorum longus and peroneus tertius. The posterior aspect of the lower end is related to structures that enter the sole from the posterior compartment of leg. From medial to lateral, they are, tibialis posterior, flexor digitorum longus, posterior tibial artery, tibial nerve and flexor hallucis longus.

Growing End

The upper end of tibia is its growing end. The large nutrient foramen points inferiorly. The nutrient artery is derived from posterior tibial artery.

Delayed Union of Tibial Fractures

The fractures of the tibia are frequent nowadays due to increase in the road traffic accidents (RTA). The tibia is comparatively slender at the junction of its upper two-thirds and lower third hence fracture at this site is very common. The union of the fracture at this site is delayed due to inadequate blood supply to the lower one-third of tibia. There are two reasons for this. The nutrient artery enters the tibia at its upper third. The fracture at the junctional site may injure the nutrient artery. Much of the blood supply to the tibia comes from the muscles attached to the shaft via the periosteum. Absence of muscle attachments in the distal third of tibia is a contributory factor for poor blood supply to its lower one-third.

Fibula

The fibula is the lateral bone of the leg. Since it does not transmit weight it is very thin. The upper end has head, neck and styloid process. The lower end projects as lateral malleolus. The tip of the lateral malleolus is lower than that of medial malleolus. On the medial surface of the lateral malleolus, there are two features, which help in holding the bone in anatomical position. A triangular articular facet is present anteriorly and the malleolar fossa is present posteriorly. The lateral surface of the malleolus is subcutaneous.

The head and neck of fibula are palpable. The common peroneal nerve can be rolled against the posterolateral surface of the neck. The nerve is injured in fracture of the neck of fibula or due to tight fitting plaster cast.

There are three borders, anterior, posterior and medial, which give attachment to anterior and posterior intermuscular septa and to the interosseous membrane of the leg. The surfaces are, anterior, lateral and posterior. The peroneal crest or median crest, which is located on posterior surface, is closely related to peroneal artery. Fibula is an ideal bone for taking pieces for bone grafting.

Growing End

The upper end of fibula is its growing end. The direction of nutrient foramen is towards the ankle. The nutrient artery is a branch of peroneal artery.

Rule of Ossification

The rule of ossification states that the secondary center that appears first fuses last or the one that appears last fuses first. In the case of fibula, the secondary center for lower end appears in first or second year and fuses with the shaft by 15 to 19 years. The center for upper end appears by third or fourth year and fuses by 17-19 years. Therefore, fibula breaks the rule of ossification. The lower end of fibula is pressure epiphysis (takes part in ankle joint) and upper end is traction epiphysis (does not take part in joint but gives attachment to biceps femoris).

Fractures of Bones of Leg

Both the bones of the leg fracture commonly in motorcycle accidents. The tibia, being more exposed is more vulnerable. The fractures of the tibial condyles will involve the knee joint also. The fractures of tibial shaft usually injure the vessels in the leg causing hemorrhage in the closed fascial compartments. This may lead to vascular insufficiency to the leg and foot. The fractures of the tibia and fibula involving the ankle joint are known as Pott's fracture. Depending on the direction of rotational forces different parts of the two bones may be fractured. Fracture of medial and lateral malleoli may occur alone or in combination. Rupture of interosseous tibiofibular ligament may cause dislocation of ankle joint. Fracture of medial malleolus may be accompanied by rupture of medial ligament (deltoid ligament) of ankle. This results in lateral displacement of talus. In typical Pott's fracture, there is fracture of medial malleolus and rupture of deltoid ligament, fracture of lower end of fibula and lateral displacement of the whole foot with the talus.

Measurement of Length of Lower Limb

Ideally, the distance from the head of the femur to the sole reflects the length of the lower limb. But, actually the anterior superior iliac spine is the upper bony point and medial malleolus is the lower bony point. The distance between these points measured in the supine position, is taken as true leg length.

Skeleton of Foot

The foot consists of 28 bones, 7 tarsal, 5 metatarsal, 14 phalanges and 2 sesamoid bones in the tendons of insertion of flexor hallucis brevis.

Tarsal Bones

These small irregular bones articulate with each other and with the metatarsal bones to form segmented levers in the foot. The talus is the weight bearing bone since it takes part in ankle joint. It is shaped like a tortoise with a body, neck and head. One special feature of talus is that it has no muscular attachments. The inferomedial part of the head of talus is supported by spring ligament. The calcaneus is the largest and most posterior tarsal bone. It forms the heel of the foot. The shelf-like projection from its medial side (sustentaculum tali) supports the talus. The cuboid is located along the lateral margin of foot. Its inferior surface bears a groove, which is converted in a tunnel for peroneus longus tendon by the long plantar ligament. The navicular bone lies along the medial margin of the foot. The tuberosity of the navicular bone projects medially and is felt along the medial margin of the foot. The medial, intermediate and lateral cuneiform bones are wedge-shaped and are part of medial longitudinal arch.

Ossification Centers of Tarsal Bones

a. Calcaneus—primary center in third month of intra-uterine life and secondary center for posterior surface (which gives attachment to tendocalcaneus) at six to eight years after birth.
b. Talus—sixth month of intrauterine life
c. Cuboid—just before birth
d. Lateral cuneiform—in the first year
e. Medial cuneiform—in the second year
f. Lateral cuneiform and navicular—in the third year.

Metatarsal Bones

There are five metatarsal bones, which are numbered from medial to lateral side. The first metatarsal is short and stout for weight bearing. The head of the first metatarsal bone makes pressure contact with the ground at the beginning of taking a step. The sesamoid bones in the tendons of flexor hallucis brevis articulate directly with the plantar surface of this bone. The second metatarsal is the longest and least mobile. The fifth bone has a tuberosity at its base, which can be palpated along the lateral margin of foot. The tuberosity receives insertion of peroneus brevis. Sometimes the pull of contraction of this muscle may fracture the tuberosity. Sometimes the tuberosity may ossify by a separate center and remain separate from the base, in which case it is known as os Vesaleus.

Fractures of the Bones of Foot

Fractures of talus and calcaneus are not common. But they may be crushed in landing on the calcaneus from a height. The tuberosity of the fifth metatarsal bone may be avulsed by trivial twisting injuries of the forefoot. Fatigue fractures (march fractures) are common in metatarsal bones. This is due to repeated small bending stresses to the bones. The second metacarpal bone is the most frequently fractured bone in young adults, who walk excessively.

Assessment of Bone Age—Skeletal Age

The bone age is an indicator of the physiological development. It is necessary to assess bone age in children in certain clinical conditions. For this, the presence of ossification centers in the bones of the limbs is studied in the radiographs of the shoulder, elbow, wrist, knee and foot regions of the child.

a. In the newborn, the X-ray of foot and knee is studied. In the full term newborn babies, usually, five ossification centers are present (all in the lower limb). Two centers are located around knee (lower end of femur and upper end of tibia) and three are located in the foot, (calcaneus, talus and cuboid). In 20% of individuals the center for head of humerus appears just before birth.
b. In infants between second to sixth months, the radiograph of shoulder shows the ossification center in the head of the humerus, which appears usually (80%) during the first six months after birth. The radiograph of the wrist reveals the ossification in the capitate by two months and in the hamate by the end of third month.
c. At the end of first year, the wrist shows ossification in the lower end of radius and hip shows ossification in the head of femur. By eighteen months, the centers for greater tuberosity and capitulum appear in humerus.
d. From third year onwards the X-rays of carpal and tarsal bones are more useful.
e. The medial epicondyle of humerus shows the center around 4 to 6 years.
f. Between the 6 to 8 or 7 to 9 years the fusion between the pubic and ischial rami takes place in the hipbone.
g. The center for trochlea of the humerus appears around 9 years.
h. The center for pisiform appears by 10 to 12 years.
i. The center for lateral epicondyle of humerus appears by 12 years.

205 Bones of Thoracic Cage

STERNUM

The sternum or the breast-bone is the axial bone located in the midline of the front of the thoracic cage. From above downwards, the three parts of the sternum are, the broad manubrium sterni, long body and a pointed xiphoid process, which projects in epigastrium of anterior abdominal wall. The xiphoid process is cartilaginous in young age but is ossified in adult. The joint between the manubrium and body is called angle of Louis or sternal angle, which is an important landmark for counting ribs in a patient. The second costal cartilage is attached at the sternal angle. The upper seven ribs articulate with sternum by their costal cartilages. Except the first, the other sternocostal joints are synovial joints. The upper border of manubrium corresponds to lower margin of second thoracic vertebra while its lower border is level with the lower margin of fourth thoracic vertebra. So, manubrium is opposite third and fourth thoracic vertebrae. The sternal angle is at the level of lower margin of fourth thoracic vertebra. The sternal body lies opposite fifth to ninth thoracic vertebrae. The xiphisternal joint corresponds to ninth thoracic vertebra.

Joints of Manubrium

a. Sternoclavicular joint is of synovial variety.
b. Manubriocostal joint (first chondrosternal joint) is between the first costal cartilage and the manubrium. This joint belongs to the unclassified variety of synarthrosis or atypical synchondrosis (also described as primary cartilaginous joint).
c. Manubriosternal joint between the manubrium and first piece of sternum is a secondary cartilaginous joint or symphysis.

Important Relations of Manubrium

Posterior surface of manubrium forms the anterior wall of superior mediastinum. Its vascular relations are the aortic arch and the three branches of aortic arch. The left brachiocephalic vein crosses in front of the three branches, hence this vein is in danger of injury during sternal puncture. On the lateral aspect, the posterior surface is related to the anterior margins of lungs and pleurae.

Important Relations of Body

The posterior surface of the body of sternum forms the anterior boundary of middle mediastinum. Therefore, it is related to the pericardium and the anterior margins of lungs and pleurae. The heart is usually approached for bypass surgery by placing a midline sternum-splitting incision from the jugular notch to the xiphoid process. In head—on collusion, the steering wheel of the car pushes through the sternum into the middle mediastinum of the driver, which may cause rupture of the heart or ascending aorta.

External Cardiac Massage

In a patient with cardiac arrest, the cardio-pulmonary resuscitation (CPR) provides the basic life support. This is done by a technique called external cardiac massage. Firm pressure is applied to the chest vertically downwards on the lower part of the sternum, which should move posteriorly for 4 to 5 cm. This may force the blood out of the heart in the ascending aorta and may act as a stimulant for contraction of the heart.

Ribs or Costae

The ribs are arched bones. The ribs are the only bones having cartilage as their part. The rib and its cartilage are in contact with each other by the continuity of the periosteum of the rib with the perichondrium of the costal cartilage. The costochondral joint belongs to the unclassified synarthroses or atypical synchondroses. The costal cartilages impart elasticity to the rib cage. The ribs articulate posteriorly with the thoracic vertebrae. They are broadly divided in true and false ribs. The first seven ribs are true because they articulate with sternum. The last five ribs are false because they do not articulate with sternum. Depending on their anterior attachments, the ribs are divided in three types.

a. The vertebrosternal ribs are the ones that connect with the sternum through their costal cartilages. The first seven ribs are vertebrosternal ribs or true ribs.
b. The vertebrochondral ribs or false ribs are connected to each other by cartilage (eight to tenth ribs).
c. The floating or vertebral ribs or false ribs (eleventh and twelfth ribs) have their anterior ends free in the abdominal wall. The tenth rib is usually floating in Japanese.

The movements of the ribs are responsible for increasing the anteroposterior and transverse diameters of thorax during inspiration. The ribs are obliquely placed one below the other in the thoracic cage in the adult. In the child, up to the age of 4-6 years, the ribs are horizontally disposed. As a result of this, the child has abdominal breathing. Afterwards, when the ribs become oblique, the respiration becomes thoracic.

The first two and last three ribs have special features hence are called atypical ribs The remaining seven ribs show similar features hence are called typical ribs. The lowest limit of the costal margin is formed by tenth rib.

Typical Rib

The posterior end of the rib bears the head, neck and tubercle. The curved shaft is long and shows the costal groove on lower part of its inner surface. The head bears two facets. The upper facet is for articulation with the body of the vertebra above and the lower one for the numerically corresponding vertebra. The neck is long and lies in front of the transverse process of the corresponding vertebra. The tubercle lies on the outer surface at the junction of the neck and shaft. The articular part of the tubercle articulates with facet on the transverse process of the numerically corresponding vertebra to form costotransverse joint. The heads of the typical ribs are related anteriorly to the sympathetic chain. The shaft of a typical rib is curved like a letter "C". A short distance lateral to the tubercle the rib is twisted and is marked by a rough line. This point is the angle of the rib, where the rib is weakest and hence liable to fracture. The fractured rib may injure the pleura and the lungs. Injury to pleura might result in pneumothorax or hemothorax. Injury to the lower ribs may injure the abdominal organs. The fracture of the left tenth rib may injure the spleen.

First Rib

a. The first rib is the shortest and the most curved rib. It is obliquely placed so that its posterior end is at a higher level compared to its anterior end, which is very broad.
b. The head of first rib has only one facet for the first thoracic vertebra.
c. The anterior relations of the neck are, the sympathetic chain, superior intercostal artery and T1 ventral ramus. The neck and its anterior relations form the posterior relations of the apex of the lung. Therefore, the cancer of lung apex (Pancoast tumor) may present as Horner's syndrome and weakness of small muscles of hand with sensory changes along the inner margin of forearm and hand.
d. The shaft is flat with superior and inferior surfaces separated by inner and outer borders. The lower surface is smooth (as it is covered with costal pleura) and has no costal groove. The inner border is marked by scalene tubercle, which provides insertion to scalenus anterior. The vascular groove in front of the scalene tubercle is for subclavian vein and the one behind it is for subclavian artery and the lower trunk of brachial plexus. Behind the groove for the artery, the superior surface provides attachment to the scalenus medius muscle. The relationship of the two scalene muscles to the neurovascular structures on the superior surface of first rib has clinical significance. The scalene triangle is a narrow triangular gap, which is bounded by the scalenus anterior and medius muscles and the groove for the artery. The subclavian artery and lower trunk in the triangle may be compressed if the scalenus anterior muscle is hypertrophied or if the cervical rib projects in the triangle. The subclavian

vein may also be compressed though outside the triangle. This produces neurovascualr symptoms in the upper limb, which are collectively known as thoracic outlet syndrome or cervical rib syndrome, or scalenus anterior syndrome.

Second Rib

This rib is longer and narrower than the first rib. Its anterior end articulates with the sternal angle. So the second rib is easy to identify in the living.

Tenth Rib

This rib has a single facet on its head, which articulates with the upper border of 10th thoracic vertebra near its pedicle.

Eleventh and Twelfth Ribs

These floating ribs have pointed anterior ends, which are tipped with cartilage. The twelfth rib is related to the costo-diaphgmatic recess of pleura. It is related to posterior surface of kidney in lumbar region. Therefore, in operations on kidney by lumbar route the last two ribs are important landmarks.

Relation of Inferior Line of Pleural Reflexion

The inferior margin of pleura starts from the lower end of anterior margin at sixth costal cartilage on left side and costoxiphoid angle on the right side. As it passes laterally, it crosses the eighth rib at the midclavicular line and the tenth rib at the midaxillary line (about 5 cm above the costal margin). It then passes deep to the eleventh and twelfth ribs to the side of the vertebral column inferior to the medial part of twelfth rib.

Costal Cartilages

The costal cartilages are of hyaline variety. They represent the unossified anterior ends of the ribs. During inspiration, they are twisted upwards. This movement of the costal cartilages stores energy, which is released during expiration. Costal cartilages provide external elastic recoil during normal quiet expiration so that the muscular effort is spared. Calcification of costal cartilages usually occurs in old age. This results in loss of elasticity of the thoracic cage, which in turn results in diaphragmatic or abdominal inspiration.

Abnormal Ribs

The costal elements of the seventh cervical and first lumbar vertebrae may grow to form a rudimentary or complete rib. When an accessory rib is present on both sides, the person will have thirteen pairs of ribs. It is rare to have both lumbar and cervical ribs in the same individual.

a. About 0.5 percent people have cervical ribs. Cervical ribs are the elongated costal elements of seventh cervical vertebra. They may be unilateral or bilateral. They may be fully developed ribs or just fibrous strand reaching the first rib beyond the scalene tubercle. Cervical rib may be symptomless but in some cases, it gives rise to pressure on the structures in relation to the superior surface of first rib causing neurovascular disturbances. It is one of the causes of thoracic outlet syndrome.
b. Lumbar ribs (Gorilla ribs) are comparatively rare. The first lumbar vertebra may show a small projection of a lumbar rib. The only importance of lumbar rib is that it may confuse the identification of vertebral levels in radiographs or it may be confused with fracture of the transverse process of the first lumbar vertebra.

Thoracic Vertebrae

There are twelve thoracic vertebrae, out of which second to eighth are typical and the first, and ninth to twelfth are atypical. All are characterized by presence of costal facets on the body.

Typical Thoracic Vertebra

The body of the vertebra is heart-shaped. On each side, it presents two costal facets, which are actually demifacets. The superior costal facets are placed on the upper border near the pedicle and the lower facets are placed on the lower border. The vertebral foramen is circular. The anterior surface of transverse process near the tip, bears a facet for articulation with the tubercle of corresponding rib. The spine is long and directed downwards and backwards. Tuberculosis of vertebral column (Pott's spine) is common in the thoracic region.

Clinical Highlights

a. Costochondritis is the painful inflammation of the synovial chondrosternal joints.
b. Flail chest is produced when there are multiple rib fractures at chostochondral junctions and near the rib angles. As a result of this, a part of rib cage remains isolated without bony support. This part shows paradoxical movements of chest wall (moves in during inspiration and moves out during expiration).
c. Stove in chest condition develops from localized crushing injury with multiple rib fractures. The affected area is depressed and becomes relatively immobile. It leads to lung complications.
d. In the fracture of ribs, pleura and lung are in danger of injury. In fracture of lower ribs upper abdominal organs like spleen and liver are likely to be injured.
e. Excision of rib is performed to gain access to the thoracic cavity. A segment of the rib is removed by incising the periosteum, which is left inside the body. In this way, the lost rib regenerates after the operation from the osteogenic layer of the periosteum.

206 Bones of Abdomen and Pelvis

LUMBAR VERTEBRAE

There are five lumbar vertebrae. They do not present costal facets and foramina in the transverse processes. The body of lumbar vertebra is quite large. The vertebral foramen is large and triangular. The transverse process shows accessory process at the root. Each superior articular process bears a rough projection called mamillary process on its posterior margin. The lower end of the spinal cord (conus medullaris) and spinal meninges are present in the vertebral canal of first lumbar vertebra. The vertebral canal of the lower four lumbar vertebrae contains the cauda equina, arachnoid mater and dura mater. The sympathetic chain is related to the sides of the anterior surfaces of the bodies of the lumbar vertebrae.

Fifth Lumbar Vertebra

This vertebra is wedge-shaped and hence produces the lumbosacral angle (normal value is 120 to 130°). The transverse processes of the fifth lumbar vertebra are strong and encroach on the body. This is the distinguishing feature of fifth lumbar vertebra. The roots of the obturator nerve and the contribution of the fourth lumbar ventral ramus to the lumbosacral trunk pass anterior to the transverse process of the fifth vertebra. These nerves may be damaged in fracture of the transverse process.

Sacrum

The sacrum consists of five fused vertebrae. It is a large triangular bone that presents markedly concave anterior or pelvic surface and convex posterior surface. Its broad base is directed above and apex is its lower end. By its base, it articulates with fifth lumbar vertebra and by its apex, it articulates with the coccyx. The base has the upper opening of the sacral canal. The supero-anterior margin of the body of first sacral vertebra projects forwards as the sacral promontory, which is useful in measuring the diameters of the pelvis. Weber's point is situated one cm below the sacral promontory and it represents the center of gravity (CG) of the body. The lower end of the sacrum shows sacral hiatus, which is the lower opening of the sacral canal. The anterior surface bears four anterior sacral foramina, which give passage to ventral rami of upper four sacral spinal nerves. The posterior rami of the upper four sacral spinal nerves emerge through the posterior sacral foramina.

Ala of Sacrum

The upper surface of the lateral mass of sacrum is termed the ala of sacrum. It is grooved by lumbosacral trunk (L4, L5) and is covered by the psoas major muscle. The ala is crossed by sympathetic chain and iliolumbar artery. The obturator nerve is said to be related anteriorly to the ala.

Important Relations of Sacrum

The pelvic surface of the first three pieces of sacrum is covered with peritoneum. The rectum is related to the pelvic surface of third, fourth and fifth pieces of sacrum. The sympathetic chains are directly related to the pelvic surface (medial to the anterior sacral foramina). The median sacral vessels and lateral sacral vessels are in contact with the bone. The superior rectal artery bifurcates behind the rectum on the third piece of sacrum.

Contents of Sacral Canal

The sacral canal contains the cauda equina, dura mater and arachnoid mater. At the lower margin of second sacral vertebra, the subarchnoid and subdural spaces terminate. The fifth sacral roots, coccygeal roots and filum terminale pierce the blind end of the dural tube. Beyond the dural tube, there is roomy extradural space in the sacral canal. The capacity of sacral canal is 25 to 30 cc.

Sacral Hiatus

The structures that emerge from the sacral hiatus are, the filum terminale, fifth sacral nerves and coccygeal nerves. The sacral hiatus is of considerable importance since it provides access to the extradural space in the sacral canal. It lies about 5 cm above the tip of the coccyx, directly beneath the upper end of natal cleft. The other method to locate the sacral hiatus is as follows. The base of the equilateral triangle is formed by a line connecting the two posterior superior iliac spines (PSIS). The apex of the triangle indicates the surface marking of the sacral hiatus.

Caudal or Sacral Anesthesia

The anesthetic solution is injected into the extradural space in the sacral canal via the sacral hiatus. The needle is inserted at the upper end of natal cleft and it will pass through skin, subcutaneous tissue, deep fascia and sacrococcygeal ligament to enter the canal. This technique is used for perineal anesthsia and for painless labor in obstetric practice.

Coccyx

The coccyx consists of four small and rudimentary vertebrae, which are fused to form a triangular bone at the lower end of vertebral column. It articulates by its base with the apex of sacrum at the mobile sacro-coccygeal joint. Its base presents two cornua that project upwards and are connected to the cornua of sacrum by intercornual ligaments. The inferior (dorsal) surface and the tip of the coccyx can be palpated in the natal cleft about 2.5 cm behind the anal orifice. Coccydynia (pain in coccyx) is usually caused by direct trauma to the coccyx.

Bony Pelvis

The bony pelvis consists of four bones united by four joints and two ligaments. The bones include the two hip bones, sacrum and coccyx. The joints are, right and left sacroiliac joints, pubic symphysis and sacrococcygeal joint. The ligaments are the sacrospinous and sacrotuberous. The pelvis houses the pelvic viscera, blood vessels and nerves. In the female, it has an important function of accommodating the growing fetus in the uterus and at the end of gestation, it forms the canal through which the fetus passes during vaginal delivery.

Joints of Pelvis

a. Sacroiliac joint is the articulation between the sacral and iliac auricular surfaces. It is a plane variety of synovial joint. Its function is to transmit the weight of body from the vertebral column to the lower limb. The surface marking of the middle of the joint is the dimple indicating posterior superior iliac spine. There are anterior and posterior sacroiliac ligaments and the interosseous sacroiliac ligament, which fill the irregularities between the articulating bones. The ligaments soften during pregnancy and hence the mobility of joint becomes slightly more. This is the reason for frequency of subluxation of the joint during or after pregnancy. The relations of the joint are clinically important. The erector spinae and gluteus maximus muscles cover the joint from posterior aspect. The psoas major and iliacus muscles cover the abdominal surface of the joint. The obturator and femoral nerves are related to this surface. The pelvic surface is in relation to lumbosacral trunk and the ventral ramus of first sacral nerve. Any of these nerves, may be involved in disease of the joint and give rise to pain in the area of the sensory distribution of the nerve concerned. The formation of common iliac vein and division of common iliac artery occurs in front of the joint. The ureter crosses the front of the joint.
b. Pubic symphysis is the joint between the two pubic bones. It is located anteriorly in the midline. It is a secondary cartilaginous joint. Very slight movements are possible in this joint, though some separation is believed to take place during childbirth.

c. Sacrococcygeal joint is a secondary cartilaginous joint between the base of coccyx and apex of sacrum. It is the mobile joint of the bony pelvis.

Complications of Pelvic Fractures

Fractures of pelvic bones are common in accidents. A heavy fall on the greater trochanter of femur may dislocate the femoral head upwards in the pelvic cavity by rupture of acetabulum. Fractures of sacrum and coccyx may occur. These fractures are complicated by soft tissue injury. The internal iliac veins and the tributaries are thin-walled and hence vulnerable to rupture causing intraperitoneal or extraperitoneal bleeding. The male urethra is in danger in fractures of pubic bone involving perineal pouches. The urinary bladder is vulnerable in both sexes as it lies just behind the pubic symphysis. Fracture of sacrum may rupture rectum and injure sacral plexus. Fracture of the bony boundaries of the greater sciatic notch may injure the sciatic nerve.

Subdivisions of Pelvis

The pelvis is divided into a false pelvis and a true pelvis by the pelvic brim, which consists of sacral promontory and linea terminalis (an arcuate line of ilium, pectineal line of the superior ramus of pubis and pubic crest). The false pelvis or greater pelvis lies above the pelvic brim. It is formed by the iliac fossa and limited above by iliac crest. The cavity of the false pelvis is part of abdominal cavity. The true pelvis or lesser pelvis is divided into inlet, cavity and outlet.

Pelvic Inlet

The pelvic inlet is the brim of the pelvis. It is an oblique plane. The bony parts taking part in it on both sides are, upper border of symphysis pubis, linea terminalis, sacroiliac joint, ala of sacrum and sacral promontory. The pelvic inlet is heart shaped in male but in female, it is transversely oval. The diameters of the inlet, are particularly important in female because it is through the inlet that the fetal head enters the true pelvis during labor.

Structures Crossing Pelvic Brim

The sympathetic chains, lumbosacral trunks, obturator nerves and ureters cross the brim to enter the true pelvis, in both sexes. The ovarian vessels and the round ligament of uterus cross the brim in the female. The vas deferens crosses in the male. The following arteries cross the brim to enter the pelvis, the internal iliac arteries, median sacral artery and superior rectal artery in both sexes. The iliolumbar branch of internal iliac artery leaves the pelvis to enter posterior abdominal wall across the brim.

Pelvic Cavity

The pelvic cavity lies between the inlet and outlet. It is continuous above with abdominal cavity and closed below by pelvic diaphragm. The reproductive, urinary and alimentary tracts in both sexes perforate the pelvic floor. The cavity is curved in such a way that it is directed at first downwards and backwards and then downwards and forwards. Its anterior wall is shorter than its posterior wall. During normal delivery the fetus passes through the pelvic cavity, so the assessment of the size of the cavity before delivery is very important.

Pelvic Outlet

The pelvic outlet is diamond-shaped. It is wider in female. Its anterior boundary is the lower margin of symphysis pubis and anterolaterally it is bounded by the conjoint ischiopubic rami, laterally by ischial tuberosities, postero-laterally by sacrotuberous ligaments and posteriorly by the tip of coccyx.

Sex Differences in Pelvis

a. The ischiopubic rami are everted in male but not in female. This difference is due to the attachment of strong crus penis and well-developed ischiocavernosus muscle.
b. The cavity of acetabulum is larger in male.
c. Preauricular sulcus is not distinct in male but prominent in female.
d. The body of first sacral vertebra is wider than ala of sacrum in male but in female the body of S1 vertebra is equal to the ala of sacrum.

e. The subpubic angle is acute in male and wider in female.
f. The pelvic inlet is heart-shaped in male and circular or transversely oval in female.
g. The pelvic outlet is smaller in male and much larger in female.
h. The pelvic cavity is shorter and more conical in male but wide and roomy in female.
i. The diameters of the pelvis are smaller in male compared to the female.

Diameters of Female Pelvis

Successful labor and delivery depend largely on compatibility of pelvic dimensions and shape with the fetal head. In cephalopelvic disproportion (CPD) normal delivery cannot take place.

Diameters of Pelvic Inlet

a. The AP diameter or true conjugate is the distance from the midpoint of sacral promontory to the inner margin of the upper border of symphysis pubis.
b. The diagonal conjugate can be measured by digital examination. It is the distance between the lower margin of symphysis pubis and the midpoint of sacral promontory. The diagonal conjugate is usually 12 cm. The anatomical conjugate can be inferred by subtracting 1.2 cm from the diagonal conjugate and obstetrical conjugate can be inferred by subtracting 2 cm from the diagonal conjugate.
c. Transverse diameter is the distance between the farthest points on the pelvic brim.
d. The oblique diameters extend from one sacroiliac joint to the opposite iliopubic eminence.

Diameters of Pelvic Cavity

a. The AP diameter is from the middle of the back of symphysis pubis to the central point of the third piece of sacrum. The pelvic cavity is most roomy at this plane.
b. The midpelvic diameter between the ischial spines is the smallest diameter of the pelvis and is the place, where difficulty is encountered during labor.

Diameters of Pelvic Outlet

a. The transverse or intertuberous diameter is the distance between the inner borders of the ischial tuberosities.
b. The AP diameter extends from the lower border of symphysis pubis to the tip of coccyx. This diameter is the longest at the outlet.

Types of Female Pelvis

a. Gynecoid pelvis is the one in which pelvic inlet is circular and its transverse diameter is maximum. It is the normal female pelvis.
b. Android pelvis is the one in which pelvic inlet is heart-shaped like that of male pelvis. This type of pelvis may cause difficulty during childbirth.
c. Anthropoid pelvis is the one in which antero-posterior diameter of the inlet is more than the transverse diameter. This type will cause difficulty in normal delivery.
d. Platypelloid pelvis (flat pelvis) is the one in which the transverse diameter is very wide compared to the AP diameter so the pelvis is anteroposteriorly compressed. This is due to deficiency of vitamin D. This is a truly contracted pelvis, were normal delivery is impossible.

207 Bones of Head and Neck

FETAL SKULL

The size and shape of fetal skull is adapted to the maternal pelvis. The non-ossified membranous areas called fontanelles join the flat bones of skull vault to each other.

Functions of Fontanelles

a. The fontanelles permit gliding movements (moulding of skull) of one bone over the other during the passage of head through the birth canal. The moulding disappears within few hours after birth.
b. The fontanelles provide for the postnatal rapid growth in the size of brain

Location of Fontanelles

There are six fontanelles that are situated at the angles of parietal bone at the time of birth. They are, anterior, posterior, right and left sphenoidal and right and left mastoidal.

a. The anterior fontanelle is the largest. It is diamond-shaped. It closes, when the child attains the age of 18 months. After the closure, its site is indicated by the bregma of adult skull.
b. The posterior fontanelle closes by the age of 2 to 3 months. The lambda of adult skull indicates its site.
c. The sphenoidal fontanelles close by 2 to 3 months and their sites are denoted by pterion.
d. The mastoidal fontanelles close by 12 months and their sites are indicated by asterion.

Clinical Highlights

By palpation at this site the pediatrician can estimate the degree of dehydration in the infants and the assess intracranial pressure in children.

Special Features of Fetal Skull

a. Frontal bone is in two halves joined by metopic suture.
b. The mandible is in two halves.
c. The jaw bones are edentulous.
d. The occipital bone is in four parts. The primary cartilaginous joint between the basilar part of occipital bone and body of sphenoid permits postnatal growth in the base of skull.
e. The temporal bone is incomplete. Its tympanic plate is absent, being represented by tympanic ring. Hence, there is no bony part of external acoustic canal in fetal skull.
f. The styloid and mastoid processes are absent.
g. The parietal tubercle or eminence is prominent. The interparietal diameter (distance between the parietal tubera) is of obstetric importance and can be assessed before delivery.
h. The paranasal air sinuses are rudimentary. The frontal sinus is absent at birth. The maxillary sinus is the first to develop and identifiable at birth as a small groove.

Caput Succedaneum

Caput succedaneum is the swelling in the fetal skull due to stagnation of fluid in the scalp layers. The swelling of caput succedaneum is diffuse because it is not restricted to any particular bone. It disappears within 24 hours. The caput succedaneum should be distinguished from cephalo-hematoma, which is the collection of blood between the pericranium and the parietal bone. It is due to rupture of the emissary vein, due to fracture of the bone in forceps delivery. The ceplalohematoma is restricted to the parietal bone. The swelling gradually subsides over a period of few months.

Adult Skull

The skull is divided in three parts, calvaria or brain box, the facial skeleton and mandible. The skull minus the mandible is the cranium. The skull consists of 22 bones of which, 8 belong to calvaria and 14 belong to facial skeleton. The cranial bones unite with each other by joints. The most common joints encountered are the sutures. The joint between the rostrum of sphenoid and the ala of vomer is a special type of fibrous joint called schyndylesis. The base of sphenoid and occipital bones unite by primary cartilaginous joint to allow for expansion of the base of the cranium. During the age of 18 to 25 this joint is ossified. The mandible, the only mobile bone of the skull articulates by paired synovial temporomandibular joints with the base of skull.

Anatomical Position of Skull

The skull is held in such a way that a transverse plane passes through the infraorbital margin and upper margin of the external acoustic meatus. This orbitomeatal plane is known as Frankfurt plane.

Norma Verticalis

The view of skull from above is norma verticalis. Norma verticalis corresponds to the calvaria or vault or dome of the skull. It is covered with scalp. The anterior part of norma verticalis is characterized by sagittal and coronal sutures. The frontal bone is separated by the coronal suture from the parietal bones. The sagittal suture intervenes between the two parietal bones. The meeting point of coronal and sagittal sutures is known as the bregma. Posteriorly the suture between the occipital bone and the parietal bones is called the lambdoid suture. The meeting point of the sagittal and lambdoid suture is called the lambda. The vertex is the highest point of the skull, when it is held in Frankfurt plane and it lies near the middle of sagittal suture.

The overall size and shape of the skull may be altered due to disorders of the brain or due to premature closure of the sutures of the vault of the skull (craniosynostosis).

a. Microcephaly is due to underdeveloped brain.
b. Macrocephaly is due to congenital hydrocephalus (excessive CSF in the ventricles of brain).
c. Anencephaly is absence of the greater part of the vault of the skull. It is due to nonclosure of the anterior neuropore of the neural tube.
d. Scaphocephaly or boat-shaped skull (frontal and occipital expansion) is due to premature closure of sagittal suture.
e. Acrocephaly or tower skull is due to premature closure of coronal suture.

Norma Occipitalis

The posterior portion of the skull is known as norma occipitalis. The lambdoid suture is a prominent landmark. The occipitomastoid suture is between the occipital and mastoid bones. The parietomastoid suture meets the lambdoid suture and the occipitomastoid suture at asterion. The external occipital protuberance is a palpable landmark at the upper limit of the median furrow at the back of neck. Inion is the most prominent point of the external occipital protuberance. The superior nuchal line extends from the protuberance on each side. The highest nuchal line, which is more arched, extends from the protuberance on either side but above it. The external occipital crest extends below the protuberance to the foramen magnum and it gives attachment to ligamentum nuchae. The inferior nuchal lines go laterally from the middle of the crest on each side.

Norma Frontalis

The facial aspect of the skull is called norma frontalis. Orbits (two bony sockets for the eyeballs) and the bony nasal aperture are the prominent features of the norma frontalis. The frontal bone is the skeletal basis of forehead. The metopic suture separates the two frontal bones upto the age of 6-8 years. The maxillae take part in forming the margins of orbit, nasal cavity and oral cavity. The body of zygomatic bone (cheekbone) forms the prominence of cheek. The nasal bones form the nasal bridge, which is located in between the two orbits. The movable mandible (lower jaw) is the lower part of norma frontalis.

The superciliary arch is a curved elevation in the frontal bone just above the medial part of the upper margin of orbit. It is more prominent in males.

The glabella is a median elevation connecting the right and left superciliary arches.

The nasion is an important landmark useful in surface marking. It is a meeting point of the frontonasal and internasal sutures at the root of the nose.

Each orbital opening is quadrangular in shape. It has four margins. The supraorbital margin is palpable. At the junction of its lateral two thirds and medial one third, it presents the supraorbital notch or foramen for the passage of suoraorbital nerve and vessels. The compression of supraorbital nerve at the foramen causes intense pain. This fact is utilized in clinical practice to determine the depth of anaesthesia or to arouse an unconscious patient. The lateral orbital margin has frontozygomatic suture, which is a palpable landmark useful in surface marking of middle meningeal artery.

The maxilla is present on either side of nasal aperture. Its anterior surface presents, infraorbital foramen and incisive and canine fossae. The canine fossa, is present below the infraorbital foramen and is used for anterior approach to the maxillary sinus through the vestibule of mouth. The infraorbital foramen gives passage to infraorbital nerve and vessels. The zygomatic bone presents zygomaticofacial foramen, through which nerve and vessels of the same name emerge. The temporal process of the zygomatic bone articulates with zygomatic process of temporal bone to form zygomatic arch, which is seen in norma lateralis.

Norma Lateralis

When viewed from the lateral side, the skull shows the opening of bony external acoustic meatus and zygomatic arch in front of it. The lateral surface of this arch is subcutaneous. The superficial temporal vessels and the auriculotemporal vessels cross the root of the zygomatic arch just in front of the auricle. The artery can be felt at this site (especially by the anesthetist, who sits at the head end of the patient during operation). The posterior end of the zygomatic arch is attached to the squamous temporal bone by two roots. There are three tubercles in relation to these roots. The tubercle at the root of the zygomatic arch (zygoma) gives attachment to lateral ligament of TMJ. The posterior end of zygomatic arch divides in anterior and posterior roots. The anterior root turns downwards and medially to form the articular tubercle, which lies in the anterior boundary of mandibular fossa. The posterior root terminates in postglenoid tubercle. The bony part of external acoustic meatus is mainly formed by the tympanic plate of the temporal bone on all sides except the posterosuperior margin, which is formed by the squamous temporal bone.

Boundaries of Suprameatal Triangle (McEwan's Triangle)

The boundaries of the triangle are, the supramastoid crest above, posterosuperior margin of the external acoustic meatus in front and a vertical tangent to the posterior margin of meatus behind. Since the triangle forms the lateral wall of the mastoid antrum, pus in the antrum can be drained through it. The cymba conchae (of auricle) indicates the position of the triangle on the surface.

Mastoid Process

The mastoid process is the projection from the lower part of the mastoid part of the temporal bone. It is absent in fetal skull and appears by the age of two years. Apart from muscular attachments, the important vascular relation of the mastoid process is the occipital artery, which grooves the bone on its inner aspect.

Temporal Fossa

The temporal fossa is the region between the temporal lines above and the zygomatic arch below. This aspect of the zygomatic bone presents a tiny zygomaticotemporal foramen.

Pterion

The pterion is situated in the floor of temporal fossa. It is an H-shaped suture, where four bones, namely, the greater wing of sphenoid, squamous temporal, frontal and anteroinferior angle of parietal meet each other. The central point of pterion is an important landmark. It is situated four cm above the zygomatic arch and 3.5 cm behind the frontozygomatic suture. This point is known as sylvian point. Cranium is very thin at this point. Its immediate deep relations are the frontal branch of middle meningeal artery and accompanying vein. Fracture or even a blow at this point may injure middle meningeal artery and give rise to extradural bleeding. It also indicates the position of the terminal part of the stem of lateral sulcus of brain.

Norma Basalis

The basal aspect of the skull is subdivided into three parts, anterior, middle and posterior.

Anterior Part

The hard palate is the prominent feature anteriorly. The bones taking part in the hard palate are, the palatine processes of the maxillae (anterior two-thirds) and the horizontal processes of the palatine bones (posterior one-third). The alveolar processes of the maxillae partially surround the hard palate. The incisive fossa is present in the midline behind the sockets of the incisor teeth. Two incisive foramina are seen in the walls of the incisive fossa. Each foramen gives passage to the greater palatine vessels from the palate to the nasal cavity and to the nasopalatine (sphenopalatine) nerves from nasal cavity to the palate. The greater palatine vessels and nerves travel in a groove on the lateral side of the hard palate from the greater palatine foramen forwards towards the incisive fossa. The lesser palatine foramen is seen in the pyramidal process of the palatine bone. It transmits nerves and vessels of the same name. The free posterior margin of the hard palate presents the posterior nasal spine in the middle.

Middle Part

a. The midline area of the middle part has following features from before backwards. The posterior margin of vomer separates the two posterior nasal apertures (choanae). Inferior margin of the vomer articulates with the superior surface of hard palate in the nasal cavity. Its superior margin splits into two alae, which articulate with the rostrum of sphenoid projecting from the body of sphenoid. The midline bar of bone posterior to the choanae is union between the body of sphenoid and the basilar part of the occipital bone. It forms the roof of nasopharynx and hence related to pharyngeal tonsil. The basilar part of the occipital bone shows a pharyngeal tubercle in front of foramen magnum. This tubercle indicates the posterior limit of the nasopharynx at the base of cranium.
b. The lateral area of the middle part shows the pterygoid process on each side. This process projects downwards behind the third molar tooth. It divides in medial and lateral pterygoid plates, which bound the pterygoid fossa posteriorly but are fused to each other anteriorly. The free posterior margin of the medial plate divides superiorly to enclose scaphoid fossa. Its lower end is prolonged downwards and laterally to form pterygoid hamulus. The greater wing of sphenoid forms the roof of the infratemporal fossa and extends in the temporal fossa to form part of its floor. The posterior margin of the greater wing and the anterior margin of petrous temporal bones bound a groove (sulcus tubae) for lodging the cartilaginous part of the auditory tube. The sulcus tubae leads laterally to the opening of the bony part of auditory tube in the petrous temporal bone.

The spine of the sphenoid projects in the infratemporal fossa and is related to 2 nerves and gives attachments to 2 muscles and 2 ligaments. It is related laterally to the auriculotemporal nerve and medially to the chorda tympani nerve. This relationship is the basis of the clinical condition in which the fracture of the spine leads to the cessation of salivary secretion in the parotid, submandibular and sublingual salivary glands. The spine gives attachments to the sphenomandibular ligament and anterior ligament of malleus in addition to tensor tympani in addition to tensor palati muscles.

In front of the spine, the foramen spinosum gives passage to the middle meningeal artery. The larger foramen ovale, which is located anteromedial to the foramen spinosum, gives passage to the mandibular nerve. The mandibular fossa is limited anteriorly by the articular tubercle. It consists of anterior articular part (squamous temporal) and posterior nonarticular part (tympanic plate). The squamotympanic fissure demarcates the two parts of the mandibular fossa.

The tegmen tympani from the petrous temporal bone projects in to the sqamotympanic fissure and divides it in petrosquamous and petrotympanic parts. The petrotympanic fissure transmits three structures, which are associated with middle ear (anterior ligament of malleus, anterior tympanic vessels and chorda tympani nerve). The tympanic part of the temporal bone is a bony plate that forms the floor and anterior wall of the external acoustic meatus. The styloid process is a long linear projection from the temporal bone. It lies anteromedial to mastoid process. Stylomastoid foramen, located between the styloid process medially and mastoid process laterally, transmits the facial nerve.

The styloid process gives attachment to three muscles and two ligaments. Its base is related to the facial nerve on its lateral aspect, which is overlapped by the parotid gland. Its medial aspect is in close relation to internal jugular vein. At times, the tip of the styloid process may reach the lateral pharyngeal wall.

Petrous temporal bone presents as a rough triangular bone between the greater wing of sphenoid in front, basilar part of the occipital bone medially and the styloid process laterally. Between the apex of the petrous temporal and the body of the sphenoid, there is an irregular gap called foramen lacerum, which is closed in life at the cranial base by a piece of fibrocartilage. A circular smooth foramen (opening of carotid canal) pierces the inferior aspect of petrous temporal for the passage of internal carotid artery, which travels in the carotid canal forwards to open in the posterior wall of the foramen lacerum. The internal carotid artery enters the middle cranial fossa through the foramen lacerum. The pterygoid canal begins in the anterior wall of the foramen lacerum and conducts the nerve and vessels of pterygoid canal to the sphenopalatine fossa.

The cartilaginous part of the auditory tube is lodged in the groove (sulcus tubae) between the petrous temporal behind and the greater wing of sphenoid in front. The upper end of the posterior margin of the medial pterygoid plate supports the cartilaginous part of the tube before the tube pierces the pharyngobasilar fascia, to enter the lateral wall of nasopharynx.

The levator palati takes origin from the inferior surface of the petrous temporal, medial to the cartilaginous part of the auditory tube and from the adjacent part of the tube. Its tendon passes inferiorly to pierce the pharyngobasilar fascia along with the auditory tube, to enter the pharynx on its way to the palate.

The tensor palati muscle takes origin from the scaphoid fossa, cartilaginous part of auditory tube and the spine of sphenoid. The tendon of the muscle travels downwards to wind round the pterygoid hamulus and enter the pharynx deep to the origin of buccinator muscle from the tendinous band (spanning the gap between the maxillary tuberosity and the tip of pterygoid hamulus).

Posterior Part

The foramen magnum is the largest foramen in the cranium. It is present in the midline in the occipital bone and connects the posterior cranial fossa to the vertebral canal. Its posterior part provides passage for medulla oblongata, and meninges. The subarachnoid space gives passage to spinal accessory nerve, vertebral arteries, posterior spinal arteries, and anterior spinal artery. The epidural space contains the internal vertebral venous plexus. Its anterior part transmits apical ligament of dens and membrana tectoria (continuation of posterior longitudinal ligament), since these structures are attached to the cranial aspect of the basisphenoid.

The lateral area of the posterior part of the base shows, condylar part of occipital bone, squamous part of occipital bone and the jugular foramen between the petrous temporal and occipital bones. The kidney-shaped occipital condyles articulate with the kidney-shaped superior articular facets of atlas. The anterior condylar canal pierces the bone anterosuperior to the occipital condyles and transmits the hypoglossal nerve. The jugular foramen lies between the petrous temporal in front and jugular process of occipital bone behind. Its anterior part transmits inferior petrosal sinus. The middle part gives passage to the ninth, tenth and eleventh cranial nerves. The internal jugular vein passes through the posterior part, which encroaches on the jugular fossa in the anterior wall of the foramen. The jugular fossa houses the superior bulb of the IJV and forms the floor of the middle ear. There are three small openings in this region, which transmit structures related to the three parts of the ear. The tympanic canaliculus is located at the junction of jugular fossa and the carotid canal. It transmits the tympanic branch of the CN IX (Jacobson's nerve) to the middle ear. The lateral wall of the jugular fossa has the opening of the mastoid canaliculus, which carries the auricular branch of the vagus nerve to the external ear. At the opening of the cochlear canaliculus (aqueduct of cochlea or perilymphatic duct), near the medial end of the jugular foramen, the subarachnoid space comes in contact with the perilymph brought through the cochlear canaliculus from the scala tympani of inner ear.

Jugular Foramen Syndrome

This syndrome consists of involvement of the ninth, tenth and eleventh cranial nerves in the jugular foramen due to tumor of glomus jugulare or neurofibroma of the nerves or extension of the intracranial meningioma through the jugular foramen or thrombosis of the superior bulb of IJV. The glomus jugulare or tympanic body (similar in structure to carotid body) is seen in the adventitia of the superior bulb of IJV.

Interior of Cranium

The interior of the cranium is divided into three cranial fossae (anterior, middle and posterior).

Anterior Cranial Fossa

The cribriform plate of the ethmoid lies in the midline in the floor of the fossa. The orbital plates of the frontal bone are present on either side. The body of the sphenoid (jugum sphenoidale) is seen posterior to the ethmoid and the lesser wings of the sphenoid form the posterior margins of the fossa on either side. The cribriform plate of ethmoid separates the nasal cavity from the anterior cranial fossa. The foramina in the cribriform plate transmit olfactory nerves from the olfactory mucosa into the anterior cranial fossa. On either side of the cribriform plate, on the frontoethmoidal suture, anterior and posterior ethmoidal foramina are present. The anterior ethmoidal nerve (continuation of nasociliary) and vessels (branches of ophthalmic vessels) enter the anterior cranial fossa through the anterior foramen and leave through the slit by the side of crista galli to enter the nasal cavity. The posterior ethmoidal foramen gives passage to posterior ethmoidal vessels only (posterior ethmoidal nerve is spent in the supply of ethmoidal and sphenoidal sinuses), which leave the anterior cranial fossa via the slit by the side of the crista galli to enter the nasal cavity. Fractures of the anterior cranial fossa may cause escape of CSF in the nose or bleeding in the orbital roof leading to black eye.

Relation to Brain

The gyrus rectus sits on each half of the cribriform plate. The olfactory bulb lies on the frontoethmoidal suture on each side. The orbital surface of the frontal lobe is in close contact with the orbital plate of the frontal bone. The free posterior margin of the lesser wing of sphenoid fits into the stem of the lateral sulcus of cerebrum.

Middle Cranial Fossa

This fossa is at a lower level compared to the anterior fossa. The overhanging free margin of the lesser wing of sphenoid is the anterior boundary of the fossa and the sloping anterior surface of the petrous temporal bone is its posterior boundary. The body of the sphenoid forms the median part of the fossa. The greater wing of the sphenoid and the cerebral surface of the squamous temporal lie in its floor. The body of the sphenoid presents the sulcus chiasmaticus in front, which connects the two optic foramina to each other. The optic chiasma does not lie in this sulcus. The optic foramen (enclosed by the two roots of lesser wing and the body of sphenoid) opens into the orbit and transmits optic nerve to the middle cranial fossa and the ophthalmic artery to the orbit. The sella turcica (Turkish saddle) is the hollowed out upper surface of the body of the sphenoid. It consists of three parts, tuberculum sellae in front, hypophyseal fossa in the middle and the dorsum sellae behind. The hypophysis is located in the hypophyseal fossa. The carotid sulcus, which is present on each side of the body of sphenoid, starts from the foramen lacerum and is limited by lingula on its posterolateral aspect. The cavernous sinus and the intracavernous part of the internal carotid artery are in contact with the carotid sulcus.

Relation to Brain

The floor of the middle cranial fossa is in contact with the tentorial surface of the temporal lobe of the cerebrum.

Superior Orbital Fissure

This fissure (bounded by the body, greater and lesser wings of sphenoid) opens anteriorly into the orbit. Its lateral part transmits lacrimal nerve, frontal nerve, trochlear nerve, superior ophthalmic vein and anastomotic branch of middle meningeal artery (which anastomoses with recurrent branch of lacrimal artery). The middle part transmits upper and lower divisions of oculomotor nerve, nasociliary nerve and abducent nerve. The inferior ophthalmic vein passes through its medial part.

Foramina in Greater Wing of Sphenoid

The greater wing of sphenoid presents foramen rotundum for maxillary nerve, foramen ovale for mandibular nerve and foramen spinosum for middle meningeal artery.

Foramen Lacerum

The boundaries of the foramen lacerum are, the apex of petrous temporal, body of the sphenoid and the adjacent greater wing. The internal carotid artery enters the middle cranial fossa through it.

Anterior Surface of Petrous Temporal Bone

The anterior surface of the petrous temporal bone presents trigeminal impression, near the apex, for the trigeminal ganglion. There are two grooves for the greater and lesser petrosal nerves, which enter the middle cranial fossa from the middle ear. The arcuate eminence (produced due to underlying superior semicircular canal) indicates the position of internal ear on the anterior aspect of petrous temporal. The thin tegmen tympani, which is lateral to the arcuate eminence indicates the position of the middle ear and the mastoid antrum behind the middle ear. The proximity of the middle ear and mastoid antrum to the middle cranial fossa is responsible for spread of infection to the cranial cavity in otitis media and mastoiditis. Fracture of the middle cranial fossa may give rise to bleeding and discharge of CSF through ear.

Posterior Cranial Fossa

The posterior cranial fossa is very large and deep compared to the other two fossae. The anterior wall of the fossa is formed by the clivus, which is sloping surface formed by fusion of the basilar part of occipital bone and the body of the sphenoid. The clivus is a primary cartilaginous joint. It is ossified (synchondrosis) by 18 to 25 years of life. The anteroposterior growth of the base of the cranium takes place at this joint. The anterior surfaces of the medulla oblongata and the pons are in direct contact with the clivus. Behind the foramen magnum the posterior fossa is walled by squamous part of occipital bone. It has a midline crest called internal occipital crest, the upper end of which is called the internal occipital protuberance. The three dural folds (falx cerebri, falx cerebelli and tentorium cerebelli) meet at this site, which is indicated on the external surface by the inion. From the internal occipital protuberance the transverse sulcus extends laterally and becomes continuous with the deep sigmoid sulcus. The mastoid antrum is very closely related to the sigmoid sinus lodged in the sigmoid sulcus.

On each side of the foramen magnum, anterior condylar or hypoglossal canal lies above the anterior part of the lateral margin of the foramen. The tuberculum jugulare is an elevation above the anterior condylar foramen. It is crossed by ninth, tenth and eleventh cranial nerves, which enter the jugular foramen. The foramen magnum communicates the posterior fossa to the vertebral canal.

Relation to Brain

The inferior vermis of the cerebellum is in contact with the vermian fossa at the lower end of the internal occipital crest. On either side of the foramen magnum the squamous part of the occipital bone is directly in contact with the cerebellar hemisphere below the transverse sulcus and to the occipital lobe of the cerebrum above the sulcus. The tonsil of the cerebellum is usually in contact with the foramen magnum.

Internal Acoustic Meatus

The posterior aspect of the petrous temporal bone presents a medial opening of internal acoustic meatus, through which facial nerve; statoacoustic nerve and labyrinthine artery enter the canal of the meatus in the petrous temporal bone. The lateral end of the meatus (fundus of meatus) contains the vestibular ganglion. A bony plate at the lateral end the meatus shows a number of foramina. Its upper part gives passage to the facial nerve in front. Through the superior and inferior vestibular areas, pass the dendrites of the bipolar neurons of the vestibular ganglion towards the inner ear. The anterior part of the lower area is called the tractus spiarlis foarminosus, which gives passage to the axons of the bipolar neurons of the spiral ganglion (which is inside the osseous labyrinth).

Clinical Highlights

a. Fractures involving the squamous part of occipital bone may cause bleeding in the muscles of the back of neck.
b. Foramen magnum anomalies are clinically important. In Arnold- Chiari malformation, there is herniation of cerebellar tonsils and medulla oblongata through the foramen magnum in the cervical vertebral canal. The herniation may block the displaced fourth ventricle causing hydrocephalus. Syringomyelia (enlargement of central canal) in cervical spinal cord may be associated with mild degree of Arnold-Chiari malformation. In this condition, it is found that the

cerebellar tonsils are located on the posterior margin of foramen magnum. A sudden increase in pressure during the acts of coughing or straining push the cerebellar tonsils into the foramen magnum and transmit the increased pressure of CSF to the central canal of spinal cord instead of the subarachnoid space. This may develop into sudden-onset syringomyelia during a bout of cough.

INDIVIDUAL SKULL BONES

Parietal Bone

The right and left parietal bones are large quadrilateral bones forming a major part of the vault of skull. Each parietal bone has four angles. Each angle forms a fontanelle in fetal skull. The anterosuperior (frontal) angle takes part in bregma, the anetroinferior (sphenoidal) angle forms the pterion, the posterosuperior (occipital) angle takes part in lambda and posteroinferior (mastoid) angle in asterion. The inner aspects of the four angles have vascular relations. The bregma and lambda are related to superior sagittal sinus. The asterion is related to sigmoid sinus and pterion is intimately related to anterior division (frontal branch) of middle meningeal artery. The parietal bones ossify in membrane.

Occipital Bone

It is a single bone occupying the back of the skull. It is characterized by presence of a large foramen called foramen magnum. The bone has three main parts, squamous (above and behind foramen magnum), basilar part (basiocciput in front of the foramen magnum) and lateral or condylar parts on each side of the foramen. There are four fossae on the internal surface. The upper cerebral fossae lodge the occipital lobes of the cerebrum and the lower cerebellar fossae house the cerebellar hemispheres. The clivus supports the medulla oblongata and pons. The inferior vermis of the cerebellum is in relation to the vermian fossa in the midline just above the posterior margin of foramen magnum. The occipital bone is related to two tonsils. Each cerebellar tonsil lies in contact with the posterior margin of the foramen magnum. The nasopharyngeal tonsil is a midline structure, which is in contact with the inferior surface of the basilar part of the occipital bone. The occipital bone articulates with adjacent bones by means of three types of articulations. The joint between the basiocciput and basisphenoid is synostosis or primary cartilaginous joint, atlanto-occipital joints are synovial and the rest of the joints with parietal and temporal bones are suture type of fibrous joints.

Frontal Bone

Frontal bone forms the anterior part of the vault of the skull. It ossifies in membrane from two primary centers, which appear one on each side in the region of frontal tuber. At birth the frontal bone is in two parts, separated by interfrontal or metopic suture. The suture fuses by eighth year. The frontal bone has two asymmetrical air sinuses inside it. The frontal air sinuses are absent at birth but are well-developed by the age of puberty. The air sinuses open in the middle meatus of nasal cavity by infundibulum. The inner aspect of the bone including the superior surface of orbital plate, is in contact with the frontal lobe of cerebrum.

Ethmoidal Bone

It is the lightest among the cranial bones. It ossifies in cartilage. It is located between the two orbits in the anterior part of the cranial base. It consists of a pair of labyrinths (containing ethmoidal air cells), cribriform plate and a perpendicular plate. The cribriform plate lies in the floor of anterior cranial fossa and in the roof of nasal cavity and gives passage to olfactory nerves. The perpendicular plate projects downwards from the undersurface of the cribriform plate in the nasal cavity to take part in the bony nasal septum. The labyrinths of the ethmoid are two masses filled with air cells, which are situated on each side of the perpendicular plate. The medial surface of the labyrinth presents superior and middle nasal conchae or turbinates, which project into the nasal cavity from the lateral wall. The labyrinth contains three groups of ethmoidal sinuses, which open in the lateral wall of nasal cavity. Thus, it must be understood that ethmoid bone contributes to the skeleton of roof, lateral and medial walls of the nasal cavity, hence, is the crucial bone of nasal cavity. The lateral surface of the ethmoid labyrinth is known as lamina papyracea because it is very thin. This forms part of the medial wall of the orbit.

Sphenoid Bone

The sphenoid resembles the butterfly or bat with outstretched wings. It has a body, a pair of greater wings, a pair of lesser wings and a pair of pterygoid processes. The body of the sphenoid contains a pair of sphenoidal sinuses, which open in the sphenoethmoidal recess of the nasal cavity. Most important relation of the superior surface of the body, is the pituitary gland. The inferior surface of the body forms the roof of the nasal cavity and that of the nasopharynx. The transnasal and trans-sphenoidal surgical approach to the pituitary gland is based on the inferior relations of the body of the sphenoid. The lateral surface of the body is closely-related to cavernous sinus and internal carotid artery. The greater wing lies mainly in the floor of the middle cranial fossa internally and in the roof of the infratemporal fossa and the floor of temporal fossa, externally. It presents foramen rotundum, foramen ovale and foramen spinosum besides other foramina for emissary veins. The lesser wings project laterally from anterior part of the body to which they are connected by two roots, which enclose the optic foramen. Its free posterior margin fits in the stem of the lateral sulcus of cerebrum. The pterygoid processes project vertically downward from the junction of greater wing and the body. The sphenoid articulates with maximum number of bones. Its inferior surface articulates with the vomer. The sphenoidal sinus is rudimentary at birth. It extends in the body of sphenoid during early childhood and attains normal size by the age of puberty.

Temporal Bone

The temporal bone is intimately related to the ear and houses a number of structures. Each bone is made of five parts, squamous, mastoid, petrous, tympanic and styloid process.

Squamous Part

Its outer surface has the grooves for middle temporal artery (a branch of superficial temporal artery). The suprameatal triangle is present on this surface. The articular part of mandibular fossa is contributed by squamous temporal bone. It gives off the zygomatic process for articulation with temporal process of zygomatic bone. The inner surface faces the middle cranial fossa and hence shows impressions of cerebral sulci and gyri and the grooves for the middle meningeal vessels.

Mastoid Part

The mastoid part encloses the mastoid air cells in the mastoid process. The medial surface of the mastoid process is marked by a vascular groove for occipital artery.

Contents of Petrous Temporal Bone

a. It houses three spaces. The middle ear and mastoid antrum are the air-filled and the internal ear is the fluid- filled space.
b. Three canals pass through the bone, carotid canal, facial canal and internal acoustic meatus. The carotid canal contains the internal carotid artery, which enters the canal at the base. The facial canal contains the intrapetrous part of facial nerve. The internal acoustic meatus contains the facial nerve, statoacoustic nerve, labyrinthine vessels and the vestibular ganglion (at the fundus).
c. Three small bony canals called canaliculi pass through the bone. The mastoid canaliculus is for auricular branch of vagus nerve. The tympanic canaliculus is for the tympanic branch of glossopharyngeal nerve. The cochlear canaliculus is for the perilymphatic duct (aqueduct of cochlea) and the prolongation of sub-arachnoid space inside it.
d. Three small bones of the middle are inside the middle ear cavity.
e. Three sensory ganglia associated with the three nerves are located inside. The geniculate ganglion of the facial nerve is located at the anterior end of the medial wall of middle ear. The spiral ganglion of cochlear nerve is inside the bony cochlea and the vestibular ganglion is at the medial blind end of the internal meatus.
f. Three branches of the facial nerve arise in its intra-petrous course, chorda tympani, greater petrosal and nerve to stapedius.
g. The lesser petrosal nerve begins in the middle ear from the tympanic plexus and leaves through the tegmen tympani.
h. Two muscles are present inside the middle ear, tensor tympani and stapedius.

Tympanic Part

This is a curved plate of bone located below the squamous part and in front of the mastoid part. It forms the floor, anterior wall and lower part of posterior wall of the bony external acoustic meatus. At its medial end it gives attachment to the tympanic membrane. Its anterior surface forms the posterior non-articular part of the mandibular fossa.

Styloid Process

It is a thin and elongated process, which projects downward, forward and laterally from the base between the tympanic plate in front and the mastoid process behind. The facial nerve crosses the lateral aspect of the base of the styloid process. The external carotid artery crosses its tip. The stylomastoid foramen is located between the styloid and mastoid processes. The styloid process gives attachments to stylopharyngeus, stylohyoid and styloglossus muscles. It also provides attachments to stylohyoid and stylomandibular ligaments.

The squamous and tympanic parts ossify in membrane and the petromastoid and styloid process ossify in cartilage. The styloid process develops from the cartilage of second branchial arch.

Temporal Bone in Newborn

The appearance of the temporal bone at birth is different than adult. The middle ear, mastoid antrum, tympanic membrane and ear ossicles are of adult size. The inner ear is of adult size. The tympanic part is represented by tympanic ring, hence, the bony external acoustic meatus is absent. The mastoid process and mastoid air cells are absent.

Maxilla

The two maxillae are the large bones, which are located one on each side of the nose below the orbit. The alveolar processes of the two maxillae form the upper jaw. Each maxilla has a body and four processes, the frontal, zygomatic, alveolar and palatine. The body is triangular in shape. Its base is directed medially towards the nasal cavity and the apex is directed laterally at the zygomatic process. It encloses a large maxillary sinus.

Sensory Nerves in Relation to Maxilla

a. The anterior wall of the bone contains canals for anterior superior alveolar nerves. On the anterior surface there is infraorbital foramen (above the canine fossa) through which infraorbital nerve comes out.
b. The posterior surface is related to the posterior superior alveolar nerves. Above the maxillary tuberosity, the maxillary nerve grooves the posterior surface.
c. The infraorbital groove on the superior surface leads from the inferior orbital fissure in to the infraorbital canal to terminate at the infraorbital foramen on the anterior surface. The groove, canal and foramen contain infraorbital nerve and vessels.

   The pain of maxillary sinusitis radiates to the upper teeth because of the close proximity of the anterior and posterior superior alveolar nerves.

Maxillary Hiatus

The medial surface of the maxilla forms part of the lateral nasal wall. It shows a large opening (maxillary hiatus) by which the maxillary sinus opens into the middle meatus of nose. The size of the hiatus is reduced by the uncinate process of ethmoid from above, descending process of lacrimal bone from above, inferior nasal concha from below and perpendicular plate of palatine bone from behind. In maxillary sinusitis, pus may fill the sinus because the maxillary hiatus is located at a higher level compared to the floor of the sinus. The position of the opening of the frontal air sinus in the middle meatus is at a higher level than that of maxillary hiatus. This favors the drainage of pus from the frontal sinus into the maxillary sinus in frontal sinusitis. Hence, the maxillary sinus is regarded as the secondary reservoir of frontal sinus. The maxillary sinus is approached through the canine fossa to drain the pus in Caldwell-Luc operation.

Mandible

The mandible is the bone of lower jaw (the shape of its body is like a horseshoe). It is the only movable bone of the cranium. It develops in membrane from the perichondrium of the cartilage of the first arch (Meckel's cartilage). The coronoid and condylar processes, however, develop in cartilage. A ramus projects from the posterior end of the body on each side and it bears the condylar and coronoid processes. The head or condyle is carried on the condylar process. Beneath the head there is a narrow neck. The mandibular head articulates with the mandibular fossa of squamous temporal bone at temporomandibular joints, where mandibular movements take place.

Relation to Salivary Glands

The mandible is related to three salivary glands. The parotid gland is related to the posterior border and adjacent lateral and medial surfaces of the ramus. The submandibular gland is in contact with the submandibular fosse below the mylohyoid line on the inner surface of the body. The sublingual gland is in contact with the sublingual fossa anteriorly above the mylohyoid line.

Nerves Closely Related to Mandible

a. The inferior alveolar nerve (a branch of mandibular nerve) enters the mandibular foramen and travels in the mandibular canal inside the mandible.
b. Lingual nerve (a branch of mandibular nerve) is in direct contact behind the posterior end of the mylohyoid line.
c. The masseteric nerves (branches of mandibular nerve) pass through the mandibular notch to reach the masseter, which is attached to the lateral surface of the ramus.
d. The auriculotemporal nerve (branch of mandibular) is related to the medial side of the neck of the mandible.
e. The mylohyoid nerve (a branch of inferior alveolar) lies in the mylohyoid groove.
f. The mental nerve comes out of the mental foramen on the outer surface of the body of the mandible.

Relation to Facial Artery

The facial artery can be palpated at the base or inferior margin of the body of mandible at the anteroinferior angle of the masseter.

Ligaments Attached to Mandible

The stylomandibular ligament, which is the thickened part of the deep cervical fascia, is attached to the angle of mandible. The sphenomandibular ligament, which is the derivative of first branchial arch gains attachment to the lingula (a bony spicule that guards the mandibular foramen). The pterygomandibular raphe is attached to the inner surface behind the third molar tooth. The lower end of the lateral temporomandibular ligament is attached to the lateral surface of neck of the bone.

Angle of Mandible

The inferior border of the ramus of mandible meets the posterior border at an angle called mandibular angle. This is typically everted in males and is inverted in females.

Age Changes in Mandible

a. At birth, the mandible is in two halves. Fusion occurs at symphysis menti by first year. The mental foramen is near the lower margin because the bone is made of only the alveolar sockets. For the same reason the mandibular canal runs near the lower margin. The jaw is edentulous. The mandibular angle is obtuse because the head is in line with the body. The coronoid process projects upward above the head.
b. In adults, the mental foramen opens midway between the upper and lower margins. The mandibular canal runs parallel to the mylohyoid line. The angle of mandible reduces because the ramus is almost vertical. There are teeth in the alveolar sockets.
c. In old age, the teeth fall and hence the alveolar sockets are absorbed. Because of this, the height of the mandible is reduced. The mental foramen and mandibular canal shift toward the upper margin. The angle of mandible becomes obtuse because of oblique disposition of the ramus.

Hyoid Bone

It is a U-shaped bone, which is an important landmark in the midline of the front of the neck. The hyoid bone consists of a body and a pair of greater and lesser horns or cornua. It lies opposite C3 vertebra, at rest. The hyoid has no articulations with other bones. It is suspended from the skull by stylohyoid ligaments. The hyoid is attached to the styloid process by stylohyoid muscle, to the mandible by mylohyoid and geniohyoid muscles, to the tongue by hyoglossus muscles, to pharynx by middle constrictor, to thyroid cartilage by thyrohyoid muscle, to sternum by sternohyoid muscles and to the scapula by omohyoid muscles. The intermediate tendon of the digastric muscle is fixed to the greater horn by a fibrous pulley. The thyrohyoid membrane passes posterior to the hyoid bone to be attached to its upper margin. A subhyoid bursa facilitates the movements of the hyoid on the thyrohyoid membrane. The hyoid bone develops from cartilages of second and third pharyngeal (branchial) arches.

Cervical Vertebrae

There are seven cervical vertebrae. All cervical vertebrae are characterized by the presence of foramen transversarium in the transverse processes. The foramina in the transverse processes of upper six cervical vertebrae transmit the second part of the vertebral artery. The first (atlas) and second (axis) cervical vertebrae do not confirm to the typical pattern. The typical cervical vertebra has a bifid spine. The anterior tubercle of the transverse process of sixth cervical vertebra is large and palpable. It is called carotid tubercle of Chassaignac. The common carotid artery can be compressed against it, medial to the anterior margin of the sternomastoid muscle. The seventh cervical vertebra has a prominent spine, which is not bifid. Hence, the seventh vertebra earns the name vertebra prominence. The tip of the spine of this vertebra is easily felt in the back of the neck. This allows the tips of the subsequent spines to be numbered. Another peculiarity of the seventh vertebra is that the vertebral artery does not pass through its foramen transversarium. Only the vertebral venous plexus passes through it.

Atlas

The atlas supports the globe of the skull. It is a ring-shaped vertebra. It has no body and no spine. It consists of large lateral masses joined anteriorly by a short anterior arch and posteriorly by a longer posterior arch. The transverse processes are long and pierced by foramen. The kidney shaped superior articular processes articulate with occipital condyles. The inferior articular processes are circular and articulate with superior articular processes of axis. The anterior arch has a facet on its inner aspect for articulation with the dens of axis, which is supported by the transverse ligament of atlas. The superior surface of the posterior arch shows a groove for the third part of the vertebral artery. From these features it is possible to hold the atlas in the anatomical position. The transverse ligament of atlas divides the large vertebral foramen in to posterior part containing spinal cord, meninges, spinal arteries and spinal accessory nerve and a smaller anterior part containing the dens of the axis. The anterior arch provides attachment to the anterior longitudinal ligament at the anterior tubercle and to the anterior atlanto-occipital membrane at the upper margin. The posterior arch provides attachment to the highest pair of ligamenta flava at its lower margin. Its posterior tubercle gives attachment to the ligamentum nuchae and to its lower margin is attached the posterior atlanto-occipital membrane.

Relations of Transverse Processes

The transverse processes are very long and hence the atlas vertebra is the widest among the cervical vertebrae. The tip of the transverse process can be felt in the living in front of and below the mastoid process (at the midpoint between the mastoid process and the angle of the mandible). The occipital artery, internal jugular vein and the spinal accessory nerve are the anterior relations of the transverse process.

Articulations of Atlas

There are two atlanto-occipital joints and three atlantoaxial joints (two lateral and one midline).

Lateral Masses

The transverse ligament of atlas is attached on each side to the tubercle on the medial surface of the lateral mass. It is a very strong ligament responsible for retaining the dens in contact with the anterior arch of atlas. From the midpoint of its upper margin a vertical band passes upward to be attached to the basilar part of occipital bone. From its lower margin a weak band passes to the posterior surface of the body of axis. Cruciform ligament of atlas is the combination of transverse atlantal ligament and the two vertical bands attached to it. The transverse ligament is stronger than the dens. In death by hanging, the dens dislocates backwards by tearing the transverse ligament and impinges on the lower medulla and upper spinal cord. This is due to atlantoaxial dislocation without fracture of dens.

Jefferson's Fracture

This is the fracture of atlas at the anterior or the posterior arch (fracture at two or three places) causing separation of the lateral masses. The spinal cord is not compressed in this fracture.

Axis

The axis is the second cervical vertebra. It is identified by the presence of a tooth-like upward projection from the body of axis. This projection is called the dens or odontoid process, which represents the body of atlas vertebra. The apex of the dens gives attachment to the apical ligament and its sides to the alar ligaments. The anterior surface of the body gives attachment to the anterior longitudinal ligament. The lower margin of the posterior surface of the body gives attachment to the posterior longitudinal ligament. The membrana tectoria, which is the upward continuation of the posterior longitudinal ligament, is attached to the posterior surface of the body.

Fractures of Axis

The dens or the pedicle of the axis may be fractured in road traffic accidents (RTA) or a fall from the height. These may be fatal injuries because of the danger of compression of the spinal cord.

a. The fracture of the dens is accompanied with rupture of the transverse ligament. This will cause dislocation of the dens posteriorly towards the spinal cord.
b. The Hangman's fracture occurs at the interarticular part of the pedicle, which is long and thin in axis because the superior articular processes are located much anteriorly compared to the inferior articular processes (this type of orientation of the articular processes is present in axis only). There is a double break in the axis, which may cause posterior dislocation of the median atlantoaxial joint.

Annexure: Instant Access Data Bank

Weights

Brain—1400 gm (males) and 1275 gm (females)
Pituitary gland—0.5 to 0.6 gm
Thyroid gland—20 to 40 gm
Lung—450 gm (right) and 375 gm (left)
Heart—300 gm
Liver—1400 to 1500 gm
Spleen—150 to 200 gm
Kidney—130 to 160 gm
Pancreas—90 to 120 gm
Suprarenal gland—5 to 6 gm
Ovary—7 gm
Uterus—30 to 40 gm
Testis—20 to 27 gm
Prostate—15 to 20 gm
Placenta full term—500 gm
Ratio of weight of placenta and the fetus—by 4th month—1:1 and by term—1:7
Ratio of the size of facial skeleton to cranial skeleton at birth—1: 8

Lengths

Small intestine—600 cm
Large intestine—150 to 170 cm
Human sperm—50 micron
Umbilical cord at term—50 to 60 cm
Transverse colon—50 cm
Spinal cord—45 cm
Thoracic duct—45 cm
Adult femur—45 cm
Vas deferens—45 cm
Pelvic colon—40 cm
Esophagus—25 cm
Ureter—25 cm
Duodenum—25 cm
Descending colon—25 cm
Root of mesentery—15 cm
Ascending colon—15 cm
Male urethra—18 cm
Trachea—12 cm
Pharynx—12 cm
Heart from base to apex—12 cm
Kidney 12 cm × 6 cm × 3 cm
Fallopian tube—10 cm
Appendix—7.5 to 10 cm (average 9 cm)
Common bile duct—7.5 to 10 cm
Uterus—7.5 cm × 5 cm × 2.5 cm
Uterine cavity (as measured by uterine sound) × 6 cm
Vagina: anterior wall—7.5 cm and posterior wall—10 cm
Cecum—6 cm long and 7.5 cm breadth (length smaller than breadth)
Left bronchus—5 cm
Right bronchus—2.5 cm
Meckel's diverticulum—5 cm
Optic nerve—4 cm
Anal canal—4 cm
Inguinal canal—4 cm
Female urethra—4 cm
Pharyngotympanic tube—3.6 to 4 cm
External acoustic meatus—2.4 cm

Capacity

Stomach—1100 to 2000 ml
Gallbladder—30 to 50 ml
Urinary bladder—250 to 500 ml
Extradural space in sacral canal—25 to 30 ml

Unique Features of Lower Limb

Longest and strongest long bone—femur
Largest sesamoid bone—patella
Largest synovial cavity—knee joint
Strongest ligament—iliofemoral
Longest muscle—sartorius
Strongest tendon—tendocalcaneus
Thickest nerve—sciatic nerve
Longest cutaneous nerve—saphenous nerve
Longest superficial vein—great saphenous vein
Largest nutrient artery to—tibia

Maximum number of ossification centers at birth is five—lower end of femur, tibial tuberosity, calcaneus, talus and cuboid.

Maximum number of sesamoid bones is six—patella in quadriceps femoris, fabella in lateral head of gastrocnemius, rider's bone in adductor longus, two sesamoid bones in flexor hallucis brevis and one in peroneus longus.

Remnants of Axis Artery of Upper Limb

Axillary artery, brachial artery, anterior interosseous artery and median artery.

Remnants of Axis Artery of Lower Limb

Inferior gluteal artery, companion artery of sciatic nerve, popliteal artery and peroneal artery.

Statistical Analysis of Nervous System

Total count of neurons in the cerebral cortex of the adult—8000 to 10,000 million.

Total count of neuroglia cells in the cerebral cortex of the adult—64,000 million.

Cerebral cortex of the size of a grain of sand contains 100,000 neurons, 2 million axons and 1 billion synapses.

Number of corticospinal fibers—2 million
Total fibers in crus cerebri—20 million
Number of ganglion cells in retina—100,000
Number of nerve fibers in optic nerve—100,000.

Index

A

B

Index

D

E

F

Index

G

H

M

N

Index

O

T

U

V

W

Z

W

Z